For Carol,

in memory of the

old times

George Hall.

SHORT PRACTICE
OF ANAESTHESIA

JOIN US ON THE INTERNET VIA WWW, GOPHER, FTP OR EMAIL:

WWW: http://www.thomson.com
GOPHER: gopher.thomson.com
FTP: ftp.thomson.com
EMAIL: findit@kiosk.thomson.com

A service of I(T)P

SHORT PRACTICE OF ANAESTHESIA

Edited by

Maldwyn Morgan MB BS FRCA
Reader in Anaesthetic Practice, Royal Postgraduate Medical School
Honorary Consultant, Hammersmith Hospital
London, UK

George M. Hall MBBS PhD FIBiol FRCA
Professor of Anaesthesia, St George's Hospital Medical School
Honorary Consultant, St George's Hospital and Atkinson Morley's Hospital
London, UK

CHAPMAN & HALL MEDICAL
London · Weinheim · New York · Tokyo · Melbourne · Madras

Published by Chapman & Hall, 2–6 Boundary Row, London SE1 8HN

Chapman & Hall, 2–6 Boundary Row, London SE1 8HN, UK

Chapman & Hall GmbH, Pappelallee 3, 69469 Weinheim, Germany

Chapman & Hall USA, 115 Fifth Avenue, New York, NY 10003, USA

Chapman & Hall Japan, ITP-Japan, Kyowa Building, 3F, 2-2-1 Hirakawacho, Chiyoda-ku, Tokyo 102, Japan

Chapman & Hall Australia, 102 Dodds Street, South Melbourne, Victoria 3205, Australia

Chapman & Hall India, R. Seshadri, 32 Second Main Road, CIT East, Madras 600 035, India

First edition 1998

© 1998 Chapman & Hall

Typeset in 10/12 Palatino by Photoprint, Torquay, Devon
Printed in Great Britain by Cambridge University Press, Cambridge

ISBN 0 412 71890 1

Apart from any fair dealing for the purposes of research or private study, or criticism or review, as permitted under the UK Copyright Designs and Patents Act, 1988, this publication may not be reproduced, stored, or transmitted, in any form or by any means, without the prior permission in writing of the publishers, or in the case of reprographic reproduction only in accordance with the terms of the licences issued by the Copyright Licensing Agency in the UK, or in accordance with the terms of licences issued by the appropriate Reproduction Rights Organization outside the UK. Enquires concerning reproduction outside the terms stated here should be sent to the publishers at the London address printed on this page.

The publisher makes no representation, express or implied, with regard to the accuracy of the information contained in this book and cannot accept any legal responsibility or liability for any errors or omissions that may be made.

A catalogue record for this book is available from the British Library

Library of Congress Catalog Card Number: 97-67258

CONTENTS

List of contributors	ix
Preface	xiii
List of abbreviations	xv

PART ONE   EQUIPMENT — 1

1 Anaesthetic machines — 3
  A. P. Adams

2 Principles of monitoring — 19
  L. B. Cook, K.K. Panikkar and M. Morgan

3 Ventilators for anaesthetic use — 47
  L. Loh

4 Anaesthetic breathing systems — 69
  D. C. White

5 Equipment for airway management — 83
  A. Davey

6 Atmospheric pollution and toxicity of inhalational agents — 101
  G. G. Lockwood

PART TWO   PREOPERATIVE ASSESSMENT — 109

7 Risk evaluation, audit and quality of practice — 111
  C. J. E. Day and S. N. C. Bolsin

8 Preoperative evaluation, scoring systems and premedication — 123
  J. P. H. Fee

9 Preoperative tests — 147
  W. J. Fawcett

10 Inherited diseases — 163
  E. O'Leary and G. M. Hall

PART THREE   SUBSPECIALTY — 183

11 Thoracic surgery — 185
  R. S. Vaughan and G. Phillips

12 Cardiac surgery S. J. George and D. Royston	203
13 Vascular surgery J. P. Desborough	233
14 Neurosurgery R. Dwyer	247
15 Genitourinary and renal surgery S. E. Hutchinson	269
16 Hepatobiliary and pancreatic surgery A. Holdcroft	287
17 Ophthalmic surgery A. P. Rubin	303
18 Ear, nose and throat surgery B. O'Donoghue	317
19 Paediatric surgery A. I. McEwan and A. E. Black	337
20 Day-care surgery D. J. Wilkinson	361
21 Dental surgery A. Chan and P. J. Flynn	371
22 Plastic surgery C. E. Blogg	387
23 Anaesthesia for radiology C. J. Peden	401
24 Endocrine surgery R. A. Mason	417
25 Trauma and orthopaedic surgery P. G. Edge and M. Fennelly	437
26 Anaesthesia for the thermally injured patient L. Davis and L. T. A. Rylah	457
27 Transplantation of liver and kidney S. V. Mallet and T. Peachey	469
28 Laparoscopic surgery A. J. Cunningham and D. J. Kelly	493
29 Epidural and spinal anaesthesia D. P. Dob and M. Morgan	503
30 Peripheral nerve blocks S. M. Geddes	521

31 Obstetric anaesthesia and analgesia 549
M. H. Nathanson and D. G. Bogod

32 Anaesthesia in the elderly 571
C. Traynor

33 Anaesthesia and obesity 587
C. S. Reilly

34 The infectious patient 597
D. A. Zideman

35 Diabetes mellitus 611
G. M. Hall and J. Dinsmore

36 Total intravenous anaesthesia 625
N. P. Sutcliffe and G. N. C. Kenny

PART FOUR   SPECIAL SITUATIONS 635

37 Post-anaesthetic recovery room 637
J. P. Millns and G. M. Cooper

38 Control of postoperative pain, nausea and vomiting 651
M. Harmer

39 The difficult airway 675
B. A. Sutton

40 Fluid therapy 697
P. G. Roe

41 Massive haemorrhage, blood clotting and replacement 717
D. Royston

42 Anaphylaxis to anaesthetic drugs 741
M. Fisher

43 Awareness in anaesthesia 753
J. Andrade and J. G. Jones

44 Cardiopulmonary resuscitation 765
M. E. Ward

45 Brain death 785
P. A. Razis and R. Rogers

46 Management of head injury 797
P. A. Razis

Index 811

CONTRIBUTORS

DR. A. P. ADAMS PhD, FRCA, FANZCA
Professor of Anaesthetics,
in the University of London, and
Honorary Consultant Anaesthetist to
Guy's and St. Thomas' Hospitals, and to
King's College Hospital
London, UK.

J. ANDRADE, PhD
Lecturer in Psychology,
University of Sheffield, Sheffield UK.

A. E. BLACK
Consultant Anaesthetist,
Great Ormond Street Hospital for Children,
London, UK.

C. E. BLOGG
Consultant Anaesthetist,
Nuffield Department of Anaesthetics,
The Oxford Radcliffe Hospital NHS Trust,
Oxford, UK.

D. G. BOGOD, FRCA
Consultant Anaesthetist,
Nottingham City Hospital,
UK.

S. N. C. BOLSIN, FRCA
Director, Division of Acute Services,
Department of Anaesthesia,
The Geelong Hospital,
Victoria, Australia.

A. CHAN, FFARCSI, FRCA
Consultant,
Intensive Care Unit,
North Middlesex Hospital,
London, UK.

L. B. COOK, FRCA
Consultant Anaesthetist,
Department of Anaesthesia,
Royal Oldham Hospital,
Oldham, UK.

G. M. COOPER, FRCA
Senior Lecturer in Anaesthesia,
University of Birmingham, and
Hononary Consultant Anaesthetist,
University Hospital Birmingham NHS Trust,
Birmingham, UK.

A. J. CUNNINGHAM, MD, FRCPC
Professor of Anaesthesia,
Royal College of Surgeons in Ireland, and
Beaumont Hospital,
Dublin, Ireland.

A. DAVEY, FRCA
Consultant Anaesthetist,
Royal Sussex County Hospital,
Brighton, UK.

L. DAVIS, FRCA
Department of Anaesthetics,
Royal London Hospital,
London, UK.

C. J. E. DAY, MRCP, FRCA
Department of Anaesthetics,
Bristol Royal Infirmary,
Bristol, UK.

J. P. DESBOROUGH, MD, FRCA
Senior Lecturer and Honorary Consultant,
St George's Hospital Medical School,
London, UK.

J. DINSMORE, MD, FRCA
Department of Anaesthesia,
St George's Hospital Medical School,
London, UK.

D. P. DOBB, FRCA
Department of Anaesthesia,
Royal Postgraduate Medical School,
London, UK.

R. DWYER, FFARCSI, MRCP
Consultant Anaesthetist,
Beaumont Hospital,
and Senior Lecturer,
Royal College of Surgeons in Ireland,
Dublin, Ireland.

P. G. EDGE, PhD, FRCA
Consultant Anaesthetist,
Royal National Orthopaedic Hospital,
Stanmore, UK.

W. J. FAWCETT, FRCA
Consultant Anaesthetist,
Royal Surrey County Hospital Trust,
Guildford, Surrey, UK.

J. P. H. FEE, MD, PhD, FFARCSI
Professor of Anaesthetics,
The Queen's University of Belfast,
Belfast, Northern Ireland, UK.

M. FENNELLY, FFARCSI
Consultant Anaesthetist,
Royal National Orthopaedic Hospital
Stanmore, UK.

M. FISHER, MD, FANZCA, FFICANZCA, FRCA
Clinical Professor,
Department of Anaesthesia,
University of Sydney,
Royal North Shore Hospital,
St Leonards, Australia.

P. J. FLYNN, FFARCSI, FRCA
Senior Lecturer and Honorary Consultant,
Anaesthetics Unit,
The Royal London Hospital,
London, UK.

S. M. GEDDES, FRCA
Consultant Anaesthetist,
Glasgow Royal Infirmary,
Glasgow, UK.

S. J. GEORGE, MRCP, FRCA
Department of Anaesthetics,
St George's Hospital Medical School,
London, UK.

G. M. HALL, PhD, FIBiol, FRCA
Professor of Anaesthesia,
St George's Hospital Medical School,
Honorary Consultant,
St George's Hospital and Atkinson Morley's Hospital,
London, UK.

M. HARMER, FRCA
Senior Lecturer,
Department of Anaesthetics and Intensive Care Medicine,
University of Wales College of Medicine,
Cardiff, UK.

A. HOLDCROFT, MD, FRCA
Senior Lecturer and Honorary Consultant Anaesthetist,
Royal Postgraduate Medical School,
London, UK.

S. E. HUTCHINSON, FRCA
Consultant Anaesthetist,
St George's Hospital Medical School,
London, UK.

J. G. JONES, MD, FRCP, FRCA
University Professor of Anaesthesia,
Addenbrooke's Hospital,
Cambridge, UK.

D. J. KELLY, MRCPI, FFARCSI
Consultant Anaesthetist,
Royal College of Surgeons in Ireland, and
St Vincent's Hospital
Dublin, Ireland.

G. N. C. KENNY, MD, FRCA
Professor,
University Department of Anaesthesia,
Chief of Anaesthesia (HCI) (Scotland),
Clydebank, UK.

G. G. LOCKWOOD
Senior Lecturer in Anaesthesia,
Hammersmith Hospital,
London, UK.

L. LOH, FRCA
Consultant Anaesthetist,
The Nuffield Department of Anaesthetics,
The Oxford Radcliffe Hospital NHS Trust,
Oxford, UK.

S. MALLET
Consultant Anaesthetist,
Royal Free Hospital,
London, UK.

R. A. MASON, FRCA
Consultant Anaesthetist,
Swansea NHS Trust, UK.

A. I. McEWAN
Consultant Anaesthetist,
Great Ormond Street Hospital for Children,
London, UK.

J. P. MILLNS, FRCA
Consultant Anaesthetist,
Birmingham Women's Hospital,
Birmingham, UK.

M. MORGAN, FRCA
Reader in Anaesthetic Practice,
Royal Postgraduate Medical School,
Honorary Consultant,
Hammersmith Hospital,
London, UK.

M. H. NATHANSON, MRCP, FRCA
Consultant Anaesthetist,
Department of Anaesthetics,
University Hospital,
Queen's Medical Centre,
Nottingham, UK.

B. O'DONOGHUE, FRCA
Consultant Anaesthetist,
The Royal National Throat, Nose and Ear Hospital,
London, UK.

E. O'LEARY, FFA, RCSI
Senior Lecturer and Honorary Consultant,
Department of Anaesthesia,
St George's Hospital Medical School,
London, UK.

K. K. PANIKKAR
Department of Anaesthetics,
Royal Postgraduate Medical School,
London, UK.

T. PEACHEY
Consultant Anaesthetist,
Royal Free Hospital,
London, UK.

C. J. PEDEN, FRCA
Consultant Anaesthetist,
Royal United Hospital,
Bath, UK.

G. PHILLIPS, FRCA
Consultant Anaesthetist,
Withinshaw Hospital,
Manchester, UK.

P. A. RAZIS, FRCA
Consultant Anaesthestist,
St George's and Atkinson Morley's Hospitals,
London, UK.

C. S. REILLY
Professor of Anaesthesia,
University of Sheffield,
Department of Surgical and Anaesthetic Sciences,
Royal Hallamshire Hospital,
Sheffield, UK.

P. G. ROE
Consultant in Anaesthesia and Intensive Care,
Addenbrooke's NHS Trust,
Cambridge, UK.

D. ROYSTON, FRCA
Consultant Cardiothoracic Anaesthetist,
Harefield Hospital,
Middlesex, UK.

A. P. RUBIN, FRCA
Consultant Anaesthetist,
Chelsea and Westminster Hospital,
London, UK.

L. T. A. RYLAH, FRCA
Consultant Anaesthetist,
Basildon and Thurrock NHS Trust,
Essex, UK.

N. P. SUTCLIFFE, MRCP, FRCA
Consultant Anaesthetist,
HCI (Scotland),
Clydebank, UK.

B. SUTTON, SRN, FRCA
Consultant Anaesthetist,
St George's Hospital Medical School,
London, UK.

R. ROGERS, FRCA
Oxford Radcliffe NHS Trust,
Oxford, UK.

C. TRAYNOR, FFARCSI
Consultant Anaesthetist,
Coombe Women's Hospital and
St James's Hospital,
Dublin, Ireland.

R. S. VAUGHAN, FRCA
Consultant Anaesthetist,
University Hospital of Wales,
Cardiff, UK.

M. E. WARD, FRCA
Consultant Anaesthetist, Chairman,
Resuscitation Council (UK) 1994–97,
Nuffield Department of Anaesthetics,
The Oxford Radcliffe Hospital NHS Trust,
Oxford, UK.

D. J. WILKINSON
Medical Director, Day Surgery Centre,
Royal Hospitals Trust,
St Bartholomew's Hospital,
London, UK.

D. C. WHITE
Honorary Consultant,
Northwick Park Hospital,
Harrow, Middlesex, UK.

D. A. ZIDEMAN, FRCA, DipIMC
Consultant Anaesthetist,
Hammersmith Hospital Trust, and
Honorary Senior Lecturer,
Royal Postgraduate Medical School,
London, UK.

PREFACE

Why publish another textbook of anaesthesia? There are already several excellent textbooks, but they have increased in size dramatically in the past 10 years so that a total pagination of 2000 is commonplace. This has been associated inevitably with a similar rapid rise in price. Most of the chapters in the major textbooks are authoritative, extensively referenced and often considered as the standard work on a particular subject. They are useful for providing a detailed account of a subject and often act as a starting point for in-depth study or as a guide to possible research. Their sheer size and expense deters many trainees, and the basic knowledge needed in a particular branch of anaesthesia is often not emphasized. In many respects, they are more valuable to the teacher than to the trainee.

In a *Short Practice of Anaesthesia* we have concentrated on the core knowledge of anaesthesia required by trainees in the UK. We hope that it will also act as a guide to current practice for senior anaesthetists. The chapters are not referenced but contain recommendations for further reading. The emphasis is on important clinical considerations in anaesthesia; intensive care and chronic pain have not been included as they merit separate and extensive coverage. Similarly, the basic scientific aspects of the specialty have been included only where they are essential to understanding clinical problems.

We thank all the authors for their contributions and appreciate the support, encouragement and professionalism of the staff of Chapman & Hall, particularly Dr Joanna Koster and Ellie Gillam. We also wish to acknowledge the technical expertise of Dr Helen Juden, copy-editor, and Helen MacDonald of Prepress Projects. The steadfast support of our secretaries, Shirley Richens and Shirley Cave, has been invaluable. Their inability to panic when the cause was lost has helped greatly to see the project to completion.

M. Morgan
G.M. Hall
1997

ABBREVIATIONS

$[K^+]_i$	intracellular potassium ion concentration	AST	aspartate transaminase
$[K^+]_o$	extracellular potassium ion concentration	ASTM	American Society for Testing and Materials
2,3 DPG	2,3-diphosphoglycerate	ATG	antithymocyte globulin
5-HT	5-hydroxytryptamine	ATLS	advanced trauma life support
A–ao$_2$	alveolar–arterial oxygen gradient	ATP	adenosine triphosphate
a.c.	alternating current	ATPD	atmospheric temperature and pressure, dry
AAGBI	Association of Anaesthetists of Great Britain and Ireland	AV	aortic value
ABI	ankle–brachial index	AV	atrioventricular
ACE	angiotensin converting enzyme	AVM	arteriovenous malformation
ACT	activated clotting time	AVN	atrioventricular node
ACTH	adrenocorticotrophic hormone (= AVP)	AVP	arginine vasopressin (= ADH)
AD	anno domini	AZT	zidovudine
ADH	antidiuretic hormone	b.p.m.	beats per minute
ADP	adenosine diphosphate	breath min^{-1}	breaths per minute
AEP	auditory evoked potential	BC	before Christ
AER	auditory evoked response	BLS	basic life support
AIDS	acquired immune deficiency syndrome	BMI	body mass index (w/h^2)
ALA	aminolaevulinic acid	BP	blood pressure
ALF	acute liver failure	BS	British Standard
ANSI	American National Standards Institute	BTPS	body temperature and pressure saturated
AO	aorta	c-AMP	cyclic adenosine monophosphate
APACHE	acute physiology, age and chronic health evaluation	C0, C1–C7	cervical vertebrae
APL	adjustable pressure limiting (valve)	C1EI	C1 esterase inhibitor
APTT	activated partial thromboplastin time	CBF	cerebral blood flow
ARDS	acute respiratory distress syndrome	CBV	cerebral blood volume
ASA	American Society of Anesthesiologists	CEN	Comité Européen de Normalisation
ASD	atrial–septal defects	CENELEC	CEN electrical section
		CEPOD	Confidential Enquiry into Perioperative Deaths
		CI	cardiac index
		CK	creatine kinase
		CKBB	CK BB isoenzyme
		CMR	cerebral metabolic rate

CMRglu	cerebral metabolic requirement of glucose	ED_{50}	median effective dose
$CMRO_2$	cerebral metabolic requirement of oxygen	EDV	end-diastolic volume
		EEG	electroencephalogram
CMV	controlled mandatory ventilation	eloHAES®	hexastarch solution
		EMG	electromyogram
CMV	cytomegalovirus	EMLA	eutectic mixture of local anaesthetics
CNS	central nervous system		
COAD	chronic obstructive airways disease	EMO	Epstein–Macintosh–Oxford (vaporizer)
COP	colloid osmotic pressure	EMRSA	epidemic MRSA
CPAP	continuous positive airway pressure	ER	extraction ratio
		ERCP	endoscopic retrograde cholangiopancreatography
CPB	cardiopulmonary bypass	ESLD	end-stage liver disease
CPP	cerebral perfusion pressure	ESPVR	end-systolic pressure–volume relation
CPR	cardiopulmonary resuscitation		
CPU	central processing unit	ESRF	end-stage renal failure
CSF	cerebrospinal fluid	EU	European Union
CT	computed tomography	FDA	Food and Drugs Administration (USA)
CTZ	chemoreceptor trigger zone		
CUSUM	cumulative sum technique	$FEF_{25-75\%}$	forced expiratory flow, mid-expiratory phase
CV	closing volume		
CVP	central venous pressure	FER	forced expiratory ratio, FEV_1/FVC
d.c.	direct current		
D5RL	dextrose 5% Ringer's lactate	FEV_1	forced expiratory volume in 1 s
DA	ductus arteriosus	FFP	fresh-frozen plasma
DBS	double burst stimulation	FGF	fresh gas flow
DDAVP	vasopressin analogue, desmopressin	FIGlu	formimino-glutamic acid
		FIO_2	fractional concentration of inspired oxygen
DHCA	deep hypothermic circulatory arrest		
		FMA	facial muscle activity
DIC	disseminated intravascular coagulopathy	FO	foramen ovale
		FRC	functional residual capacity
DISS	diameter indexed safety system	FVC	forced vital capacity
DO_2	diffusing capacity of oxygen	G	gauge, as in 25 G needle
DS	degree of substitution	GA	general anaesthesia
DTS	dipyridamole thallium scintigraphy	GCS	Glasgow coma scale
		Gd-DTPA	gadopentate dimeglumine (MRI constrast medium)
DVT	deep vein thrombosis		
E	expiration	GIK	glucose–insulin–potassium (regimen)
EAA	excitatory amino acids		
EACA	tranexamic acid	GIP	gastric inhibitory peptide
EAR	enclosed afferent reservoir	GTN	glyceryl trinitrate
ECF	extracellular fluid	GTT	glucose tolerance test
ECG	electrocardiogram	H_1	histamine receptor
ECMO	extracorporeal membrane oxygenation	H_2	histamine receptor
		HAES®	pentastarch solution

HANE	hereditary angioneurotic oedema	LA	left atrium
HbA	adult haemoglobin	LAD	left anterior descending artery
HbAS	symptomless sickle cell disease	LBB	left bundle branch
		LCAR	lung compliance and airways resistance
HbC	an abnormal haemoglobin	LD_{50}	median lethal dose
HBeAg	hepatitis Be antigen	LMA	laryngeal mask airway
HbF	fetal haemoglobin	LV	left ventricle
HbS	sickle cell haemoglobin	LVAD	left ventricular assist device
HBsAg	hepatitis B surface antigen	LVEDP	left ventricular end-diastolic pressure
HbSS	homozygous sickle cell disease		
HBV	hepatitis B virus	LVSWI	left ventricular stroke work index
HCV	hepatitis C virus		
HDV	hepatitis D virus	MAC	minimal alveolar concentration (of anaesthetic gas)
HELLP	haemolysis, elevated liver enzymes and low platelets (syndrome)		
		MAO-A	type A monoamine oxidase
		MAOI	monoamine oxidase inhibitor
HES	hydroxyethyl starch	MAP	mean arterial pressure
HIV	human immunodeficiency virus	MBC	maximal breathing capacity
		MH	malignant hyperthermia
HMMA	hydroxymethyl mandelic acid	MI	myocardial infarction
HTL V1	human T-cell leukaemia virus	mIGB	meta-iodobenzylguanidine
I	inspiration	MLR	multiple logistic regression
i.m.	intramuscular	MODY	maturity onset diabetes of the young
i.u.	international units		
i.v.	intravenous	MRI	magnetic resonance imaging
IAPP	islet amyloid polypeptide	MRSA	methicillin-resistant staphylococcus aureus
ICF	intracellular fluid		
ICP	intracranial pressure	MUGA	multiple uptake gated acquisition (scan)
IDDM	insulin-dependent diabetes mellitus		
		MV	mitral valve
IEC	International Electro-technical Committee	MVO_2	mixed venous oxygen saturation
		MVV	maximal voluntary ventilation
IgE	immunoglobulin E	MW	molecular weight (relative molecular mass)
IHD	ischaemic heart disease		
IMA	internal mammary artery	NCEPOD	National CEPOD
IPPV	intermittent positive pressure ventilation	Nd-YAG	neodymium-yttrium-aluminium-garnet laser
ISO	International Organization for Standardization	NDNMB	non-depolarizing neuromuscular blocking drug
IVC	inferior vena cava	NIBP	non-invasive blood pressure
IVCT	*in vitro* contracture test	NIDDM	non-insulin-dependent diabetes mellitus
IVRA	intravenous regional anaesthesia		
JR	junctional reservoirs	NIST	non-interchangeable screw threads
KTP	potassium tintanyl phosphate (laser)		
		NMB	neuromuscular blocking drugs
L1, L2	lumbar vertebrae	NMDA	*N*-methyl-D-aspartate

NSAID	non-steriodal anti-inflammatory drugs	PP cells	pancreatic polypeptide cells
NYHA	New York Health Association	PRST	arterial pressure, heart rate, sweating and tear (score)
OER	oxygen extraction ratio	PT	prothrombin time
OIB	Oxford Inflating Bellows	PTA	percutaneous transluminal angioplasty
OKT3	monoclonal anti-T cell antibody	PTH	parathyroid hormone
OLV	one-lung ventilation	PV	pulmonary vein
OMV	Oxford Miniature Vaporizer	PVC	poly(vinyl chloride)
OSAS	obstructive sleep apnoea syndrome	PVR	pulmonary vascular resistance
p.p.m.	parts per million	RA	right atrium
p.s.i.	pounds per square inch	RAE	Ring–Adair–Elwin tubes
PA	pulmonary artery	RAST	radioallergosorbent test
$Paco_2$	partial pressure of arterial carbon dioxide	RBB	right bundle branch
PAF	platelet aggregating factor	RCA	right coronary artery
PAO_2	partial pressure of alveolar oxygen	RCA	Royal College of Anaesthetists
Pao_2	partial pressure of arterial oxygen	Rcof	ristocetin cofactor
		RES	reticuloendothelial system
PAOP	pulonary artery occlusion pressure	RIA	radioimmunoassay
		RNV	radionuclide ventriculography
PAWP	pulmonary artery wedge pressure	ROC	receiver operating characteristic
		ROP	retinopathy of prematurity
P_B	barometric pressure	RQ	respiratory quotient (0.8)
PBG	porphobilinogen	RV	residual volume
PCA	patient-controlled analgesia	RV	right ventricle
PCC	prothrombin complex concentrate	RVAD	right ventricular assist device
		s.c.	subcutaneous
Pco_2	partial pressure of CO_2	SAH	subarachnoid haemorrhage
PCV	packed cell volume (haematocrit)	Sao_2	saturation of arterial haemoglobin with oxygen (measured by tonometry)
PCWP	pulmonary capillary wedge pressure	SIMV	synchronized intermittent mandatory ventilation
PDA	patent ductus arteriosus	SpEP	spinal evoked potential
PDPH	post-dural-puncture headache	Spo_2	oxygen saturation measured by pulse oximetry
PE	pulmonary embolism		
$PE'co_2$	partial pressure end-tidal CO_2	SR	spontaneous respiration
$PE\,co_2$	partial pressure expired CO_2	SV	stroke volume
PEEP	positive end-expiratory pressure	SVC	superior vena cava
PEFR	peak expiratory flow rate	Svo_2	saturation of venous haemoglobin with oxygen
PET	positron emission tomography		
PFS	preferential flow system	SVR	systemic vascular resistance
Pio_2	partial pressure of inspired oxygen	t-PA	tissue plasminogen activator
		T1, T2	thoracic vertebrae
PONV	postoperative nausea and vomiting	T_3	tri-iodothyronine

T_4	thyroxine	TURP	transurethral resection of the prostate
TBW	total body water		
TCD	transcranial Doppler ultrasound	TV	tidal volume
TCI	target controlled infusions	URTI	upper respiratory tract infection
TENS	transcutaneous electrical nerve stimulation	VATS	video-assisted thoracic surgery
		VF	ventricular fibrillation
THF	tetrahydrofolate	VIP	vasoactive intestinal peptide
TIPS	transjugular intrahepatic portosystemic shunt	$V_{O_{2max}}$	maximal oxygen consumption
		VRE	vancomycin-resistant enterococcus
TIVA	total intravenous anaesthesia		
TLC	total lung capacity	VSD	ventricular–septal defects
TOE	transoesophageal echocardiography	VT	ventricular tachycardia
		vWF	von Willebrand factor
TSH	thyroid stimulating hormone	WHO	World Health Organization

PART ONE
EQUIPMENT

ANAESTHETIC MACHINES 1

A. P. Adams

Continuous flow anaesthetic machines are often generically called Boyle's machines after Dr H.E.G. Boyle, of St Bartholomew's Hospital, who did a lot of work in this field. However, this is a misnomer as Boyle did not invent the anaesthetic machine, having obtained the idea from Gwathmey in the USA and Geoffrey Marshall, a physician at Guy's Hospital, London. In recent years machines have become more complex and now incorporate electronic technology allowing professional needs to be re-examined. The new generation of anaesthetic machine incorporates four main functions: dosing, ventilation, monitoring and data management. Dissatisfaction with the anaesthesia workplace has been likened to the inadequate cockpit conditions in aeroplanes: there is concern about safety, incompatibility and inflexibility. These workplaces are unacceptable today to both patients and anaesthetists. This chapter discusses the anaesthetic machine and its place in the concept of the anaesthetic workstation.

STANDARDS GOVERNING ANAESTHESIA MACHINES AND ASSOCIATED EQUIPMENT

Besides International and European Standards most countries have their own National Standards for anaesthetic equipment. The present standard in the UK is BS 4272 Part 3, 1989 (with amendments 1990). The EU (European Union) standards are those of CEN (Comité Européen de Normalisation) which corresponds with the ISO (International Organization for Standardization). In Europe, CEN has produced a draft standard (prEN 740) for the anaesthetic workstation, which is expected to supersede all European national standards for anaesthetic machines, including BS 4273:3, although it will not become effective until 1997 at the earliest. Meanwhile, ISO is also working on a new draft standard for the anaesthetic workstation (ISO/DIS 8835:1), which will eventually supersede the existing ISO 5358 standard for the basic anaesthetic machine.

CONTINUOUS-FLOW MACHINES

The anaesthetic machine has been described as 'an accident waiting to happen'. Recent technological advances and the need to eliminate human error factors associated with present anaesthetic apparatus have led to attempts to design safer anaesthetic machines and to automate functions such as record keeping and monitoring. Failure to ensure adequate oxygenation accounts for the great majority of serious accidents seen in anaesthesia and equipment should be designed to minimize the chances of hypoxia and for education in the understanding and correct use of equipment. The safety features which may be expected on anaesthetic machines manufactured in the last ten years include:

Short Practice of Anaesthesia. Edited by M. Morgan and G. M. Hall. Published in 1997 by Chapman & Hall, London. ISBN 0 412 71890 1

- oxygen supply pressure failure alarm
- low oxygen pressure N_2O 'cut-off' or fail-safe
- oxygen percentage monitor
- single oxygen flow control knob which is touch coded
- oxygen flowmeter at extreme right (USA and Canada)
- central gas supply pressure gauges
- colour coded flow meters and control valves
- oxygen/nitrous oxide ratio monitor/controller
- locking common gas outlet (no longer standard in the UK)
- pin-index safety system (indexed cylinder yokes)
- indexed pipeline inlet connectors: NIST (non-interchangeable screw threads) in the UK or DISS (diameter indexed safety system) in the USA
- disconnect alarm on ventilator

GAS SUPPLIES

Medical gas cylinders

Great confusion concerning cylinders occurred during the Second World War since different colour standards were in use by different countries and armies. International agreement (BS 1319, (1976), BS 1319C (1976) and ISO 32 (1977)), led to a great improvement. Nevertheless, several countries still do not conform to the ISO standard; for example, although the ISO colour for an oxygen cylinder is all white, it is still green in the USA and black cylinder with a white shoulder in the UK.

Medical gas cylinders must be properly secured and stored when not in use on the anaesthetic machine. Serious accidents can happen to patients and hospital personnel if an unrestrained cylinder falls, or is damaged. A survey in the USA showed that 1.2% of 14 500 cylinders delivered had potentially hazardous irregularities. The dangers of medical gas delivery systems are not the result of a lack of regulations but the result of lack of compliance with existing regulations by gas suppliers and hospitals. Fractures of the cylinder or disconnection of the cylinder from the valve stem converts the cylinder into a lethal torpedo.

Pin-index system

Although the tragedy of the 'wrong cylinder' or 'wrong gas' has been known for years and was portrayed in the British film *Green For Danger* (1946), it continues to occur. The classical situation was when a nitrous oxide cylinder could be coupled to the oxygen yoke of an anaesthetic machine. The pin-index or non-interchangeable flush fitting system (BS 1319; ISO 407) was introduced to prevent the coupling of cylinders of anaesthetic gases to the wrong manifold or inlet on the anaesthetic machine (BS 1319 (1955)). The system consists of six possible pin positions on the yoke and six possible hole locations on the cylinder valve. Each gas is identified by two pin positions, allowing ten possible combinations. Pin diameters are identical and their positions are numbered from one to six. Even with this system, however, incorrect connection of cylinders (or pipeline gas sources) to yokes with the connecting block in an upside-down position, has occurred. The pins should be inspected since they can become loose in the yoke and ingenious methods have been used to circumvent the system or less subtle manoeuvres such as forcibly removing the indexing pins. The yoke is often termed a 'hanger yoke' since the cylinder hangs in the yoke supported only by the locating pins and the pressure of the tightening handle. Suppliers of medical gases protect the stem of the cylinder valve outlet with an rigid plastic seal.

Medical gas pipeline supplies

Pipeline supplies of medical gases are more secure than the use of supplies from cylinders. The NIST system as used in the UK and the DISS in the USA have replaced the facility for a user-detachable pipeline on the anaesthetic machine itself which has led to cross-over accidents.

A piped oxygen system is not a guarantee against supply failure. The 'tug test' is a test where, after connecting the pipeline probe to the piped gas outlet, the anaesthetist tugs or pulls on the flexible pipeline to check that the probe remains fully engaged. This test must always be carried out as part of the pre-use check on anaesthetic machines; there have been instances of an incorrectly located probe, which visually appears to be correctly positioned and delivering gas, becoming disengaged during later use. There have also been occasions when a pipeline was thought to be connected, but the probe was in fact incorrectly located, the oxygen instead being supplied from a cylinder which had been left open. When the cylinder eventually emptied, the impression was given that pipeline failure had occurred. Interruption or obstruction of gas pipelines is uncommon, although many instances go unreported: the author is aware of several recent incidents where workmen have accidentally drilled through pipelines. Incidents have occurred when pipelines have been disconnected inadvertently. Machines equipped for pipeline operation must have at least one reserve cylinder of oxygen.

Gas pipelines of copper (prescribed in most standards) are preferable to potentially kinkable flexible hoses. If the latter are used they should be exposed throughout their length and should connect to fittings which are easily visible on the exterior of the machine. In modern equipment the pressure gauges can be permanently fitted to the yokes which are themselves an integral part of the apparatus, and permanent metal tubing with different screw connectors and colour coding for each gas should be used to connect the appropriate pressure reducing valves and flowmeters. The requirement to provide a reserve cylinder of oxygen is now included in International and National standards, and a device to warn if the pipeline supply is shut off for any reason.

VALVES AND GAUGES

Before the cylinder is connected to its yoke it should be 'cracked' (i.e. opened only slightly) to blow away any dust or other potentially inflammable foreign material adhering to the valve. The appropriate flowmeter needle valve should be turned on before this is done in order to prevent any sudden build up in pressure. The valves of cylinders must be opened 2½ turns. Marginal opening of such valves has resulted in failure to deliver sufficient oxygen when the pressure has fallen only slightly. Cylinder valves should be opened slowly to prolong the time during which adiabatic compression of the gas between the cylinder valve and the high-pressure side of the reducing valve, and the consequent production of heat, occurs. In this way heat of compression is dissipated and the establishment of a shock wave and flash fire prevented: a flash fire in a British anaesthetic machine of an obsolete design occurred due to failure of the non-return valve in the yoke used for the pipeline supply. The flowmeter needle valve is then reset. Complacency regarding the risk of fires and explosions in the operating room is unwarranted, even by those who do not use flammable agents. A cylinder valve should not be overtightened during closure lest damage to the lead seal between the valve body and the cylinder neck occurs.

Pressure gauges of the Bourdon type are universally fitted to anaesthetic machines. It has been argued that they are unnecessary in the case of nitrous oxide cylinders because they only give an indication of pressure and not necessarily of the contents of a cylinder.

Nevertheless, an N_2O cylinder nearly empty containing just gas and no liquid will still deliver gas for 20–40 min, during which time a pressure gauge provides very useful information. Gauges fitted to machines using centrally supplied piped gases should indicate the line pressure. In the design of the machine it is important that the gauge is clearly marked 'pipeline' or 'cylinder' as appropriate to minimize confusion. Gauges must be easily visible and should be positioned close to the relevant cylinder. ISO 5358 lays down that the contents gauge shall be provided with a scale marked '0, ¼, ½, ¾, full', of which the 0–¼ segment shall be coloured red.

One-way or backflow check valves

These are usually placed next to the inlet yoke but their position in the system may vary. Their function is to prevent loss of gas from an empty yoke and to prevent inadvertent transfilling between paired cylinders. Leakage of gas through the yoke when empty cylinders are changed should draw attention to defective check valves.

Pressure reducing valves (regulators)

Pressure reducing valves not only reduce the delivered pressure to a safer lower valve but also regulate the lower pressure so that it remains constant despite changes in the supply pressure, e.g. as a cylinder empties. This obviates the need for continuous minor adjustments of the flowmeter needle valve. Pressure regulators are only needed where the cylinder gauge pressure exceeds 10 kPa × 100; hence, they are not used for attached pipeline supplies. The exact set pressure is just below the pipeline pressure. The set valve is 400 kPa in the UK, 50 p.s.i. (333 kPa) in the USA and 310 kPa in France.

High-pressure gas flows through the inlet ports, through the inlet filter and reaches the control valve which restricts the flow into the low pressure chamber formed in the body below a flexible but stiff diaphragm. As soon as the pressure in this chamber reaches a predetermined value, the diaphragm is forced against the action of a control spring thereby drawing the needle valve onto the valve seating obstructing the flow of gas. Conversely, if the pressure in the chamber falls, the spring pushes the diaphragm against the gas pressure, opens the needle valve and permits a greater flow. The working pressure of the regulator is set by adjusting the tension of the spring. A pressure relief valve is also incorporated into the body so that if the diaphragm should rupture the anaesthetic machine is not subjected to a dangerous pressure. The intermediate pressure region of the anaesthetic machine includes components which receive gases at the reduced pressure, i.e. after passage through the pressure reducing valve or from the pipeline inlet connections which connect the machine to the medical gas pipeline systems.

Some anaesthetic machines have a second-stage oxygen regulator, located downstream from the oxygen source, adjusted to a precise value (e.g. 15–30 p.s.i. (100–200 kPa)). This regulator supplies a constant pressure to the oxygen flowmeter control regardless of fluctuations in the pipeline pressure.

Flowmeter needle valves

The gearing ratio of the control governing these needle valves varies according to different manufacturers. The control should enable the Rotameter™ float to travel the length of the tube with the minimum number of turns, yet fine adjustments should be readily possible. The name of the gas should be clearly marked and the control knobs should be colour coded: oxygen is singled out by the standards as distinctive by touch and made more prominent than the other controls. Each float and corresponding glass flowmeter tube is etched with an individual identification number.

The flowmeter needle valve control is usually positioned before the Rotameter. Because the Rotameter is calibrated by a 'free-flow' method, resistance encountered later (small calibre pipework, vaporizer, ventilators) may affect the absolute calibration though not the concentrations of gases.

FLOWMETERS AND RESTRICTORS

Flowmeters

The Rotameter is the most popular type of flowmeter and a precision of ±2.5% of reading over a 10:1 ratio of flow range is readily achieved. Extended ranges of flow can be obtained without major scale compression by a change in taper as in the 9 inch tubes. An arrangement of two flowmeters in series is used where very low flows are required, such as in closed circuit anaesthesia, but is confusing as the anaesthetist may fail to appreciate which range he is using; this was a particular problem in the past when more than one flowmeter control was provided for the specific gas. Flowmeters for the same gas should never be arranged in parallel and there should be only one flow control per gas. The space between the float and the tube is very small and so the vertical alignment must be correct and dirt excluded if the float is to rotate freely. The calibration should be permanently etched onto the tubes. Failure to see the float clearly at the extreme ends of the tube has resulted in accidents. Although a wire stop incorporated at the top of all Rotameters will prevent the float reaching the top, this problem has recurred. Illumination of the bank of flowmeters by soft lighting is helpful, although the anaesthetist should never be expected to work in a totally darkened room.

The simple 'left-to-right' flowmeter sequence is shown in Figure 1.1. Should a crack develop in the carbon dioxide or cyclopropane tube, or the seating of the tube or its connections become faulty, it is possible for

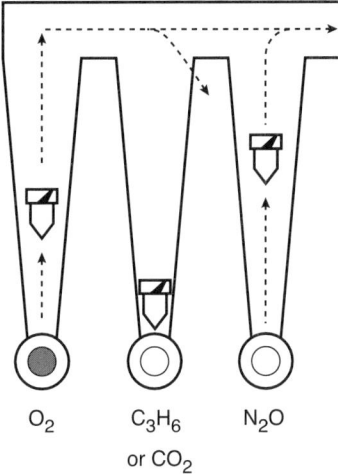

Figure 1.1 Conventional left-to-right flowmeter sequence as originally used in the UK. (Reproduced with permission from Adams, A.P. and Newton, N.I. (1996) Anaesthetic machines, in *International Practice of Anaesthesia* (eds C. Prys-Roberts and B.R. Brown), Butterworth-Heinemann, Oxford, pp. 2/147/1–18.)

oxygen to leak from the system at that point leaving the resulting hypoxic anaesthetic mixture to flow to the patient. This can also occur if an empty yoke is not blanked and its backflow check valve is faulty. Oxygen may easily leak through this if there is no pressure regulator to act as a 'stop'. The best solution is to interchange the positions of the oxygen and nitrous oxide flowmeters, but this simple expedient has been resisted in the UK on grounds of cost. Instead, a baffle is used to divert the oxygen to be last in sequence (Figure 1.2). However, the arrangement in North America with 'oxygen on the right' (Figure 1.3) is not completely foolproof and continuous monitoring of the oxygen concentration of fresh gas mixtures with an in-line oxygen analyser is recommended. The American National Standards Institute (ANSI) has described a pin-indexing system for flowmeters to eliminate the possibility of installing a flowmeter calibrated for nitrous oxide in place, say, of an oxygen flowmeter. The part

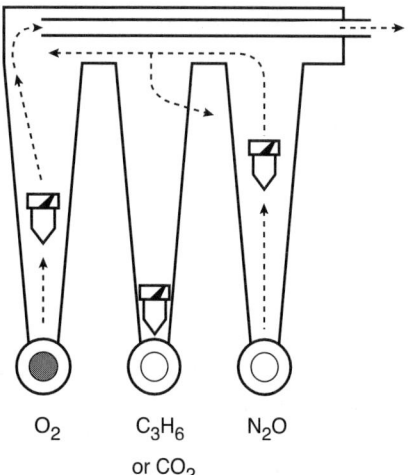

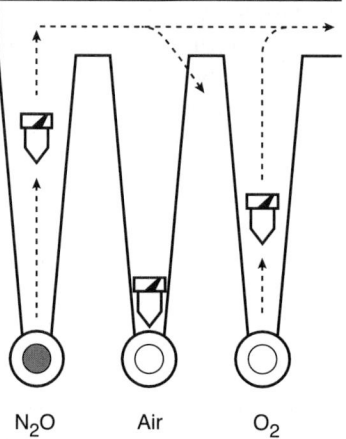

Figure 1.2 Conventional left-to-right flowmeter sequence as used in the UK. One way of diverting the oxygen away from a cracked or badly seated flowmeter tube is to use a baffle. (Reproduced with permission from Adams, A.P. and Newton, N.I. (1996) Anaesthetic machines, in *International Practice of Anaesthesia* (eds C. Prys-Roberts and B.R. Brown), Butterworth-Heinemann, Oxford, pp. 2/147/1–18.)

Figure 1.3 Flowmeter sequence used in the USA and Canada with oxygen 'on the right'. (Reproduced with permission from Adams, A.P. and Newton, N.I. (1996) Anaesthetic machines, in *International Practice of Anaesthesia* (eds C. Prys-Roberts and B.R. Brown), Butterworth-Heinemann, Oxford, pp. 2/147/1–18.)

of the anaesthesia machine downstream of the flowmeters is termed the low pressure region since the pressure is only slightly above atmospheric.

Flow restrictors

These are incorporated in modern anaesthetic machines operating at a working pressure of 300–400 kPa. The restrictors are placed at the entry point of the pipelines to protect the flowmeters from damage when the pipelines are connected. They may also be placed on the outlet or downstream side of vaporizers (or incorporated into the vaporizer), thus keeping the vaporizers slightly pressurized and hence making them less susceptible to variations in their output concentration from back-pressure ('pumping') effects within the patient circuit.

Filters

A system of sintered bronze filters is located proximal to the chain of critical units such as check valves, pressure gauges, reducing valves and flowmeter needle valves to protect against foreign material being introduced into gas lines.

SAFETY DEVICES

Oxygen failure alarm

The basic requirement is to give an adequate and appropriate warning of impending oxygen failure and secondarily to cut off or divert the flow of other gases. Reliance should not be placed on outside sources of power such as batteries nor on the pressure of other gases such as N_2O. The alarm should be on the reduced side of the oxygen supply line. The unit should 'fail-safe', be tamperproof and be unaffected by back-pressure developed by anaesthetic ventilators. The requirement (ISO and ASTM (American Society for Testing and

Materials) standards) is for a primary audible alarm of 7 s duration: in addition secondary oxygen failure protection devices may come into operation. There are several different types of alarm available.

Direct oxygen flush valve (emergency oxygen bypass)

The entry of the oxygen bypass should always be downstream of the vaporizers (Figure 1.4). This position avoids throttling of the supply by restrictions and also avoids passage through the vaporizers. The flow of oxygen delivered when the bypass control is operated should not be less than 35 $l\,min^{-1}$ nor more than 75 $l\,min^{-1}$. The bypass control should be of a design that prevents accidental operation and hence the risk of pulmonary barotrauma. Many cases of awareness during surgery have resulted from the control being inadvertently left on. Instances where the control has been operated accidentally have resulted from mechanical interference by the valve or bag mount attached to a closely positioned Cardiff swivel on the common gas outlet. For these reasons the supply of emergency oxygen should only flow as long as the anaesthetist holds down the control. However, in some machines the bypass control can be locked on to deliver a constant supply of gas leaving the anaesthetist's hands free should he/she desire it; this feature is no longer offered as standard on new anaesthetic machines.

Safety valves

Two types of valve are desirable. The pressure limiting valve limits the pressure within the breathing system to 6–8 kPa to minimize the risk of barotrauma to the patient. Anaesthesia machines must be fitted with vents to prevent the possibility of dangerously high gas pressures developing. The pressure relief valve opens at 35–40 kPa to protect the anaesthetic machine, e.g. the flowmeters and their seals, in the event of an occlusion to gas flow at the common gas outlet. Even vaporizers have 'exploded' as a result of high pressure in the system. In the event of a failure of the oxygen supply, the entrainment of atmospheric air in the spontaneously breathing patient may be permitted by an inlet valve built into the device for shutting off the supply of N_2O. Both these requirements are demanded by BS 4272 Part I (1968) which relates to anaesthetic machines of the on-demand type supplied with nitrous oxide and oxygen from separate containers. However, the entrainment of air by the patient is often of no value in some kinds of breathing system (e.g. circle and Bain systems) because of the high resistance of the long narrow bore delivery tube.

VAPORIZERS

Detachable vaporizers, introduced in 1972 as the SelectaTec™ system, are now almost universal. Awareness or hypoventilation during anaesthesia may result from leaks usually as a result of a missing O-ring seal, the presence of foreign bodies, a deranged mechanism, or failure of the anaesthetist to check that the vaporizer is correctly locked on to the backbar of the machine.

There have been several reports of high concentrations of vapour being delivered when a traditional freestanding vaporizer is used and the gas flow reversed through it by incorrect connection. The coloured key specific indexing system for filling vaporizers was introduced by Fraser Sweatman in the late 1960s. This is analogous to the pin-index system used for coupling medical gas cylinders to their yokes on the anaesthetic machine. However, mirrored matching indexing collars have been incorrectly fitted at the factory to bottles of liquid anaesthetic so the system is not completely foolproof. Vapour from an 'upstream' vaporizer should not be able to contaminate another on the 'downstream' side. For example, if halothane should

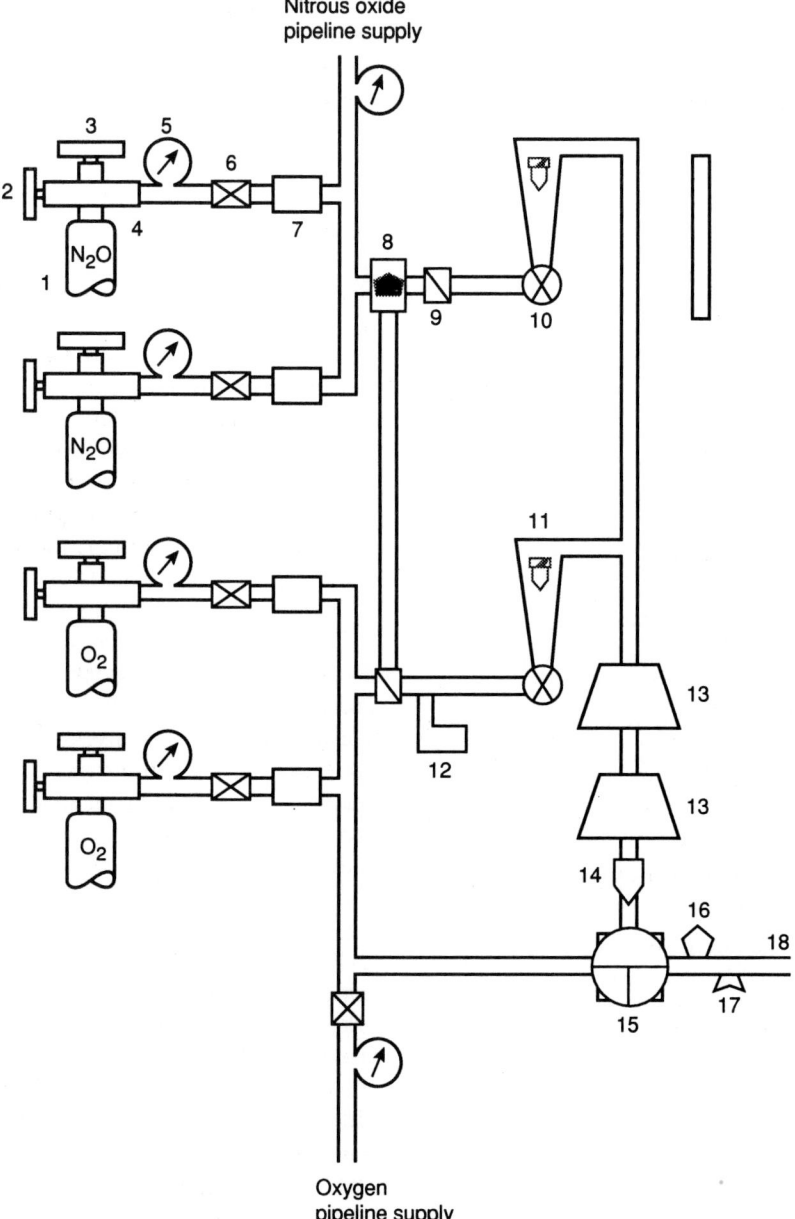

Figure 1.4 Sequence of components of a continuous flow anaesthetic machine: 1, gas cylinder(s); 2, hand screw to tighten cylinder in yoke; 3, hand wrench to open cylinder valve; 4, pin index yoke; 5, cylinder pressure gauge; 6, backflow check valve; 7, pressure reducing valve; 8, nitrous oxide cut-off; 9, flow restrictor; 10, flowmeter needle valve; 11, flowmeter; 12, oxygen failure alarm; 13, vaporizer(s); 14, one-way valve; 15, emergency oxygen control; 16, safety 'blow-off' valve; 17, safety air inlet valve; 18, common gas outlet from anaesthetic machine. (Reproduced with permission from Adams, A.P. and Newton, N.I. (1996) Anaesthetic machines, in *International Practice of Anaesthesia* (eds C. Prys-Roberts and B.R. Brown), Butterworth-Heinemann, Oxford, pp. 2/147/1–18.)

contaminate a 'downstream' methoxyflurane vaporizer a high concentration of halothane may subsequently be delivered from the methoxyflurane vaporizer. This could be prevented through a parallel arrangement of vaporizers. However, accidents may occur through faulty parallel switches or the anaesthetist not being aware which vaporizer was in use. Modern vaporizers, e.g. the Ohmeda Tec series versions 4 onwards, incorporate a mechanical interlock to prevent more than one agent being delivered.

The protection of vaporizers by flow restrictors has been mentioned. The pin-index system for vaporizers to prevent filling with the wrong liquid agent is a valuable safety feature. It is important to check that gases flow in the correct direction through vaporizers: the correct direction is usually indicated by an arrow. Many vaporizers will deliver twice the indicated concentration of agent should inadvertent reversal of direction of flow occur and the error is greater as the flow of gas is increased. Versions of the Oxford Miniature Vaporizer (OMV) are available for gas flow in either direction.

DRAW-OVER AND PORTABLE ANAESTHETIC MACHINES

Modern methods of providing analgesia to mothers in labour has led to the withdrawal of draw-over inhalers for obstetric purposes in the developed world. Nevertheless, such simple systems are used in very many countries where resources are inadequate or almost nonexistent, and the EMO (Epstein–Macintosh–Oxford) vaporizer still continues in production.

Portable anaesthetic equipment is used in dental, work, domiciliary obstetrics minor surgery, and civil disasters as well as in military situations. It is unfortunate that many anaesthetists do not have the opportunity to become experienced in using this type of equipment because the apparatus is not usually in everyday hospital use.

Systems centred on the use of a low-resistance draw-over vaporizer together with a means of applying intermittent positive pressure ventilation (IPPV) such as the Oxford Inflating Bellows (OIB) or a bag resuscitator are well established. Although ambient air is the carrier gas the addition of oxygen or anaesthetic gases may be made. The bellows *must* be placed between the vaporizer and the patient: this prevents the bellows being used to pressurize the vaporizer which could otherwise easily happen. The EMO vaporizer has received worldwide acceptance as a simple thermocompensated anaesthetic apparatus. The OMV using halothane and placed in series with an EMO vaporizer greatly facilitates the induction of ether anaesthesia. Versions of the EMO and OMV are available for different volatile anaesthetic agents.

The best known portable system is the Tri-Service unit used by the three British Armed Forces. This comprises two Penlon OMV 50 vaporizers in series plus plastic corrugated tubing, valves and a self-filling bellows for IPPV; this arrangement gave good service in the Falklands campaign in the South Atlantic.

CHECKING THE ANAESTHETIC MACHINE

A thorough pre-use check of the anaesthetic machine is absolutely vital. Anaesthetists are required to rely heavily on memory for essential facts when carrying out routine and emergency procedures. In contrast, airline pilots do not rely solely on memory but use standard checklists. Many anaesthetists are not correctly trained in the checking of their machines before use. The importance of training in checklist procedures is emphasized as an integral part of training in anaesthesia. Checklists for anaesthetic machines have been published by various bodies. Checklists are often prepared by commercial companies for specific anaesthetic machines. Many manufacturers include very detailed check procedures (often known as Operation Verification

CHECKING THE ANAESTHETIC MACHINE

This pictorial check (*Anaesthesia* 1993; **48**: 183-185) is derived and extended from *Checklist for Anaesthetic Machines: a recommended procedure based on the use of an oxygen analyzer* published July 1990 by the Association of Anaesthetists of Great Britain & Ireland, 9 Bedford Square, London WC1B 3RA. The original document must have been read previously. Easy modifications may be made if there is no pipeline supply or a varying numbers of cylinders.

1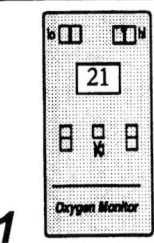

Set up oxygen analyzer according to instructions

Attach the sensor to the common gas outlet

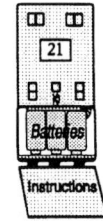 **2**

3 **Medical Gas Supplies**
- Anaesthetic machine disconnected from pipelines
- Remove all unwanted cylinders
- Check remaining cylinders correctly seated and turned 'off'
- Empty yokes blanked
- All vaporizers 'off'
- Electrical supply 'on'
- Open ALL flowmeter control valves

4 Turn O_2 cylinder ON

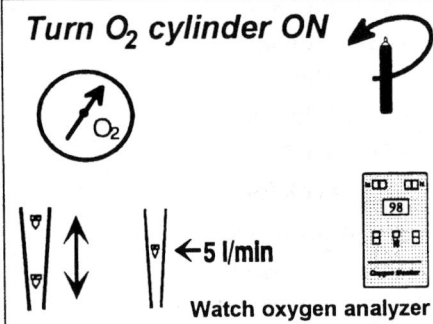

←5 l/min

Watch oxygen analyzer

5 Turn N_2O cylinder ON

5 l/min

Turn O_2 cylinder OFF

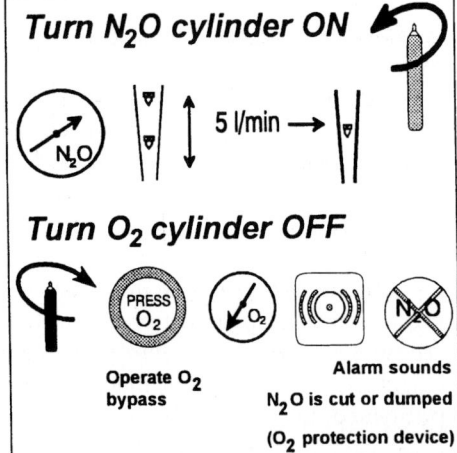

Operate O_2 bypass

Alarm sounds
N_2O is cut or dumped
(O_2 protection device)

6 Connect oxygen pipeline

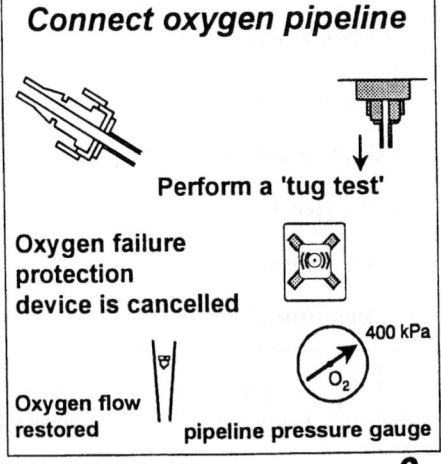

Perform a 'tug test'

Oxygen failure protection device is cancelled

Oxygen flow restored

400 kPa

pipeline pressure gauge

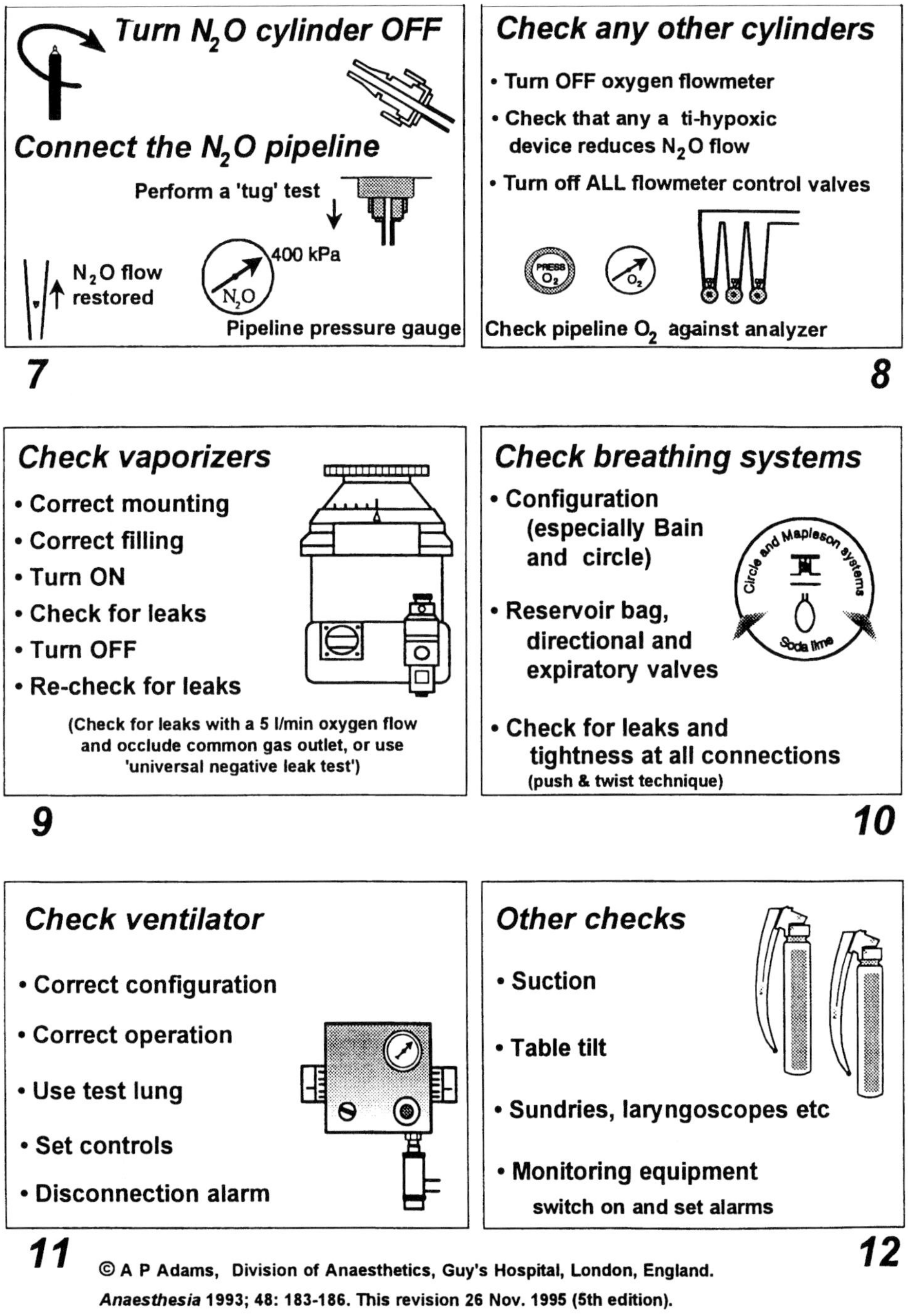
Turn N2O cylinder OFF
Connect the N2O pipeline
Perform a 'tug' test
400 kPa
N2O flow restored
N2O
Pipeline pressure gauge
7
Check any other cylinders
• Turn OFF oxygen flowmeter
• Check that any a ti-hypoxic device reduces N2O flow
• Turn off ALL flowmeter control valves
PRESS O2
O2
Check pipeline O2 against analyzer
8
Check vaporizers
• Correct mounting
• Correct filling
• Turn ON
• Check for leaks
• Turn OFF
• Re-check for leaks
(Check for leaks with a 5 l/min oxygen flow and occlude common gas outlet, or use 'universal negative leak test')
9
Check breathing systems
• Configuration (especially Bain and circle)
• Reservoir bag, directional and expiratory valves
• Check for leaks and tightness at all connections
(push & twist technique)
Circle and Mapleson systems
Soda lime
10
Check ventilator
• Correct configuration
• Correct operation
• Use test lung
• Set controls
• Disconnection alarm
11
Other checks
• Suction
• Table tilt
• Sundries, laryngoscopes etc
• Monitoring equipment
switch on and set alarms
12
© A P Adams, Division of Anaesthetics, Guy's Hospital, London, England.
Anaesthesia 1993; 48: 183-186. This revision 26 Nov. 1995 (5th edition).

Figure 1.5 Pictorial check for anaesthetic machines. © A.P. Adams, 1996. (Reproduced with permission from Adams AP, Morgan M, *Anaesthesia*, 1993, **48**: 183–185.)

Procedures) in their service manuals intended for use by service engineers which may take up to one hour to complete: these checks are not designed for daily use.

Many published checking procedures take a considerable time to perform and although this may not be resented by passengers in the case of preflight checks by aircrew, there does appear to be a demand for quick checks by staff in the case of anaesthesia: this is yet another instance of the anaesthesia workplace sacrificing safety for expediency. The oxygen concentration monitor is an essential tool for checking out the anaesthetic machine and its use is demanded by the check system issued by the Association of Anaesthetists of Great Britain & Ireland (AAGBI) in 1990. A pictorial checklist based on the AAGBI checklist is available (Figure 1.5) and may be personalized according to the equipment a particular institution possesses by modifying the images. This checklist is the most appropriate way of being sure that there is no crossover (the so-called 'wrong gas' effect) between the oxygen supply, the nitrous oxide supply and (where fitted) a compressed air source. This device will also detect contamination of the pipeline oxygen supply as has happened from the retrograde filling of the pipeline with gases other than oxygen due to faulty blender devices in other parts of the hospital, or frank contamination of the liquid 'oxygen' source. The AAGBI checklist is not designed to be specific to any particular anaesthetic machine. Although it may not be possible to apply such checks to every conceivable type of anaesthetic machine it is applicable to the vast majority of machines in present use in the UK. It aims to strike the right level of checking so that it is not so superficial that the value is doubtful or so detailed that the procedure is impracticable. The problem of checking the anaesthetic machine has been approached from a novel viewpoint which is to base the checks on using the oxygen analyser attached to the common gas outlet of the anaesthetic machine. This approach will detect situations such as incidents where an oxygen medical gas cylinder was refilled with nitrogen, or where contamination of the liquid oxygen reservoir with nitrogen had occurred; existing checks relying on visual identification of colour markings to avoid crossover would not detect these dangerous situations. The AAGBI checklist was surveyed in a teaching hospital: the most frequent problems were the poor reliability of some oxygen analysers, absent ventilator disconnection alarms and absent oxygen failure alarms on some older machines. No problems were detected during anaesthesia which were missed by the checklist. The mean time to complete the checklist for one machine was under 9 min. Faults were found in 60% of the machines checked; 18% of these were deemed to be serious.

In the USA, the Food and Drug Administration (FDA) produced a new checklist in 1993. In particular, their approach is to test for leaks by a 'universal negative leak test'. The machine master switch, the flow control valves and the vaporizers are turned off. A rubber suction bulb is attached to the common gas outlet and squeezed repeatedly until it is fully collapsed. The machine is leak free if the hand bulb remains collapsed for at least 10 s. A leak is present if the bulb reinflates in this time. The test must be repeated with each individual vaporizer turned on.

Despite the wide publicity regarding the need to perform checks before use of the anaesthetic machine, accidents continue to occur. In 1993 the UK Department of Health issued yet another hazard warning, drawing attention to their previous report concerning maintenance-induced faults, and has now insisted that the checking of anaesthetic equipment is an audited activity within the user's department. This action followed a serious accident which occurred because the gas pipelines had been transposed inside the machine during servicing. The anaesthetic machine had not been adequately checked after servicing by the engineer or before being used on the patient by hospital staff. The AAGBI check would have discovered the problem.

An electronic checklist has been developed which expands the concept to include additional protocols and problem-solving checklists in addition to the pre-anaesthesia checklist. Advantages claimed for the electronic, rather than paper, approach are that support in the form of 'on line help' is available to explain the checklist or provide insights for decision making, the documentation is legible and useful in medicolegal respects. However, the concept of comprehensive electronic checklists needs to be evaluated further.

CLASSIFICATION OF ANAESTHETIC MACHINES

Anaesthetic machines were originally classified as either the continuous flow (plenum) type or the intermittent flow (on-demand) type. The latter type are now almost obsolete. Developments in the continuous flow type may be classified as follows.

FIRST GENERATION

The first generation of anaesthetic machines were essentially gas driven units which did not have the ability to measure easily the concentration of gases and vapours which were dispensed. Thus the underlying philosophy was that the machine should be built on the basis of accurate engineering to produce known concentrations of gases and vapours such that its performance could be relied upon.

SECOND GENERATION

The second generation of machines incorporated an electrical power supply, which primarily enabled the anaesthetic machine to monitor its own function by means of integral monitors such as oxygen analysers, disconnection alarms, etc. This concept introduced the term 'anaesthetic workstation'. Once an electrical power supply was an accepted feature of the anaesthetic machine, made possible by the discontinuance of inflammable agents, it was possible initially to provide power sockets on the machine for monitors, and subsequently to build the monitors into the machine itself. This has paved the way for integrated monitors which may have a common alarm system which can be prioritized. Furthermore, a compatible automated chart recording system and data collection can be incorporated. Hence the second generation machine was a safety-oriented refinement of the original concept and this describes the majority of anaesthetic machines in use today. The provision of an integrated electrical power supply enables the machine to be provided with the following.

- Machine monitors, including sensing the oxygen and vapour concentration delivered at the common gas outlet.
- Monitors of lung ventilator function and breathing system with associated alarms, including airway pressure, minute and tidal volumes, frequency of ventilation, etc.
- Monitors of the breathing system: airway pressure; minute and tidal volumes; frequency and associated alarms. In addition end-tidal carbon dioxide and volatile agent concentration may be monitored as well as inspired oxygen and nitrous oxide.
- Patient monitors: ECG, pulse oximetry, non-invasive blood pressure (NIBP), temperature, etc. Also, the facility for invasive arterial and central venous pressure monitoring.

Monitors may be integrated with common alarm systems and facilities for automated chart recording and data collection.

THIRD GENERATION

The third generation of anaesthetic machine which is just becoming available involves a completely new concept for the workstation which takes advantage of the rapid growth in electronics and microprocessor control. The general concept includes the following.

- The machine no longer functions on conventional pneumatic principles.
- It no longer requires the conventional layout and may even be keyboard operated.
- Depends on sophisticated self-monitoring and alarms to warn of malfunction.
- The monitoring system – for the anaesthetic machine and for the patient – embraces the anaesthetic machine itself and is the most sophisticated aspect of the anaesthetic workstation.
- These machines use electronics and fluid logic systems to control the passage of gas and vapour as well as providing an integral method for automatic ventilation of the lungs.

This class of system is likely in the future to incorporate a feedback system to control the activity of the machine according to the patient's response. Economy may be effected by use of closed systems with resultant environmental pollution control. In such machines (Engström, Physioflex) the liquid anaesthetic does not need to be poured into the vaporizer; the bottle is merely screwed into a yoke on the back of the machine. The liquid is siphoned, exact amounts of vapour produced and added to the gas stream by microprocessor control. The new Engström Elsa machine has much of the traditional look about it: the anaesthetist adjusts controls to alter gas flows and vapour concentration. Information is passed to him in the form of a simulated flowmeter or vaporizer dial by means of a bar-graph or dial display. The anaesthetist readily understands the layout of the machine, without having to understand the actual way in which it functions.

In the Physioflex® machine there is no attempt to simulate any of the traditional format. The heart of the machine is a series of microprocessors and the display is a conventional computer visual display monitor. The input of medical gases and vapours is from pipelines and the bottles of liquid anaesthetic screwed to their attachments. When the machine is switched on it performs a self-check and then information on the screen indicates how to set it up. The machine can be programmed for the individual anaesthetist, or operating list. Requirements are entered at the keyboard. The user enters basic data such as the weight of the patient and what kind of anaesthetic is to be used. The computer analyses this information and monitors itself and the patient's responses. There is a fully integrated patient monitoring system with prioritized alarms, automated chart recording and data collection. The patient is connected to a closed circle breathing system through which a high constant flow of gas of about $70 \, l \, min^{-1}$ is circulated. This means that changes in gaseous or vapour composition are instantly transmitted to the patient. A charcoal filter is used to remove vapours if it is necessary to suddenly reduce the vapour concentration in the breathing system. The concept may be difficult to embrace, although a person coming newly into anaesthesia who had never seen or used the traditional anaesthetic machines would have no problem. Advances like this must be tempered with the thought 'what happens if there is a power cut or the computer fails?' Obviously a reliable and adequate back-up system must come into force. The developmental effort behind these anaesthetic workstations is immense.

THE ANAESTHESIA WORKSTATION

Experience in industry has clearly shown that the organizational structure of the work environment significantly affects safety. Current anaesthesia equipment does little to support the anaesthetist in his various tasks where the best human performance and vigilance are vital. His daily tasks have been compared with those of a systems manager, where the patient represents a dynamic system. The anaesthetist gathers and records data from the system, interprets the data to detect deviations from the desired state, and then controls the system to maintain a steady state. The anaesthesia workplace is filled with discrete items of equipment which collect data from the patient and from the machine. The data may be displayed over a wide area and may be presented in a less than optimum manner. The anaesthetist thus performs a complex task in a difficult and poorly designed workspace. Part of the reason for this problem may be lack of appreciation of the importance of team dynamics, human–machine and human–environment interactions in optimizing monitoring performance, or insufficient study of operating room requirements. Often, anaesthetic considerations are forced to the back of the queue for economic reasons. One step towards improving this state of affairs is the development of the anaesthesia workstation. The proposed role of this workstation would be: to provide a central and uniform format for the display of information; to aid in providing control of the selected variables; to aid in the detection of unexpected events; and to prepare a record of the anaesthetic. A prototype anaesthesia workstation has given promising results. Proposals for improving the anaesthetic workplace include the following.

- There should be ergonomic improvements to the anaesthetist's workplace so that he can perform well, adequate space and automation of repeated and relatively less important activities.
- Vital information about the patient's condition must be provided in a position where it will dominate the anaesthetist's attention.
- Information about medications, infusions, transfusions, etc. can be located on the left-hand side of the anaesthetist.
- All other devices can be located beside the anaesthetist or even behind him, as they are of minor importance.
- The most useful alternative to the present arrangement would be to position the information panels of primary and secondary monitoring devices to the immediate right, or on the right- and left-hand sides of the anaesthetist at an angle of 15–30° each. These information panels should be arranged so they can be monitored using movable screens which may be tilted.
- The most important of the patient's vital signs should be monitored by means of warning devices which can easily identify the exact problem and not cause confusion.
- The problem of fatigue must be taken into consideration in establishing optimal anaesthesia workplaces in the future.

Equipment standards are now being formulated particularly with respect to mandatory monitoring of volatile anaesthetic agents and the interrelationships of monitors and their alarms with anaesthesia machines. The work on anaesthetic workstations started in the USA but almost simultaneously was taken up by the ISO and CEN. There is considerable overlap in both committees to some extent as the major anaesthetic manufacturers are all multi-national companies. The current standards specifically exclude patient monitoring such as pulse oximeters, ECG, NIBP, etc. as these are chosen by clinical practice. The basic concept of the anaesthetic workstation is that each workstation is operated with 'delivery system' devices (an 'actuator' that delivers either energy or drugs), and specific associated devices designed for protection against the hazards from the delivery of this energy or substance to the patient. The intent is that for every specific delivery system (actuator) there will be a specific hazard protection device associated with it, e.g. when a ventilator is in use, a pressure monitor with a high pressure alarm (the hazard protection device) also must be in use. However the draft standards prohibit any monitor controlling an actuator: the 'closed loop' is only permitted if an independent monitor is provided in addition. Development of the new workstation standard is almost complete and is expected to be submitted soon to the national delegations within the ISO committee on anaesthesia. The European Community will adopt, or very closely adapt, an existing ISO standard. In many cases the ISO standards are very similar, if not identical, to current USA (ASTM F-29) standards.

The prioritization of alarms is included in the anaesthesia workstation standard. The alarm characteristics of monitors should be grouped into three categories:

- high priority, indicating a condition requiring urgent and immediate attention
- medium priority, requiring prompt action on the part of the anaesthetist
- low priority, a signal indicating a condition of which the anaesthetist must be aware, but may or may not respond to (e.g. warning of low battery condition).

Usually these monitors have both audible and visual alarms, the audible alarms serving to capture the anaesthetist's attention and indicating the degree of urgency with which he should respond, while the visual alarm confirms the alarm and indicates the probable site or cause of the alarm condition. It is possible for a central monitor to process, integrate and announce these alarms and this is to be preferred. Multiple alarms sounding simultaneously can be distracting and counterproductive when urgent action is required. A single central alarm-cancelling button is preferable to locating individual alarms.

Standardization of alarm signals (both visual and auditory) has been agreed, the auditory signals being designed to be recognizable in terms of priority, but not too alarming in themselves. ISO standards are in the course of publication and CEN will follow.

FURTHER READING

Adams, A. P. (1992) Safety in anaesthetic practice, in *Recent Advances in Anaesthesia and Analgesia*, (eds R. S. Atkinson and A. P. Adams) 17th edn, Churchill Livingstone, London, pp. 1–24.

Adams, A. P. and Morgan, M. (1993) Checking the anaesthetic machine – checklists or visual aids? *Anaesthesia*, **48**, 183–186.

AAGBI (1990) *Checklists for Anaesthetic Machines. A recommended procedure based on the use of an oxygen analyzer.* Association of Anaesthetists of Great Britain & Ireland, London.

BS 1319. (1976) *Specification for medical gas cylinders, valves and connections.* British Standards Institution, Milton Keynes.

BS 1319C. (1976) *Chart of colours for identification of the contents of medical gas cylinders.* British Standards Institution, Milton Keynes.

Davey, A., Moyle, J. B. T. and Ward, C. S. (1992) *Ward's Anaesthetic Equipment*, 3rd edn, W. B. Saunders, London.

Feldman, J. M., Blike, G. and Cheung, K. H. (1992) New electronic checklists aim at decreasing anesthesia errors. *Anesthesia Patient Safety Foundation Newsletter*, **7**, 1–2.

International Standard IEC 601–2–13. (1st edn 1989). *Medical electrical equipment. Part 2: Particular requirements for the safety of anaesthetic machines.* Bureau Central de la Commission Electrotechnique Internationale, Geneva, Switzerland.

Russell, W. J. (1992) The anaesthetic machine, circuits and gas supplies: recent developments, complications and hazards. *Current Opinion in Anaesthesiology*, **5**, 799–805.

PRINCIPLES OF MONITORING 2

L. B. Cook, K. K. Panikkar and M. Morgan

GENERAL PRINCIPLES: CARDIORESPIRATORY

L. B. Cook

The first documented general anaesthetic was administered in 1846. Although other patients must surely have succumbed in the interim, the first death attributed solely to anaesthesia occurred two years later. Fifteen year old Hannah Greener had been 'crying continually and wishing she were dead, rather than submit' to the removal of an ingrowing toenail. Shortly after induction she had a cardiac arrest. This illustrates two points. Firstly, disasters can and do happen to young fit patients during the most minor procedures. Secondly, since the earliest years of anaesthesia, mishaps have been uncommon. Our own mistakes being rare, we must learn from the errors of others.

We may also hope to learn from their wisdom. One of the first dedicated anaesthetists, Joseph Thomas Glover, claimed in 1871 to have administered over 11 000 anaesthetics without a death. He explained his success simply. 'It is my habit ... to watch the pulse as well as the breathing ...'. This 'habit' would have prevented most anaesthetic mishaps to date.

Vital though clinical observation still is, it no longer suffices, because advances in anaesthesia have multiplied the things that can go wrong. The anaesthetic machine, for example, introduced the problems of disconnections, hypoxic mixes and barotrauma. Muscle relaxants made modern surgery possible, but also brought awareness and recurarisation. As anaesthetic techniques develop, new problems emerge and the need for monitoring changes

HUMAN BEINGS AND MACHINES

The first and main monitor is always the anaesthetist, who can monitor the whole of the patient's condition and follow the course of the surgery, anticipating problems and correcting them when they occur.

By contrast, even the most sophisticated electronic monitors are inherently limited. They can only monitor one aspect of the patient's condition. They require power, need maintenance, occasionally develop faults and are prone to error. Their advantage is immunity to stress, boredom, distraction and fatigue. People cannot be completely vigilant at all times. A correctly set monitor saves lives by drawing attention to a problem before it is too late to correct it. In addition, some monitors provide information which is not otherwise obtainable. Examples include inspired and

Short Practice of Anaesthesia. Edited by M. Morgan and G. M. Hall. Published in 1997 by Chapman & Hall, London. ISBN 0 412 71890 1

expired oxygen, carbon dioxide and vapour concentrations.

RISK AND BENEFIT

The benefit of using a monitor lies in its ability to warn of adverse events. There are several considerations. How important is the event? How preventable? How likely? How good is the monitor at detecting this particular event? Good in this context means how early does it warn, how sensitive is it (how reliably does it pick up the event) and how specific is it (how often does it alarm when the event has not occurred).

Monitoring may impose direct risks. These are appreciable with a pulmonary artery catheter, for example and minimal with an oximeter. Monitors also carry indirect risks, because they may distract and confuse. Distraction is inevitable; while zeroing the arterial line one cannot observe the chest movement. Each additional monitor distracts attention from the patient and from other monitors. Confusion occurs when the information the monitor provides is misinterpreted. A normal looking ECG trace, for example, may delay recognition that the patient has become pulseless.

It is not appropriate to attach every available monitor to each patient. Rather, we choose monitors to enable us to detect and treat likely adverse events. For a cardiac cripple undergoing major surgery this may require direct measurement of systemic and pulmonary artery pressure, an unacceptably dangerous mode of monitoring for healthy patients having lesser surgery. Some monitors, however, are so useful and so safe that they should be used in all patients. These form the core of safe practice and are described next.

MINIMAL MONITORING STANDARDS

All patients undergoing anaesthesia are at risk. Most disasters stem from failure to recognize some simple problem, for example a ventilator disconnection. Most such problems can be detected by relatively simple, safe, monitoring, which is therefore recommended for all patients.

The first set of standards to be published was that of the Harvard Medical School System in 1986. The American Society of Anesthesiologists endorsed a similar set of recommendations the following year. The Association of Anaesthetists of Great Britain & Ireland published its own recommendations in 1988 and these were revised in 1994. The summary is reproduced in Table 2.1.

Particularly important is that monitoring begins before induction and continues until after recovery, with the anaesthetist present throughout. Monitoring is clinical observation supplemented by a variety of techniques including oximetry, capnography and electrocardiography, as well as intermittent determinations of blood pressure.

This represents the minimal acceptable provision of care for anaesthesia in the developed world. Medicolegally and ethically it would be difficult to defend a practice which fell short of these standards.

EVIDENCE

The scientific basis of modern medicine is the randomized controlled clinical trial. With death rates from anaesthesia already low, there is no prospect of using such a trial to prove the case for monitoring. What evidence we have is anecdotal.

When minimal monitoring standards were introduced, anaesthesia-related deaths declined (and anaesthetists' insurance premiums fell). However, the death rate was probably falling anyway. Monitoring was substandard in many cases where an anaesthetic mishap occurred. Does this prove that improved monitoring will prevent such episodes? No, because it might be that bad

Table 2.1 Recommendations for standards of monitoring during anaesthesia and recovery

1. The Association of Anaesthetists of Great Britain and Ireland strongly recommends that the standard of monitoring used during general anaesthesia should be uniform in all circumstances irrespective of the duration of anaesthesia or the location of administration.
2. An anaesthetist must be present throughout the conduct of general anaesthesia.
3. Monitoring should be commenced before induction and continued until the patient has recovered from the effects of anaesthesia.
4. These recommendations also apply to the administration of local anaesthesia, regional analgesia or sedation where there is a risk of unconsciousness or cardiovascular or respiratory complications.
5. The anaesthetist should check all equipment before use. Monitoring of anaesthetic machine function during the administration of anaesthesia should include an oxygen analyser with alarms. During spontaneous ventilation, clinical observation and a capnometer should be used to detect leaks, disconnections, rebreathing and high pressure in the breathing system. Measurement of airway pressure, expired volume and carbon dioxide concentration is strongly recommended when mechanical ventilation is employed.
6. A pulse oximeter and capnometer must be available for every patient.
7. It is strongly recommended that clinical observation of the patient should be supplemented by continuous monitoring devices displaying heart rate, pulse volume or arterial pressure, oxygen saturation, the electrocardiogram and expired carbon dioxide concentration. Devices for measuring intravascular pressures, body temperature and other parameters should be used when appropriate. It is useful to have both waveform and numerical displays.
8. Intermittent non-invasive arterial pressure measurement must be recorded regularly if invasive monitoring is not indicated. If neuromuscular blocking drugs are used, a means of assessing neuromuscular function should be available.
9. Additional monitoring may be required in certain situations. These recommendations may be extended at any time on the judgement of the anaesthetist.
10. A printed record of monitoring measurements provides a contemporaneous record during emergency situations and allows the anaesthetist to concentrate on managing the patient.
11. When handing over to recovery staff, anaesthetists should issue clear instructions concerning monitoring during postoperative care. Monitoring of oxygen saturation is strongly recommended for all patients and temperature monitoring is recommended for patients at risk of hypothermia.
12. Standards for monitoring during transfer of sedated, anaesthetized or unconscious patients should be as high as during the administration of anaesthesia. All patients should have oxygen saturation, electrocardiogram and arterial pressure monitored. Other monitors may be appropriate in certain circumstances.
13. For interhospital transfers, a specialist retrieval team based at the receiving hospital can have advantages.

anaesthetists use fewer or inappropriate monitors, so the inadequate monitoring reflects generally substandard care, which causes the poor outcome.

The most compelling evidence is our own experience. Most anaesthetists would admit to having failed to notice a potentially life threatening event until some monitor (or other person) warned them. In this respect our experience parallels that of the aviation industry. No airline has randomized its aircraft to have or not have radar, black boxes or landing lights. Few of us would fly with the airline that did.

MONITORING THE RESPIRATORY SYSTEM

Most preventable anaesthetic mishaps are caused by failure of oxygenation. It is easy to see why. The patient is connected to the anaesthetic machine via a whole series of push-fit connectors, any of which can come adrift. Many breathing systems are a lashed-together ramshackle confusion of valves, con-

Table 2.2 The reservoir bag

Observation	Interpretation	Possible causes
Does not fill	No gas	Disconnection Low fresh gas flow into circle system Fresh gas fail
Bulging	Gas outflow obstruction	Expiratory valve closed Valve stuck Faulty scavenging
Pulsation synchronous with heartbeat	Airway clear	Apnoea with cardiac pulsation
Small movement and little patient effort	Respiratory depression	Vapours and anaesthetic drugs
Small movements with obvious patient effort	Obstruction	Anywhere between alveolus and bag
Easy to squeeze Refills slowly	Leak	Valve open Bag leak Oesophageal intubation
Difficult to squeeze Refills slowly	Increased resistance	Kinked tube Bronchospasm Other obstruction
Difficult to squeeze Refills rapidly	Reduced compliance	Endobronchial intubation Relaxants wearing off Surgeons leaning on chest Steep head down Diaphragm packed/splinted Pneumothorax Pulmonary oedema

nectors and tubes. Equipment, acquired piecemeal over the years, offers any number of ways to deliver the wrong gas mix, or no gas at all. It is a tribute to the skill and vigilance of anaesthetists that disasters are not more common. Even one, however, is one too many.

CLINICAL MONITORING

Generations of anaesthetists have emphasized the importance of the clear airway and adequate ventilation. These are still the most important guarantors of patient safety and most accidents result from failure to ensure them. With no equipment at all, some observations can be made. Is the chest moving? Can air be felt issuing from the mouth or nose? Can respiration be heard? If so, does it sound obstructed or gurgling?

An anaesthetic breathing system adds a powerful monitor, the reservoir bag. A great deal can be deduced both from watching the bag move and from squeezing it (Table 2.2). A kinked tube, for example, produces a characteristic feel. The increased resistance means it requires more pressure to squeeze the bag. In expiration, gas leaves the lungs slowly so the bag hangs limply. A fall in compliance (e.g. due to endobronchial intubation) feels very different. The inflating pressure is also high but the bag springs back into the ventilating hand in expiration. This is why hand ventilation is recommended when a ventilation problem is suspected. It is also why many still prefer hand ventilation for neonatal anaesthesia, where the patient is often totally obscured and inaccessible.

Nowadays we may readily monitor the volumes breathed in and out, the pressures generated by a ventilator and the nature of the gases inspired and expired. Wonderful though these technologies are, they *supplement* and do not replace basic clinical monitoring.

PRESSURE AND FLOW

If the patient is breathing spontaneously, then watching the reservoir bag confirms an adequate tidal volume. Similarly, during hand ventilation, disconnections and airway problems are immediately apparent. Usually, however, intraoperative ventilation is delegated to a machine. Here the potential for mishap is great, so it is mandatory to monitor the airway pressures and preferably the expired tidal volume as well.

Ventilator disconnect alarms are among the cheapest and most useful monitors. They provide no information which is not available from squeezing the bag or looking at the ventilator pressure gauge. They simply check, over and over, that ventilation is still occurring.

In the simplest devices, the alarm sounds if during a 10 s interval the airway pressure fails to reach the preset threshold (commonly 7–10 cmH$_2$O). A different alarm sounds if the airway pressure exceeds a preset maximum (30–40 cmH$_2$O). More complex alarms allow the apnoea time and the airway pressure limits to be varied. Normally, the pressure threshold should be set to a little lower than the patient's peak airway pressure and the high pressure alarm to around 10 cmH$_2$O higher than the patient's peak pressure.

The pressure sensor should be sited in the inspiratory limb of the ventilator tubing. If sited in the expiratory limb, the device would still detect disconnection and ventilator failure. However, it would fail to detect high pressure due to obstruction in the expiratory limb upstream of the sensor site.

Expired minute ventilation may be measured close to the patient or at any point in the **expiratory** limb of many ventilators and circle systems. In spontaneously breathing patients, continuous measurement of minute ventilation supplements clinical observation and provides a useful alarm for hypoventilation. In patients attached to ventilators clinical observation is less reliable (there is no reservoir bag) and measurement of expired ventilation is a vital indicator of continuing ventilation.

The first practical monitor of expired tidal volume was Wright's respirometer. This directs the expired gas at a tangent to a vane, which rotates, turning the needle on the gauge via a series of gears. These devices are still widely used for intermittent measurement of tidal volume. Electronic versions consist of a spirometer head within the breathing system, connected to a display and alarm unit. Within the spirometer head the rotating vane cuts a beam of light, producing a stream of electrical impulses from a light sensor. These are summed by the display unit to produce values for tidal volume and total ventilation. These devices can (and should) be set to alarm if the total ventilation falls below a safe level.

Rotating vanes are only one of the many ways available to measure expired gas flow. Pneumotachographs measure the pressure drop across a resistance, which is proportional to flow (Ohm's law). A hot wire suspended in the gas flow loses heat; the higher the flow, the more current required to heat the wire to constant temperature. This is the basis of the hot wire anemometer (though nowadays the 'wire' is often a silicon bridge on a microchip). Other devices simply measure the pressure exerted on a flap protuding into the gas flow or the pressure difference between

Table 2.3 Gas and vapour monitoring

Gas constituent	How measured	Why measured
Carbon dioxide	Infrared spectroscopy Mass spectroscopy Raman spectroscopy Chemical indicators	Tracheal tube position Visual indicator of gas exchange Adequacy of ventilation Early warning of many problems

Oxygen	Paramagnetism
	Chemical
	    Fuel cell
	    Polarographic
	Mass spectroscopy
	Raman spectroscopy
		Adequate oxygen in mix
		
		In low flow systems, increasing oxygen suggests driving gas is contaminating breathing system

Nitrogen	Mass spectroscopy Raman spectroscopy	Accumulates in low flow systems Research purposes
Nitrous oxide	Infrared spectroscopy Mass spectroscopy Raman spectroscopy	In low flow systems, concentration unpredictable. Too high, suggests oxygen too low Too low, suggests contamination of breathing system
Anaesthetic vapours	Infrared spectroscopy Mass spectroscopy Raman spectroscopy Piezo absorption	Guard against awareness (especially in low flow systems) Avoid accidental overdose

orifices facing into and away from the gas flow (the Pitot effect).

Ideally, all patients attached to ventilators should have both airway pressure and expired total ventilation monitored continuously. Many modern ventilators provide this monitoring automatically. Some will not function without it. Of the two, pressure monitoring is usually the more informative. This is because, in the operating theatre environment, most ventilators deliver a preset volume. In the absence of leaks and disconnections, the patient will receive a known tidal volume and changes in the patient characteristics will show up as changes in airway pressure. In patients breathing spontaneously, however, the airway pressure is not useful and continuous monitoring of the expired minute ventilation is a useful guard against hypoventilation.

GASES AND VAPOURS

A major advance in recent years has been the ability to monitor the concentration of individual gases breathed in and out. Apart from the rather rudimentary 'sniffing the mix' to see if a vapour is present, this information is not available through clinical observation.

Both oxygen and carbon dioxide concentrations should be measured throughout anaesthesia. Table 2.3 summarizes how and why various gases may be measured.

Oxygen

Delivery of a hypoxic gas mix is disastrous, so the inspired oxygen concentrations should be monitored throughout anaesthesia. A bonus is that a rising inspired oxygen concentration may warn of contamination of a breathing system with driving gas from the ventilator, with risk of awareness.

Oxygen is commonly measured by a galvanic or paramagnetic device which may be sidestream (within the capnograph) or mainstream (within the breathing system). The latter may conveniently be sited between the common gas outlet and the Magill or Bain breathing system. When a low flow system is used, the oxygen concentrations within the circle are lower than those in the fresh gas inflow. The analyser must be sited within the circle, not at the common gas outlet. If attached between the common gas outlet and a Manley ventilator, the device will over-read by approximately 10–15% because of back pressure. It is better placed in the ventilator inspiratory limb.

The working principles of oxygen analysers are described in a subsequent section.

Carbon dioxide

Carbon dioxide is the end product of aerobic metabolism. Produced in the tissues, it is transported by the cardiovascular system to the lungs and voided in the expired air. A normal capnogaph trace is a welcome sight, because it suggests that aerobic metabolism is present and the cardiorespiratory system is functioning. Absence of carbon dioxide strongly suggests that something is deeply wrong. For example, following intubation, if ventilation fails to produce a normal capnograph trace, the tube should be assumed to be in the oesophagus.

A normal expired breath consists of a volume from the trachea followed by a volume of alveolar gas. The boundary between these two volumes is quite sharp and the alveolar gas is relatively homogeneous. This explains the normal capnograph trace (Figure 2.1): a sharp rise in carbon dioxide content is detected when the alveolar gas reaches the sampling point and a clear plateau is seen for the remainder of the expiration. The end-tidal partial pressure of carbon dioxide in this phase is close to that in arterial blood, if alveolar deadspace small. In healthy patients, therefore the capnograph provides an extremely useful indication of the adequacy of ventilation.

Very different traces are frequently seen, some of which are shown and explained in Figure 2.1. They result from different respiratory patterns, some anaesthetic breathing systems and lung disease. Most of these traces do not yield reliable estimates of arterial P_{CO_2}.

When disaster strikes, the capnograph may give valuable clues to its nature. The flat line of apnoea is obvious and should be immediately recognized. Rare, but diagnostic, is the rapid rise of carbon dioxide in malignant hyperthermia. Failure of the cardiorespiratory systems causes characteristic traces, some of which are shown in Figure 2.2.

GAS ANALYSERS

The concentration of an individual gas or vapour is measured by exploiting some attribute which is not shared with other gases in the mix. Most commonly used is the ability to absorb radiation at some frequency, usually within the infrared spectrum. This is the basis of infrared spectroscopy. Oxygen does not absorb infrared radiation but may be measured by its behaviour in magnetic fields (paramagnetism) or by its ability to accept electrons. Two properties, the mass of the molecule and its Raman spectrum, allow analysis of all gases and vapours.

Infrared spectroscopy

Gases and vapours in the anaesthetic mix look colourless because they do not absorb light within the visible spectrum. Light at longer wavelengths, however, is strongly absorbed by those gases and vapours whose molecules are asymmetric and contain at least two different atoms. All that is required to detect such a gas is to find a wavelength of

26 *Principles of monitoring*

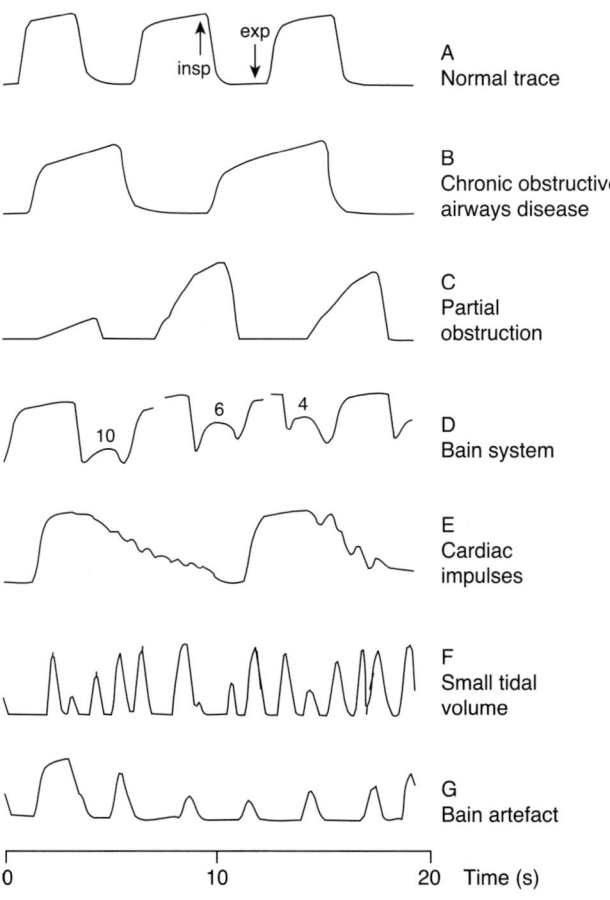

Figure 2.1 In the normal capnograph trace (A), when expiration starts (marked exp) the first volume expired is deadspace. Carbon dioxide is not detected until alveolar gas reaches the sampling point. There is a brisk upstroke and a well defined plateau, because alveolar air is homogeneous. Inspiration (insp) produces an immediate fall in carbon dioxide concentrations.

The plateau slopes in chronic lung disease (B) because fast alveoli are well ventilated, have low carbon dioxide tensions and empty early in expiration whereas slow alveoli have higher carbon dioxide tensions and empty later. When the airway is partially obstructed (C), turbulence mixes deadspace and alveolar gas before it reaches the sampling point, so the upstroke in carbon dioxide is slow.

The Mapleson D system (D) is shown with 10, 6 and 4 l min^{-1} of fresh gas inflow. The first gas inspired is fresh gas but when inspiratory flow exceeds fresh gas inflow, gas is drawn from the outer limb of the circuit. This produces the characteristic inspiratory 'hump', more pronounced with lower fresh gas flows.

Cardiac oscillations (E) are seen during expiratory pauses. Each heartbeat sends a volume of blood into the alveoli, causing a small jet of gas to be ejected from the trachea. Capnographs may misinterpret these oscillations as breaths or as a high inspired carbon dioxide tension.

When the tidal volume only just exceeds the anatomical deadspace the natural variation in the respiratory pattern means a variable amount of alveolar gas reaches the sampling site in each breath, giving pattern (F).

A similar pattern (G) results when the fresh gas flow is high in Mapleson D and E systems, because the jet of fresh gas dilutes the gas issuing from the trachea. In (G) the Bain system was connected after the first (normal) breath.

Only in traces A, D, and E does the trace afford a good estimate of alveolar carbon dioxide tension.

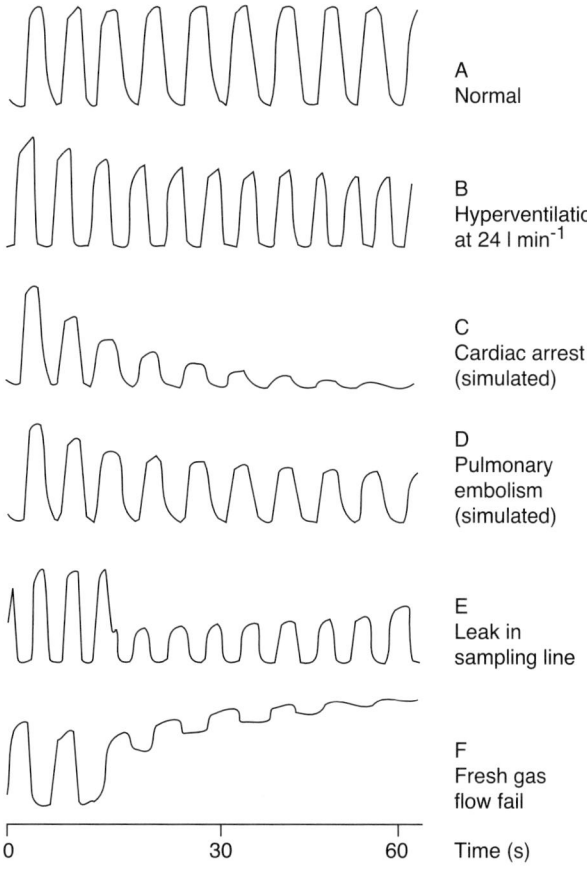

Figure 2.2 Changes in capnograph traces: (A) shows a normal capnograph trace; even gross hyperventilation (B) produces a relatively slow fall in end-tidal carbon dioxide tension, as the large reservoirs of this soluble gas are washed out slowly. Cardiac arrest (C) means that no further carbon dioxide is delivered to the alveoli and the store within the lungs is depleted by each new breath. Pulmonary embolism (D), whatever the nature of the embolus, results in a sudden increase in alveolar deadspace. The carbon dioxide within the unperfused alveoli is rapidly washed out and the end-tidal carbon dioxide tension stabilizes at a new level, less than that in arterial blood. Sudden falls in end-tidal carbon dioxide (E) are artefacts, usually due to leaks in the sampling system (in this case a cracked water-trap). When fresh gas fails there is gross rebreathing (F).

light which is strongly absorbed by that gas and no other.

There are many different ways to construct a functional infrared gas analyser. Common to them all is that light is shone through the sample to be analysed and the amount absorbed is proportional to the concentration of the gas of interest. All must also have a reference, to compensate for variation in the light source and photodetector. This can be arranged in two ways. The light beam may be divided into two, one traversing a reference gas, the other the sample to be analysed. Alternatively two frequencies of light may be shone through the sample, one strongly absorbed and the other not absorbed by the gases present. Either way, the ratio between the absorbtion of the reference and the measuring beam is used to calculate the measured concentration.

In a common design, a rotating disk called a chopper lies between the light source and the sample chamber. The chopper contains filters allowing a narrow range of light wavelengths to pass. To measure the concentrations of (say) carbon dioxide, filters are chosen to produce two wavelengths, one strongly absorbed by carbon dioxide and one not absorbed by any gas likely to be present. As the chopper rotates, a flash of first one then the other light passes through the sample to the photodetector. The machine compares the output from the photodetector at each wavelength. In use, this ratio is independent of the actual brightness of the light source, but varies with the concentration of carbon dioxide within the sample chamber. Nowadays the chopper will have many such pairs of filters, each designed to measure the concentration of a specific gas or vapour.

Zeroing to room air is usually done automatically when first switched on and at intervals thereafter. The machine thus 'knows' the ratio between the outputs of the photodetector for each pair of filters when there is no gas of interest in the sample chamber. Calibration is performed weekly or even less often, because in modern analysers calibration drift is very slow. It involves using a gas (supplied by the manufacturer of the analyser) with known concentrations of the gases and vapours to be analysed. With the machine in calibration mode the sampling line is connected to the can of calibration gas and a couple of breaths delivered. The machine electronically compares its own reading of the concentration of the constituents with the actual concentrations (stated on the container), updating its parameters as necessary.

Paramagnetism

This effect allows rapid accurate measurement of oxygen concentration. Individual oxygen molecules have magnetic moments due to their unpaired electrons. In a magnetic field, these moments line up, strengthening the field. The effect is that oxygen is attracted into powerful magnetic fields. This may be measured in different ways. In one arrangement a miniature dumb-bell containing nitrogen lies between the poles of an electromagnet. Outside the dumb-bell is the gas to be analysed. When the electromagnet is activated, oxygen is attracted into the field displacing the dumb-bell. The torsion on the axis of the dumb-bell is proportional to the oxygen concentration. In another method, a pulsed magnetic field is applied to twin coils, one containing a reference gas (usually air) and the other the gas to be analysed. The pressure difference between the two coils is directly proportional to the difference in oxygen content.

Galvanic and polarographic cells

Oxidation (in chemical terms, accepting electrons) is the reason oxygen is essential to life. Fuel cells (galvanic cells) are batteries, producing an electric current from the transfer of electrons in such reactions. The partial pressure of oxygen determines the number of oxygen molecules which diffuse across a membrane into the cell to take part in reactions. The more oxygen, the more current produced.

Commonly used is the oxidation of lead

$(2Pb + O_2 \rightarrow 2\ PbO)$.

How does this reaction produce an electric current? The answer lies in separating the oxidation into two reactions, one producing and one consuming electrons. The lead electrode is in a solution of hydroxide ions. It can be oxidized

$(2Pb + 4\ OH^- \rightarrow 2\ PbO + 2\ H_2O + 4e^-)$

provided the hydroxide ions are plentiful and the electrons produced can be disposed of. The latter flow round a circuit (being measured en route) to the inert electrode. Here they are accepted by oxygen, regenerating the hydroxide ions consumed at the other electrode

$$(4e^- + 2 H_2O + O_2 \rightarrow 4 OH^-).$$

Thus the lead only gets oxidized if oxygen diffuses into the cell, but the molecules which diffuse in are not the ones which end up forming lead oxide, at least not initially.

Similar to fuel cells are polarographic oxygen sensors, widely used in blood gas analysers. Again the number of oxygen molecules is measured by the current produced but an external voltage is applied to drive the reaction.

The mass spectrometer

Mass spectroscopy measures the relative abundance of different molecules, differentiating between them on the basis of their mass. Inside the spectrometer, a very high vacuum is maintained. A tiny sample of the gas to be analysed is allowed to leak into a chamber within the machine, where it is bombarded with electrons. The charged molecular fragments (ions) thus produced are accelerated by an electrical field towards the detectors. En route to the detectors, they are deflected by a powerful magnetic field. The more massive the ion, the less it is deflected by a given magnetic field, allowing ions of different mass to be discriminated. Strictly, it is the mass to charge ratio that is measured, as some ions have a charge greater than unity. In some machines the magnetic field is kept constant and the number of ions falling on different detectors is measured. Alternatively, just one detector is used and the magnetic field varied instead. Analysis is rapid, so breath to breath analysis of all gases is possible.

A problem is that some molecules have the same mass. In particular, nitrous oxide and carbon dioxide both have a mass of 44. This is overcome by measuring the abundance of a range of fragments (e.g. carbon, mass of 12) from which the relative contributions of carbon dioxide and nitrous oxide may be deduced. Mass spectrometers intended for respiratory system monitoring are pre-programmed with the 'signatures' of common gases and vapours and carry out this process automatically.

Raman spectroscopy

The Raman effect was described in 1928 but has only recently been used to provide practical respiratory system monitoring. When monochromatic light (from a laser) is shone through any transparent substance, most of the light passes straight through. However, a small amount (the Raman spectrum) is absorbed and re-emitted at a different wavelength and in a different direction. This light represents the results of elastic collisions between photons and the gas molecules. Different gases emit characteristic Raman spectra. All gases and vapours found in the anaesthetic mix may be accurately measured in this way. Monitors exploiting the Raman effect are accurate and reliable, but somewhat expensive.

Other methods

The methods already discussed account for the majority of gas analysers in use. However, there are other possibilities. A remarkably simple device includes a filter impregnated with a chemical that changes colour on contact with carbon dioxide. These single-use devices allow semi-quantitative capnography and are useful for resuscitation and patient transfer. Refractive indices differ among gases and vapours and allow accurate measurement of their concentrations, a technique too cumbersome for routine use. Analysers have been used which exploit the effect of vapours on the elasticity of rubber, or the effect of their absorption on the vibration of crystals.

MONITORING THE CARDIOVASCULAR SYSTEM

CLINICAL OBSERVATION

Simple observation provides much vital information, which in many cases is otherwise unavailable. Examples include: whether the patient looks well perfused, flushed, cyanosed or pale; the capillary refill; the colour of the conjunctivae; the skin temperature, and turgor; the characteristic mottled appearance of skin in limb ischaemia; the rash of anaphylactoid reactions. If at all possible, part of the patient should be left exposed to permit this essential monitoring.

Palpation of a pulse provides useful information, not least whether it is present. Likewise inspection of the neck veins may suggest low, normal or high central venous pressure. Auscultation of the heart, especially via an oesophageal stethoscope is also useful and is under-used.

THE ECG

Electrocardiography has two functions. The more important is to monitor the cardiac rhythm. The other is to detect ischaemic changes. In addition, changes in the ECG may raise suspicion of electrolyte imbalance, hypothermia, pulmonary embolism and other problems.

The electrocardiograph is essentially a voltmeter, measuring the potential difference between two points. Muscles and nerves generate potentials, but these usually average out to zero (they do affect the ECG sometimes, for example in shivering). The heart differs because its electrical activation starts at a focus and spreads in a defined direction. Thus atrial depolarization spreads away from the sino-atrial node and ventricular depolarization spreads down the bundle of His into the ventricles. This spread of depolarization leads to changing potential differences over the whole trunk.

A normal ECG trace does not indicate that there is a cardiac output. However, when there is clinical evidence that the cardiac output is inadequate, the ECG is vital in diagnosing why. It should be monitored in all patients throughout anaesthesia.

PULSE OXIMETRY

Pulse oximetry allows continuous display of a peripheral pulse waveform as well as continuous measurement of oxygen saturation. It has supplanted such techniques as transcutaneous oxygen tension measurement and should be used during all anaesthetics. In addition, it has proved invaluable in intensive care units, paediatric and neonatal units and in the accident and emergency department. Other applications include diagnosis of sleep apnoea syndromes and postoperative monitoring.

Oximetry is extraordinarily safe. Among the very rare problems reported are distal sensory loss and skin necrosis as a result of pressure at the probe site, usually in neonates or debilitated intensive care patients. Probes can malfunction, overheat and cause burns.

Working principles

Deoxygenated blood looks very dark because it strongly absorbs light in the visible spectrum. Oxygenated blood, however, absorbs little red light, so looks bright red. The absorbtion of light is also known as **extinction** and the ability of blood to absorb light of a given frequency is its **extinction coefficient**.

This colour difference is exploited by the co-oximeter, which pre-dated pulse oximeters by many years. Light of two different wavelengths is shone through a blood sample; the ratio of the amount absorbed at each wavelength allows the oxygen saturation to be calculated accurately. (Modern co-oximeters use many different wavelengths and can also measure carboxyhaemoglobin, methaemoglobin and other haemoglobin variants.)

The pulse oximeter uses a convenient tissue bed, commonly the finger or earlobe instead of a blood sample. Two different wavelengths of light are shone through the tissue bed to a photodetector. Most of the blood within the tissue bed lies in the veins and capillaries, so the simple ratio of the transmission of each wavelength will merely reflect the mean saturation of all the blood in the tissue bed. So how can the oximeter measure the saturation of blood only in the arterial tree?

The solution is that only the arterial blood is pulsatile. The volume and oxygen saturation of blood in the capillaries and veins are assumed to be constant over short periods (as is the absorbtion of light by bone, muscle, skin, etc.). When a pulse arrives at the tissue bed, the arterioles expand to accommodate the extra volume of blood, shrinking again as the blood runs off into the venous system. This extra volume of blood within the arterioles provides an additional barrier to the light traversing the tissue bed. How much of a barrier it is depends upon how strongly it absorbs light of that frequency. For example, if the arterial haemoglobin is predominantly oxygenated then the extra volume of blood arriving during a pulse will absorb relatively little red light but proportionately much more infrared light.

Thus the difference in light transmission over some short period is due to the pulsatility of the arterial system. The ratio of the difference in red light transmission to the difference in infrared light transmission depends only on the colour of the blood in the arterial tree. This is what we wish to know.

The pulse oximeter repeats a cycle of a burst of first one wavelength of light, then the other, measuring the amount of each which reaches the photodetector. The wavelengths used are usually 660 nm (red) and 940 nm (infrared) and are generated by light emitting diodes within the probe. Typically this cycle is repeated 25–60 times each second and a ratio obtained thus:

$$R = \frac{\text{red light transmitted now} - \text{red light transmitted last cycle}}{\text{infrared light transmitted now} - \text{infrared light transmitted last cycle}}$$

In practice the oximeter uses a weighted moving average of the ratio over a few seconds to calculate the displayed saturation. Different manufacturers use different algorithms for this conversion, aiming to minimize the effect of artefact while still allowing a rapid response to genuine changes in saturation.

Pitfalls

Poor contact between the probe and the skin may lead to falsely low readings, as may nail polish. Artefacts caused by motion and surgical diathermy may be misinterpreted as arterial pulsation, giving grossly inaccurate results. This is usually obvious because the displayed waveform is clearly not arterial. Poor arterial pulsation (e.g. in the shocked patient) may make the method inaccurate or unusable. In these patients, a tissue bed such as the tongue, lip or nasal septum may allow a trace to be obtained.

A less common source of error is flicker caused by artificial light reaching the photodetector. The effect is reduced by synchronizing the oximeter cycling rate with mains frequency (50 Hz in the UK, 60 Hz in North America). Probes should still be shielded from ambient light.

The volume of blood in the venules is assumed to be constant. This assumption is invalid if there is venous pulsation, as in complete heart block (cannon waves) or tricuspid regurgitation.

Abnormal haemoglobins may absorb different amounts of the frequencies used, giving erroneous results. Fortunately, the absorbtion of light by most haemoglobin variants is sufficiently close to that of HbA that pulse oximetry may be used as normal. This is true for fetal haemoglobin (HbF) (so oximetry gives reliable results in neonates) and for the haemoglobin (HbS) found in sickle cell anaemia. Rare abnormal haemoglobins (e.g. haemoglobins Hammersmith and Koln) do cause gross errors in oximetry. Acquired abnormal haemoglobins also cause errors. Carboxyhaemoglobin is perceived as oxyhaemoglobin so may falsely elevate the calculated saturation. Methaemoglobin has an absorbtion similar to haemoglobin that is 85% saturated, so the displayed saturation will tend towards 85% when large amounts are present. Various dyes absorb light and may transiently produce very odd results when injected intravenously.

Bilirubin does not significantly affect the accuracy of pulse oximetry and neither does skin colour.

BLOOD PRESSURE

Perfusion of vital organs requires an adequate systemic blood pressure. Anaesthesia, surgery, the patient's underlying condition and adverse events may all affect blood pressure, which should therefore be monitored in all patients. In most patients, intermittent non-invasive readings are sufficient. Continuous direct measurement of blood pressure requires an arterial cannula, but is invaluable for some patients and procedures.

Non-invasive techniques usually produce good estimates of systolic blood pressure, but less accurate diastolic and mean pressures. Intra-arterial monitoring reliably measures mean blood pressure but systolic and diastolic pressures can be very inaccurate.

There are differences in pressure among arteries. The mean pressure is a little lower in distal arteries than in the aorta and proximal arteries. However, the systolic and diastolic pressures are usually higher distally than centrally, because the shape of the waveform changes as the pulse traverses the arterial tree. Within the aorta the pulse waveform is broad, becoming thinner and taller as it moves distally. (Just as the broad swell in mid-ocean becomes the tall wave that reaches the beach).

Table 2.4 summarizes reasons why pressure in a given artery may not accurately reflect systemic arterial pressure. The site where blood pressure is monitored should usually be chosen so as to avoid such problems.

Non-invasive blood pressure monitoring

Arteries are elastic and may be occluded by applying a pressure greater than that of the blood pressure. Intermittent measurement of blood pressure requires a cuff to apply pressure over the artery and some means of detecting arterial occlusion. A variant on the technique, the Finapres apparatus, allows continuous measurement and is described briefly.

All such methods rely on the pressure in the cuff being effectively transmitted to the artery. For this reason, the cuff must be applied so that the bladder lies over the artery. It should fit snugly, and be applied to the skin, not over clothing. If the cuff is too narrow, the pressure transmitted to the artery will be less than that within the bladder, giving falsely high blood pressure readings. It is recommended that the width of the cuff be at least 120% of the diameter of the limb. Some obese patients have conical upper arms, so the cuff slides down over the elbow. In such cases the cuff is better applied to the forearm instead.

The sphygmomanometer

Every doctor and nurse will have used this device. If used correctly, it is the most accurate of the non-invasive blood pressure methods, especially for determining diastolic pressure. It is too cumbersome for routine intraoperative use but may be used in recovery areas. The cuff is made of a strip of

Table 2.4 Errors in blood pressure (BP) monitoring

Problem	Cause	Example
Artery chosen does not reflect systemic BP	Anatomical site	Distal arteries: higher systolic and diastolic pressures Lower mean pressures
	Hydrostatic	Pressure in dependent arteries increased
	Obstruction upstream	
	Extrinsic	Patient position, retraction, cervical ribs
	Within the wall	Previous arterial surgery (angiography, trauma) Atheroma/spasm
	Within the lumen	Thrombus
Non-invasive BP problems	Problems with cuff	Too small or wrongly applied Conical arm Clothing, jewellery, dressings
	Difficulties detecting pulsation	Small volume pulse Arrhythmias Motion, vibration, noise
Invasive BP problems	Occlusion	Kinking, thrombus
	Transducing system problems	Height Zeroing Calibration Damping and resonance

inelastic cloth containing a single bladder. The pressure within the cuff is displayed by a column of mercury or an aneroid gauge. The cuff is inflated rapidly to 30 mmHg above the pressure at which the pulse disappears. It is then deflated slowly while the operator listens over the artery for the Korotkov sounds.

The oscillotonometer

This device is suitable for intraoperative use. It consists of an aneroid gauge connected to a special cuff, containing two bladders. As a pulse moves down the arm, the pulsation is transmitted to the proximal, then the distal bladder. A lever on the instrument switches it between two modes. In the resting state, it simply displays the pressure in the bladders. Depressing the lever connects one bladder to the inside and one to the outside of the measuring bellows, so the gauge displays (magnified) the difference between the pressure in the bladders, rather than the actual pressure within them. Cuff deflation only occurs in this mode, via a small leak governed by a knob next to the lever.

The instrument should be zeroed before use. The bulb is squeezed to inflate the cuff to a pressure above the expected systolic pressure. The lever on the instrument is then depressed. When the needle starts to flicker, it indicates that the pressure in the cuff equals systolic pressure. The lever **must** be released in order to read this pressure. When the lever is depressed again, the pressure within the cuff continues to fall. Pulsation of the needle increases to a maximum, then suddenly tails off. Releasing the lever at this point provides an (unreliable) estimate of diastolic pressure.

Automated blood pressure monitoring

Early devices sought to replicate the manual methods, detecting the pulsation either with double cuffs or various probes positioned over the artery. Improved electronics now allows a simpler approach, which is the basis of most modern devices. A cuff with a single bladder is used. The cuff is automatically inflated to a preset pressure (typically around 180 mmHg). The cuff is then deflated in small steps (3–8 mmHg). When the pressure in the cuff falls to less than systolic pressure, pulsation is transmitted to the cuff. A transducer within the machine measures both the absolute pressure and the magnitude of any such transmitted pulsations. As the cuff is deflated further, these increase to a maximum, then decrease to a constant. The pressure at which pulsation is first detected is the systolic pressure. The algorithms used to derive mean and diastolic pressure differ among machines and these measurements are less reliable than the systolic pressure. The pressure at which transmitted pulsation is maximal is close to the mean arterial pressure. Diastolic pressure is close to the pressure at which the magnitude of transmitted pulsation becomes unaffected by further decreases in cuff pressure.

Useful though these devices are, they have some disadvantages. There is a danger of misinterpreting movement or extraneous noise as pulsations of the artery. To avoid this, most machines look for two or three similar beats at each cuff pressure. However, if the patient has an irregular heart rhythm, consecutive beats are often not similar. In these patients the machine may fail to find a blood pressure or be very inaccurate. Similarly, in patients who are poorly perfused the machine may fail to read. Worse, lacking any pulse from the patient it may generate an artefact, reporting a grossly raised blood pressure in a hypotensive patient! Often these artefacts produce an impossibly narrow pulse pressure (e.g. 190 mmHg systolic, 180 mmHg diastolic) and this is a valuable clue to the falsity of the reading.

Automated versus manual blood pressure measurement

Automatic measurement of blood pressure is convenient. It frees the anaesthetist for other tasks, ensures the pressure is actually checked regularly and eliminates observer bias. Often a printout is provided and the machine may store previous readings allowing the trend in pressures to be easily seen. These are major advantages. Sadly, these machines frequently fail when faced with profoundly shocked patients and those with arrhythmias, precisely the patients in whom we most wish to know the blood pressure.

The primitive manual oscillotonometer is portable and fast. Because the needle flicker is visible, the anaesthetist can distinguish between artefact (which is not in time with the ECG and oximeter traces) and genuine arterial pulsation. This allows pressures to be measured in circumstances where the automated recorder fails.

The Finapres

This device is mainly used for research purposes. It consists of a cuff applied to a finger, inflated by a very rapidly responding pump. A light shines through the finger pulp to a photodetector. As a pulse arrives at the finger, the extra blood decreases the transmission of light to the photodetector. The machine pumps air into and out of the cuff to keep the optical signal constant. The pressure in the cuff thus varies throughout the cardiac cycle, to keep the flow constant, and produces a good approximation to an arterial waveform. Under laboratory conditions it is reasonably accurate.

Direct blood pressure monitoring

Many peripheral arteries may be readily cannulated. This remarkably safe technique allows beat-to-beat monitoring of blood pressure. It is indicated where major haemodynamic changes are anticipated. Examples include major vascular, cardiac, thoracic, trauma and major cancer surgery. Other indications include the very fragile patient, in whom any haemodynamic derangement may be poorly tolerated and induced hypotension, especially when this is to be profound. A benefit is that blood samples may be readily obtained.

The pressure is translated into an electrical signal by a transducer. Many of these devices are descendants of the strain gauge, in which applied pressure stretches a wire, changing its electrical resistance. The wire is incorporated in an electrical circuit (Wheatstone bridge) which takes a constant input voltage and returns a voltage dependent on the resistance of the wire. Microelectronics has revolutionized these devices, which are now usually accurate, reliable and cheap enough to be disposable. The output from the transducer is displayed as a waveform on a screen.

Transducers small enough to be inserted into arteries have been described but are not in routine use. Instead the transducer is connected to the arterial cannula via a length of narrow-bore plastic tubing, filled with saline from a pressurized bag. This is the cause of almost all the adverse sequelae of the technique and of most of the errors in measurement. Ports on the connecting tubing may be wrongly used to inject drugs and offer a route for infection. They must be clearly labelled and no-one should touch any part of the cannula, tubing or transducer without first washing their hands.

Zeroing and calibration

Before any reading is believed the transducer should be seen to be at the correct height (i.e. at the same level as the left atrium) and should read zero when exposed to atmospheric pressure. Most errors stem from overlooking these two points. Calibration can be conveniently checked when preparing to insert the cannula. The fluid-filled manometer tubing is connected to the transducer and the open end held 1 m higher; the transducer should read 75 mmHg. With modern transducers, calibration seldom drifts, but can readily be re-checked as described.

If there is a clear path between the artery and the transducer and there is no flow then the mean pressure within the transducer must equal that in the artery. A correctly zeroed and calibrated transducer will display an accurate mean arterial pressure. Systolic and diastolic pressures may still be inaccurate, because they are influenced by damping and resonance within the system.

Damping and resonance

Damping results when the measuring system can not respond fast enough to changes in the pressure being monitored, so the peaks and troughs are smoothed out. At its most extreme, it produces a flat line representing mean pressure.

The opposite of damping is resonance, which produces elevated systolic and depressed diastolic pressures. The cause is 'ringing' within the tubing, like the distortion heard when listening to someone shouting at the other end of a tunnel.

Examples of damped and resonant waveforms and their causes are shown in Figure 2.3. Air bubbles cause both damping and resonance, in an unpredictable way. It is frequently possible to correct many of the causes to provide acceptable estimates of systolic and diastolic pressures, and deliberate damping may be used to compensate for resonance. However, where possible therapy should be directed by mean pressures.

CENTRAL VENOUS PRESSURE

Measurement of central venous pressure (CVP), used correctly, is valuable where large blood losses, fluid shifts or changes in cardiac

36 *Principles of monitoring*

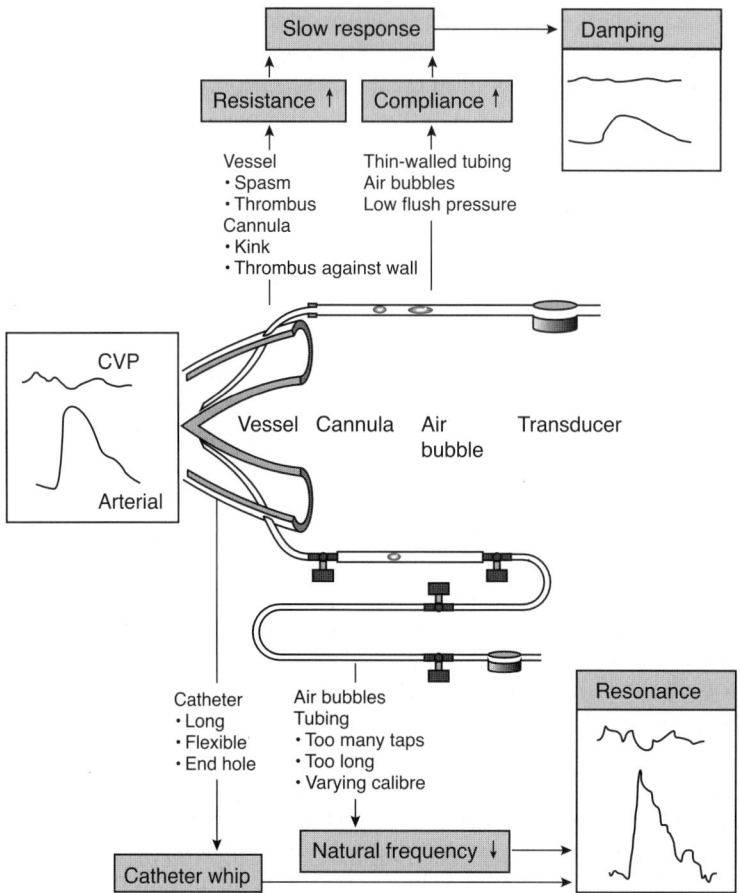

Figure 2.3 Damping and resonance. The waveforms on the left show the actual pressures within the vessels. The upper part of the diagram depicts damping. The tubing and transducer are not completely rigid, they have a small compliance. For the pressure within the transducer to rise, a tiny volume must therefore enter the system along the arterial cannula. If the compliance is high the volume which must enter is increased. If the resistance is high, it takes longer for any given volume to enter. Thus both compliance and resistance may slow the response of the system. During systole, the pressure in the artery increases rapidly. If the system responds slowly, the pressure within the transducer does not reach peak arterial pressure before the latter starts to fall again. The peak of the systolic pressure is therefore not displayed and the damped waveforms are sketched at the top right.

Resonance (bottom) is the opposite of damping. The system from transducer to cannula has a natural frequency at which it 'rings'. Frequencies within the arterial waveform close to this frequency are amplified. Usually the natural frequency is high, so only the highest frequencies within the arterial waveform are affected. These are seen when the pressure is changing most rapidly. The effect is to exaggerate the systolic upstroke and the diastolic downstroke (bottom right). Long tubing, too many taps and air bubbles lower the natural frequency, exacerbating resonance. Catheter whip is a separate problem, causing a similar trace. The tip of the catheter is shaken by the vessel, superimposing artefact on the pressure trace. Usually re-siting the cannula cures the problem.

performance are possible. It offers a guide to cardiac filling pressures, giving early warning of fluid overload. It is vital that the transducers (or saline manometer) be correctly sited and zeroed. If transduced, a clear CVP waveform (as in Figure 2.4) should be obtained before the pressures are believed, as falsely high readings may be generated by semi-occluded catheters or those which impinge on the vessel wall.

The pressure obtained can only be interpreted in the context of other information. For example, a low blood pressure associated with a falling CVP suggests the need for fluid, whereas the same blood pressure with a rising CVP suggests cardiac failure and the need for inotropes. More informative still is a fluid challenge; if this restores the blood pressure and the CVP, then fluid was the answer. If the CVP and blood pressure rise transiently only to fall again, then not enough fluid has been given. If the CVP rises and stays high without improvement in blood pressure then further fluid is contraindicated.

Pitfalls of the technique are many. Apart from the many well-documented complications of insertion techniques, it is easy to misinterpret the information gained. Partly this is because the filling pressures of the right heart are monitored, whereas the blood pressure is dependent on left heart performance. High central venous pressures may be recorded despite hypovolaemia in pneumothorax or cardiac tamponade.

It is a mistake to treat the CVP. Fluid prescriptions such as 'normal saline to keep CVP 5–10 mmHg' are rarely justified. A better alternative is normal saline to keep mean BP >75 mmHg and urine output >30 ml h^{-1} and CVP <10 mmHg.

PULMONARY ARTERY CATHETERIZATION

Since its introduction in 1970 this technique has been surrounded by (mostly undeserved) mystique and controversy. It provides three different types of information: pressures, cardiac output and mixed venous oxygen saturation. A catheter is introduced into a large vein and a balloon at its tip inflated. The balloon is pulled by the blood flow through the right heart into the pulmonary artery, where it wedges in a branch, occluding a segment of the pulmonary circulation. The balloon is then deflated. The traces obtained during this process confirm the catheter position and are sketched in Figure 2.4.

Pulmonary artery pressures are occasionally useful in their own right, but usually the important pressure measured is that with the balloon inflated, the pulmonary artery wedge pressure (PAWP). This affords an estimate of left atrial pressure (Figure 2.4). However, when pulmonary venous resistance is increased, the wedge pressure may be considerably higher than left atrial pressure. Common causes of such discrepancies include positive pressure ventilation, positive end-expiratory pressure, congested lungs and cardiac surgery.

Wedge pressure can be very helpful in assessing cardiac filling and monitoring fluid and inotrope therapy in difficult cases. As with central venous pressure, the information obtained must not be treated in isolation but combined with clinical and other assessment.

Thermodilution cardiac output entails rapidly injecting a bolus of 'cold' saline via the proximal (right atrial) lumen of the catheter. The temperature of the blood in the pulmonary artery is measured continuously via a thermistor near the catheter tip. The higher the cardiac output, the more blood traverses the heart during the injection (diluting the cold saline), so the smaller the measured temperature drop. It is important that the volume and temperature of injectate match those expected by the cardiac output computer, or gross errors will result. Lesser errors include injecting slowly, erratically or via other ports.

Mixed venous oxygen saturation gives an indication of the adequacy of cardiac output

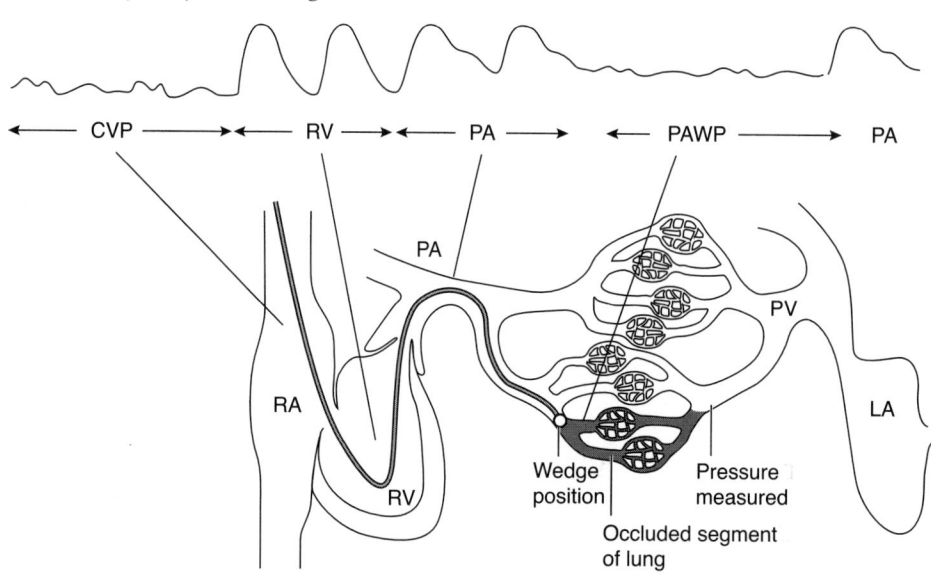

Figure 2.4 The pulmonary artery catheter. The circulation is shown schematically. The trace encountered when inserting the catheter is sketched (top). A central venous trace (CVP) is encountered first. As the catheter advances, it enters the right ventricle (RV) and the trace changes dramatically. When it enters the pulmonary artery (PA) the diastolic pressure rises. Finally it wedges in a branch of the pulmonary artery and the trace changes to the pulmonary artery wedge pressure (PAWP), also called pulmonary artery occlusion pressure (PAOP). Deflating the balloon should restore the pulmonary artery (PA) trace. In health the normal values for these pressures are: CVP 0–6 mmHg, RV 15–25/0–6 mmHg, PA 15–25/5–15 mmHg, PAWP 4–12 mmHg.

When the catheter is wedged it occludes a segment of pulmonary circulation (shaded). If there is no flow through this segment, there can be no pressure difference across it and the pressure measured is at the point indicated. Normally the resistance in the pulmonary veins (PV) is trivial, so this pressure equates to left atrial pressure.

to meet the body's oxygen needs. It may be measured either by aspirating a blood sample from the distal lumen or by using an oximetric catheter.

MEASURING BLOOD FLOW

Cardiac output is currently measured by thermodilution techniques, using a pulmonary artery catheter. However, less invasive methods are becoming available. Cardiac output can be estimated from the velocity of blood in the descending aorta, which may be measured with a Doppler ultrasound probe in the oesophagus. A variant is to use the velocity of blood in the pulmonary trunk, measured by a tracheal probe. Other methods include thoracic bioimpedance and are mainly used for research purposes.

MONITORING PERFUSION OF INDIVIDUAL ORGANS

Global measures of cardiovascular performance may conceal poor flow to individual organs. The brain is particularly at risk during surgery on its vasculature. Perfusion may be monitored by keeping the patient awake and talking, but this is not always feasible. During carotid surgery, stump pressure may be measured. This is the pressure cephalad of the clamp; low pressures despite adequate systemic pressure suggests flow through the collateral vessels is inadequate. Other techniques include transcranial Doppler ultrasound of cerebral blood vessels, jugular venous oxygen saturation measurement and near-infrared spectroscopy to monitor brain oxygenation.

Myocardial ischaemia may be detected electrocardiographically or deduced from a fall in cardiac performance (falling blood pressure and rising central pressures). Neither is specific for ischaemia.

Gut ischaemia may contribute to the problems of shock. (It is postulated that redistribution of blood away from the gut damages the integrity of the gut mucosa, allowing toxins and bacteria to leak into the circulation.) Gastric intramucosal pH reflects the adequacy of gut blood flow and may be estimated by tonometry. A saline-filled balloon is inserted into the stomach (or rectum). The partial pressure of carbon dioxide in the saline comes to equal that in the gut lumen, itself equal to that in the gut mucosa. A sample withdrawn from the balloon is simply passed through a conventional blood gas analyser. The measured partial pressure of carbon dioxide is combined with the arterial bicarbonate concentration in the Henderson–Hasselbach equation to yield an estimate of the intramucosal pH.

TRANSOESOPHAGEAL ECHOCARDIOGRAPHY

Pulmonary artery and central venous catheters are used to answer vital questions. How well is the heart beating? And is it full or empty? Visualizing the heart via an oesophageal ultrasound probe provides the same information and much more. The technique is not yet widely used but shows enormous potential. All four cardiac chambers are shown, allowing continuous observation of the filling status and contractility of both left and right ventricles. Estimates of end-diastolic volume and stroke volume are readily obtained. Regional dyskinesia is detectable and allows early diagnosis of myocardial ischaemia.

Other applications of the technique will revolutionize medical intensive therapy. With experience the probe may be manipulated to bring the cardiac valves, coronary vessels and even coronary bypass grafts into view. As well as cardiac chambers, the aorta, venae cavae and pulmonary arteries may be visualized, as may abnormal communications between them. Blood flow may be examined by Doppler techniques and colour mapping allows superimposition of the flow information on the anatomical views.

The method is not entirely without risk. Manipulating the probe may traumatize the oesophagus and the probe may cause burns. Rarely arrhythmias and haemodynamic compromise may follow probe insertion. Operator expertise is required to place the probe and interpret the images, especially from the more obscure views. The equipment is currently very expensive. However, the technique has already proved its value in cardiac surgery and will surely find an increasing role in managing sick patients in both the operating theatre and the intensive care unit.

SPECIAL SITUATIONS

Conscious sedation and local analgesia are alternatives to general anaesthesia. It must be emphasized that the same standards of care apply as to general anaesthesia. Verbal contact with the patient is an extremely important monitor. Indeed, the point at which it is lost marks the end of sedation and the beginning of anaesthesia.

During patient transfer, portable monitors are now available which allow ECG, oximetry and capnography to be measured. These should have a fully charged battery and preferably a spare battery as well. The anaesthetist must be in a position to monitor the adequacy of ventilation, which frequently dictates that the patient be intubated. Suffi-

DEPTH OF ANAESTHESIA, TEMPERATURE, NEUROMUSCULAR FUNCTION

K. K. Panikkar and M. Morgan

DEPTH OF ANAESTHESIA

A clinically simple and effective method of monitoring depth of anaesthesia remains one of the main goals of anaesthetic research. The problem of monitoring arose following the introduction of muscle relaxants. Before this time, surgery was performed under deep anaesthesia with spontaneous ventilation and depth was measured using Guedel's signs (strictly speaking only applicable to ether anaesthesia in the absence of premedication). These signs are abolished by the use of muscle relaxants, with the result that awareness is always a possibility. A number of methods have been used to detect awareness and monitor the depth of anaesthesia, but the final solution remains elusive.

CLINICAL SIGNS

The paralysed patient can only respond via the autonomic nervous system. Increased sympathetic activity with tachycardia, hypertension, pupillary dilatation and sweating are indicative of too light a level of anaesthesia, but the former two can be caused by other factors while the latter might be abolished by anticholinergic drugs.

ELECTROENCEPHALOGRAM (EEG)

This is of little use in the practical setting because of difficulties in recording and interpretation of findings. The EEG changes are agent specific and affected by such things as Pa_{O_2}, Pa_{CO_2}, blood glucose, electrolytes and temperature. Attempts have been made to simplify the process by reducing the number of electrodes and traces, but instruments such as the cerebral function monitor and cerebral function analysis monitor have had little success. Anaesthesia causes a shift in the EEG principal frequencies to the lower end of the spectrum and display of the median frequency of most of these low frequencies, the spectral edge, has been used in attempts to monitor anaesthetic depth. Again, this is agent specific and has met with little success as a routine monitor.

AUDITORY EVOKED POTENTIALS

Auditory stimuli in the form of a large number of 'clicks' are presented binaurally and the EEG over the mastoid process recorded. The waveforms are the result of impulses passing through the auditory pathways; they are averaged and a single waveform produced. Increasing depth of anaesthesia results in delays in transmission (latency) and decreased amplitude. Surgical stimulation can antagonize these changes, indicating arousal. This is currently the most promising method of monitoring depth of anaesthesia.

OESOPHAGEAL CONTRACTILITY

The lower end of the oesophagus consists of smooth muscle and its spontaneous activity can be measured with a balloon catheter. This activity is suppressed in a dose-dependent manner by anaesthetic agents. However, the changes are not consistent and there is wide interindividual variability. It is also affected by smooth muscle relaxants, anticholinergic agents and oesophageal pathology.

FRONTALIS EMG

The frontalis muscle receives some autonomic innervation via the facial nerve. There is a reduction in tonic EMG activity with loss of consciousness and an increase in amplitude with surgical stimulation. The method has proved unreliable and was affected by use of neuromuscular blocking drugs.

ISOLATED FOREARM TECHNIQUE

In this simple method, a tourniquet is inflated around an arm before administration of the muscle relaxant. At intervals the patient is told to move this arm. Many patients appear to move the arm on command, but virtually none recall the event; this has been termed amnesic awareness. This has limited its usefulness as a method of routinely monitoring depth of anaesthesia.

TEMPERATURE MONITORING

Man is homeothermic and maintains his body temperature within limits of $\pm 2°C$ despite very large variations in ambient temperature. Maintenance of this temperature is necessary for optimal cellular and enzymatic activity and deviation from this ideal temperature will impair these functions.

Body temperature is a balance between heat production and heat loss and is controlled by complex physiological mechanisms. Basal metabolism forms heat, although this is not produced uniformly throughout the body, but mainly in the muscles, liver and glands. The body's main mechanism for increasing heat production is increased muscular activity, either voluntarily or by shivering. Heat is lost from the body by the processes of radiation, conduction, convection and evaporation. Anaesthesia inhibits thermoregulation and there is a tendency for heat loss to be increased particularly during prolonged surgery with open body cavities. In certain types of surgery, body temperature is deliberately decreased. In some pathological conditions, e.g. malignant hyperthermia, hypothalamic dysfunction and sepsis, temperature increases, occasionally to such an extent as to be lethal. The maximum body temperature that is survivable in humans is 42–43°C but no such figure can be accurately stated for low temperatures.

Monitoring of body temperature is therefore an important part of patient management during anaesthesia and surgery. It should be used routinely during major surgery and where indicated, however minor the procedure, if a condition such as malignant hyperthermia is expected.

CORE TEMPERATURE

The body can be regarded, in a very simplified manner, as consisting of a central warm core in which the temperature varies only between very narrow limits and a peripheral region where there are various temperature gradients. The core consists of the cranium, thorax and abdomen and the temperature here is not directly affected by changes in temperature of the peripheral tissues. Strictly speaking, the core temperature is that of the hypothalamus. Sites which are usually regarded as indicating core temperature are the nasopharynx, tympanic membrane, and oesophagus.

Because of the propensity to lose heat during major surgery, efforts must be made to prevent this. Low ambient temperature is one of the major causes of heat loss and efforts must be made to prevent the environmental temperature in the operating room from falling to less than 23°C. Below this, decreases in body temperature of 0.3°C h^{-1} have been reported. Other measures include use of heat and moisture exchangers in the breathing system, warming blankets and mattresses and blood warmers for intravenous infusions.

TYPES OF THERMOMETER

Because of the nature of surgery and problems of accessibility, thermometers used in anaesthesia are usually remote reading. Those using the thermocouple, thermistor or resistor principles are most frequently used; rapid response with a continuous display are the necessary requirements. Thermometers using a liquid crystal display may be useful for skin temperature measurement.

SITES OF TEMPERATURE MONITORING

Oesophageal

This is one of the most convenient sites in the unconscious patient and is taken as an indication of myocardial or aortic temperature. It is important that the thermometer be inserted into the **lower quarter** of the oesophagus, which is at least 24 cm below the corniculate cartilages in adults. Any higher and the temperature may be decreased due to ventilation with cold gases.

Nasopharyngeal

This site is uncomfortable in conscious subjects and erroneous readings may result due to cooling by leakage of gases from the trachea or by the tip lying in poorly conducting secretions.

Tympanic membrane

This approximates closely to hypothalamic temperature, but it is uncomfortable to maintain probes in position in the conscious subject. Trauma can occur to the aural canal and tympanic membrane during insertion and anticoagulation is a contraindication to its use. A thermometer which measures infrared emissions from the tympanic membrane is now available and is non-invasive.

Rectal

This is the most unreliable site of measurement of core temperature and should only be used when other sites are not available. The probe might enter faeces, which acts as an insulator. The recorded temperature may be up to 0.5°C higher than core temperature due to bacterial fermentation. If the probe is inserted too far, then an erroneously low temperature might be recorded due to cool blood returning from the legs. It cannot be used during pelvic operations. During cooling and rewarming, e.g. during cardiopulmonary bypass, rectal temperature lags behind oesophageal temperature.

Skin

Skin temperature is widely dependent on blood flow. The probes are in the form of loops or flat discs, but application to the skin may alter the recorded temperature. The axilla is the most stable area for measurement of skin temperature, and is usually 0.5–1.0°C lower than core temperature. Skin temperature is used in assessment of the effectiveness of sympathetic blockade and peripheral perfusion in conjunction with a core temperature measurement.

Pulmonary artery

Many such catheters now incorporate a temperature probe, which gives an accurate measurement of core temperature.

Bladder

This has been used as an assessment of core temperature using thermistor tipped urinary catheters and it correlates well with pulmonary artery temperature if urine flow is high.

MONITORING NEUROMUSCULAR FUNCTION

Neuromuscular blocking drugs are an integral part of modern anaesthetic practice, but their misuse results in one of the commonest causes of anaesthetic-related mortality due to inadequate restoration of muscle power at the end of anaesthesia. There is a very wide variation in response to neuromuscular relaxants and monitoring their effects should be routine in order to prevent overdosing and to ensure adequate reversal.

CLINICAL ASSESSMENT

This can be done in a number of ways. Tests can be made of muscle strength by asking the patient to open their eyes, protrude the tongue, cough and assessing their grips on the anaesthetist's hand. Lifting the head off the pillow and sustaining it for 5 s simulates tetanic stimulation. However, all these tests require patient cooperation which might not be possible at the end of an operation.

Measurement of minute volume, vital capacity, maximum inspiration and inspiratory force can indicate adequate neuromuscular function, but all these measurements can also be affected by centrally acting drugs such as opioids, intravenous and inhalational anaesthetics. Screening for adequate diaphragmatic activity is not feasible at the end of surgery.

EVOKED RESPONSES

The most suitable method of monitoring the effects of neuromuscular relaxants is to stimulate an accessible nerve in order to evoke a response in the appropriate muscles. Any nerve can be stimulated, but the 'gold standard' is the ulnar nerve at the wrist and the response of the adductor pollicis muscle. The evoked response can be assessed in a number of ways.

- Visual, which is the most unreliable.
- Tactile, by holding the thumb and feeling the response. This is much more reliable than merely observing the response and is the most widely used method clinically.
- Mechanomyography. A force transducer is used to measure the response of the thumb.
- Electromyography. A single summed action potential is recorded from an electrode placed over the belly of the appropriate muscle, e.g. adductor pollicis.
- Accelarography. The acceleration of the thumb in response to stimulation is measured using a piezoelectric wafer. The electrical potential generated is proportional to the acceleration and as the mass of the system is constant, the force can be calculated (Newton's second law).

NERVE STIMULATION

Electrical stimulation

When an electrical impulse of sufficient current density is applied to a nerve, the latter depolarizes and produces an action potential. After such a potential, the nerve is resistant to further stimulation for 0.5–1.0 ms: this is the refractory period. For the observed muscle response to be meaningful clinically and to quantify reliably the response to neuromuscular relaxants it is essential that the nerve is depolarized once in response to a stimulus, that the same number of fibres are stimulated on each stimulus and that direct stimulation of muscle is avoided. If the duration of a single stimulus exceeds the refractory period or a non-square pulse wave is used, the nerve may be stimulated as the current is switched off and repetitive nerve stimulation may occur. Thus the optimal duration of a single stimulus is 0.2 ms.

To ensure that the same number of nerve fibres are stimulated on each occasion, a supramaximal stimulus is used. This is achieved with a current 10–20% above that necessary to stimulate all the fibres in the nerve. A current of 40 mA will provide supramaximal stimulation of the ulnar nerve at the wrist in the vast majority of subjects; very occasionally 60 mA will be needed.

Stimulating electrodes

ECG surface electrodes can be used in conjunction with stimulation of the ulnar nerve at the wrist. Adequate skin contact is essential and the skin should be cleaned with alcohol, slightly abraded and excess hairs removed. The smaller surface area of paediatric ECG electrodes increases current density and allows more accurate electrode placement and hence a lower current.

Magnetic stimulation

Magnetic nerve stimulation is currently being investigated and early studies indicate that it is a useful technique for evaluating residual neuromuscular blockade. It has the advantage that single twitch stimulation is not painful.

PATTERNS OF NERVE STIMULATION

Whatever the pattern of stimulation, the stimuli must always be supramaximal in intensity.

Single twitch

Single twitch stimuli at a rate of 0.1–0.15 Hz may be used, but at least 75% of receptors must be occupied before there is a reduction in twitch height. With non-depolarizing drugs the response diminishes on increased rate of stimulation due to occupancy of presynaptic receptors which serves to reduce the mobilization of acetylcholine in the nerve terminal. For single twitch stimuli to be of use in the quantification of the degree of neuromuscular blockade, it is necessary for a control twitch height to be established before the neuromuscular blocking drug is given.

Train of four

Four stimuli are given at a rate of 2.0 Hz repeated every 12–20 s. Following a depolarizing block, during onset the four twitches decrease in size at the same rate and during recovery the increase occurs in the same manner. After a non-depolarizing drug the fourth twitch disappears first, then third and so on. During recovery, the first twitch reappears before the second, etc. The pattern is shown in Figure 2.5.

Train-of-four stimuli are the most widely used to quantify the degree of non-depolarizing blockade. The fourth twitch (T4) disappears at about 75% depression of T1, T3 at 80–85% and T2 at 90% and therefore a rough estimate can be obtained of the degree of block according to the number of twitches present. Non-depolarizing block can usually be easily reversed when two twitches are present. A T4/T1 ratio of 70% correlates well with clinical recovery from neuromuscular block.

Monitoring neuromuscular function 45

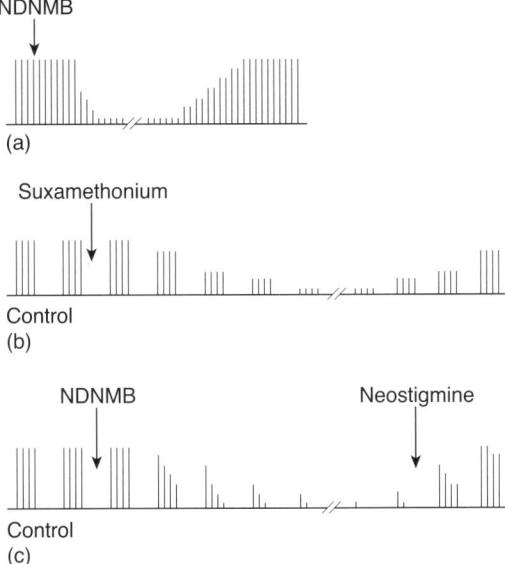

Figure 2.5 Diagram of (a), twitch response (b), train-of-four response to suxamethonium and (c), train-of-four response to a non-depolarizing neuromuscular blocking drug (NDNMB). Note that fade occurs with the latter type of drug but not with the depolarizing drug suxamethonium. (Reproduced with permission from Hunter, J.M. (1992) Clinical use of neuromuscular relaxants and monitoring of neuromuscular transmission, in *Anaesthesia*, 2nd edn. (eds W.S. Nimmo, D.J. Rowbotham and G. Smith), Blackwell Scientific Publications, Oxford.)

Train-of-four stimuli are used as the fourth twitch at a rate of 2 Hz is always the most maximally depressed.

Tetanus

This is repetitive high frequency stimulation and the accepted rate is now 50 Hz. Under normal circumstances, muscle response is maintained, but if neuromuscular transmission is impaired by non-depolarizing drugs, the response cannot be sustained and fade occurs. Very small degrees of block can be detected by tetanic stimulation, but it is pain-ful and not tolerated by conscious patients. Fade also occurs in conditions such as myasthenia gravis and the myasthenic syndrome; it is not a feature of depolarizing block.

Following a tetanic stimulation, there is increased mobilization of acetylcholine. If a single twitch is applied within 5 s of a tetanus in a patient who has had a non-depolarizing drug, then the resulting twitch response is much greater than the twitch immediately before the tetanus. This is post-tetanic facilitation; it does not occur with depolarizing block.

Post-tetanic count

This is a method of assessment of dense non-depolarizing block. If the response to train of four is completely abolished, the anaesthetist does not know if the first response is about to appear or whether this will take some time. A 5 s 50 Hz tetanus is applied followed by 1 Hz stimulation starting 3 s after the tetanus. The number of twitches that result is inversely related to the density of the block. A count of 10 twitches usually coincides with the appearance of the first twitch of a train of four.

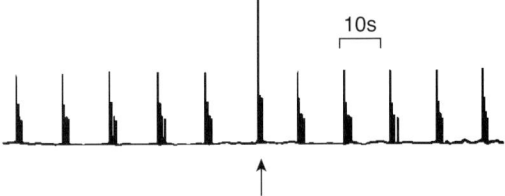

Figure 2.6 Response to double-burst stimulation following a non-depolarizing neuromuscular blocking drug. Note that the degree of fade is much greater than following train-of-four stimulation and would be much easier to appreciate tactically. (Reproduced with permission from Engback, T., Østergaard, D. and Viby-Mogensen, J. (1989) Double burst stimulation (DBS): a new pattern of nerve stimulation to identify residual neuromuscular block. *British Journal of Anaesthesia* **62**: 274–8.)

Double-burst stimulation

This was designed because of difficulty in assessing clinically by feel the ratio of T4/T1 in the train of four, where it is not possible to assess this ratio when it is greater than 50%; 70% is necessary for return of adequate neuromuscular function. Three pulses of 50 Hz stimulation are applied and repeated 750 ms later. Comparing the resultant contractions tactically is much easier than when a train of four is applied (Figure 2.6).

FURTHER READING

Association of Anaesthetists of Great Britain & Ireland (1989) Recommendations for standards of monitoring during anaesthesia and Recovery.

Bennett, D. (1993) *Cardiac Arrhythmias*, 4th edn, Butterworth/Heineman, Oxford.

Blitt, C. D. Monitoring in anaesthesia and critical care medicine.

Buck, N., Devin, H. B. and Lunn, J. N. (1989) The report of a confidential enquiry into perioperative deaths.

Davey, A., Moyle, J.T.B. and Ward, C.S. (1992) *Anaesthetic Equipment*, 3rd edn, WB Saunders, London.

VENTILATORS FOR ANAESTHETIC USE 3

L. Loh

Ventilators are mechanical devices which cause the bulk movement of gas in and out of the lungs and take over or assist the function of the respiratory muscles. They are used in a variety of circumstances.

In emergency situations of acute respiratory failure these devices are termed resuscitators and are usually simple portable pieces of equipment often manually operated. In the intensive care unit they are frequently highly sophisticated, versatile machines with several modes of operation which incorporate monitors and alarms. The ventilators used in the operating theatre vary widely in sophistication. They are used not only to provide ventilation but also to conduct anaesthetic gases and vapours to the alveoli and the pulmonary circulation to produce anaesthesia. In this chapter the discussion is confined to ventilators used for anaesthesia. However, the principles described can often be applied to ventilators for intensive care use.

The description of a ventilator can be divided into two parts. One describes the basic mechanism which produces the gas flow and, equally importantly, the phasic switch on and off of the flow and enables one to predict the behaviour of the machine under various circumstances and also to understand the interaction of the machine with the patient. These can be termed the **functional characteristics** of the ventilator. The other part of the description is the interface between ventilator, anaesthetic machine and the operator including its controls, modes of operation, monitors, alarms and so on. These are the **operational characteristics** of the ventilator.

THE FUNCTIONAL CHARACTERISTICS OF A VENTILATOR

Pulmonary ventilation can be achieved by intermittently generating a pressure difference between the airway and the outside of the chest wall (which includes the thorax and abdomen). In the case of negative pressure ventilation, using devices such as the iron lung and cuirass ventilator, a negative pressure is applied over the thorax and abdomen and the airway remains at ambient pressure. In the case of positive pressure ventilation, a positive pressure is applied to the airway and the surface of the chest wall is at ambient pressure; this is the commonest mode of ventilation for anaesthesia.

The volume change in the lung at each inspiration is determined by the pattern of gas flow into the lung and the duration of that flow.

$$\text{volume} = \text{flow} \times \text{time} \tag{3.1}$$

The total ventilation which occurs over a period of time depends on volume change and the frequency of the respiratory cycle.

$$\text{ventilation} = \text{tidal volume} \times \text{frequency} \tag{3.2}$$

Ventilation is thus determined by flow, time and breath frequency. Flow is a function of

---

Short Practice of Anaesthesia. Edited by M. Morgan and G. M. Hall. Published in 1997 by Chapman & Hall, London. ISBN 0 412 71890 1

the pressure difference generated and resistance to flow

$$\text{flow} = \frac{\text{pressure difference}}{\text{resistance}} \quad (3.3)$$

and pressure difference is determined by the volume/pressure characteristics of the lungs and chest wall or total thoracic compliance.

$$\text{compliance} = \frac{\text{volume change}}{\text{pressure change}} \quad (3.4)$$

It can be seen that the ventilation achieved by a mechanical ventilator may be dependent not only on the characteristics of the ventilator but also on the characteristics of the patient's lung compliance and airways resistance (LCAR) and it is important to know how a particular ventilator will behave in the face of changes in LCAR. Ventilators have been classified in various ways (e.g. stable and unstable, volume pre-set and pressure pre-set) but the most discriminating classification has been that outlined by Mushin *et al*. In this classification the respiratory cycle is divided into four parts (Figure 3.1): how the inspiratory flow is produced; how inspiratory flow is terminated and the expiratory phase begun (1→E cycling); how the expiratory flow is produced; and how the expiratory phase is terminated and the inspiratory flow initiated (E→I cycling).

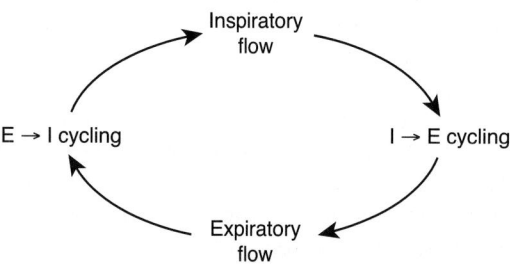

Figure 3.1 The division of the respiratory cycle for the purposes of the functional analysis of ventilator performance.

INSPIRATORY FLOW PRODUCTION

The two basic methods of producing a flow have been termed **pressure generation** and **flow generation** and they are to a degree dependent on the power available to develop pressure. If only a relatively low pressure can be developed then the flow that results will be affected by changes in the downstream airway pressure. For example, in Figure 3.2(a) a bellows containing gas is pressurized by a weight which generates a constant pressure (P_1) in the bellows unless the bellows is empty. When the tap is opened the bellows is connected to the lung. Since the pressure in the bellows (P_1) is greater than the pressure in

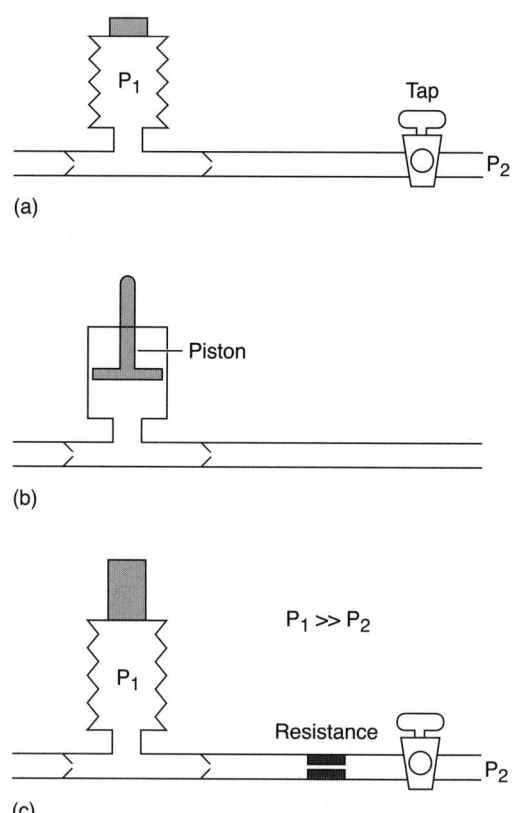

Figure 3.2 Basic methods of flow production during inspiration: (a) pressure generation; (b) flow generation, piston driven by a powerful motor; (c) high pressure–high resistance flow generation.

the airway (P_2) gas will flow from the bellows into the lung. However, as the lung inflates the pressure in the airway increases and the pressure difference between P_1 and P_2 decreases. Therefore flow will decrease progressively until P_1 and P_2 are equal when flow will cease (Equation 3.3) or until inspiratory flow is terminated by some cycling device. The pattern of flow is dependent on the lung and chest wall compliance and airways resistance. In this example the driving pressure is a constant pressure produced by the weight on the bellows. However, a bellows pressurized by a spring would produce a decreasing pressure as the bellows volume decreased and the spring became less taught. In this case the inspiratory flow would depend on the interaction between the bellows and the spring as well as the patient's lung characteristics. Both these mechanisms of producing a flow are termed **pressure generators**. A pressure generator may be defined as a mechanism which produces a pattern of flow which is dependent on the patient's lung compliance and airways resistance.

In contrast, the device in Figure 3.2(b) is a piston which is driven by a powerful motor and the pattern of flow out of the piston is governed by the motor. Any impedance to flow is easily overcome by the development of a higher pressure in the airway. This is a form of **flow generator** which may be defined as a mechanism which produces a pattern of flow which is independent of the patient's lung compliance and airways resistance. The pattern of flow would depend on the pattern of drive of the piston.

Figure 3.2(c) shows a bellows which is loaded to a high pressure (P_1) by a very heavy weight. The difference between P_1 and P_2 is large and if the bellows were to be connected directly to the airway, the inspiratory flow would be very high and the bellows would empty rapidly and completely into the lung and possibly produce harm. However, if a high resistance were to be interposed between the high pressure source and the patient, the flow would be reduced to a manageable level (Equation 3.3) and the duration of flow could then be controlled by a switch mechanism. This would make the system a reasonable ventilator. The changes in airway pressure (P_2) would be small compared to the difference between P_1 and P_2 so that flow would be hardly altered by changes in patient lung compliance or airways resistance and, by definition, this ventilation system would be classified as flow generator. Provided P_1 and resistance remains unchanged the pattern of flow during inspiration would be constant (constant flow generator). However, subtle changes in resistance could produce variations in flow pattern (variable flow generator). Any high pressure gas source which has a flow restrictor is likely to behave as a flow generator.

There are three ways in which a flow generator can be modified to behave as a pressure generator: gas entrainment, gas leakage and gas compression. If a flow generator is used to entrain air or other gas using, for example, a Venturi system, then the ventilator is then converted to a pressure generator since the downstream pressure (the change in airway pressure) will affect the amount of gas entrainment and thus the total flow pattern is influenced by the patient's lung characteristics.

Similarly, if there is a leak or blow-off valve in the system, the flow that the patient receives will vary according to the size of the gas escape which in turn is dependent on the airway pressure. Thus a flow generator with a leak behaves as a pressure generator.

During the inspiratory phase some of the gas delivered by the ventilator is compressed within the volume of the breathing system itself. This volume of compressed gas will be dependent on the volume and elasticity of the breathing system and on the pressure developed in the system at end inspiration. This gas compression modifies the flow to the patient and is dependent not only on the compliance of the patient's lung but also on the compliance of the breathing system itself.

Having discussed the ways in which inspiratory flow is produced, we have now to describe how inspiratory flow is terminated. From Equation 3.1, it is clear that it is the duration of flow that determines tidal volume.

CYCLING FROM INSPIRATION TO EXPIRATION

There are four basic ways in which inspiratory flow is terminated and the expiratory phase initiated: time cycling; pressure cycling; volume cycling; and flow cycling.

Time cycling

This occurs when the duration of the inspiratory phase is predetermined by a control on the machine. A *pressure generator* which is time cycled in inspiration will deliver a tidal volume which changes with LCAR since the flow pattern varies. A time cycled *flow generator*, however, will deliver the same tidal volume irrespective of LCAR since pattern and duration of flow are unchanged.

Pressure cycling

In this case inspiratory flow is terminated when a predetermined pressure is reached either in the machine or in the airway. This pressure is set by a control on the machine. A *pressure generator* which is pressure cycled will deliver a variable tidal volume, since not only is the inspiratory flow pattern but also the point during inspiration at which the cycling pressure is reached dependent on LCAR. In the case of a *flow generator* which is pressure cycled, again the time taken to reach the cycling pressure is going to depend on LCAR and thus tidal volume will vary according to LCAR.

Volume cycling

With this method of cycling the inspiratory phase is terminated when a predetermined tidal volume has been delivered from the machine. A *pressure generator* which is volume cycled will vary the *duration* of the inspiratory phase according to LCAR. Although the tidal volume delivered will remain the same, the change in inspiratory phase duration may alter total respiratory cycle time and therefore frequency, so that minute ventilation may change with LCAR. A *flow generator* which is volume cycled will not alter inspiratory duration despite changes in LCAR.

Flow cycling

This is not commonly used but the machine terminates inspiration when a predetermined flow has been reached. This form of cycling was mainly used with *pressure generators* when flow progressively decreased with lung inflation. When a predetermined low flow was achieved the machine cycled into expiration. Here again the volume delivered would vary since the pattern of inspiratory flow and the duration of the inspiratory phase varied with LCAR. With some sophisticated ventilators the flows in both the inspiratory and expiratory limb of the ventilator can be monitored continuously and by comparing the two flows the start of inspiration and expiration can be determined. This can be used to control ventilator function. This is flow cycling related to spontaneous respiratory effort rather than LCAR.

EXPIRATORY FLOW PRODUCTION

Most ventilators allow expiration to occur passively and the flow during expiration is determined by the elastic recoil of the lung and chest wall together with the airway and apparatus resistance. By definition, this is *pressure generation* in expiration. Some older ventilators can generate a negative pressure in the airway in expiration and at some phase during expiration the machine controls expiratory flow. When this occurs then expiratory flow is produced by *flow generation*. However, the application of a negative pressure during expiration is seldom used nowadays as it has been shown to encourage atelectasis in the lungs. Expiratory flow through a restrictor or threshold resistor in order to produce positive end-expiratory pressure (PEEP) is still classified as pressure generation.

CYCLING FROM EXPIRATION TO INSPIRATION

The majority of ventilators cycle from expiration to inspiration using time cycling. Either the inspiratory and expiratory phases are timed or the total cycle time or frequency is determined by the machine. Several machines also have the facility to recognize an inspiratory effort by the patient and employ this to initiate the inspiratory phase. This can be termed **patient cycling** or **patient triggering**. In this case cycling is either through a slight decrease in airway pressure due to an inspiratory effort or through flow cycling as mentioned above. It is believed that flow cycling has the advantage over pressure cycling in that it is more sensitive, faster responding and requires less patient work. However, such sophistication is not usually seen in ventilators used for anaesthetic purposes at the present time.

The ventilator classification as described above enables one to predict the behaviour of a ventilator when used with changing or different conditions of LCAR and gives one an insight into the intricacies and problems of ventilator design. Many ventilators use combinations of flow and pressure generation and cycling in different ventilatory modes. A ventilator might be a time cycled flow generator in controlled mandatory ventilation mode, but use a mixture of flow generation and pressure generation and with time, pressure or flow cycling when in synchronized intermittent mandatory ventilation (SIMV) mode with inspiratory pressure support.

Ideally a functional analysis of the performance of a ventilator should be documented and available for inspection from the manufacturer. This would show tracings of the flow, pressure and volume changes obtained when the machine is made to work against a variety of compliance and resistance combinations relevant to the machine's sphere of use, i.e. using lung models simulating adult, paediatric or neonatal patients. The functional characteristics of the ventilator can thus be demonstrated and the ventilators limitations defined.

OPERATIONAL CHARACTERISTICS

Mechanical ventilators come in all shapes and sizes to suit many different environments and pockets. Some are simple bag squeezers and others are versatile, microprocessor controlled machines with built in monitoring and alarms. Some are stand alone ventilators, others are an integral part of the anaesthetic machine. A number of these operational characteristics will be discussed in a general fashion here and then a few production ventilators used for anaesthesia will be described in more detail.

POWER SOURCE

The energy used to inflate the lungs during artificial ventilation can be derived from compressed gas or electrical sources. Perhaps the most common energy source is the potential energy stored in compressed gases either from pipeline supplies, portable gas cylinders or from electrically driven gas compressors. The pressurized gas can be used to lift a weighted bellows as in the Manley Pulmovent when the force of gravity is used to drive the gas into the lungs (Figure 3.3(a)). Alternatively, the compressed gas can expand a spring-loaded bellows and the potential

52 Ventilators for anaesthetic use

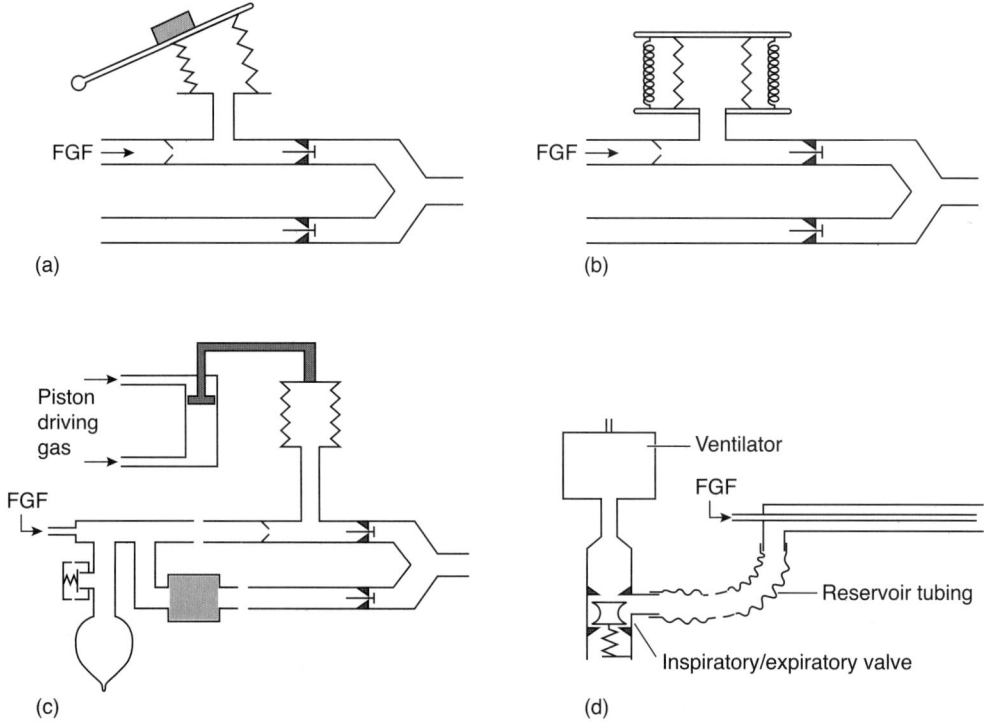

Figure 3.3 Some common methods of ventilation for anaesthesia: (a) weight operated bellows; (b) spring operated bellows: (c) pneumatically driven bellows, note this system can be easily converted to a circle system with CO_2 absorber; (d) ventilator acting as a pneumatic piston with a Bain system. FGF=fresh gas flow.

energy in the stretched spring is used to inflate the lungs as in the Manley Servovent or Siemens Servo 900 (Figure 3.3(b)). In these cases the fresh gas from the anaesthetic machine is used to expand the bellows during the expiratory phase and is then also delivered to the patient's airway during inspiration. In the case of the Penlon Oxford ventilator (Figure 3.3(c)) a separate pressurized gas source is used to drive a bellows back and forth and this is entirely separated from the respired gas. The Penlon Nuffield 200 ventilator on the other hand is often used with a Mapleson D system (Bain system) (Figure 3.3(d)) with the compressed gas which powers the ventilator acting as a pneumatic piston moving gas through a reservoir tube. This driving gas is capable of mixing with respired gas of the patient breathing system. Other anaesthetic ventilators use pressurized gas to compress a bag or bellows housed in a rigid container (bag-in-bottle) (Figure 3.4) In this instance the driving gas and the respired gas are separated.

Many anaesthetic ventilators are constructed with a bellows or piston directly driven by an electrical motor. In older generations of anaesthetic machines these motors were moderately heavy and large. They were usually floor standing (Cape–Waine) and had the anaesthetic equipment attached to the ventilator. The more modern motor driven ventilator can now be made with a small but efficient stepper motor, which is microprocessor controlled and much more versatile than its predecessor and conveniently incor-

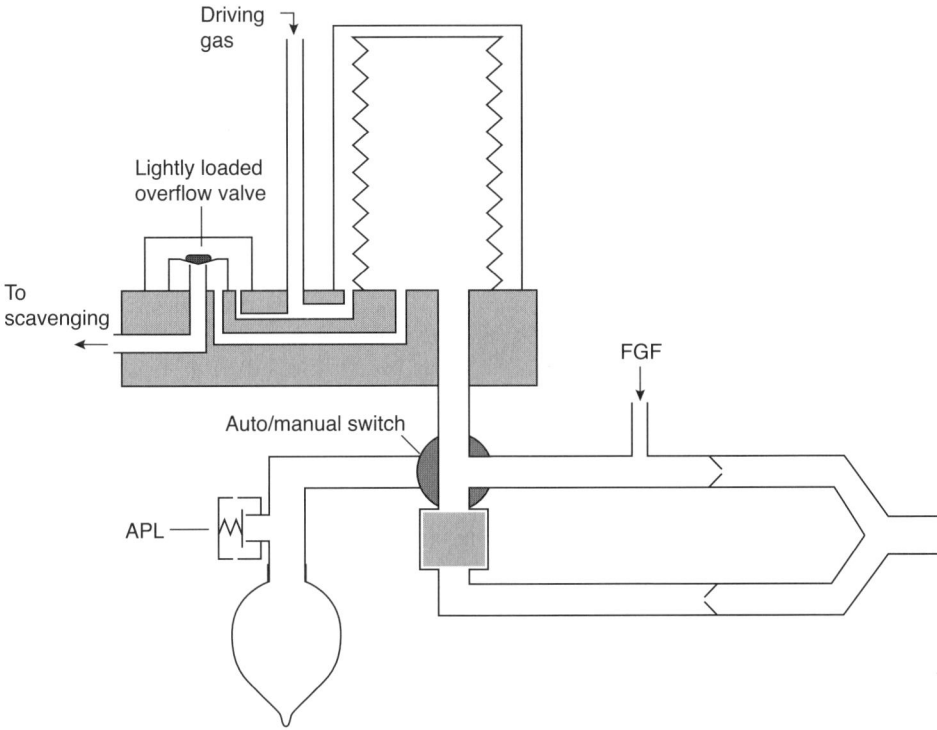

Figure 3.4 Typical bag-in-bottle with circle absorber system. FGF=fresh gas flow; APL=adjustable pressure limiting valve.

porated into the anaesthetic machine (e.g. Drager Cato).

Most modern operating theatres have piped oxygen or air available as a readily accessible source of power for ventilators. This is a relatively cheap source of power if one discounts the capital outlay and maintenance costs of the gas storage and pipeline system. Gas powered ventilators tend to be smaller, lighter and cheaper than their electrically driven counterparts.

The use of gas cylinders on anaesthesia machines poses major problems. The cylinders are costly to hire. They create a problem with storage space and can be a hazard to personnel if inappropriately secured. They present more work for portering staff. The cylinders can empty of gas unexpectedly and thus be a hazard to patients unless they are frequently checked. The use of a ventilator which has a high gas consumption is therefore not appropriate on anaesthetic machines dependent on gas cylinders.

Electrical air compressors can be used to power some gas driven ventilators and thus substitute for a pipeline system. However, the extra bulk and weight of a compressor may not be convenient. Electrically driven ventilators thus have an advantage in areas where there is no pipeline supply.

BREATHING SYSTEM

The operational characteristics of the ventilator will also determine the type of breathing system used. It will be appreciated that those machines which employ the fresh gas flow to expand the bellows as in Figure 3.3(a) and 3(b) are suited to non-rebreathing systems. The fresh gas flow required is equal to the minute ventilation and these ventilators are sometimes termed **minute volume dividers**. The expired gas is not recycled and the consumption of anaesthetic gases and vapours is considerable. These machines could be made to drive partial rebreathing circle absorber systems, but would require a separate driving gas source with a calibrated Rotameter™ in addition to the anaesthetic gas system. The majority of other ventilators can be used with partial rebreathing or circle absorber systems as illustrated in Figures 3.3(c), 3(d) and 4. The T-piece breathing system, commonly used in the form of a Bain system (Figure 3.3(d)) can be used with any ventilator attached to the expiratory limb. In this configuration the volume and length of the expired limb is important as the ventilator driving gas mixes with the gas in the expiratory limb and may contaminate and dilute the gas ventilating the lungs if this conducting tubing volume is too small. The lower the fresh gas flow and the larger the tidal volume the more important this becomes.

In the same way any ventilator can be used to drive a circle absorber system by joining the patient connection port of the ventilator to the reservoir bag port of the circle system provided a sufficient length of tubing is interposed between the ports. This tubing again ensures that the ventilator gas does not contaminate the respirable gas in the circle system.

BAG-IN-BOTTLE SYSTEM

The bag-in-bottle system separates the ventilator driving gas from the respired gas usually in a circle absorber system. When the ventilator pressurizes the inside of the bottle, not only is the bag compressed but the overflow valve of the circle system is also closed (Figure 3.4). The overflow valve is usually slightly loaded so that it opens only after the bag has filled in expiration. It may open to atmosphere as in Figure 3.4 or it may open into the inside of the bottle, in which case the spilled anaesthetic gas exits through the ventilator expiratory system (Figure 3.14).

The bag is commonly a concertina bellows which gives an indication of the volume delivered out of the system. The importance of the visual indication of volume change depends on the availability of other measurements of the volume delivered. Some concertina bellows are compressed downwards and others are compressed upwards. When the bellows is compressed downwards during inspiration, during upward refilling the weight of the bellows itself increases the pressure in the breathing system. The overflow valve is further loaded so that it does not open until the bellows is filled. This inevitably creates a small (2–4 mbar) PEEP. The advantage of this arrangement, however, is that any significant leak in the breathing system is indicated by a failure of the bellows to fill adequately.

Due to its weight, a concertina bellows which fills downwards in expiration tends to generate a small negative pressure in the breathing system. This may be disadvantageous since outside air may be drawn into the system if there is a significant leak in the breathing system and, as the bellows movement may be relatively unchanged, this leak may go undetected.

Some bellows are filled fully at end expiration and are only partially emptied during inspiration (Figure 3.4). Others are completely compressed at end inspiration and are limited in their expansion by an adjustable platform in order to give the required tidal volume (Figure 3.14).

As a general rule, a bellows in which the tidal volume is limited as in Figure 3.14 and which is emptied completely at end-inspiration can be driven by any ventilation system. All that is required is that the pressure developed in the bottle is sufficient to empty the bellows in the required time. The pressure in the bottle can be considerably higher than that in the airway at end-inspiration since this pressure is not transmitted to the rest of the breathing system when the bellows is empty. On the other hand, a system which only partially empties the bellows has to accurately control the flow of driving gas to the bottle and cycle from inspiration to expiration after the appropriate volume has been displaced out of the bellows. A further implication of bellows design is discussed in the following section on the internal compliance of the ventilator.

INTERNAL COMPLIANCE

During the inspiratory phase the pressure in the breathing system increases and the gas which is delivered by the ventilator (the swept volume, Figure 3.5) may be distributed in three ways. The majority of the gas volume is conducted to the patient's lung and airways providing tidal ventilation. Some of the gas may be lost through leakage out of the breathing system and a proportion of the delivered gas will be compressed within the volume of the breathing system itself. The volume of compressed gas with each breath will be determined by the end-inspiratory pressure and the volume of the breathing system and also its elasticity or expandability. The relationship of the volume of gas compressed and the pressure in the system is called the *internal compliance* of the ventilator.

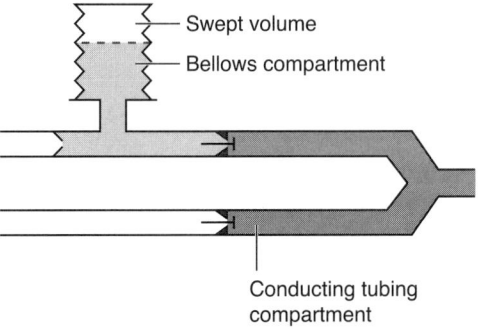

Figure 3.5 Diagram showing internal compliance of the bellows and conducting tubing compartments. The change in volume of the bellows during an inspiration is called the **swept volume**.

This too can be subdivided into the internal compliance of the bellows compartment, if present and the internal compliance of the tubing system.

With most ventilator systems the internal compliance value lies between 2 and 10 ml mbar^{-1}. An adult being ventilated with a swept volume of 700 ml and a frequency of 12 min^{-1} should have a minute volume of 8400 ml. If the internal compliance of the breathing system were 3 ml mbar^{-1} and the end-inspiratory pressure was 15 mbar then the compressed gas volume would be 45 ml per breath. The actual tidal volume the patient received would be 655 ml and over 12 breaths the total loss due to gas compression is 540 ml. This is not a significant volume in an adult, but should the internal compliance value be 6 ml mbar^{-1} then, of the 8400 ml swept minute volume, 1080 ml would be lost in gas compression. The greater the compliance figure and the higher the end-inspiratory pressure the more gas is compressed in the breathing system and the less actual ventilation the patient receives. This becomes very significant when dealing with babies or young children. Here the tidal volumes are small and the airway pressures comparatively high, so that if the above ventilator system were to be used in a child with a swept volume of 200 ml and end-inspiratory pressure of 15 mbar, the compressed volume per breath would still be 45 ml as with the adult, but a much larger proportion of the swept volume. For this reason most adult ventilators are not suitable for small children and babies and ventilators with low internal compliance (small internal volume, shorter, narrower and less elastic tubing) are preferred. A few sophisticated, microprocessor controlled ventilators can compute the compressed gas volume and compensate for it.

Ventilators using bellows which are only partially compressed during inspiration may have a large internal compliance in the bellows compartment. The smaller the tidal volume the larger the residual volume left in the bellows and the greater the compressed gas volume. This arrangement may not be suitable for paediatric work unless pressure controlled ventilation is used and alternative methods of measuring the adequacy of ventilation are employed.

The internal compliance of the ventilator system can be measured in various ways and if one knows the compliance value then the volume loss to the patient can be calculated and compensated for. Measuring the expired tidal volume on the expiratory limbs of the breathing systems is unreliable since both true expired tidal volume and compressed gas volume will be measured by the spirometer in this position. The best index of actual patient ventilation is to measure tidal volume at a site between the patient and the ventilator tubing connection.

One rough way of measuring the internal compliance of the breathing system is to block the tubing Y-piece and any other source of gas leakage and set the ventilator to deliver a small known tidal volume into the system and note the end-inspiratory airway pressure. Dividing the tidal volume by the pressure will give the internal compliance. When the system is connected to the patient the volume of gas compressed can then be calculated from the actual end-inspiratory pressure and this derived compliance value. Some modern ventilators make an assessment of internal compliance and calculate and deliver a tidal volume to compensate for this. Although usually the internal compliance of the breathing system is not a major problem, it does explain why the ventilatory requirements are often considerably in excess of that predicted by the Radford Nomogram.

The end-inspiratory pressure in the airway is determined by the lung compliance and this end-inspiratory pressure in turn determines the volume of compressed gas in the ventilator conduction system. If the internal compliance of the conduction system is high then the actual gas flow and tidal volume delivered at each breath to the patient is also dependent on the patient's lung compliance. This means that a ventilator which is constructed as a flow generator in inspiration will behave more as if it were a pressure generator if the internal compliance of the system is high.

It may be thought that the above discussion is somewhat academic for these days as ventilation is usually closely monitored and guided by end-tidal carbon dioxide measurements. Nevertheless, unless these physical considerations are understood one cannot truly appreciate the consequences of equipment design and account for the variations in performance between different systems.

THE EFFECT OF FRESH GAS FLOW ON TIDAL VOLUME

In many anaesthetic ventilators, the pressurized flow of fresh anaesthetic gases and vapours is continuously delivered to the patient during inspiration and will be in addition to that volume of gas displaced by the ventilator mechanism. The tidal volume the patient receives is thus dependent on the fresh gas flow and the ventilator output. This is clearly seen when using a T-piece system and ventilating a reservoire tube (Figure 3.3d) or a bag in a bottle circle system (Figure 3.4). Changes in fresh gas flow will thus change total ventilation unless adjustments are made to the ventilator output as well. Often these changes can only be detected by measuring tidal volume at the patient airway. Some ventilators have been designed to overcome this problem by decoupling the fresh gas flow during inspiration (Drager Cato) or by taking into account the fresh gas flow during inspiration when computing the bellows volume displacement required to deliver the set tidal volume (Datex-Engstrom).

MODES OF VENTILATION

The majority of anaesthetized patients who require artificial ventilation are ventilated because they have been given muscle relaxants to assists surgery. Controlled mandatory ventilation (CMV) is all that is required and the versatility of the intensive care ventilator is a luxury. A simple, inexpensive but reliable workhorse is sufficient for the majority of surgical patients with normal lungs and chest wall. There are, however, some patients who would fare better with more sophisticated ventilators. Critically ill patients who are in intensive care and have been treated with special ventilation modes may be better managed with the same modes in the operating theatre. But it might be difficult to justify the purchase of such versatile machines for routine use in anaesthesia in all operating theatres.

There are some types of surgery in which PEEP may be desirable. For example, during a thoracotomy it may be desirable to apply PEEP in order to maintain the volume of the dependent lung. With the patient in the sitting posture during neurosurgery, PEEP in combination with a G-suit can be useful to maintain a high cerebral venous pressure to prevent venous air embolism. The smooth transition from CMV to spontaneous ventilation may be assisted by SIMV or inspiratory pressure support. These modes are now easier to incorporate into anaesthetic ventilators with the advance in microprocessor controlled machines.

MONITORING AND ALARMS

Patient safety is enhanced by monitoring not only the patient's physiological parameters but also the proper functioning of the anaesthetic equipment and the composition of the respired gases. Many anaesthetic ventilators are an integral part of the anaesthetic machine and its monitors and alarm systems. Most modern systems monitor inspiratory and expiratory airway pressure, tidal and minute volume, oxygen, carbon dioxide and anaesthetic gas and vapour concentration. Even continuous spirometry is now available in the operating theatre.

Having outlined some of the functional and operational characteristics of ventilators for use with anaesthesia, the following section describes the workings of three ventilators in more detail. The ventilators have been chosen because they not only illustrate some of the features described above but also because they have been relatively recently introduced and represent examples of current technology.

THE MANLEY MULTIVENT (PENLON)

The Manley Multivent has been designed by the late Dr Roger Manley for use primarily to 'free up' the hands of a hard pressed anaesthetist with possibly only a basic training in anaesthesia. It is designed to have few and simple controls and be capable of ventilating patients over 20 kg with relatively normal lungs. A further primary aim is to make economical use of electricity and compressed gases. It needs to be supplied with mains electricity for only 1–2 hours per week and requires a volume of driving gas (air or oxygen) of only 10% of the minute volume. It is electrically controlled either by mains power or a rechargeable battery so it is suited to conditions where the electrical power supply is unreliable. The design is simple, robust and requires minimal maintenance. The cost of the ventilator is reasonable. In field trials in Africa and India it has proved to be reliable and easy to use.

There are two models of the Manley Multivent. The O-model (Figure 3.6), which has the bellows mechanism and electrical controls closely connected together, is not for use with flammable anaesthetic agents. The E-model has the electronic control module raised above the bellows by more than 25 cm so that ether or other flammable agents can be used safely.

The ventilator has an inspiratory bellows

58 *Ventilators for anaesthetic use*

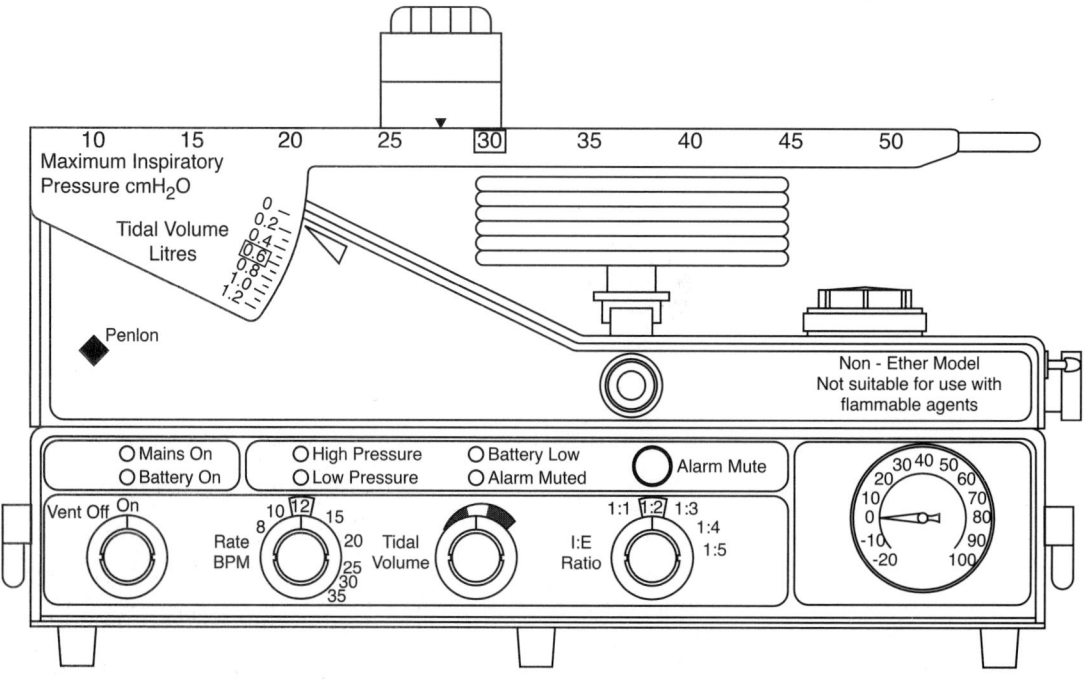

Figure 3.6 Drawing of front view of the Manley Multivent. (Reproduced by courtesy of Penlon.)

attached to a rigid pivoted arm with a sliding weight to vary the inspiratory pressure in a similar fashion to the Manley Pulmovent. The pressure can be varied in the range 10–50 mbar, so the machine acts as a constant pressure generator during inspiration. Flow during expiration is through pressure generation. The timing of the respiratory phases is electronically controlled. It is thus time cycled from inspiration to expiration and from expiration to inspiration. The rigid arm is raised by a thruster rod which is pneumatically driven by a pressurized gas source. This gas source could be compressed air or oxygen. Compressed air at 4 bar, derived from a DeVilbis oxygen concentrator, can be used to drive the bellows and the oxygen from the concentrator can be used to supplement the inspired air. As mentioned above, the required flow of this driving gas is about one tenth of the minute ventilation. If cylinder oxygen is available then this can be used to drive the bellows and this same oxygen can then be diverted to enrich the inspired air. Therefore oxygen enriched air can be drawn through a draw-over vaporizer into the inspiratory bellows and delivered to the patient through a single outlet tube and non-rebreathing Laerdal valve (Figure 3.7). Alternatively the machine can be used to ventilate a circle or T-piece system.

THE PNEUMATIC SYSTEM

The pneumatic system is shown in Figure 3.7. A pressurized gas source at 20–100 p.s.i. is required to lift the inspiratory bellows. The gas passes first through a filter and then a pressure regulator which reduces the pressure to a constant 20 p.s.i. A flow restrictor then creates a high pressure–high resistance flow generator system which maintains flow fairly constant in the face of varying loads on the

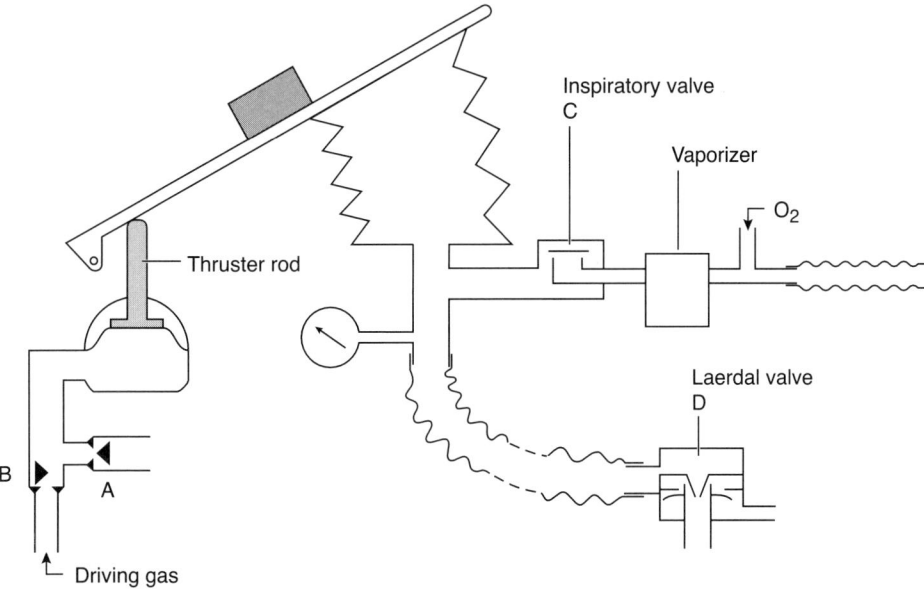

Figure 3.7 Diagram of the pneumatic system of the Manley Multivent.

thruster rod depending on the position of the weight on the bellows. With solenoid valve B open and valve A closed, the gas flows into the pneumatic thruster rod chamber during the expiratory phase and raises the thruster rod and the bellows at a relatively constant rate and causes the inspired gas to pass via one way disc valve C into the bellows. The non-rebreathing valve D prevents gas being drawn back along the patient outlet tube. The tidal volume control on the front panel of the electronic unit determines the duration of the drive gas flow and, therefore, the volume drawn into the bellows, by controlling the time that valve B remains open. When valve B closes there is a phase when both valves (A and B) are closed and the bellows is held in a stationary position and the tidal volume can be determined on the tidal volume scale on the proximal part of the rigid arm of the bellows (Figure 3.6). This scale is only intended as a guide and tidal volume is best measured at the patient airway with a respirometer. The setting of the respiratory rate and I:E ratio control (O model only) then determines the opening of valve A (time cycling from expiration to inspiration). When valve A opens, the bellows starts to empty, the pressure increases in the patient system and valve C closes and valve D opens to the patient. Inspiratory flow is determined by the weight on the bellows (the pressure generator) and the patient's LCAR. The position of the weight should be adjusted so that the bellows empties completely before the start of the expiratory phase. The start of expiration is also determined by the setting of the rate and I:E ratio controls (E model has fixed I:E ratio of 1:2) and is achieved by the opening of valve B and the closing of valve A. The bellows starts to rise, the pressure in the patient system falls and valve D allows the patient to exhale to atmosphere. Valve D in Figure 7 is illustrated as a Laerdal valve but could equally be an Ambu E1 or Ambu Mk 3 non-rebreathing valve or similar. The driving gas exiting through valve A during inspiration can be ducted to the gas intake reservoir and used as part of the fresh gas which is particularly useful if the driving gas is oxygen.

THE ELECTRONIC SYSTEM

Incoming mains power in the range 88–264 V a.c. can be used to power the ventilator's electronic circuits. A resettable fuse protects the printed circuit boards from spikes and surges and an electronic filter smoothes the supply and it is reduced to 19–57 V a.c. A power supply unit then produces a rectified 25–80 V. 14.8 V is used to charge the battery. If the incoming mains voltage is inadequate to trickle charge the battery, the mains supply is switched off and the battery takes over until 88 V a.c. mains power is reinstated. The valves A and B are latching solenoids which require very little power to operate and the rest of the electronic components also consume very little power. Thus the charged battery will work for a minimum of 100 h. A one hour recharge of the battery is sufficient for 50 h use. A battery low indicator lights up when one hour of operation remains. The system has high and low pressure switches. The high pressure switch is preset to 58 mbar and sets off a high pressure alarm if this pressure is exceeded. The low pressure alarm is PEEP referenced. This means that a PEEP reference solenoid valve closes off a small reservoir at end expiration. The pressure in this reservoir, is then used as a reference pressure for the low pressure alarm system. If the airway pressure during the inspiratory phase is more than 5 mbar above the PEEP reference pressure then the low pressure switch is closed and the low pressure alarm is inhibited. If for any reason the 5 mbar pressure difference is not exceeded, the low pressure switch opens and a visual and audible alarm is activated. The audible alarm can be muted for 1 min.

When the ventilator is first switched on, a two second test cycle is performed which checks all visual and audible alarms and indicators.

MANUAL OPERATION

When electrical power is exhausted or switched off or if the driving gas supply fails, the drive gas release valve A is automatically in the open state and the thruster rod is in its lowest position. Thus the bellows arm can be manually operated. In this mode it is possible to generate airway pressures up to 60 mbar which is the blow-off pressure of the inspiratory pressure relief valve.

This ventilator can be used both for anaesthesia and intensive care although it is recognized that it cannot cope with low compliant lungs or high airways resistance. It is simple in design but has the virtue of providing controlled mandatory ventilation with oxygen enriched air either from cylinder oxygen or an oxygen concentrator. The power requirements are low and the electronic controls will function on the rechargeable battery for a long time. Maintenance is simple. The manufacturers recommend the use of a preventative maintenance kit every 12 months and a full service 5 yearly. Periodically it requires the cleaning and changing of the O-rings of the inspiratory valve and lubrication of the thruster rod assembly. The inspiratory valve block is precision machined and should be liquid sterilized but the rest of the patient breathing system is autoclavable.

E-MODEL

This not only differs from the O-model by having the electronic unit separated from the pneumatic unit to reduce any fire risk, but the E-model also has in addition an ether isolating diaphragm which separates the breathing system gas from the electronic pressure sensing system and yet allows pressure change to be transmitted adequately. The E-model also has the I:E ratio fixed at 1:2.

The Divan (Drager) 61

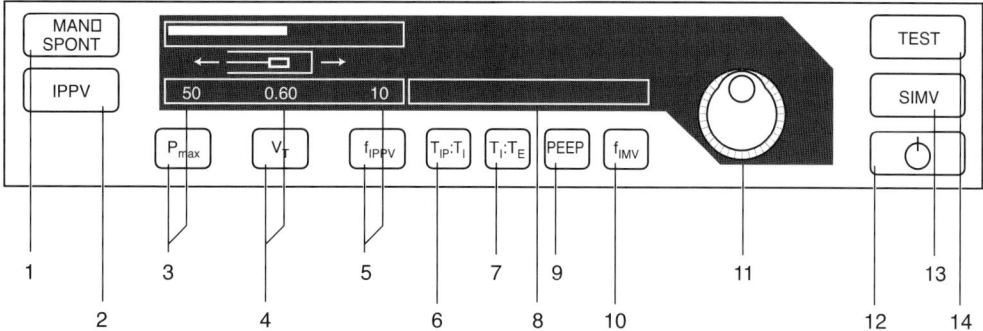

Figure 3.8 Drawing of front panel of Divan ventilator showing softkeys which control ventilator function. (Reproduced by courtesy of Drager.)

1. MAN/SPONT
2. IPPV
3. P_{MAX} (mbar)
4. V_T (ml)
5. f_{IPPV} (min^{-1})
6. $T_{IP} : T_I$
7. $T_I : T_E$
8. Display messages
9. PEEP
10. f_{IMV} (min^{-1})
11. Rotary knob
12. Standby
13. SIMV
14. TEST

THE DRAGER DIVAN (DIGITAL VENTILATOR ANAESTHESIA)

The Drager Cato Anaesthetic Workstation has an integral ventilator named the Divan. It sits neatly under the worktop and has a front panel with a number of soft keys to call-up and display any particular function (Figure 3.8). This function can then be adjusted to the required value using a single rotary knob. The function value is confirmed by pressing the rotary knob.

Above and behind the worktop is an electroluminescent screen showing the ventilation parameters. This is a very sophisticated display system giving graphical and digital information about the breathing system gases from the anaesthetic gas and vapour analyser, pressures in the airway and alarm information. When the workstation is first switched on the machine initiates an automatic self-test and the information is displayed on this screen. The machine then goes into standby mode until a ventilation mode is selected. The screen has three main configurations. The standard screen (Figure 3.9) shows selected waveforms and relevant digital information. Other information can be called up through

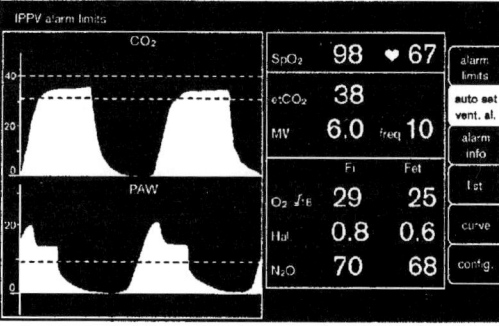

Figure 3.9 Standard airway monitoring screen on Drager Cato Anaesthetic Workstation.

the soft keys at the side of the screen. Data and Trend screens can also be displayed. Using the soft keys and another rotary knob, the alarms can be set and the screens specifically configured. The Cato also has a Parameter Box which receives inputs from the patient monitoring leads and which interfaces with a second monitor screen to complete the monitoring system.

The anaesthetic ventilator is a piston–cylinder unit driven by mains electrical power. The piston movement is determined by a stepper motor which is software controlled from the front panel. A major advantage of such a system is that the set tidal volume can be delivered with great precision and the tidal volume has a range of 20 ml to 1400 ml. The ventilator can thus cope with patients from neonates to large adults. However, there is a P_{max} control which limits the maximum pressure developed and this can be used to provide pressure controlled ventilation in neonates if required. The pattern of flow and the timing is also precision controlled with a frequency range (f_{IPPV}) of 6 to 60 min^{-1} and an I:E ratio ($T_I:T_E$) from 2:1 to 1:3. The machine will also deliver an end-inspiratory plateau from 0 to 60% of the inspiratory time (T_{IP}/T_I). This system can generate a PEEP of 0–20 mbar. SIMV is available as well. The patient trigger is set at 0.5 mbar below the set PEEP level.

The ventilator is thus a flow generator in inspiration, a pressure generator in expiration and is time cycled except during SIMV when it is pressure cycled from expiration to inspiration.

The whole system is controlled by two computers. One interfaces with the operation unit (front panel), registers the required settings and primarily controls the stepper motor and valves. Both computers receive information concerning the piston displacement, piston and airway pressures and information from the valves. The two computers communicate, feed back information to servo-control the system and activate alarms (Figure 3.10).

THE BREATHING SYSTEM

The valves and interconnecting channels of the breathing system are cut into a compact aluminium block which reduces the volume of the system and thus the internal compliance. The system is designed to be used with a 1.5 l carbon dioxide absorber at low fresh gas flow with a high efficiency in the use of fresh gas. There is fresh gas decoupling

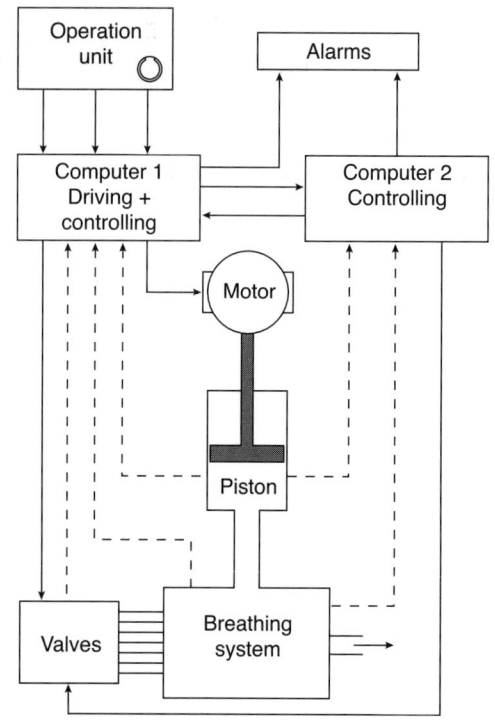

Figure 3.10 The Divan ventilator control system block diagram. (Reproduced by courtesy of Dräger.)

so that during inspiration the fresh gas flow does not alter the volume of gas delivered.

Figure 3.11 shows the breathing system and the pneumatically operated, computer controlled valve positions. At the start of inspiration the fresh gas decoupling valve (A) is closed as are valves B, C and D on the expiratory side. The ventilator piston forces the gas through the absorber via the inspiratory disc valve (I) to the patient. At the start of expiration the fresh gas decoupling valve then opens and expired gas flows through the PEEP valve and expiratory disc valve (E), pushing the gas remaining in the expiratory limb through the absorber and into the fresh gas reservoir/manual ventilation bag. The piston then moves back drawing gas from the expired limb and from the fresh gas reservoir bag (again through the absorber). At the end

The Divan (Drager) 63

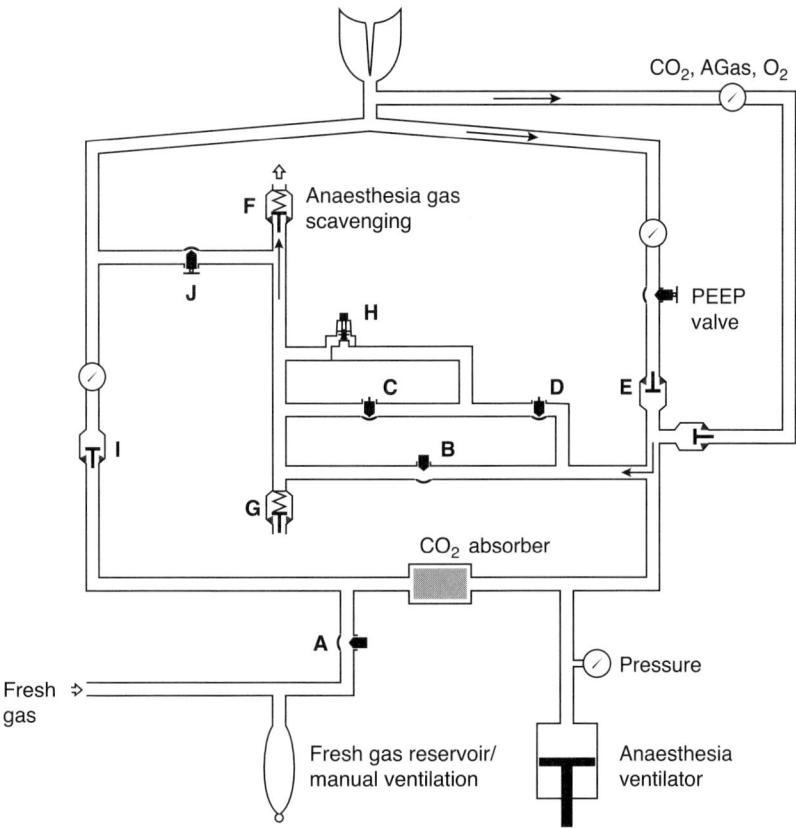

Figure 3.11 The Divan ventilator pneumatic system diagram. Valve positions during expiration. (Reproduced by courtesy of Drager.)

of the piston stroke, any further expired gas from the patient or displaced by the fresh gas flow is then diverted through valve B to the gas scavenging system. Some of the expired gas can pass through the absorber three times before being recycled to the patient.

During spontaneous ventilation valve A is open, valve B is closed and the excess gas is diverted via valves C and D to valve F and the scavenging system. Should the fresh gas flow be inadequate, air can be drawn in through an intake valve G set to open at −2 mbar. With manual ventilation, when the pressure in the system increases valve C closes and the gas is spilled via valve D through the adjustable pressure limiting (APL) valve (H) to valve F. There is a high pressure limiting valve (J) set at 80 mbar. Figure 3.11 also shows that gas aspirated from the airway for the gas analyser is returned to the system. This is particularly important during minimal flow applications. The PEEP valve is pneumatically controlled and is closed during inspiration and opens fully during expiration until the set PEEP value is reached. This valve is also used in a reversed-flow test and leak test. The maximum pressure in the system can be limited between 10 and 80 mbar to produce pressure limited ventilation. If the pressure limit is set low, the ventilator acts as a pressure generator.

During the start up test procedure it is possible to measure the internal compliance of the system (usually about 3 ml mbar^{-1} and the tidal volume can be automatically corrected for loss due to gas compression. Changing the patient conducting tubing to smaller volume tubing would make this system very suitable for neonatal anaesthesia because of its inherent low internal compliance.

A lot of thought has been put into designing this ergonomic, user friendly ventilator. It has a wide sphere of use, is compact and autoclavable. Any problems with the hardware can be easily remedied by replacing the faulty units. It interfaces with a sophisticated monitoring system to provide a safe and reliable anaesthesia system.

DATEX-ENGSTROM AS/3™ ANAESTHETIC DELIVERY UNIT (ADU)

The Datex-Engstrom AS/3™ Anaesthesia Delivery Unit is an anaesthetic machine which incorporates an anaesthetic gas delivery system with integral ventilator together with full anaesthetic, respiratory and cardiovascular monitoring using the latest technology. The anaesthetic ventilator is designed for use with all patient breathing systems and has facilities for spontaneous ventilation, manual ventilation or controlled mandatory ventilation with PEEP. At first glance the ventilator seems to be a conventional bellows-in-bottle system, but on close investigation there is a significant increase in sophistication in the delivery of anaesthetic gas, control of ventilation and monitoring of respiratory parameters.

CENTRAL ELECTRONIC CONTROLS

The central processing unit (CPU), a back-up processor and the printed circuit boards are placed in a gas tight box behind the main display screen. The CPU controls functions, set by the operator via the display screen, such as tidal volume, respiratory frequency, I:E ratio, inspiratory pause, PEEP and sigh function and the alarm levels. Using feed back from pressure and flow signals the CPU drives the valves and stepper motors which govern the ventilator functions. All the electronic components are within an electromagnetic interference-shielded frame. All relevant information is shown in graphical and digital form on a screen with a user friendly control.

On start up, the CPU organizes a self-check and performs a leak test and computes the internal compliance of the ventilator system. The CPU uses this compliance value together with information about the fresh gas flow (TV_{FGF}) to compensate for gas compression within the breathing system (TV_{COMPL}) and to deliver the required tidal volume (TV_{SET}).

$$TV_{SET} = TV_{BELLOWS} + TV_{FGF} - TV_{COMPL}$$
$$= TV_{DELIVERED}$$

THE PNEUMATIC SYSTEM

The bellows assembly

The bellows system is conventional (Figure 3.4) with a concertina bellows attached to a valve block and enclosed in a clear plastic cover. During the inspiratory phase the driving gas enters the bellows chamber, compressing the bellows and pressurizing and closing the overflow valve. During expiration the bellows fills with breathing system gas until it is fully expanded and then the overflow valve opens allowing further breathing circuit gas to be expelled to the scavenging system. The auto/manual switch separates the bellows and manual systems and, when switched to manual, connects the APL valve and manual reservoir bag with the patient system. This switch also starts and stops the ventilator.

The driving gas system

Oxygen and air supplies entering from the back of the anaesthetic machine are directed to a driving gas selecting unit (Figure 3.12). The primary driving gas is air or oxygen depending on the model ordered. However, if

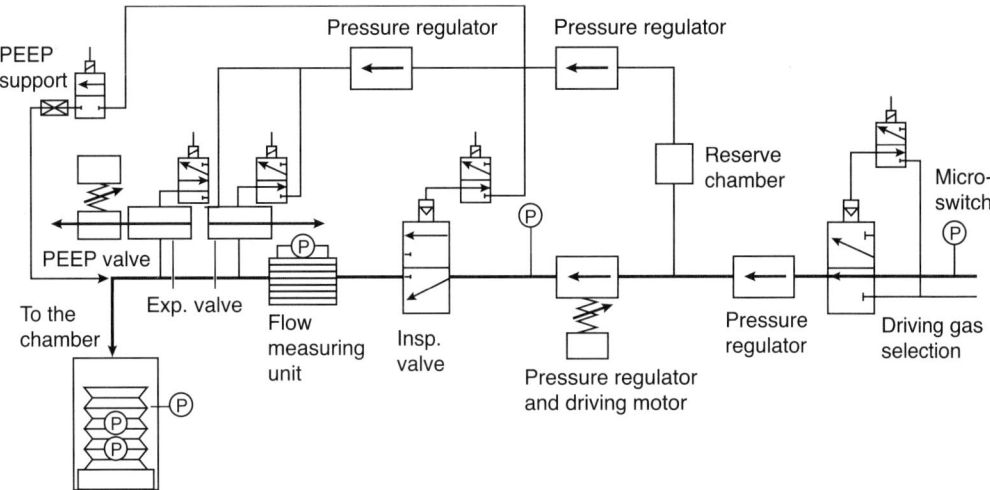

Figure 3.12 Diagram of the pneumatic system of the Datex-Engstrom AS/3 Anaesthesia Delivery Unit ventilator. (Reproduced by courtesy of Datex-Engstrom.)

air is the primary driving gas and the air pressure falls below 2.7 bar, the system automatically selects the oxygen supply to drive the bellows. The driving gas pressure is reduced by a pressure regulator and the flow is split into two paths. One gas supply serves the pneumatically driven but electronically controlled inspiratory and expiratory valves and the PEEP support system and the other constitutes the driving gas supply to the bellows chamber. The latter driving gas then passes through a motor-driven pressure regulator which controls the inspiratory flow, through the inspiratory valve and then, via a sensor which measures the flow, the gas enters the bellows chamber. The flow signal is fed back to the CPU which thus servo-controls the driving gas pressure regulator to achieve the required flow.

During the inspiratory phase the PEEP and expiratory valves and the PEEP support valve are closed. At end inspiration the inspiratory valve closes and there is a short end-inspiratory pause before expiration.

At the beginning of expiration, the expiratory valve opens. The driving gas in the bellows chamber then exits via the expiratory valve to room air. If PEEP is desired, the pressure level required is determined by the operator through the control panel. In this case both the PEEP and expiratory valves are open at the start of expiration. The PEEP support valve, which allows a flow of $6\,l\,min^{-1}$ to enter the driving gas system, is also open. When the pressure in the breathing system falls to the required PEEP level (measured close to the patient circuit connector), the main expiratory valve closes and the PEEP support gas flow then exits through the PEEP valve, the pressure in the system being servo-controlled by the motorized PEEP valve to maintain the desired PEEP level.

The ventilator is thus a flow generator in inspiration, a pressure generator in expiration and time cycled from inspiration to expiration and from expiration to inspiration.

Fresh gas control unit

Oxygen, air and nitrous oxide (N_2O) are supplied to the gas distribution block and thence to the fresh gas control unit (Figure 3.13). The gases, having been filtered and their pressures reduced through pressure regulators,

Ventilators for anaesthetic use

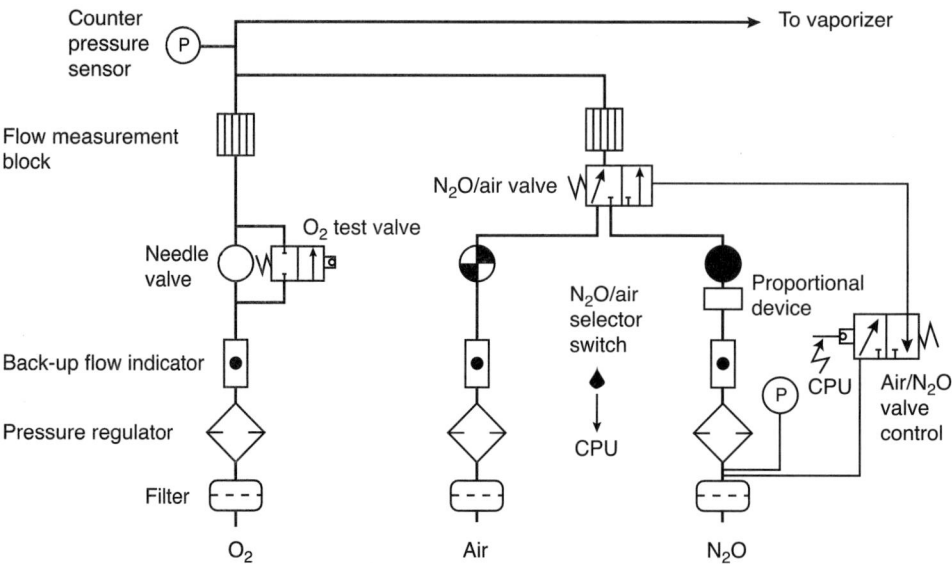

Figure 3.13 Diagram of the fresh gas flow control system of the Datex-Engstrom AS/3 Anaesthesia Delivery Unit ventilator. (Reproduced by courtesy of Datex-Engstrom.)

pass through visible Rotameters to mechanical needle valves which the operator controls from the front panel.

A N_2O air selector switch allows the operator to choose either N_2O or air to be mixed with oxygen in the fresh gas flow. If N_2O is selected then an electronically driven proportional device limits the N_2O flow to a maximum of 75% of the total flow, assuring a minimum of 25% oxygen. If air is selected, the ratio of air to oxygen is unlimited.

The oxygen flow is continuously monitored with a flow measuring device (a laminar flow differential pressure transducer) as is the flow of either air or N_2O. The two flow signals are registered in the CPU. The flows are mixed and pass through a counter-pressure sensor into the vaporizer unit. The flow measurement units have each a zeroing device which corrects for zero drift and, with the information from the counter-pressure sensor, allow the CPU to calculate an accurate fresh gas flow value. This value is then used in the equation above to compute the bellows displacement in the delivery of the set tidal volume. The flow signals also enable gas composition to be calculated. Standard vaporizers and back bar or the Datex electronically controlled vaporizer system options are available.

The Datex electronically controlled Aladin cassette vaporizers are lightweight units of the plenum type. One vapour at a time can be slotted into the fresh gas flow system. The CPU automatically identifies the cassette in use. The vapour concentration required is determined by the user with the vapour control knob on the front panel close to the vaporizer and displayed on the screen. The temperature of the anaesthetic liquid is continuously monitored. Using an electronically driven proportional valve on the outlet side of the liquid chamber flow, the CPU then adjusts the ratio of the bypass flow and liquid chamber flow to deliver the required concentration. The CPU takes into account the total gas flow, temperature of the liquid in the cassette and saturated vapour pressure of the anaesthetic agent at that temperature in calculating the cassette flow. A further flow transducer measures the bypass flow. The ratio of the bypass and cassette flow is used to servo-control the system. The continuous measurement of the liquid temperature means that the vaporizer unit does not need a large heat sink to keep the temperature stable and can thus be made much lighter. In addition, since the control of the concentration is exterior to the vaporizer cassette, the cassette is of simple, robust design, requiring no maintenance.

PAEDIATRIC AND NEONATAL VENTILATION

Although the Drager Divan has been mentioned as a ventilator which can deliver tidal volumes as small as 20 ml, the majority of adult ventilators have difficulty delivering tidal volumes of less than 200 ml. Some systems can be modified to deliver smaller tidal volumes and the modifications depend on whether the flow generator characteristics of the ventilator are to be maintained or not.

MODIFICATION TO MAINTAIN FLOW GENERATOR CHARACTERISTICS

Use of smaller bellows

By changing the bellows to one which has a smaller cross sectional area, the volume delivered per linear displacement is reduced and this improves the accuracy of volume displacement if this is determined by visual displacement of the bellows. The residual volume in the bellows at end inspiration is also decreased which helps reduce the internal compliance of the bellows compartment.

Reduction of internal compliance of tubing compartment

By using shorter, narrower and more rigid tubing the internal compliance of the breathing system is reduced and this makes the volume delivered to the patient more predictable.

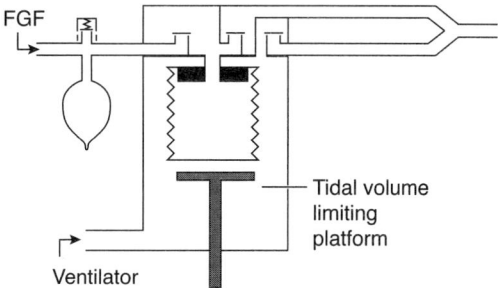

Figure 3.14 Diagram of the Cape paediatric attachment. The adjustable platform determines tidal volume. The solid block at the top of the bellows reduces the residual gas volume of the bellows compartment. FGF=fresh gas flow.

Separate paediatric attachment

The ageing Cape–Waine ventilator has a paediatric attachment which is a bag-in-bottle arrangement (Figure 3.14). The bellows is completely emptied at end inspiration and tidal volume is determined by the position of the adjustable volume limiting platform. Fresh gas is drawn from a reservoir as the bellows fills downwards. The system can be positioned close to the patient which allows the use of short, narrow tubing. The bag in the bottle can be compressed by any adult ventilator and the pressure developed in the bottle is immaterial provided it is sufficient to compress the bellows completely.

CONVERSION OF THE VENTILATOR TO A PRESSURE GENERATOR

Increase internal compliance

In the past the internal compliance of the breathing system has been deliberately increased to produce a parallel compliance which increased the gas compressed in the breathing system and reduced the actual tidal volume delivered to the child. The end-inspiratory pressure in the system determined the tidal volume. This system was cumbersome and is not used nowadays.

Introduction of a leak

The Penlon Nuffield 200 ventilator is a time cycled flow generator which can be modified for paediatric use. In this case the normal inspiratory and expiratory valve is replaced by the Newton valve which allows a leak to occur in inspiration. This converts the system into a pressure generator and the inspiratory pressure is controlled by the flow control on the ventilator. The inspiratory pressure thus determines the tidal volume generated but this tidal volume will also be dependent on lung compliance and airway resistance.

Pressure controlled ventilation

Some ventilators are capable of providing pressure controlled ventilation when the maximum airway pressure can be adjusted by the operator. Under these circumstances, a flow generator behaves as a pressure generator (see Drager Divan). This may be advantageous in paediatric and neonatal ventilation as the maximum airway pressure can be limited to prevent barotrauma and in addition, a pressure generator can cope with small leaks in the breathing system such as may occur when using uncuffed tracheal tubes.

VENTILATION WITH A T-PIECE

The T-piece breathing system is often used in small children and babies. It has the advantage that it can be made of narrow lightweight tubing with small, lightweight connections and low apparatus deadspace. Any suitable ventilation system can be used with it and it is easy to convert to manual ventilation or spontaneous ventilation.

The T-piece can be used in two ways for IPPV. (a) A ventilator substitutes for the reservoir bag of a Mapleson D system and produces bulk flow of gas towards the patient along the expiratory limb during inspiration. The Nuffield 200 with Newton valve is commonly used in this way. (b) The expiratory limb of the T-piece is intermittently occluded by a mechanical valve so that the fresh gas flow is diverted to the patient. In this case the inspiratory flow is produced by flow generation and the tidal volume is determined by the fresh gas flow and the duration of the inspiratory occlusion. The flow of fresh gas is thus relatively high compared with other systems. But since this is small compared to adult flow requirements, most anaesthetists regard the extra cost as insignificant.

The problem with the various modifications for paediatric anaesthesia is that actual minute ventilation cannot easily be measured. However, the routine monitoring of end-tidal carbon dioxide makes this less of a problem these days and ventilation can be adjusted according to the CO_2 value. With convenient spirometry at the airway becoming available as well, the problems of monitoring ventilation may diminish.

FURTHER READING

Mushin, W. W., Rendell-Baker, L., Thompson, P. W. and Maplesmon, W. W. (1980) *Automatic Ventilation of the Lungs*, 3rd edn, Blackwell Scientific, Oxford.

Radford, E. P. (1955) Ventilation standards for use in artificial respiration. *Journal of Applied Physiology*, **7**, 451.

ANAESTHETIC BREATHING SYSTEMS 4

D. C. White

An anaesthetic breathing system is the assembly of tubes, valves and reservoirs through which gas is conveyed from the anaesthetic machine to the patient. The term 'circuit' is to be discouraged since it is, in most cases, inaccurate. The performance of the system, in particular the flow of fresh gas it requires to eliminate CO_2, is determined by the relative positions of the various components of the system. Gas enters the system from the common gas outlet of the anaesthetic machine and any surplus gas escapes from the system via a spring loaded valve. This is termed the adjustable pressure limiting valve (APL) (also pop-off, Heidbrink or dump valve). The term 'expiratory valve' is best avoided because it could also be used for one of the valves within a circle system. In some systems (T-pieces) the surplus gas escapes via an open expiratory limb. In the completely closed system there is no surplus gas.

Before discussing the details of these systems and their use it is necessary to review the respiratory requirements which must be met by the systems in clinical practice. Ventilation of the lungs has two major functions, the delivery of oxygen to the respiratory epithelium which lines the pulmonary alveoli and the removal of CO_2 which has diffused into the alveoli. Oxygen consumption of mammals may be calculated (in ml min^{-1}) from body weight as kg$^{3/4}$ × 10 (Brody's law). This gives a figure of 242 ml min^{-1} O_2 for a 70 kg subject. However, oxygen requirements are reduced by 15–30% during anaesthesia and are also diminished by increasing age. The figure of 200 ml min^{-1} O_2 for a 70 kg subject is a more realistic approximation for clinical practice. Knowledge of the oxygen consumption per minute is only of immediate significance during completely closed circuit anaesthesia where it must be provided with some accuracy; however it does regulate CO_2 production. The removal of CO_2 is the second of the respiratory functions mentioned above and this must now be briefly discussed.

The total capacity of the lungs of the customary 70 kg subject is 6 l, of which about 4.8 l can be exchanged by a maximal effort (vital capacity), leaving 1.2 l of residual volume. Normal breathing exchanges only about 500 ml, the tidal volume (V_T), which lies in the middle of the vital capacity range. When the tidal volume enters the lungs they already contain 2.2 l of gas containing CO_2. This important volume is the functional residual capacity (FRC) made up of the residual volume already mentioned plus the expiratory reserve volume. The FRC is much larger than V_T and consequently the effect on the composition of the alveolar gas of the coming and going of V_T is relatively slight. The FRC can be seen to lie as a buffer zone of gas tensions between the blood and the atmosphere and all the respiratory regulatory mechanisms are directed to the maintenance of alveolar gas tensions. The mean alveolar CO_2 tension is 40 mmHg (5.3 kPa), or 5.2% (ignoring small

---

Short Practice of Anaesthesia. Edited by M. Morgan and G. M. Hall. Published in 1997 by Chapman & Hall, London. ISBN 0 412 71890 1

changes due to anaesthesia). If the oxygen uptake is 200 ml min^{-1} and the respiratory exchange ratio is 0.8 then it can be calculated that the CO_2 production is 160 ml. This 160 ml is diluted in the FRC. It can be calculated that to maintain the alveolar CO_2 at 5% an alveolar ventilation of 3.2 l min^{-1} is required. The figures given above must be taken as examples only. During anaesthesia a number of variable factors may affect the situation. Among these variables is the decrease in FRC produced by anaesthesia and increase in shunt, i.e. blood passing through the lungs without exposure to alveolar gas.

Mammalian ventilation consists of drawing in fresh gas containing oxygen and expelling gas containing CO_2 and diminished O_2 from the alveoli of the lungs. In addition to the gas actually entering and leaving the alveoli a further volume must be drawn or pumped in to fill the passageways leading from the outside world to the alveoli. These passageways are in the nose, pharynx, larynx, trachea and bronchi leading to the alveoli. No gas exchange takes place in these passageways, called the anatomical dead space, which have a volume of about 130 ml. It approximates to the body weight in pounds. In addition, not all the alveolar gas comes fully into equilibrium with the pulmonary blood (alveolar dead space). Under normal circumstances and over quite a range of tidal volumes one third of each tidal volume occupies dead space, i.e. it takes no part in gas exchange. The first part of each V_T which enters the alveoli at the beginning of each breath is alveolar gas (containing CO_2). It is the last part of the previous expiration. To produce the alveolar ventilation of 3.2 l min^{-1} given above, a $\dot{V}_E$ of 4.8 l min^{-1} would be needed. ($\dot{V}_E$=expired minute volume)

The anatomical dead space is approximately halved by tracheal intubation; any part of an anaesthetic breathing system which is in series with the pharynx and trachea in which no gas exchange process takes place also becomes part of the dead space, the 'apparatus dead space'. The alveolar CO_2 is regulated by the ratio between dead space and alveolar ventilation. If the minute volume is fixed (artificial ventilation) then alveolar CO_2 is regulated by the dead space. If the patient is breathing spontaneously then increases in dead space by raising alveolar CO_2, increase the minute volume to compensate for this and restore CO_2 equilibrium. Clearly it is important to reduce dead space in breathing systems to a minimum unless it is being used to control CO_2 when V_T is fixed.

FLOW REQUIREMENTS IN BREATHING SYSTEMS

Figure 4.1 shows the changing gas flows during a respiratory cycle in an anaesthetized patient. The peak inspiratory flow in anaesthetized patients does not normally exceed 30 l min^{-1} and 20 l min^{-1} is an average figure. Gas flow from the Rotameter, or other gas mixing apparatus of the anaesthetic machine, is at a steady flow of much less than this and so it is necessary to incorporate in the breathing system an elastic reservoir bag to accommodate these high momentary flows. A 2 l rubber reservoir bag, if overfilled, will expand to more than 144 l before bursting. Under these circumstances the pressure in the bag does not rise above 4 kPa (30 mmHg) and the bag therefore has a pressure limiting function. Less commonly a demand valve can be used instead of a reservoir bag and a gas mixing device may be incorporated; this is described as an intermittent flow machine.

RESISTANCE IN BREATHING SYSTEMS

All breathing systems impose some increased resistance on respiratory gas flow and it is important that this should be minimized because of its adverse physiological effects. The subject is not easy to discuss in a quantifiable manner for a number of reasons. One is the complex nature of the transition from laminar flow (pressure gradient determined

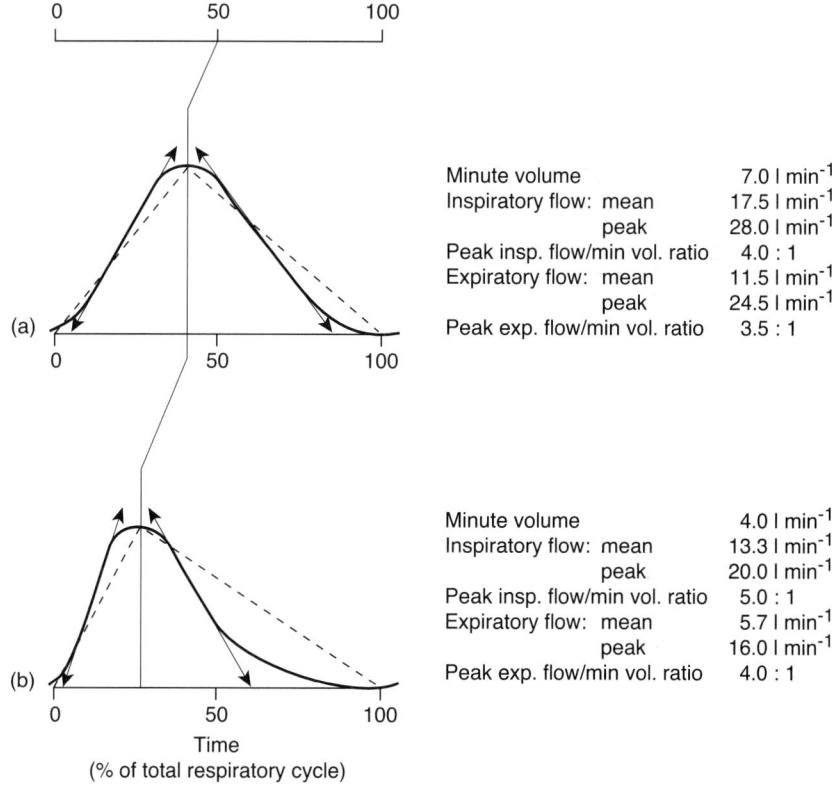

Figure 4.1 Respiratory waveforms of (a) conscious subject and (b) anaesthetized patient breathing spontaneously. Mean flow rates are shown by broken lines and peak flow rates by arrows. (Reproduced with permission from Nunn, 1987.)

by Poiseuille's law, viscosity dependent and directly proportional to flow) to turbulent flow (pressure gradient and density dependent and proportional to square of gas flow).

Despite this complexity it is useful to record features in breathing systems which tend to produce turbulent flow. These are high gas flows and rough walls or projections into the gas stream, sharp angles and branches and abrupt changes in diameter of tubing: these must all be eliminated or minimized.

Resistance to flow is measured by the pressure drop across the resistor (tubing, valve orifice, etc.) expressed usually in cmH$_2$O. It is considered that the highest permissible resistance to respiratory gas flow is one producing a 2 cm pressure difference when the gas flow is 20 l min^{-1}. This flow corresponds to the peak flow in the anaesthetized patient and also the minimum resistance of a standard APL (Heidbrink) valve. By this standard the resistance to flow of all usual pieces of anaesthetic equipment is acceptably low, e.g. that of a 9 mm tracheal tube being below 1 cm of water and that of the standard corrugated tubing ('elephant' tubing) is extremely low. This tubing, corrugated to prevent kinking on bending, is commonly used in breathing systems and has been for the past 90 years. It has an internal diameter of about 20 mm. The rough corrugated wall of this tubing may increase resistance to flow and it has been found that if smooth walled tubing of only

15 mm internal diameter is used it has acceptably low resistance for breathing systems, but in kink resistant (armoured) form is more expensive than standard tubing which in plastic form is now semi-disposable.

CLASSIFICATION OF BREATHING SYSTEMS

Anaesthetic breathing systems may be conveniently classified as follows.

- Systems incorporating soda lime or other substances able to remove CO_2 from gas mixtures passed through them. Gas flow in these systems may be circular or to-and-fro.
- Non-rebreathing systems in which each inspired breath is entirely fresh gas and the whole of each breath is expired from the system. Gas flow in these systems is one-way only except at the junction with the patient's airway.
- Partial rebreathing systems in which gas flow may be circular, but usually is to-and-fro. Note that rebreathing is not of physiological significance if extra CO_2 does not enter the alveolus with each breath. By extra CO_2 is meant CO_2 in addition to that expired into the dead space at the end of each breath (and reinspired into the alveolus at the beginning of inspiration). Note also that if the fresh gas flow (FGF) into these systems is sufficiently high they will become non-rebreathing. To reach this state the FGF will have to equal or exceed the peak inspiratory flow.

These three types of system are considered in detail below.

CO_2 REMOVAL SYSTEMS

These anaesthetic breathing systems employ canisters containing granules of soda lime or other alkaline compounds to remove CO_2. Systems using CO_2 absorption can operate with much lower FGFs than other systems; this results in a lower usage of expensive

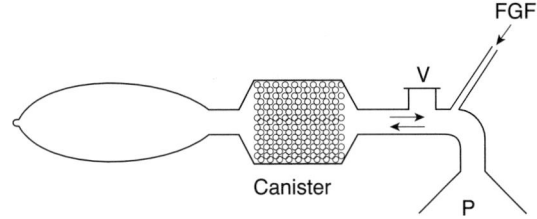

Figure 4.2 To-and-fro CO_2 absorption system (Water's canister).

liquid inhalational agents (usage is proportional to FGF). This potential economy of operation has resulted in increased interest in these systems recently.

To-and-fro systems (Figure 4.2) have no valves, the canister in which the absorption of CO_2 takes place must be placed close to the airway because the tubing between patient and canister is deadspace. This is not always convenient and brings the strongly alkaline soda lime close to the airway. As the soda lime is used up, there is a gradual increase in deadspace. The canister for to-and-fro absorption of CO_2 is designed so that when it is packed with soda lime of optimum granule size (1.5–5 mm in diameter) the intergranular space approximates in volume to the tidal volume. This is to allow the tidal volume of expired gas to rest in the canister during the expiratory pause which occurs during the normal ventilatory cycle. The removal of CO_2 by soda lime is so rapid (a contact time of 0.16 s reduces CO_2 from 5 to 0.5%) that this rest in the soda lime is not necessary. Smaller canisters, less clumsy than the standard, can therefore be used effectively, although having a shorter life.

The standard Water's canister holds about 500 g of soda lime and this has a theoretical life of 4 h under normal conditions. In practice the duration of efficient CO_2 absorption is about 90 min.

In circle systems (Figure 4.3) gas is directed around the system by two valves usually mounted on top of the large absorption can-

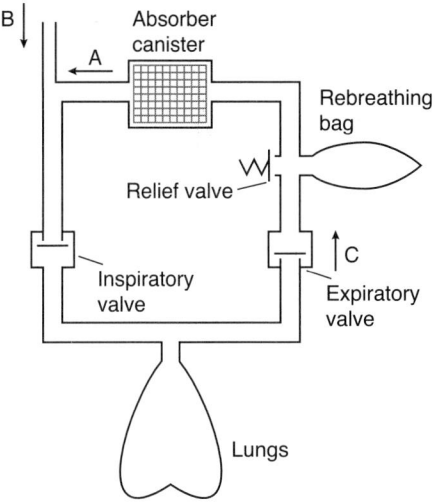

Figure 4.3 Components of anaesthesia circle systems.

ister (1–2 kg). The only deadspace is that within the T-piece connecting the patient to the double tubing of the circle so the canister can be mounted in a vertical position on the machine. The large canister allows a time of about 8 h between refills. In practice the life of the soda lime depends on the fresh gas flow; if this is above basal then gas will be lost from the system via the APL and CO_2 will be lost with it thus reducing the load on the soda lime. This assumes that the APL is placed before the soda lime on the expiratory side of the circle. This is usually the case.

Now that continuous CO_2 monitoring is widely available, the duration of active life of soda lime is not of such great interest. As soon as the inspired CO_2 is seen to rise above about 0.2% the soda lime requires to be changed. This facility has not always been available so soda lime usually has an indicator incorporated with it. A colour change gives indication of exhaustion and this can be seen through the transparent wall of the canister. This does not compare in accuracy with direct measurement of CO_2.

If a circle system is used with basal gas flow (completely closed) the order in which the five components of the system (two valves, APL, reservoir bag and FGF entry port) are arranged is of little importance. However, as the FGF rises the performance of the system comes to depend to some extent on the relative positions of the components. Since there are five components this is a subject of potential complexity. The optimum position for the APL during spontaneous breathing is at the T-piece connecting the patient to the circle. However, this is inefficient for controlled ventilation since fresh gas would be lost. As described above, a position for the APL on the expiratory side before the canister of CO_2 absorbent is an acceptable compromise. It is important that the APL valve should not be between the FGF inlet and the patient as this would result in loss of fresh gas.

The chemical reaction (hydroxide to carbonate) by which soda lime takes up CO_2 generates heat. The temperature inside the canister may reach 60°C but usually does not exceed 48–50°C. This may cause some breakdown of anaesthetic agents with possible formation of toxic substances. Attention is therefore being directed to finding alternative methods of removing CO_2. One possibility is the use of zeolites. These are natural or synthetic aluminium silicates of the alkaline metals which have an unusual honeycomb structure bearing a negative charge and having the ability to act as molecular sieves, retaining one component of a gas mixture passed through them. Which gas is retained depends on the precise dimensions of the cavities within the specific zeolites. Zeolites can be regenerated by heating or subjecting to reduced pressure.

NON-REBREATHING SYSTEMS

These systems employ non-rebreathing valves (Figure 4.4). These are devices having three ports attached to the body of the valve which permit gas to be drawn (or pumped) in at one port, entering and leaving the lungs through

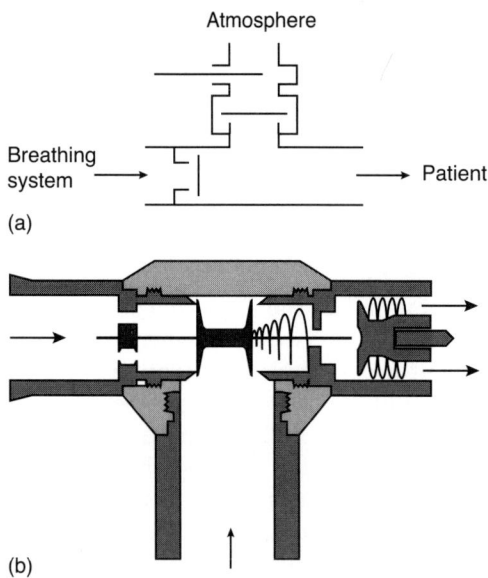

Figure 4.4 Non-rebreathing valve (Ruben).

a second port and directing the expired gas out through the third port. The fresh gas supply must be able to deliver the peak inspiratory flow and this may be achieved by mounting a reservoir bag on the inspiratory side. The FGF must be equal to or exceed the patient's minute volume ($\dot{V}_E$). Alternatively non-rebreathing valves may have a low resistance ('breath through') vaporizer attached to the inspiratory port by suitable tubing so that anaesthetic and air is breathed in on inspiration. This is called a draw-over system.

An alternative to the reservoir bag is the demand valve (Figure 4.5). This is a type of reducing valve capable of delivering a high gas flow at low pressure in response to a sub-atmospheric pressure applied to its inspiratory port by the patient's inspiratory effort. Two demand valves may be used together to constitute a gas mixer (N_2O and O_2) and a vaporizer having a low resistance to gas flow such as the Goldman or Oxford Miniature Vaporizer (OMV) may be placed between the demand valve(s) and the non-rebreathing valve. This is an intermittent-flow anaesthetic machine, commonly used for dental anaesthesia.

Demand valves are capable of delivering much higher flows than those required for anaesthetized patients and consequently are suitable for attachment to Entonox cylinders (50/50 N_2/O_2) for use in obstetric analgesia and postoperative physiotherapy.

PARTIAL REBREATHING SYSTEMS

The standard descriptive classification of these systems is that of Mapleson (1954) and this is given in the first column of Figure 4.6. Each system is discussed individually below. As can be seen these are single tube systems so that gas flow is bi-directional during the respiratory cycle. The most important functional attribute of these systems is how great a flow of fresh gas they require to maintain normocarbia. As will be seen, this depends not only on the morphology of the system, but also whether it is used with spontaneous or controlled ventilation. The FGF requirement for each system and mode of ventilation is given in column 3 of Figure 4.6, it is expressed as a fraction of the minute volume ($\dot{V}_E$). These figures should be regarded as guidelines only. The performance of these systems is changed by quite small modifications. The shape of the respiratory wave form, in particular the duration of the expiratory pause, also affects those systems in which a relatively low FGF accumulates in a reservoir tube or bag.

Understanding of the working of these systems is helped by considering the functional classification of Miller (1988) in which the performance (gas economy) of each Mapleson system is explained by reference to the position of the reservoir bag. This can be on the afferent side of the system (bringing fresh gas to the patient) or the efferent side (conveying it away). As already mentioned, the systems illustrated in column 1 of Figure 4.6 combine afferent and efferent functions in one tube, but they can be redrawn in twin-tube ver-

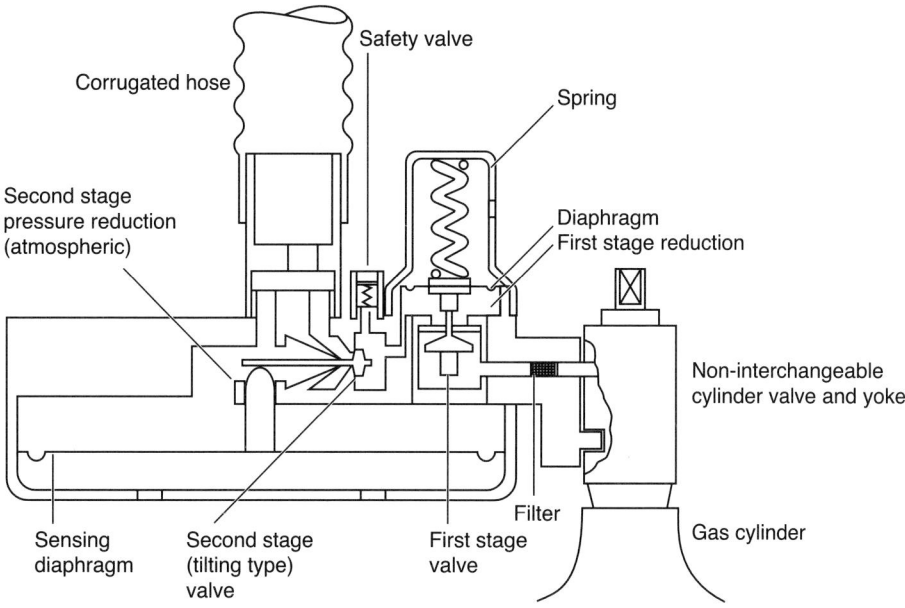

Figure 4.5 Demand valve. (Reproduced by courtesy of Ohmeda Ltd.)

sions in which these functions are separated. This has been done in column 2 of Figure 4.6. This assists explanation of Miller's classification and is not an entirely academic exercise since some of these twin-tube versions have advantages in clinical practice. All twin-tube systems can be made coaxial and those which have been used clinically are also described below.

MAPLESON A SYSTEMS

This system, described by Dr Ivan Magill in 1928, is characterized by efficiency in gas requirements for normocarbia during spontaneous breathing. As can be seen from Figure 4.6, the volume between the patient's airway and the APL valve is apparatus dead space. As expiration begins this dead space gas together with dead space gas from the patient (containing no CO_2) passes back along the corrugated tube. The FGF from the anaesthetic machine, unable to pass along the tube inflates the reservoir bag and the pressure in the system rises until the APL valve opens (1–2 cmH$_2$O). The gas which now escapes from the valve is alveolar gas containing CO_2. It is expelled by elastic recoil of the patient's lungs. When inspiration starts the pressure falls and the APL valve closes. The gas now drawn into the patient's airway is firstly CO_2 free dead space gas which has been remaining in the system, followed by fresh gas from the reservoir bag and anaesthetic machine.

This system thus preferentially expels CO_2 containing alveolar gas and preserves CO_2 free deadspace gas for rebreathing. This mode of operation is characteristic of systems having a reservoir in the afferent limb (AR systems). This relationship is made clear in the twin-tube version of the Mapleson A (Figure 4.6 column 2).

The exact amount by which $\dot{V}_F$ can be reduced below $\dot{V}_E$ when using this system depends on circumstances. $\dot{V}_F/\dot{V}_E = 0.7$ was found to be adequate for normocarbia. Other investigators have used slightly different criteria to define the onset of CO_2 rebreathing. $\dot{V}_F/\dot{V}_E = 0.8$ gives a FGF of 4.8 l for a 70 kg patient having a $\dot{V}_E$ of 6 l (figures cited as

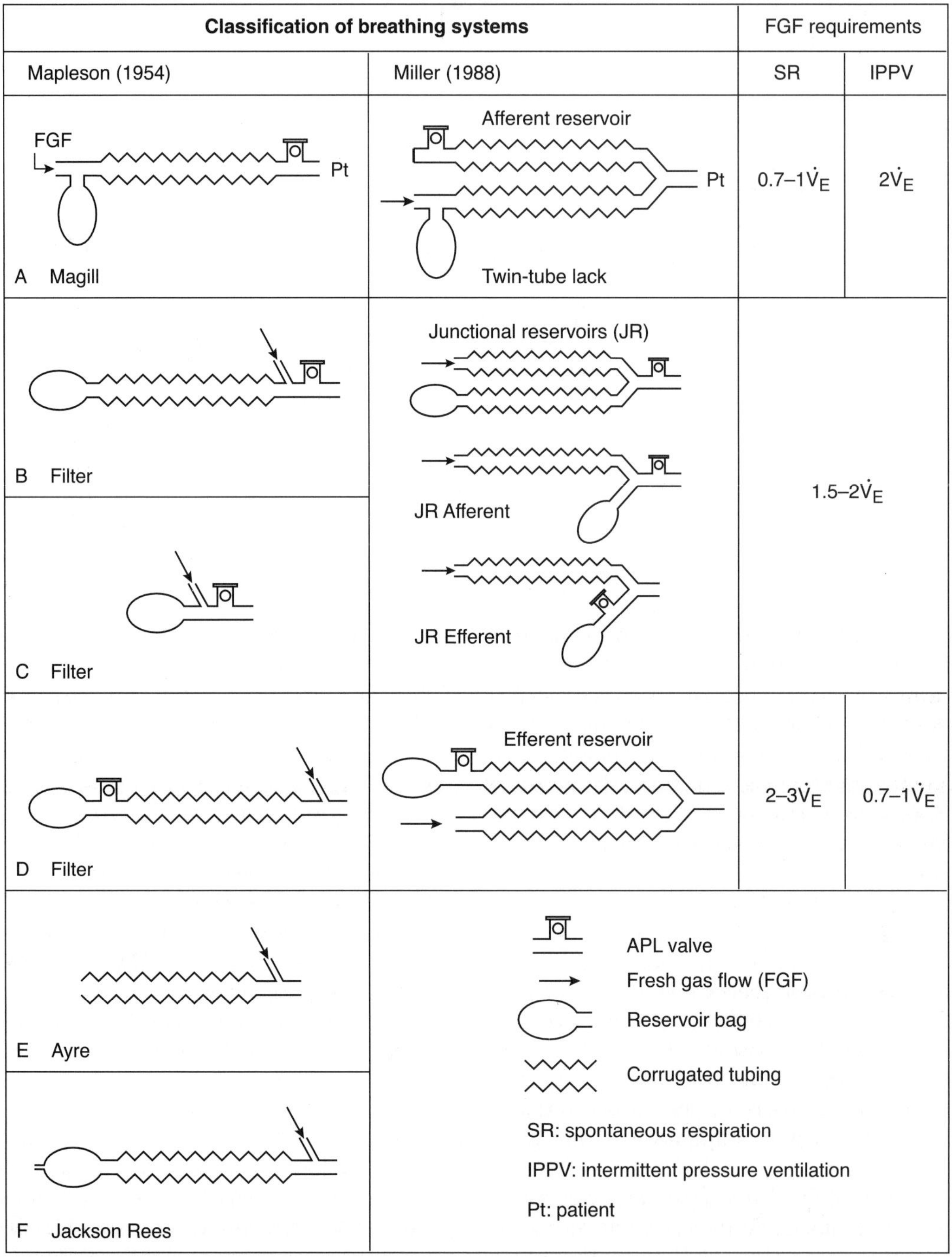

Classification of breathing systems		FGF requirements	
Mapleson (1954)	Miller (1988)	SR	IPPV
A Magill	Afferent reservoir / Twin-tube lack	$0.7\text{--}1\dot{V}_E$	$2\dot{V}_E$
B Filter	Junctional reservoirs (JR)	$1.5\text{--}2\dot{V}_E$	
C Filter	JR Afferent / JR Efferent		
D Filter	Efferent reservoir	$2\text{--}3\dot{V}_E$	$0.7\text{--}1\dot{V}_E$
E Ayre			
F Jackson Rees			

Legend:
- APL valve
- Fresh gas flow (FGF)
- Reservoir bag
- Corrugated tubing
- SR: spontaneous respiration
- IPPV: intermittent pressure ventilation
- Pt: patient

Figure 4.6 Classification of partial rebreathing systems.

examples using Radford nomogram). This figure works well in practice, fine tuning to minimize FGF is not worthwhile because ventilatory volumes vary during surgery.

The foregoing relates to spontaneous breathing. If the Mapleson A system is used to control ventilation by squeezing the reservoir bag a very different state of affairs prevails. During inspiration the pressure in the system is above atmosphere and, as well as entering the lungs a variable amount of fresh gas is lost through the APL valve and to maintain normocarbia a $\dot{V}_F/\dot{V}_E = 3$ may be needed, i.e. 18 l min^{-1} for our 70 kg patient example.

The antithesis of the Mapleson A system is the Mapleson D and this is discussed below.

MAPLESON B AND C SYSTEMS

These systems are characterized by having a blind limb and are not much used in clinical practice. Their gas flow requirements for normocarbia lie between the A and D systems. Conway (1985) found experimentally that a B system could be made to work with moderate efficiency (FGF of 0.8–1.2 $\dot{V}_E$) for spontaneous breathing if CO_2 containing gas could be prevented from entering the closed limb. To do this required critical adjustment of $\dot{V}_D/\dot{V}_E$ and tidal volume, quite impractical for clinical use.

The C system might be considered even less efficient than the B because there is no tube to maintain the separation of the dead space and alveolar gas and all the expired gas is mixed in the reservoir bag. However, the system, usually in the form of a Water's to-and-fro system without the canister, is very convenient for short term manual inflation of the lungs before intubation or for chest physiotherapy.

These systems are classified by Miller (1988) as junctional reservoir systems and this is appropriate to their gas flow requirements (1.5–2 V_E). The junctional reservoir may be on the afferent or efferent side; gas flow requirements are not greatly affected.

MAPLESON D, E AND F SYSTEMS

These are all T-piece systems characterized by having the fresh gas flow enter between the patient and the expiratory limb which terminates in a reservoir bag and APL (D), an open end (E) or a reservoir bag with a controllable leak in the tail (F). The fresh gas flow requirements of these systems are similar, but systems E and F have been chiefly used for paediatric anaesthesia.

The functioning of the D system has been extensively studied. The results of these studies can be summarized by saying that the D system is inefficient during spontaneous breathing and requires a FGF of $\dot{V}_F/\dot{V}_E$ of 2 (more in the coaxial version, see Bain system below). But for controlled ventilation a FGF of $\dot{V}_F/\dot{V}_E$ of 1 is adequate for normocapnia.

During spontaneous breathing with the D system the preservation of the dead space portion of the expired volume is lost and there is preservation of the alveolar gas portion. This is the reverse of the situation obtaining with the A system and a higher FGF is necessary to flush out the system. If the FGF equals or exceeds the peak inspiratory flow then clearly this will suffice to prevent rebreathing of CO_2, but in practice a lower flow can be used because during the time that the inspiratory flow is less than FGF a surplus of fresh gas accumulates in the system which can be enough to prevent CO_2 rebreathing during the time that the inspiratory flow exceeds FGF. This is helped if there is an appreciable end-expiratory pause.

The separation of dead space and alveolar portions of expired gas, which is the basis of all these gas economies, is lost during controlled ventilation. Because of the more abrupt gas movements expired and fresh gas mixes in the system so that there is always some CO_2 rebreathing. The non-linear relationship between $\dot{V}_F$ and $\dot{V}_E$ during controlled ventilation with a T-piece system is shown in Figure 4.7 which shows the theoretical relationship between P_{CO_2}, FGF and

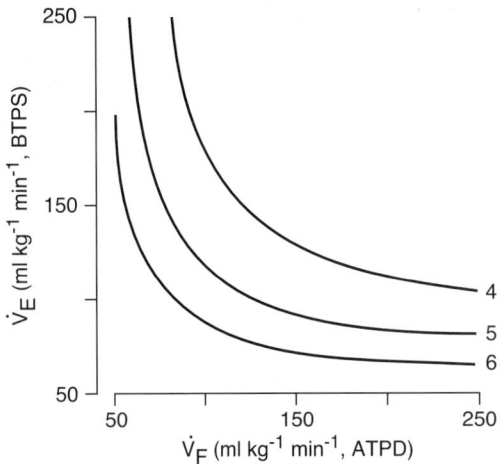

Figure 4.7 Curves to show the inter-relationships of P_{CO_2}, FGF and ventilation when controlled ventilation is carried out using a T-piece system. The three curves are CO_2 isopleths at P_{CO_2} values of 4, 5 and 6 kPa. (Reproduced with permission from Conway 1985.)

ventilation. The distance between the CO_2 isopleths (representing 4, 5 and 6 kPa) shows that at high FGF the P_{CO_2} depends chiefly upon ventilation, but at low FGF it is the FGF which regulates P_{CO_2}. These relationships can be used in clinical practice to adjust P_{CO_2} with considerable precision (controlled rebreathing).

The Mapleson E system uses a T-piece for spontaneous breathing with intubated patients. It was first described (for paediatric use) by Philip Ayre in 1937 following a fatality in which a child's lungs were inflated at gas supply pressure. It has the advantages of simplicity and of having no valves. To prevent air entering the patient's lungs the volume of the expiratory limb (reservoir) should exceed the tidal volume. The original Ayre's T-piece had an internal diameter of 10 mm, considerations of resistance to peak flow make it acceptable up to the age of about 5 years. Gas flow requirements are the same as for the D system.

To permit controlled ventilation with the Ayre's T-piece Jackson Rees described a modification in 1950 which is the F system. A bag is attached to the end of the expiratory limb. Gas escapes from the tail of the bag and the overflow can be controlled by the operator to keep enough gas in the bag to permit inflation of the lungs. A simple device which, together with the Ayre's T-piece, has gained world-wide use.

COAXIAL SYSTEMS

A coaxial system – two tubes, one inside the other and sharing a common long axis – was used in a twenty foot length to feed anaesthetic gases to and from an unconscious subject (Dr E. A. Pask) floating in an Oxford swimming pool. This was done in wartime tests of life jacket design by Macintosh and Pask.

THE BAIN SYSTEM

In 1972 two Canadian anaesthetists, Bain and Spoerel, described a coaxial system (Figure 4.8a) which is a version of the Mapleson D system described above. The system is 1.8 m long, longer than the standard (1 m) Magill (A) system, but of the same 22 mm diameter corrugated tubing. The inner tube is of narrow bore (5 mm) and is for gas delivery only, which gives the outer tube sufficient volume to act as a reservoir (Mapleson E). The addition of a bag and APL valve converts it to a D system.

The advantages of this system are that it removes the APL valve from close proximity to the patient, where it may be covered by towels, and puts it on the machine at the fresh gas outlet where it is accessible for adjustment and scavenging. The absence of a valve at the patient's end makes it light and convenient to use. The other big advantage of this system is that, for controlled ventilation, a small and cheap ventilator such as the Penlon or Pneupac can be attached instead of the reservoir bag. The ventilator drives a

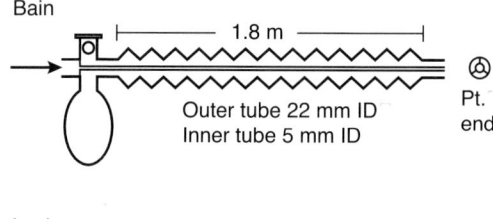
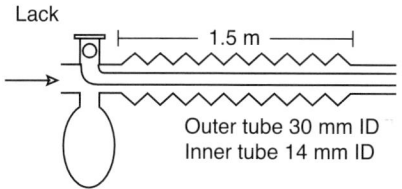
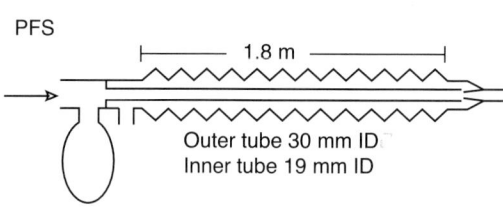

PFS: preferential flow system (Miller & Couper 1983)

Figure 4.8 Coaxial systems: (a) Bain, (b) Lack, (c) preferential flow system.

'piston' of gas (air or oxygen) up and down a piece of corrugated tubing (the trunk) which is attached instead of the reservoir bag. The trunk must have a capacity greater than the tidal volume so that gas driving the ventilator does not reach the patient.

This method of ventilation has the advantages mentioned when discussing the Mapleson D system. It permits good inflation of the lungs, desirable to prevent intraoperative pulmonary collapse, without hypocapnia (controlled rebreathing) and is economical in anaesthetic gas usage.

The chief drawback to the Bain system is the high fresh flow requirement when used with spontaneous ventilation. There has been some controversy in the past on this subject. One reason for this is that although the coaxial and non-coaxial versions of the D system behave similarly during controlled ventilation they differ when used with spontaneous breathing, as the coaxial system requires a higher FGF than the twin tube version. It is considered that this is because the stream of fresh gas, emerging from a small orifice and directed towards the patient's airway and against the expiratory gas flow produces turbulent flow within the system which prevents the separation of expired and fresh gas necessary for economy. Because of this a FGF of 2–3 $\dot{V}_E$ is recommended for normocarbia with spontaneous breathing.

A potential hazard with coaxial systems is detachment of the internal tube. This has occurred with Bain systems and results in the patient's subjection to a large dead space. It is helpful to have the outer tube made of transparent or semi-transparent material and the inner tube deeply coloured so that its continuity and placement can be clearly seen. These precautions are desirable for all coaxial systems.

THE LACK SYSTEM

The Bain system gained widespread use despite its high FGF requirement during spontaneous breathing. To overcome this problem and make the system as easy to scavenge as the Bain, a coaxial version of the A system was described by Dr J. A. Lack in 1976 (Figure 4.8b). The original design required some modification, but the Lack system now functions as well as the conventional Magill system. The length is 1.5 m, the inner tube, unlike the Bain, must have a low resistance to gas flow since expiration takes place through it. It is of 14 mm internal diameter and this necessitates the outer tubing being of 30 mm diameter since the patient breathes in through the annular space between inner and outer tubes. An overall resistance to flow of 1.3 cmH$_2$O at 30 l min^{-1} gas flow has been reported for this system, which is an acceptable figure. Although the gas economy figures for the Lack are the same as those for the

Magill (A) it is not actually identical in its configuration since it has a long expiratory limb with an APL at the end. It has been claimed that the twin-tube (parallel) version of the Lack (Figure 4.6) is slightly more efficient in gas economy than the conventional A system (Magill) and this may be because of the better separation of expiratory and inspiratory gas flow at the Y-piece connecting the patient to the system in the twin-tube version.

The coaxial Lack system, although it functions well, has not been so widely used as the Bain; it is slightly more bulky and cannot easily be adapted to controlled ventilation.

Another coaxial system which has been tested clinically is the preferential flow system (PFS). This is a coaxial system in which fresh gas, after passing the reservoir bag T-piece (i.e. an afferent reservoir), enters an inner tube of large bore (19 mm) inside an outer tube of 30 mm bore. The resistance to flow is therefore considerably less in the inner tube than the outer. As shown in Figure 4.7c a flow directing jet (9 mm) projects into the gas delivery tube. During expiration dead space gas is preferentially directed into the inner tube (and then preserved) until the pressure builds up to expire alevolar gas into the outer tube. Experimentally the PFS was shown to be as economical as the Mapleson A during spontaneous breathing and to have a lower resistance to expiration.

Coaxial tubing can be conveniently used to replace the double tubing of circle systems. Tubing used for this purpose must be of Lack specification.

A–D SWITCHES

Considerable ingenuity has been expanded on designing switches or taps which will rapidly convert an A system to or from a D system. The best known of these is the Humphrey ADE system, a well engineered tap with a two-position control lever which attaches to the fresh gas outlet and gives either a twin-tube Lack or twin-tube Mapleson D (or E) system.

ENCLOSED AFFERENT RESERVOIR

In addition to the various taps which have been described for switching between A and D systems the enclosed afferent reservoir (EAR) system was devised by Miller in 1988. A diagram showing the principle of the system is given in Figure 4.9. As can be seen it is basically a twin tube Lack system having the (afferent) reservoir bag A enclosed in a bottle connected to the expiratory limb. At the end of the expiratory limb is an APL and another bag or ventilator for generating IPPV. The important valve is located in the expiratory limb as shown. During spontaneous breathing the system functions as a twin tube Lack but when an above-atmospheric pressure is produced by squeezing bag B (IPPV) then valve V closes and bag B is compressed, inflating the patients lungs without the loss of fresh gas which accompanies this action with the A system. Expiration occurs in the same way with both forms of ventilation.

It has been shown that this system (and a similar one using the PF system described above) are economical with gas as shown by $\dot{V}_F/\dot{V}_E < 1$ in both modes of ventilation. However, the system is bulky and quite complex. It is difficult to see that it has any advantage over a well designed switch such as the Humphrey ADE

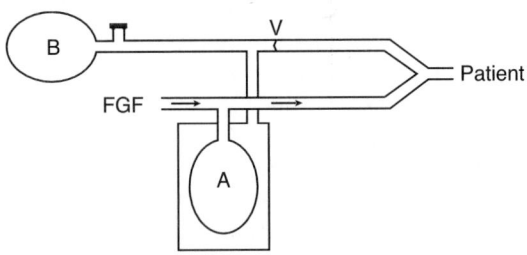

Figure 4.9 Principle of enclosed afferent reservoir system. (Reproduced with permission from Criswell *et al.* 1990.)

FILTERS

A variety of filters are manufactured and advocated for use in breathing systems. They must be mounted close to the airway and will increase deadspace. The filters are intended to humidify inspired gas and keep bacteria out of the breathing system. In closed and low flow systems there is usually too much water, not only does it condense out on the expiratory side, but the reaction of soda lime with CO_2 generates water. A case can be made for humidifying inspired gas with high gas flow systems if the patient is intubated, but the benefits of doing this for routine anaesthesia have not been demonstrated.

Studies have shown that bacteria can lodge in breathing systems but the use of bacterial filters does not affect the incidence of postoperative chest infection. All studies agree that breathing systems are not a source of cross-infection under normal circumstances. In cases where infection is clearly a risk (e.g. open tuberculosis) systems must be fully sterilized, or better still, a disposable system should be used.

FURTHER READING

Conway, C. M. (1985) Anaesthetic breathing systems. *British Journal of Anaesthesia* **57**, 649–657.

Cook, L. B. (1996) The importance of the expiratory pause. *Anaesthesia*, **51**: 453–460.

Criswell, J., McKenzie, S., Day, J., Disley, W., Bruce, E. and Soni N. (1990) The Bain, ADE, and enclosed Magill breathing systems. *Anaesthesia*, **45**, 113–117.

Humphrey, D. (1983) A new anaesthetic breathing system combining Mapleson A, D and E principles. *Anaesthesia*, **38**, 361–372.

Mapleson, W. W. (1954) The elimination of rebreathing in various semi-closed anaesthetic systems. *British Journal Anaesthesia*, **26**, 323–332.

Miller, D. M. (1988) Breathing systems for use in anaesthesia. *British Journal of Anaesthesia*, **60**, 555–564.

Miller, D. M. and Couper, J. L. (1983) Comparison of the fresh gas flow requirements and resistance of the preferential system with those of the Magill system. *British Journal Anaesthesia*, **55**, 569–574.

Miller D. M. and Miller J. C. (1988) Enclosed afferent reservoir breathing systems. *British Journal Anaesthesia*, **60**, 469–475.

Murphy P. M., Fitzgeorge R. B. and Barrett R. F. (1991) Viability and distribution of bacteria after passage through a circle anaesthetic system. *British Journal Anaesthesia*, **66**, 300–304.

Nunn J. F. (1987) *Applied Respiratory Physiology*, 3rd edn. Butterworths, London, p.67.

Voss T. J. V. (1967) The adaptation of ventilators for anaesthesia. *South African Medical Journal*, **1**, 107910–82.

Voss T. J. V. (1985) The ultimate circuit not another circuit. *Anaesthesia and Intensive Care*, **1**, 98.

EQUIPMENT FOR AIRWAY MANAGEMENT 5

A. Davey

When a general anaesthetic is administered to a patient, relaxation of muscles within the pharynx often leads to upper airway obstruction and this can, in turn, result in hypoxia. Much of the art of anaesthesia lies in the ability of a practitioner to overcome this and secure and maintain the airway under a wide variety of conditions, many of which are imposed by the nature of the operation to be carried out. This art also includes the ability to supply respirable gas to the patient's airway via apparatus which is leak free so ensuring that a known concentration and volume is being administered, and that this can also be delivered under pressure if required, for control of ventilation. Crucial to this ability has been the development of a wide range of devices (listed below).

FACEMASKS (Figure 5.1)

Facemasks are designed to fit over the patient's nose and mouth providing a leak free seal between the patient's airway and the rest of the anaesthetic apparatus. This is achieved by contouring the edges of the mask (Figure 5.1a–c), as well as fitting it with a flap (Figure 5.1a) or a cylindrical inflatable cuff (Figure 5.1b). The body of the mask may have a wire gauze incorporated into the material which allows its shape to be changed to fit an individual face. Facemasks also come in a variety of sizes to cater for anatomical differences

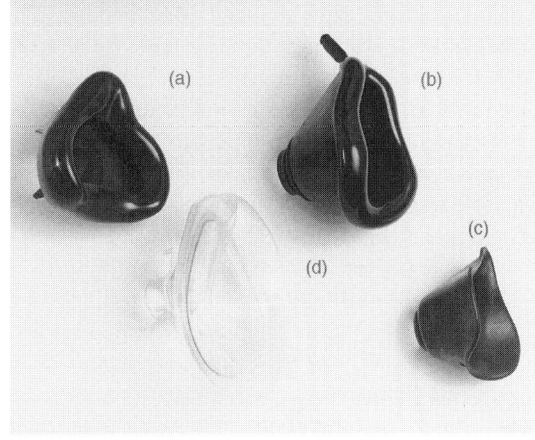

Figure 5.1 Facemasks: (a) contoured neoprene mask fitted with a flap; (b) fitted with an inflatable rim; (c) paediatric mask with small internal volume; (d) clear plastic disposable mask with inflatable rim.

between patients allowing a practitioner to choose a 'best fit'. Those for neonates and infants are designed to have as small an internal volume as possible so as to minimize respirable deadspace (Figure 5.1c) and the problem of rebreathing exhaled gases.

Masks may be made of neoprene, polycarbonate or plastic. Neoprene masks can be made malleable and are autoclavable but are opaque. Those made of polycarbonate (autoclavable) or plastic (disposable) are rigid but transparent and allow the early detection of

Short Practice of Anaesthesia. Edited by M. Morgan and G. M. Hall. Published in 1997 by Chapman & Hall, London. ISBN 0 412 71890 1

84 *Equipment for airway management*

vomit should this misfortune occur (Figure 5.1d). Also, respiration can be confirmed by the appearance of condensation inside the mask. The transparent ones may also appear less threatening to anxious patients and small children.

It is useful to stock a variety of masks in different sizes as no one type is guaranteed to fit every face. A good fit is essential to prevent dilution of inhaled gas with room air and to allow positive pressure ventilation without a leak. Poor fits occur more frequently in edentulous patients and in those with beards. The cheeks of the former usually sag away from the mask edges producing a leak which may be solved by selecting a smaller mask or inserting an oral airway. Beards often prevent a good seal around the edge of the mask and a leak free fit may be achieved with a bigger mask often held on with two hands.

The body of the mask is fitted with a 22 mm International Organization for Standardization (ISO) female connection to a breathing system. Where this is made of an elastic material (neoprene or silicone), repeated use can cause wear and eventually produce either a leak or a potential for accidental disconnection. Masks which are reused should be regularly checked and discarded before this occurs.

AIRWAYS

The relaxation of pharyngeal muscles in an anaesthetized supine patient causes the tongue and epiglottis to fall back against the posterior pharyngeal wall, occluding the laryngeal inlet and obstructing the upper airway. This occurs more easily in those patients in whom this space is already reduced by a large tongue, a small lower jaw, large tonsils or a short fat neck. Simple elevation of the jaw often relieves the obstruction but may require the insertion of a device which separates these structures and creates an artificial airway. The latter may be inserted via the mouth (oropharyngeal airway) or nose (nasopharyngeal airway).

OROPHARYNGEAL AIRWAY (Figure 5.2)

The most popular oropharyngeal airway is the Guedel pattern as shown in Figure 5.2. This consists of a stiff plastic hollow tube which is C shaped so as to resemble the normal airspace within the oropharynx. It is produced in various sizes, (neonate to large adult). The right size should, when inserted through the mouth, pass between the tongue and the posterior pharyngeal wall so that its tip lies just above the epiglottis, displacing it

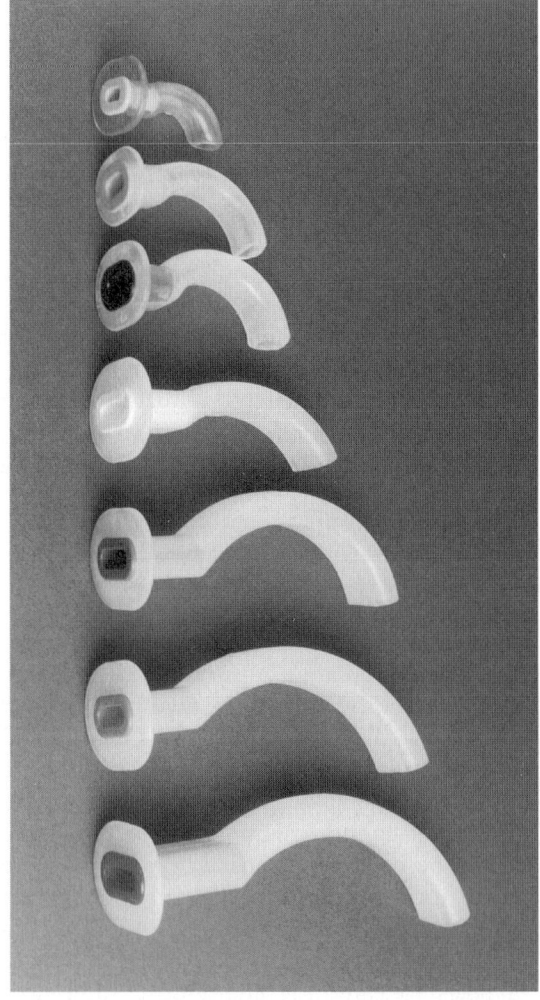

Figure 5.2 Guedel airways: sizes 000, 00, 0, 1, 2, 3, 4.

anteriorly along with the tongue. The proximal end, which fits between the patient's lips and teeth has a straight section with a flange to limit its insertion and this is reinforced to prevent collapse should the patient bite on it. The devices are usually colour coded and numbered for size.

Inserting the airway

The airway should only be inserted into a patient whose pharyngeal reflexes have been sufficiently depressed by topical or general anaesthesia. Failure to do this will result in gagging, retching or laryngospasm which can be both professionally embarrassing and dangerous to the patient! It should be well lubricated with a water based gel and inserted so that its curvature follows that of the tongue. Alternatively, it can be inserted with its curvature facing the opposite direction and when half way in, rotated around to its normal position and fully inserted.

Inserting the airway and maintaining its position can occasionally be difficult. It often appears to snag about three quarters of the way in. This is usually overcome by lifting the angles of the lower jaw forward with the middle fingers of both hands and gently pushing on the flange with both thumbs. Once inserted, it may be partially pushed out if the patient's jaw is unsupported and allowed to fall back. It may also become dislodged in patients with marked anterior displacement of their upper teeth. When the lower jaw is supported, the lower teeth act as a fulcrum for the action of the upper teeth on the airway. Downward pressure by the upper teeth pushes the bite section downwards and lifts the tip out of the posterior pharynx.

Inappropriate use of these airways may produce significant morbidity. Damage to the front teeth occurs only too frequently, as a result of excessive pressure on the airway due to postoperative masseter spasm or over enthusiastic jaw support. Porcelain bridges and crowns are more easily damaged than normal healthy teeth and the presence and state of the former should be recorded in the preoperative notes. The simple expedient of inserting a rubber dental prop between the patient's molar teeth could significantly reduce this problem.

NASOPHARYNGEAL AIRWAY (Figure 5.3)

Made from soft tubular plastic, polyurethane or latex rubber, nasopharyngeal airways can be inserted through the nares and passed along the floor of the nose and down into the oropharynx to just above the epiglottis, to provide a patent airway. The proximal end is flanged to limit the depth of insertion so that it does not impinge on the larynx, pass down the oesophagus or disappear past the nares making its retrieval a test of a practitioner's ingenuity! The distal end is bevelled and may have a hole cut into the wall opposite this so that should the bevel become blocked with mucus during the insertion, airway patency will be maintained. As with oral airways, they are produced in a range of lengths and internal diameters (measured in millimetres) for different sizes of patient.

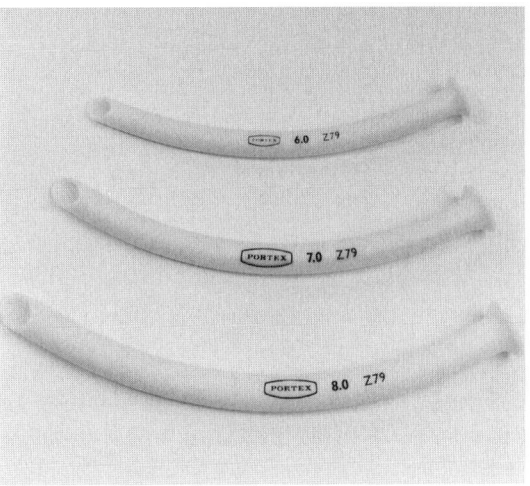

Figure 5.3 Nasopharyngeal airways: sizes 6, 7, 8 mm internal diameter.

They are most useful in patients with limited jaw opening, awkward or fragile dentition or where the oral airway is frequently displaced by a marked overlapping bite. However, complications do occur with their use. They may traumatize the septal mucosa, nasal polyps or adenoidal tissue producing an epistaxis which will compromise the airway. Hence they should not be used where there is evidence of a coagulopathy.

THE LARYNGEAL MASK AIRWAY (Figure 5.4)

The laryngeal mask airway (LMA) fulfils the function of a traditional facemask and airway in one device. The distal end consists of a miniaturized mask surrounded by an inflatable tubular cuff which provides a snug fit over the laryngeal inlet. The back of the mask is attached to a wide bore tube which passes out through the mouth terminating in a 15 mm ISO male tapered connection for attachment to a breathing system. The tube is guarded by bars at its point of entry into the mask to prevent the epiglottis falling into it and occluding its lumen. The inflatable cuff is supplied by a narrow bore inflation tube which includes a self sealing inflation valve.

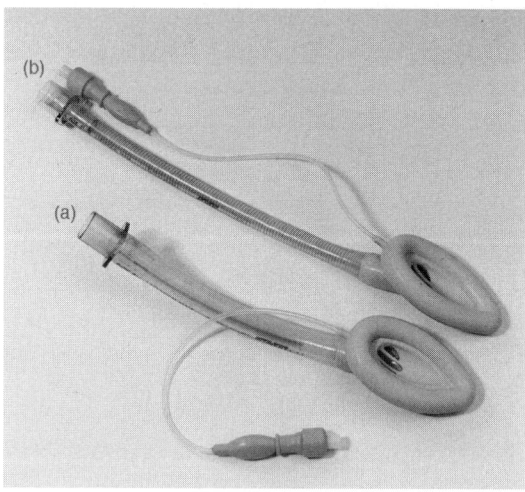

Figure 5.4 Laryngeal mask airway: (a) standard airway; (b) reinforced airway.

The device is made from silicone so that it can be autoclaved and reused to the manufacturer's recommended maximum of 40 times.

There are currently two versions of the airway. In the standard version the tubular breathing channel is made from thick wide bore silicone. An alternative version is available in which the breathing channel is made from thinner, narrower and longer tubing which is reinforced with a steel spiral to provide added flexibility without kinking. This version is designed for use in head and neck surgery where the reduced diameter of the tube improves intra-oral surgical access and the extra length and flexibility improves facial access. The standard airway is supplied in six sizes. The manufacturer's recommendation is that size 1 should be used for neonates up to 6.5 kg; size 2 for patients from 6.5 to 20 kg; size 2½ for patients between 20 and 30 kg; size 3 for children and small adults; size 4 for average sized adults and size 5 for large adults. Discretion should be used in cases where the predicted size does not fit. For example, a large adult may have a smaller than expected pharynx whereas an elderly patient may well have one larger than expected.

The LMA should only be inserted in a patient whose pharyngeal reflexes have been sufficiently depressed by general anaesthesia. Propofol is ideal in this respect. It can also be inserted following application of topical analgesia to the pharynx.

Inserting the LMA (Figure 5.5)

Before insertion, the LMA should be checked and prepared. The cuff is firstly inflated to 50% more than the filling volume and checked for leaks. It is then deflated with the concave part of the mask pressed against a hard surface. The deflated cuff becomes folded backwards notably at its tip. The airway is held using the gloved index finger and thumb of one hand close to the mask whilst the operator's other hand extends the pa-

which the mask portion, with its opening facing forward and back part well lubricated, is inserted. The airway is then pushed with one firm movement so that it slides smoothly around the palate and posterior wall of the pharynx avoiding collision with the epiglottis. The fingers are withdrawn and the tube pushed further in until a resistance is felt. This is usually the point of full insertion. Without holding the tube, the cuff is then inflated with the recommended volume (4 ml for size 1; 10 ml for size 2; 14 ml for size 2½; 20 ml for size 3; 30 ml for size 4; and 40 ml for size 5). This allows the LMA freedom to move into its correct anatomical position. Correct placement is confirmed thus. In a spontaneously breathing patient breathing should be non-stridorous and the reservoir bag of the breathing system should show a normal excursion. In an apnoeic patient, squeezing the reservoir bag should produce normal chest movements with an applied pressure no greater than 2 kPa (20 cmH$_2$O). A small leak is permissible; a large leak or an inflation pressure higher than expected will usually indicate the possibility of either a misplacement or breath holding by the patient. Only the recommended amount of air should be used to inflate the cuff as under- or over-inflation may fail to provide the correct shape, and therefore anatomical fit, for the mask.

This method has limitations if the operator has small hands or if the patient is large and modifications of the technique have been described. For example, the standard airway can be gripped close to the connector rather than the mask whilst the operator's other hand extends and elevates the patient's head by cradling the occiput. The airway is inserted into the mouth and pushed with one firm movement so that it slides around the palate and posterior wall of the pharynx until a resistance is felt. If using the reinforced airway, the tubular section may not be stiff enough to allow it to be pushed into the pharynx with this method; stiffening it with a

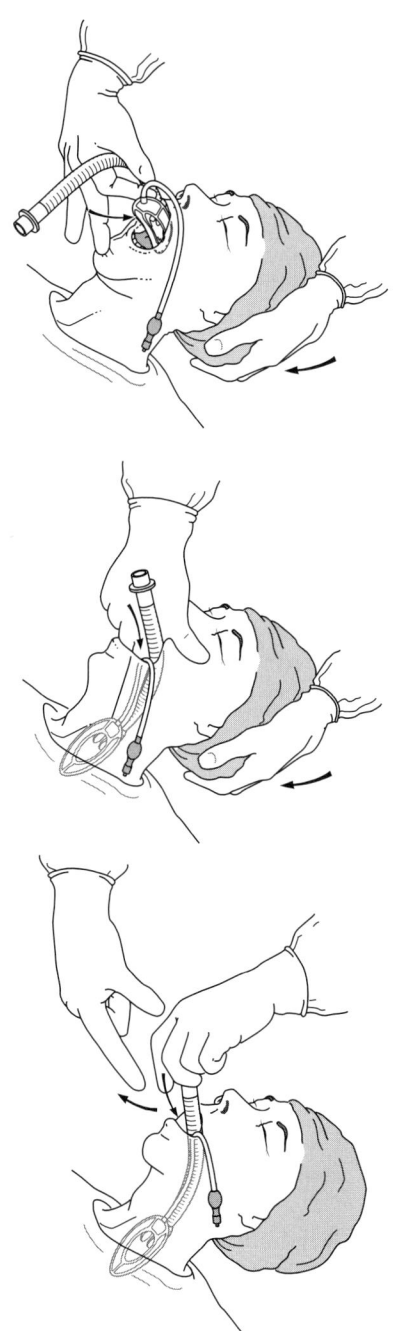

Figure 5.5 Method of insertion of the LMA.

tient's neck by cradling the occiput. This manoeuvre opens the patient's mouth through

malleable introducer or smaller tracheal tube has been described.

Partially inflating the cuff is popular, as is elevating the jaw during the insertion, either by an assistant pulling forwards on the angles of the jaws or by inserting a gloved thumb behind the lower front teeth and pulling forwards and upwards to make insertion easier. This is especially true in patients with receding jaws, high arched palates or limited neck movement. A technique in which the mask is inserted with the bowl facing cephalad with late rotation into the correct position has been described. This appears to be very useful in children.

Although the device was originally designed to maintain the airway in spontaneously breathing patients, leak free positive pressure ventilation is possible in most instances where the peak inflation pressure required is less than 2.5 kPa (25 cmH_2O). Best results are achieved by prolonging the inspiratory phase and slowing the inspiratory flow so as to reduce peak pressures. Although this feature allows its use in many instances where controlled ventilation with a tracheal tube would have been chosen, it is more easily dislodged than a tracheal tube and in its present form does not protect the larynx from regurgitated gastric contents. It would be therefore inadvisable to use it in situations where access to the airway to readjust its position or substitute it for a tracheal tube is difficult. Similarly, its use should be avoided where regurgitation is potentially possible as in those patients with full stomachs.

Removal of the LMA

The airway should be left *in situ* until the patient regains consciousness. It is well tolerated during emergence from anaesthesia providing a clear airway unless the patient develops trismus and bites on it. It is for this reason, as well as the fact that the device can be damaged (which can be very expensive!) that a bite block should always be inserted. This should be placed between the upper and lower molars on one side of the jaws so as to wedge them open. The patient should be left undisturbed until protective reflexes have returned. Swallowing is an early indication that this so. The device is only removed when the patient can open the mouth on command. Earlier removal may allow saliva, which can accumulate behind the mask during the operation, to enter the larynx and produce spasm, a coughing fit or retching as well as causing loss of airway patency.

Indications for use of the LMA

Despite the provisos above, the laryngeal mask airway has become deservedly popular throughout the world as an extremely useful aid to airway maintenance in a wide variety of circumstances. It may be used in place of a conventional mask and pharyngeal airway in anaesthesia:

- with the added benefit of releasing anaesthetic 'hands' to deal with other equipment;
- securing a more reliable airway, especially with patients placed in unusual positions (such as on the side), or in remote situations such as in MRI or CT scanner suites or in postoperative recovery rooms;
- offering a lower resistance to respiration.

It may be used in place of a tracheal tube:

- for head and neck surgery including procedures inside the mouth, dispensing with the need to used muscle relaxant drugs usually required for tracheal tube placement;
- for predicted difficult intubation where conventional laryngoscopy could be traumatic or where dental damage might occur or where neck movement should be minimized as in unstable neck fractures;
- for failed intubation as an alternative airway especially in an emergency;
- in balanced anaesthesia using controlled ventilation where intubation may elicit un-

desirable cardiovascular responses, (as in patients with severe ischaemic heart disease) or coughing and/or raised intra-ocular pressure in patients having ophthalmic procedures (somewhat controversial);
- by paramedical staff in emergencies, i.e. cardiorespiratory arrests, especially where such staff are not regularly trained in tracheal intubation or the art of ventilating a patient with a facemask.

The LMA has been used as an aid to difficult intubation. A suitably sized, uncut, cuffed tracheal tube may be inserted through the LMA so that its tip projects just beyond the protective bars of the mask. The LMA is then inserted in the normal manner and when *in situ*, the tracheal tube is advanced into the larynx, the cuff inflated and the connector attached to a breathing system. The LMA is left in position for use as a postoperative airway. Successful placement of the tube may be assisted and confirmed by the use of a flexible fibreoptic laryngoscope.

TRACHEAL TUBES

There are situations where the devices discussed above do not provide either adequate or sufficiently secure a passage between the lungs and the anaesthetic apparatus. For example, in a patient with a hiatus hernia or a full stomach, gastric contents may enter the pharynx and subsequently the lungs. Similarly, any intra-oral or nasal bleeding or surgical debris if allowed into the pharynx in sufficient quantity, may do the same. Furthermore, should high inflation pressures be required to ventilate the lungs, a significant proportion of the tidal volume may be lost down the oesophagus. Not only does this reduce lung ventilation, but the gastric distension produced increases the likelihood of reflux with subsequent tracheal soiling.

A tracheal tube is a device which overcomes these problems. Most commonly it is inserted through the mouth and through the larynx into the trachea. It may be of sufficient diameter that it fits snugly into the larynx with only a minimal leak (mainly in neonates, infants and small children) or the tracheal portion may be surrounded by an inflatable cuff which is filled to seal the space between the tube and tracheal wall. It may also be inserted through the nose and passed down the nasopharynx and into the larynx when surgical access to the oropharynx is required. Here, the size of tube required is limited by the size of the nares and reduced accordingly.

Tracheal tubes are provided in a range of sizes, designs and materials.

SIZE

The size of a tube is designated by its internal diameter in millimetres. The widest diameter tube that can be easily passed should be used so as to minimize its resistance to gas flow and reduce the work of breathing. However, it should not be so big that it damages the tracheal mucosa by pressing too tightly against it. Tubes are usually supplied in lengths longer than required and are often cut to the appropriate size for an individual patient so as to prevent the tip entering a main bronchus and ventilating only one lung. A shorter tube also has a reduced resistance to gas flow which may be important in neonates and infants where resistance is already compromised by tubes with small diameters. However, some practitioners do not cut tubes but fix them to the face so that they cannot normally be inserted further.

MATERIAL

The tube should be made from a material which is non-toxic and preferably non-flammable. It should be sufficiently elastic to allow bending without kinking but strong enough to have a thin wall which resists collapse from external pressure or torsion. If the tube is designed to be reused then the material should withstand repeated autoclaving as a means of sterilization. It should also preferably be transparent so that any foreign object may easily be seen. Most commonly, tubes are made from polyvinyl chloride (PVC) and are for single use only. However, when cold they are quite stiff and are not ideal for atraumatic nasal insertion even when pre-warmed. This has led to the development of polyurethane tubes which are softer. Silicone is used less commonly because although it is soft, it is expensive; however, it does have the advantage in that it will withstand autoclaving and so can be reused. Red rubber and latex have been the traditional materials for tubes but these have almost disappeared from common use with the move to single use items in clinical practice.

DESIGN

A typical tube is shown in Figure 5.6. It usually has a pre-formed curve which vaguely conforms to the anatomical shape of the pharynx. This aids insertion and ensures that when the tube, is further flexed when *in situ*, it is unlikely to kink. The distal end is cut obliquely (bevelled) so that the aperture faces to the left when held in the operator's right hand. When inserted into the larynx, the bevel allows the tip of the tube to be seen passing between the vocal cords. There may be a hole in the wall (a Murphy eye) opposite the bevel. This is designed to provide a secondary port for gas movement in and out of the tube should the bevel become blocked or wedged against the tracheal wall. The tube carries a number of markings one of which is a longitudinal line of radio-opaque material so that correct placement can be verified radiographically if required. The distance from the tip of the bevel is also marked (in centimetres) on the wall, along with the internal diameter and a stamp carrying the initials Z 79-IT which confirms that the material used in the construction has been deemed 'implant tested' and so non-toxic.

TRACHEAL CUFF

The inflatable tracheal cuff which surrounds the tube shaft at its distal end provides a seal between the tube and the tracheal wall. It is filled by injecting gas through a self sealing valve, into a pilot balloon and pilot line which is usually incorporated within the wall of the tracheal tube. The cuff prevents any con-

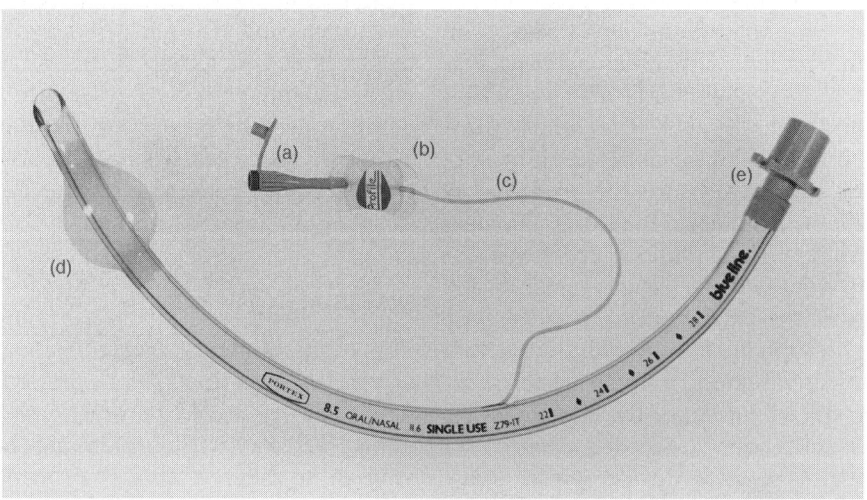

Figure 5.6 A standard disposable tracheal tube made from clear PVC: (a) inflation valve; (b) pilot balloon; (c) pilot tube; (d) cuff; (f) 15 mm ISO connector.

tamination of the lungs from aspiration of pharyngeal contents and allows the lungs to be ventilated without any loss of gas. The cuff may be made from an elastic material (latex, rubber or neoprene) which fits snugly to the tube and which when inflated expands to meet the tracheal wall. If the cuff is thick walled to make it robust and durable, it will require a high pressure to inflate (high pressure cuff) and usually expands as a spherical shape. It would normally be inflated so that only the widest circumference touches the trachea providing a seal, the contact area of which is small.

Further inflation increases the area of seal but at the expense of transmitting the high cuff pressure to the wall. This may cut off the blood supply to the underlying mucosa and produce ischaemia and necrosis. The cuff wall may be made much thinner to avoid this but as a result may be easily damaged if snagged against teeth, instruments, intubation guides or bony spurs in the nasopharynx. Alternatively, the cuff may be made from a large volume of a thin non-elastic material (PVC) which, when inflated, would be larger than required. When it is inflated to provide a seal *in situ*, there is a large area of contact between the tracheal wall and the cuff before the material is fully stretched. The pressure can therefore be kept low enough (low pressure cuff) so as not to occlude mucosal blood flow. However the cuff should only be inflated to a pressure (around 2.5 kPa/25 cmH$_2$O) which would normally prevent a gas leak during assisted ventilation as well as preventing potential pharyngeal aspirate from forcing its way past the cuff into the lungs. If overfilled, the material will be stretched to the limit of its compliance at which point the pressure will increase dramatically to levels above that of the blood flow to the underlying mucosa.

Overfilling may inadvertently occur due to diffusion of anaesthetic gases into the cuff. Nitrous oxide in particular readily diffuses through most cuff materials until its partial pressure equilibrates on each side. The speed at which this occurs depends on the permeability of the material, its thickness and the concentration of the nitrous oxide impinging on the cuff.

There are a number of ways of controlling the pressure increase. The cuff may be filled with an identical concentration of the anaesthetic gas mixture in use or with sterile water so that diffusion cannot occur. A manometer may be attached to the inflation line to monitor the pressure which can then be released when it rises excessively. Alternatively, there are a number of devices which can be fitted to the inflation line to automatically control it. The Mallinckrodt Lanz system (Figure 5.7a) has a pilot balloon which allows the nitrous oxide to diffuse to the atmosphere. The Mallinckrodt Brandt device (Figure 5.7b) has a large compliant pilot balloon which exerts a constant pressure on the cuff. Any increase in volume due to diffusion in the latter is passed on to the pilot cuff which is able to expand to absorb it.

A cuff, if excessively inflated, may herniate around and over the bevel of the tube or it may inflate asymmetrically pushing the bevel against the tracheal wall. It may even cause

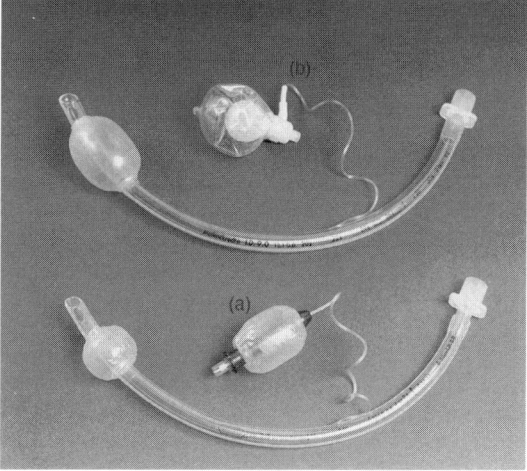

Figure 5.7 (a) Mallinckrodt Lanz system; (b) Mallinckrodt Brandt system for controlling cuff pressure.

inward herniation of the tube wall under the cuff so reducing its lumen.

CONNECTORS

The tracheal tube is attached to the other components of a breathing system via a male to female tapered connection. The tube houses the male taper which normally has the ISO size of 15 mm (Figure 5.8a).

The early pioneers in anaesthesia produced connections in a variety of shapes and sizes designed mostly to streamline the fit and so improve surgical access to the head and neck of a patient. This function has largely been incorporated into the design of the various specialist tracheal tubes (see below), allowing a single size of connection to be developed. A smaller size of 8.5 mm is becoming popular for use in neonates as this reduces the weight of the components (Figure 5.8c).

The part of the connector which fits into the lumen of the tracheal tube is made slightly bigger so that the tube material has to be stretched to fit. This produces a secure connection which can often only be broken by cutting the tube. This principle is important where manufacturers supply the tube and connector separately as too small a connector may separate from the tube probably at the most inopportune moment!

CATHETER MOUNTS

Although the tracheal tube can be connected directly to a breathing system, the relative bulkiness of the latter in such close proximity to the face may interfere with surgical access, the preparation of the operating field, or it may drag on the tube causing it to change position. A 'catheter mount' or 'tracheal tube adapter' is a short piece of narrow bore corrugated breathing hose (usually 15 mm) with ISO connections at each end which allows the breathing system to be connected a short distance away from the patient's face (Figure 5.8b and d). Where it is attached to the tracheal tube, it often has a right angled swivel to reduce any torsion, and may also have a port with a detachable cap so that suction catheters can be passed into the trachea. The device increases the apparatus deadspace of the breathing system, which although probably insignificant in adults, may be significant in the very young.

SPECIALIST TRACHEAL TUBES

Paediatric tubes

The size and shape of the larynx and cricoid cartilage in the very young requires special consideration when designing a tracheal tube for use in this age group. The smallest part of the upper airway is the cricoid not the larynx as in adults. As the diameter of the cricoid is already small, intubation with a tube will reduce the airway even further. This reduction is kept to a minimum by choosing materials with a higher tensile strength such

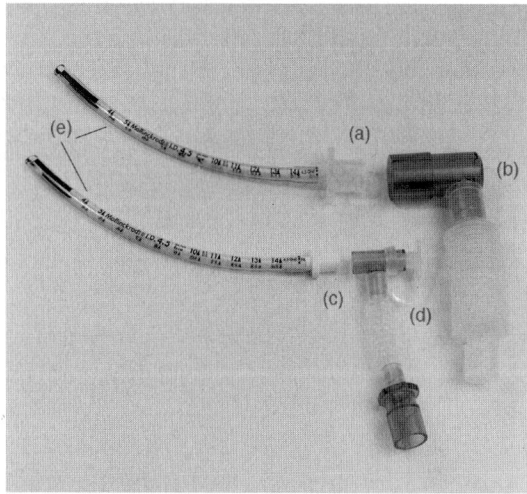

Figure 5.8 Tracheal tube connectors and catheter mounts: (a) 15 mm ISO male tapered connection; (b) catheter mount with a 15 mm ISO female tapered connection; (c) 8.5 mm paediatric male tapered connection; (d) catheter mount with a 8.5 mm female tapered connection; (e) 4.5 mm PVC uncuffed paediatric endotracheal tube.

as PVC rather than rubber so that the walls of the tube may be made as thin as possible whilst still avoiding the risk of kinking (Figure 5.8e). Plain tubes are preferred as they provide a wider internal diameter than cuffed tubes of similar size. The latter have thicker walls in order to resist collapse under the cuff segment when the cuff is inflated. However, as the cricoid is circular, a suitably sized plain tube, being also circular, will provide a snug fit so the cuff can be dispensed with. Too tight a fit will produce tracheal mucosal ischaemia resulting in oedema on extubation. This may reduce the airway diameter to such extent that it may cause severe respiratory embarrassment. Ideally, there should be a small leak around the tube when positive pressure of approximately 2.5 Pa (25 cmH$_2$O) is applied. The correct diameter is often made by selecting from a range around that predicted by various charts or formulae, one of which is dividing the patient's **age** by **4** and adding **4**. A formula that determines the approximate length of an tracheal tube required is **age** divided by **2** plus **12** with the proximal end of the tube at the incisors

RAE pre-formed tubes (Figure 5.9)

These tubes (named after their inventors: (Ring, Adair and Elwin) have two distinct patterns. The oral tube is U-shaped so that the connection is sited below the chin so improving surgical access to the face. The nasal version is shaped like a figure '7' so that the 'horizontal' portion lies against the patient's forehead. It is used to improve surgical access in intra-oral procedures. The main disadvantage of both designs is in the fixed length of the intra-oral section. This is rarely too short but is occasionally too long and can enter a main bronchus. Although it may be withdrawn into the trachea, the pre-formed curve no longer fits the face snugly and securing the tube becomes difficult. Furthermore, the acute curvature impedes the passage of fibrescopes and suction catheters.

Reinforced tubes (Figure 5.10)

These tubes are made from soft materials such as latex, silicone or thin PVC into which is embedded a reinforcing spiral of either steel or nylon. They are therefore very flexible and difficult to kink and are especially valuable in all head and neck surgery where they can resist compression by surgical instruments or extreme neck flexion. They are also valuable in maintaining the airway in patients placed prone.

However as they are floppy, they are more difficult to insert. Most commonly, a lubricated malleable stylette is inserted into the lumen to shape it or it may be passed over a bougie which has first been inserted into the trachea. These tubes cannot be shortened as the reinforced portion cannot be stretched to accommodate the connectors. In fact the connectors are usually permanently bonded to the tube by the manufacturer. Those that are supplied for both oral and nasal use are long and if inserted too deeply via the oral route will result in endobronchial intubation.

Microlaryngeal tubes (Figure 5.11)

These are narrow bore tubes (internal diameters 4–6 mm) which when inserted allow better visibility and surgical access to the

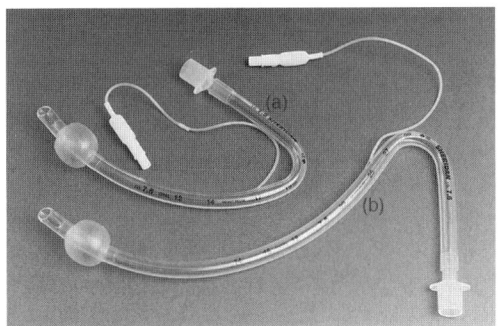

Figure 5.9 RAE pre-formed cuffed tracheal tubes: (a) oral and (b) nasal.

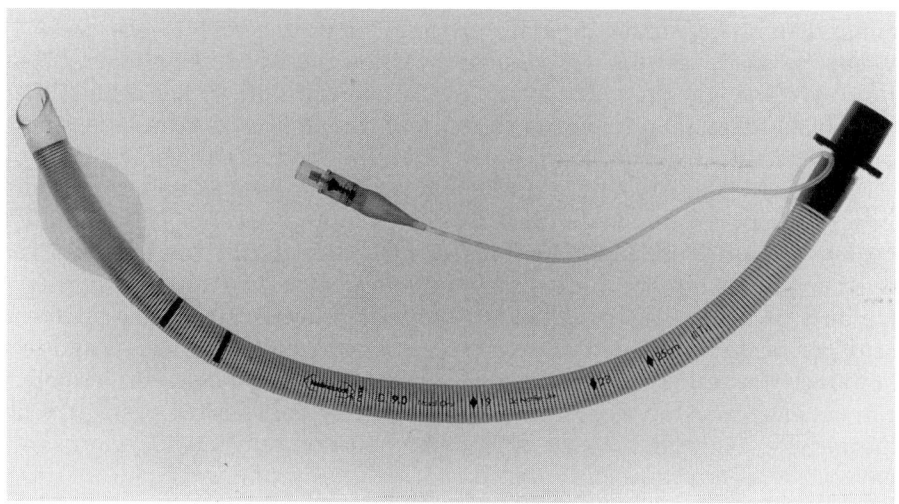

Figure 5.10 Reinforced oral/nasal cuffed tracheal tube.

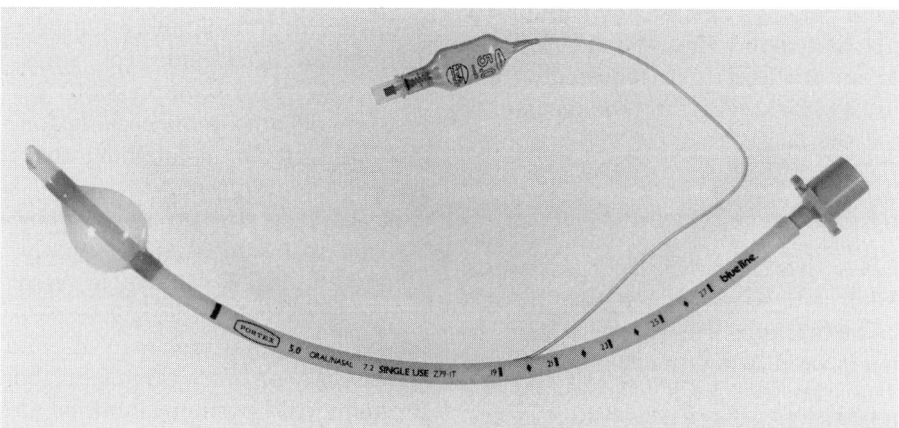

Figure 5.11 Microlaryngeal tube.

larynx and surrounding tissue. They are fitted with a standard size cuff for a tracheal seal in adults. The narrow bore may provide too great a resistance for all but the briefest bouts of spontaneous respiration so that in most instances controlled ventilation is employed. Exhalation is prolonged so sufficient time should be allowed for this, otherwise a stepwise increase in end exhalation volume will occur resulting in a Valsalva effect.

Tracheostomy tubes (Figure 5.12)

The distance between a tracheal stoma and the carina in a patient is both variable and often short. Tubes placed in the trachea via a

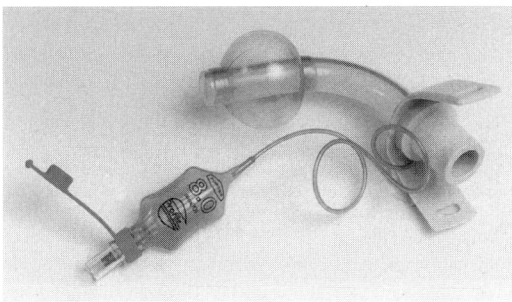

Figure 5.12 Tracheostomy tube.

tracheostomy are therefore designed to be non-bevelled, short in length and with the cuff bonded closer to the tip of the cube to prevent accidental endobronchial intubation. They are also pre-formed into a right angle to prevent kinking with neck flexion

Laryngectomy tubes (Figure 5.13)

The bulk of a tracheostomy tube with a catheter mount can obscure the surgical field around a tracheostomy. The laryngectomy tube overcomes this by having a proximal end which is long enough to dispense with a catheter mount and a distal end which has a pre-formed U-shaped curve to retain the properties of a tracheostomy tube.

Oxford pattern tubes (Figure 5.14)

This tube is pre-formed into a right angle so that it conforms to the anatomy of the oropharyngeal airway when the patient's head is placed in the neutral position. As a result, it is less likely to kink when the neck is flexed (as is common during some neurosurgical operations). Also, the wall of the original red rubber version was made thicker than other comparable patterns to increase resistance to kinking. This would have made a suitably sized tube too bulky to fit the trachea and so the distal part was tapered. The shape of the tube can be made less curved by inserting a stylette so as to make them easier to insert.

The bevel is cut so that it faces backwards rather than to the left as with most other tracheal tubes. This causes the tip to pass

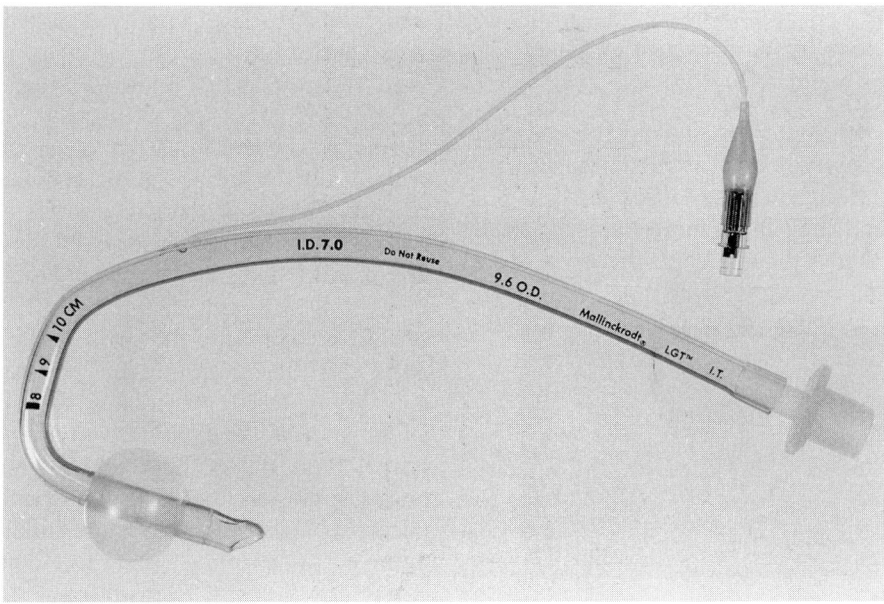

Figure 5.13 Laryngectomy tube.

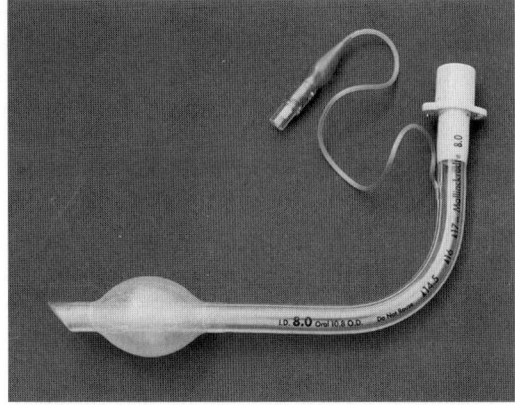

Figure 5.14 Oxford pattern tube.

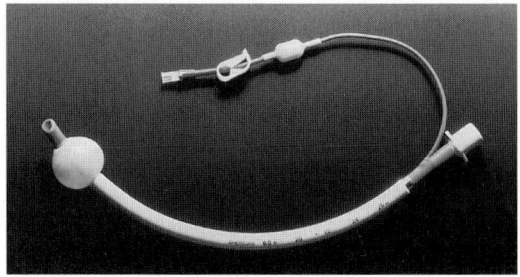

Figure 5.16 Sheridan laser tube.

through the glottis in the mid-line and so is less likely to snag on the vocal cords. However, if an anterior hernia developed in the cuff of an older reusable rubber tube, the bevel could lie against the tracheal mucosa and become blocked, especially if (ironically) the neck were flexed. As a result, some anaesthetists would cut off the bevel prior to using them.

Tubes for use in the presence of lasers
(Figures 5.15 and 5.16)

Conventional materials used in the construction of tubes will burn if hit with sufficient energy by a carbon dioxide, Nd–YAG or KTP laser beam. They burn more fiercely (plastic more so than rubber) in the presence of gas mixtures enriched with oxygen and nitrous oxide and can seriously injure patients. To avoid this, tubes can either be made from materials that reflect laser beams such as metal (Norton tube, Mallinckrodt Laser-flex tube, Figure 5.15) or from conventional materials (usually rubber) which are shielded by spirally wound aluminium foil (Xomed Laser-Shield II, Rusch Lasertubus) or copper foil (Sheridan Laser Trach, Figure 5.16). The foil is stippled (to disperse deflected beams), and to prevent damage *in situ*, is covered with a protective spongy material. The latter, being also porous, is normally soaked in saline which absorbs laser energy should the beam accidentally hit it.

As the cuff has to remain elastic, it cannot be similarly protected as the tube. Stray laser beams can burn holes in it causing it to deflate and possibly ignite. These problems may be in part solved by the use of double cuffs (Mallinckrodt Laser-flex, Figure 5.15) and foam filled cuffs (Bivona Fome-cuf). In the former should the first cuff burst, the second will provide the seal. Also if both the cuffs are filled with sterile water rather that air, the material is unlikely to ignite. The water should be dyed with methylene blue which then stains the trachea when a cuff bursts, giving a clearer indication that this has occurred. Foam filled cuffs are inflated when open to atmosphere and are deflated by extracting air prior to insertion. *In situ*, they are re-inflated and should remain so in the event of a cuff puncture. However, if this

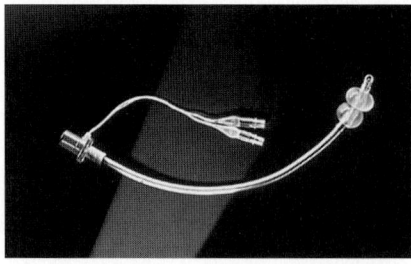

Figure 5.15 Mallinckrodt Laser-flex endotracheal tube.

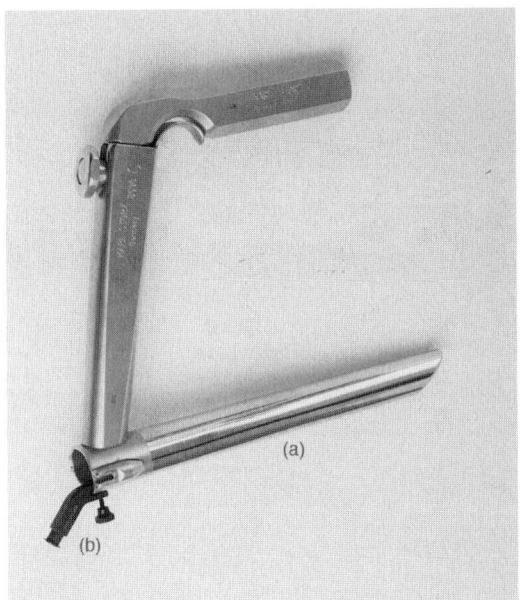

Figure 5.17 (a) Rigid laryngoscope; (b) with Venturi injector.

occurs they can be difficult to remove as they may not be easily deflated.

Because of the materials used, all these tubes have thick walls and as they must not be so bulky as to obscure surgical access, a suitably sized tube will have a smaller than usual internal diameter. This may provide too great a resistance for spontaneous respiration and assisted ventilation is often required.

Laser surgery to the airway can be performed without any tube *in situ*. A rigid straight bladed operating laryngoscope (Figure 5.17) may be inserted into a suitably anaesthetized patient so that its tip lies just above the cords. An injector is attached to the side of this through which high pressure oxygen is passed as a jet. This behaves as a Venturi device, entraining air to provide suitable ventilation provided that the injection pressure is adequate. This can be adjusted via a pressure regulator in the injection system. This method provides the best surgical access although the Venturi may not always develop adequate pressure to ventilate obese patients.

A compromise may be to intermittently pass a cuffed tracheal tube down the operating laryngoscope to supplement ventilation.

LARYNGOSCOPES

As the larynx is hidden behind the tongue, a device is normally required which displaces the latter to provide a direct view for the insertion of a tracheal tube. This task is normally performed by a rigid laryngoscope which consists of a blade which is passed behind the tongue, a light source which is attached to the blade and a handle which contains the power supply to the light source (Figure 5.18).

The components

The blade can be either curved or straight and is available in various lengths and designs to cater for the variation in anatomy between patients. The tip is made bulbous so as not to traumatize any pharyngeal structures. It is attached to the handle at a right angle when

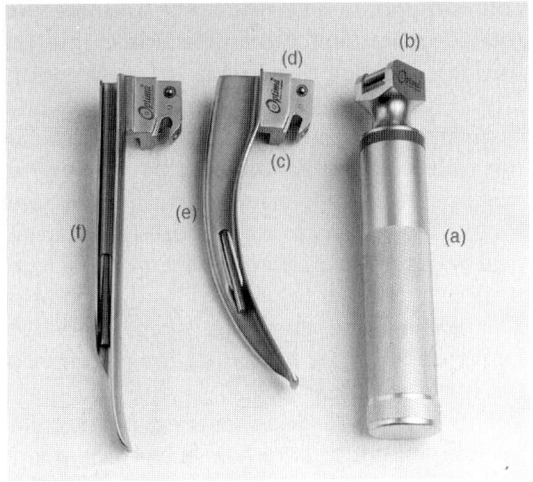

Figure 5.18 (a) Laryngoscope handle with (b) pin for accepting (c) hook and (d) locking bar. (e) Macintosh curved pattern; (f) Miller straight pattern blades with 'hook on' connection and fibreoptic light bundles.

ready for use, this being the most efficient angle for holding the handle and exerting the required force to displace the tongue and lower jaw away from the posterior pharynx. The blade and handle may be made from a single moulded piece of plastic or if made from metal, from separate components. The latter allows the blades to be detached so that different sizes can be used with the same handle. Most commonly, the detachable blade is fitted with both a hook, which fits around a pin on the handle and a bar. When the blade is extended around the pin into its working position, the bar slots firmly into a close fitting matching recess on the handle, locking the blade into position. A light source is attached to the blade close to the tip to illuminate the larynx. This may be a very small electric bulb or a fibreoptic bundle which transmits light from a bulb in the handle. In both versions the light is switched on when the blade is locked in position.

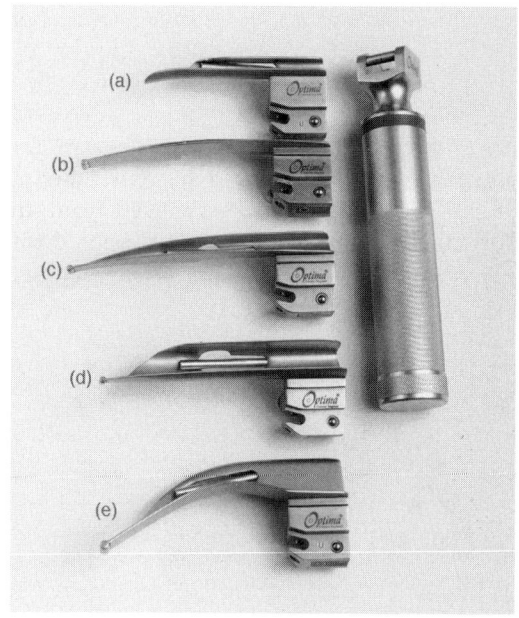

Figure 5.19 Paediatric laryngoscope blades: (a) Millar (b) Robertshaw (c) Seward (d) Oxford (e) Macintosh.

Insertion

With the lower cervical spine flexed by suitable support behind the neck and the jaw rotated upwards, the curved blade is inserted through the mouth and passed conventionally behind and to the right of the tongue displacing it to the left until the tip reaches the vallecula. The handle is gripped firmly in the operator's left hand and the jaw and tongue lifted away from the posterior pharyngeal wall (taking care not to lever on the front teeth) to expose the larynx and epiglottis. This manoeuvre creates a space which is larger on the right hand side for insertion of the tracheal tube.

The straight blade is inserted in a similar fashion except that when the epiglottis is exposed the blade is passed behind it so that the tip lies just at the laryngeal inlet. It is particularly useful in an adult with long and floppy epiglottis. However it may also be used in a manner similar to the curved blade. Straight blades also provide a better view in the very young and Figure 5.19 provides examples of the more popular blades and sizes.

CONFIRMATION OF CORRECT PLACEMENT OF TRACHEAL TUBES

If a tracheal tube is not placed in the trachea it will lie in the oesophagus with disastrous consequences to the patient if unrecognized and a high index of suspicion should always accompany all but the easiest of attempted insertions.

Following an easy intubation in a slim patient, a correctly placed tube will normally provide visible bilateral expansion of the thorax at a low inflation pressure with assisted ventilation. However, it would be foolish to rely on this sign alone. Confirmation should always include auscultation of the apices and bases of both lungs. Even this may be masked in an obese patient or one with bronchospasm or where the tube may be marginally in one main bronchus. Further confirmation should always be sought by looking for carbon dioxide in the exhalate though this may be unreliable in a patient with little or no blood flow to the lungs for whatever reason. (It should be remembered that carbon dioxide can be retrieved from an oesophageal intubation if there has been difficulty in providing ventilation when expired gases can be forced into the stomach prior to intubation.)

A simple yet novel test has been described by Wee for determining the placement of a tracheal tube. It relies on the fact that air may be aspirated from a tube in the trachea but not from one placed in the oesophagus. The wall of the oesophagus is normally collapsed and will be sucked into the lumen of a tracheal tube if aspiration through the latter is attempted. The trachea, however, is filled with air and held open by rings of cartilage and so will allow air to be aspirated from it.

Wee's oesophageal detector device, as originally described, consists of a 15 mm (female) tracheal tube adapter, a corrugated rubber catheter mount and a 50 ml bladder syringe which are connected in sequence. This has been simplified by Nunn to two components; a tracheal tube adapter and the bulb of an Ellick's evacuator (Figure 5.20). Both devices must be airtight and so should be tested before use. In the latter, this is done by squeezing the bulb to evacuate most of the air, occluding the adapter and confirming that the bulb remains collapsed. In use, the bulb is firstly squeezed and then attached via the adapter to the tracheal tube. If the bulb remains collapsed when released, the tracheal tube must be in the oesophagus. If it expands immediately, then the tube is in the trachea.

A recent but novel method of identifying tracheal intubation uses a portable, battery powered device (Penlon Scoti, Figure 5.21) which when connected to the tracheal tube emits a continuous sound wave down it to excite the gas just beyond the tip. It analyses and differentiates between those acoustic

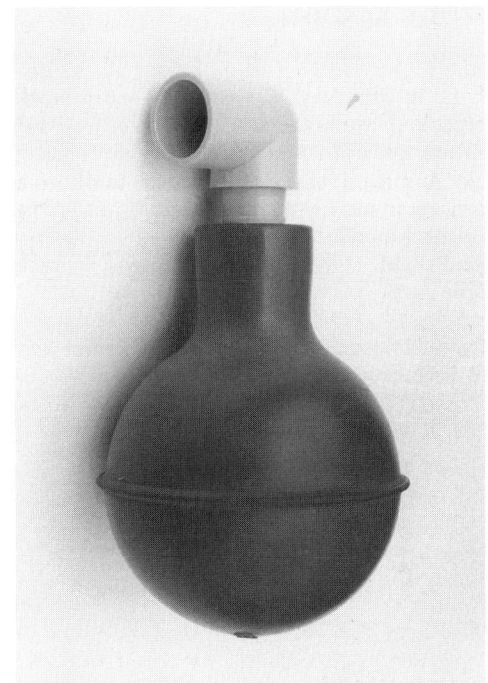

Figure 5.20 Oesophageal detector device.

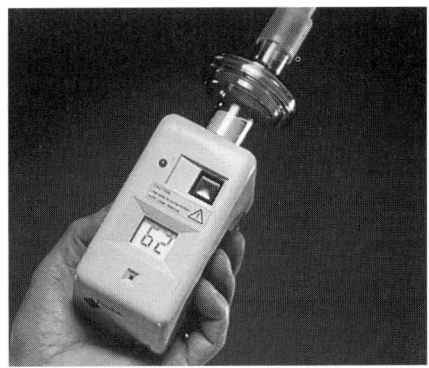

Figure 5.21 Penlon Scoti device.

properties of the gas in the trachea (which is an open tube), with those in the oesophagus (which is a closed tube). Both audible and visual confirmation of placement are displayed on the device.

FURTHER READING

Bolder, P. M., Healy, T. E. J., Bolder, A. R., Beatty, P. C. W. and Kay, B. (1986) The extra work of breathing through adult endotracheal tubes. *Anaesthesia and Analgesia*, **65**, 853–859.

Brain A. I. J. (1983) The laryngeal mask: a new concept in airway management. *British Journal of Anaesthesia*, **55**, 801–804.

Chandler, M. (1986) Pressure changes in tracheal tube cuffs. *Anaesthesia*, **41**, 287–293.

Clark, A. D. (1958) Potential dead space in an anaesthetic mask and connecters. *British Journal of Anaesthesia*, **30**, 176–181.

Editorial (1991) The laryngeal mask airway. *Lancet*, **338**, 1046–1047.

Jephcott, A. (1984) The Macintosh laryngoscope. *Anaesthesia*, **39**, 474–479.

Leach, A. B. and Alexander, C. A. (1991) The laryngeal mask: an overview. *European Journal of Anaesthesia*, **4** (suppl.), 19–31.

Nunn, J. F. (1988) The oesophageal detector device. *Anaesthesia*, **43**, 804.

Seegobin, R. D. and van Hasselt, G. L. (1984) Endotracheal cuff pressure and tracheal mucosal blood flow: endoscopic study of effects of four large volume cuffs. *British Medical Journal*, **288**, 965.

Sosis, M. (1990) Hazards of laser surgery. *Seminars in Anaesthesiology*, **9**, 90–97.

Wee, M. Y. K. (1988) The oesophageal detector device. *Anaesthesia*, **43**, 27–29.

ATMOSPHERIC POLLUTION AND TOXICITY OF INHALATIONAL AGENTS

G. G. Lockwood

This chapter deals with the toxic effects of nitrous oxide and volatile anaesthetics administered to patients, the effect of occupational exposure to trace concentrations of these drugs and their potential to pollute the atmosphere.

NITROUS OXIDE TOXICITY

The toxic effects of nitrous oxide arise entirely from its irreversible inactivation of vitamin B_{12} by the oxidation of Co^+ to Co^{2+} within the molecule. Intracellular B_{12} is a cofactor for methionine synthase, generating methionine and methyl-tetrahydrofolate (methyl-THF) from homocysteine and THF. The turnover of methionine is twice its dietary intake and so its synthesis is essential. Methionine is needed for protein synthesis and as a precursor of S-adenosyl methionine, which is a methyl donor in many reactions, including the transformation of noradrenaline to adrenaline, the synthesis of arachidonic acid and myelination. S-adenosyl methionine is also involved in the generation of active formate which coverts THF to 10-formyl-THF. This enters a metabolic path resulting in donation of a carbon group to convert deoxyuridine into deoxythymidine, which is essential for DNA synthesis. This pathway can also be fed by 5-formyl-THF (folinic acid). The toxic effects of nitrous oxide arise from the disruption of DNA and myelin synthesis and these are manifest clinically in the reproductive, haemopoietic and central nervous systems.

A relatively non-invasive test is available to determine the folate status in the body. Histidine is metabolized to formimino-glutamic acid (FIGlu) and thence, if THF is available, to glutamic acid. THF deficiency is shown by increased excretion of FIGlu in response to an ingested load of histidine. Some patients show a positive FIGlu test the day after breathing 70% nitrous oxide for more than 90 min and all show a positive result after 4 h. This subclinical abnormality clears in 2 days. The deoxyuridine suppression test is more invasive because it requires bone marrow aspirate. Deoxyuridine in external solution is taken up by normoblasts in culture and converted intracellularly to thymidine, which then suppresses the uptake of external, radioactive thymidine. Normoblasts that are folate or B_{12} deficient cannot synthesize thymidine and continue to take up the extracellular thymidine.

A megaloblastic anaemia has been reported following repeated exposure of patients or chronic abusers to nitrous oxide. It has also been reported following a single exposure to nitrous oxide in patients with pre-existing vitamin B_{12} deficiency or who are severely ill.

Short Practice of Anaesthesia. Edited by M. Morgan and G. M. Hall. Published in 1997 by Chapman & Hall, London. ISBN 0 412 71890 1

Vitamin B_{12} is found in animal products, so strict vegetarians may have a sub-clinical deficiency and be at risk. Breathing 50% nitrous oxide for 5–6 h will produce bone marrow changes or abnormal deoxyuridine suppression tests in normal people. In the 1950s, when nitrous oxide was used in the management of patients with tetanus, agranulocytosis developed after 4 days. If repeated exposure to nitrous oxide is necessary then 30 mg of folinic acid, twice daily immediately before anaesthesia and for 3–4 days afterwards, should maintain DNA synthesis and prevent bone marrow changes. There is no doubt that nitrous oxide can be a very dangerous drug and it has even been evaluated as an adjuvant to methotrexate in the treatment of animal leukaemia, though it has not found a place in the treatment of the human disease.

Nitrous oxide is teratogenic in small laboratory rodents, causing birth defects, reduced fertility, increased spontaneous abortion rates and reduced birth weight. Exposure *in utero* or early in extrauterine life has caused behavioural abnormalities lasting up to 3 weeks. These are disturbing facts but they must be put in context. The dose given to these animals is commonly (though not exclusively) large, often 70% inspired nitrous oxide for several hours or days. The half life of vitamin B_{12} deactivation in human patients breathing 70% nitrous oxide is 46 min, but rat B_{12} is inactivated 10 times faster. The animal exposures therefore correspond to extremely lengthy procedures in humans. Such operations are rare during pregnancy and most procedures, such as cervical cerclage, are particularly brief. The outcomes of pregnancies following such procedures is unaffected by the use of nitrous oxide. No effect of nitrous oxide given during egg collection could be demonstrated on the outcome of an *in vitro* fertilization programme. The fetus may be protected by the short duration of administration and the relatively inefficient transfer across the placenta. It has been found that methionine synthase activity in human placenta is normal after a Caesarean section using nitrous oxide. In fact, there is no evidence of effects on the reproductive system of patients anaesthetized with nitrous oxide.

Neurological symptoms following anaesthesia and surgery have been caused by acute (i.e. nitrous oxide induced) or chronic vitamin B_{12} deficiency. Patients have complained of numbness, paraesthesiae, weakness and difficulty walking, all starting some weeks after anaesthesia. Marked improvement or complete recovery has followed administration of cyanocobalamin. Animal work suggests that orally administered methionine would also be helpful, but folinic acid is not appropriate because it only restores DNA synthesis and not the methylation capacity necessary for myelin synthesis. Similar symptoms have been found in chronic abusers although recovery is less certain. The blood of people suffering neurological symptoms from nitrous oxide may be normal.

In summary, the only toxic effects of anaesthetic concentrations of nitrous oxide in humans are in the haemopoietic system, where a few hours anaesthesia normally produces some effect and, if prolonged or repeated over several days, reliably produces a life-threatening condition. This serious problem is largely preventable with folinic acid and must be balanced against the undoubted virtues of nitrous oxide. It is a well-tried agent with a good safety record except during very long administrations and most anaesthetists continue to use it. Even in patients undergoing bone marrow transplants, a particularly vulnerable group, no adverse effects could be ascribed to nitrous oxide. Nonetheless, it would seem prudent to administer folinic acid to cover long anaesthetics (perhaps greater than 12 h) and to protect the critically ill or B_{12} deficient patients and to consider treatment with cyanocobalamin in the postoperative period.

VOLATILE ANAESTHETIC TOXICITY

The volatile anaesthetics in current practice are extremely safe drugs with virtually no direct toxicity to any organ. In spite of this there has been great attention paid to hepatic and renal injuries following anaesthesia with these drugs. These are thought to be caused by the products of their biodegradation. It is now also realized that the products of degradation of these drugs by soda lime may be volatile and have toxic effects when inhaled.

Halothane undergoes oxidative and reductive metabolism in the liver. Approximately 20% of the absorbed dose of halothane (which may be several grams) is metabolized, mainly through the oxidative path. The products of this degradation include trifluoroacetic acid and bromide and are benign. The reductive path generates chlorodifluorethylene, chlorotrifluoroethane and inorganic fluoride. The first two are toxic to the kidney and liver respectively, but only at much greater concentrations than are seen clinically. They are volatile, but their presence is more easily assumed by using the simpler assay of serum fluoride as a marker. The reductive pathway becomes more important during hypoxia, in the obese and after enzyme induction with barbiturates. Gamma irradiation decomposes halothane to a hepatotoxic butene compound. This presents a theoretical risk during anaesthesia for certain radiotherapy procedures which has yet to be reported in practice.

The anaesthetic ethers are metabolized much less than halothane and they follow an oxidative path. Phenobarbitone, phenytoin and isoniazid all increase their metabolism, but not usually to a clinically significant extent. The exception is the combination of isoniazid and enflurane which, in about half the population (the fast acetylators), results in a significant increase in enflurane metabolism. Enflurane, isoflurane and desflurane all produce trifluoroacetic acid in decreasing amounts, but sevoflurane uniquely does not generate this metabolite. No identified organic metabolite of the ethers is significantly toxic; degradation products following exposure to soda lime are discussed later.

LIVER

Anaesthetic toxicity has focused on the liver because of 'halothane hepatitis'. Hundreds of cases of severe hepatitis following halothane anaesthesia were reported within 5 years of its widespread use. The US National Halothane Study was set up in 1966 to investigate a possible causal relationship between halothane and subsequent hepatitis, but in spite of its huge size (856 000 anaesthetics, one-third using halothane) the results were inconclusive. The difficulties of such a study may be appreciated more in the light of another American study which investigated the hepatic function of 7620 apparently healthy patients admitted for elective surgery in a New York hospital. Eleven ASA I patients had their operation cancelled because of abnormal laboratory tests and three went on to develop overt viral hepatitis with jaundice, an incidence of 1:2500. Some workers continue to deny the existence of halothane hepatitis, others argue over its incidence and aetiology. The following is a possible interpretation of the evidence.

Halothane anaesthesia is usually associated with an acute, mild and clinically insignificant impairment of hepatic function, sometimes described as Type I halothane hepatitis. The phenomenon becomes more marked if halothane is administered repeatedly. It may be due to reactive intermediate products of the reductive metabolism of halothane but local hypoxia (due to impaired splanchnic perfusion during anaesthesia) must contribute *per se*. Although perfusion can be reduced by anaesthetics, particularly halothane and enflurane, surgery has a more profound effect. Serum transaminases are characteristically elevated and these enzymes are found particularly in the centrilobular hepatocytes which are most at risk from hypoxia. The onset of this mild hepatitis is relatively rapid (within 3 days of anaesthesia) but it is usually self limiting. Similar changes may follow anaesthesia with the ethers to a lesser extent.

The classical picture of halothane hepatitis (Type II) has an incidence of perhaps 1 in 10 000. It typically occurs in a middle aged woman who has been administered halothane on a number of occasions. There may have been minor reactions such as pyrexia or subclinical hepatitis on previous exposures. One or two weeks after her last exposure she develops a pyrexia and minor gastrointestinal symptoms before severe jaundice and hepatic failure ensue. There is commonly eosinophilia and serum autoantibodies may be present. The disease carried a high morality of 30–50% and seems quite distinct from the common postanaesthetic liver dysfunction. In view of this distinction and the presence of autoantibodies, an immune aetiology has been proposed. Molecules of halothane and its metabolites are too small to generate an immune response, but trifluoroacetic acid tends to bind covalently to tissue protein at lysine residues. This is usually of no consequence but a very small minority of patients develop autoantibodies to the trifluoroacetic acid–protein complexes. The resultant autoimmune hepatitis is slow in onset, but is severe and commonly fatal. Trifluoroacetic acid is produced in lesser amounts by biodegradation of enflurane, isoflurane and desflurane and exceedingly rare cases of autoimmune hepatitis resulting from enflurane have probably occurred. Isoflurane and desflurane seem safe. Sevoflurane metabolism does not generate trifluoroacetic acid; the main organic metabolite is hexafluoroisopropanol, which is less reactive than trifluoroacetic acid and rapidly glucuronidated. It is therefore unlikely *a priori* that sevoflurane is hepatotoxic. Hepatitis following sevoflurane has been reported, but causation is unproved.

There can be little doubt that halothane anaesthesia does cause hepatic injury, but it is not usually apparent clinically. Severe halothane hepatitis is too rare to be able to base guidelines on firm evidence, but the recommendation of the Committee on Safety of Medicines that halothane anaesthesia should not repeated within 3 months and that it is contraindicated by a history of unexplained pyrexia or jaundice after any previous exposure, seems to be as good advice as any.

KIDNEY

In the early 1970s an association was made between methoxyflurane anaesthesia and high output renal failure. Metabolism of this drug produced plasma concentrations of inorganic fluoride greater than 100 μmol l^{-1} which were present for long periods postoperatively, causing the nephrotoxicity. Methoxyflurane has been withdrawn, but other anaesthetics release fluoride during their metabolism. Reductive degradation of halothane releases fluoride, but no more than 10 μmol l^{-1} plasma fluoride has been measured. This will not cause renal injury although renal failure may develop during halothane hepatitis. Enflurane metabolism following almost 1.0 MAC-hour anaesthesia in volunteers produced plasma fluoride concentrations of up to 33 μmol l^{-1} and a mild vasopressin resistant polyuria for a few days. In general, enflurane nephrotoxicity is not considered to be a clinical problem, but because isoniazid increases enflurane metabolism to fluoride, its administration may be considered a contraindication to prolonged enflurane anaesthesia. The minimal metabolism of isoflurane and desflurane means these drugs have no potential for renal injury.

Sevoflurane is metabolized to fluoride with plasma concentrations of 50 μmol l^{-1} recorded. No impairment of renal function has been demonstrated, however, which may be because the rapid elimination of sevoflurane ensures that the elevated concentration of fluoride is transient. It has also been suggested that the methyl-ethyl-ether anaesthetics undergo metabolism in the kidneys themselves, resulting in local tissue concentrations higher than expected from plasma measurements, whilst sevoflurane is exclusively metabolized in the liver. Whatever the explanation, sevoflurane does not cause impairment of renal function. The kidneys seem not to be at risk from modern volatile anaesthetics. Though very sensitive tests (e.g. alanine aminopeptidase excretion, a marker of proximal tubular injury) may be abnormal in the postoperative period, this is as likely to be due to the surgery as the anaesthetics used.

OTHER SYSTEMS

Enflurane has a direct toxic effect on the central nervous system, producing convulsions when used in high concentrations during hyperventilation. The effect terminates on withdrawal of the drugs with no long-term sequelae, but enflurane should be avoided in known epileptics. The metabolism of halothane releases bromide ions which are excreted very slowly through the kidneys and may cause somnolence after prolonged anaesthesia. General anaesthetics depress all body functions reproducibly, including white blood cell phagocytosis and the beating of respiratory tract mucosal cilia. Such effects are limited to the duration of anaesthesia and have not been shown to influence outcome adversely.

CARBON DIOXIDE ABSORBERS

Soda lime and Baralyme present extreme chemical environments and it is not surprising that some degradation of anaesthetics occurs. In clinical use the methyl-ethyl-ethers are remarkably stable in soda lime and volatile breakdown products are not found. Halothane is known to be degraded to chloro-bromo-difluoro-ethylene, producing concentrations of up to 0.05% (500 p.p.m.). The LD_{50} for this compound in mice is only 250 p.p.m., but the widespread use of halothane in closed systems without clinical effects attributable to this degradation product has led to this potential problem being largely ignored. The same attitude cannot be taken with new drugs, and the decomposition of sevoflurane in soda lime has attracted great attention. The most important degradation product has been labelled Compound A: Compound B is much less volatile, and Compounds C, D and E are only produced when the soda lime is hotter than occurs in clinical practice. Compound A is toxic to lungs and kidneys and an LC_{50} of 490 p.p.m. has been determined in rats following a 3 h exposure. The highest concentration found during human anaesthesia with sevoflurane has been less than 70 p.p.m. and is generally less when soda lime rather than Baralyme is used as the absorbent. Zeolites can absorb CO_2 without reacting with soda lime and may be used more in the future. No adverse effects attributable to Compound A have been found in humans anaesthetized with sevoflurane using circle systems.

Soda lime is supplied with a water content of 15%. If it is allowed to dry then its pattern of reactivity changes: desflurane becomes significantly degradable and carbon monoxide is produced; 30% carboxyhaemoglobin has been recorded in a patient during desflurane anaesthesia using a soda lime canister that had been dried by a low flow of dry medical gases throughout the preceding weekend. This potentially lethal source of toxicity can be easily avoided by using fresh soda lime at the start of each day; the absorption of CO_2 creates water which prevents drying during clinical use.

LOCAL POLLUTION

In order to discuss operating theatre pollution one needs to know the extent of the problem. The easiest way to quantify it is to take random samples of ambient gas and pass them through an appropriate gas analyser which will provide a number, usually quoted in parts per million or p.p.m. (1% is equivalent to 10 000 p.p.m.). This value would have little relevance to exposure risk because it is derived from a single sample chosen arbitrarily in space and time whilst pollutants vary through the day and throughout any particular operating theatre. This is best demonstrated by a thermal camera looking across the theatre at a heated screen which is an infrared source: anaesthetics absorb infrared energy and so show up as dark clouds. The technique identifies source of spills and inadequacies in their removal by scavenging and ventilation systems and makes it clear that air samples must be taken repeatedly throughout the day from many locations within the operating theatre. A better system is to sample continuously into a small collector that staff can carry on them as this gives a better estimate of mean inspired anaesthetic concentration. In a naturally ventilated environment without scavenging, concentrations of nitrous oxide may increase to 3000 p.p.m. Such situations arise particularly in dental surgeries. In a well ventilated operating theatre the concentrations may be one tenth of this, reduced further to 30 p.p.m. nitrous oxide by the use of a cuffed tracheal tube (or, presumably, a laryngeal mask airway), low flow systems and scavenging. When used, volatile agents are normally present at 1–2% of the nitrous oxide in concentrations. In general, human studies can only examine the effect of breathing a multiply-polluted atmosphere whilst working in operating theatres where stress and exposure to X-rays, pathogenic organisms and chemicals such as sterilizing solutions and bone cement may have an additional effect that is impossible to control exactly. It is possible to investigate the effects of trace concentrations of particular anaesthetics on animals, but their relevance to humans is not always clear.

Studies of female rats have shown that continuous exposure to 1000 p.p.m. nitrous oxide during pregnancy reduces litter size. Clinical concentrations are required to cause teratogenicity and at least part of these effects may be due to a reduction in uterine blood flow as a result of pharmacological actions of nitrous oxide. Exposure to trace concentrations of nitrous oxide have impaired spermatogenesis in rats, but other workers have failed to show effects at higher concentrations. Trace concentrations of volatile agents have not been implicated and there is virtually no evidence of mutagenesis or carcinogenesis from exposure to any inhaled anaesthetic agent in current use. Evidence of similar effects in humans has been sought.

Early epidemiological studies on spontaneous abortion rates prompted anxiety over operating theatre pollution, but in retrospect their evidence is not strong and may be due to reporting bias and poor choice of controls. A study of the Swedish Medical Birth Rate Registry failed to link nitrous oxide exposure with fetal morbidity or mortality. A study of male anaesthetists found normal sperm with no change after one year of occupational exposure. This may be reassuring in view of the animal experiments, but two epidemiological studies have found an increased incidence (approximately 30% above controls) of malignancy amongst nurse anaesthetists and among female, but not male, operating department staff. These results are in contrast to the laboratory evidence, which raises the possibility that a different, non-anaesthetic environmental agent may be causative. Other studies have failed to show an increase in cancer mortality or any evidence of mutagensis amongst anaesthetists.

In view of the clear effects of clinical concentrations of nitrous oxide on vitamin B_{12} activity, the possibility of a similar specific effect of trace concentrations has been examined. Anaesthetists whose mean nitrous oxide exposure lay between 50 and 160 p.p.m. had normal FIGlu tests. No abnormalities have been shown in peripheral blood films or serum methionine concentrations of operating theatre staff. The evidence for toxicity amongst dental workers is much stronger. Those most exposed may show abnormalities of bone marrow and peripheral blood. Female dental assistants have an increased incidence of spontaneous abortion and reduced fecundity, both correlating with exposure. This correlation with inhaled dose may explain the rather weak evidence found for these effects among operating department staff whose exposure to nitrous oxide and other pollutants is much less. There have also been cases of neurological symptoms due to vitamin B_{12} deficiency among dentists, some of which seem to be related to nitrous oxide pollution.

There is evidence of enzyme induction in anaesthetists which may be due to occupational inhalational of volatile anaesthetics. Antipyrine clearance was increased in one study of anaesthetists but not in another when scavenging was in routine use. Anaesthetists have been shown to have increased urinary D-glucaric acid excretion, another marker of liver enzyme function. Both results imply that occupational exposure to anaesthetic may cause enzyme induction, but other environmental causes cannot be excluded and there is no suggestion that the effect is injurious to health.

Possible pharmacological effects of trace concentrations of anaesthetics (i.e. impaired mental function) were reported in the 1970s. 500 p.p.m. and 50 p.p.m. nitrous oxide were both shown to produce impairment of reaction time in volunteers, with or without halothane in concentrations of 1–15 p.p.m.; 15 p.p.m. nitrous oxide with 0.5 p.p.m. halothane did not produce demonstrable effects. These studies have not proved repeatable and clinical studies have also failed to demonstrate an acute impairment of mood or performance due to work in operating theatres. The weight of evidence is therefore against such an effect.

Thus it seems that the only evidence for an adverse effect of anaesthetic pollution on attending staff is from large exposures to nitrous oxide amongst dentists and their assistants. This may be preventable by improved ventilation in the dental suite. Recommended maximum exposures vary e.g. in the USA, 25 p.p.m. nitrous oxide, 0.5 p.p.m. halothane. In the UK, under the current regulations of the Control of Substances Hazardous to Health (COSHH), the maximum permissible levels of pollution expressed as 8 h time-weighted averages are: N_2O, 100 p.p.m.; enflurance and isoflurane, 50 p.p.m.; halothane 10 p.p.m. Levels for sevoflurane and desflurane have not yet been set. These levels are much less than have been shown reproducibly to be harmful and can only be achieved with scavenging low flow breathing systems and minimal leak around the airway (which implies the use of a cuffed tracheal tube or laryngeal mask airway). Against this ideal must be put the risk of patient injury from scavenging systems. Active scavenging has emptied breathing systems and accidentally occluded scavenging has prevented expiration and may cause barotrauma. Modern systems are safer, but if they are used their function should be tested as part of the routine check of the anaesthetic machine. It is reasonable to strive to minimize workplace pollution, but it must be remembered that there is clear evidence of the harm scavenging equipment can cause patients and only indirect evidence of the harm it is designed to prevent.

GLOBAL POLLUTION

Over the last two decades it has become accepted that the ozone layer is thinning and that a hole may develop in it over the South Pole according to the season. The ozone layer is a region of the atmosphere above the stratosphere at a height of 20–25 km where diatomic oxygen, bombarded by extra-terrestrial ultraviolet radiation, forms triatomic ozone molecules. This reaction absorbs the radiation, so the ozone layer is a shield protecting us from high energy radiation. Chlorine-containing chemical pollutants in the atmosphere react with the ozone, converting it back to diatomic oxygen. Halothane, enflurane and isoflurane all contain chlorine. Could they be contributing to the destruction of the ozone layer?

There are several reasons why this concern is unwarranted. In the first place the quantity of volatile anaesthetic agents spilled into the atmosphere is tiny compared to the quantities of chlorofluorocarbon refrigerants. Secondly, it can take five years for molecules to diffuse to the ozone layer, for although we live in a turbulent part of the atmosphere (the troposphere) the stratosphere above is cold and cloudless, with strong steady winds which have little vertical component. During their ascent anaesthetics are likely to have been destroyed by radiation and reactive radicals and any free chlorine would be washed back to earth as dilute hydrochloric acid in rain. Desflurane may be more stable but, like sevoflurane, it is halogenated exclusively with fluorine and is thus blameless in this situation. Nitrous oxide is more likely to complete the journey to the ozone layer and it too can catalyse the conversion of ozone to diatomic oxygen, but it also binds avidly to free chlorine and so, in a polluted atmosphere, nitrous oxide may actually benefit the ozone layer. However, the contribution to atmospheric nitrous oxide pollution by anaesthetics is less than 2% of the release from nitrate fertilizers on farms and from car exhausts.

The greenhouse effect is due to an increase in the insulating layer of infrared-absorbing gas in the atmosphere. On a planetary scale, the earth absorbs high energy photons and radiates photons in the infrared region, i.e. heat. Without an atmosphere the planet would have a surface temperature of $-15°C$, but water vapour, carbon dioxide and, to a lesser extent, methane, nitrous oxide and ozone in the atmosphere absorb infrared radiation and reflect some back. They form an insulating jacket. Any extra insulation around the planet will cause it to warm up, which would lead to ecological changes. All anaesthetic agents can absorb infrared energy, but quantitatively nitrous oxide is much the most important. However, as stated before, the contribution towards global nitrous oxide pollution by the anaesthetic community is small, and furthermore the contribution towards the greenhouse effect by all nitrous oxide is small compared to that of carbon dioxide and water vapour. Anaesthetists need not tax their consciences over their part in atmospheric pollution.

FURTHER READING

Armstrong, P. J. and Spence, A. A. (1993) Toxicity of inhalational anaesthesia: long-term exposure of anaesthetic personnel – environmental pollution. *Ballière's Clinical Anaesthesiology*, **7**, 915–935.

Baird P. A. (1992) Occupational exposure to nitrous oxide – not a laughing matter. *New England Journal of Medicine*, **327**, 1027.

Brown, B. R. and Gandolfi, A. J. (1987) Adverse effects of volatile anaesthetics. *British Journal of Anaesthesia*, **59**, 14–23.

Nunn, J. F. (1987) Clinical aspects of the interaction between nitrous oxide and vitamin B_{12}. *British Journal of Anaesthesia*, **59**, 3–13.

Ray, D. C. and Drummond, G. B. (1991) Halothane hepatitis. *British Journal of Anaesthesia*, **67**, 84–99.

Westhorpe, R. and Blutstein, H. (1990) Anaesthetic agents and the ozone layer. *Anaesthesia and Intensive Care*, **18**, 102–104.

PART TWO
PREOPERATIVE ASSESSMENT

RISK EVALUATION, AUDIT AND QUALITY OF PRACTICE

C. J. E. Day and S. N. C. Bolsin

RISK EVALUATION

INTRODUCTION

The desire for accurate risk prediction has been an intellectual challenge for doctors for many years. The proliferation of possible treatments in the last few decades has made it vital to select the right treatment for each patient. Unfortunately, many decisions have to be based on figures for population risk: for example, the risk of dural tap during insertion of an epidural needle is about 1%. Ignorance of a patient-specific risk for an uncommon complication is a small problem, but this does not apply when the complication is more serious as in cardiac surgery. Clearly the mean mortality rate of 3–4% would be a gross underestimate of risk for a patient with unstable angina and cardiogenic shock who undergoes cardiac surgery.

Thus, accurate prediction is desirable for patient information, but it is also important for research and health care planning. Research in subjects such as intensive care medicine is made difficult by many compounding variables that affect outcome. Only if these are allowed for, is it possible to know whether differences in outcome are due to the treatment or the case mix. Inclusion of risk stratification into a trial methodology greatly increases the power of the study.

Health care resources worldwide are finite and scarce; this makes optimal utilization of these resources extremely important. The methods described in this chapter can be used to estimate the duration of a patient's stay in the intensive care unit (ICU). Within a cardiac surgical unit this information could be used to help plan operating lists, to avoid cancellation of operations because no ICU bed is available.

It is apparent that accurate risk prediction is already useful, but is likely to become even more important. In this section we aim to highlight some of the established systems of risk evaluation and discuss some of the methods available.

ASA PHYSICAL STATUS

In 1961 Dripps and colleagues modified the original classification system sponsored by the American Society of Anesthesiologists (ASA) to produce the familiar five stage grading (Table 7.1). This system has been widely used for a long time, there is general agreement that it has some predictive ability for operative mortality, but less agreement that it predicts anaesthetic mortality (where chance misadventure has a relatively greater effect). The greatest agreement is that there are marked interobserver differences in allocating scores. It is noteworthy that most studies report mortality rates of 50% or less for grade V, despite the definition being patients not

---

Short Practice of Anaesthesia. Edited by M. Morgan and G. M. Hall. Published in 1997 by Chapman & Hall, London. ISBN 0 412 71890 1

American Society of Anesthesiologists
classification of physical status

	Description
	Healthy patient with no systemic disease processes
II	Mild systemic disease – no functional limitations, e.g. mild diabetes, treated hypertension, heavy smoker
III	Severe systemic disease – with functional limitation, e.g. ischaemic heart disease with limited exercise tolerance
IV	Severe systemic disease that is a constant threat to life, e.g. chronic bronchitis with dyspnoea at rest
V	Moribund patient not expected to survive 24 h with or without operation

expected to survive 24 h with or without an operation.

GOLDMAN RISK INDEX

Goldman and colleagues made a retrospective analysis of 1001 patients in 1977 and described an additive sum score to determine cardiac risk in patients after non-cardiac surgery. They identified a variety of variables by discriminant function analysis, that had significant independent relations with postoperative outcomes. Each factor was given a weight (Table 7.2) and the weights were added to produce the score for an individual patient. The scores were arbitrarily stratified and they showed that there was an increased incidence of both death and serious cardiac events with increasing score. However, the score was never successfully validated in a new population despite several attempts.

APACHE SCORE

The APACHE score was developed in 1981 by William Knaus to predict outcome of intensive care patients. The number of variables was reduced to form APACHE II, which is the most commonly used scoring system in

Table 7.2 The Goldman Cardiac Risk Index for non-cardiac surgery: the presence of the variable in a patient's history or examination leads to the points being added to the patient's score

Variable	Points scored
Age >70 years	5
Myocardial infarction within last 6 months	10
Raised central venous pressure or S_3 gallop	11
Important aortic stenosis	3
Non-sinus rhythm	7
>5 premature ventricular contractions per min before surgery	7
Pa_{O_2} <60 or Pa_{CO_2} >50 mmHg or $[K^+]$<3.0 or $[HCO_3^-]$ <20 mmol l^{-1} or urea >18 mmol l^{-1} or creatinine >240 µmol l^{-1} or abnormal liver function or patient bedridden from non-cardiac cause	3
Intraperitoneal, intrathoracic or aortic operation	3
Emergency operation	4

Points total 0–5 = Group I
6–12 = Group II
13–25 = Group III
26–53 = Group IV

intensive care units today. It has three components: acute physiology score (AP), age (A) and chronic health evaluation (CHE).

Each physiological variable is weighted on an integer scale, 0–4: higher scores are given for greater deviation from the normal range (Table 7.3). Age is stratified and awarded points and the definitions of severe organ insufficiency are very strict, as shown in Table 7.3. For each system insufficiency two chronic health points are awarded if the patient has had an elective operation, and five if the patient has had an emergency operation or has not had an operation. All these points are summed to obtain the APACHE II score.

There has been a further development to form the APACHE III score. This has been reported to offer improved prediction. It also features direct downloading of physiological variables from monitoring systems. Unfortun-

Table 7.3 The APACHE II score is obtained by adding the acute physiology, age and chronic health points from this table

Acute physiology points

Physiological variable	High abnormal range				0	Low abnormal range			
	+4	+3	+2	+1	0	+1	+2	+3	+4
Rectal temperature (°C)	≥ 41	39–40.9		38.5–38.9	36–38.4	34–35.9	32–33.9	30–31.9	≤ 29.9
Mean arterial pressure (mmHg)	≥160	130–159	110–129		70–109		50–69		≤ 49
Heart rate (b.p.m.)	≥180	140–179	110–139		110	70–109		40–69	≤ 39
Respiratory rate (b.p.m.)	≥ 50	35–49		25–34	12–24	10–11	6–9		≤ 5
Oxygenation									
$F_{IO_2}>0.5$ $(A-a)D_{O_2}$	≥500	350–499	200–349		<200				
Pa_{O_2} if $F_{IO_2}<0.5$					> 70	61–70		55–60	≤ 55
Arterial pH	≥ 7.7	7.6–7.69		7.5–7.59	7.33–7.49		7.25–7.32	7.15–7.24	≤ 7.15
Sodium (mmol l^{-1})	≥180	160–179	155–159	150—154	130–149		120–129	111–119	≤110
Potassium (mmol l^{-1})	≥ 7	6–6.9		5.5–5.9	3.5–5.4	3–3.4	2.5–2.9		≤ 2.5
Creatinine (mg 100 ml^{-1})	≥ 3.5	2–3.4	1.5–1.9		0.6–1.4		<0.6		
Hematocrit (%)	≥ 60		50–59.9	46–49.9	30–45.9		20–29.9		≤ 20
White cell count (10^3 mm^{-3})	≥ 40		20–39.9	15–19.9	3–14.9		1–2.9		≤ 1
Glasgow coma score (GCS)					Score=15−GCS				

Age points

Age (years)	Points
≤44	0
45–54	2
55–64	3
65–74	5
≥75	6

Chronic health points (must have been present before hospital admission: score 2 or 5, see text)

Liver	Biopsy proven cirrhosis and documented portal hypertension; episodes of gastrointestinal bleeding due to portal hypertension; or previous encephalopathy
Cardiovascular	New York Heart Association Class IV
Respiratory	Severe exercise restriction; chronic hypoxia, hypercapnoea or polycythemia; or pulmonary hypertension >40 mmHg
Renal	Receiving chronic dialysis
Immunocompromised	Known immunosuppressing drug therapy or immunosuppressive disease in an advanced stage

ately the underlying algorithm has not been made public by the developers, so the program functions as a 'black box'. This lack of transparency combined with the licensing costs of using the system have prevented its widespread use.

DEFINITIONS

Outcome

Outcome is a measure of the status of a patient after medical intervention that we are interested in predicting; it is important that it is clearly defined. It may be **continuous**, such as duration of treatment; **ordinal**, such as the New York Heart Association classification of functional impairment; or **categorical** such as good or bad.

Explanator

This is any patient variable that is used to predict the outcome. Explanators can also be continuous, ordinal or categorical. They must be clearly defined and selected so their measurement is reproducible.

Training data

The development of a predictive model requires a data set that has known explanatory variables and known outcomes. In general terms the modelling process attempts to define a linkage between the explanatory and outcome variables.

Model

This is the mathematical linkage between the explanators and the outcome. A simple example that illustrates these terms is:

$$Y = m X + c \qquad (7.1)$$

Where

Y is the outcome variable
X is the explanator.
m is a parameter
c is a constant term

Models like this are used in every day anaesthetic practice, for example when determining the appropriate size of a tracheal tube for a child:

tube diameter = $0.25 \times$ age (years) + 4.5

Multivariate analysis

Life is never as simple as the example above, and several explanatory variables may have an effect on the outcome. Any analysis that utilizes more than one explanatory variable at the same time is termed **multivariate**.

Independence

Variables are independent if they are not correlated. For example duration of surgery and duration of anaesthesia are likely to be highly correlated and not independent.

Validation data

The model should be tested on a different data set (test or verification data) to see if it is generally applicable. No part of this data should have been used to develop the model.

TYPES OF MODEL

Multiple regression

This type of model can be used when the outcome variable is continuous and has a normal distribution. The model form is shown in Equation 7.2. A linear combination of the explanatory variables is derived by selecting the regression coefficients so that there is the closest agreement possible with the outcome variable.

$$Y = m_1 X_1 + m_2 X_2 + \ldots + m_i X_i + c \qquad (7.2)$$

Where

Y is the outcome variable
X_1 to X_i are the explanators
m_1 to m_i are the parameters, one for each explanator
c is a constant term

This model is widely available as part of statistical packages, but its use in risk evaluation is limited by two factors. First, most risk evaluation problems do not have a continuously distributed outcome variable. Second, the explanatory variables are assumed to have a multivariate normal distribution. This is commonly not the case, many explanatory variables are categorical (e.g. gender, presence of a disease etc.).

Multiple logistic regression

This type of model although similar to multiple regression has some important differences that account for its widespread use in risk evaluation. Multiple logistic regression (MLR) is used when the outcome variable is binary (e.g. alive or dead, good or bad etc.). There is no requirement for the explanatory variables to be normally distributed, indeed they can be categorical, ordinal, continuous or a combination of these types. This makes the model very flexible and applicable to clinical problems where explanatory variables may be of various types.

The output from the model is a predicted probability, for each patient, of being in one of the outcome groups (Equation 7.3). This has advantages and disadvantages. The model may predict that a patient has a 20% chance of dying. Thus if ten such patients were treated, two of them would be expected to die (0.2 × 10). The 20% figure may also be useful for the patient when they are asked to give informed consent. However, if the patient has a 20% chance of vomiting do we give an antiemetic? To answer this question we will need a threshold, or cut-off, value. The threshold can be determined empirically by the clinician, statistically (e.g. to minimize the number of incorrect classifications) or economically ('if we can afford to treat X patients we will only treat those with a risk greater than Y'). Threshold selection can have a profound effect on the predicted outcome.

$$\hat{p} = \frac{e^{\text{logit } p}}{(1 + e^{\text{logit } p})}. \quad (7.3)$$

Where

logit $p = \beta_0 + \beta_1 X_1 + \beta_2 X_2 + \ldots + \beta_i X_i$
$\hat{p}$ Predicted probability
β_0 is the intercept
β_1 to β_i the parameter estimates for each variable X

Discriminant analysis

Discriminant analysis is a multivariate statistical method that is similar to multiple regression, but the outcome variable is categorical. In contrast to MLR, discriminant analysis is not limited to two outcome groups. The output of the model is a class membership and not a probability of class membership. Like multiple regression, there is an assumption that the explanatory variables have a multivariate normal distribution. It is likely that discriminant analysis is more sensitive to violations in this assumption, which may account for its infrequent use in medical studies.

Bayesian model

Bayes' Theorem is a potentially powerful tool for predicting outcome. One of its attractions is that it is conceptually simple and may be regarded as a formalization of clinical diagnosis. It has limited application because it is mathematically tedious and there is no commonly available computer software to perform Bayesian analysis.

The training data set is used to form a 'conditional probability matrix', this is a 'database' of the frequency of each class of explanatory variable in each class of outcome variable. From this it follows that all the variables (outcome and explanatory) have to be categorical.

A simple statement of Bayes' Theorem is:

posterior odds = prior odds
  × likelihood ratio   (7.4)

The terminology is best explained by considering a 2 × 2 contingency table for outcome Y_0 or Y_1 with a variable X that can be either present $(X+)$ or absent $(X-)$ (Table 7.4)

The odds for an event with a $k\%$ chance of happening are $k : (100 - k)$.

Table 7.4 A 2×2 contingency table for outcome Y (which may be 0 or 1), with explanatory variable X (which may be present (+) or absent (−))

	X+	X−	
Y_0	A	B	A+B
Y_1	C	D	C+D

The prior odds are the odds before taking into account variable X. Thus they are $(A + B)(C + D)$.

The posterior odds are the odds after taking variable X into account, they are A/C if X is positive and B/D if X is negative.

The likelihood ratio if X is positive is

$$\frac{A \times (C + D)}{C \times (A + B)}.$$

It can now be seen that Equation 7.4 becomes:

$$\frac{A}{C} = \frac{(A + B)}{(C + D)} \times \frac{A(C + D)}{C(A + B)}$$

The more general form of Bayes theory is unfortunately more complicated to write mathematically, but is still conceptually simple (Equation 7.5). If there are now several mutually exclusive outcomes $Y_1, Y_2, \ldots Y_i$ and several independent categorical variables $X_1, X_2, \ldots X_j$ then Bayes theory states:

posterior odds = prior odds × likelihood ratio for X_1 × likelihood ratio for X_2 × $\ldots$ × likelihood ratio for X_j (7.5)

This statement may be used for most problems. The only assumption is that the explanators are independent which may not apply in many clinical situations. The consequence of non-independent explanators is unreliable estimation of the overall risk. It is also very time consuming to perform the calculation.

Neural networks

Neural networks have been developed by computer scientists and mathematicians. They are increasingly used for prediction in financial markets, weather forecasting and medicine.

A neural network is a collection of neurodes, arranged in layers and interconnected. A simplified representation can be seen in Figure 7.1. The general form consists of an input layer, an output layer and one or more hidden layers between. A neurode may be connected to any other neurode in an adjacent layer.

The basic processing unit is the neurode. Each neurode has a series of inputs and the ability to produce an output. The relationship between the input and output is the neurode's function, it may be a simple threshold (if the summed inputs are above a certain threshold the neurode fires) or more complex.

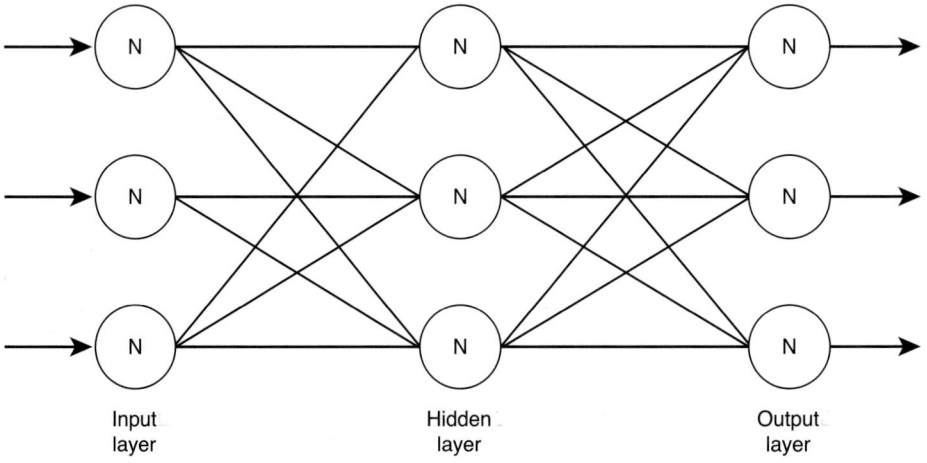

Figure 7.1 Fully connected neural network: N represents a neurode. All neurodes are arranged in layers.

Each connection between neurodes has a weight or weighting function to modify the output of the preceding neurode before it acts as an input to the next neurode.

An 'untrained' network initially has random weights assigned. The training process involves repeatedly offering each data set to the input layer and determining the error of the output (i.e. multiple iterations). The weights are then adjusted in such a way as to minimize the error term. The number of iterations may need to be very large (10^5). This process of adjustment is repeated for each iteration to produce an optimum agreement between known explanators and outcome in the training data. It has the advantage of no prior distributional assumptions about the data, but it requires a lot of computer power and much skill in controlling the optimization process.

COMPARISON OF MODELS

Having developed a predictive model it is important to know how successful it is in predicting the outcome. If several different models are to be compared then the same test must be applicable to all of them. There are several terms that recur frequently when comparisons are made, and they are best illustrated by considering a 2 × 2 contingency table of observed outcome against predicted outcome (Table 7.5).

Logistic regression will produce, for each patient, a continuously distributed probability of a given class membership. A threshold value may then be selected (this does not have to be 0.5) and those above the value are assigned to one group, and those below are assigned to the other. The members of each group may have been correctly, or incorrectly, assigned, thus there are four mutually exclusive categories that can be represented in a 2 × 2 contingency table (Table 7.5). There are many terms to describe the categories created by this division, the essential ones for this discussion are listed below.

true positive	E
true negative	H
false positive	F
false negative	G
sensitivity	$E/(E + G)$
specificity	$H/(F + H)$

The values of these terms are dependent upon the threshold value. This may be illustrated graphically as shown in Figure 7.2a. The X-axis represents the probability of a bad outcome, and the Y-axis the frequency. The left hand curve represents the probabilities from a group who had a good outcome and the right hand curve is a group who had a bad outcome. The groups overlap, so wherever the threshold is set some of the patients will be incorrectly classified. If the threshold is set at 0.05 (line (a) Figure 7.2a) then all the patients will be predicted to have a bad outcome, thus the sensitivity will be 100% but the specificity will be 0%. As the threshold is increased (towards line (b) Figure 7.2a) the sensitivity will decrease and the specificity will increase.

The sensitivity and specificity at one threshold level offer limited information about this distribution. The receiver operating characteristic (ROC) curve is a plot of sensitivity against '1 − specificity' for all possible thresholds. They are used to describe how 'separable' the groups are by the model, or the discriminating ability of the model. Figure 7.2b represents a typical ROC curve that could have come from the data in Figure 7.2a. The greater the area enclosed by the curve (i.e. the closer it gets to the top left corner),

Table 7.5 Contingency table of predicted outcome against actual outcome. The letters E–H represent the frequency for that particular cell

	Good outcome	Bad outcome
Predicted Good	E	F
Predicted Bad	G	H

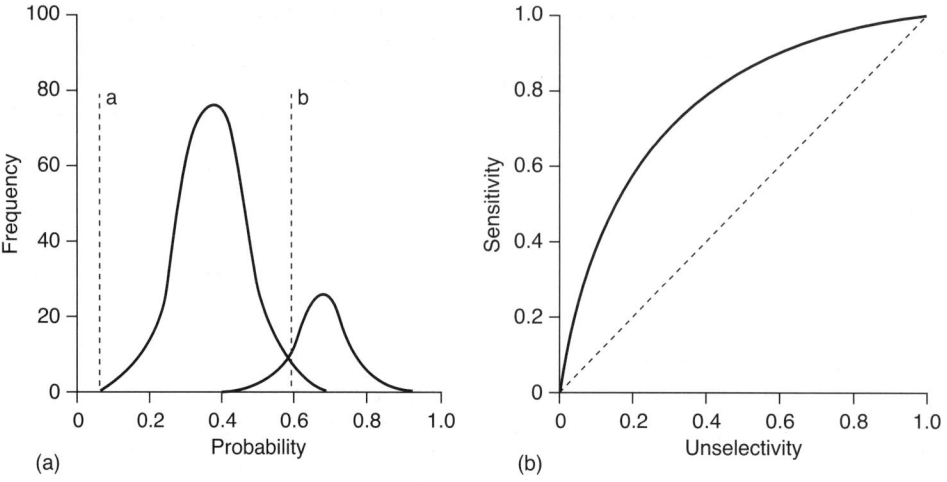

Figure 7.2 (a) Frequency distribution of the predicted probability of a bad outcome, the curve on the right represents those patients who had a bad outcome. The one on the left represents those patients who had a good outcome. (b) Receiver operating characteristics (ROC) curve or plot of sensitivity versus unselectivity for the distributions shown in (a). This gives an indication of the ability of the predictive model to separate the data into good and bad outcomes.

the greater is the discriminating ability of the model.

ROC curves display more information than sensitivity and specificity at a single threshold, but there is some debate about how to compare ROC curves for two different models. The area under the ROC curve is commonly used as a summary for the ROC curve.

THE FUTURE OF RISK EVALUATION

The progress in computer-aided data collection is likely to encourage routine use of predictive models. It is likely they will be used not only as diagnostic and prognostic aids, but also for health service planning and optimizing resource utilization. Risk stratification of outcome data is an important step forward in comparison of practice between units. This is desirable, not because of political fashion, but because identification of true differences in outcome highlights areas for research that are more likely to yield dividends. It is naive not to recognize the potential of risk stratified outcome for monitoring performance, but because the results need careful interpretation and background understanding, the responsibility for monitoring cannot be delegated to non-clinicians. It is vital that the methods involved, and their weaknesses, are understood by the profession so that poor outcome is not incorrectly attributed to practice or treatment. The medical profession generally, and anaesthetists in particular, need to retain self regulation and should embrace any mechanism that helps maintain standards.

AUDIT

'The systematic critical analysis of the procedures for diagnosis, care and treatment; examining the use of associated resources and evaluating the effect that care has on the outcome and quality of life of the patient'. (Department of Health definition in the white paper *Working for Patients* 1989)

The *Working for Patients* document published by the UK Government in 1989 contained specific references to the monitoring and improvement of medical and hospital practice by the use of medical audit. Early attempts to define the nature and implications of this type of audit led to the expenditure of *c.* £6 million by 1994 with expressions of concern from political and central sources. In the same year medical audit was extended to clinical audit, which introduced the concept of the professions allied to medicine becoming involved with doctors in the audit process. Whether this extension has strengthened this process is not yet clear.

If doctors and health professionals are to be encouraged to monitor the performance of other doctors how are these performances to be measured, and by what standards are they to be judged? This question introduces important, but ill-defined, performance indicators for assessment of medical practice, which were probably the goal of audit as referred to in the *Health of the Nation* document.

Cardiac surgery and anaesthesia have been the first specialties to practise detailed outcome research and to develop increasingly sophisticated methods of risk adjustment. Cardiac surgery has probably been the area chosen for this type of analysis for two reasons: firstly, the increasing provision of cardiac surgery per head of population in western healthcare systems and second, the high cost of these interventions both individually and collectively. The results of these analyses have been of varied structure and value. The early data collections used only simple analyses to extrapolate previous experience to future prediction. Recently more sophisticated methods have been used to improve the predictions.

The attempts to regulate hospital and surgeon activity in New York State by the application of such technologies has led to a well-publicized debate. In New York they have completed the full 'audit cycle' of setting objectives, auditing present practice, making changes in areas of underachievement and re-auditing.

In the UK the development of the Audit Programme of the Association of Anaesthetists of Great Britain & Ireland has attracted less debate, but has achieved considerable success. Data have been retrieved electronically from over 25% of the adult cardiac centres in the UK allowing the construction of a database of more than 6000 patients. Thus, it has been possible to produce a risk-adjusted, mortality rate for each participating centre and compare this to the average national mortality rate. These data are fed back to the contributing centres by anonymous, secure (password protected) computer disc for local information. The comparative data are included in a multi-media presentation containing a personal introduction by the Chief Medical Officer and sections on the statistics used in the analyses and the development of the Audit Programme. The programme will also produce an annual report.

CEPOD AND NCEPOD

In 1977 the Association of Anaesthetists of Great Britain and Ireland (AAGBI) was funded by the Nuffield Provincial Hospitals Trust to undertake an audit of deaths associated with anaesthesia. The results of the enquiry were published in 1982 and led to the introduction of a pilot confidential enquiry into deaths occurring in hospitals, within 30 days of anaesthesia and surgery, and involved both anaesthetists and surgeons. The pilot took place in three Health Districts (Bloomsbury, Darlington and Exeter) and was then extended to three Health Regions (North East Thames, Northern and South Western) and was entirely voluntary. This extension was funded by the Nuffield Provincial Hospitals Trust and the King Edward's Hospital Fund for London. The CEPOD project (Confidential Enquiry into Perioperative Deaths) involved all deaths occurring in hospital within 30 days of surgery being notified to an enquiry assessor in strict confidence. Deaths at home were not notified to the enquiry, and maternal deaths and deaths after cardiac surgery were not considered. Details of included deaths were then obtained by volunteer local organizers, again in strict confidence. The CEPOD organizers had already obtained an undertaking from the Secretary of State that the information provided to CEPOD would be privileged, and not disclosed to litigants or open to subpoena at any stage in the future. The cause of death was then investigated by the assessors and the contribution of various factors (e.g. equipment, staffing, expertise, anaesthesia, surgery) was determined.

The enquiry, headed by the visionary Dr John Lunn, produced reports in 1982 and 1987 with the first national report in 1990 followed by reports in 1992 and 1993. The thorough confidential background, anonymous nature and independent assessments made by the enquiry had a considerable impact. Early recommendations concerned monitoring standards in anaesthetic rooms and operating theatres, which were quickly endorsed by the AAGBI. In 1989 the enquiry was extended nationally and included a special examination of the care of children under 10 years of age. Since then different specialist areas have been examined in considerable detail including lower limb amputation, oesophagectomy, pulmonary resection, prostatectomy, coronary artery bypass graft, hysterectomy and primary elective hip replacement.

Key recommendations of the National Confidential Enquiries into Perioperative Deaths NCEPODS have covered: Anaesthetic sub-specialty staffing and case mix, Surgical sub-specialty unit staffing and case mix, emergency operating times and daytime emergency operating theatres. One of the recurrent themes of the reports has been the failure to achieve 100% completion of data forms when deaths are notified to the responsible consultant surgeon and anaesthetist.

The original pilot study undertaken by the AAGBI is now a national Audit involving the following professional bodies:

- Faculty of Public Health Medicine of the Royal College of Physicians of the UK
- Faculty of Dental Surgery of the Royal College of Surgeons of England
- Association of Anaesthetists of Great Britain and Ireland
- Association of Surgeons of Great Britain and Ireland
- Royal College of Obstetricians and Gynaecologists
- Royal College of Surgeons
- Royal College of Anaesthetists
- Royal College of Pathologists
- Royal College of Radiologists
- College of Ophthalmologists

The most striking, but unavoidable, shortcoming of the enquiry has been that, although most deaths were reported and therefore investigated, no assessment of the total number of procedures carried out was made. That is the numerator of the fraction of deaths occurring after anaesthesia and surgery for any procedure was known, but the denominator was not.

The overall number of operations has been calculated from hospital activity databases.

QUALITY OF PRACTICE

TRAINING AND THE ASSESSMENT OF QUALITY

The Chief Medical Officer has recently proposed changes to postgraduate training in medicine and these have been publicized following the production in April 1993 of *Hospital Doctors – Training For The Future*. The Calman Report, as it became known, recommended widespread changes to postgraduate training in all specialties in the UK. The Royal College of Anaesthetists (RCA) has published a document *Specialist Training in Anaesthesia, Supervision and Assessment* which proposes a 6 year training programme incorporating all the basic elements of the present system of training, but in a more compact and modular format. The document also suggests that the use of training log books will form an integral part of the assessment of training in anaesthesia and the use of computer databases for storing this information is the next logical step. The RCA has participated in the development, by anaesthetists, of a computerized log book for the Psion 3a pocket organizer. The program is available and its use is becoming more widespread.

The application of industrial quality control methods to this type of information has already been proposed and one analysis, the cumulative sum technique (CUSUM), is particularly suited to training. It has been demonstrated that CUSUM may have a role to play in training in anaesthesia, especially when accurate numerical data is stored in a training log book. The results can be of value in the assessment of both trainee and trainer.

The technique allows preset target rates of success to be identified before data collection and progress towards the targets to be monitored. The use of 80% and 95% confidence limits are helpful in that if the number of cumulative failures crosses these lines, a significant departure from the agreed target has occurred. Deviation from a preset achievement path is identified objectively and early in the training process. This triggers an agreed response by both the trainee and the trainer.

Once data collection is achieved in training it is a logical step to continue the collection and incorporate the analysis into one aspect of a continuing professional development programme. This may not be acceptable to trained clinicians, but would be accepted by those used to such routine data collection and familiar with the benefits conferred.

The participation of consultants in this type of activity along with the more conventional educational conferences and NCEPOD enhances the credibility of the specialty in its claims to be committed to the continued improvement of patient care.

PROFESSIONAL PERFORMANCE AND ETHICAL RESPONSIBILITIES

Concerns about the under performance of a pathologist working at an orthopaedic hospital led to a report in August 1995 from a committee chaired by the Chief Medical Officer. The report *Maintaining Medical Excellence*, accepted that poorly performing doctors represented a very small minority of those in practice in the UK, but reiterated current advice from both the Department of Health and the General Medical Council. This important advice was stated in the recommendations and conclusions.

'... doctors not only have an ethical responsibility for themselves and their patients, but they also have a professional responsibility to ensure that concern about colleagues is brought to the attention of the appropriate authority. Patient safety must take precedence over all other concerns, ...'

'We consider that the professional responsibility to monitor the standard of colleagues professional performance needs to be reinforced to all doctors.'

CONCLUSIONS

The present trends in audit and quality assurance may be regarded as a formalization of longstanding professional objectives. The increased allocation of resources to audit provides an opportunity to establish regional and national audit programmes that may encourage uniformly high standards of medical practice. It is important that clinicians remain at the centre of audit, quality control and risk evaluation if the full potential of these processes is to be realized. Clinicians can only remain at the centre if they understand the methods on which it is based.

FURTHER READING

Campling, E. A., Devlin, H. B., Hoile, R. W. and Lunn, J. N. (1993) *The Report of the National Confidential Enquiry into Perioperative Deaths 1991/1992*. NCEPOD, 35–43 Lincoln's Inn Fields, London.

Goldman, L., Caldera, D. I. *et al.* (1977). Multifactorial index of cardiac risk in non-cardiac surgical procedures. *New England Journal of Medicine*, **297**, 845–850.

Green, J. and Wintfeld. N. (1995). Report cards on cardiac surgeons – assessing New York State's approach. *New England Journal of Medicine*, **332**, 1229.

Hair, J. F., Anderson, F. E., Tatham, F. L. and Black, W. C. (1992) *Multivariate Data Analysis with Readings*, 3rd edn. Macmillan Publishing Company, New York.

Hannan, E. L., Kilburn, H. *et al.* (1994). Improving outcomes of coronary artery bypass surgery in New York State. *Journal of the American Medical Association*, **271**; 761.

Knaus, W. A., Draper, E. A, *et al.* (1985). APACHE II: A severity of disease classification system. *Critical Care Medicine*, **13**; 818.

Metz, C. E. (1978). Basic principles of ROC analysis. *Seminars in Nuclear Medicine*, **8**: 283.

PREOPERATIVE EVALUATION, SCORING SYSTEMS AND PREMEDICATION

J. P. H. Fee

PREOPERATIVE EVALUATION

The evaluation of patients before operation is an essential preliminary. It is the only opportunity for the anaesthetist to judge whether or not a patient is fit for anaesthesia and surgery and, if not, to institute appropriate therapy. It also serves as an opportunity for the anaesthetist to establish trust with the patient and to explain anaesthetic management. Unfortunately, the modern approach favouring fast throughput of cases often conflicts with good preoperative evaluation. Formerly, it was usual for a patient scheduled for major surgery to be admitted to hospital some days in advance for evaluation and investigations. Except before major surgery, this would now be unusual in many hospitals, preoperative evaluation often being performed at a clinic some weeks in advance. It is at this clinic that routine ECG, radiography, blood and urine investigations are arranged. Although it is desirable for anaesthetists to provide this service, modern conditions demand that their time is concentrated in the operating theatre and so the responsibility for preoperative assessment is gradually devolving to nurses. The anaesthetists who work in institutions which provide this type of preoperative assessment must satisfy themselves that the nurses to whom these duties are delegated are adequately trained and supervised. Agreed protocols and good communication are the keys to success. Any problems which come to light must be referred to the anaesthetist well in advance of the operation so that arrangements can be made for the anaesthetist to see and examine the patient. Failure of communication at this stage risks last minute cancellation the evening before operation with disappointment and frustration for the patient and wasted operating time. Whether or not a preoperative assessment clinic is available, the anaesthetist should visit the patient in hospital before operation. This is a courtesy and also an opportunity to check that the patient's condition has not changed since the evaluation. In circumstances where no such evaluation has taken place the anaesthetist will rely on the house officer's routine history and examination to identify major areas of concern which might affect the conduct of the anaesthetic.

MEDICAL HISTORY

This is the most instructive part of the preoperative evaluation, a fact which is often poorly appreciated by junior doctors. The objective is to form an estimate of the patient's functional reserve with particular emphasis on cardiovascular and respiratory systems. Particular attention should be paid to pre-existing conditions such as ischaemic heart disease, uncontrolled hypertension, asthma, chronic obstructive airways disease and endocrine, rheumaticalogical, haematological or neuromuscular disorders. Neurological conditions such as multiple sclerosis and Parkinson's disease also have implications for anaesthetic management. Routine questioning about exercise tolerance, orthopnoea, dizzy spells or blackouts may reveal much useful information. It is important that patients are asked about any recent weight loss or change in bowel habit. Details of medication, cigarette and alcohol consumption and the family history ('reactions' or 'allergies' to anaesthetics, malignant hyperthermia cholinesterase deficiency, porphyria) should be sought. The anaesthetist must develop a concise history-taking method which allows pertinent questions to be asked about all body systems. Records of previous anaesthetics should be checked routinely when available. The anaesthetist should confirm from the patient that to the best of their knowledge there were no untoward incidents during any previous anaesthetics. Any hint of possible difficulties should be investigated and the relevant anaesthetic records obtained.

PHYSICAL EXAMINATION

It is normally not necessary for the anaesthetist to conduct a full systematic examination and he should concentrate on those aspects which might impinge on his care. The examination will necessarily be focused on the cardiovascular and respiratory systems. Particular attention should be paid to any conditions which might create problems with laryngoscopy and tracheal intubation. These include: advanced dental caries, dental crowns, bridges and inlays, operation scars involving the neck and chest, instability or rigidity of the cervical spine (rheumatoid arthritis, ankylosing spondylitis), Down's syndrome, arthritic conditions affecting the range of movement of the temporomandibular joint. Prominent upper incisors and receding mandible (micrognathia) signal a possibly difficult tracheal intubation.

The precordium should be examined and any thrills noted. The heart sounds should be identified and particular attention paid to any murmurs or bruits. The jugular venous pulse should be inspected. Heart rate and rhythm and the condition of the peripheral pulses are useful indicators of underlying disease. Bradycardia of < 50 b.p.m. or tachycardia of > 100 b.p.m. in an adult or any irregularity in rhythm should be investigated by ECG (see below). The anaesthetist should ensure that the arterial blood pressure has been measured and is within a normal range. Higher systolic values are permitted in the elderly than in younger adults provided the diastolic pressure does not exceed 100 mmHg at rest. The anaesthetist should be aware that spurious readings may occur when patients are settling in following admission to hospital or during the examination itself. It is, therefore, important that when hypertension is suspected on a single measurement the patient be allowed to rest and the measurement repeated on several occasions.

Cyanosis, dyspnoea, finger clubbing, nicotine staining and a barrel chest all point to severe respiratory disease. Chest percussion may reveal hyper-resonance in the presence of emphysema. Auscultation of the chest may reveal bronchospasm, crepitations, pleural rubs, or bronchial breathing. All of these are indicators of significant acute and/or chronic respiratory disease which, inevitably, will increase the risks of complications in the perioperative period.

There is no place for routine chest radiography. It may, however, be useful as a back-up investigation for patients with suspected or established cardiorespiratory disease and as a screen for recent immigrants from countries where tuberculosis is endemic.

It is essential that the preoperative evaluation (with the correct date and time) is recorded in the patient's notes. Any difficulties encountered in obtaining old records or the results of investigations should also be recorded. Although the onus is clearly on the anaesthetist to ensure that patients are adequately prepared for anaesthesia, it is acknowledged that time is limited and that the assessment of relatively fit patients will be brief and to the point.

ROUTINE INVESTIGATIONS

Haematology

The need for routine investigations before elective surgery has been challenged. The widespread practice of performing large numbers of biochemical tests using automated equipment is now seen to be largely pointless. Patients who are physically fit and who are attending hospital for routine minor or body surface surgery will rarely need haematological or biochemical investigations. Those who are suffering from systemic illness are in a different category, but even for these only those investigations which are necessary should be performed. The majority will require baseline measurements of haemoglobin, haematocrit and white cell count. It has been traditional to take $10\ g\ dl^{-1}$ as the minimum acceptable haemoglobin concentration for surgery, but lower values may be acceptable, particularly when there is little risk of blood loss. However, with an ageing population, often in a poor state of nutrition, it is probably best to aim for a figure of $10\ g\ dl^{-1}$. Co-existing cardiac and respiratory disease are relevant factors. Apart from haemoglobin concentration, oxygen delivery is dependent on blood flow and the optimal haematocrit figure at which both transport (cardiac output) and flow are best matched is approximately 30%. The hazards of HIV infection acquired from transfused blood have increased the risk of homologous blood transfusion and there is a need to develop facilities for autologous blood donation and perioperative blood salvage. Haematological investigations for sickle cell trait are mandatory for all patients of African ancestry. Coagulation screening should be performed on patients with bleeding or clotting diatheses, or who are jaundiced, or who are taking anticoagulant or thrombolytic therapy.

Electrolytes

There is little consensus as to which tests are truly necessary and it is difficult to identify, beyond a few very obvious ones, in what way abnormal results might dictate changes in anaesthetic management. Biochemical derangements are unlikely in young patients who are reasonably fit and active. Plasma sodium, potassium, calcium and urea concentrations should, however, be checked in the elderly and in circumstances where the clinical condition of the patient suggests that these may be abnormal, e.g. Addison's disease. As indicated above, biochemical investigations may be performed some weeks or months before the date of operation and it is not normally necessary to repeat these unless the overall condition of the patient has changed or there has been a long delay. Up-to-date electrolyte checks, however, will be required in patients with known renal dysfunction, diabetes mellitus or who are receiving diuretic treatment. Persistent diarrhoea, vomiting, leaking fistulae and severe burns will inevitably cause extensive derangement of plasma electrolytes and these must be corrected before operation.

Disorders of acid–base balance are unusual in the elective patient but, if present, must be investigated and corrected. There is a high rate of false positive results from random blood glucose estimations and urinalysis is to be preferred as a screen for diabetes mellitus.

Electrocardiography

Electrocardiography is advisable in patients over 50 years of age presenting for major surgery. Its principal objective is to serve as a baseline against which future changes can be compared but it is also necessary in order

Table 8.1 Categories of patients in whom preoperative electrocardiography is recommended before major operations

Aged >50 years
Ischaemic heart disease
Valvular heart disease
Cardiomyopathy
Hypertension
Diabetes mellitus >40 years
Thyroid disease
Electrolyte imbalance
History of arrhythmias
Hyperlipidaemia
Peripheral vascular disease
Cardioactive medication

to rule out an acute myocardial event or arrhythmia.

Preoperative electrocardiography is also advised in a number of other circumstances (Table 8.1).

MEDICAL CONDITIONS AFFECTING ANAESTHETIC MANAGEMENT

It is difficult to think of a medical condition which does not have implications for the conduct of anaesthesia. However, only the more commonly encountered conditions will be mentioned here and the reader is referred to the relevant chapter for a fuller exposition.

Cardiovascular disease

With few exceptions, anaesthetic drugs have a depressant effect on the cardiovascular system. Volatile agents reduce both cardiac output and systemic vascular resistance with a consequential decrease in arterial blood pressure. Some anaesthetic drugs increase heart rate with an attendant increase in myocardial oxygen requirements. Regional anaesthesia involving blockade of the thoracolumbar sympathetic outflow will have a profound effect on both afterload and preload. Neither general nor regional anaesthesia should be contemplated in a patient with severe cardiac disease unless there is an overwhelming need for surgery.

Left ventricular failure

Elective surgery is contraindicated in patients with acute left ventricular failure. Goldman's Multifactorial Index (see Table 7.2) indicates that these individuals are at extremely high risk. Crepitations, a third heart sound, gallop rhythm and raised jugular venous pulse are associated with marked decompensation. Anaesthesia can, however, be considered in patients whose left ventricular failure has been successfully treated with diuretics, angiotensin converting enzyme inhibitors and inotropes, but care must be taken to maintain adequate cardiac output and coronary perfusion pressures. Whereas a great deal of effort has gone into identifying those at high risk due to ischaemic heart disease, less attention has been paid to the optimization of ventricular function before subjecting patients to the insults of anaesthesia and surgery.

Ischaemic heart disease

The condition of the arterial vessels can be judged by the severity of anginal pain, intermittent claudication and usage of coronary artery vasodilators, e.g. glyceryl trinitrate. Silent angina may, however, be more common and perhaps more dangerous than the other sort. Transient ischaemic attacks may be secondary to advanced disease of the carotid vessels. In many circumstances it may be preferable to correct the vascular conditions either by bypass grafting or endarterectomy before proceeding to other forms of elective non-cardiac surgery.

A recent myocardial infarction is a contraindication to non-urgent surgery and outcome is improved after six months' postponement. The incidence of myocardial infarction in patients with severe vessel disease after non-cardiac surgery is up to 6% in those who have not had bypass grafting compared to about 1% when coronary artery bypass grafting has been performed. The mortality in unoperated patients, about 2.4%, is much higher than that in patients who have had bypass grafting, i.e. 0.5%. Although these appear compelling figures, the benefits of bypass grafting may be exaggerated in that those who survive that procedure are also likely to survive after non-cardiac surgery. Patients with severe angina, aortic stenosis, cardiomegaly, mitral incompetence and atrial or ventricular arrhythmias are likely to experience a higher incidence of severe complications in the perioperative period.

Hypertension

Major non-urgent surgery should not be contemplated in patients with diastolic arterial blood pressures which consistently exceed 120 mmHg. These patients should be referred for urgent investigation and control. Providing the anaesthetist is aware of possible drug interactions, particularly with β-adrenoceptor blockers and providing the mean blood pressure is maintained at or near preoperative values, anaesthesia does not constitute a significant hazard in this group of patients. Ephedrine is the vasopressor of choice for the treatment of hypotensive episodes and labetalol is favoured by many for the control of hypertensive crises/episodes.

Cardiac pacemakers

A patient with a cardiac pacemaker should not be anaesthetized unless the anaesthetist is fully aware of the type of device involved and knows what to do if it ceases to function properly. It is essential that adequate documentation, including previous notes and investigations, are available for consultation some days before the planned operation. This allows time for discussion with the cardiologist concerned.

Virtually all newly implanted pacemakers are programmable in terms of rate, output and sensitivity. They may sense R-waves in the ventricle or P-waves from the atrium (single chamber type) or both (dual chamber type) (Table 8.2). These devices may be programmed to trigger a ventricular impulse under certain circumstances or they may be more sophisticated. A fully automatic dual pacemaker may have four modes involving continuous atrioventricular pacing. Other devices may respond to alterations in physical activity or body temperature and some may be switched between one or more modes. Pacemakers which respond to preload are not yet available clinically, although devices which automatically defibrillate or convert ventricular tachyarrhythmias are now available.

The most likely cause of malfunction during anaesthesia is interference with the pacemaker signal due to electrocautery. This is particularly true of the devices which respond to tachyarrhythmias. In general, the dia-

Table 8.2 Coding system for cardiac pacemakers

1st letter: Chamber paced	2nd letter: Chamber sensed	3rd letter: Mode of response	4th letter (optional); Programmable features	5th letter (optional): Arrhythmia treatment
A=atrium	A=atrium	T=triggered	P=programmable	B=burst
V=ventricle	V=ventricle	I=inhibited	M=multiprogrammable	N=normal
D=double	D=double	D=double	O=not programmable	S=scanning
	O=none	O=not applicable	R=rate modulated	E=external

thermy pad should be placed in such a way that the electrical current does not vector across the heart. Bipolar cautery should be used – with this, the current passes between the tips of the cautery forceps, rather than from the cautery tip through the body to the distant pad. If there is an automatic defibrillation facility in the pacemaker this should be deactivated before the start of surgery to prevent inappropriate triggering. The anaesthetist must be confident of deactivating this mode and generally this is achieved using a magnet positioned over the pacemaker. Switching-off is confirmed by a change in the audible tone of the device. The anaesthetist should remember to reactivate the pacemaker when the patient returns to the recovery area.

Respiratory disease

Acute or chronic diseases of the lungs and bronchi reduce respiratory reserve. Virtually all intravenous and inhalation anaesthetic agents have a depressant effect on respiration either through an action on the pontine respiratory centre or peripherally through their relaxant effects on skeletal muscle. The use of muscle relaxants in such patients will also impair the contractility of the skeletal muscle even when apparently well reversed at the end of an operation. Ciliary action in the bronchi is impaired both by the action of inhaled drugs and also as a result of the inevitable trauma caused by tracheal intubation.

For these reasons patients with respiratory conditions are often best anaesthetized using local anaesthetic techniques. In general these have less effect on respiratory function, except in circumstances where motor blockade affecting respiratory muscles occurs, e.g. thoracic epidural block. However, general anaesthesia is unavoidable for thoracic, neurosurgical, otorhinolaryngological and upper abdominal surgery. Pre-existing respiratory disease will inevitably result in a high incidence of anaesthetic related morbidity and mortality, even in the hands of the most skilful and experienced anaesthetist. The primary objectives of the preoperative evaluation should be to: assess suitability for surgery, identify those most at risk of perioperative complications, and optimize function.

Asthma

The incidence of asthma is increasing worldwide although the reasons for this are unclear. It is a condition in which there are periods of acute exacerbation followed by periods of remission. It is difficult to weigh the risk of anaesthesia for an individual patient against the preoperative severity of the disease. In common with all types of respiratory illness it is imperative to optimize the patient's condition before non-urgent surgery, particularly if general anaesthesia is required. The majority of asthmatic patients with moderate disease will be receiving long-term treatment with β_2-agonists (salbutamol, terbutaline or isoprenaline), sodium cromoglycate, ipratropium, theophylline or steroids. In refractory cases it will be necessary to try alternative bronchodilator therapy and any active infection should be aggressively treated with antibiotics and chest physiotherapy. The anaesthetist should be aware of the danger of provoking arrhythmias by inadvertent overdosage when administering aminophylline or other bronchodilators to patients already receiving these types of drugs.

Patients who continue to have severe bronchospasm despite all efforts to relieve it are one of the most testing challenges for the anaesthetist. If necessary the patient should be referred to a physician with an interest in asthma. General anaesthesia should only proceed when there are facilities for postoperative ventilation and support.

Chronic obstructive airways disease

This group of conditions is characterized by increased sputum production, airway narrowing and diminished responsiveness to carbon dioxide. Loss of alveolar architecture in emphysema will increase the physiological dead space and diminish the area of healthy tissue which is available for gas exchange. Many of these individuals will be heavy cigarette smokers and the associated impairment of ciliary activity will increase the likelihood of retained secretions, lung collapse and infection in the postoperative period. Polycythaemia secondary to chronic hypoxia is frequent and there may be a high proportion of haemoglobin bound to carbon monoxide as carboxyhaemoglobin. Patients with chronic productive cough should not have surgery postponed unless there is evidence of acute superimposed infection. Providing the patient is apyrexial, has a normal white cell count and has no evidence of active infection on chest radiography there would seem little purpose in deferring surgery. A short period of smoking abstinence would not appear to be worthwhile although studies have shown that longer periods of about 2 months markedly reduce the incidence of postoperative respiratory complications. Chronic respiratory conditions are frequently associated with right-sided heart failure and this should be treated with diuretics and digoxin.

Investigations

In planning the anaesthetic management of patients with significant respiratory disease it is useful to have objective measures of respiratory function. Spirometry is the key investigation. A vital capacity of less than 80% of the predicted value can be taken as abnormal and may be due to pulmonary fibrosis, pneumonia, or surgical removal of lung tissue. Other non-pulmonary conditions may limit the depth of inspiration, e.g. neuromuscular disease, pain or drugs. Obstructive conditions such as asthma and bronchitis reduce expiratory flow. Normal patients can exhale at least 70% of the forced vital capacity in 1 s (FEV_1/FVC %) after a maximal inspiration and values of less than this indicate airway obstruction of increasing severity.

Peak flow is a measure of the maximum flow achieved at any point during forced expiration and can be measing easily using a portable meter. In healthy men below 40 years of age peak flow is at least 500 l min^{-1}: less than 200 l min^{-1} suggests that coughing will be inefficient and that postoperative chest complications are likely. This test is more convenient than spirometry but is more dependent on patient effort than the FEV_1 measurement. Such tests, including arterial blood gas estimations, may assist in gauging fitness for operation and be useful as yardsticks against which to judge progress. Chest radiography is mandatory to establish the presence of active infection, fibrosis, lung cysts, bullae and neoplasia.

Endocrine disorders

Diabetes mellitus

This is a systemic disease with long-term effects on arteries, kidneys and peripheral nerves. During anaesthesia it is essential to maintain good control of blood glucose so that any risk of unobserved hypo- and hyperglycaemia can be minimized. The severity of the disease and the nature of the surgical intervention will have a major bearing on how best this control can be achieved in the perioperative period.

Patients with diabetes are best operated on in the morning so that the fasting period can be kept to a minimum and good liaison with the preoperative evaluation clinic is essential in these circumstances. Insulin-dependent diabetics scheduled for complex surgery should be admitted to hospital at least 48 h in advance of operation for assessment by a diabetologist. These patients will have to discontinue their long-acting insulin treatment and a new regimen of short-acting insulin will have to be substituted. Control of blood glucose is most difficult in the early postoperative period after major surgery and should be supervised by a diabetologist. Anaesthetists' working patterns do not normally allow time to provide close supervision and it is inappropriate for a junior surgeon to carry the responsibility alone.

Non-insulin dependent diabetes can be controlled by diet with or without oral hypoglycaemic drugs. As far as these patients are concerned, particularly if they are only scheduled for minor surgery, it will only be necessary to omit the morning dose of hypoglycaemic agent, check the fasting blood glucose concentration and ensure that there is no significant amount of glucose in the urine.

The choice of anaesthetic must take into account the nature of surgery and preoperative renal and cardiovascular function. Whatever technique is chosen the anaesthetist should be aware of the problems associated with autonomic neuropathy. Diabetic patients often exhibit considerable cardiovascular instability during regional and general anaesthesia and are known to have increased requirements for intraoperative vasopressors. Although diabetics are said to be susceptible to infection there is little good evidence that this is really the case. Nevertheless, all diabetic patients should be screened preoperatively for signs of acute infection using urinalysis, white cell count and chest radiography. In all but the most urgent circumstances any infection should be treated before operation. Strict asepsis should be employed during all interventions, particularly spinal or epidural block, central venous cannulation and tracheal intubation.

The association between diabetes, peripheral vascular disease and coronary artery disease is well known and some diabetic patients will have had previous bypass operations. Others may be symptomless or on treatment with β-adrenoceptor blocking drugs, nitrates, etc. All diabetics aged over 40 years of age should have electrocardiography performed preoperatively to identify ischaemia and exclude the possibility of a recent infarction.

Clinical nephropathy is present in about 20% of diabetics (both insulin and non-insulin dependent) after 20 years duration of disease and the proportion increases with increasing age. Nephropathy in insulin-dependent diabetics is associated with a relative mortality some 10–20 times that of age-matched comparators without proteinuria. The impairment of function varies in its severity from those who have established chronic renal failure to those with no obvious loss of function, with an intermediate group identifiable by a blood urea of above 12 mmol l^{-1} and/or a creatinine concentration of above 180 mmol l^{-1}. Patients in this category are at risk of acute renal failure secondary to hypotension, hypoxia or the administration of drugs with intrinsic nephrotoxic potential, such as aminoglycoside antibiotics, non-steroidal anti-inflammatory drugs and some diuretics.

A full description of the anaesthetic management of the diabetic patient can be found in Chapter 35.

Obesity

Some 10 to 15% of the UK population are thought to be overweight. Those defined as 'morbidly obese' (ideal body weight plus 45 kg) are most at risk from anaesthesia and surgery. Obese patients present a greater technical challenge than those of average build. The siting of venous and arterial cannulae, visualization of the glottis and maintenance of a clear airway may all be difficult. Hiatus hernia is common and there is a higher risk of regurgitation and aspiration of stomach contents even in the fasting state. Difficulty in the identification of anatomical landmarks may render regional block well-nigh impossible.

Surgery itself will be much more difficult and may be prolonged and the anaesthetist should be prepared for additional blood losses.

One of the most critical aspects of obesity is its effect on the mechanics of breathing. The weight of the omentum and anterior chest wall in the supine position will make breathing virtually impossible in severe cases. In order to prevent desaturation, positive pressure ventilation may be necessary for even the shortest procedure. Weaning from ventilatory support in the postoperative period may present considerable difficulties and there is an increased risk of deep venous thrombosis, pulmonary embolus, atelectasis and chest infection after operation.

Fatty infiltration of the heart and liver carries a poor prognosis and obese patients are at greater risk of drug-related renal and hepatic toxicity. Except in the gravest emergency obese patients should be strongly advised to lose weight before surgery. In circumstances where weight loss has not been achieved they must be informed of the greater risk of complications and even death. The likelihood of a period of postoperative ventilatory support should be explained beforehand.

Neurological diseases

Parkinson's disease

This is a common neurological condition in elderly patients and the extent to which the disease constitutes a risk depends on its severity. General and regional anaesthesia are usually tolerated well in those whose symptoms are well controlled with L-dopa and other anti-Parkinsonian medication. Severely affected patients are, however, difficult to mobilize postoperatively and are prone to respiratory complications. Only in circumstances where life is at risk should surgery be contemplated in these cases.

Epilepsy

Well-controlled epileptic patients do not present a particular hazard in respect of anaesthetic management. Standard anaesthetic techniques can be employed, but the anaesthetist should ensure that any medication continues up until the day of operation and restarts as soon as possible thereafter.

The majority of epileptic patients will be taking long-term medication with barbiturates and/or phenytoin, the enzyme inducing properties of which may reduce the duration of effects of anaesthetic and other drugs, e.g. warfarin.

Rare neurological diseases

Specialized anaesthetic management is required for patients with myopathies and neuropathies such as myasthenia gravis or the Guillain–Barré syndrome. The same principles in respect of preoperative preparation apply with particular attention being paid to the respiratory system. Any infection must be treated with antibiotics and chest physiotherapy so that the patient's condition may be optimized. A period of postoperative ventilatory support is usual and patients and their relatives should be advised of this possibility.

Although there is little evidence to support it, regional block may be inadvisable for medicolegal reasons in patients with multiple sclerosis, neuropathies, myopathies, Parkinson's disease and other neurological conditions. There is always a risk of relapse of a neurological illness irrespective of the anaesthetic technique employed. Whatever technique is chosen, however, the anaesthetist must be able to justify a particular method and in these circumstances detailed contemporary notes are essential.

Rheumatoid arthritis and ankylosing spondylitis

Although not strictly a neurological disease, advanced rheumatoid arthritis affecting the neck may be associated with neurological symptoms. The anaesthetist must be aware of the risks of instability of the upper cervical vertebrae and take steps to ensure that no further neurological damage occurs as a result of his interventions. Assessment by a neurologist is an essential prerequisite and the anaesthetist must be satisfied that the patient's preoperative neurological status is clearly recorded in the notes. The hazards associated with manipulation of the neck should be explained to the patient and only an anaesthetist with appropriate experience should accept responsibility for this type of case. Rheumatoid arthritis may also affect the temporomandibular joint making laryngoscopy and tracheal intubation impossible using conventional methods; the larynx might also be affected in the rheumatoid process. Ankylosing spondylitis may also affect the cervical vertebrae, the resulting rigidity making it impossible to align the head and neck for tracheal intubation. Here again, good communication between the preoperative assessment clinic and the anaesthetist is essential if delays and disappointments are to be avoided.

Renal diseases

The severity of renal impairment may vary from those dependent on renal dialysis to those with slightly elevated plasma urea and creatinine concentrations. Impairment may be on the basis of glomerular disease (nephrotic syndrome) or tubular dysfunction (uraemic). The majority of patients will be on low sodium or other diets and taking treatment for hypertension or other associated conditions. Particular care should be taken to avoid precipitating acute on chronic failure as a result of hypotension, nephrotoxic drugs (including NSAIDs) or hypoxaemia. Excess electrolyte and water loads should be avoided in patients with chronic renal failure.

Thorough biochemical and haematological screening should be carried out before operation and hyperkalaemia or other major electrolyte derangements should be corrected, if necessary using haemodialysis. The anaesthetist should be aware that these patients may be hypoalbuminaemic and lower doses of protein bound drugs may suffice. Drugs which are excreted exclusively by the renal route should be avoided.

Recipients of renal allografts may present for surgery. These patients will be receiving long-term treatment with steroids and/or immunosuppressive drugs and strict asepsis should be followed for any invasive procedure.

Gastrointestinal disorders

Disturbed function may arise because of obstruction, disorders of motility and malabsorption. The anaesthetist will be concerned with all of these at different stages of his care. Obstructive conditions involving the oesophagus (stricture) or stomach (pyloric stenosis) increase the risk of pulmonary aspiration during induction of anaesthesia even in the fasted patient. Hiatus hernia is associated with regurgitation of stomach contents. This may occur at any time in the perioperative period but particularly when the patient is in the supine position. Obstruction involving the remainder of the alimentary tract most commonly arises as a result of bands or adhesions. Carcinoma may be responsible in older age groups and intussusception or volvulus in infants and young children. Retrograde peristalsis may occur and large amounts of faeculent material may accumulate in the stomach. In these circumstances it is vital that gastric drainage be provided using continuous suction. In cases where there is extensive loss of fluid and/or electrolyte due to diarrhoea, vomiting, fistulae or drainage tubes, the patient's acid–base and electrolyte status should be checked and corrected before the operation. Hourly urine output and central venous pressure should be monitored when major surgery is planned. When there is active bleeding blood should be crossmatched in advance. In all cases where there is risk of pulmonary aspiration tracheal intubation is mandatory.

Liver disease

Alcohol related cirrhosis is a common cause of liver dysfunction and is associated with significant postoperative morbidity and mortality. The galactose elimination test offers an objective measure of the integrity of the hepatocyte although other more pertinent parameters such as clotting time are perhaps a better guide to suitability for operation. Patients with gross coagulation abnormalities are unsuitable for surgery until these have been corrected, usually by administration of fresh frozen plasma, cryoprecipitate, etc. In common with patients suffering from cardiovascular or respiratory conditions these patients should be under the care of an appropriate specialist so that their overall condition can be optimized before non-urgent surgery. Avoidance of encephalopathy is a prime objective and sterilization of the gut is advisable. Stones, strictures and swellings may affect the hepatic or bile ducts causing varying degrees of obstruction and jaundice. When preparing jaundiced patients for surgery the anaesthetist must check the coagulation screen and correct any abnormalities. Vitamin K supplementation is a wise precaution in those with obstructive lesions due to malabsorption arising from impaired emulsification of fat.

Viral infections

Hepatitis B and HIV may be transmitted by contact with body fluids. Recent concern has been expressed about the possible transmission of hepatitis C and other infections such as tuberculosis in breathing systems. Patients whose lifestyle exposes them to higher risk should be counselled before operation and with their agreement should be tested for the presence of infection or, failing that, treated as though infected. It must be accepted, however, that a large number of infected patients will not be readily identified. It is important that staff take all possible steps to avoid contracting infection, including hepatitis B vaccination.

DOCUMENTATION

The previously casual approach to the keeping of a written record of the preoperative evaluation is no longer acceptable. In the absence of a contemporary note the anaesthetist may find it difficult to persuade a court of law that he visited a patient before operation, particularly if the patient claims he did not. Details of the relevant past history, drug therapy, previous anaesthesia (including the date and technique) and dental state should be recorded. When a particular technique has been discussed with a patient and a choice made, the reasons for following a particular course should be clearly stated.

Questionnaires are a useful method of acquiring information in the day care facility and all anaesthetic departments should ensure that a standard form is available for the purpose. The anaesthetist must not only be aware of the patient's present and past state of health but be in a position to show that he knew if challenged.

In some circumstances, e.g. emergencies or split-site commitments, it may not be possible for the anaesthetist to make the usual preoperative evaluation. In the case of split-site working it is essential that the anaesthetist has a system in place for informing him about patients. This will require close cooperation with those responsible for preoperative evaluation.

Written consent is mandatory before general anaesthesia and surgery except in life-threatening emergencies. The patient has a fundamental right under common law to grant or withhold consent before examination or treatment and if the patient is treated without consent doctors and hospitals may be sued. Some patients now expect a fuller explanation of the risks and problems associated with anaesthetic techniques and drugs. If the anaesthetic carries a substantial risk the patient must be informed of this so that his consent can be given with full knowledge. In circumstances where a patient refuses the recommended anaesthetic technique the anaesthetist may be prepared to take this into account in recommending an alternative. However, the anaesthetist should never be tempted to use a technique which he knows is unsuitable for a particular case and must be prepared to refuse to proceed.

Patients who are in shock, in pain, who cannot understand English or who have a mental disability may not be capable of giving informed consent. In these circumstances consent to proceed must be obtained from parents, next of kin, guardians or a court of law before an operation can take place.

Although it is not yet a legal requirement it may be necessary in future to obtain consent for the participation of medical students in the anaesthetic care of patients.

CHILDREN

The law recognizes that young people over the age of 16 years may consent to any surgical treatment and it is not necessary to obtain separate consent from the parent or guardian. For children under the age of 16 years, in the vast majority of cases, parental consent will be obtained although a child of this age may consent on his own account provided that the doctor is satisfied that the child has sufficient understanding of what is involved. In circumstances like these the doctor should make detailed notes of the factors he used when making his assessment of the child's capacity to give valid consent. Rarely, the parents may refuse to consent to urgent or life-saving treatment and in those circumstances the child may be made a ward of court.

BLOOD TRANSFUSION

Patients may refuse blood transfusions for religious or other reasons. Although such refusal need not be a bar to major surgery involving significant amounts of blood loss the patient must be left in no doubt of the need for the transfusion proposed. The decision on whether or not to proceed with a particular operation in these circumstances is a matter for the individual anaesthetist or surgeon to consider. Provided the patient is willing to accept the additional risks, surgery may be performed. Detailed notes should be kept of all discussions and if possible these should be witnessed by an independent party. In the case of a minor it may be necessary to apply to the courts for permission to proceed with a blood transfusion.

FASTING

The disastrous consequences of pulmonary aspiration of stomach contents during general anaesthesia have been recognized as a hazard since the early days of anaesthesia. On Snow's recommendation surgery should be delayed for 4–6 h after a meal, this interval being based on the presumed gastric emptying time. Following the introduction of intravenous induction agents, muscle relaxants and tracheal intubation, successive reports on the causes of maternal deaths implicated general anaesthesia and in particular aspiration of gastric contents as the major factor affecting mortality during Caesarean section. This focused a great deal of attention on the need for a prolonged period of fasting even in non-obstetric patients and for many years it has been the rule that anaesthesia should be delayed until a minimum of 4 h since the previous meal. In practice this often meant that fasting commenced at 10 or 11pm the night before operation and continued on for some considerable period afterwards. The need to provide simple instructions which could be applied to all patients meant that little account could be taken of the needs of particular individuals.

It is quite clear that a fast exceeding 4 h in generally healthy patients does not reduce the volume or acidity of gastric contents at induction of anaesthesia. Many fasting patients have gastric fluid volumes of more than 25 ml with pH < 2.0. There is now clear evidence that a light breakfast within the 4 h period need not increase gastric pH or volume at induction. Other investigations have shown that clear fluids may be safely taken up to 2 h before operation and may actually reduce both gastric volume and acidity compared with fasting controls. These findings will be welcome news for the vast majority of young reasonably healthy patients but traditional fasting regimens should be maintained in the elderly in the absence of suitable data.

PREPARATION FOR THEATRE

The medical staff are responsible for ensuring that the patient is correctly identified and that the operation to be performed corresponds with that recorded in the notes and on the consent form. It is essential that operating lists are drawn up in time for the anaesthetist to check on his preoperative ward round. The nursing staff should ensure that the patient is wearing an identity band with the correct details and that lipstick and cosmetics have been removed. Relevant notes, including the consent form, radiographs and scans, should be available for consultation in theatre. There is no good reason for removal of dentures until the last possible moment and some anaesthetists prefer that these be left in place during anaesthesia.

CONCURRENT MEDICATION

Psychoactive drugs

Tricyclic antidepressants

These drugs act by blocking the reuptake of noradrenaline into nerve terminals. In so doing, the action of noradrenaline, adrenaline and other directly acting sympathomimetic drugs is enhanced. Their anticholinergic properties can induce sinus tachycardia, atrial ectopic beats or more dangerous arrhythmias and they will potentiate the effects of atropine and hyoscine. Tricyclic antidepressants have a high affinity for cardiac muscle and are negative inotropes. They delay conduction by their quinidine-like, membrane stabilizing action and this may be seen on the ECG as prolonged PR, QRS and QTc times, the latter increasing the risk of sudden ventricular fibrillation. Severe cardiovascular side effects are a feature of overdosage.

Monoamine oxidase inhibitors

Newer drugs are selective for the MAO-A subtype of the monoamine oxidase enzyme, and although probably not any more effective than older MAOIs, are less likely to interact with foods or other drugs. The most serious interaction occurs with pethidine, which, when given to a patient on an MAOI, is characterized by hypertension, hyperthermia, sedation or coma and sometimes convulsions. This picture is unlikely with other opioids unrelated to pethidine although data are scarce. Apart from this there are no serious interactions with the commonly used anaesthetic agents. Discontinuation of MAOIs may induce severe anxiety, agitation, sleeplessness and paranoid psychosis. By careful choice of anaesthetic drugs it is usually preferable to continue treatment. Marked hypertension results following administration of indirect acting sympathomimetics, e.g ephedrine in the presence of the original MAOIs, but this is unlikely with the newer type of drug.

Anticonvulsants

The barbiturates and phenytoin are well known inducers of hepatic enzymes and this property may increase the dosage requirements of many drugs. They are also thought to induce resistance to non-depolarizing muscle relaxants although the mechanism of this is unclear. The benzodiazepines do not cause significant enzyme induction and there are no clinically important interactions with drugs used in anaesthesia.

Alcohol

Chronic long-term ingestion leads initially to induction of hepatic enzymes which enhance the metabolism of alcohol itself in addition to other drugs. In some individuals cirrhosis develops and the functional reserve of the liver is reduced. Conversely, acute intake of alcohol inhibits microsomal enzymes and enhances the effects of drugs. Pharmacodynamic alterations may also occur with chronic alcohol abuse which may be the result of adaptive changes in cell membrane lipids or proteins leading to tolerance. Alcoholic patients are tolerant of the central nervous system effects of anaesthetic drugs but not the cardiovascular and respiratory depressant effects.

Cardiovascular drugs

Calcium channel antagonists

These drugs act by depressing cardiac conduction (slowing sinoatrial node discharge, prolongation of atrioventricular node refractoriness, slowing of atrioventricular conduction). They exert a direct negative inotropic effect and induce vasodilation of both coronary and systemic arteries and arterioles. The potential for depression of cardiac function is usually offset by afterload reduction and this is most obvious in the case of nifedipine which is the most potent negative inotrope in the group.

The volatile anaesthetics may interact adversely with calcium channel blockers. Both halothane and enflurane have direct cardiac inhibitory effects similar to those of verapamil and diltiazem. In contrast, the peripheral vascular effects of isoflurane resemble the dihydropyridines (nifedipine and nicardipine) which are principally vasodilators. Conduction in the heart has been shown to be affected by both isoflurane and halothane but there are few data on interactions with the newer agents.

Nifedipine, nicardipine and nimodipine are vasodilators whose effects may be intensified when combined with similarly acting drugs such as sodium nitroprusside or glyceryl trinitrate.

The cardiotoxic effects of bupivacaine may be accentuated in patients receiving treatment with calcium channel or β-blocking drugs.

β-adrenoceptor blocking drugs

These drugs are indicated for the treatment of hypertension, angina and migraine. Side effects include bronchospasm, cardiac failure, hypoglycaemia, bradycardia, heart block, inter-mittent claudication and Raynaud's phenomenon.

Bradycardia, hypotension and bronchospasm are the main hazards in patients who are scheduled for anaesthesia. Continuation of treatment up to and including the day of operation improves preoperative cardiovascular stability and avoids any risk of rebound effect due to abrupt withdrawal. Bradycardia may occur in patients receiving volatile anaesthetic agents, particularly halothane and following neostigmine. Although bronchospasm is not an intrinsic property of these drugs, β-adrenoceptor blockade increases the reactivity of the airway and the likelihood of bronchospasm during instrumentation.

Angiotensin converting enzyme (ACE) inhibitors

Captopril, enalapril and their congeners act on the renin angiotensin system and inhibit the formation of angiotensin II, a powerful vasoconstrictor. These drugs are used for treating renovascular hypertension and congestive cardiac failure. It is usually recommended that ACE inhibitors are continued in the perioperative period and they may improve haemodynamic stability during operation, particularly during aortic aneurysm repair and coronary artery bypass grafting. Conversely, there is evidence that ACE inhibitors may predispose to hypotension during anaesthesia and that they reduce cerebral blood flow during this. In general, it is advisable to continue these drugs up to and including the day of operation.

Clonidine

Clonidine is an antihypertensive drug with a central α_2-agonist action combined with weaker peripheral α_1-antagonist activity. It would seem to modify the pressor response to laryngoscopy and tracheal intubation and it improves the pressor responses to indirectly acting vasopressors such as ephedrine. It is recommended that clonidine treatment be continued up to and including the day of operation.

Corticosteroids

Prolonged treatment may cause suppression of the pituitary–adrenal axis with an impaired response to stresses induced by surgery and anaesthesia. Preoperative biochemical tests (the insulin hypoglycaemia test of hypothalamic–pituitary–adrenal function; the adrenocorticotrophic hormone stimulation test of adrenocortical function) may be used to identify patients who are unable to mount a cortisol response to stress. However, this form of testing is complex and despite impairment of the stress response many patients do not require steroid supplementation during the perioperative period. If supplementation is considered necessary hydrocortisone 100 mg may be given intravenously at induction for patients undergoing minor operations, continuing with 100 mg i.m. six hourly for three days for those undergoing major surgery.

Other regimens involving approximately one quarter of these doses have also been used successfully.

Antibiotics

The aminoglycoside, polymyxin, lincosamide and tetracycline antibiotics possess neuromuscular blocking activity. These drugs may potentiate the action of non-depolarizing muscle relaxants such as tubocurarine, pancuronium, vecuronium and atracurium. The anaesthetist should be aware of treatment with these compounds and should be prepared to use lower doses of muscle relaxants than normal in conjunction with train-of-four stimulation or similar monitoring.

SCORING SYSTEMS

A number of systems have been devised which attempt to quantify the risks of anaesthesia *per se* and of complications in particular organs and tissues. When the preoperative evaluation has been completed all patients should be graded according to the American Society of Anesthesiologists (ASA) classification (Table 7.1) and this should be recorded in the notes. Other systems are used to grade the degree of risk specifically in cardiac disease, notably those of Goldman (Table 7.2) and the New York Heart Association (Table 8.3). The risk of non-cardiac surgery varies from almost nil in ASA I patients to 75% in the highest risk category (Table 8.4).

The general applicability of using preoperative ischaemia to identify those at risk of postoperative cardiac morbidity has been challenged; it would appear that postoperative ischaemia in the 48 h after operation is a better correlate with adverse cardiac outcome

Table 8.3 New York Heart Association classification of angina

Grade	Physical status
I	Ordinary physical activity, e.g. walking or climbing stairs, does not cause angina. Angina with strenuous or rapid prolonged exertion at work or recreation.
II	Slight limitation of ordinary activity. Walking or climbing stairs rapidly, walking uphill, walking or stair climbing after meals, in cold, in wind, or when under emotional stress, or only during the few hours after awakening. Walking more than two blocks on the level and climbing more than one flight of ordinary stairs at a normal pace and under normal conditions.
III	Marked limitation of ordinary physical activity. Walking one or two blocks on the level and climbing one flight under normal conditions and at a normal pace. Comfortable at rest.
IV	Inability to carry on any physical activity without discomfort: anginal syndrome may be present at rest.

Table 8.4 The probability of cardiac complications in different types of patients derived using the multifactorial cardiac risk index. (Adapted from Goldman (1988))

Type of patient	Approximate risk of major cardiac complications for this type of patient (%)	Approximate risk of major cardiac complications for this type of patient as adjusted using multifactorial index (%)[a]			
		Class I	Class II	Class III	Class IV
Minor surgery	1	0.3	1	3	19
Unselected consecutive patients >40 years who have major non-cardiac surgery	4	1.2	4	12	48
Patients who have abdominal aortic aneurysm surgery or who are older than 40 years and have high-risk characteristics that require medical consultations before major non-cardiac surgery	10	3	10	30	75

[a]Calculated by multiplying the prior odds of complications by the likelihood ratio for each case

than any other factor. It would seem that, at best, the present scoring systems can serve only as a guide as to the advisability of surgery in an individual patient.

PREMEDICATION

At a time when anaesthesia and surgery have become safer and more effective than ever before it is ironic that a considerable number of patients remain fearful. These fears may be rational and be related to past unpleasant experiences or the nature of the present illness. Those with malignancy or suspected malignancy are particularly anxious and fearful of the future. Patients may be afraid of not waking up again, or of not being properly asleep. Less rational are the fears of needles, masks and other equipment. The first objective of premedication should be to minimize

Table 8.5 Secondary objectives of premedication

Treatment of pain
Prevention of acid aspiration
Prevention of undesirable autonomic reflexes
Prevention of thrombus formation
Antibiotic prophylaxis
Amnesia
Painless venepuncture in children (EMLA cream)

EMLA = eutectic mixture of local anaesthetics

Table 8.6 Recommended doses of drugs for premedication

	Route	Dose
Anxiolytics		
Diazepam	Oral	10–20 mg
	i.v.	10–20 mg
Temazepam	Oral	10–30 mg
Midazolam	i.v.	2.5–5 mg
	(Oral	10–20 mg)[a]
Oxazepam	Oral	15–30 mg
Lorazepam	Oral	2.5–5 mg
	i.v.	2–4 mg slowly diluted in normal saline
Zopiclone	Oral	7.5 mg
Analgesics		
Morphine	i.v.	5–10 mg
Pethidine	i.v.	25–75 mg
Anti-emetics		
Prochlorperazine	i.m.	1.5 mg
	rectal suppository	25 mg
Cyclizine	i.m., i.v.	50 mg
Hyoscine	Oral	0.5–1.0 mg
	i.m., i.v.	0.2–0.4 mg
Droperidol	i.m., i.v.	0.3–5 mg (see text)
Metoclopramide	i.m., i.v.	10 mg
Vagolytic		
Atropine	Oral	1.5–2.0 mg
	i.m., i.v.	0.4–0.6 mg
Children		
Temazepam elixir	Oral	1 mg kg^{-1}
Diazepam syrup	Oral	0.2 mg kg^{-1}
Papaveretum +hyoscine	i.m.	0.25 mg kg^{-1} +0.005 mg kg^{-1}
EMLA cream[b]	Topically to dorsum of both hands and/or both antecubital fossae	1–2 h preoperatively

[a]Not available in UK or USA
[b]EMLA: eutectic mixture of local anaesthetics
Timing: intramuscular and oral drugs should be given 1–1.5 h before operation

these feelings and induce a state of tranquillity. Secondary objectives are shown in Table 8.5.

The shift towards day-care surgery has impeded effective premedication. As a consequence many patients arrive at the day-care facility in a markedly anxious state. The organization of these facilities frequently makes it impossible for the anaesthetist to interview the patient before he/she appears in the anaesthetic room. This precludes any opportunity for the anaesthetist to provide reassurance: well known to be the best form of premedication.

Unpremedicated, anxious patients require larger doses of induction agents if awareness during instrumentation of the airway is to be avoided. Recommended doses of drugs commonly used for premedication are listed in Table 8.6.

ANXIOLYSIS

The benzodiazepines comprise a large number of lipophilic compounds exhibiting anxiolytic, sedative, amnesic and anticonvulsant properties. They differ mainly in their pharmacokinetic profiles, some having a short duration of action and others being slowly eliminated. They are well absorbed after oral administration, plasma concentrations peaking by 90 min. Therapeutic doses in young healthy patients have few cardiovascular or respiratory side-effects, but at higher doses and in the presence of hypovolaemia these drugs may cause hypotension or respiratory arrest. The response to benzodiazepine drugs

Temazepam

This drug had, until recently, displaced diazapam as the standard oral anxiolytic for use before operation. Its main advantages are its very rapid absorption from capsules and elixir and its short elimination half-life (Table 8.7). It has no hypnotically active metabolites and no specific disadvantages, although it cannot be formulated as a parenteral preparation on account of its insolubility. The standard dose of temazepam varies from 10 to 30 mg in adults and approximately 1 mg kg^{-1} as the elixir in children aged 3–12 years.

As a result of problems with abuse, temazepam is now a Schedule 3 category drug and must be stored in a locked cabinet. Although a register is not a requirement some hospitals have decided to apply the same conditions to temazepam as for a Schedule 2 controlled drug such as morphine.

Diazepam

Like temazepam this drug is rapidly absorbed when given by mouth and has a pronounced anxiolytic action. It has a marked anterograde amnesic effect following a standard intravenous dose (10 mg) or after higher doses by mouth. Like the other benzodiazepines it has an unpredictable anxiolytic and sedative action and it frequently results in a hangover effect due to its long elimination half-life (Table 8.7). This latter effect is accentuated by the presence of active metabolites (N-desmethyldiazepam, temazepam, oxazepam). The standard dose of diazepam is 10 to 20 mg by mouth in adults and 0.2 mg kg^{-1} as the syrup in children.

The intravenous preparation consists of the active drug emulsified in a soya bean oil preparation (Diazemuls). This preparation may be used to provide sedation and anxiolysis before operation in the very nervous but only where there are suitable nursing and monitoring facilities.

Lorazepam

This drug shares many of the properties of the other benzodiazepines but it has some unusual features. The onset of action is delayed after both intravenous and oral dosing and it has a duration of action of almost 6 h. Its amnesic properties are more pronounced than those of other benzodiazepines and it has a markedly sedative effect.

The half-life is intermediate between that of diazepam and temazepam (Table 8.7) but its clinical action is longer than either of these. Lorazepam is probably best reserved for tense, agitated patients before high-risk surgery, when night sedation in a dose of 2.5 to 5 mg by mouth followed by a repeat dose on the morning of operation is often very effective.

Table 8.7 Pharmacokinetic values of some of the more widely used benzodiazepines

	Oral bioavailability (%)	β half-life, $t_{\frac{1}{2},\beta}$ (h) (range)	Volume of distribution, V_d (l kg^{-1}) (range)	T_{max} (h) mean (range)
Diazepam	100	31–47	0.9–1.2	1.0 (0.5–1.5)
Temazepam	80	5–15	1.3–1.5	0.8
Midazolam	48	1.5–3.5	0.8–1.1	0.7
Lorazepam	93	10–20	1.0–2.0	2.3 (1.0–3.0)
Flunitrazepam	85	15	3.3	—
Oxazepam	97	5–15	0.7–1.7	2.0 (1.0–4.0)

Midazolam

Midazolam shares the general properties of the other members of its class, but unlike most of these it is water soluble and is sometimes used as an intravenous premedicant in day-care patients. Although it is approximately twice as potent as diazepam it undergoes a significant amount of first pass metabolism (Table 8.7) and must be given in a relatively high oral dose. Midazolam is commercially available in tablet form in some European countries but not in the UK or USA. It has a short duration of action, short elimination half-life and negligible amounts of active metabolites are produced. The drug is painless on intravenous injection and is not associated with venous complications. For these reasons midazolam is widely used as intravenous sedation for dentistry, invasive investigations and a variety of endoscopic procedures.

Zopiclone

Although not a benzodiazepine this drug acts on the benzodiazepine receptor complex and has similar pharmacological properties. It is said not to induce dependence. The drug is well absorbed after oral administration and it is a useful sedative/anxiolytic with a short duration of action. Its main disadvantage is a persistent bitter or metallic taste.

VAGAL BLOCK

It is rarely necessary to prescribe vagolytic premedication in adults. The drying of secretions was once a primary indication but the advent of intravenous induction agents and less irritant volatile anaesthetics has made this unnecessary except in children. Atropine may be given by mouth with other drugs before operation or, when required to prevent bradycardia, intravenously at induction of anaesthesia. It should be given cautiously to patients with ischaemic heart disease to avoid inducing tachyarrhythmias. In contrast, hyoscine does not have a pronounced chronotropic action and is usually employed for its antisialogogue, anti-emetic and amnesic effects (see below). It may cause confusion in the elderly.

Glycopyrrolate, unlike atropine and hyoscine, does not cross the blood–brain barrier and so lacks central nervous system effects. It is rarely used for premedication. The doses of the commonly used anticholinergic drugs are given in Table 8.6.

ANALGESIA

Opioids

Although once popular, opioid analgesics are unsuitable for routine premedication mainly because of their respiratory depressant properties. In the presence of pain, however, morphine (0.2 to 0.3 $mg^{-1} kg$) or pethidine (1.5 $mg^{-1} kg$) are effective by intramuscular injection but should be combined with an anti-emetic. When short-acting opioid analgesics are used to supplement anaesthesia these should be given at induction when their depressant actions are of minor importance. There is no reliable evidence that the pre-emptive administration of opioid or other analgesics is effective as a means of preventing postoperative pain although the amount of general anaesthetic necessary is reduced by about 10%. Unfortunately, premedication with opioid drugs delays recovery and increases the incidence of postoperative nausea and vomiting. In general, apart from pethidine, opioids have a tonic effect on smooth muscle and should be avoided in asthmatic patients. Pethidine 50–100 mg slowly intravenously is suitable for the treatment of biliary and ureteric colic.

Non-steroidal anti-inflammatory drugs (NSAIDS)

These drugs, despite their well known side effects, are widely used in anaesthetic practice. Preoperative administration is often convenient and, with the patient's agreement, rectal administration is probably preferable to the oral route particularly in the fasted state. Diclofenac sodium 100 mg may be given by suppository 1 to 4 h before operation and this may be repeated after 12 h. There are abundant data demonstrating the opioid sparing effects of NSAIDs and when given to reasonably healthy patients for a few days the risk of complications would seem to be low. There are few reliable data comparing the incidence of complications in different compounds. NSAIDs are contraindicated in patients who are dehydrated, or who have dyspeptic symptoms, a history of peptic ulceration, hiatus hernia, acute or chronic renal failure, bleeding or coagulation disorders, or who are taking steroid medication.

ANTACIDS

The routine use of saline antacids to neutralize gastric acid has, for many years, been a routine precaution in obstetric anaesthesia. This form of protection has disadvantages, notably an increase in gastric volume, unreliable effect on gastric pH and, in the case of sodium bicarbonate, the formation of large volumes of carbon dioxide. However, antacids are usually acceptable to the patient, have little effect on the fetus or on the progress of labour and are inexpensive.

The discovery of histamine (H_2) receptors on acid secreting gastric parietal cells and the subsequent development of drugs which blocked them altered the pattern of acid prophylaxis in obstetric patients. This now consists of combined H_2 receptor antagonist and antacid therapy. Ranitidine is preferred to cimetidine on account of its lack of interactions with other drugs and its more prolonged antisecretory effect.

Acid prophylaxis is mandatory in non-obstetric patients who are at high risk of pulmonary aspiration. These include patients who are obese or who have a history of hiatus hernia, heartburn, dyspepsia or peptic ulcer disease. In these circumstances acid prophylaxis with ranitidine 150 mg by mouth should be commenced the night before operation and repeated in the morning. Omeprazole is a more recent drug which reduces gastric acid secretion by inhibiting adenosine triphosphatase. As a proton pump inhibitor it blocks the final common pathway of acid release and has a longer duration of action than H_2 receptor antagonists.

PREVENTION OF NAUSEA AND VOMITING

Nausea and vomiting are common and sometimes highly distressing complications occurring in up to 40% of all patients. Risk factors are listed in Table 8.8. Prophylactic antiemetic treatment, although often poorly effective, is advisable for those at risk or who have experienced severe symptoms after previous operations. The areas of the brain concerned with vomiting include the reticular formation, the nucleus tractus solitarius, and the dorsal nucleus of the vagus. Physiologically, these areas act as a 'vomiting centre' which receives afferent impulses from elsewhere in the central nervous system (chemoreceptor trigger zone (CTZ) in the floor of the fourth ventricle

Table 8.8 Risk factors for postoperative emetic complications

Fear, anxiety
Unpleasant smells, tastes
Gastrointestinal pathology
Female gender
Ophthalmic, gynaecological surgery
Pregnancy
Drugs: opioids, digitalis glycosides, levadopa, NSAIDs
Labyrinthine disorders
Ingested toxins
Uraemia
Movement
Blood transfusion
Cancer chemotherapy
Radiation

Table 8.9 Recommendations for endocarditis prophylaxis for 'at risk' procedures under general anaesthesia

Drug	Dose	Route	Timing	Indication
Amoxycillin	**Adults** 1 g +500 mg	i.m. in 2.5 ml 1% lignocaine Oral	at induction 6 h after induction	Dental, genitourinary, obstetric, ENT and bowel procedures in patients at no special risk
	Children <5 years ¼ adult dose **Children 5–10 years** ½ adult dose			
Gentamicin	**Adults** 120 mg	i.v.	at induction	Procedures as above. 'High risk' patients with prosthetic valves or who have had bacterial endocarditis previously
Amoxycillin	500 mg	Oral	6 h after induction	
Gentamicin	**Children <5 years** 2 mg kg^{-1}	i.v.	at induction	
Amoxycillin	125 mg	Oral	6 h after induction	
Gentamicin	**Children 5–10 years** 2 mg kg^{-1}	i.v.	at induction	
Amoxycillin	250 mg	Oral	6 h after induction	
Clindamycin	**Adults** 300 mg 150 mg	i.v. i.v. or oral	at induction over 10 min 6 h after induction	As above but for patients allergic to penicillin. Not recommended for genitourinary or bowel procedures
	Children <5 years ¼ adult dose **Children 5–10 years** ½ adult dose			
Vancomycin	**Adults** 1 g	i.v. infusion	over 2 h	For genitourinary and bowel procedures in penicillin allergic patients
Gentamicin	120 mg	i.v.	at induction	
Vancomycin	**Children <10 years** 20 mg kg^{-1}	i.v. infusion		
Gentamicin	2 mg kg^{-1}	i.v.		

close to the area postrema, cerebral cortex, vestibular and cerebellar nuclei). The 'vomiting centre' also receives impulses from the gastrointestinal tract. Essentially, emetic responses can be modified by blocking: central cholinergic (muscarinic) receptors (cholinergic pathways, vestibular nerve nucleus); dopamine receptors in the CTZ/area postrema; or 5-HT (5-hydroxytryptamine) receptors in the CTZ/area postrema.

Anti-emetic drugs may be given as part of the premedication or at the time of induction of anaesthesia in the hope of reducing the incidence of nausea and vomiting in the post-operative period. The class of drugs used for this purpose and their pharmacology is described in Chapter 38.

ANTIBIOTIC PROPHYLAXIS

Patients scheduled for surgery with valvular or congenital heart disease or who have a prosthetic heart valve are at risk of bacterial endocarditis. This is most likely during procedures involving the mouth, teeth, genitourinary or gastrointestinal tracts which may cause a transient bacteraemia. A selection of penicillin and non-penicillin regimens suitable for the prevention of bacterial endocarditis is shown in Table 8.9. Prophylactic antibiotics are also prescribed by surgeons in order to prevent operative infection during bowel surgery or when foreign material is to be implanted (prosthetic joints, arterial grafts). It is essential to ensure that the patient is questioned about possible allergies to antibiotics (and other drugs) beforehand and that this information is recorded in the notes.

ANTITHROMBOTIC PROPHYLAXIS

It is usual to restrict this form of prophylaxis to patients who are at high risk of developing deep venous thrombosis (Table 8.10). However, some surgeons and anaesthetists prescribe low dose heparin for all patients undergoing major operations. In recent years there has been a trend towards low molecular weight heparin (enoxaparin) which is said to have a more sustained and reliable action. Heparin should not be prescribed for patients with bleeding or clotting abnormalities, before ophthalmic or neurosurgery, or for those with hypertension, peptic ulceration or oesophageal varices. The prophylactic regimen may consist of heparin 5 000 units by subcutaneous injection 8 to 12 hourly beginning the evening before operation. Alternatively, low molecular weight heparin (enoxaparin) 20 mg can be given subcutaneously 1–2 h before surgery followed by 20 mg daily for 7 to 10 days. For patients at very high risk these doses may be doubled. Other alternatives include dextran 70 in saline solution 500 ml at induction of anaesthesia and daily thereafter for two days. Monitoring coagulation is usually unnecessary during prophylactic therapy.

Neither the progesterone-only contraceptive pill nor hormone replacement therapy appear to constitute significant risks and specific antithrombotic prophylaxis is unnecessary in the absence of other risk factors.

Table 8.10 Risk factors for deep venous thrombosis

Obesity
Previous thrombosis
Bed rest, immobility
Dehydration
Pain
Malignant disease
Pelvic, lower limb surgery
Arterial, cardiac surgery
Cigarette smoking
Polycythaemia
Oestrogen-containing contraceptive pill

ALPHA ADRENOCEPTOR AGONISTS

These drugs are of considerable theoretical interest in anaesthesia and are currently being investigated. Clonidine 0.2 mg by mouth has similar anxiolytic properties to temazepam 20 mg. Although these drugs have analgesic and sedative actions they cannot be recommended for routine premedication because of their tendency to cause hypotension. Dexmedetomidine is believed to have a more specific action than clonidine and is currently being studied in humans.

FURTHER READING

Berry, F. A. (1991) Preoperative fasting. *Current Opinion in Anesthesiology*, **4**, 359–362.

Bilous, R. W. (1996) Diabetic nephropathy. *Prescribers' Journal*, **36**, 78–84.

Deroy, R. and Graham, T. R. Pacemakers and anaesthesia. *Current Anaesthesia and Critical Care*, **6**, 171–179.

Goldman, L. (1988) Assessment of the patient with known or suspected ischaemic heart disease for non-cardiac surgery. *British Journal of Anaesthesia*, **61**, 38–43.

Goldman, L., Caldera, D. L., Nussbaum, S. R. et al. (1977) Multifactorial index of cardiac risk in non-cardiac surgical procedures. *New England Journal of Medicine*, **297**, 845–850.

Haagensen, R. and Steen, P. A. (1988) Perioperative myocardial infarction. *British Journal of Anaesthesia*, **61**, 24–37.

Juste, R. N., Lawson, A. D. and Soni, N. (1996) Minimizing cardiac anaesthetic risk: the tortoise or the hare? *Anaesthesia*, **51**, 255–262.

Mangano, D. T. (1990) Perioperative cardiac morbidity. *Anesthesiology*, **72**, 153–184.

Mangano, D. T. and Goldman, L. (1995) Preoperative assessment of patients with known or suspected coronary disease. *New England Journal of Medicine*, **333**, 1750–1756.

Muir, A. D., Reeder, M. K., Foëx, P. et al. (1991) Preoperative silent myocardial ischaemia: incidence and predictors in a general surgical population. *British Journal of Anaesthesia*, **67**, 373–377.

PREOPERATIVE TESTS

W. J. Fawcett

The function of preoperative tests is to provide information additional to that already obtained from the history and examination. They should only be used when they add significantly to this information. Preoperative tests should be reserved for patients in whom the results from the tests would change the patient's management (such as the timing of surgery or the anaesthetic technique) or add further to the evaluation of the perioperative risk.

The prime objective of preoperative assessment is to determine physiological reserve, especially that of the cardiovascular and respiratory systems, and therefore the bulk of routinely used tests are cardiorespiratory. Considerable perioperative demands may be placed on these systems, particularly following major surgery. The cardiovascular system may have to cope with large changes in fluid balance and there may be changes in respiratory function that last several days postoperatively. Thus, patients in whom there is limited cardiorespiratory reserve will require further careful evaluation with preoperative tests.

Preoperative tests may be divided into two categories: those for further investigation of the patient with a known medical condition and those used as a screening procedure to detect silent and important abnormalities in the wider population.

In the past it was common practice to screen patients with tests such as the electrocardiogram, chest X-ray, haemoglobin and electrolytes and urea estimations. The incidence of significant abnormalities found by such screening is low (0.1–0.5%) and rises, not surprisingly, with age. These abnormalities generally have no effect on mortality or morbidity; indeed widepread screening has not been shown to have any effect on improving outcome. Moreover, a number of normal patients lie outside the commonly accepted limits. With a normally distributed variable, 5% of patients lie outside the mean ± two standard deviations. These false positive patients may then have surgery unnecessarily delayed and be subjected to further tests, adding to already considerable expense. Also with many tests it is unclear what age or gender of patients need to be screened. The ideal screening test is one which has high specificity (a high pick up rate of those with the disease) and sensitivity (a high rejection rate of those without the disease) in looking for a condition which is common, serious and not readily detectable from the history and examination. There are few, if any, tests that approach this ideal.

Thus, in recent years the widespread practice of screening patients has decreased as it adds little to the patient's overall preoperative assessment and it is not cost effective. A rational approach would be to question not only which test is to be ordered, but also whether or not any test should be ordered.

Short Practice of Anaesthesia. Edited by M. Morgan and G. M. Hall. Published in 1997 by Chapman & Hall, London. ISBN 0 412 71890 1

CARDIOVASCULAR SYSTEM

Nearly 20 years ago, Goldman described a multifactorial index of cardiac risk for non-cardiac surgical operations and, despite several modifications of his original index, a number of factors clearly influence cardiac risk in non-cardiac surgery. Two very important clinical entities are those of ischaemic heart disease (IHD) and left ventricular dysfunction, with recent myocardial infarction and congestive cardiac failure of particular importance. Also of importance are valvular heart disease, hypertension and cardiac arrhythmias. Cardiovascular tests are therefore used to determine baseline function, detect and quantify abnormalities, and assess risk.

ELECTROCARDIOGRAPHY (ECG)

Resting 12 lead ECG is one of the most commonly requested preoperative investigations, both as a further investigation of patients known to have cardiac disease, and as a screen for the population as a whole.

The incidence of ECG abnormalities for both symptomatic and asymptomatic patients increases approximately exponentially with age. As a screening procedure for the general population, however, the pickup rate for significant abnormalities (i.e. those that influence anaesthetic management) is very low. Although a case was made for screening all men over the age of 30 and women over 40 by the American Medical Association, usual practice in the UK would probably restrict these tests to those of 60 years of age or over.

The ECG is important in two main clinical areas: rhythm and conduction disturbances and IHD. Whilst there is overlap between the two areas, as IHD may be the underlying factor causing arrhythmias or heart block, a number of patients will have primary rhythm or conduction abnormalities that require treatment before surgery. Rapid tachyarrhythmias such as atrial fibrillation, flutter or atrioventricular nodal rhythm will require preoperative control to a resting ventricular response rate of below 80–90 b.p.m. Bradyarrhythmias (such as complete heart block), particularly if associated with syncope, will require preoperative pacing. Asymptomatic bifasicular block (right bundle branch block with left anterior or posterior hemiblock) would not usually require pacing, but if this coexists with second degree heart block, many would establish central venous access and have pacing facilities on hand should a deterioration to complete heart block occur. One caveat is that a 12 lead ECG gives only a snapshot of the cardiac electrical activity at that time it was taken, so that paroxysmal arrhythmias for example may not be detected.

More importantly, the ECG is commonly used for patients with suspected or known IHD. There are several pitfalls with this. Although ECG abnormalities are common in patient with IHD, up to a third of patients with 75–100% occlusion of a major coronary artery have a normal ECG. Moreover, there are many ECG abnormalities associated with myocardial ischaemia such as rhythm and conduction abnormalities, pathological Q waves, poor R wave progression, ST depression or elevation and T wave changes. Also, there may be other factors that make interpretation of the ECG difficult. In particular analysis of the ST segment is complicated by bundle branch block, pacing, left ventricular hypertrophy, digoxin therapy and electrolyte abnormalities. Overall, in patients with IHD, although many have found the 12 lead ECG a sensitive (although non-specific) indicator of cardiac outcome, others have failed to find it predictive. Perhaps its most useful role is in the detection of previously unrecognized myocardial infarction, both acute and chronic, when the anaesthetic technique may be modified or further investigations ordered.

It is unclear how often ECGs should be repeated before surgery. It seems that new changes are not infrequent: up to half of abnormalities may arise within a two year period. Thus, it seems prudent to arrange new ECGs where indicated before all surgery irrespective of the date of the last test. Previous recordings may then be used for comparison.

In summary, a 12 lead ECG is usually requested as screening procedure for patients over the age of 60, or in patients under this age with symptoms or signs of cardiac disease. Its usefulness depends on correct interpretation by the anaesthetist. A patient with an abnormal ECG may require further investigation or treatment before surgery. A normal ECG may be found in patients in whom there is a high risk of cardiac complications, such as those with severe IHD or ventricular failure. Further data are required to establish its place as an accurate predictor of morbidity and mortality.

EXERCISE ECG

It might be anticipated that an exercise ECG would provide further indication of cardiovascular reserve. Indeed, for high risk patients such as those undergoing vascular surgery, there are a number of studies demonstrating that there is a positive predictive value for postoperative myocardial infarction (MI) with this investigation, although the history and resting ECG may have been normal in a third of patients. In contrast, when the exercise ECG is used as a screening test for major non-vascular surgery, it has been shown to have little or no predictive value for postoperative MI. Although the exercise ECG may be useful in identifying high risk patients, there are a number of problems. Firstly, the cardiovascular changes of an exercise test (particularly tachycardia) have little in common with those occurring in the perioperative' period, when changes such as hypertension, hypoxaemia and hypercoagubility may play a major role. In addition, some patients, such as those with intermittent claudication or severe arthritis, may be unable to perform an exercise test. However, the overall benefits of this procedure need emphasizing. It is cheap, safe (the mortality is probably less than 1 in 10 000) and useful in both confirming the diagnosis, and to some extent the prognosis, of patients with IHD. In particular, severe ischaemia is suggested by early onset of severe ST depression, subnormal increases in heart rate or blood pressure, and arrhythmias. It may also provide an indication of the haemodynamic thresholds of ischaemia.

There are a number of more recently described tests, some of which are suitable for patients who are unable to exercise. These include ambulatory ECG monitoring, dipyridamole thallium scintigraphy, radionuclide ventriculography to calculate ejection fraction and the use of dobutamine and other agents for stress echocardiography.

AMBULATORY ECG MONITORING

This is a useful test which may prove to have a better predictive value than the exercise ECG. Patients are monitored preferably for 48 h. The presence of significant ST depression (>1 mm, lasting in excess of 1 min) appears to correlate with postoperative infarction rates, although more recent studies show a lower predictive value. However, although preoperative ischaemia may be a major factor in determining postoperative problems, one weakness of ambulatory ECG is its inability to detect the patients at lower risk, such as those aged less than 70 years, or who do not have IHD or diabetes. Further difficulties with this technique include obtaining a stable baseline, ST changes that result from changes in posture, and ventricular arrhythmias. Overall, ambulatory ECG monitoring has demonstrated that silent ischaemia is common and may be as important as symptomatic ischaemia as an indicator of cardiac events. It may also have role as a predictor of long-term outcome. Further studies are required to confirm its usefulness as a preoperative predictor of cardiac events.

DIPYRIDAMOLE THALLIUM SCINTIGRAPHY (DTS)

DTS works on the principle that following administration of thallium-201, which is taken up by perfused myocardium, imaging the heart will leave a perfusion deficit ('cold spot') in areas of absent or poor perfusion, such as myocardial infarction or ischaemia. Although a sensitive test, isolated thallium imaging lacks specificity. When thallium imaging is performed during conditions of increased coronary blood flow the test becomes much more specific. Whilst exercise may be used to produce an increase in blood flow, in patients who are unable to tolerate this a similar effect can be achieved with the use of coronary vasodilators such as dipyridamole (or more recently adenosine) before the administration of the thallium. A perfusion deficit may be identified as either a fixed defect over areas of myocardial infarction or as a transient defect (reperfusion or redistribution defects), in which an image will appear some 3–4 h later, in areas of viable myocardium perfused by stenosed coronary arteries. Sometimes later imaging at 18–24 h or a second dose of thallium may be required to differentiate between fixed and redistribution defects.

Overall DTS is both sensitive and specific for the detection of coronary artery disease and so for risk stratification following non-cardiac surgery. A number of studies over the last ten years have suggested DTS to be a reliable predictor of postoperative cardiac outcome, with only one major study confounding this finding. Moreover, when DTS is combined with clinical data, the predictive value is improved still further. Eagle has assessed patients for the presence or absence of a number of clinical markers. These were Q waves on the ECG, ventricular ectopics, age >70 years, a history of angina or diabetes.

The data have had a major impact on the assessment of middle-risk patients. If patients had one or two clinical markers and a positive DTS, there was a 30% cardiac ischaemic event rate, whereas in patients in whom there were one or two markers but a negative DTS there was only a 3% cardiac ischaemic event rate (and no mortality): the same rate as for those with no clinical factors. On the other hand, patients with either none of these risk factors or with three or more risk factors were at very low or high risk respectively, regardless of the DTS result, and indeed the DTS test was probably unnecessary. Another refinement in the use of DTS is the quantitative assessment of redistribution rather than a purely qualitative assessment (i.e. presence or absence), which may also increase its predictive value.

DTS is not without its risks. It may precipitate angina, MI and, in about 1 in 2000 cases, death. It may also cause bronchospasm and is thus contraindicated in patients with asthma and chronic obstructive airways disease. In addition, it requires delayed imaging at 3–4 h and possibly at 24 h. There are, moreover, a few reported failures in the detection of severe coronary artery disease, notably in patients with severe triple vessel disease and no normal myocardium to contrast reperfusion. This will result in a failure to predict cardiac events following vascular surgery.

The bulk of published data relates to patients scheduled for vascular surgery and there is little evidence to support its use for patients undergoing other surgical procedures.

RADIONUCLIDE VENTRICULOGRAPHY (RNV)

Patients with depressed left ventricular function and/or advanced signs of congestive cardiac failure have consistently been demonstrated to have an increased cardiac risk. Both Goldman and Larsen identified clinical markers of ventricular failure as the highest scoring factor in predicting adverse cardiac outcome. RNV assesses ventricular function in terms of ejection fraction. A commonly used indicator of poor left ventricular function is an ejection fraction of <35%. Early studies appeared to identify patients who were at increased risk from myocardial infarction when undergoing vascular surgery but, perhaps surprisingly, more recent studies have questioned its predictive value, even after exercise. In the largest study to date, Baron has shown RNV to be predictive of postoperative left ventricular failure, but not an independent predictor of postoperative myocardial infarction, prolonged ischaemia or death. Other studies suggest that a low ejection fraction is associated with a poorer long-term survival.

ECHOCARDIOGRAPHY

Another way of assessing ventricular function is by echocardiography. It gives information on ventricular filling, ejection and contractility. In addition, myocardial ischaemia is associated with characteristic appearances within the ventricular wall termed segmental wall motion abnormalities. A more important assessment of left ventricular function is its response to exercise or pharmacological stress. Exercise echocardiography has a sensitivity similar to, or perhaps better than, exercise ECG in the diagnosis of IHD, particularly when there is single vessel disease. However a major problem is the necessity for experienced echocardiographers, particularly with the artefacts caused by the movement of exercise. Stress echocardiography, using pharmacological agents such as dobutamine, dipyridamole or adenosine appears to be a suitable alternative. Dobutamine stress echocardiography involves observing patients for either worsening of pre-existing wall motion abnormalities or development of new segmental wall motion abnormalities during a dobutamine infusion. The results of dobutamine stress echocardiography appear to be encouraging, with a superior predictive value compared with ambulatory ECG, DTS and RNV, although the numbers of published studies are small to date. Moreover, the trend so far is that, unlike the aforementioned tests, the predictive value of dobutamine stress echocardiography is increasing in recent studies. For example, it has been demonstrated that after a negative test patients experienced no cardiac complications, whereas the complication rate was approximately 40% in those in whom the test was positive. Furthermore, over 80%, of patients with a positive test had >50% luminal narrowing in one or more coronary arteries and preoperative intervention (coronary artery surgery or angioplasty) resulted in an uneventful perioperative period.

Dobutamine stress echocardiography is not without adverse effects; life-threatening arrhythmias may occur, although overall it appears to be safe without serious complications due to myocardial ischaemia, is relatively quick (it usually takes less than 1 h) and may be performed as an outpatient procedure.

Vasodilators such as dipyridamole and adenosine have been used successfully with echocardiography and are reported as highly specific and sensitive tests for the diagnosis of IHD and for the prediction of perioperative cardiac events. Further data are awaited on these agents, but dipyridamole in particular appears to offer excellent positive (78%) and negative (99%) predictive values for patients suffering cardiac events after vascular surgery.

OTHER TESTS

No mention has been made of one of the most commonly requested investigations for patients with cardiovascular disease, the chest X-ray. There are, surprisingly, few data to support its use. It adds little to the assessment of the patient with uncomplicated, known or suspected, IHD, but in those patients with an enlarged heart or who have interstitial or alveolar pulmonary oedema, there are characteristic X-ray changes and these warrant further investigation. Clinical indices, perhaps supplemented by echocardiography or RNV will provide greater information in terms of assessment, response to treatment and prognosis for patients with poor left ventricular function. A further problem is that some chest X-ray appearances, such as those of pulmonary oedema, can lag several days behind the clinical situation. A chest X-ray may be a useful baseline for changes expected in the postoperative period, such as for ventilated patients or patients undergoing thoracic surgery or major upper abdominal surgery. Overall, in many cases it is unlikely to change anaesthetic management or to help in quantifying perioperative cardiac risk. An enlarged heart will be a starting point for further evaluation, particularly for patients scheduled for major surgery.

For some years intensivists have focused on oxygen delivery as a predictor of postoperative outcome. There are a few studies in which patients have been investigated by the use of a pulmonary artery catheter before undergoing major surgery and where measuring and manipulating variables such as pulmonary capillary wedge pressure, cardiac output and O_2 delivery with combinations of fluids and inotropes or vasoactive drugs, has resulted in dramatically improved outcome for high-risk patients. For example, patients with an O_2 delivery in excess of 600 ml min^{-1} m^{-2} had a 75% reduction in mortality, compared with those who did not. A drawback is the heterogeneous group of patients included in such studies. Further data are awaited to confirm the value of measuring and optimizing haemodynamic and oxygen transport variables. However, these studies are of interest in that they document the sequence of testing, intervention and its effect on outcome.

SUMMARY

With a large number of tests described for investigating a patient with known or suspected cardiac disease, a practical approach is required. Careful clinical assessment, with history and examination, cannot be overemphasized. Together with a resting ECG, those patients who appear to be at high risk from cardiac events (infarction or death) as calculated by one of the major cardiac risk indices such as Goldman or Larsen need further evaluation. This would include those who have or have had ventricular failure, IHD (myocardial infarction or angina) or who are old and, to a lesser extent, those with diabetes or renal impairment. Another major factor is the proposed surgery, with vascular surgery widely accepted as posing a high risk of peroperative ischaemia. Patients who are identified as at low risk by this approach probably do not benefit from further investigation, particularly if they have good exercise tolerance. Patients recognized to be at higher risk, either from their underlying condition, or from the proposed surgery, need further investigation to attempt to quantify the risk. Further tests include an exercise ECG in patients who can exercise, or ambulatory ECG, or pharmacological stress testing in those who cannot (if available).

With those patients who are at high risk of perioperative events, aggressive intervention such as coronary artery surgery may then be warranted, although coronary artery surgery carries it own mortality (1–2%) and the overall benefits of this are still debated. Another approach would be to subject these patients to intense, perioperative monitoring and treatment.

This is an evolving subject and there are several areas of current interest. Eagle's study suggests that the combination of clinical risk factors, as well as some form of stress testing, may prove to yield the best prognostic data. There are a number of encouraging results particularly from stress echocardiography, and although a number of other tests appear to have declined in predictive value over the past few years, this may be a reflection of improved perioperative management. Finally, with the realization that postoperative myocardial ischaemia and not preoperative ischaemia is the strongest predictor of perioperative morbidity, emphasis will undoubtedly shift from the preoperative tests to postoperative therapies for patients with cardiac disease.

RESPIRATORY SYSTEM

A major problem in evaluating respiratory system investigations is that large studies in patients with severe respiratory disease are lacking. Nevertheless, there are two main areas that need to be addressed: the assessment of the patient for non-thoracic surgery and that of the patient undergoing thoracic surgery.

NON-THORACIC SURGERY

For patients undergoing non-thoracic surgery, there are a number of areas of interest concerning preoperative investigations. First, which patients should be subjected to preoperative respiratory investigations? Second, what influence does general or regional anaesthesia have in terms of outcome in patients with respiratory disease? Finally, are there predictive values for patients who will require postoperative respiratory support in the postoperative period?

Chest X-ray

There are a number of tests available for investigating the respiratory system. The most commonly requested is probably the chest X-ray. The usefulness of this test is a contentious issue. Some argue that it adds little to overall assessment that is not detected from preoperative history and examination. Others argue that it is a useful investigation that should be applied to all patients over the age of 60 years and patients with any cardiorespiratory disease. There are, however, very little data on how chest X-ray appearances are related to postoperative outcome. Indeed, many studies emphasize the variation in criteria for ordering chest X-rays both within and between anaesthetic departments, that the vast majority of abnormalities were not unexpected, and that only rarely was surgery postponed or the anaesthetic technique significantly altered as a direct result of the chest X-ray. The Royal College of Radiologists recommends that preoperative X-rays are performed on patients with acute respiratory symptoms, those with possible metastases, those with cardiorespiratory disease who have not been X-rayed in the preceding 12 months and immigrants from countries where tuberculosis is endemic. There is no mention of age or type of surgery.

There are certain chest X-ray appearances that would nevertheless affect anaesthetic management. Pneumothoraces and large pleural effusions should be drained and extreme caution exercised in the use of intermittent positive pressure ventilation in the presence of bullae. Deviation or compression of the trachea should alert the anaesthetist to possible airway difficulties, and areas of pulmonary collapse and consolidation should be investigated and treated, if possible before surgery.

Spirometry

Spirometry is, in one from or another, available in almost every hospital. Commonly measured variables include forced vital capacity (FVC) which is the exhaled volume recorded following a maximal inspiratory effort. The FVC is usually decreased with restrictive defects (pneumonia, pulmonary oedema or fibrosis) or in respiratory muscle weakness or embarrassment such as myopathies, abdominal distension and pain. The FVC is conventionally subdivided into the

FEV$_1$ (exhaled volume recorded in 1 s) and this figure is then expressed as a ratio of the FVC: the FEV$_1$/FVC ratio or forced expiratory ratio (FER). Usually diseases associated with airway obstruction have a decreased FER, whereas restrictive diseases have a preserved FER. Normal spirometry is usually defined as an FVC of >80% predicted, with FER >90% predicted. An obstructive defect is defined as an FVC of >80% predicted, with FER <90% predicted; a restrictive defect as an FVC of <80% predicted and FER >90% predicted. Other tests include peak expiratory flow rate (PEFR) which is a widely available measurement of airway obstruction (and the response to bronchodilators) and the maximal voluntary ventilation (MVV) sometimes termed maximal breathing capacity (MBC). There are a number of other tests that are usually available within a modern respiratory function laboratory. These include flow–volume loops for elucidating the site and extent of airway obstruction (such as intrathoracic or extrathoracic), measurement of total lung capacity (TLC), residual volume (RV), diffusing capacity for carbon monoxide (Dco) and closing volume (CV), but in general these measurements are not so useful for preanaesthetic assessment in terms of their predictive value for postoperative complications.

There are a number of published criteria for guidelines for preoperative spirometry. Generally these include patients for upper abdominal or thoracic surgery, patients with evidence of chronic respiratory disease (heavy smokers, dyspnoea or persistent cough) and the morbidly obese. In spite of this, the majority of publications focus not on the value of the tests, but more on anaesthetists' failure to adhere to these guidelines.

Arterial blood gas analysis

Arterial blood gas analysis is a useful adjunct for patients with significant respiratory disease. It should be performed with the patient at complete rest and be preceded by the use of local anaesthetic to the sampling site (usually the radial artery) as hyperventilation induced by the pain of the procedure will have a significant impact on the results. Arterial blood gas analysis is useful for determining the severity of gas exchange abnormalities and providing guidelines for postoperative management. The arterial partial pressure of oxygen (Pao$_2$), together with a calculation of the alveolar partial pressure of oxygen (PAO$_2$) enables the alveolar–arterial oxygen gradient (PAO$_2$ − Pao$_2$) to be determined. The PAO$_2$ is estimated by calculating first the inspired oxygen partial pressure (PIO$_2$) from barometric pressure (PB):

$$P\text{IO}_2 = (P\text{B} - 6.2)\ F\text{IO}_2\ (\text{kPa})$$

and then using the alveolar gas equation:

$$P\text{AO}_2 = P\text{IO}_2 - P\text{aCO}_2/RQ,$$

where RQ is the respiratory quotient, and is usually taken as 0.8. For a healthy patient breathing air, the PAO$_2$ is estimated as follows:

$$\begin{aligned}P\text{AO}_2 &= P\text{IO}_2 - P\text{aCO}_2/0.8 \\ &= 20 - 5.3/0.8 \\ &= 13.4\ \text{kPa}\end{aligned}$$

Following this estimation and knowing the Pao$_2$, the PAO$_2$ − Pao$_2$ can be calculated. A marked gradient may be caused by any right to left intracardiac shunt and by a severe decrease in cardiac output, but in the absence of these, it reflects the degree of ventilation–perfusion mismatch. It is noteworthy that correct interpretation of Pao$_2$ requires knowledge of the FIO$_2$ and PaCO$_2$. As shown above, a grossly elevated PaCO$_2$ will cause hypoxaemia in a patient breathing room air. If the PAO$_2$ − Pao$_2$ is normal (less than 1 kPa) it implies that the hypoxaemia is due to elevated PaCO$_2$ and not to a shunt.

The arterial partial pressure of carbon dioxide (PaCO$_2$) is also of great importance. Retention of carbon dioxide e.g. PaCO$_2$ > 8 kPa in patients with chronic lung disease implies that respiratory drive is lost centrally and driven by hypoxaemia at the peripheral chemoreceptors. In this case, a high inspired oxygen in the perioperative period will depress and ultimately stop respiration.

Finally, the pH is noted. In patients with long standing respiratory disease, the pH is usually about normal, with respiratory acidosis compensated by a metabolic alkalosis. Marked pH abnormalites are commonly due to acute disturbances, usually in Pa_{CO_2}.

Evaluation of tests

There are a number of factors which place patients with lung disease undergoing non-thoracic surgery at added risk of pulmonary complications. Patients undergoing upper abdominal surgery are at highest risk, with those having peripheral surgery at less risk. In addition, obesity, age and smoking also place the patient at increased risk. There are, however, little data on how preoperative tests may improve assessment of patient risk.

In 1962 it was demonstrated that of all the tests available, a peak expiratory flow rate (PEFR) of less than 200 l min^{-1} was the best predictor of the development of postoperative complications, although FEV_1 and FVC were also significantly reduced preoperatively in these patients. Later studies confirmed this and demonstrated that an FER of <65%, an FVC of <70–75% predicted and a MVV finding of less than 50% predicted, were also significant in this regard. If there was no improvement in these tests after preoperative treatment (bronchodilators and/or physiotherapy) then the patient was deemed to be at further risk. In one of the largest studies to date, Nunn looked at 42 patients with severe chronic obstructive airways disease, in whom the FEV_1 was in the range 0.3–1 l. It was demonstrated that the best predictors of the need for postoperative ventilation were first a Pa_{O_2} of less than approximately 7 kPa or 70% of normal, and second, dypsnoea at rest. They found that other factors including age, upper abdominal surgery, regional anaesthesia, FEV_1, FER, and Pa_{CO_2} added nothing to the predictive value. They emphasize that a large battery of tests for patients undergoing non-thoracic surgery is unnecessary and the benefit unproven, and agree with Gass and Olsen's review that there is no test result which absolutely contraindicates surgery.

THORACIC SURGERY

In contrast to patients undergoing non-thoracic surgery, patients undergoing thoracic surgery have been the subject of many studies over the last forty years. A posteriorantero chest X-ray is useful to determine the anatomy of the trachea and bronchi, which may be of value in predicting difficulty in the passage of an endobronchial tube. Respiratory function tests and in particular FEV_1, FVC, FER, MVV, PEFR as well as RV and D_{CO} are commonly advocated, as is arterial blood gas analysis. There are two further areas of testing that may be undertaken, those of split lung function studies and exercise testing.

Split lung function studies

Split lung function studies, which may be used to quantify ventilation and perfusion in both lungs, allow the impact of a proposed lung resection to be estimated. The earliest form of split lung function studies involved placement of a double lumen tube in awake patients and measuring exhaled volumes from each lung in a technique termed bronchospirometry. Patients were tested in both the supine and left and right lateral positions. During lateral positioning both ventilation and perfusion shift to the dependent lung, permitting the contribution of each lung to total lung function to be quantified. It was for this type of testing that Carlens originally described the use of a double lumen tube. A less invasive assessment of split lung spirometry, termed radiospirometry, quantifies differential lung function following the administration of isotopes such as xenon-133 by counting activity over each lung. Using these techniques postoperative lung function can be calculated from the equation:

predicted postoperative FEV_1 = preoperative FEV_1 × percentage function of remaining lung tissue

In addition to tests of ventilation, it has been appreciated for many years that a major limiting factor affecting mortality and morbidity following lung resection was the disturbance in pulmonary blood flow resulting in pulmonary hypertension and right ventricular failure. Exercise limitation in many of these patients was due to reduced cardiac output. Thus a number of studies have evaluated the impact of temporary unilateral pulmonary artery occlusion on mean pulmonary artery pressures in an attempt to characterize these changes. The method involves measuring pulmonary artery pressures and Pa_{O_2} at rest and exercise, both before and during total balloon occlusion of the pulmonary artery on the diseased side. Unfortunately the procedure carries a technical failure rate of about 25% and is of historical interest only. Radioperfusion tests, using iodine-131 or technetium-99m provide information on differential lung perfusion.

Exercise testing

Exercise testing has assumed growing importance in the past 10 years. The emphasis of preoperative testing for patients undergoing lung resection has been to combine assessment of both ventilatory and cardiovascular reserve; this is achieved by exercise testing. In particular, it mimics the increase in pulmonary blood flow that occurs to remaining lung tissue after resection. Generally, there is a breath-by-breath measurement of airflow and gas exchange together with pulse oximetry, during a bout of exercise, such as cycle ergometry. A commonly measured endpoint is that of maximal oxygen consumption ($\dot{V}_{O_2 max}$). Moreover exercise testing can, in theory, separate cardiac from respiratory limitation. In spite of the relative simplicity of the technique there are a number of unresolved problems. In particular, there is no agreed protocol for exercise testing, which makes it difficult to compare studies. Some have used maximal, and others have used submaximal work rates, and the work rate may be constant, or incremental, in nature.

Evaluation of tests

Of the many tests available for patients scheduled for thoracic surgery which provide the best prognostic information? Forty years ago it was demonstrated that patients whose MVV was less than 50% of predicted and with an FVC of less than 70% had a 40% mortality following resection, or lung collapse, for pulmonary tuberculosis. A number of subsequent studies have agreed with the figure of 50% MVV, and in addition, patients with an FVC and FER of less than 50% predicted, an FEV_1 of less than 2 l, RV/TLC of greater than 50% and a D_{CO} of less than 50% predicted, had a poor prognosis after pneumonectomy. Of interest, patients with a nonspecifically abnormal ECG had a mortality of 46%. Some have applied absolute, rather than percentage values, and patients with an FVC of less than 1.7 l, RV greater than 3.3 l and a TLC greater than 7.9 l, an RV/TLC greater than 47%, an FEV_1 less than 1.2 l or 35%, all have a high risk for lung resection.

For patients in whom a calculation of postoperative FEV_1 is made (such as those having undergone split lung function studies), an estimated FEV_1 of 0.8–1 l is widely regarded as the minimum compatible with a reasonable level of daily activity. Others have chosen to quote a predicted value of less than 30% of normal as a cut-off point. In addition, a preoperative Pa_{CO_2} in excess of 6 kPa is regarded by several workers as placing patients for lung resection at greater risk.

The crucial effects of pulmonary hypertension and cor pulmonale have been specifically addressed in a number of studies. It appears, pooling the available data, that a resting pulmonary artery pressure of greater than 22 mmHg, rising to greater than 32 mmHg during temporary unilateral pulmonary artery occlusion and in excess of 35 mmHg during exercise with occlusion, with a concomitant Pa_{O_2} of less than 6 kPa, are associated with increased mortality after lung resection. A more straightforward estimation is that of pulmonary vascular resistance (PVR), which if rising during exercise to greater than 190 dyne s cm^{-5} predicts a high mortality (100% in one study).

Formal, non-invasive, exercise testing has an evolving role in the prediction of post-thoracotomy complications. In one striking study those patients with a $\dot{V}_{O_2\,max}$ of less than 15 ml kg^{-1} min^{-1} experienced a 100% complication rate, 15–20 ml kg^{-1} min^{-1} a 66% complication rate, and greater than 20 ml kg^{-1} min^{-1} a 10% complication rate. Of particular interest, the classical respiratory function tests were not significantly different between the two groups. Whilst several other studies demonstrate a predictive role for exercise testing and in particular estimation of $\dot{V}_{O_2\,max}$, this still awaits confirmation and acceptance.

CARDIAC SURGERY

In spite of considerable data on lung surgery, there are very few data on patients undergoing cardiac surgery. Although patients with decreased spirometric lung function studies have been shown in one study to have a longer stay in intensive care, the majority of the complications necessitating this extra stay were non-pulmonary. It would appear that the high quality of immediate postoperative care that is widely available in cardiac surgical units overrides the influence of poor postoperative function, with other factors determining postoperative morbidity and mortality.

In summary, despite the wealth of investigations that are available for the assessment of the respiratory system of patients undergoing non-thoracic surgery, there is no single test which contraindicates surgery, and the estimated risks of the surgery must be clearly weighed against the benefits. There is very little information attempting to resolve whether regional or general anaesthesia is preferable in patients with severe lung disease, or what are the predictors for postoperative respiratory support.

In spite of some compelling evidence for the predictive value of a number of preoperative tests for patients scheduled for lung resection, the poor survival rate from carcinoma of the bronchus must also be borne in mind, with surgery offering the only chance of long-term survival.

OTHER TESTS

THE AIRWAY

Assessment of a patient's airway is an essential part of any preoperative visit. There are two main areas of interest: the prediction of difficult tracheal intubation and the unstable cervical spine.

There are a number of bedside tests available for predicting difficult intubation, but a major problem is that they are approximately only 80% specific and sensitive: combining tests may improve the situation (such as Mallampati's test, and thyromental distance). Although X-rays of the mandible and cervical spine have been advocated to describe anatomical features that are associated with difficult intubation, there are no large scale predictive studies to support their use. A number of radiological features are described, in particular loss of the atlanto-occipital or atlanto-axial gaps, which limit head extension. It is widely believed that failure of extension at C0–C1 (and to a lesser extent C1–C2) is an important cause of difficult intubation. More recently, however, it has been argued that head extension is limited by the tectorial membrane, (a prolongation of the posterior longitudinal ligament) and not by abutment of bones, so the use of radiographical markers may be misleading. A second radiographical measurement is that of the posterior mandibular depth. When increased, it is associated with a difficult intubation. It is usually expressed as a ratio of the effective mandibular length, whereby if the mandibular length is less than 3.6 times the length of the posterior mandibular depth, direct laryngoscopy is difficult and vice versa.

Overall, there is no single test that is reliable in predicting a difficult intubation. There are a number of factors, other than bony structures, that are important in determining ease of laryngoscopy and intubation, such as size of the soft tissues (particularly the base of the tongue), mobility of the temporomandibular joint, thyromental distance, body weight and presence of protruding teeth. Thus, although radiological tests may help in theory, their place is largely unproven and it is impractical to screen all patients at risk.

A separate area is that of the unstable neck following trauma, or associated with joint or bone disease such as rheumatoid arthritis. Here, cervical spine X-rays are required and should be scrutinized for joint space, loss of bony alignment and bone destruction. Of particular importance in rheumatoid arthritis is neck flexion, where the odontoid peg may move posteriorly and compress the spinal cord and/or the vertebral arteries. If the distance between the anterior margin of the odontoid peg and the posterior margin of the anterior arch of the axis is greater than 3 mm on flexion X-rays, then the patient is at risk of spinal cord damage. It is noteworthy that patients with Down's syndrome are at risk of cervical cord damage even with normal X-rays.

HAEMATOLOGY

The most commonly requested blood test is a full blood count and, in particular, the haemoglobin concentration. Like many of the cardiovascular and respiratory investigations, the concept of physiological reserve is vital for any patient undergoing surgery. In the case of haemoglobin, the oxygen carrying reserve is relevant. For the body as a whole, oxygen delivery is defined as:

$$Hb(g\ 100\ ml^{-1}) \times Sao_2(\%) \times CI\ (l\ min^{-1} m^{-2}) \times 0.134$$

where Sao_2 is arterial oxygen saturation, and CI is cardiac index. This is expressed in ml min^{-1} m^{-2}, and ignores dissolved oxygen. Following oxygen extraction in the tissues, the oxygen content of blood returning to the heart is calculated as follows:

$$Hb(g\ 100\ ml^{-1}) \times Svo_2(\%) \times CI\ (l\ min^{-1}\ m^{-2}) \times 0.134$$

where Svo_2 represents mixed venous oxygen saturation. Oxygen consumption is thus given by:

$$Hb \times (Sao_2 - Svo_2) \times CI \times 0.134$$

Given figures of an Sao_2 of 100% and an Svo_2 of 75%, the oxygen extraction ratio (OER) is 25%. However, OER varies markedly between tissues, with some like the heart having a high OER (over 60%), and the skin having a low OER (approximately 10%). There is a limit for oxygen extraction, around 65%, below which, hypoxia and acidosis are inevitable consequences. Thus, if there is a low haemoglobin there will be considerably less reserve for tissue oxygenation, particularly for tissues with high OERs. Should any of the other factors in the oxygen delivery equation fall, such as cardiac output or Sao_2, this deficit would be exaggerated. This lack of reserve is present even though oxygen transport and OER may be satisfactory at rest due to compensatory changes such as decreased viscosity, increased cardiac output and increased 2,3 diphosphoglycerate values which shift the oxygen dissociation curve to the right, and aid oxygen transfer at the tissues. Moreover, in patients with IHD, anaemia will cause a compensatory increase in cardiac output and this in itself may precipitate myocardial ischaemia. Coupled with the marked increase in oxygen demands that may occur following major surgery, these patients will clearly be at risk from anaemia which is not offset by the small improvement in flow afforded by the reduced viscosity.

Who are the patients, therefore, to benefit from preoperative haemoglobin estimations? Certainly, all patients who are to undergo surgery involving the risk of significant blood loss (greater than 10% of circulating blood volume) should undergo this test to dictate if, and when, transfusion should occur. Other patients include those with IHD, and patients in whom anaemia is a likelihood, such as those with severe renal impairment, long-standing blood loss from any cause, or chronic disease associated with anaemia, e.g. rheumatoid arthritis. Finally, general screening might include those in whom anaemia is a reasonable possibilty such as infants, women of child bearing potential, and patients over 60 years of age. However there are patients one would anaesthetize for minor procedures without a preoperative haemoglobin estimation in whom the likelihood of blood loss is minimal (cystoscopy, cataract surgery), where one is confident of maintaining CI and Sao_2 in the knowledge that there is a modest reduction in oxygen requirements under general anaesthesia.

In adults, some argue that anaemia is usually detectable from a careful history and examination and that screening provides a low pick up rate. This, coupled with the uneventful outcome of minor operations on anaemic patients, has led some anaesthetists not to screen adult patients. However, few anaesthetists ask patients about menorrhagia, for example, and detection of anaemia clinically is not always reliable. Thus, a more prudent approach would be to screen all women and patients over the age of 60 years, particularly as it is a cheap and simple test. Definitive studies in this area are lacking.

In children there are two large studies (2000 patients or more) confirming that the incidence of anaemia (haemoglobin <10 g dl^{-1} is 0.5%, rising to about 1.9% in children from lower socioeconomic groups. All patients had uneventful general anaesthetics and there is now a substantial body of opinion recommending that haemoglobin estimations in children are reserved for children deemed to be at risk, and that general screening is abandoned.

Other commonly requested blood tests include sickle testing which is generally regarded as essential for patients of Afro-Caribbean origin. Other patients at risk include those from areas of India and the Middle East. A positive sickle test should then be followed by haemoglobin electrophoresis. This is of value in quantifying the percentage of haemoglobin-S (HbS), the response to treatment such as exchange transfusion (where an HbS level <30% is the usual target before surgery) and the detection of other abnormal haemoglobins such as HbC. The absence of anaemia, or symptomatic sickle cell disease, does not remove the requirement for sickle testing. A minority of anaesthetists are prepared to undertake minor surgery without a sickle test, but as the disease carries a significant morbidity and mortality, this approach cannot be defended, particularly in view of the simplicity of the test. It should be remembered that the result from testing infants under the age of 3 months is unreliable, as fetal haemoglobin remains the predominant haemoglobin type at this age.

Clotting tests are generally requested by anaesthetists in those patients thought to be at risk from complications of central neural blockade. General consensus dictates that clotting should be normal and the platelet count should be in excess of 100×10^9 l^{-1}. It is worth noting that platelet function, and not count, is a more important consideration. However, there are little data to support the use of the bleeding time for patients who have recently ingested aspirin. Moreover, obstetric data on the use of low-dose aspirin for pre-eclampsia suggest that these patients are not at increased risk of extradural haematoma.

BIOCHEMISTRY

Biochemical testing is usually directed towards the diagnosis of Na^+ and K^+ abnormalities (particularly the latter) and assessment of renal function. Again there are no absolute criteria, but it is prudent to test all patients at risk (e.g. those on diuretic therapy) and to screen the elderly, perhaps those over the age of 65 years. The diagnosis of diabetes is also relevant and will be dealt with under urine testing.

Hypokalaemia

Hypokalaemia (serum $K^+ < 3.5$ mmol l^{-1}) has generally been regarded as a reason for postponing surgery pending potassium supplementation, because of the risk of arrhythmias in general and ventricular arrhythmias in particular. Evidence of how preoperative potassium concentration therapy is related to outcome is conflicting. Potassium is a predominantly intracellular cation (98%) and serum potassium values are a poor reflection of total body potassium. Moreover, the ratio of intracellular to extracellular potassium concentration ($[K^+]_i/[K^+]_o$) plays a major role in determining the resting membrane potential of excitable cells, according to the Nernst equation:

$$E = 60 \log \frac{[K^+]_o}{[K^+]_i}$$

or, more usefully,

$$E = -60 \log \frac{[K^+]_i}{[K^+]_o}$$

$[K^+]_i/[K^+]_o$ is usually 39/1, giving a resting membrane potential of -95 mV. Electrophysiological studies on the heart have demonstrated that hypokalaemia causes an increase in the slope of phase 4 diastolic depolarization, enhancing automaticity, as well as a slowing of conduction and a unidirectional block, favouring the development of reentrant arrhythmias. Clinically there are a number of important considerations. If the onset of hypokalaemia is acute (e.g. following vomiting and/or diarrhoea) then $[K^+]_i/[K^+]_o$ is likely to be disrupted with significant, electrophysiological cardiac changes. However, with a chronic onset of hypokalaemia (diuretic therapy, hyperaldosteronism) and both intracellular and extracellular depletion, $[K^+]_i/[K^+]_o$ will be unchanged, and so little risk for the onset of arrhythmias. A second consideration is the setting in which hypokalaemia occurs. In patients who have suffered acute myocardial infarction, there appears to be an inverse relationship between the incidence of arrhythmias and $[K^+]$, although the methodology in many of these studies has been questioned. Of the studies involving hypokalaemia and intraoperative arrhythmias, the evidence is more controversial. Ignoring animal studies, clinical data suggest that intraoperative ventricular arrhythmias are related more to conditions such as congestive cardiac failure and digoxin therapy than to hypokalaemia. Even in these groups of patients, hypokalaemia and diuretics did not increase the incidence of arrhythmias. A number of authors have emphasized that potassium replacement may be hazardous. This is unsurprising as an abrupt decrease in the $[K^+]_i/[K^+]_o$ ratio can occur.

Taking into account the available data, the following approach is suggested. In patients with moderate chronic hypokalaemia, $[K^+]$ of 3.0 mmol l^{-1} or more, no action need be taken. However, patients at risk of myocardial ischaemia treated with digoxin, who have ventricular dysfunction, electrocardiographic evidence of hypokalaemia or ventricular arrhythmias, or who are scheduled for major vascular and cardiac surgery, should have their serum [K$^+$] elevated to a minimum of 3.5 mmol l^{-1} before surgery. Furthemore, only oral potassium treatment should be used for asymptomatic patients. Hypokalaemia has recently been expertly reviewed by Wong and colleagues.

Renal function

Preoperative detection of renal impairment is important in patients undergoing major surgery, particularly cardiac, vascular and thoracic surgery. Postoperative renal failure has a mortality of 50–100%, despite advances in intensive care, renal replacement, haemodynamic manipulation and antibiotics. In a review of 28 studies, containing over 10 000 patients, Novis demonstrated that an increased serum creatinine, urea or known renal dysfunction were consistent factors in the aetiology of postoperative renal failure. Other factors of lesser predictive value included poor left ventricular function, advanced age (the definition of which varied between studies), active bacterial endocarditis, emergency surgery and vascular disease. Unfortunately, no two studies contained the same definition of preoperative renal impairment, renal failure or normal creatinine values in the elderly. Knowledge of preoperative renal dysfunction enables anaesthetists to undertake specific action to avoid further deterioration in function by the use of renal-dose dopamine, mannitol and optimization of haemodynamic variables, such as cardiac filling pressures, cardiac output and mean arterial pressure, and avoidance of nephrotoxic agents. The efficacy of such measures is still unproven despite being widely practised. Notwithstanding this, it is prudent to investigate all patients considered at risk in the above groups, particularly those with suspected renal impairment, or poor left ventricular function, or over 65–70 years old.

Urinalysis and diabetes mellitus

Testing the urine is probably the most widely used screening test for patients attending hospital. It may alert staff to the presence of renal disease and previously undiagnosed diabetes mellitus. The latter is important as the morbidity and mortality of diabetic patients undergoing surgery is several times higher that of others. Indeed, in both Eagle's and Larsen's study diabetes was an independent, significant predictor of cardiac risk in non-cardiac surgery. The presence of silent myocardial ischaemia in diabetics who have autonomic dysfunction is a well recognized entity. While it is tempting to speculate that tight perioperative control of blood glucose reduces that risk, this awaits confirmation in large studies. There seems no reason to deviate from the accepted practice of screening all adult patients' urine for glycosuria and to follow this up with appropriate serum estimations, but in common with all screening tests, its overall impact on management or postoperative outcome is likely to be minimal.

SUMMARY

The use of preoperative investigations needs constant reappraisal. Screening of the healthy adult and paediatric population is not worthwhile in terms of outcome and cost. Screening of the elderly population (>60 years) for baseline ECG, haemoglobin and biochemistry is nevertheless an accepted part of the pre-anaesthetic assessment and will continue, probably justifiably, because patients in this age group have poor physiological reserve. For the majority of patients, however, appropriate investigations should be targeted to those who are deemed to be at risk from either their medical status, or because of the surgery involved: in particular vascular surgery. Future studies in this area need to focus on how preoperative investigations and the consequent interventions affect patient outcome.

FURTHER READING

Baron, J. F., Mundler, O. and Bertrand, M. (1994) Dipyridamole-thallium scintigraphy and gated radionuclide angiography to assess cardiac risk before abdominal aortic surgery. *New England Journal of Medicine*, **330**, 663–669.

Eagle, K. A., Coley, C. M., Newell, J. B. *et al.* (1989) Combining clinical and thallium data optimises preoperative assessment of cardiac risk prior to vascular surgery. *Annals of Internal Medicine*, **110**, 859–866.

Edwards, N. D. and Reilly, C. S. (1994) Detection of perioperative myocardial ischaemia. *British Journal of Anaesthesia*, **72**, 104–115.

Fleischer, L. A. and Barash, P. G. (1992) Preoperative evaluation for noncardiac surgery: a functional approach. *Anesthesia and Analgesia*, **74**, 586–598.

Gass, G. D. and Olsen, G. N. (1986) Preoperative pulmonary function testing to predict postoperative morbidity and mortality. *Chest*, **89**, 127–35.

Goldman, L. (1995) Cardiac risk in noncardiac surgery: an update. *Anesthesia and Analgesia*, **80**, 810–820.

Mantha, S., Roizen, M. F., Barnard, J. *et al.* (1994) Relative effectiveness of four preoperative tests for predicting adverse cardiac outcomes after vascular surgery. *Anesthesia and Analgesia*, **79**, 422–433.

Novis, B. K., Roizen, M. F., Aronsen, S., and Thisted, R. A. (1994). Association of preoperative risk factors with postoperative renal failure. *Anesthesia and Analgesia*, **78**, 143–149.

Nunn, J. F., Milledge, J. S., Chen, D. and Dore, D. (1988) Respiratory criteria of fitness for surgery and anaesthesia. *Anaesthesia*, **43**, 543–551.

Wong, K. C., Schfer, P. G., and Schultz, J. R. (1993) Hypokalemia, and anesthetic implications. *Anesthesia and Analgesia*, **77**, 1238–1260.

# INHERITED DISEASES

E. O'Leary and G. M. Hall

Inherited diseases affecting anaesthetic management are quite rare. The objective of this chapter is to present an overview of the more common diseases presenting for surgery. The pathophysiology, common presenting problems, and overall anaesthetic management will be discussed.

HAEMOGLOBINOPATHIES

The haemoglobinopathies are a group of genetic diseases due to abnormalities of a single gene. The function of haemoglobin itself may be altered leading to inadequate oxygen delivery and carbon dioxide removal in spite of apparently adequate amounts of haemoglobin. Common haemoglobinopathies include sickle cell trait and disease, HbAS / HbSS, and the thalassaemias: alpha (α) and beta (β).

SICKLE CELL SYNDROME

Sickle cell disease is a qualitative disorder of structurally abnormal haemoglobin. The term sickle cell syndrome encompasses a spectrum of disease ranging from the almost symptomless sickle cell trait (HbAS genotype) to the most severe homozygous (HbSS genotype) sickle cell disease. HbSS is frequently lethal, and homozygotes rarely live more than 2 years when it occurs in populations with low standards of living, limited access to medical care and with a high prevalence of other diseases. HbS was first discovered in 1959 and its gene frequency varies proportionately with malaria prevalence. Epidemiological data seem to confirm that heterozygotes suffer from malaria less frequently and less severely than normal individuals, the so called 'heterozygote advantage'. Homozygous sickle cell disease is most frequently found in persons of equatorial African origin, e.g. Cameroons, Zaire, Uganda and Kenya. The abnormality in sickle cell disease results from substitution, at position 6 in the β chain, of glutamate by valine, with normal alpha chains. Normal adult haemoglobin is made up of two α and two β subunits. Each subunit contains one haem group located within each chain. The major function of haemoglobin is to transport O_2 from the lungs to the tissues. The oxygenated form of HbS appears almost identical to the oxygenated form of HbA with respect to structure and function. In HbSS, the mutant Hb is susceptible to polymerization, or aggregation, when the red cell is deoxygenated during its normal transit in the circulation. This results in altered erythrocyte properties leading to impaired cell flexibility, premature red cell destruction and tissue damage secondary to microvascular occlusion. The extent of the aggregates formed is determined by the intracellular haemoglobin concentration as well as O_2 saturation, temperature, 2,3 DPG (2,3-diphosphoglycerate) and intravascular pH.

Short Practice of Anaesthesia. Edited by M. Morgan and G. M. Hall. Published in 1997 by Chapman & Hall, London. ISBN 0 412 71890 1

Individuals with sickle cell anaemia lead a very precarious existence which is usually dotted with periods of haemolytic crises and intercurrent infections, commonly pulmonary, renal or bone. If adult life is reached, the disease follows a more benign course. Sickling of cells, with occlusion and haemolysis, is responsible for many of the clinical manifestations of this disease. The following systems may be involved.

Cardiovascular system

Cardiomegaly associated with the severe anaemia is present in the majority of patients and in one study 76% had radiologically enlarged hearts. The cardiac enlargement is due also partly to multiple thrombi in vessels of the pulmonary circulation with resulting cor pulmonale progressing to cardiac failure.

Respiratory system

Lung infarcts are common leading to a loss of functional pulmonary tissue. This in turn gives rise to a fall in arterial oxygen saturation of the blood particularly on exertion. There is a shift of the oxygen dissociation curve to the right, which readily liberates oxygen to the tissues from the sickle cell haemoglobin when required.

Liver

Due to repeated crises, the activity of the liver is increased to deal with the haemolysed blood. The liver tends to be enlarged in young children and often liver function tests are abnormal. Jaundice is common and pigment stones may form in the gall bladder. Repeated blood transfusions may cause iron to be deposited as haemosiderin in the liver, later resulting in cirrhosis.

Kidneys

The kidneys may also sustain infarcts due to thrombi. Albuminuria is common as is microscopic haematuria, though gross haematuria is rare. The kidneys are unable to excrete very concentrated urine, but renal failure is rare.

Brain

Hemiplegia, facial weakness, sensory and motor disturbances, headache, vomiting and convulsions have all been reported.

THALASSAEMIAS

Thalassaemias constitute a quantitative deficiency in the amount of normal haemoglobin produced. Alpha and beta thalassaemias are a major public health problem in the Mediterranean, Middle East, India, the Far East, tropical Africa and the Caribbean. They are characterized by deficient synthesis of α and β chains respectively. The α-globin gene cluster is found on chromosome 16 and the β-globin gene cluster is found on chromosome 6. Accurate diagnosis requires DNA analysis. Most α-thalassaemia syndromes are silent and result from underproduction of α-globin chains in fetal Hb (HbF) and adult Hb (HbA). The major clinical syndromes resulting from α-thalassaemia are Hb Bart's hydrops fetalis syndrome and HbH disease. Hb Bart's hydrops fetalis syndrome is usually associated with complete absence of α-globin chain synthesis. These infants almost always die *in utero*, or shortly after birth. Predominant features of HbH are anaemia, jaundice, hepatosplenomegaly and presence of HbH. Splenectomy often improves symptoms.

Heterozygotes for β-thalassaemias are clinically asymptomatic and these are referred to as thalassaemia minor. Homozygotes have severe disease, are transfusion dependent, and are referred to as thalassaemia major (or Cooley's anaemia). Homozygotes are normal at birth as HbF (no β chains) forms the majority of haemoglobin at this stage. However, in the first year of life, as HbF decreases, anaemia develops because of inadequate β-globin synthesis and patients present with pallor and failure to thrive. Regular blood transfusions are required for survival, although splenectomy at 8–9 years old will reduce the transfusion requirements. Chelation therapy with desferrioxamine is necessary to prevent iron overload, with its attendant problems.

ANAESTHETIC MANAGEMENT

Patients with sickle cell trait do not present an increased risk for anaesthesia. In these patients 30–50% of the patient's haemoglobin is HbS and the remainder is HbA. The red blood cells have a normal life span and affected persons generally are neither anaemic or symptomatic. However, sickling crises may occur in heterozygotes under hypoxic conditions. A report in the *Canadian Journal of Anaesthesia* in 1987 documented the case of a HbAS patient who sustained a cardiac arrest and died during a Caesarean section delivery under general anaesthesia. The mechanism for this cardiac arrest may have been the delivery of a large volume of hypoxaemic, acidotic blood with sickled cells resulting from severe, concealed, aortocaval compression during the operation.

Patients with HbSS or sickle thalassaemia are in a different risk category. In patients presenting for surgery, preventive measures are designed to avoid conditions such as infection, cold, acidosis and dehydration. Vascular occlusive accidents in the brain may occur resulting in cerebral lesions. Hemiplegia, facial weakness, sensory and motor disturbances, headache, vomiting and convulsions have been reported.

Preoperative management

A careful history and physical examination must be carried out and the cardiopulmonary status should be thoroughly investigated because of cardiac and pulmonary complications in these patients. Laboratory investigations include full blood count, serum urea, creatinine and electrolytes, coagulation profile, ECG and chest X-ray. A blood smear for the presence of sickle cells, haemoglobin electrophoresis to determine the amount of haemoglobin S and a reticulocyte count should also be carried out.

Preoperatively, any evidence of infection or dehydration should be corrected. Anaemia is treated by transfusion if haemoglobin is less than 7 g dl^{-1}: the ideal haematocrit, is 25–30% as greater values predispose to sickling through increased viscosity. The use of exchange transfusion in these patients remains controversial. Some centres recommend that for most surgical procedures exchange transfusion should be carried out using buffy-coat free, packed red blood cells to reduce the haemoglobin S fraction to less than 40%.

Intraoperative management

Intraoperative management includes the principles common to the administration of all general anaesthetics, but adherence to them is more crucial in this patient population. The actual choice of anaesthetic agents used does not seem to be of particular importance. Sickle cell crisis may occur under anaesthesia, as the red cells are very sensitive to reduced oxygen tension. It is very important to avoid any degree of hypoxia such as may be caused by respiratory depression or obstruction. Large doses of premedicants, breath-holding during the induction, and hypoventilation due to any cause, should be avoided where possible. Supplemental oxygen is mandatory throughout the operative period and pulse oximetry is useful as an indication of the adequacy of treatment. Fluid therapy should be guided by the measurement of central venous pressure if possible. The patient should be hyperventilated to avoid acidosis and sickling. Treatment with alkalis has been advocated in an effort prevent acidosis and sickling, but the inability of this technique to reverse established sickling has made this form of therapy unpopular.

Postoperative management

Prevention of hypoxia, acidosis, hypotension, stasis and hypothermia should be continued into the immediate postoperative period. Supplemental oxygen should be given for 24 h postoperatively and adequate oxygenation should be ensured by measuring O_2 saturation. The incidence of postoperative respiratory infection is high, and is a leading cause of morbidity. Hypoxaemic episodes are always a threat and may precipitate a sickling crisis. Postoperative physiotherapy helps prevent the development of such complications.

Treatment of sickle cell crisis

The following guidelines have been advocated for the treatment of a sickle cell crisis:

- patients should managed in the intensive care unit
- oxygen therapy: either by face mask, or by intubation and ventilation
- hydration: adequate intravenous fluids must be administered
- infection must be looked for as a precipitating cause, and actively treated when present
- patients may need opiates for the control of severe pain (usually pethidine)
- partial exchange transfusions are helpful in reducing the amount of haemoglobin S and thus improving the symptoms
- the use of sodium bicarbonate remains controversial, but is sometimes tried

THE PORPHYRIAS

The porphyrias are a group of inborn errors of metabolism caused by inherited enzyme defects in the haem biosynthetic pathways resulting in overproduction of intermediate compounds called porphyrins. Each porphyria is characterized by a specific enzyme defect with altered patterns of synthesis and excretion of porphyrins which accumulate, and are linked to clinical manifestations. They may be classified as acute, or non-acute, porphyrias. The non-acute are largely dermatological conditions which present clinically as cutaneous photosensitivity. Most forms are inherited as Mendelian autosomal dominants except for the rare congenital porphyria, which is recessive. Prevalence of each type of porphyria varies; for example, in Europe, the carrier frequency for the gene for acute intermittent porphyria is 1:10 000 whereas variegate porphyria occurs in 1:400 white South Africans.

ACUTE PORPHYRIAS

The acute porphyrias: acute intermittent porphyria, variegate porphyria, hereditary coproporphyria and plumboporphyria, are of most importance since attacks of these may be life threatening. Abdominal pain, limb weakness and various neuropsychiatric features are the hallmarks of an acute presentation. Apart from acute intermittent porphyria, all acute and non-acute porphyrias demonstrate photosensitive skin changes. The attacks vary in duration and intensity, and usually are followed by complete remission. The porphyrias are termed pharmacogenetic disorders in that commonly used drugs can precipitate an attack. Some drugs, usually hepatic enzyme inducers, are known precipitants of acute porphyrias in patients, while others may be identified as porphyrinogenic in animal models. Barbiturates, sulphonamides, oral contraceptives and enzyme-inducing anticonvulsants and antidepressants (e.g. phenytoin, carbamazepine, phenobarbitone, amitriptyline) are most commonly involved. There is strong evidence that attacks may be induced by endogenous hormonal changes: they are four times more common in women. Attacks are rare before puberty, and after the menopause, and there have been associations with menstruation, pregnancy and the use of the contraceptive pill.

Pathogenesis

The agents that precipitate attacks are inducers of amino laevulinic acid (ALA) synthase and hepatic cytochrome P450. Massive induction of P450 synthesis depletes the intracellular haem pool resulting in production of excessive ALA which is channelled into subsequent enzymic steps. Individuals with impaired enzymes are unable to handle this excessive load resulting in overproduction and increased excretion of porphyrins and/or porphyrin precursors and a decrease in haem formation. The increased excretion of porphyrin precursors in the acute porphyrias is due to the decreased activity of porphobilinogen (PBG) deaminase. However, the link between the molecular abnormalities and clinical manifestations of the porphyrias remains elusive.

Clinical features

Acute intermittent porphyria

Acute intermittent porphyria is the most common of the acute porphyrias with reduction in the activity of PBG deaminase. The affected gene is on chromosome 11 and attacks are more common in women, with the highest risk in the age range 20–40 years for women and 30–50 years for men. Most patients present with persistent or colicky abdominal pain, which may radiate to the back, and vomiting and constipation. Relief of constipation may herald the onset of recovery. Diarrhoea occurs in 10% of cases. Hypertension and tachycardia are the commonest signs and examination often reveals abdominal tenderness. The presentation may be difficult to differentiate from the acute abdomen, especially in the accident and emergency department.

A neuropathy occurs in two thirds of cases with symmetrical weakness mainly involving limb and girdle muscles. Upper limbs and proximal muscles are the worst affected, and truncal muscle weakness may lead to respiratory embarrassment or paralysis resulting in death. Distal limb involvement may lead to permanent deformity. Upper motor neurone lesions may develop, and rarely the cerebellum and basal ganglia are involved. The presentation of porphyria as an atypical psychiatric disorder, such as atypical psychosis and schizoaffective disorder has been noted. An associated hyponatraemia may indicate the syndrome of inappropriate antidiuresis in severe attacks. Transient renal impairment may also be seen during the attack. Less commonly, there may be urinary retention and early onset, chronic renal failure. Cardiovascular features occur in 70% of cases. The usual manifestations are sinus tachycardia and systemic hypertension which may persist after the acute phase of the attack. In an acute attack, urine when passed becomes dark on standing due to porphobilinogen polymerizing to ruroporphyrin and a brownish red pigment porphobilin. The key investigation is the examination of urine for excess PBG. A bedside test is its reaction with an acidic solution of *p*-dimethyl amino benzaldehyde which gives a red compound, not extractable by chloroform. Positive tests should be confirmed by specific, quantitative measurement of urinary PBG. In remission, urinary PBG excretion declines, but rarely to normal.

Hereditary coproporphyria

This is caused by decreased coproporphyrinogen oxidase activity leading to excess coproporphyrin in the urine and elevated ALA synthase. Genetic studies show the defect is located on chromosome 9. Hereditary coproporhyria is a milder disease than acute intermittent porphyria but respiratory paralysis and fatalities do occur. The principal biochemical abnormalities found in the acute stage are increased urinary ALA, PBG, and coproporphyrin 111 excretion.

Variegate porphyria

Common in South Africa, this is caused by proporphyrin oxidase deficiency. Clinical features are similar to hereditary coproporphyria, except for the more severe skin photosensitivity with scarring. On exposure to light, the urine shows a dark, port wine discoloration.

Management

General

Patients should be well informed about precipitating factors and be given a booklet of 'unsafe drugs'. A Medic-Alert bracelet should be worn at all times in case of the need for emergency anaesthesia.

Management of the acute attack

Setting Management of acute attacks is best carried out in an intensive care unit where vital signs can be closely followed. Respiratory muscle involvement may necessitate controlled ventilation.

Fluid balance The importance of adequate fluid balance and nutrition in the acute attack rests with the fact that carbohydrate is known to prevent the induction of ALA synthase by porphyrinogenic drugs. The recommendations for feeding are that at least 1500–2000 kcal per 24 h is required. If the patient is unable to continue with oral feeding due to vomiting, feeding may then be carried out with a nasogastric tube, or even with parenteral feeding.

Symptomatic therapy Adequate analgesia should be given to control pain and this may include intravenous, opiate infusion. Vital signs must be carefully monitored during the infusion. Hypertension and tachycardia may complicate an acute attack and are thought to be the result of sympathetic overactivity. Treatment with β-blocking drugs has been advocated.

Sedatives and tranquillizers have been used to control psychotic symptoms and chlorpromazine has been found useful.

Seizures require the use of anticonvulsants, but most commonly used agents are porphyrinogenic. Sodium valproate and diazepam are not porphyrinogenic in man and diazepam can be used safely in the acute attacks to control seizures.

Haem therapy Haematin, an intravenous haem precursor, has been used for over 20 years to treat acute attacks. It acts by reducing the overproduction of porphyrins and precursors by a negative feedback inhibition of ALA synthase. Its disadvantages are instability in solution, harmful effects on coagulation, and thrombophlebitis.

Others Cimetidine has been shown to cause a 50% reduction in hepatic ALA synthase activity in an animal model. Some studies have shown a marked improvement in neurological symptoms.

Menstruation may precipitate acute attacks, and suppression of ovulation by LHRH analogues will prevent attacks precipitated by gonadal, endocrine factors.

Skin lesion occurrence from photosensitivity is related to the amount of exposure to sunlight. Barrier sunscreens may be of some use and excess sunlight should be avoided.

Anaesthetic management

Drug-induced, acute attacks may be life-threatening and some commonly used anaesthetic drugs are highly dangerous in porphyria. Many anaesthetic drugs are listed as potentially porphyrinogenic, but often the evidence is tenuous. The pitfalls in diagnosis require emphasizing, as laboratory screening may not necessarily exclude porphyria unequivocally. It has been suggested that the only defence for the anaesthetist is to treat all patients who have a family history of porphyria, or who have signs and symptoms suggestive of porphyria, as potentially at risk irrespective or age or biochemical status.

Induction agents

Induction of anaesthesia has yielded major problems when anaesthetizing the porphyric patient. The barbiturates have long been contraindicated. Propanidid was generally accepted as the induction agent of choice, but was withdrawn from the market due to its high incidence of anaphylactic reactions consequent on its Cremophor formulation. Etomidate is also potentially porphyrinogenic, as was althesin before it was withdrawn from practice. Ketamine has just one report implicating it as the cause of a porphyric crisis in a patient postoperatively. However, some of its other side-effects militate against it being routinely used as an induction agent. Propofol, the newest of the induction agents, lacks porphyrinogenic potential in an animal model, and this has been confirmed in a controlled, clinical trial in patients with variegate porphyria. There has been just one case report of increased levels of urinary porphyrin concentration following its administration. It appears that propofol can now fill the gap created by the withdrawal of propanidid as a safe induction agent. The benzodiazepines do not act consistently in porphyric patients. Acute attacks have been reported following the use of diazepam, chlordiazepoxide, flunitrazepam and nitrazepam, while experimental data have suggested that they are non-porphyrinogenic. Indeed, diazepam has been used safely for the management of porphyric crises; lorazepam and midazolam appear to be safe.

Volatile agents

Enflurane is considered potentially porphyrinogenic as a result of work done in animal models, although no acute attack in humans has been ascribed to it (it has been used safely in the management of porphyric patients).

The use of halothane is contentious, as there are some experimental data contraindicating its use and also adverse clinical reports. However, the general consensus is that halothane may be the safest of the inhalational agents so far.

There is not enough evidence available on isoflurane to date, and until proof exists to the contrary, it must be regarded as unsafe.

Neuromuscular blocking drugs

Suxamethonium and tubocurare are known to be safe, but there has been a suggestion that pancuronium may be harmful. Alcuronium has also been classified as unsafe by some authorities. Most of the other neuromuscular blocking drugs have been used without any adverse effects.

Narcotic analgesics

Morphine and fentanyl are safe in the management of these patients. Pentazocine and tildine are known to be unsafe. Pethidine, although it has been implicated in an acute attack, has a long record of safety.

Local anaesthetics

There is no evidence to support the contention that any of the local anaesthetics, either amides or esters, have induced an acute attack of porphyria. Lignocaine has been found to be porphyrinogenic in animals, but it has been used frequently in humans without any adverse effects.

The objective in the management of the hereditary porphyrias is to avoid any drug that has clinically significant porphyrinogenicity. The anaesthetic approach must consist of a detailed pre-anaesthetic evaluation; particular attention should be paid to the neurological examination, arterial pressure and heart rate, intravascular volume status, serum electrolytes, blood creatinine concentration and respiratory system function.

COAGULATION DISORDERS

CLASSIFICATION OF HAEMOSTATIC DEFECTS

The most common congenital disorders are von Willebrand's disease (deficiency of platelets) and haemophilia A and B (abnormalities in the clotting mechanism). The remaining patients do not have any demonstrable lesion of platelets, or clotting mechanisms, and appear to bleed as a result of vascular abnormalities. A clinical distinction can frequently be made between bleeding due to clotting defects, and bleeding due to diminished number and/or function of platelets. Patients with clotting defects usually present with abnormal bleeding in the deep tissues, that is muscles or joints. On the other hand, patients with platelet abnormalities usually present with superficial bleeding, that is bleeding into the skin and from the epithelial surfaces of the nose, uterus and other organs.

NORMAL HAEMOSTASIS

Normal haemostasis involves the interaction of plasma and tissue factors with platelets and the vessel walls. Primary haemostasis results from vasoconstriction and the formation of a platelet plug; coagulation forms a fibrin clot; fibrinolysis removes fibrin.

Normally, vascular endothelial cells secrete prostacyclin, a vasodilator and inhibitor of platelet aggregation. Damage to the endothelium of a blood vessel brings blood into contact with the underlying collagen fibres. Endothelial cells secrete von Willebrand factor which permits platelets to adhere to one another and collect at the defective site on the endothelium. The platelet plug seals the hole, especially in smaller injuries, and serotonin is released which causes local vasoconstriction. At the same time, the actual process of clotting is set off by two further mechanisms: an extrinsic system triggered by tissue factors such as tissue thromboplastin which is set free when a tissue is damaged, and an intrinsic system activated by contact between clotting factor XII and the collagen fibres. Both systems can activate either singly, or in combination with plasma factor X which initiates the common pathway. This eventually cleaves prothrombin to thrombin which in turn converts fibrinogen to fibrin. Fibrin monomers aggregate to form a soluble fibrin clot.

TESTS FOR CLOTTING DEFECTS

Intrinsic system

Activated partial thromboplastin time (APPT)

This will remain normal until the factor concentrations are less than 30% of normal. Citrated plasma is obtained and to this is added a mixture of kaolin and phospholipid followed by calcium. The time taken for the mixture to clot is measured. Prolongation of the APPT is almost always due to deficiency of factors VIII and IX.

Whole blood clotting time

Venous blood is allowed to clot in a glass tube at 37°C. This normally takes from 5–11 minutes and is a simple, but insensitive, test for the integrity of the intrinsic system. It will only detect major deficiencies of factors VIII and IX and is rarely performed.

Extrinsic system

Prothrombin time (PT)

This test is carried out by adding factor III (tissue thromboplastin) together with calcium to citrated plasma. The name is a misnomer as prolongation of the prothrombin time may result from deficiencies of I, II, V, VII and X. The PT is chiefly sensitive to deficiency of factors V, VII and X, platelet deficiency does not affect it.

Clotting defects conveniently fall into two groups: in the first group are those patients with acquired deficiencies of several factors (II, VII, IX, X) resulting from treatment with coumarin drugs, vitamin K deficiency and liver disease. Three of these factors lie in the extrinsic system and the specific test for this system is the prothrombin time (PT). In the second group of patients, there is a congenital defect of one of the clotting factors; 80–90% of patients in this group have factor VIII deficiency (haemophiliacs) 10–20% have factor IX deficiency, and less than 1% have a deficiency of one of the other eight factors. In practice, nearly all of the congenital defects lie in the intrinsic system and these can be detected by the APPT.

HAEMOPHILIA (FACTOR VIII DEFICIENCY, HAEMOPHILIA A)

Haemophilia A is caused by the X linked deficiency of factor VIII. Deficiency of factor VIII results from an abnormality in the factor VIII gene which is found on the long arm of the X chromosome. This disease is almost entirely confined to males (XY), since the normal X chromosome in heterozygous females usually ensures adequate factor VIII production. The prevalence of this disorder is about 1 in 10 000 males. Factor VIII circulates in the plasma in a non-covalent complex with von Willebrand factor (vWF), a property that enhances factor VIII synthesis, protects it from proteolysis and concentrates it at sites of active haemostasis. In addition, factor VIII has coagulant activity only when combined with vWF. In haemophilia, it has been found that although factor VIII coagulant activity is depressed, vWF concentrations are within normal limits.

Haemophilia A is a clinically heterogeneous disorder. Patients may have severe haemophilia (no detectable factor VIII) or have moderate (1–4% of normal factor VIII level) or mild (5–25% of normal level) disease.

Clinical features

Severe haemophiliacs have spontaneous bleeds into joints and, less frequently, muscles. The knees, elbows and ankles are the most commonly affected joints. If not properly treated, bleeding into joints can result in crippling deformity. Haematuria, epistaxis and gastrointestinal bleeding are less common. At least one quarter of all deaths are due to intracranial bleeding. The severity of bleeding and mode of presentation is related to the factor VIII concentration.

Diagnosis

Abnormal APPT

The diagnosis is strongly suggested by a laboratory finding of a normal extrinsic clotting system (normal PT) and a prolonged activated partial thromboplastin time (APPT). Confirmation can be obtained by showing that the addition of plasma from a known case of factor VIII deficiency to the patient's plasma does not correct the clotting defect.

Factor VIII concentration

Measurement of factor VIII concentration gives the definitive diagnosis.

Treatment

In the case of a spontaneous or post-traumatic bleed, treatment should always be given at the earliest sign. If an operation is planned, prophylactic treatment should be given. Treatment consists of factor VIII in a concentrated form to maintain plasma factor VIII coagulant activity between 5 and 100% of normal, depending on the severity of the injury, or the extent of the proposed surgical procedure. Two types of concentrated factor VIII preparation are available, cryoprecipitate and freeze-dried factor VIII preparation.

Cryoprecipitate is made by freezing and slow-thawing of plasma and is relatively impure. It has about 100 units of factor VIII per 10 ml bag and one unit of factor VIII per kg raises plasma activity by 2%. Therefore, in a 70 kg patient 3500 units of factor VIII are required to raise the plasma activity from 0 to 100%.

Cryoprecipitate has been mainly replaced by the highly purified, but more expensive freeze-dried material. Other advantages are that it can be stored in a domestic refrigerator and that adequate amounts can be injected in a small volume. Freeze-dried factor VIII preparations are derived from large pools of plasma, and several preparations used in the past have contained the human immunodeficiency virus (HIV). This virus has been eliminated from current preparations by using donors who do not have HIV antibodies, and by heat treating the final product at 80°C for 72 h, a process known to kill the virus.

Recombinant factor VIII is now available as an isolate from the cell culture of heterologous mammalian cells. This was developed in response to HIV infection within the haemophiliac population. The concerns raised about recombinant factor VIII relate primarily to cost, as it is highly efficacious, safe and is a major improvement on earlier factor VIII products.

The amount of factor VIII required for patients undergoing dental extraction can be reduced by treatment with the antifibrinolytic agent, tranexamic acid. The vasopressin analogue, desmopressin, may also be used to increase factor VIII clotting activity in mild or moderate haemophilia.

FACTOR IX DEFICIENCY (HAEMOPHILIA B, CHRISTMAS DISEASE)

About 20% of patients with haemophilia have factor IX deficiency. The clinical features and inheritance are identical to factor VIII deficiency, but in general the disease is milder. The diagnosis can be made by assaying factor IX level. Normal individuals have a factor IX level of 60–150%. The most serious bleeding problems require treatment to achieve factor IX levels of about 70–100% by infusion of factor IX. For less serious injuries, levels of 30–50% will usually suffice. Factor IX deficiency may be treated with fresh frozen plasma or purified factor IX. Freeze-dried factor IX is available and should be administered intravenously as soon as spontaneous or post-traumatic bleeding starts. Factor IX, molecular weight 56 000, has a volume of distribution twice that of factor VIII. Thus 1 unit of factor IX per kg raises plasma factor IX by only 1%. To increase the factor IX level from 0% to 100% in a 70 kg patient, requires 7000 units of factor IX. Factor IX has a longer half-life in plasma (24 h) than factor VIII (12 h) and hence can be given at less frequent intervals.

Cryoprecipitate does not contain factor IX, and desmopressin does not increase factor IX in plasma, so neither are useful in the treatment of Christmas disease.

VON WILLEBRAND'S DISEASE

This was first described by von Willebrand in 1926. It is characterized by excessive bleeding presenting in infancy, and differs from haemophilia in that the defect is not sex-linked. The gene responsible for this defect is found on chromosome 12. Most patients are heterozygous for the von Willebrand gene. Spontaneous bleeding is usually confined to mucous membranes and skin and takes the form of epistaxis and ecchymoses. Severe haemorrhage following surgical procedures is not uncommon. The cause of bleeding is the failure of the platelets to form a haemostatic plug, and this failure results either from a reduction in, or a complete lack of, von Willebrand factor (vWF). vWF is a glycoprotein present in plasma, platelets and vessel walls and has a dual function. First, it acts as a carrier for factor VIII, one factor VIII molecule is associated with about 1000 vWF subunits; second, it is an adhesive molecule which binds platelets to subendothelial tissues in an injured vessel wall. As vWF acts as a carrier for factor VIII, the reduction in vWF in this disease results in a reduction in factor VIII concentration (usually measured as clotting activity) which may be as low as 5–30% normal, similar to that found in mild haemophilia. Thus, the excessive bleeding in the disease is due both to factor VIII deficiency as well as to the failure of the platelet adherence.

Clinical features

Bleeding episodes usually start in early childhood. Typical symptoms include mucous membrane bleeding, bleeding from tonsils, bruising after minor trauma, excessive blood loss following dental extraction, tonsillectomy or other surgical procedures. It is inherited in an autosomal dominant or recessive manner. In most patients the diagnosis can be made on the basis of clinical symptoms, autosomal inheritance and usual laboratory tests. In typical cases of von Willebrand's disease, bleeding time is prolonged; the platelet count is usually normal.

The following investigations should be carried out.

Bleeding time

The bleeding time remains the best clinical screening test for the estimation of platelet function. The Ivy bleeding time technique is the most reliable method for assessment of the functional integrity of primary haemostasis. It is estimated by making a small wound in the skin of the forearm after applying a blood-pressure cuff to the upper arm and inflating to 40 mmHg. The depth of the wound is standardized. The average time that elapses until bleeding ceases is then measured. The normal range is 2–4 min. Since the wound only damages small vessels, haemostasis is mainly dependent on the formation of a platelet plug, hence the bleeding time is prolonged when platelet numbers are reduced. It is almost always normal in the presence of clotting defects.

vWF:Ag in plasma

vWF:Ag is decreased in von Willebrand's disease. This may be measured by an electro-immunoassay technique.

Ristocetin cofactor (Rcof) activity

Ristocetin, an antibiotic, causes platelet aggregation in normal blood, but not in blood from a patient with von Willebrand's disease. This abnormality is corrected both *in vivo* and *in vitro* by normal plasma, haemophilia A plasma, and isolated factor VIII related protein. Rcof activity is usually reduced in all types of von Willebrand's disease.

Reduced factor VIII clotting activity

This should also be measured in suspected von Willebrand's disease.

Treatment

The aim of therapy is to correct the vWF-dependent prolonged bleeding time. When a factor VIII abnormality is present, it should also be corrected.

Desmopressin (DDAVP)

This should be considered in all mild and moderately affected patients. DDAVP induces release of vWF from storage sites. The recommended dosage is 0.3–0.4 µg per kg body weight which increases vWF concentration two to three fold. An intranasal spray has been available since 1986 and peak concentrations are reached in 60 min.

Fresh frozen plasma/cryoprecipitate

The treatment of bleeding episodes in patients with von Willebrand's disease has long relied on the use of cryoprecipitate, containing five to ten times more vWF than plasma. The risk of viral contamination exists with cryoprecipitate as no safe method of virus inactivation is yet available. Fresh frozen plasma can only be used in patients in whom more intensive treatment is not required.

Factor VIII/vWF concentrates

Some recently available factor VIII concentrates are able to correct the bleeding defect in von Willebrand's disease. These concentrates are virus inactivated and are now preferred in the treatment of patients with von Willebrand's disease. The recommended dosage for severe bleeding or as treatment before surgery in a patient with von Willebrand's disease is 40–60 units per kg body weight.

INHIBITORS OF COAGULATION

Prevention of uncontrolled, massive, intravascular coagulation is accomplished by several mechanisms. As noted, prostacyclin from normal vascular endothelium maintains vasodilatation, inhibits platelet aggregation and exposure of the phospholipid platelet factor 3. Normal blood flow dilutes and washes away activated coagulation factors which are preferentially removed from the circulation. Antithrombin 111, protein C and protein S are naturally occurring anticoagulants. Antithrombin 111 complexes with thrombin and other clotting factors clearing them from the circulation.

Antithrombin III

Congenital antithrombin III deficiency is usually inherited as an autosomal dominant characteristic. Antithrombin is mainly an inhibitor of thrombin and its action is markedly potentiated by heparin. Carriers may suffer from recurrent deep venous thrombosis, superficial thrombophlebitis and pulmonary embolism.

Protein C and protein S

These are two other inhibitors of coagulation and are vitamin K-dependent substances. Activated protein C inactivates factors V and VIII; it also promotes fibrinolysis. Protein S potentiates the effects of activated protein C.

Some individuals have a hereditary deficiency of protein C with about 50% of normal levels. They are particularly prone to develop superficial thrombophlebitis and cerebral vein thrombosis.

The prevalence of protein S deficiency is about 1 in 20 000 and a proportion of heterozygotes for this defect suffers from recurrent venous thromboembolism.

C1 ESTERASE DEFICIENCY

Hereditary angioneurotic oedema (HANE) or C1 esterase inhibitor deficiency (C1EI), is inherited as an autosomal, dominant trait. About 85% of patients have low levels of normal C1EI, whereas the remaining 15% have normal C1EI values, but these are functionally inactive. The incidence is estimated at 1 in 10 000. The first component of the complement system is in an inactive state in the serum. It is activated under certain conditions, setting off the complement cascade. The enzyme C1EI regulates the first step in the complement cascade. A deficiency of this enzyme leads to an uncontrolled activation and accumulation of vasoactive substances C2, C3 and C5. These substances produce oedema by increasing vascular permeability. Attacks may be complicated by incapacitating cutaneous swelling, life-threatening upper airway obstruction, and severe gastrointestinal colic.

CLINICAL MANIFESTATIONS

HANE is characterized by recurrent, circumscribed, non-pitting, subepithelial oedema. It may involve any part of the body, but usually affects the extremities. Typically, there is no pain or pruritus involved beyond that caused by distension of the skin and subcutaneous tissue. Urticaria associated with angioedema usually indicates a diagnosis other than HANE.

Visceral involvement may occur independently and is manifested by colicky, generally severe, abdominal pain followed by watery diarrhoea. The diarrhoea is caused by intraluminal fluid in the oedematous gut. Severe vomiting may also be a cause of dehydration. On examination, the abdomen may be tender, but is seldom rigid. Mortality may be as high as 25% in patients with HANE and is due to the predisposition, in certain patients, to complete airway obstruction caused by laryngeal oedema.

Urinary bladder retention, pleural effusions, and mild chest discomfort may also be infrequently associated with the condition. The central nervous system can be involved with severe headaches, hemiplegia and seizures possibly due to localized brain tissue oedema.

Menstruation has been reported to lead to an increase in the number of attacks. Most patients improve after menopause. Interestingly, during pregnancy it has been reported that fewer or no attacks occur; also no relapse of angioedema occurs at parturition, despite the trauma to the birth canal.

The term 'angioneurotic oedema' was initially used as patients affected responded to emotional affliction with an episode of angioedema. A recent evaluation of a large number of patients with HANE showed no increase in psychiatric disorders. The increase in neurotic behaviour described by some researchers may well be caused by anxiety created by an awareness of the life-threatening nature of the disease, the unexplained episodes of oedema and the painful abdominal symptoms.

The most commonly identified precipitating factors include dental manipulation, concomitant illness, tonsillectomy, and accidental trauma, although in about half of reported cases no cause has been identified.

TREATMENT

There are three stages of therapy in patients with C1EI deficiency: treatment of acute attacks; maintenance therapy; and short-term prophylactic regimens.

Acute attacks

The most immediate concern is alleviation of airway obstruction. This may require intubation and ventilation, or even necessitate surgical intervention with a tracheostomy. Adrenaline, antihistamine agents and corticosteroids have all been advocated for use in the acute attack, but very often patients do not respond satisfactorily to such treatment. Infusions of fresh frozen plasma have been reported to be beneficial in the treatment of life-threatening attacks of HANE. However, it carries the potential risks of infectious disease transmission and an anaphylactoid reaction.

A concentrate of purified C1EI exists and is considered more appropriate than fresh frozen plasma. During an acute attack, 500–1000 units are infused and mucosal oedema begins to resolve within 30 min to 2 h of injection. To date, this is not approved for medical use in the USA.

Maintenance therapy

Long term therapy has been suggested for those patients with a history of frequent, partial, laryngeal obstruction, or episodes of facial and neck swelling. The prophylactic agents that have been used include antifibrinolytic medications, hormonal agents and purified C1EI concentrates. Two antifibrinolytic drugs, ε-aminocaproic acid (EACA) and its analogue, tranexamic acid (Cyclokapron) have been used in the past. These agents are known to inhibit C1 activation, although the exact mechanism of action remains unclear. Hormonal agents used include methyltestosterone, and the synthetic agents danazol and stanozolol. These have been shown to cause increased levels of C1EI. Long-term replacement with purified C1EI concentrate has been suggested to be safe and clinically beneficial in a selected group of patients who may have reactions to the other available drugs.

Short-term preventive measures

Short-term improvement may be obtained by administering danazol daily for 5–10 days before surgical trauma. In the past infusions of fresh frozen plasma have been advocated before surgery.

ANAESTHETIC MANAGEMENT

Patients presenting with HANE are of grave concern to the anaesthetist as laryngeal oedema poses a great danger to the patient. Recommendations include the avoidance of general anaesthesia as pressure or trauma of oral, nasal or tracheal airways may result in life threatening respiratory obstruction. Local or regional techniques are preferred, but general anaesthesia by mask and even endotracheal intubation has been described. Nasotracheal intubation is generally considered more dangerous than orotracheal, and should be avoided.

For elective cases, short-term prophylaxis has been achieved with administration of danazol for as little as ten days before surgical procedures. The dose of danazol that prevents HANE attacks is variable, does not correlate with body mass, and must be empirically determined in each patient. As much as 600 mg per day by mouth may be required.

Fresh frozen plasma (FFP) contains C1EI and can be used prophylactically within 24 h of surgery. For every 2 units of FFP infused, C1EI level increases by 2.5 mg dl^{-1}. Moreover, an acute attack can be terminated by using FFP. Concentrate of C1EI may be preferable to FFP as it eliminates the risk of hepatitis. However, the plasma half-life is short, about 4 days, and the enzyme is also very expensive.

In the emergency situation, concentrates of C1EI are recommended as is the use of FFP. Clinical improvement occurs within 20–40 min of infusion of FFP.

MARFAN'S SYNDROME

Marfan's syndrome is an autosomally dominant, inherited, connective tissue disorder with a prevalence of 1 in 10 000 of the population. Fibrillin, a glycoprotein, is reduced, or defective, in tissues affected in Marfan's syndrome. It is an essential component of the elastic elements in the extracellular matrix. The fibrillin gene is located on the long arm of chromosome 15. The diagnostic criteria for Marfan's syndrome were established in 1988, and include involvement of at least two of the three systems classically affected plus a family history. The clinical features of Marfan's syndrome occur most commonly in the cardiovascular, ocular and skeletal systems, but the lungs and central nervous system can also be involved.

CARDIAC SYSTEM

Mitral valve prolapse is the commonest cardiac defect occurring in this syndrome, although severe mitral regurgitation may also be a problem. Death is common in the fourth decade of life, and is usually due to aortic root dilation and dissection. Specific measures to retard the aortic root dilation include avoidance of contact sports and isometric exercises. The regular use of beta blocking drugs has been shown to impede this dilation, and atenolol is often prescribed for patients with dilated aortic roots and for those who have had previous aortic root surgery.

Marfan patients should have an annual echocardiography to assess aortic root size. Once the aortic root is 6 cm in diameter prophylactic surgery is recommended. Elective surgery has a mortality of 2–5% but the long-term survival of patients who have prophylactic surgery is significantly improved.

OCULAR SYSTEM

Lens dislocation is the commonest ocular abnormality and affects more than 70% patients. Retinal detachment at unusual sites occurs in about 10% patients and these may be difficult to repair. Children with this syndrome should have annual ophthalmic examinations as they may not realize what normal vision is.

SKELETAL SYSTEM

Disproportionate length of long bones, or arachnodactyly, is one of the diagnostic signs. Scoliosis is the main skeletal complication and should be regularly monitored by an orthopaedic surgeon and surgery performed if necessary. A high arched palate is also often present and may make intubation difficult. Joint laxity is a common feature.

ANAESTHETIC MANAGEMENT

Patients with Marfan's syndrome usually present for the management of complications of their disease, but they may also present for unrelated surgery. The risk of sudden death in these patients is high, despite seeming healthy. Preoperative management includes a history, physical examination, chest X-ray and ECG, specifically documenting the presence of arrythmias, heart failure and aortic or mitral regurgitation. Preoperative echocardiography has been advocated to evaluate the heart and aorta. Antibiotic prophylaxis for bacterial endocarditis is given, even in the absence of valvular disease. Beta blocking therapy should normally be continued throughout surgery.

Before induction, the patient should be positioned to place minimal stress on joints and other connective tissues. The insertion of an arterial canula is an advantage where cardiac disease has been identified preoperatively. Intubation, if necessary, should be performed gently to avoid dislocation of the temporomandibular joint. The haemodynamic response to laryngoscopy and intubation should be attenuated to avoid aneurysm dissection, or heart failure secondary to increased oxygen consumption. There are no contraindications to any particular anaesthetic drugs in the intraoperative management of these patients, but vigilance and skill are of utmost importance. Intermittent positive pressure ventilation may lead to pneumothorax, even at what would normally be considered safe inflation pressures.

CHOLINESTERASE VARIANTS

Plasma cholinesterase (EC 3.1.1.8), sometimes known as pseudocholinesterase or butyrylcholinesterase, is present in most tissues in the body, except red blood cells, and is capable of hydrolysing many esters. Cholinesterase, like albumin, is synthesized in the liver and has a plasma half-life of about 5–8 days. The physiological importance of circulating cholinesterase is unknown, but it may play a role in lipid metabolism. The anaesthetic importance of this enzyme is related to its action in hydrolysing the depolarizing neuromuscular blocking drug, suxamethonium. A new non-depolarizing muscle relaxant, mivacurium, is also metabolized by cholinesterase. Prolongation of action of suxamethonium will occur in the presence of an abnormal genetic variant of cholinesterase 'suxamethonium apnoea'. Paralysis may persist for up to 2–3 h in homozygous patients and can be an important anaesthetic complication. Low circulating concentrations of the normal enzyme occur commonly in a variety of diseases (see below), but rarely cause important prolongation of action of suxamethonium until values are < 1000 units 1^{-1} (normal range 3000–10 000 units 1^{-1}).

GENETICS

Cholinesterase synthesis is controlled by two allelic genes and the normal genotype is given by $E_1^u E_1^u$ where u indicates the usual gene. There are at least three other alleles and these are described by E_1^a, E_1^f and E_1^s to indicate the atypical, fluoride-resistant and silent gene respectively. Inheritance follows an autosomal codominant pattern. Differentiation between the genotypes is made by the use of two inhibitors of cholinesterase activity, dibucaine and fluoride. These tests were described over 30 years ago and have been validated in thousands of patients. For example, a normal patient $E_1^u E_1^u$ has a dibucaine number of around 80, whereas a homozygous patient with the atypical gene $E_1^a E_1^a$ has a dibucaine number of less than 30. Heterozygote patients ($E_1^u E_1^a$) have an intermediate dibucaine number, such as 50–60. The fluoride-resistant gene is identified by using fluoride as the inhibitor and the silent gene shows virtually no enzymatic activity. Other variants are known to exist, in particular E_1^j and E_1^k, and occasionally it is still not possible to accurately genotype all patients referred for testing. The common genotypes found in patients sensitive to suxamethonium are $E_1^a E_1^a$ and $E_1^a E_1^s$.

MANAGEMENT OF SUXAMETHONIUM APNOEA

If spontaneous respiration fails to occur after the administration of suxamethonium, ventilation of the lungs must be maintained and unconsciousness guaranteed. Apnoea due to other causes **must** be excluded by the use of a nerve stimulator. The diagnosis cannot be confirmed without assessing neuromuscular transmission. Treatment usually consists of waiting for normal synaptic function to return, which may take as long as 3–4 h. The infusion of fresh frozen plasma and a purified form of human cholinesterase have been reported, but are unnecessary.

After operation a careful history of drug therapy, previous anaesthetics and even a family history must be taken. A blood sample for cholinesterase activity and genotyping must be sent to a specialized centre. If an abnormal genotype is found, this must be stated prominently in the patient's notes and other members of the family tested. All affected individuals should wear a Medic-Alert bracelet.

Although the use of suxamethonium is slowly declining, other drugs are being developed that are dependent on circulating cholinesterase to terminate their action. A knowledge of genetic cholinesterase variants is still required.

CAUSES OF DECREASED CIRCULATING CHOLINESTERASE ACTIVITY

- inherited: rare genetic variants
- physiological: pregnancy and puerperium
- diseases: liver disease
  burns
  carcinoma
  acute and chronic infection
  renal failure
  uraemia
  hypothyroidism
  myocardial infarction
- iatrogenic: chemotherapy
  radiotherapy
  oral contraceptives
  ecothiopate eye drops
  plasmapheresis
  organophosphorus poisoning

MALIGNANT HYPERTHERMIA

Malignant hyperthermia (MH) is a rare complication of general anaesthesia which results from an abnormal increase in muscle metabolism following the use of all volatile anaesthetics and suxamethonium. There is often a family history of anaesthetic problems and the genetic basis of MH was recognized in the first case-report in 1960. It is inherited as an autosomal dominant characteristic. The primary defect in MH is an abnormal increase in intracellular $[Ca^{2+}]$ probably resulting from a defect in the sarcoplasmic reticulum or sarcolemma/sarcoplasmic reticulum junction. The raised $[Ca^{2+}]$ is responsible for the three cardinal features of MH: heat production, glycogenolysis with lactic acidosis and muscle rigidity. The incidence of MH is low, perhaps as infrequent as 1:50 000 in adult practice, but an increased incidence is found in males, children and young adults and in patients with congenital musculoskeletal disorders. The preponderance of MH in male patients is not related to its inheritance, and may reflect the increased muscular development in young, male adults.

GENETICS

MH susceptibility was reported to map to chromosome 19 in several families in the early 1990s. The locus for the MH gene, 12–13.2q, is similar to that of the ryanodine receptor gene. The importance of this observation lies in the knowledge that ryanodine selectively binds to the calcium-release channel of the sarcoplasmic reticulum suggesting the site of the defect in MH. Although this relationship between the ryanodine receptor gene and the MH gene is extremely consistent in porcine MH, in the human syndrome several families have been reported in which linkage to chromosome 19 could not be found. This suggests that MH is heterogeneous and that a simple DNA-based blood test will not be easily developed.

A variety of other disorders, particularly myopathies, have been linked to MH susceptibility and it is hoped that increased knowledge of the inheritance of these problems will clarify their relationship to MH. At present, the only myopathy that predicts MH susceptibility is central core disease. The gene for this condition is also situated on chromosome 19 close to the MH gene. Muscular dystrophies, myotonic dystrophy, hyperkalaemic periodic paralysis, neuroleptic malignant syndrome, heat stroke and even sudden infant death syndrome, have all been linked with MH usually on the basis of a positive *in vitro* contracture test (IVCT). Most attention has been given to the dystrophies, as there have been several reports of 'MH-like' syndromes occurring during anaesthesia. Hyperkalaemia is a prominent feature of these syndromes, with less acidosis and hypermetabolism than usually found in MH, suggesting that the volatile agents have induced primarily a large increase in sarcolemmal permeability.

PREOPERATIVE DIAGNOSIS OF MH SUSCEPTIBILIITY

The preoperative diagnosis of MH is not easy but the patient often gives a family history of problems, and even death, associated with general anaesthesia. An increased circulating creatine kinase (CK) concentration may be found in MH-susceptible patients, but unfortunately this enzymatic test is of limited value. Creatine kinase values are raised in a variety of myopathic disorders, so the test is not specific, and it is known that some MH-susceptible patients have normal CK concentrations. At present, the most accurate method of diagnosing MH is to use IVCT of a muscle biopsy to halothane and caffeine. This can only be undertaken in specialized centres and the test has been standardized in Europe. Following exposure to caffeine and halothane in carefully controlled conditions, the patient is described as MHS (susceptible), MHN (normal), or MHE (equivocal). MHE patients respond positively to either halothane or caffeine, but not both. The validity of the IVCT has been disputed, but it probably errs on the side of safety and yields some false-positive data.

CLINICAL PRESENTATION

All volatile agents can induce MH in susceptible patients and this includes the recently introduced drugs such as desflurane and sevoflurane. The response to the use of suxamethonium is abnormal in some MH-susceptible patients. Instead of muscle fasciculations followed by relaxation, there are vigorous fasciculations with failure of relaxation. In particular, masseter spasm occurs which may make endotracheal intubation difficult. The occurrence of masseter spasm should be treated as an important warning sign, as approximately 50% patients are found to be MH-susceptible on subsequent IVCT. The key feature of the management of patients with masseter spasm is to avoid the use of volatile anaesthetics. A 'safe' technique should be used (see below).

Apart from the occurrence of masseter spasm, there are no obvious signs of the onset of MH. The main clinical indicators are:

- abnormal response to suxamethonium
- tachycardia and/or arrhythmias
- tachypnoea
- increased use of soda-lime
- muscle stiffness
- possibly peripheral cyanosis

The metabolic signs of MH are much more obvious than the clinical signs and the increased use of physiological monitoring during anaesthesia has helped in the early detection of MH. The metabolic disorders reflect the massive, uncontrolled stimulation of muscle metabolism:

- acidosis, both respiratory and metabolic
- hyperkalaemia
- haemoconcentration
- hyperglycaemia
- hyperthermia

Usually the earliest sign of the onset of MH is increased CO_2 production which is reflected in a marked increase in end-tidal CO_2 concentration at constant volume ventilation. Together with a tachycardia this should alert the anaesthetist to the possibility of MH. Confirmation is usually obtained by arterial gas analysis and in established MH a severe acidosis, both respiratory and metabolic, and often hyperkalaemia are found. Once the diagnosis of MH has been confirmed, treatment must be started immediately.

TREATMENT OF ESTABLISHED MH

The treatment of MH can be considered as specific therapy with dantrolene and general management of the other metabolic and physiological problems: acidosis, hyperkalaemia, haemoconcentration, arrhythmias and hyperthermia. The following guidelines have been shown to be effective.

- stop volatile agent, terminate surgery
- hyperventilate with 100% O_2, maintain unconsciousness
- correct metabolic acidosis (100 mmol $NaHCO_3$)
- dantrolene 1 mg kg^{-1} i.v. every 10 min until MH controlled
    assess therapy by
        arterial gas analysis
        tachycardia
        muscle stiffness
        temperature
- establish additional monitoring, if required
- correct hyperkalaemia and rehydrate
- correct tachycardia/arrhythmias if persistent
- cool if necessary
- induce diuresis when rehydrated
- measure serial CK values and urinary myoglobin

It is imperative that dantrolene is administered as soon as possible after MH has been diagnosed; most patients only require a total dose of 1–2 mg kg^{-1} i.v.

ANAESTHESIA FOR SUSCEPTIBLE PATIENTS

If MH susceptibility is known, or suspected, then a 'safe' anaesthetic technique is required. This means avoiding the administration of suxamethonium and volatile agents and also using a 'clean' anaesthetic machine. A 'clean' machine is obtained by removing the vaporizers, changing all the disposable tubing and then flushing with O_2 at the maximal flow rate for 6 min.

Regional or general anaesthesia may be used. All local anaesthetic drugs are safe and regional anaesthesia is particularly appropriate in MH-susceptible patients. For general anaesthesia, the common intravenous induction agents are safe, as are all the non-depolarizing neuromuscular blocking drugs, and the opioids and nitrous oxide. Therefore, a technique of i.v. induction, opioid, non-depolarizing muscle relaxant and ventilation with N_2O in O_2 is appropriate. Full monitoring must be undertaken and may include the intravascular measurement of arterial pressure and central venous pressure. Prophylactic dantrolene is not recommended because it causes persistent muscle weakness that cannot be ameliorated and its effects are unpredictable.

OTHER INHERITED MYOPATHIES

There are many rare, inherited myopathies which occasionally intrude into anaesthetic practice. The most common are the muscular dystrophies and the myotonias.

MUSCULAR DYSTROPHIES

These can be classified as follows.
- X-linked: Duchenne
  Becker
  Emery–Dreifuss
- autosomal dominant: facioscapulohumeral
  distal
  ocular
- autosomal recessive: severe
  mild limb girdle

Duchenne dystrophy is associated with the most severe anaesthetic problems, although fatal complications have also been reported with Becker dystrophy. Cardiac involvement and weakness of respiratory muscles is uncommon, except in Duchenne dystrophy.

DUCHENNE DYSTROPHY

This severe form of dystrophy presents with rapidly progressive muscle weakness, initially of the thighs and pelvis. The weakness eventually involves all muscles and patients die from respiratory failure or cardiac disease.

Preoperative evaluation must pay particular attention to the respiratory and cardiovascular systems. Respiratory muscle weakness is common and diaphragmatic failure can occur. ECG abnormalities are frequent: a hypertrophic cardiomyopathy and mitral valve prolapse may be present.

An 'MH-like' syndrome has been reported during general anaesthesia in patients with Duchenne dystrophy. Arrhythmias are common, particularly during induction of anaesthesia, and respiratory problems in the postoperative period must be expected.

Regional anaesthesia is particularly appropriate, but can be difficult in anxious children. Suxamethonium is contraindicated because of the risk of hyperkalaemia, arrhythmias and cardiac arrest. Many patients with Duchenne dystrophy have been successfully anaesthetized with volatile agents such as halothane. However, it is prudent to restrict the use of volatile agents to short anaesthetics (up to 30 min duration) and use a 'safe' technique (see above) for more prolonged surgery. Full monitoring is mandatory and, if there is any doubt about respiratory function on completion of surgery, elective pulmonary ventilation should be undertaken in the early postoperative period.

MYOTONIAS

There are three familial myotonias: dystrophia myotonica, myotonia congenita and paramyotonia. They are inherited in an autosomal dominant pattern. Whereas the muscular dystrophies are characterized by destruction and dysfunction of the muscle, the myotonias are diseases of the muscle membrane. The typical abnormality is delayed muscle relaxation following contraction in response to a variety of simple stimuli such as touch and cold. The underlying pathophysiology is an abnormality in the chloride channel in the muscle membrane. The sustained contraction cannot be prevented, or treated, with non-depolarizing neuromuscular blocking drugs, or regional anaesthesia.

Dystrophia myotonica or myotonic dystrophy

This syndrome does not usually present until middle age and the myotonia is associated with muscle wasting and weakness. The weakness is progressive and so causes some problems that are similar to the dystrophies.

Preoperative evaluation must include careful assessment of respiratory and cardiovascular function. The administration of suxamethonium is contraindicated, because a prolonged contraction occurs. Non-depolarizing neuromuscular blocking drugs can be given and a peripheral nerve stimulator must be used to monitor neuromuscular transmission. The use of neostigmine is controversial; it is helpful if it can be avoided. The use of regional anaesthesia avoids some of the problems associated with drugs given for general anaesthesia, but muscle relaxation is not guaranteed. Direct injection of local anaesthetic drugs into muscle has been used to try to treat myotonia, dantrolene is of little value. Careful evaluation is necessary in the early postoperative period to prevent respiratory problems.

Myotonia congenita

This occurs typically in infants of mothers with dystrophia myotonica and muscle weakness is the main problem. Most patients develop the adult form of the disease in the first decade of life but may require surgery for paediatric problems such as herniotomy, talipes or other congenital problems.

Suxamethonium should not be used, and sensitivity to non-depolarizing neuromuscular blocking drugs has been described. An 'MH-like' syndrome has been reported occasionally, but such patients are negative on subsequent IVCT. Regional anaesthesia is ideal, otherwise monitoring of neuromuscular function is essential.

FURTHER READING

Symposium (1988) Malignant hyperthermia. *British Journal of Anaesthesia*, **60**, 251–319.

Donaldson, V. H. and Bissler, J. (1991) C1 inhibitors and their genes: an update. *Journal of Laboratory and Clinical Medicine*, **119**, 330–333.

Furie, B., Limentani, S. A. and Rosenfield C. G. (1994) A practical guide to the evaluation and treatment of haemophilia *Blood*, **84**, 3–9.

Huisman, T. H. J. (1993) The structure and function of normal and abnormal haemoglobins *Baillière's Clinical Haematology*, **6**, 1–25.

Jensen, N. F., Fiddler, D. S. and Striepe, V. (1995) Anesthetic considerations in porphyrias. *Anaesthesia and Analgesia*, **80**, 591–599.

Katz, J., Benumof, J. and Kadis, L. (1990) *Anesthesia and Uncommon Diseases*, 4th edn.

Whittaker, M. (1980) Plasma cholinesterase variants and the anaesthetist. *Anaesthesia*, **35**, 174–197.

Yao, F. F. and Artusio, F. (1993) *Anesthesiology: Problem-Oriented Patient Management*, 3rd edn.

PART THREE
SUBSPECIALTY

THORACIC SURGERY

R. S. Vaughan and G. Phillips

The major problem in the development of thoracic anaesthesia was that of the open pneumothorax. When the chest is open, inspiration results in an increase in negative pressure in the intact pleural cavity and air moves from the collapsed lung, which becomes smaller, into the intact lung; this is accompanied by a shift of the mediastinum towards the intact side. The reverse occurs on expiration. This movement of air between the lungs was originally termed 'pendeluft' or pendulum air. The net results are increased deadspace, decreased Pa_{O_2}, increased Pa_{CO_2}, increasing acidosis, decreased venous return and decreased cardiac output; death was the inevitable result. The problem was solved by tracheal intubation and intermittent positive pressure ventilation (IPPV). Chest drainage and underwater seals also ensured that the chest could be closed.

Excess secretions and their control, which was a major problem for the pioneers of thoracic anaesthesia, have now been largely solved by the decline in tuberculosis, use of antibiotics and vigorous preoperative physiotherapy. The main concerns are now those of the management of one-lung anaesthesia and postoperative complications.

PREOPERATIVE ASSESSMENT

Assessment of lung reserves is mandatory, especially when lung resection is a strong possibility. The patient should be exercised, the development of tachycardia, arrhythmias and undue breathlessness being ominous signs. Attempts should be made to stop patients smoking for at least 2 weeks preoperatively because of an associated increase in postoperative morbidity. Most patients are in the older age groups and may be receiving a variety of drugs. In general, all therapy is continued throughout the perioperative period.

Treatment of malignant tumours with bleomycin can be problematical, as its use has been associated with pulmonary interstitial disease. An increased inspired oxygen concentration in these patients may induce lung injury and the F_{IO_2} may have to be limited to a maximum of 0.3.

INVESTIGATIONS

The standard haematological and biochemical tests for patients undergoing major surgery must be available. Arterial blood gas analysis is important for two reasons. First, they give the baseline readings and second, can indicate a shunt with a decreased Pa_{O_2} whilst breathing air and altered levels of Pa_{CO_2}. If there are signs of myocardial ischaemia, coronary artery surgery may be required before thoracic surgery as there is considerable myocardial strain during one-lung anaesthesia and after pneumonectomy. Lung function tests must be available. Particular attention is paid to the ratio of the forced expiratory volume in one second (FEV_1) to the forced vital capacity (FVC). A figure of above 75% is considered normal. The right lung makes up approximately 60% of the total lung volume and the left 40%. Each lung is divided into lobes, three on the right and two on the left. If each lobe is considered to be approximately equal in volume, each lobe contributes 20% to the total lung volume.

There have been considerable advances in imaging. Traditional views on chest X-ray have been augmented by computed tomography (CT) scanning and occasionally magnetic resonance imaging (MRI). These images give a comprehensive view of the pathology and have possibly resulted in a more selected group of patients presenting for thoracotomy. A barium swallow is performed for oesophageal lesions.

ASSESSMENT

A decision has to be taken as to whether the patient will survive thoracic surgery with a reasonable quality of life. This is based on a number of observations.

- If all the results are within normal ranges, there should be no problem.
- A 50% rule can be applied. If all the ratios of the observed to the predicted investigations are greater than 50%, the patient will probably withstand a thoracotomy. This may not be true under all circumstances.
- If there is an area of consolidation clinically and on the chest X-ray, there is a degree of shunting and the Pao_2 will be lower than normal while breathing air. When this consolidated area is removed, this shunt will disappear.
- If a consolidated lobe is present, the tests will reflect a decrease in lung volume. The remaining lobes provide approximately equal volumes towards the total lung volume. For example, if one lobe is consolidated, the remaining lobes each constitute approximately 25% of the total lung volumes. If one lung is collapsed or consolidated, the tests are primarily those of the remaining lung. These are used to give an indication of the postoperative lung volumes.
- If a small lesion in a single lobe is to be removed, that lobe continues to contribute approximately 20% to the total lung volume. When that lobe is removed, the lung will function initially on 80% of its original volumes.

To prevent the patient from becoming a respiratory cripple after surgery, it is a reasonable rule of thumb to have a postoperative vital capacity roughly equal to three times the preoperative tidal volume. By and large, this means a minimum vital capacity of around 25 ml kg^{-1}. It is relatively easy therefore, to calculate the possible consequences of a lobectomy or pneumonectomy given the preoperative findings and the postoperative requirements.

Many patients receive preoperative chemotherapy through a Hickman line to treat certain malignancies of the oesophagus. This line can also be used to replace any nitrogen lost due to the disease process and correct both fluid and electrolyte balances thus generally improving the preoperative status.

PREMEDICATION

There has been a change in practice in recent years with a greater emphasis on anxiolysis, but the choice of premedication lies mainly with the preference of the anaesthetist. In children, an anticholinergic drug is indicated to counteract any parasympathetic stimulation. In patients over 55 years old, there has been a tendency to give digitalis preoperatively to prevent the onset of atrial fibrillation. Such a change in rhythm can produce pulmonary oedema which, if it occurs during one-lung anaesthesia, can cause serious problems. The use of atropine has also decreased except where awake intubation is considered, as it dries secretions leading to a decrease in ciliary movement.

DIAGNOSTIC PROCEDURES

BRONCHOSCOPY

Advances made in instrumentation have enabled anaesthetist and surgeon to share the airway relatively safely. The stress response to bronchoscopy is at least equal to that of tracheal intubation and can be prolonged, so it is advisable to use pharmacological agents to attenuate or abolish this response. Each patient has an intravenous line established and minimum monitoring applied before anaesthesia is induced.

Adults

Local anaesthesia

Diagnostic bronchoscopy can be performed under sedation and local anaesthesia. With fibreoptic instruments, either the nasal or oral route can be used. Sedation is usually achieved with benzodiazepines orally followed by agents such as fentanyl and midazolam given intravenously. A number of methods are available for local anaesthesia.

- If access through the nose is required, cocaine is still used because of its vasoconstrictor properties. This is usually applied as cocaine paste. This technique is gradually being superseded by the application of more recent local anaesthetic agents usually with adrenaline.
- The 'spray as you go' technique.
- Bilateral block of the superior laryngeal nerves.
- A cricothyroid puncture. This is increasingly the preferred technique as it enables the local anaesthetic agent to be distributed all over the upper respiratory tract.

To perform a cricothyroid puncture, a wheal is produced in the skin over the cricothyroid membrane using 1 ml of 1% plain lignocaine. A needle, attached to a syringe containing 4 ml of 4% plain lignocaine, is introduced through the skin at right angles to the neck between two fingers placed on either side of the cricothyroid membrane. A click is felt as the needle penetrates the membrane and enters the trachea. Aspiration is performed and air bubbles confirm tracheal placement. The local anaesthetic agent is injected at the end of expiration, as the next breath must be inspiration. This is followed by coughing which distributes the local anaesthetic agent above and below the cords. Some anaesthetists divide the injection volume into two: 2 ml followed around 2 min later by another 2 ml.

General anaesthesia

There are several techniques available. Most methods start with pre-oxygenation for at least 5 min. An intravenous injection of an opioid drug such as alfentanil or fentanyl is followed by induction of anaesthesia with propofol and then a programmed continuous propofol infusion plus a muscle relaxant. Suxamethonium was at one time considered to be the relaxant of choice but its use has declined with the development of the short acting nondepolarising drugs. Following muscle relaxation, the lungs are ventilated with 100% oxygen using a Storz ventilating bronchoscope (Figure 11.1). Another method would be to ventilate the lungs with a volatile agent in oxygen. A Saunders injector can also be used with this bronchoscope but its use is decreasing.

At the end of the procedure, residual muscle relaxation is reversed and the bronchoscope removed when adequate spontaneous ventilation returns. The patient is turned into the left lateral, head-down position and returned to the recovery ward breathing humidified oxygen.

An additional consideration is the lung biopsy followed by bleeding. Postoperatively, the patient is turned into the lateral position with the **affected side down** until recovery

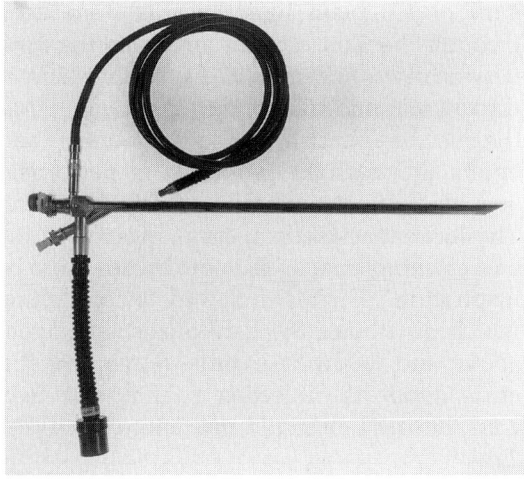

Figure 11.1 A Storz ventilating bronchoscope. (Reproduced from R.S. Vaughan (1996) Endobronchial intubation, in *Difficulties in Tracheal Intubation*, 2nd edn, (eds. I.P. Latto and R.S. Vaughan) Saunders, London.

has taken place and the patient is able to cough properly. This tends to prevent contamination of the good lung. If the biopsy is followed by massive bleeding, the main bronchus leading to the bleeding area needs to be packed and an endobronchial tube introduced into the other bronchus. A thoracotomy is then usually necessary to stop bleeding.

Children

Local anaesthesia is rarely feasible in children.

General anaesthesia

The general anaesthetic techniques and equipment used in children are similar to those used in adults although volatile agents are more popular than intravenous infusions. A Jackson–Rees modification of an Ayre's T-piece is attached to the ventilating arm of the Storz bronchoscope.

Bronchoscopy for foreign bodies

Anaesthesia can be induced either intravenously or using an inhalation agent such as halothane or sevoflurane. A muscle relaxant, usually atracurium, is given and the lungs artificially ventilated using a volatile agent in oxygen until full muscle paralysis is achieved. In children, the vocal cords are exposed by the anaesthetist so that the correct size bronchoscope can be introduced directly into the trachea. This reduces delay and possible trauma. Thereafter, the techniques are similar to those in the adult.

There are two contraindications to this method. Occasionally, following the inhalation of a foreign body, particularly a peanut, a valvular mechanism can develop at a bronchial level. During inspiration, the bronchus dilates but it is prevented from attaining the original diameter at the end of expiration. This mechanism allows a volume of gas to enter the distal lung but not all is able to leave. The lung distal to the obstruction gradually increases in size, reduces the efficiency of respiration and eventually causes mediastinal shift. This is best confirmed by chest X-rays taken at the end of inspiration and expiration. Under these circumstances, nitrous oxide must be avoided as it can rapidly increase the size of the obstructed segment by diffusion. Similar considerations apply in the presence of a lung cyst or pneumothorax. IPPV is also contraindicated because of the high risk of causing a pneumothorax. Thus, an inhalation technique using a volatile agent in oxygen is used.

If, during removal, the foreign body slips out of the holding instrument and obstructs the trachea, it should be pushed back into one or other bronchus. Adequate ventilation is re-established before another attempt is made at removal.

OESOPHAGOSCOPY

It must always be assumed that there is debris proximal to an oesophageal lesion with the possibility of regurgitation and inhalation. A rapid-sequence induction and passage of a reinforced tracheal tube should be used. The reinforced tube prevents obstruction to ventilation due to compression by the rigid oesophagoscope. During the procedure muscle relaxation must be monitored with a nerve stimulator as coughing could lead to oesophageal perforation. Consequently, many anaesthetists wait until the effects of suxamethonium disappear, then give a short acting non-depolarizing drug before allowing the investigation to proceed. With a flexible instrument, oesophagoscopy can be performed under sedation and local anaesthesia. The tracheas of all patients should be extubated in the head-down position at the end of the procedure.

MEDIASTINOSCOPY

Mediastinoscopy is performed for diagnostic purposes to obtain a biopsy of a mediastinal mass. Some of these masses are extensive and can cause tracheal compression, which presents clinically as expiratory and inspiratory stridor. Blood vessels can also be stretched over the mass and appear to the naked eye as an integral part. It is therefore possible accidentally to biopsy a blood vessel which can be followed by complete transection and massive haemorrhage into the mediastinum. If there is only venous access in the arm, resuscitation can be difficult and occasionally impossible, as blood and other fluids simply pour into the mediastinum. Consequently, many anaesthetists also have a large cannula in a foot vein. Good venous access is essential and crossmatched blood must be available in the operating theatre for this procedure.

It is essential to monitor the blood pressure in the right arm as the mediastinoscope can completely obstruct the flow of blood through the right common carotid artery. Some anaesthetists recommend direct arterial monitoring. The technique for mediastinoscopy is similar to that for oesophagoscopy, although an inhalation induction is favoured by some. The patient should be relatively awake before extubation as they are sat up as quickly as possible and transferred to the recovery area breathing humidified oxygen. If heavy bleeding occurs, anaesthesia is maintained and the mediastinium is packed, while the operating theatre staff prepare for further surgery through a right thoractomy or a median sternotomy.

In patients with myasthenia gravis or the myasthenic syndrome, muscle relaxants were traditionally avoided. However, recent work supports the use of carefully monitored muscle relaxation with the newer shorter acting non-depolarizing agents.

THORACOSCOPY

Thoracoscopy is used for inspection of the thoracic cavity, open lung biopsy, surgical removal of lung tissue, thoracic sympathectomy and oesophageal surgery.

The patient is prepared for a major thoracic procedure. A double lumen endobronchial tube is used with the bronchial lumen placed in the bronchus of the lung which is not to be collapsed. When the patient has been placed in the lateral position, the lung on the side which is to be inspected is collapsed using the same technique as for lung resection. Occasionally carbon dioxide is insufflated under pressure through a Verres needle inserted through the chest wall into the side where the procedure is to be performed. During insufflation, it is essential that the tracheal lumen of the double-lumen tube is open to the atmosphere, otherwise a tension capnothorax can occur. It can also occur if the lung has adhesions which prevent it collapsing. Ventilation to the dependent lung continues throughout. The major dangers associated with a tension capnothorax are decreased venous return, decreased cardiac output and hypotension. Hypoxia and hypercarbia can also occur. Should a tension capnothorax develop, the carbon dioxide is let out rapidly.

Damage to major organs can lead to significant haemorrhage; a formal thoracotomy is then required and blood must be available before the investigation commences. Damage to the recurrent laryngeal nerves can also occur, causing difficulties with postoperative coughing and ventilation. At the end, an underwater seal is established and a chest X-ray taken in the recovery ward.

MAJOR OPEN PROCEDURES

These require the presence of an experienced anaesthetist. Pre-induction monitoring includes ECG, blood pressure cuff, pulse oximetry and the insertion of a large intravenous cannula. Additional monitoring usually includes an intra-arterial cannula, central venous pressure, FIO_2 measurement, expired tidal volume measurement and inflation pressures. Oesophageal temperature and urinary output should be monitored.

The internal jugular veins can be cannulated using a percutaneous technique but the needle should be introduced on the **same side as the proposed surgery** as it is possible to produce a pneumothorax. A nasogastric tube is passed as gastric emptying is delayed for at least 24 h after major chest surgery.

Anaesthetists should **always** perform a bronchoscopy before endobronchial intubation to check the bronchial anatomy, particularly on the right side, as the origin of the right upper lobe bronchus is variable, and occasionally it may arise directly from the trachea. A right sided tube is used for a left sided procedure and vice versa. Some anaesthetists use a left sided tube for operations that do not involve lung resection.

INDUCTION OF ANAESTHESIA

Anaesthesia is induced in a similar fashion for bronchoscopy. If there is oesophageal obstruction or gastro-oesophageal incompetence, a rapid-sequence induction is indicated.

INTRODUCTION OF A DOUBLE LUMEN ENDOBRONCHIAL TUBE

The technique is given in Table 11.1. The checking procedures may be augmented using a fibreoptic bronchoscope which is passed through each lumen of the endobronchial tube to check that each distal orifice is opposite the appropriate bronchial orifice. Furthermore, some anaesthetists use pressure–volume loops, before and after intubation, to confirm correct positioning. Once the patient has been turned into the lateral position the checking procedures must be repeated. Anaesthesia is continued using a relaxant technique with other agents preferred by the individual anaesthetist.

ONE-LUNG ANAESTHESIA

The following data are recorded before surgery starts: minute volume, FIO_2, respiratory rate, expired tidal volume, SpO_2, end tidal carbon dioxide levels and results of arterial blood gas analysis. It is these parameters that are usually altered when the non-dependent lung is collapsed. Although there is no universal agreement about the best method of providing one-lung anaesthesia, a popular technique is based on the 25% method. The respiratory rate is increased by 25%, for example from, 12 to 15 breaths per minute. This usually results in a decrease in the expired tidal volume of around 20–25% depending on the compliance of the dependent lung. The minute volume remains unchanged. The FIO_2 is increased to at least 0.5.

Several factors influence gas exchange during one lung anaesthesia.

Factors affecting the dependent lung

The pressures on the dependent lung include: the weight of the mediastinum, the abdominal contents pushing the diaphragm upwards, solid props under the axillary area, chest pieces preventing the hemi-thorax from

Table 11.1 Technique for the introduction of a double lumen endobronchial tube

1. The double lumen tube is passed through the cords under direct vision with the tip of the tube in the antero-posterior plane. Once the tracheal (or anchor) cuff has passed beyond the vocal cords and the laryngoscope removed, the following manoeuvres are performed.
2. The complete tube is turned through 90° **towards** the bronchus to be intubated so that the distal tip lies against the appropriate lateral tracheal wall.
3. The patient's head is turned **away** from the bronchus which is to be intubated.
4. The tube is advanced until the anaesthetist feels a resistance as the tracheal portion of the tube abuts against the carina.
5. The proximal ends of the double lumen tube are connected to the breathing system using a purposely designed catheter mount.
6. The tracheal cuff is inflated until an air-tight seal is made. Air entry to both sides of the chest is confirmed with a stethoscope.
7. The catheter mount attached to the tracheal lumen of the double lumen tube is clamped so that no fresh gas flow from the breathing system can enter the lung ventilated through this lumen, i.e. the non-dependent lung.
8. The suction port distal to the clamp is opened to the atmosphere.
9. The dependent lung is ventilated through the bronchial lumen. The only way that gas can escape through the tracheal lumen is to leak past the bronchial cuff.
10. The bronchial cuff is gradually inflated until no leak is audible.
11. The ventilation to the dependent lung is confirmed using the traditional guidelines.
    (a) Looks good: only one side of the chest moves, i.e. the dependent lung.
    (b) Feels good: there is no undue decrease in compliance as the dependent lung is inflated.
    (c) Sounds good: this is the most reliable of these traditional guidelines. Air entry to each lobe must be confirmed with a stethoscope.
12. Check position of the tube with a fibreoptic bronchoscope.
13. Finally, the ventilation to the non-dependent lung is confirmed after removing the clamp and reconnection at the suction port. One-lung ventilation in the non-dependent lung can also be checked along similar lines.

expanding, and the downward force of the surgical manipulations. Pressure in this lung should be kept as low as possible as the higher the pressure, the greater the resistance to blood flow. The net result would be an increase in blood flow to the non-dependent lung thus increasing shunting.

It is essential constantly to monitor the key parameters which are the pressures required to ventilate the dependent lung, expired tidal volumes, oxygen saturation and end-tidal carbon dioxide levels. The latter usually reads lower than the Pa_{CO_2} as there is dilution by fresh gas coming out of the dependent lung which has not participated in respiratory exchange. Therefore, arterial blood gases are checked half hourly.

Secretions accumulate in the dependent lung as gravity acts against the normal lymphatic drainage. The longer the operation, the greater the changes in compliance. Ventilation patterns may, therefore, have to change. During this period, there is a requirement for an increased F_{IO_2} due mainly to an increase in shunting. Although 100% oxygen can be used throughout, micro-alveolar trapping and collapse can occur thus increasing the percentage shunt. Micro-alveolar collapse may be detrimental in the postoperative period.

Factors affecting the non-dependent lung

The major factor affecting blood flow through the collapsed non-dependent lung is the hypoxic pulmonary vasoconstrictor reflex. The Pa_{O_2} in the non-dependent lung decreases causing constriction of the pulmonary vessels supplying that area. This is a local protective reflex which diverts blood to areas which have a higher alveolar oxygen concentration. Maximum vasoconstriction is obtained when the following parameters are within normal physiological ranges: Pa_{O_2} of 10–15 kPa, an end-tidal carbon dioxide of 5–6 kPa and a pulmonary artery pressure of 20–25 mmHg.

Some anaesthetists maintain an end-tidal carbon dioxide just above normal as it causes pulmonary and peripheral vasodilatation. Myocardial work and oxygen consumption are therefore reduced as is the tendency towards arrhythmias. It could be argued that an increased Pa_{CO_2} could oppose pulmonary vasoconstriction.

Factors that can reduce the hypoxic pulmonary vasoconstriction reflex are inhalational anaesthetic agents and continuous intravenous infusions of some drugs such as vasodilators. A continuous infusion of propofol does not inhibit this reflex. If the Pa_{O_2} decreases when all the enhancing mechanisms are working to a maximum, a number of manoeuvres can be tried to increase oxygenation. The I:E ratios and times can be altered while the inspired and expired tidal volumes can also be manipulated.

If hypoxia continues, the following should be tried.

- Insufflation of oxygen into the non-dependent lung.
- Application of positive end-expiratory pressure (PEEP) to the dependent lung. Theoretically, this can increase the percentage of blood shunted to the non-dependent lung.
- Continuous positive airway pressure (CPAP) applied to the upper lung can improve oxygenation, but this does not help in the elimination of carbon dioxide.
- Both PEEP and CPAP can be applied simultaneously.
- High frequency ventilation to the non-dependent lung, which increases Pa_{O_2} and decreases Pa_{CO_2}.

These manoeuvres increase the movement of the non-dependent lung which can cause surgical difficulties, but this is not important if there is any compromise in the patient's condition. It could also be argued that two-lung ventilation should be restored.

Any secretions that have accumulated in the bronchus of the non-dependent lung during surgery should be sucked out. This prevents the dissemination of secretions into the areas which are to be re-inflated, particularly important if there has been a previous infection. The remaining lobes (or lung) are reinflated.

UNDERWATER SEAL

Before chest closure, drains must be inserted. If the patient has had a pneumonectomy, one drain is inserted. If a lobectomy has been performed, two chest drains are inserted, the first to remove any fluid from the thoracic cavity and the second to remove the remaining air. Each chest drain is connected to an underwater seal.

An underwater seal requires a wide-based circular jar which gives a large volume of water. The drainage tube from the chest is connected to a long glass tube, the end of which is placed about 2 cm below the surface of the water, so that there is a little resistance to air and fluid coming out of the drains. Should a deep inspiration occur, there is also sufficient volume of water to prevent air being sucked back into the chest cavity. Some centres use the Heimlich one-way valve.

Occasionally, **after lobectomy,** when the remaining lobe or lobes are not re-expanding the underwater seals are connected to suction apparatus which can produce a maximum negative pressure up to 20 cmH$_2$O. Suction apparatus must *never* be attached to an underwater seal after a pneumonectomy. If suction is applied the mediastinum shifts, venous return decreases due to kinking of the large central veins and cardiac output decreases. Cardiac arrest can follow.

Underwater seals are checked to be working at the end of the operation by inflating the lungs and noting that gases bubble out through the water. These underwater seal jars are usually changed 24 hourly after lobectomy but are usually removed after pneumonectomy.

TERMINATION OF ANAESTHESIA

Anaesthesia is discontinued, the lungs are ventilated with 100% oxygen ensuring that any collapsed lobes (or occasionally lung) are reinflated and the neuromuscular blockade reversed. Before extubation is performed, suction is applied to both lumens of the endobronchial tube and the pharynx. The endobronchial tube is usually removed with the patient in the lateral position. Oxygen is continued through a facemask. If the patient has had a lobectomy, he/she remains on the same side, i.e. with the operated side uppermost. This encourages the remaining lobe(s) to re-expand. Those patients who have had a pneumonectomy are usually nursed with the operated side lowermost to remove the weight of the mediastinum on the remaining lung.

When consciousness returns, the patient is sat up at 45° provided that all the parameters are within acceptable ranges. Some anaesthetists prefer to continue artificial ventilation in the intensive care unit for several hours until the patient is fully warm, pain-free and conscious. Thereafter, the management is similar to those extubated in the operating theatre.

In patients who have had major gastro-oesophageal surgery, the body temperature has usually decreased as two large cavities have been exposed to the atmosphere. Thus, it is common practice to remove the endobronchial tube, replace it with an orotracheal tube and transfer the patient to the intensive care for postoperative ventilation. Their tracheas are either extubated sometime later or the following morning.

PAIN RELIEF

Pain relief is essential. Several methods can be instigated by the surgeons during operation. Both intra- and extra-pleural catheters can be placed so that local analgesic agents can be used. Cryo-analgesia has now been discontinued due to the long-term complications. The main methods are discussed in Chapter 38.

POSTOPERATIVE CARE

Although the postoperative care should be considered as a whole, it is reasonable to discuss each system separately. When the patient arrives in a high dependency unit (or step down unit) after discharge from the recovery room, the following monitoring is applied: ECG, pulse oximetry and blood pressure. In many cases, the arterial pressure is transduced directly, as is central venous pressure.

Cardiovascular system

Preoperatively, the total cardiac output passed through both pulmonary arteries. After pneumonectomy, the same volume of blood volume has to pass through one. This is associated with an initial increase in the pulmonary artery pressure. However, physiological vasodilation reduces the pulmonary artery pressure very quickly. Fluid replacement has to be carefully controlled particularly after right pneumonectomy as the left lung is smaller and has less capacity for blood vessel recruitment.

If there is continued fluid overload, right ventricular failure or pulmonary oedema may ensue. As the pulmonary artery pressure increases, it can exceed the oncotic pressure of the blood resulting in an outflow of fluid into the lung tissues. Some of the lymphatics will have also been damaged and therefore it is possible that the total amount of fluid that has come out of the circulation will not be removed. Consequently, increasing dyspnoea occurs due to decreases in compliance. Occasionally, frank pulmonary oedema occurs which is associated with very high mortality rates.

Respiratory system

The Sp_{O_2} should be constantly monitored and periodically, arterial blood gases should be measured to confirm adequate gaseous exchange. It is not uncommon to find that although the oxygen tensions can be kept at a satisfactory level, the Pa_{CO_2} is sometimes elevated. If pain relief is not adequate both the Pa_{O_2} and the Sp_{O_2} can decrease and the P_{CO_2} can increase. Adequate pain relief and physiotherapy are essential during this period to enable effective coughing and clearance of secretions.

Urinary output

An output of 0.5 ml kg^{-1} h^{-1} is reasonable. If it should decrease below this level, fluid replacement should be reviewed and additional measures instituted, e.g. diuretic therapy.

Gastrointestinal system

A nasogastric tube is usually left *in situ* for at least 24 h which reduces the incidence of nausea, vomiting and possible inhalation of gastric contents.

Chest drains

The drains are removed at different times depending on the surgical procedure. Following pneumonectomy the chest drain is removed around 24 h after operation. After lobectomy, they are removed when basal drainage ceases and the swing seen in the second drain is very small. They are removed after the patient has taken a full inspiration. A chest X-ray is always taken after the last drain has been removed.

Deep vein thrombosis

Several therapeutic measures are used to prevent deep vein thrombosis. Subcutaneous heparin may be used, but has been cited as a contraindication to the insertion of an epidural catheter (see Chapter 20). Compression stockings may be applied preoperatively and retained for at least four or five days. Colloid solutions, particularly dextrans, and regular physiotherapy also have parts to play.

SPECIAL CASES

BRONCHOPLEURAL FISTULA

A bronchopleural fistula exists when there is direct contact between the respiratory conducting passages, the lungs, or both, with the pleural cavity. The major causes are trauma and surgery.

The traumatic bronchopleural fistula usually presents as acute dyspnoea, subcutaneous emphysema and physical signs compatible with a pneumothorax. The chest X-ray confirms the diagnosis. A fluid level may be seen as there may have been damage to blood vessels. Initially, the patient breathes oxygen enriched humidified air, is resuscitated and has an underwater seal established.

Fistulae sometimes follow thoracic surgery and are usually due to infection. The bronchial stump breaks down and the pleural cavity fills with air and fluid, which inevitably becomes infected. Once infection has become established, it is extremely difficult to close any bronchus surgically. An underwater seal is placed in the pleural cavity for drainage. The major surgical difference is that the traumatic case can usually be repaired very quickly. There are however, reports of acute ruptures following surgery being successfully repaired before infection supervenes. The sur-

Special cases

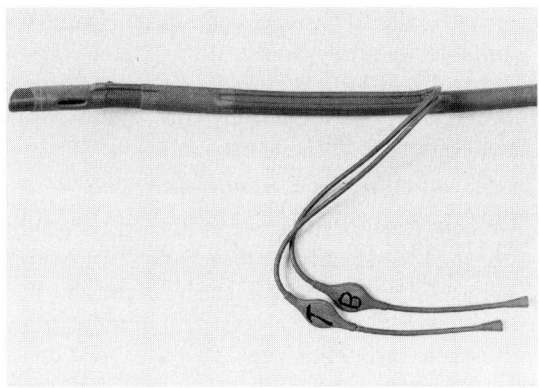

Figure 11.2 A Gordon Green (right) single lumen endobronchial tube.

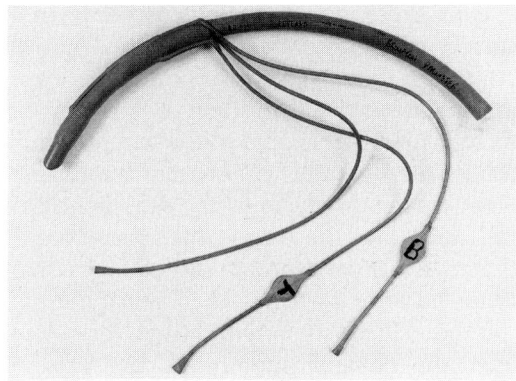

Figure 11.3 A Brompton Pallister (left) single lumen endobronchial tube.

gical infected case is usually closed much later by thoracoplasty.

Anaesthesia

The general principle governing the anaesthetic management is that whichever endobronchial tube is used to maintain the airway, it should be inserted under direct vision into the bronchus of the intact lung. The main single lumen endobronchial tubes are the Gordon Green type (Figure 11.2) for the right side and a Brompton Pallister type for the left (Figure 11.3). These are inserted mounted on a special intubating bronchoscope.

The main advantages of single lumen tubes are that they are specifically designed to be placed in the appropriate bronchus and have an internal diameter similar to a tracheal tube. However, they can kink at a tracheobronchial level or at the back of the pharynx. There are few anaesthetists nowadays who have the skill and necessary experience to use these specialized tubes. Thus, double-lumen tubes are frequently used. As the anatomy of the bronchial tree may be abnormal due to the bronchopleural fistula, these tubes are introduced under direct vision as their size and relative rigidity can cause further damage.

Induction techniques

The patients are premedicated with a benzodiazepine. They are placed in the semi-recumbent position with the good side slightly elevated. This position prevents any fluid in the pleural cavity spilling into the good lung, i.e. prevents 'flooding'. There are three possible techniques.

Sedation and local anaesthesia The sedation and local anaesthesia techniques are similar to those used for awake bronchoscopy. When judged to be adequate, 100% oxygen is continued for at least 5 min before intubation is attempted.

Inhalation anaesthesia Anaesthesia is induced, with the patient semi-recumbent with the good side uppermost, by gradually increasing the concentrations of an inhalation agent (usually halothane) until the patient is deeply anaesthetized, though still breathing spontaneously. The traditional teaching is that no muscle relaxants should be given until the airway is fully secured and the fistula isolated.

Intravenous induction followed by suxamethonium This technique has been used successfully. The major danger is that if the endobronchial tube cannot be correctly

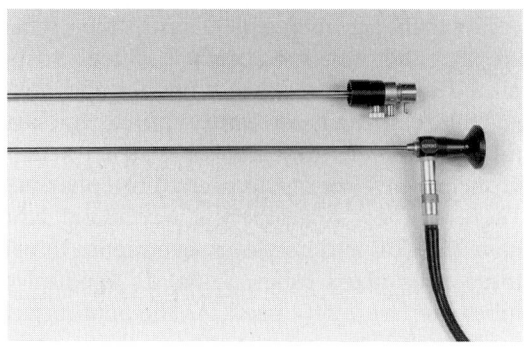

Figure 11.4 Storz Hopkins intubating bronchoscope: the telescope is protected by the stainless steel cylinder which also supports the endobronchial tube.

placed, oxygenation is impossible as gas will pass preferentially through the fistula rather than into the functioning lung. Hence, this technique is very rarely used.

Intubating techniques

Two techniques are used.

The rigid intubating bronchoscope A rigid intubating bronchoscope (Figure 11.4) is used to introduce a single lumen endobronchial tube into the appropriate bronchus. The bronchoscope is removed and the bronchial cuff is inflated until there is no air leak; the tracheal cuff is then inflated. The correct position is confirmed by auscultation and with a flexible fibreoptic bronchoscope.

The non-rigid fibreoptic intubating bronchoscope The fibreoptic bronchoscope is passed through the bronchial lumen of a double lumen endobronchial tube and into the appropriate bronchus. The tube is 'rail loaded' over the bronchoscope which is then removed with the tube held firmly at the mouth. The tracheal lumen is clamped and the bronchial cuff is gradually inflated until no leak is either audible or seen as leaking through the drainage apparatus from the opposite pleural cavity during ventilation. The tracheal cuff is inflated. The position is checked by auscultation and a fibreoptic bronchoscope, then secured.

A recent development is the Nazari tube (Figure 11.5). This is akin to a coaxial breathing system whereby the inner tube is guided into the bronchus of the dependent lung using a fibreoptic bronchoscope. Another option is the Univent tube which is a single lumen tracheal tube with a moveable bronchus blocker (Figure 11.6). The blocker is introduced under direct vision using a fibreoptic bronchoscope.

Once these tubes are confirmed to be in the correct position, patients are turned into the lateral position with the affected side uppermost. The correct position of the tube is reconfirmed. At the end of the surgical procedures, underwater drains are established. After thoracoplasty, one tube drains the pleural cavity and the second the space between the muscle layers and the skin: this is usually removed after 24–48 h. (The drainage tube in the thoracic cavity is withdrawn very slowly over the ensuing months as the proximal areas granulate and heal.) Muscle relaxation is reversed and the patient is again turned (but this time, with the affected side down) and allowed to regain consciousness with the endobronchial tube *in situ*. Once spontaneous ventilation is judged to be adequate, the tube is removed and the patient breathes humidified oxygen. Thereafter, the management of either type of bronchopleural fistula follows that seen after lobe or lung removal.

TRACHEAL STENOSIS

Tracheal stenoses are seen following long-term intubation, are associated with tumours of the tracheal wall and those which cause external compression. The latter can be removed through a sternotomy or a right

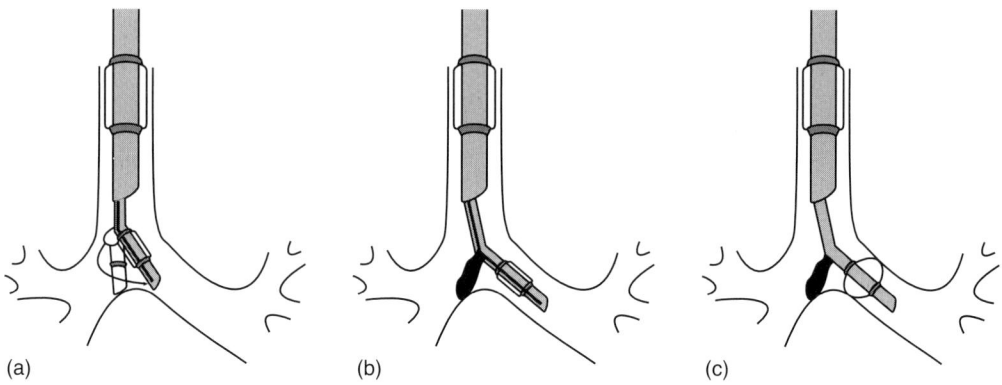

Figure 11.5 The Nazari tube. (Reproduced from S. Nazari *et al.* (1986) *Anaesthesia*, **41**, 519.)

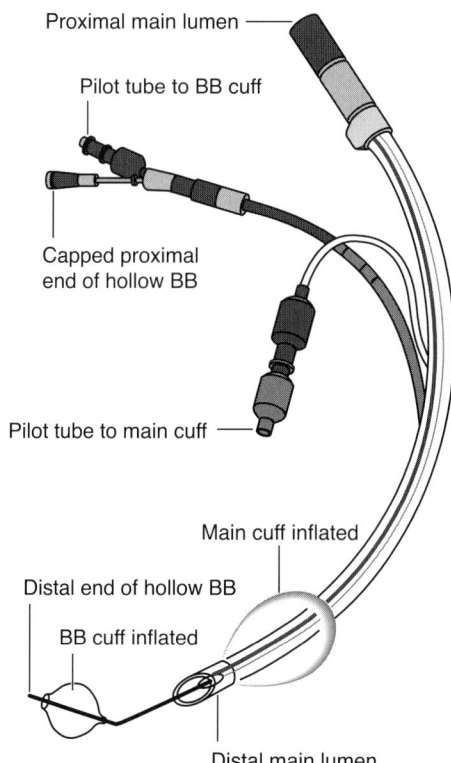

Figure 11.6 A Univent tube. (Reproduced with permission from J.L. Benumof (1995) *Anaesthesia for Thoracic Surgery* Saunders, USA.)

thoracotomy. Where tracheal resection is required, the procedure is highly specialized. The patient usually presents with increasing asthmatic like symptoms followed by the development of an inspiratory stridor. The diagnosis is made using direct fibreoptic bronchoscopy, a CT scan and occasionally MRI.

The main anaesthetic principle is that no muscle relaxants should be used until the airway has been fully secured. Hence, intubation with a reinforced tracheal tube under direct vision is accomplished either with sedation and local anaesthesia or following an inhalation induction. It is accepted that 50% of the trachea can be resected in adults but only 33% in children. Surgeons cannot interpose a conduit in the trachea as it rapidly becomes infected. Hence, end-to-end anastomosis is the only option.

The trachea can be anastomosed around the tracheal tube. Alternatively the trachea or bronchi can be intubated after the trachea has been divided distal to the tumour. Ventilation of the lungs is accomplished using either standard methods or high frequency jet ventilation into both bronchi. With the latter technique, the main danger is contamination of the lungs with blood. Cardiopulmonary bypass can be used, although increased bleeding is a problem. Whatever method is chosen, at the end of the operation the chin is sutured to the chest to prevent neck extension which could cause disruption of the anastomosis. Extubation is performed over a gum elastic bougie in case rapid re-intubation is required. The main complications are collapse of the lower lobes, pneumonia and occasionally surgical damage to the recurrent laryngeal nerves which can cause vocal paralysis and respiratory difficulties. Finally, where the tracheal tumour is not amenable to surgical resection, either laser therapy or stents can be used.

LUNG TRANSPLANTATION

Since the first successful lung transplant was performed in 1983, single and double lung transplants have become a recognized treatment for end-stage respiratory failure. Initially, single lung transplantation was seen as suitable only for patients with restrictive lung disease, most commonly fibrosing alveolitis or sarcoidosis. It was thought that in patients with end-stage obstructive lung disease due to emphysema (including α-1 anti-trypsin deficiency), the high compliance of the recipient's remaining lung would compromise the function of the transplanted lung. During inflation, the remaining lung would expand considerably, causing the mediastinum to move towards the transplanted lung thereby preventing it from expanding. However, experience has shown that this happens in only a few patients and generally, the results are satisfactory.

Single lung transplants are also possible in patients with primary pulmonary hypertension. There were initial fears of flooding of the vascular bed of the transplanted lung due to of the high pulmonary artery pressure. Although these patients often have a stormy intra- and postoperative course they ultimately do well. In secondary pulmonary hypertension, a single lung transplant may also be suitable if the cardiac lesion can be corrected. The main advantage of using single, rather than double, lung or heart–lung transplants is that more patients can be treated from the limited number of organ donors available, bearing in mind that only

Table 11.2 Donor selection criteria

Age <55 years
Non-smoker (preferably)
No pulmonary disease
No thoracic trauma or previous surgery
Pao_2 >39 kPa whilst breathing 100% O_2+5 cmH_2O PEEP
No history of aspiration
No chest infection
(Negative sputum cultures if intubated >24 h)
Clear chest X-ray
HIV, Hep B and Hep C negative

Table 11.3 Recipient selection criteria

Age <60 years
Life expectancy <18 months
No other systemic illness or organ failure
No previous major thoracic surgery
Low maintenance dose of steroids
Non-smoker
No alcohol or drug abuse
Psychosocial stability
Adequate nutritional status
Potential for rehabilitation
Cooperative with medical instructions

about 20% of multi-organ donors have lungs suitable for transplantation.

Patients with chronic infective lung disease, usually due to cystic fibrosis, continue to need replacement of both lungs in order to prevent cross infection of the donor lung. Initially, the two lungs were transplanted as a single unit with a tracheal anastomosis. Currently, bilateral sequential single lung transplants are performed using bilateral bronchial anastomosis. This produces better anastomotic healing and preserves more of the normal innervation of the bronchial tree so that the cough reflex is retained. Heart–lung transplantation is now reserved for patients with secondary pulmonary hypertension and an uncorrectable cardiac lesion. The criteria for donor and recipient selection are set out in Tables 11.2 and 11.3.

PREOPERATIVE ASSESSMENT

Organ preservation techniques for lungs are such that the maximum ischaemic time should not exceed 4 h, though longer times are inevitable for double lung transplants. The logistics of organ procurement means that organs are usually retrieved late in the evening and the operations are carried out as emergencies.

The recipient may live at some distance from the hospital and frequently there is very little time between admission and the start of the operation; preoperative assessment can therefore only be brief. These patients present all the problems of emergency anaesthesia superimposed on end-stage pulmonary and cardiac failure. Fortunately, they will have had base-line respiratory and cardiac function tests performed at the initial assessment. It is thus only necessary to assess whether there has been a significant deterioration and whether any acute illness has supervened. Premedication is usually a benzodiazepine. Patients are given 4 l min^{-1} oxygen by mask, though those with CO_2 retention need controlled low-percentage oxygen. A dose of 2 mg kg^{-1} of azathioprine is given orally.

ANAESTHETIC TECHNIQUE

In the anaesthetic room ECG, blood pressure and oxygen saturation monitoring are commenced. A wide-bore intravenous cannula and an arterial cannula are inserted. The team wait to hear whether the donor organs are suitable before inducing anaesthesia. Where there has been previous surgery and a prolonged period of haemostasis is anticipated, the operation may start before the donor organs are removed.

Anaesthesia is induced using a mixture of etomidate, midazolam and fentanyl or alfentanil with the objective of maintaining cardiovascular stability. Muscle relaxation is obtained using pancuronium or vecuronium, but where a difficult intubation is anticipated, suxamethonium may be preferred. The dose of muscle relaxant is chosen to ensure good muscle power at the end of the operation so that early extubation will be possible. A double-lumen endobronchial tube is inserted into the contralateral lung for single lung transplantation, while a left-sided double-lumen tube is preferred for sequential double lung replacement. This protocol may have to be modified if anatomical abnormalities are present. It is not necessary to use more than the usual aseptic technique for intubation. For small patients, single-lumen tracheal tubes are used as they also help in the removal of tenacious secretions. Patients who have copious secretions invariably need cardiopulmonary bypass (CPB) to enable the excision of both lungs simultaneously thereby preventing soiling of the implanted lungs. If this is not a problem, or if bilateral lung transplantation is being carried out for fibrosis or emphysema, CPB may not be necessary.

After intubation, a pulmonary artery catheter is inserted via an internal jugular vein and a triple lumen catheter inserted into a subclavian vein under sterile conditions. A urinary catheter and a nasopharyngeal temperature probe are inserted. Ceftazidime and flucloxacillin (or vancomycin) are given intravenously together with an initial dose of 500 mg methylprednisolone.

For single lung transplantation the patient is placed in the lateral position with the operation side uppermost. The upper leg is extended to permit access to the femoral vessels should CPB become necessary. In double lung transplants, the patient remains supine but the arms are strapped to a bar above the patient's face so that a bilateral transverse thoracotomy incision can be made.

In the operating theatre, a trial of one-lung ventilation is performed. This is normally well tolerated in patients with emphysema unless there is considerable air-trapping. In patients with fibrotic lungs, it may be impossible to achieve acceptable levels of Pa_{O_2} and Pa_{CO_2} without high intrathoracic pressures which may compromise venous return. If this cannot be overcome using inotropic drugs, CPB may be necessary.

Once the pulmonary vessels have been exposed, the artery supplying the lung which is to be removed is snared. The pulmonary artery and the central venous pressures are measured to see if the right ventricle is unacceptably compromised by any increase in pulmonary vascular resistance. All patients with primary pulmonary hypertension and some of those with other pathologies will develop right ventricular decompensation during this manoeuvre. It may be possible to reduce pulmonary vascular resistance using an infusion of prostaglandin or enoximone together with noradrenaline to maintain the systemic vascular resistance, but CPB is often required.

An infusion of dopamine is started to increase urine flow as the transplanted lung, having no lymphatic drainage, easily becomes oedematous. Intravenous infusions are kept to a minimum. Frusemide and mannitol are given as necessary.

Anaesthesia is maintained with low concentrations of an inhalation agent, usually enflurane, or with a low-dose infusion of propofol. A high concentration of oxygen is frequently needed to maintain oxygenation, particularly on one-lung ventilation. As nitrous oxide is poorly tolerated due to its myocardial depressant effect, air is used as the carrier gas.

If CPB becomes necessary, a dose of 300 units kg^{-1} of heparin is administered to achieve an activated clotting time (ACT) of at least 500 s. High-dose aprotinin is used in all double and most single lung transplants to reduce bleeding. The ACT is maintained above 750 s if aprotinin is used.

When the transplanted lung has been anastomosed, it is ventilated and reperfused. A further dose of 500 mg methyloprednisolone is given. The cold potassium-rich fluid from the lung is washed into the circulation and may cause short-lived bradycardia and hypotension. Ventilation and perfusion to the new lung are usually well matched and there is often a dramatic decrease in pulmonary artery pressure with an increase in oxygen saturation. However, in some patients there may be signs of reperfusion lung injury and oxygenation remains poor.

If bilateral sequential lung transplants are being performed and CPB has not been necessary for implantation of the first lung, a period of 5–10 min is allowed for ventilation-perfusion adjustment. If this is satisfactory, the second lung is excised and replaced. At the end of CPB, protamine is administered and the chest is closed. An epidural catheter may be inserted extrapleurally under direct vision for postoperative pain relief.

POSTOPERATIVE MANAGEMENT

At the end of the operation the trachea is reintubated with a single-lumen tracheal tube. A fibreoptic bronchoscopy is performed to remove any secretions and to inspect the bronchial anastomosis(es). After admission to the intensive care unit, the lungs are ventilated until the patient is awake enough to breathe spontaneously and to be extubated. Positive end-expiratory pressure (PEEP) of 5 cmH_2O is applied to the lungs without emphysema to minimize atelectasis. If there are no complications, the tracheas of most patients are extubated later on the day of surgery.

Pain relief is provided by epidural or extrapleural infusions of bupivacaine. Epidurals are inserted when the bleeding has settled postoperatively and clotting is normal. Opioid administration must be reduced to a minimum as many patients are abnormally sensitive to their respiratory depressant effects.

Postoperatively patients are treated with cyclosporin. Steroids and azathioprine are continued. They continue to receive antibiotics together with antifungal and antiviral prophylaxis.

COMPLICATIONS

Early

Transplant patients are subject to the usual postoperative complications of thoracotomy, namely bleeding, cardiovascular instability, sputum retention and impaired renal function. They may also exhibit the reperfusion syndrome which may require several days of ventilation with high inspired oxygen concentrations, PEEP and stringent measures to reduce lung water.

Some patients with emphysema will exhibit air-trapping postoperatively because the compliance of the remaining lung is much greater than that of the donor lung, particularly in the first few hours after surgery. This may result in marked mediastinal shift and gross impairment of myocardial function (pulmonary tamponade). These patients require reintubation with a double-lumen tube. The donor lung is ventilated using PEEP while continuous positive airway pressure is applied to the native lung to maintain oxygenation. Once the donor lung is functioning normally, the tube can be removed and usually, there are no further problems. Occasionally it may be necessary to perform a lung reduction procedure on the native lung. These patients are also at risk of further episodes of air-trapping if the compliance of the transplanted lung becomes impaired.

Patients with cystic fibrosis pose special problems as they have a multisystem disease of which respiratory failure is only a part. They are frequently severely malnourished and healing is therefore impaired. They also harbour multiply-resistant organisms requiring the use of more toxic antibiotics.

Damage to phrenic or recurrent laryngeal nerves may make weaning from the ventilator difficult or impair the patient's cough effort. Fortunately most of these injuries recover.

Late

When lung transplantation was first performed, dehiscence and strictures at the site of the bronchial anastomoses were common complications. Better techniques have ensured that these problems are less common, but it is still occasionally necessary to use intra-bronchial stents to treat postoperative strictures. These are introduced with either a fibreoptic or rigid bronchoscope using a routine general anaesthetic technique.

Obliterative bronchiolitis is the most serious long-term complication of lung transplantation and if untreated, it leads to an inexorable deterioration in lung function within 1–2 years following diagnosis. It is thought to be due to chronic rejection and optimal anti-rejection therapy can slow the process, but inevitably there is a cost in terms of morbidity and mortality from infection and secondary malignancies.

FURTHER READING

Benumof, J. L. (1995) *Anesthesia for Thoracic Surgery*, 2nd edn. W. B. Saunders, Philadelphia.

Boscoe, M. J. (1993) Anaesthesia for heart–lung transplantation. *Current Opinion in Anesthesiology*, **61**, 106–112.

Davis, R. D. Jr. and Pasque, M. K. (1995) Pulmonary transplantation. *Annals of Surgery*, **2211**, 14–28.

Gothard, J. W. W. (1994) *Anaesthesia for Thoracic Surgery*, 2nd edn. Blackwell Scientific Publications, Oxford.

Jenkinson, S. and Levine, S (1994) Lung transplantation. *Disease-a-Month* **401**, 1–38.

Vaughan, R. S. (1996) Endobronchial intubation, in *Difficulties in Tracheal Intubation*, 2nd edn. (eds I. P. Latto and R. S. Vaughan), W. B. Saunders, London.

CARDIAC SURGERY 12

S. J. George and D. Royston

Operating theatres for cardiac surgery may seem daunting to trainee anaesthetists, but the principles of anaesthesia still apply, tailored to a specialist surgical field. Cardiopulmonary bypass (CPB) makes cardiac anaesthesia unique, wherein the lungs and the airway, normally protected ferociously, are now redundant, and a new vocabulary is used to enable close communication between the anaesthetist, surgeon and perfusionist.

PREOPERATIVE ASSESSMENT

As with all surgery, preoperative anaesthetic assessment is required for evaluating risk, planning anaesthesia, patient education and consent. The lesion, intended surgical approach and any general medical condition (diabetes mellitus, thyroid disease, sickle status etc.), should be established. Specific attention should be paid to the coronary arteries, ventricular function and valvular function (Table 12.1) and further investigations undertaken where necessary. Significant disease of the respiratory, renal or central nervous system may predispose to prolonged postoperative recovery with the increased likelihood of extended ventilatory support, renal support and perioperative stroke, respectively. The use of aspirin preoperatively, anticoagulation, or a bleeding diathesis may delay haemostasis after operation and this can be treated promptly with appropriate agents. Additionally, a previous sternotomy and its postoperative course should be noted.

Premedication varies, but some aims that may be accomplished include: anxiolysis (temazepam, morphine/hyoscine), amnesia (lorazepam), aspiration protection (ranitidine, metoclopramide), topical analgesia for children, and prevention of bradycardia (atropine). Supplementary inhaled oxygen should be considered if respiratory depressant drugs are given. Appropriate sedation can be essential in facilitating a safe induction. An anxious patient responds with hypertension and tachycardia, and in a child, crying and coughing can give rise to a pulmonary hypertensive crisis. On the other hand, an oversedated patient may become hypoxaemic or hypercapnic before arrival in the anaesthetic room. Table 12.2 highlights some risk factors with their relative weighting.

MONITORING

NON-INVASIVE MONITORING

The simplest and cheapest monitoring for both ischaemia and arrhythmias remains the ECG. A variety of different systems are available, with varying levels of software and configuration. Cardiac theatres may have modern equipment enabling the use of advanced soft-

Table 12.1 Preoperative assessment

Examination	Coronary arteries	Ventricular and valvular function
History and examination	Angina, exercise tolerance, medications Previous myocardial infarction Palpitations	NYHA class, exercise tolerance, syncope, orthopnoea, fatigue Medications, rate, blood pressure, cardiomegaly Added sounds Right heart signs
Electrocardiography and chest X-ray	Arrhythmias, previous infarction, atrial rhythm, bundle branch block Exercise tolerance stage attained	Cardiomegaly, hypertrophy and dilatation Aneurysms Lung fields
Echocardiography	Wall motion abnormalities	Ejection fraction Wall motion Valve function
Catheter study and others	Site of lesions Likely number of grafts Left mainstem involvement	MUGA (multiple uptake gated acquisition) scan, PET (positron emission tomography) etc.

Table 12.2 Risk assessment. (Reproduced with permission from Parsonnet *et al.* (1989) *Circulation*, **79** (Suppl 1) 3–12. A method of uniform stratification of risk for evaluating the results of surgery in acquired adult heart disease

Variable	Risk factor	Assigned weight
Age (years)	70–74	7
	75–79	12
	>80	20
Sex	Female	1
Coronary arteries	Coronary artery bypass graft and valve surgery	2
Left ventricular function (ejection fraction)	30–49%	2
	<30%	4
	Left ventricular aneurysm	2
	Intra-aortic balloon pump	10
Valve surgery	Mitral (additional PA >60 mmHg)	5 (8)
	Aortic (pressure gradient >120 mmHg)	5 (7)
Concomitant disease	Diabetes	3
	Hypertension	3
	Morbid obesity	3
Reoperation	First	5
	Second	10
Emergency surgery		10
Other organ failure	Dialysis dependency	10
	Catastrophic states	10–50

ware including trends, ST segment changes and arrhythmia recall. Pulse oximetry, capnography, a urinary catheter and a temperature probe are standard.

SEMI-INVASIVE MONITORING

Echocardiography, especially with Doppler capability, allows direct assessment of the structure and dynamics of the heart. Transoesophageal echocardiography, TOE, allows continuous monitoring, without interfering with surgery, of regional and global myocardial function and can also assess the surgical repair (mitral valve and congenital repairs).

INVASIVE MONITORING

Invasive arterial cannulae are mandatory in most instances, for both pressure monitoring and assessment of blood gases. This 'gold standard' may be fraught with inadvertent errors. In particular, inconsistent positioning of the transducers, arterial vasoconstriction from inotropic drugs and a peripheral–central gradient from hypothermia or hypovolaemia. Internal jugular venous cannulation monitors right-sided pressures and where there are no intervening, confounding factors, (valvular or pulmonary dysfunction), may also reflect left ventricular (LV) filling. Where the central venous pressure (CVP) cannot reliably reflect filling or where therapy is dependent on cardiac output, vascular resistances or oxygen delivery, a pulmonary artery catheter may be inserted. In addition, newer monitoring modes may be useful including, mixed-venous oxygen saturation and right ventricular, (RV) ejection fraction estimation. Where pulmonary capillary wedge pressure (PCWP) cannot be relied on to give a reflection of left ventricular end diastolic pressure (LVEDP), especially in children postoperatively, a left atrial catheter may be placed surgically.

ANAESTHESIA

The mortality associated with routine cardiac anaesthesia has declined, and concomitantly a variety of techniques have developed. A technique used in routine surgery is described, and some of the alternatives are discussed. Specific variations are described in the relevant sections.

Premedication of morphine (0.1–0.2 mg kg^{-1}) and hyoscine (0.02–0.04 mg kg^{-1}) is given i.m, 1 h before operation. On arrival in the anaesthetic room, cannulae (usually 20 G arterial and 14 G peripheral) are inserted under local anaesthesia and O_2 given. Anaesthesia is induced with fentanyl 10 µg kg^{-1}, pancuronium (0.1–0.2 mg kg^{-1}) and a sleep dose of etomidate (0.1–0.2 mg kg^{-1}). Appropriate antibiotics may be administered. Anaesthesia is maintained with a 50:50 O_2/N_2O mix and 0.5% isoflurane. Peri-induction hypertension is managed by increasing the concentration of volatile agent and an infusion of nitrates, and hypotension with vasoconstrictors (methoxamine) or inotropic drugs. After anticoagulation with heparin (300 units kg^{-1}), and surgical insertion of aortic and atrial cannulae the bypass circuit is connected and CPB is commenced. Myocardial protection follows and hypothermia is induced. Ventilation is discontinued when left ventricular output ceases. During CPB, an infusion of propofol, or benzodiazepine, is used to maintain anaesthesia. On completion of surgery, the patient is warmed and cardiac pulsation restarts. When an adequate cardiac output is generated, cardiopulmonary bypass is discontinued and the aortic and atrial cannulae removed. Anticoagulation is reversed with protamine to correct the activated clotting time (ACT) and, following haemostasis, the sternum and skin are closed. The patient is transferred, still ventilated, to the intensive care unit.

There are many variations of this technique. In the early days of cardiac anaesthesia high doses of opiates were used with prolonged ventilation, and the advantages of a stable perioperative period, few hypertensive episodes and minimal, myocardial oxygen demand. However, the increased need for ventilation, significantly raises costs and may extend the duration of hospital stay. An alternative 'low' dose opiate technique has been described above, with the aim of early tracheal extubation. The advantages of early tracheal extubation include a faster recovery and reduced costs. However, hypertension and compromised ventilation increase myocardial oxygen demands, whilst the heart is recovering from CPB. The use of thoracic epidural analgesia with light general anaesthesia has been described, with the advantages of early extubation, lower opiate requirements, better oxygenation and lung expansion, and minimal incidence of an extradural bleed during CPB.

The volatile anaesthetic agents affect different aspects of cardiac physiology, and their effects are amplified on the damaged ventricle. All of the agents in use, including halothane, isoflurane and enflurane, have a cardiac depressant effect. The newer agents, desflurane and sevoflurane, although less thoroughly studied appear to be equivalent to isoflurane. The effect of nitrous oxide is controversial, but it probably has a weak cardiac depressant action that is countered in the intact individual by sympathetic stimulation. All volatile agents induce relaxation of the systemic vasculature and decrease systemic vascular resistance. The net haemodynamic effect is a reduction in arterial pressure with a variable influence on heart rate. The negative inotropic effect of the volatile anaesthetic agents reduces myocardial oxygen demand, but with decreased flow through the coronary vessels. Furthermore, tachycardia may reduce the time available for diastolic filling of the left coronary system.

In the late 1960s, high-dose opiate analgesia (morphine) was noted to be haemodynamically stable, and was used in cardiac anaesthesia to obtund noxious stimuli. Currently, shorter acting agents (fentanyl and sufentanil), are more commonly used. Both morphine and alfentanil have vasodilating properties at the doses used. Chest wall rigidity may be a problem if neuromuscular blocking agents are not given promptly with the opioid.

If there is difficulty in weaning off CPB with persistently low-output, cardiac failure may be secondary to residual myocardial depression from cardioplegia, incomplete myocardial protection, coronary spasm or an inadequate surgical repair. Damage may affect the right or left ventricles. Further management is described in the section relating to the compromised ventricle.

When the core temperature is above 36°C, there is adequate oxygenation and ventilation with minimal acidosis and blood loss is less than 200 ml h^{-1}, the trachea is extubated. Following a further period of satisfactory assessment the patient may be transferred to the general ward.

CARDIOPULMONARY BYPASS (CPB)

Cardiopulmonary bypass is the method of maintaining organ perfusion despite cardiac standstill. The technology is relatively new, 30 years old, and despite the large insult to physiology, major complications have been relatively few, allowing an increase in surgical procedures.

Essentially, venous return is drained from the venae cavae by gravity to a reservoir, which also drains blood, via suction, from the surgical field (Figure 12.1). Blood is then pumped (either by centrifugal or by roller pumps), through fine, hollow fibres of the oxygenator, where blood is separated from gaseous oxygen by a membrane (other designs bubble oxygen through the blood). The oxygenator receives an oxygen–air mix that may pass through a vaporizer. Next blood passes through a temperature chamber (and in some designs a defoaming chamber) where heated water is used to vary the tem-

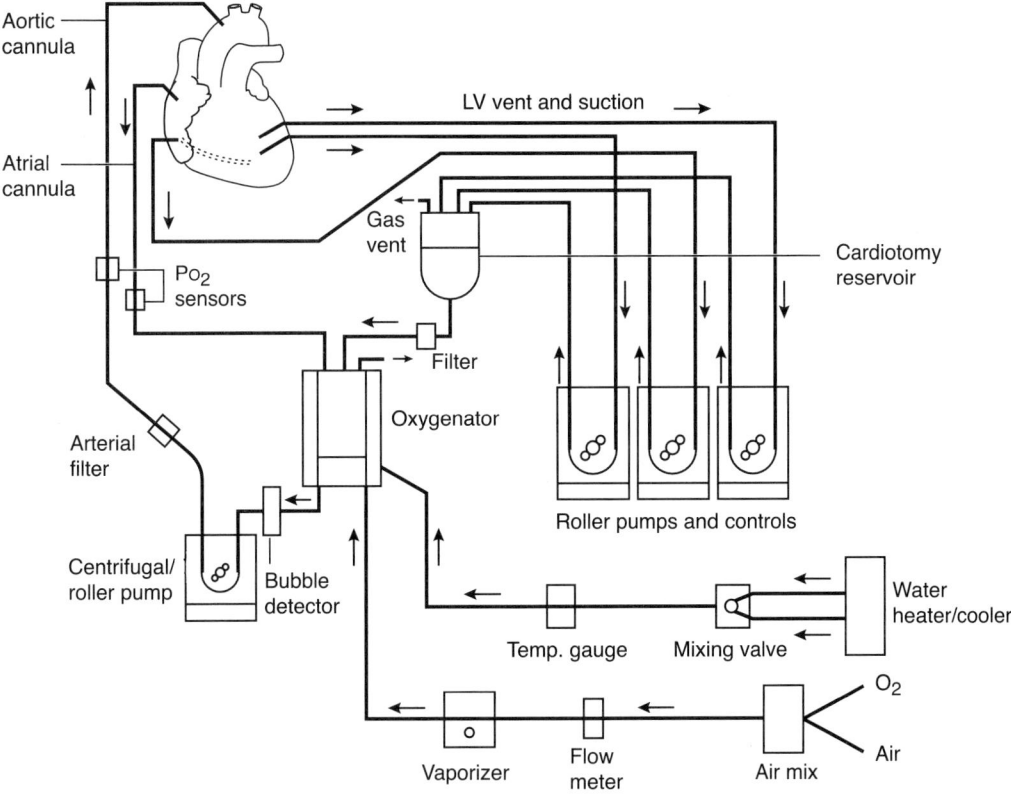

Figure 12.1 Schematic representation of the cardiopulmonary bypass circuit. (Reproduced from Reed, C.C. and Stafford, T.B. (1985) *Cardiopulmonary Bypass* 2nd edn. Houston Medical Press, USA.)

perature of the blood. Finally, oxygenated blood passes through the aortic cannula, via an inline filter, to the proximal ascending aorta.

Generated flow is limited by the amount of blood drained (preload), and systemic pressure is determined by the peripheral vascular resistance (afterload). Venous drainage may be compromised by kinked tubing, inappropriate position of cannulae, or blood loss to the pleura or the floor. The afterload is manipulated pharmacologically, by either introducing volatile agents or vasodilators (glyceryl trinitrate, phentolamine) to reduce arterial pressure, or by vasoconstrictors to increase pressure (methoxamine, metaraminol).

The perfusionist aims to preserve the circuit by ensuring adequate reservoir levels and aortic flow, and maintaining arterial pressures. The arterial oxygen tension can be varied by the oxygen–air mix, and the Pa_{CO_2} by the flow rate of gases. Increasing acidosis suggests inadequate perfusion, and may require increased flow, pressure or the addition of bicarbonate. Regular monitoring of the blood gases, K^+ concentration, anticoagulation (ACT), temperature and haemodynamic pressures is mandatory. Glucose and haemoglobin measurement may be warranted.

HYPOTHERMIA

Hypothermia is almost invariably used with CPB. Debate continues as to whether acid–base balance is best achieved by observing a pH stat or an alpha stat approach. The basis of understanding the debate is to recognize that as temperature falls, less water dissociates into H^+ and OH^-. That is, the H^+ ion concentration falls (pH rises). In the alpha stat method this rise in pH is effectively ignored (i.e. the pH at 37°C is used without correction for temperature), and the ratio of dissociated ions (specifically the **alpha** of imidazole dissociation) is maintained. The pH stat method aims to maintain normal pH at *in vivo* temperature, usually by adding CO_2 to the oxygen–air mix. It is interesting to note that cold blooded animals use an alpha stat approach at cold temperatures, while hibernating mammals use a pH stat approach. Insufficient data about outcome are available and currently both approaches are used.

WEANING FROM CPB

Weaning commences after adequate rewarming of the circulation. As the heart rewarms, spontaneous contractions return. If an abnormal rhythm occurs, this may require d.c. cardioversion or pacing. The lungs are re-expanded and ventilated. When the blood gases, haemoglobin concentration and temperature are satisfactory, gradual reduction of pump flows is attempted. If an adequate cardiac output is maintained the pump flows are terminated and the cannulae removed. Anticoagulation is reversed with protamine sulphate, and haemostasis achieved. Following the insertion of mediastinal and pleural drains, the sternum and then skin are closed.

DEEP HYPOTHERMIC CIRCULATORY ARREST

In situations where pump flow to the brain cannot be guaranteed (aortic arch surgery), or where the structures involved are so small that even low flows compromise the surgical field (children < 10 kg), circulatory arrest may be used with protection of the major organ systems by deep hypothermia: deep hypothermic circulatory arrest. This technique can provide up to 30 min of operative time. The patient is cooled to 15–18°C and the head and the heart covered with icepacks to prevent warming. Blood is then drained to the reservoir, and all cannulae removed allowing maximal surgical access.

MYOCARDIAL PROTECTION

During cardiopulmonary bypass, with the coronary arteries not perfused, the myocardium must be protected from ischaemia and hypoxia. Morbidity increases with myocardial damage; the effect is proportionately greater on previously impaired myocardium. Approaches to minimize damage include; limitation of demand (hypothermia, cardioplegia, speed of surgery), maintaining supply (continuous blood cardioplegia, intermittent reperfusion), increasing cardiac metabolic reserve (glucose–insulin–potassium, glutamate infusions, ischaemic preconditioning) and limitation of reperfusion injury (controlled reperfusion, free-radical scavengers).

INTERMITTENT AORTIC CROSS-CLAMP AND VENTRICULAR FIBRILLATION

Normal flow through the coronary arteries is maintained and the aorta is cross-clamped when the surgeon requires a still field. Ventricular fibrillation is then induced by contact with a fibrillator. The period of ischaemia is kept to a minimum, and myocardial O_2 requirements are reduced by hypothermia of 28–32°C. Coronary circulation is then reinstituted by release of the cross-clamp and either spontaneous or electrical conversion of ventricular fibrillation. Protection relies on the myocardial ability to withstand brief periods of ischaemia. The avoidance of depressant drugs and ischaemic preconditioning of the myocardium are relative advantages of this technique.

Table 12.3 Cardioplegic solutions. (Reproduced with permission from Mazer, C.D. (1993) Perspectives on intraoperative myocardial protection. *Current Opinion in Anaesthesiology,* **6**, 86.)

Delivery	Solutions	Additives	Reperfusion	Perfusion
Ante or retrograde	Blood or crystalloid	O_2, Glucose	Unmodified	Hypothermic
Intermittent or continuous	St Thomas or Buckberg	K^+, Mg^{2+}, Ca^{2+}	Controlled	Normothermic
	Fremes or Hamburg or Roe	Mannitol, buffers, membrane stabilizers β-blockers, Ca antagonists		Deep hypothermic circulatory arrest

CARDIOPLEGIA

Myocardial quiescence can be induced chemically by direct injection into the coronary arteries of a cardioplegic solution (Table 12.3). This allows more time for surgery and reduces myocardial O_2 requirements during the period of relative ischaemia. Commonly, cardioplegic agent (10–20 ml kg^{-1}) is infused into the aortic root (or in aortic regurgitation/aortic surgery, directly into the coronary arteries). Where the coronary arteries are severely diseased or left ventricular hypertrophy is present, the cardioplegic agent may be infused retrogradely, through the coronary sinus.

LIMITATION OF DEMAND

Hypothermia is by far the commonest technique to limit demand. V_{O_2} decreases exponentially with temperature, so that at 27°C, V_{O_2} is 40% of normal. Factors that may increase demand include ventricular dilation (surgeons may use a vent through the ventricular wall to collapse the left ventricle), and ventricular fibrillation (requiring d.c. version). Drugs within the cardioplegic solution reduce myocardial demand by their negative inotropic action.

CARDIAC RESERVE

Normal myocardium can utilize almost any substrate to provide energy, including glucose, fatty acids and lactate. In hypoxic conditions, however, only anaerobic glycolysis is available. Enhancing cardiac reserve is therefore attractive. A number of agents have been employed including glutamate, aspartate, thyroxine and digoxin. The most studied is the glucose–insulin–potassium regimen to enhance myocardial glycogen stores. Close monitoring of blood glucose is required, as hyperglycaemia may compromise neurological and myocardial cells during ischaemia.

LIMITING REPERFUSION INJURY

Cell death releases toxic cell constituents which build up in non-perfused areas. Reperfusion then leads to transport of these toxins to cells downstream causing further injury. Techniques to avoid this include continuous coronary perfusion and controlled reperfusion. Many of the toxins are free radicals, and scavengers of these have been shown to be of benefit. Free radical scavengers may be included in the premedication (allopurinol), or added to cardioplegic solution (mannitol).

VENTRICULAR DYSFUNCTION

Significant ventricular dysfunction requires careful preparation and attention, as deterioration may be swift, requiring a rapid response. Dysfunction may be restricted to either ventricle, but because of the structural relation, between the ventricles, deterioration in one invariably affects the other.

PATHOPHYSIOLOGY

Left ventricular dysfunction may be in discrete areas, (ischaemia), or global (cardiomyopathy). Essentially, the pathophysiological sequelae are the same, but estimates of function may be inaccurate in discretely damaged ventricles, if an unrepresentative region is analysed.

In an ischaemic area, myocytes at the centre die: infarcted myocardium. This leads to oedema and local toxin release, compromising blood flow and function of a larger area, which becomes dysfunctional and unresponsive to inotropic drugs. This area is potentially retrievable with resolution of oedema and toxin clearance, and is referred to as **stunned myocardium**. Postoperative recruitment of stunned myocardium may allow an initially struggling myocardium to function adequately. In a chronic situation, areas of myocardium may have sufficient blood supply to survive, although unable to produce ATP or perform a contractile function. These areas, depending on the extent of vascular deprivation, may be recruitable with inotropic stimulation. If blood supply is restored to these areas referred to as **hibernating myocardium**, the myocytes may recover and be fully functional following regeneration of the necessary enzymes. That is, stunned myocardium is acutely dysfunctional and may resolve in hours to days, whereas hibernating myocardium is subject to chronic ischaemia and may recover in weeks to months.

The haemodynamics of the left ventricle are well represented by the pressure–volume relations (Figure 12.2).

MEASUREMENT OF VENTRICULAR FUNCTION

The ventricular cycle can be described in four phases, as seen from the pressure–volume relation. Ventricular deterioration in any of these stages can cause global dysfunction. Ease of measurement has led to the ejection fraction becoming synonymous with left ventricular function. Ejection fraction can be maintained by compensatory increases in end diastolic volume etc., and is dependent on the volume load of the ventricle, so not always reflecting contractility. Other 'load independent' measures of contractility may be more useful, but are less easily performed routinely.

Anaesthesia in these patients allows little margin for error, as the ventricle has poor reserve, and myocardial damage has a proportionately greater effect. Postoperative dysfunction may be predicted from preoperative status. Smooth induction of anaesthesia and initiation of CPB, with optimal myocardial preservation and swift surgery is the ideal. A short duration of CPB, avoiding intricate, time-consuming surgical procedures is often the better strategy. The addition of inodilators (enoximone) to the CPB reserve, before weaning, may produce a beneficial increase in contractility. Similarly, a recuperative period on CPB, with myocardial perfusion at normal temperatures, may allow the myocardium time to recover. Persistent myocardial dysfunction, with resultant low cardiac output, may follow weaning off CPB.

MANAGEMENT

Limitation of deleterious factors such as hypoxia, acidosis, arrhythmias and hypothermia, precedes the use of drugs (Table 12.4). Drugs include the sympathomimetic amines (adrenaline, noradrenaline, dopamine), phosphodiesterase inhibitor inodilators (amrinone, enoximone), digitalis and vasodilators (hydralazine, nitrates: reducing arterial impedance and diastolic filling). Failure of drug support may necessitate mechanical support. Assessment of cardiovascular function and titration of inotropic drugs is helped by the use of a pulmonary artery catheter and transoesophageal echocardiography.

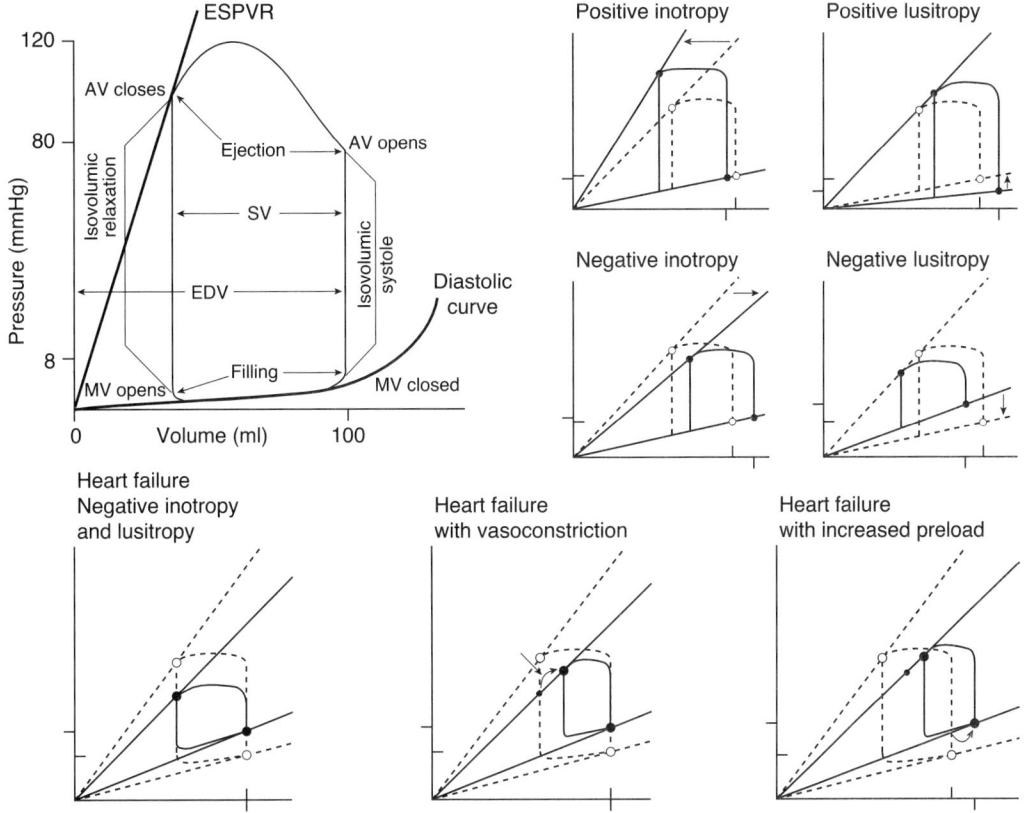

Figure 12.2 Schematic representation of pressure–volume loops and changes under different influences: ESPVR=end-systolic pressure–volume relation, EDV=end-diastolic volume. The top left loop shows the four phases of the cardiac cycle: I, isovolumic contraction; II, ejection; III, isovolumic relaxation; and IV, ventricular filling. The four loops to the right show the response with inotropic or lusitropic (diastolic) changes. The bottom three loops describe the response of the failing heart to maintain systolic pressure by increasing afterload and filling. (Reproduced with permission from: Katz, A.M. (1991) Heart failure, in *The Heart and Cardiovascular System* (eds Fozzard et al.) Raven Press, New York, p. 339.)

INTRA-AORTIC BALLOON COUNTER-PULSATION

This is a means of supporting diastolic pressure (enabling better flow through the coronary arteries) and reducing arterial resistance to left ventricular output (allowing better organ perfusion) (Figure 12.3). An inflatable balloon is introduced, via the femoral arteries, to lie within the descending aorta below the left subclavian artery and above the renal arteries. The balloon, attached to a pneumatic pump, is electrically driven, timing systole and diastole from the ECG, the arterial pressure trace or the aortic pressure wave. In diastole the balloon is inflated, and with a competent aortic valve supports diastolic pressure, exaggerating the dichrotic notch. In systole, the balloon is deflated reducing arterial resistance and improving cardiac output. The patient is weaned from intra-aortic balloon pulsation by reducing the frequency of inflations, and decreasing the amplitude of balloon inflation. The risk of peripheral thromboses necessitates anticoagulation. Dramatic improvement in haemodynamics and

Table 12.4 Assessment and treatment of hypotension after cardiopulmonary bypass

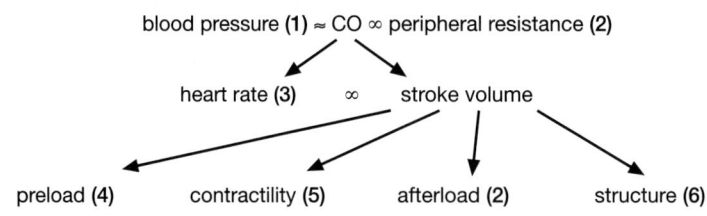

	Causative factor	Assessment and treatment
1	Spurious reading	Incorrectly positioned, or zeroed, transducers
		Peripheral – central gradient: measure aortic pressures directly
2	Peripheral resistance and afterload	Vasoconstriction for left ventricle: methoxamine, noradrenaline
		Pulmonary vasodilation for right ventricle: prostacyclin, inhaled NO
3	Rate and rhythm	Chronotropic agents: isoprenaline, adrenaline
		Pacing: d.c. version to revert to sinus rhythm
4	Volume status	Assess heart by eye, CVP, PCWP, TOE
		Hypovolaemia: crystalloid, colloid, blood
		Hypervolaemia: vasodilators (GTN), diuretics, volume removal
5	Decreased contractility	Ensure oxygenation and ventilation
		Assess with eye, TOE, and raised PCWP
		Treat with inotropes: dopamine, adrenaline, inodilators, assist devices, transplantation
6	Structural disorder	Assess with TOE → further surgery
		Valve disruption, unexpected lesions (new shunts), tamponade

renal function, allowing a decrease of inotropic support, may be seen.

ASSIST DEVICES

A variety of assist devices are available for the augmentation of flow, using external power sources including electrical and pneumatic driven apparatus. These devices frequently consist of an inflow from the atrium to a centrifugal or roller pump, from which blood is pumped to the outflow tract. Assist devices may be for the right (right ventricular assist device, RVAD), or the left ventricle (LVAD) or both. Extracorporeal membrane oxygenation (ECMO) has been used with some success in children. This is a rapidly developing field and is dependent on better materials and fewer complications and may, where left ventricular function is minimal, provide a bridge to transplantation.

RIGHT VENTRICLE

The right ventricle has a pyramidal cavity with the posteroinferior portion receiving venous return through the tricuspid valve, and the anterosuperior portion leading to the pulmonary outflow tract and pulmonary valve. Blood supply, via the right coronary artery, is not restricted to diastole. The ventricle develops pressures of 25 mmHg systolic normally, is thin walled compared to the left ventricle and unable to withstand acute rises in pulmonary vascular resistance (PVR). These increases may be seen with pulmonary emboli, ARDS, idiosyncratic reactions to protamine and in the transplanted heart with high-recipient pulmonary resistance.

As the septum forms the wall of both right and left ventricles, there is significant ventricular interaction. Distension of the right

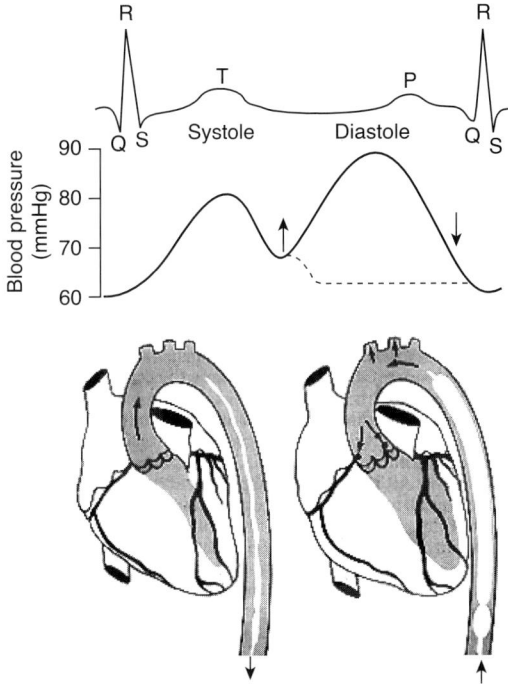

Figure 12.3 Schematic illustration of the intra-aortic balloon pump. (Reproduced from Bolooki, H. (ed.) (1984) *Clinical Application of the Intra-aortic Balloon Pump*. Futura Publishing.)

ventricle reverses the normal curve of the interventricular septum towards the left ventricle. This impedes left ventricular diastolic function and consequently stroke volume.

The management of right ventricular failure is predominantly by volume loading and reduction of PVR. The highly compliant ventricle responds well to volume loading. Occasionally, inotropic drugs and assist devices (pulmonary artery balloon pump and RVAD) may be required. Treatment of high PVR includes hyperventilation and oxygenation. Specific drugs for decreasing the PVR, include prostacyclin and inhaled nitric oxide. Inhaled nitric oxide is clinically limited to the pulmonary vasculature by rapid inactivation by haemoglobin. Specific action on ventilated alveoli improves pulmonary vascular resistance and pulmonary shunting.

HAEMATOLOGICAL ASPECTS

ANTICOAGULATION

The highly thrombogenic nature of the cardiopulmonary bypass circuit necessitates anticoagulation for safe CPB. Heparin has been the only effective anticoagulant for this purpose. Heparin is a heterogeneous mixture of proteins that combine with antithrombin III, enhancing its action of inactivating active coagulation cascade proteins. The individual protein molecular weights vary and its action is best quantified in international units (i.u.), and not weight in milligrams. Monitoring of the anticoagulant status is done by determining the activated clotting time (ACT; blood added to diatomaceous earth and the time for clot formed to hold a magnet against its field).

The safety of heparin is remarkable, even in large doses, although two problems regarding its use remain: heparin resistance and heparin-induced thrombocytopenia. Resistance to heparin may occur because of previous heparin therapy, patients on the extreme of the normal distribution of heparin sensitivity, and antithrombin III deficiency. Most patients respond to increased heparin dose. Antithrombin III deficiency is treated by increasing the supply of antithrombin III, easily achieved with two units of FFP.

Many patients show clinically insignificant thrombocytopenia in response to heparin therapy. Rarely, an idiosyncratic, probably immune-mediated, catastrophic thrombocytopenia may occur, because of unrestricted platelet activation leading to thrombotic complications.

Protamine had been used to prolong the action of insulin, and a possible, similar use with heparin was investigated. Surprisingly, the activity of heparin was neutralized by the binding of the cationic protamine to the anionic heparin. Inactivation is weight-for-weight equivalent (as opposed to units of activity). This remarkable discovery allowed

Table 12.5 Blood conservation strategies. (Reproduced with permission from Strang T.I. and Whitaker D.K. (1994) Blood conservation strategies. *Current Opinion in Anaesthesiology,* **7**, 53–58.)

Preoperative	Intraoperative	Postoperative
Autologous predonation	Protease inhibitors: aprotinin	Desmopressin
Acute normovolaemia Haemodilution	Plasminogen inhibitors: tranexamic acid	Blood salvage
Erythropoietin	Blood salvage	Permissive anaemia
Platelet-rich infusion		Erythropoietin

an almost 'on–off' control of anticoagulation. However, protamine is not without problems, including a histamine-induced vasodilation and hypovolaemia, and an idiosyncratic response of severe pulmonary vasoconstriction. Methods to overcome the hypotension include, maximal vasodilation and volume loading before protamine, and slow infusion. Idiosyncratic reactions may be managed by either using alternative heparin inactivation (heparinase), or allowing spontaneous heparin degradation and accepting the consequential blood loss.

HAEMOSTASIS

Postoperative bleeding may be due to many factors, most commonly inadequate surgical haemostasis. No systemic manoeuvre can compensate for leaking grafts or vessels speared by sternal wires. However, haemostatic disturbance is common after bypass, secondary to preoperative aspirin and warfarin, thrombolytic therapy, thrombocytopenia and platelet dysfunction secondary to CPB, fibrinolysis and disseminated intravascular coagulation secondary to inadequate anticoagulation during CPB, dilution of clotting factors or residual heparin.

Empirical reversal of heparin is usually sufficient for adequate haemostasis. Where bleeding continues, haemodynamic support with colloids and blood is necessary, and concomitantly diagnosis proceeds and surgical causes are eliminated. Diagnostic methods available in the operating theatre include the ACT and thromboelastography. Additional laboratory-based tests of platelet count, clotting screen, fibrinogen and fibrin degradation products are undertaken. If there are no surgical causes, the following may be used to correct the haemostatic profile: more protamine, platelets, FFP, cryoprecipitate and aprotinin, dependent on the results of tests.

Failure of haemostasis can lead to prolonged blood loss. Where there is a surgical cause of bleeding, reoperation will be necessary. Despite the presence of mediastinal drains, blood loss may present as cardiac tamponade requiring urgent drainage.

BLOOD CONSERVATION

With the increasing recognition of the risks of donated blood, different strategies (Table 12.5) have developed to minimize the use of blood and blood products. Acceptable haemoglobin values remain a matter of debate, as a permissive anaemia may avoid transfusion.

Two different pharmacological methods currently used include inhibition of fibrinolytic activity (tranexamic acid, EACA) and serine protease inhibitors (aprotinin). The use of aprotinin in high doses has revolutionized blood loss in the at-risk patients, e.g. repeat operations, post-thrombolysis. With aprotinin use, ACT is kept above 750 s, as aprotinin increases ACT *per se*.

COMPLICATIONS

RESPIRATORY

Respiratory disease is not uncommon amongst cardiac surgical patients. Cardiac surgery impairs respiratory function by a variety of methods including the sternotomy, high doses of opiates, myocardial dysfunction with pulmonary oedema, pleural effusions and phrenic nerve damage. Pre-existing respiratory disease (vital capacity <15 ml kg^{-1} or FEV$_1$ < 1.0) predisposes to the need for prolonged ventilatory support.

The management of postoperative respiratory dysfunction does not differ greatly from conventional methods, including standard ventilatory modes of positive end-expiratory pressure, pressure support, continuous positive airway pressure and finally, if necessary, tracheostomy. Reduced respiratory reserve also means that the lungs are less able to cope with dysfunction in other organs, especially the heart, kidneys and brain. Repeated need for ventilation may be a manifestation of cardiac dysfunction (arrhythmias, paroxysmal myocardial ischaemic episodes or inadequate valve function), or attempts to wean patients off renal support.

RENAL COMPLICATIONS

Significant deterioration in renal function occurs in 1–4% of patients after CPB. The causes are usually multifactorial, including drugs (gentamicin, cyclosporin), hypotension, low cardiac output and microemboli. The use of a low-dose dopamine infusion in the routine cardiac patient, has not proven to be of benefit, although little work has been done in patients with pre-existing renal dysfunction. The necessity for haemofiltration is associated with 70% mortality in adults.

CENTRAL NERVOUS SYSTEM

Neurological complications following routine cardiac surgery are devastating, with an incidence of 1% for a severe stroke. Other complications include cortical blindness, optic atrophy, and psychoses. Thirty five per cent of patients, develop subtle neuropsychological and cognitive changes, or show reappearance of primitive reflexes, that persist for over a year. These signs may not be identified by coarse 'end of the bed' neurological assessment. Monitoring tools for cerebral function include the EEG, jugular venous saturation and transcranial Doppler, although these have not gained widespread clinical use. Cerebral dysfunction may be secondary to inadequate perfusion, emboli or metabolic factors.

Perfusion

Adequate cerebral perfusion is dependent on the mean arterial pressure (MAP), adequate cerebral artery perfusion, venous drainage (CVP), and cerebral metabolic oxygen requirement (CMRO$_2$). Controversy remains about the ideal value of MAP, although most centres aim to maintain MAP at 50–60 mmHg. Increasing pressure compromises the surgical field as the site becomes more bloody. A history suggestive of carotid artery disease, or hypertension, requires a higher MAP. Poor placement of the aortic cannula may compromise pump flow into either carotid artery, or decrease venous drainage from the superior vena cava. Assessment at the commencement of CPB, and intermittently thereafter, to ascertain equality of pupil size, facial engorgement and CVP should detect this phenomenon. CMRO$_2$ can be decreased with barbiturates, calcium channel blocking agents or hypothermia, although their efficacy in improving outcome is controversial.

Emboli

Thrombi, air emboli and atheroma within the major vessels, may give rise to microinfarctions resulting in subtle neurological dysfunction, or major infarctions leading to stroke. Strategies to minimize these risks include the use of membrane oxygenators (avoiding physical compression of blood and the initiation of the coagulation cascade), the use of hollow fibre oxygenators (avoiding direct blood–oxygen interfaces reducing micro air emboli), the introduction of in-line arterial filters before aortic entry of the blood, and the use of TOE to guide aortic cannula placement away from plaques and allow effective de-airing of the cardiac chambers before weaning from CPB.

Metabolic

Metabolic factors may also influence neurological outcome. The most clearly accepted of these include hyperglycaemia and persistent acidosis, which adversely affect outcome in the presence of ischaemia. Other factors include hypercalcaemia and hypoglycaemia.

Awareness

About 1% of patients on close questioning are aware during CPB. Although this was first highlighted with the increasing use of high-dose opiate techniques, its presence has been associated with a wide variety of anaesthetic regimens. Most cases are not associated with pain, or accompanied by haemodynamic signs of tachycardia, hypertension, sweating and pupillary dilatation. Surgical outcome is not affected, but severe psychological sequelae may ensue. The incidence may be minimized by the sustained alertness of the anaesthetist, and by audit postoperatively with questions that elicit the presence of awareness in a minor form. In addition, the use of benzodiazepines and scopolamine aid amnesia, and a history of narcotic and alcohol abuse should modify the technique used to take account of greater drug tolerance and enhanced disposition.

MYOCARDIAL REVASCULARIZATION

Myocardial revascularization emerged in the 1960s as a treatment for coronary artery disease. It has become increasingly common and concomitantly less risky; mortality has stayed the same despite low-risk patients having angioplasty instead and an increasingly older surgical population.

Left coronary flow is mainly diastolic (Figure 12.4), as in systole, compression of vessels restricts flow. Locally, autoregulation maintains blood flow at 60–120 mmHg. A high P_{CO_2}, $[H^+]$ $[K^+]$, and temperature, and hypoxaemia vasodilate coronary vessels. Further pharmacological vasodilatation can be achieved with high dose nitrates, nitroprusside and adenosine. In addition, α and β receptors in the coronary vessels respond to the autonomic nervous system and circulating catecholamines. Other humoral influences on vasomotor tone include, vasopressin, atrial natriuretic peptide and prostacyclin.

Anaesthesia for myocardial revascularization varies between institutions, and the technique described above may be successfully used. (Figure 12.5). Critical left main stem stenosis is notorious for its susceptibility to episodes of hypotension. Once blood flow through the stenosis is restricted, cardiac arrest is inevitable and resuscitation is largely unsuccessful. It is imperative, therefore, to maintain coronary perfusion pressure, by avoiding drugs that cause a sudden drop in arterial pressure and so maintaining diastolic pressure until CPB.

Perioperative myocardial ischaemia predisposes to postoperative myocardial infarction. Detection is primarily based on the ST segment changes of the ECG. By detecting new wall motion abnormalities, TOE is a more sensitive detector of ischaemic episodes. Other variables such as the appearance of a v wave on the wedge trace, or haemodynamic changes may be useful. Ischaemic episodes should be treated with attempts to reduce oxygen demand and increase supply (Table 12.6). Increased myocardial demand may be due to hypertension, tachycardia and inappropriate use of inotropic drugs. Decreased supply may result from ventilatory problems, inadequate revascularization (distal disease, poor flow) and coronary spasm. Once ventilatory and haemodynamic influences are

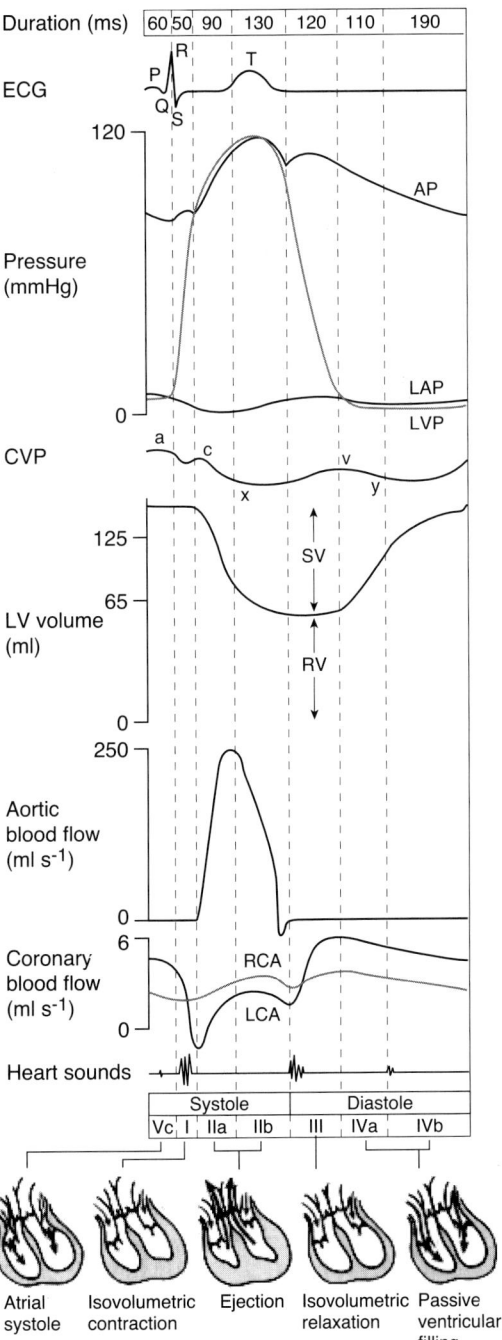

Figure 12.4 The cardiac cycle. (Reproduced with permission from Despopoulous, A. and Silbernagl, S. (1991) *Colour Atlas and Physiology*, 4th edn, Thieme, Stuttgart, p. 163.)

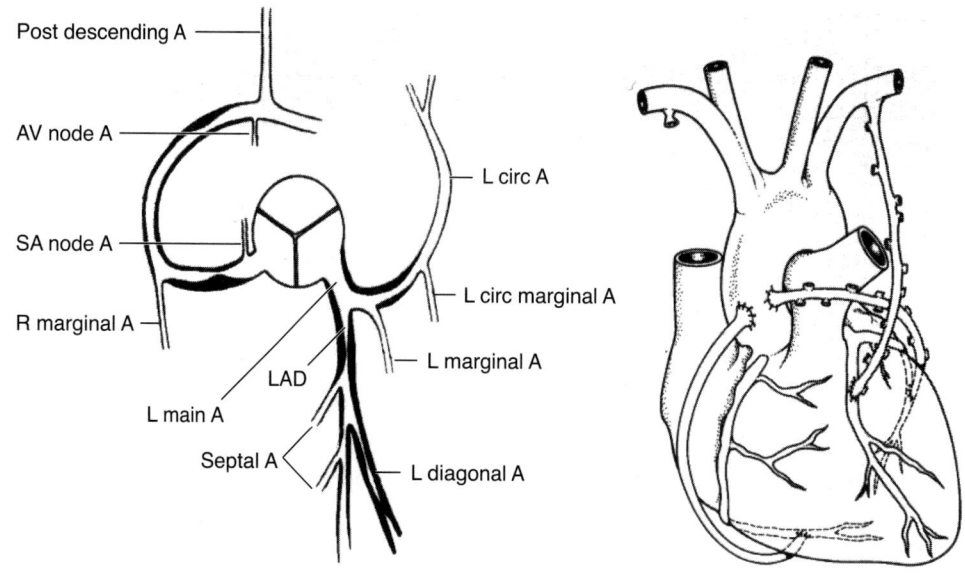

Figure 12.5 Diagram of the coronary arteries, and common stenotic regions. Also illustrated is an internal mammary artery graft to the left anterior descending artery and two venous grafts to the circumflex and the posterior descending artery. (Reproduced with permission from Willerson, J.T. et al. (1982) *Ischemic Heart Disease*. Raven Press, New York, p. 135 and Marks, C. and Marks, P.H. (1993) *Fundamentals of Cardiac Surgery* Chapman & Hall Medical, London, p. 70.)

Table 12.6 Influences on myocardial oxygen supply and demand

Supply	Demand
O_2 carrying capacity (Hb, Po_2, Sao_2)	Heart rate
Coronary blood flow	Contractility
Diastolic phase	Wall tension/afterload
Viscosity	
Resistance (vasomotor tone) (Autoregulation, Metabolic, Autonomic, Humoral)	

addressed, coronary vasodilators (glyceryl trinitrate, calcium antagonists) and β-blocking drugs (decrease demand and reduce rate) may be used. Intra-aortic balloon counterpulsation may improve coronary perfusion by diastolic pressure support. If ischaemia is secondary to poor pump function, further assist devices may be required. Isoflurane (and desflurane) have a weak, direct, coronary vasodilator effect. The theoretical possibility of the 'coronary steal' phenomenon (Figure 12.6), where a vasodilator may increase flow to well perfused areas at the cost of flow to ischaemic areas, was demonstrated in 1978, although the clinical significance in man is not proven.

VALVE SURGERY

Cardiac valve disease (Figure 12.7) has become much less common with the reduction in incidence of rheumatic fever. Abnormalities may still arise from congenital variants, ischaemic heart disease or other infectious sources. Anaesthetists should be aware not only of the acute pathophysiological changes, but also of chronic compensatory hypertrophic or dilation changes, and ventricular function (Figure 12.8, Table 12.7). Antistaphylococcal antibiotics (vancomycin,

Valve surgery

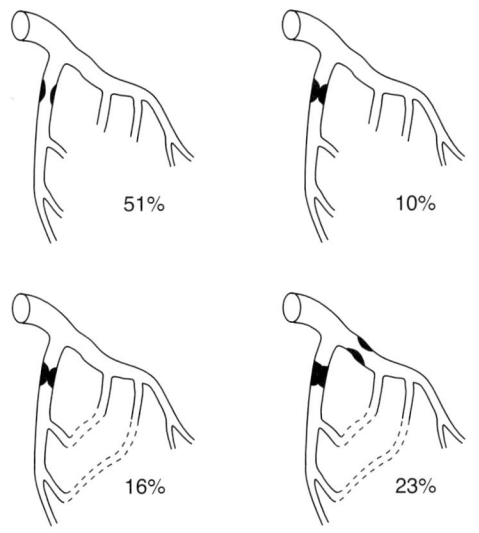

Figure 12.6 Coronary Artery Surgery Study (CASS) Registry: review of coronary angiograms delineating variant patterns. The lower right configuration predisposes to steal. (Reproduced with permission from Buffington, C.W. *et al.* (1988) The prevalence of steal prone anatomy in patients with coronary artery disease. *Anesthesiology*, **69**: 721.)

fucidin) should be included in the antibiotic regimen.

AORTIC VALVE

This is a tricuspid valve, the sinuses of which give rise to the two coronary arteries. Anatomic variants (bicuspid or tetracuspid valve), or infection, may predispose to stenosis. A wide variety of disorders, such as rheumatoid arthritis, Marfan's Syndrome or infection, may give rise to aortic regurgitation.

The most common procedure is replacement of the valve with a mechanical prosthesis, a bioprosthesis (biological valves supported by mechanical rings) or a homograft valve (cadaveric donor valves). Repair may be attempted with ultrasonic decalcification or individual leaflet repair.

Aortic stenosis

The hallmark of aortic stenosis is the pressure overload on the left ventricle. The need to work against a stenosis, increased afterload,

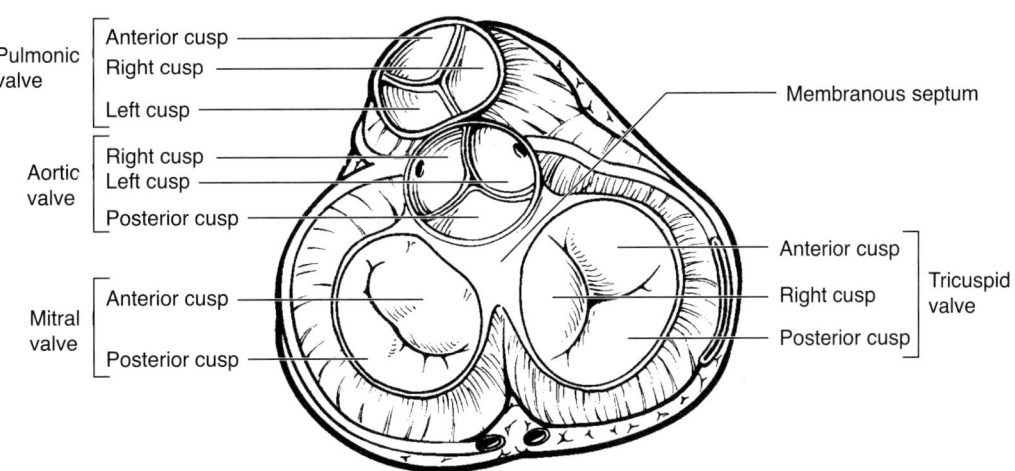

Figure 12.7 Anatomy of the cardiac valves showing their relative positions. (Reproduced with permission from Kambam, J. (ed.) (1992) *Cardiac Anesthesia for Infants and Children*, Mosby, St Louis, MO, p. 290.)

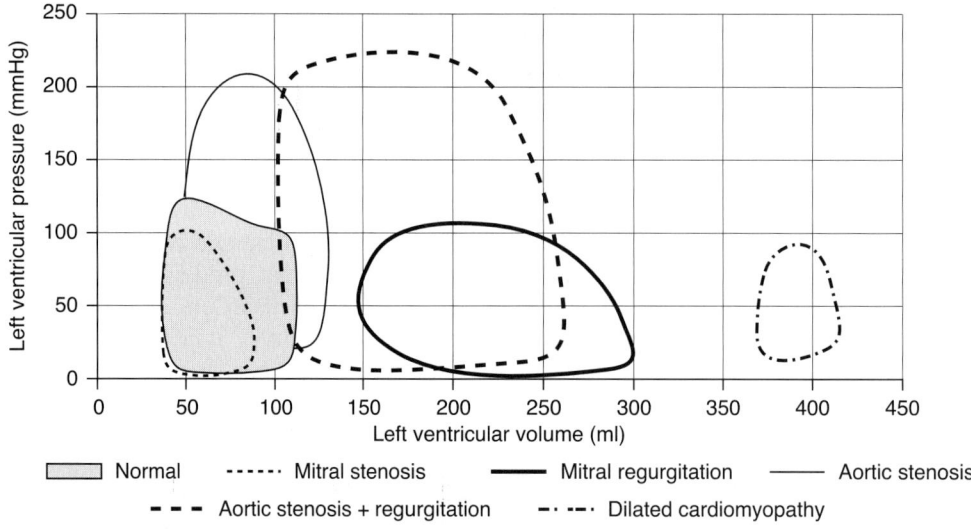

Figure 12.8 Pressure–volume loops in different pathological situations. (Reproduced from Dodge, H.T. Haemodynamic aspects of cardiac failure.)

Table 12.7 Recommended anaesthetic strategies in left sided valvular lesions

	Heart rate (1/diastolic time)	Preload (volume)	Systemic vascular resistance (afterload)	Pulmonary vascular resistance
Aortic stenosis	↓ (Sinus)	↑	↑	↔
Aortic regurgitation	↑	↑	↓	↔
Mitral regurgitation	↑	↔	↓	↓
Mitral stenosis	↓	↑	↔	↓
Mixed lesions	Treat dominant lesion and assess response to change			

leads to concentric left ventricular hypertrophy and an inability to increase stroke volume.

The normal aortic valve area is 2.6–3.5 cm², which in critical aortic stenosis may be reduced to 0.4 cm². The hypertrophied ventricle is able to generate much greater peak systolic pressures. Diastolic compliance is reduced and diastolic filling dependent on the positive push of atrial systole. Left ventricular hypertrophy and increased afterload lead to increased myocardial O_2 demand. Supply is restricted, as increased peak pressures with left ventricular hypertrophy cause coronary flow to be exclusively diastolic and additional coronary vessel disease is common.

The more critical the stenosis, the more the attention to detail ensures a smooth operative course. The onset of CPB is best achieved with slow sinus rhythm, a well filled ventricle and afterload (vascular resistance) maintained. On CPB, the increased susceptibility to ischaemia may warrant retrograde, coronary sinus cardioplegia.

After CPB, the afterload is corrected, but compensatory mechanisms may require a year to remodel, and left ventricular hypertrophy with decreased diastolic compliance persists. Additional oedema or surgical damage may compromise the conducting system (which lies close to the aortic valve) making it prone to dangerous arrhythmias. The hypertrophied ventricle may cause ST depression, independent of ischaemia. Central venous pressure and PCWP as measures of preload, may significantly underestimate volume status, because the ventricle is stiff and requires higher diastolic pressures. Direct volume data, such as from TOE may be useful.

Aortic regurgitation

This is characterized by left ventricular volume overload with compensation by dilation and increased compliance, accommodating a large increase in volume with minimal change in pressure. Smooth induction of CPB is best obtained with tachycardia and vasodilation to reduce afterload.

A faster rate, by decreasing the available diastolic time reduces regurgitation and increases cardiac output. Similarly, by decreasing vascular impedance and maintaining a high-normal left atrial pressure, proportionally more of the stroke volume is directed forward. Regurgitation is usually operated on late in the course of the disease, and myocardial dysfunction is often present making it susceptible to depressants drugs.

Regurgitation across the valve means that cardioplegic agents injected into the aortic root will simply regurgitate into the left ventricle. Therefore, cardioplegic agents are usually given directly into the coronary vessels. After operation, again the volume status may not be reflected by the PCWP until there is remodelling of the ventricle.

MITRAL VALVE

The mitral valve is a bicuspid valve, consisting of an anterior and a posterior leaflet. Competence of the valve is also dependent on a competent ring, chordae tendinae and the papillary muscles. Valve dysfunction is predominantly secondary to rheumatic infection, a prolapsing leaflet or myocardial ischaemia leading to an enlarged ring, ruptured chordae or papillary muscles.

Mitral regurgitation

The pathophysiology of mitral regurgitation leads to a volume-loaded left ventricle. However, in mitral disease, impedance to systole is reduced by the additional regurgitant pathway. This leads to an enlarging left atrium, the development of pulmonary hypertension, and the left ventricular volume overload causes chamber dilatation. The surgical procedures include mitral valve repair with leaflet or chordae repair and a ring annuloplasty, or mitral valve replacement.

Smooth induction of CPB is best achieved with a relative tachycardia, adequate circulating volume and reduced arterial impedance. Mitral valve surgery is notorious for its associated mortality and difficulty weaning off CPB. This may be secondary to intrinsic myocardial dysfunction or the combination of pulmonary hypertension and right sided failure.

The compensatory mechanisms that are present whilst the defective valve is in place may actually deteriorate with the positioning of an intact valve. Right ventricular failure and pulmonary hypertension may be overcome by the use of high doses of vasodilators such as glyceryl trinitrate, inodilators such as enoximone, specific pulmonary vasodilators prostaglandin E_1 or inhaled nitric oxide, or ultimately a right ventricular assist device.

Mitral stenosis

This is almost invariably secondary to rheumatic fever. From a normal 4–6 cm^2, the valve area can decrease to 0.4 cm^2 in severe mitral stenosis. Progressive left atrial enlargement is accompanied by episodic pulmonary oedema, dyspnoea and atrial fibrillation. Pulmonary hypertension, with episodes of haemoptysis and right ventricular enlargement and failure, may ensue.

Repair may be possible with commisurotomy, or else valve replacement is undertaken. Cardiac output is best maintained by avoiding tachycardia (allowing adequate time for left ventricular filling) and maintaining preload. Pulmonary vascular resistance should be kept low to avoid right ventricular failure. Weaning from CPB may be difficult with the right ventricle unable to overcome high pulmonary vascular pressures. The use of specific pulmonary vasodilators, prostacyclin or inhaled nitric oxide, may be useful. Chronic left ventricle underfilling may also have led to myocardial dysfunction and an inability to manage the higher left ventricular preload.

Valve dysfunction is not usually isolated to one valve and additional lesions such as those involving the tricuspid, are common. An assessment of the dominant lesion is required and flexible strategies needed should the heart respond unexpectedly.

RE-OPERATIONS

The deterioration with time, of replacement valves and revascularization procedures, may necessitate further replacement or revascularization. These repeat sternotomies have twice the usual incidence of complications after surgery, with further risks imposed if the procedure is an emergency or due to infection.

There is greater blood loss intraoperatively necessitating a large (8–12 G), intravenous cannula. Catastrophic haemorrhage may occur from a large vessel, on opening the chest. There is an increased likelihood if a bypass graft lies in the midline (clips on chest X-ray), the ascending aorta or an aneurysm is close to the midline (chest X-ray, CT scan), and gross cardiac enlargement is present. Specific investigations, (CT scan and angiography) may help in delineating the anatomy before surgery. Mediastinal repair during the

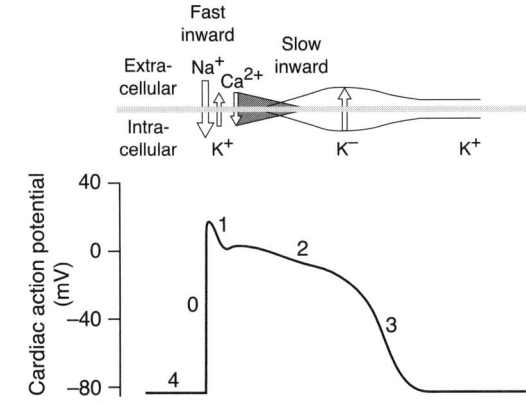

Figure 12.9 The cardiac action potential. (Reproduced with permission from Raddle, I.C. and Macleod, S.M. (1993) *Paediatric Pharmacology and Therapeutics*, 2nd edn. Mosby, St Louis, MO, p. 208.)

previous operation leaves fibrous adhesions which bleed profusely when cut. High dose aprotinin effectively diminishes the amount of bleeding.

Immediate availability of external defibrillation is prudent, as the myocardium is more prone to ventricular fibrillation and adequate access for internal defibrillation may not have been achieved.

CARDIAC ARRHYTHMIAS AND PACING

Myocardial cells have an inherent slow depolarization giving rise to rhythmic action potentials (Figure 12.9). Further specialized cells depolarize faster, propagating the action potential to the rest of the myocardium by a system of specialized cells: the conducting system (Figure 12.10).

Arrhythmias are generated by altered automaticity (unstable myocytes which depolarize faster) or by altered conductivity (unstable pacemaker cells in the conducting system, altering its pacemaker function). Perioperative factors may induce arrhythmias by unmasking borderline unstable myocytes. These factors include the volatile anaesthetic

Cardiac arrhythmias and pacing 223

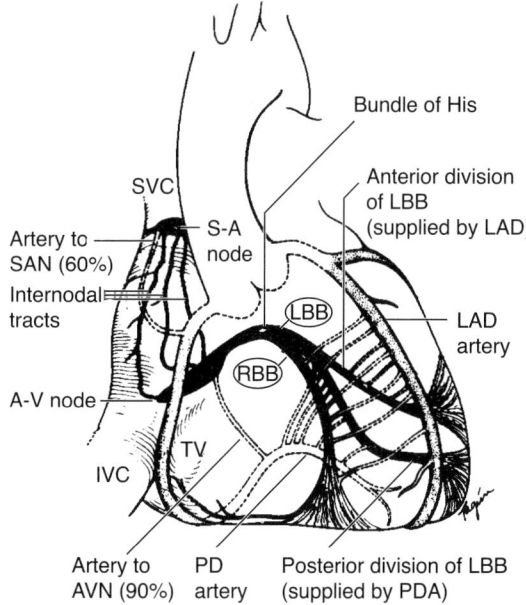

Figure 12.10 The conducting system and its blood supply. (Reproduced with permission from Harthorne, J.W. and Pohost, G.M. (1976) Electrical therapy of cardiac arrhythmias, in *Clinical Cardiovascular Physiology.* (ed. H.J. Levine), Grune and Stratton, New York, p. 854.)

agents, electrolyte disturbances (K^+, Ca^{2+}, Mg^{2+}), Po_2, Pco_2, temperature, autonomic disturbance and myocardial ischaemia. After these factors have been addressed, the management of acute arrhythmias is commonly undertaken with lignocaine, amiodarone, digoxin or cardioversion.

Patients with abnormal electrophysiology may present for anaesthesia for corrective procedures including pacemaker insertion, ablation of unstable areas and implantable defibrillator insertion. They may also present for incidental surgery with a pacemaker *in situ*.

In general, corrective or diagnostic procedures do not require CPB. Preoperative assessment of the arrhythmias and their treatment is essential, as they may be induced by anaesthesia. Concomitant left ventricular dysfunction may be significant. Most drugs used in anaesthesia in low dosage have minimal effects on electrophysiology, although droperidol should be avoided.

Pacemakers are widely used in the treatment of cardiac arrhythmias, causing some patients to become symptomless. Before anaesthesia the underlying diagnosis and need for pacing should be determined. Assessment of the pacemaker includes time of placement (<4 weeks prone to dislodge, battery lasts 6–12 years), when last checked (usually yearly), evidence of malfunction (palpitations, syncope etc.), type of pacemaker (see Table 8.2) and its response to a magnetic field. Usually, a magnet inactivates the sensing mode and converts to fixed rate pacing (newer, programmable pacemakers may respond differently). Monitoring of the paced patient must include a pulsatile component (pulse oximetry or invasive arterial pressure) as the ECG may not correlate with cardiac output. Postoperative care should include a check to confirm no change of pacemaker function.

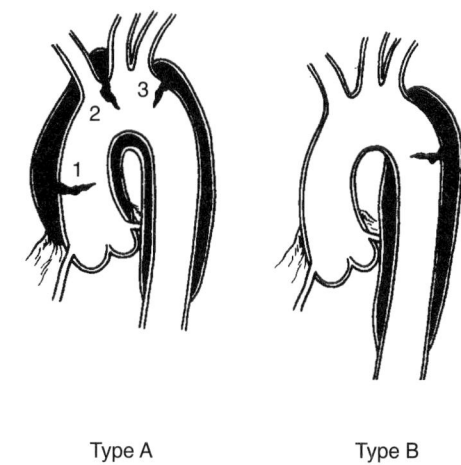

Figure 12.11 Thoracic aortic aneurysms. Stanford classification: Type A, hospital mortality decreases from 72% to 32% with surgery; Type B, hospital mortality increases from 27% to 33% with surgery. (Reproduced with permission from Miller, D.C. *et al.* (1979) Aortic dissections. *Journal of Thoracic and Cardiovascular Surgery*, **78**, 367.)

224 Cardiac surgery

The use of electrocautery increases the risks of oversensing and microshock generation down the pacemaker lead. Although avoidance of the electrocautery is ideal, in practice a careful, precautionary approach is undertaken. This involves the use of good quality, leak-free, bipolar electrocautery and monitoring of the pulse pressure. If unipolar electrocautery is used, its grounding plate should be as far away from the pacemaker as possible (15 cm). A magnet, if appropriate, may permit easier management during troublesome electrocautery, or other electromagnetic interference.

THORACIC AORTIC DISEASE

The thoracic aorta may require surgery either because of coarctation or secondary to intimal lesions leading to dissection, aneurysm or rupture (Figure 12.11). These lesions are frequently repaired by replacement of the dis-

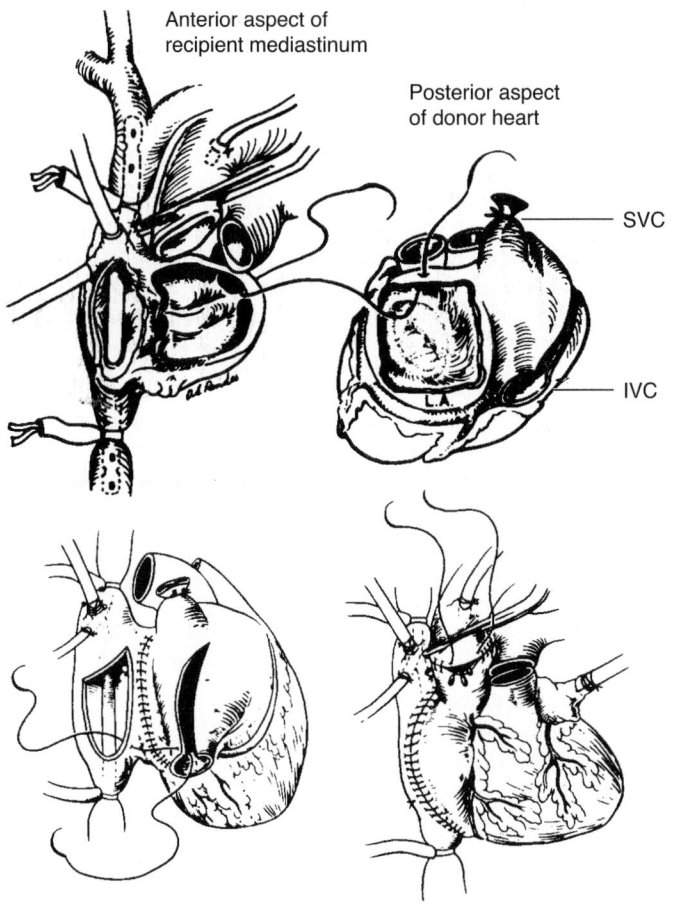

Figure 12.12 Illustrative view of cardiac transplantation. (Reproduced with permission from Raney, A.A. et al. (1982) The technique of cardiac transplantation, in *The Heart* 5th edn. (ed J.W. Hurst et al.) McGraw-Hill, New York, p. 1924.)

eased segment by a tubular graft. If a dissection has tracked proximally to involve the aortic valve, resuspension or replacement of the aortic valve may be necessary. Reoperation for patients with bleeding diatheses is more common. Brain and spinal cord injuries with paraplegia are recognized complications.

CPB is maintained through atrial drainage and femoral artery cannulation. Where the carotid arteries are involved deep hypothermic circulatory arrest will be used. If CPB is not employed, one-lung ventilation is essential for surgical access.

HEART AND LUNG TRANSPLANTATION

Transplantation with an appropriate sized heart as replacement (orthotopic), a smaller sized heart as a support (heterotopic), single or double lungs, or the heart and lungs together, has become a common procedure in cardiac transplant centres. The widespread acceptance of the concept of brain death in the 1960s, allowed transfer of a beating heart, and established technical aspects of heart transplantation (Figures 12.12 and 12.13). Further understanding of the immunological

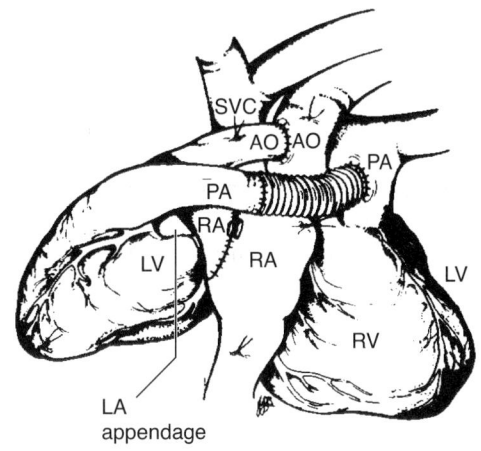

Figure 12.13 A method of heterotopic transplant, frequently used with high pulmonary vascular resistance. (Reproduced with permission from Novitzky, D., Cooper, D.K.C. and Barnard, C.N. (1983) The surgical technique of heterotopic heart transplantation. *Annals of Thoracic Surgery*, **36**: 481.)

response and its successful suppression with cyclosporin in the 1980s (Table 12.8) led to increasing success with subsequent extension to heart–lung and lung transplantation.

Table 12.8 An immunosuppressive regimen. (Reproduced with permission from Braunwald E. (ed.) (1992) *Heart Disease*, 4th edn, Saunders, Philadelphia, PA, p.528.)

	Preoperative	Postoperative	Comments
Cyclosporin	6 mg kg^{-1}	6–10 mg kg^{-1} day^{-1} (oral)	Avoid where creatinine increased
Steroids	Methylprednisolone 500 mg	Prednisone 0.4–1 mg kg^{-1} day^{-1}	Methylprednisolone 1 gm t.d.s.×3 days used for acute rejection
Azathioprine	2 mg kg^{-1} day^{-1} (oral)	2 mg kg^{-1} day^{-1} (oral)	
OKT3 (Monoclonal anti-T cell antibody)		5 mg day^{-1} for 2 weeks	Rescue for rejection after failure of high dose, pulsed steroids
ATG (rabbit or horse) Antithymocyte globulin		15 ml per day for 1–2 weeks	For rescue after failure of steroids and OKT3
Rejection confirmed by endomyocardial biopsy or bronchoscopic lung biopsy			

THE DONOR

The donor organ has to withstand the sequelae of brain death, CPB, cold transport, a new environment with different pulmonary and systemic vascular resistances, no cardiac innervation, immunosuppressive therapy and the recipient's reaction. Obviously, donor selection and management are crucial. Donor organs are commonly obtained away from the transplant centre, and the heart preserved with cardioplegia flush (either crystalloid or blood) with the lungs preserved commonly with a cold flush and vasodilators in the pulmonary artery. Transport is in an ice pack, and ischaemic times are kept to less than 4 h if possible.

THE RECIPIENT

Recipient selection needs to recognize not just the physical contraindications of irreversible pulmonary hypertension, irreversible renal or hepatic failure, and active infection, but also the psychological factors of a stable family environment, compliance with medication and an emotionally stable, well-motivated individual. With appropriate selection, the dismal prognosis of 40% mortality at one year for end-stage cardiac failure can be improved to 80–90% survival with cardiac transplantation, and 70% survival at 5 years, with an improved quality of life.

ANAESTHESIA

Anaesthesia from induction to CPB has to manage a poor left ventricle, and usually a previous sternotomy. After CPB the patient has a donor heart coping with a new environment. The patients are usually well motivated and adjusted, and an anxiolytic premedication is often unnecessary. They may be on very high doses of inotropic drugs or diuretics and vasodilators, and may also have required mechanical support. In addition, secondary to poor cardiac output, renal and hepatic failure may be present. Recipients are often only given short notice and should be treated as having a full stomach.

Induction of anaesthesia and management to CPB is similar to that for the compromised

Table 12.9 Congenital heart disease. (Reproduced with permission from Braunwald E. (ed) (1992) *Heart disease*, 4th edn, Saunders, Philadelphia, PA, p.888.)

Lesion	Frequency of lesions (%)	Operative surgery	Considerations
Ventricular-septal defect	30	Patch or direct closure	Left-to-right shunt, right ventricular overload
Atrial-septal defect	10	Patch or direct closure	Left-to-right shunt, right ventricular overload
Patent ductus arteriosus	10	Ligation	Left-to-right or right-to-left shunt
Pulmonary stenosis	7	Repair±Fontan procedure	Pressure overload, underdeveloped right ventricle
Coarctation	7	Excision and anastomosis	
Aortic stenosis	6	Valvotomy	Pressure overloaded left ventricle
Tetralogy of Fallot	6	Patch closure of ventricular-septal defect and refashioning of right ventricular outflow tract	Right-to-left shunt with dynamic right ventricular outflow tract obstruction
Transposition of great arteries	4	Jatene: arterial switch Senning: atrial switch	Coronary arteries may be anomalous

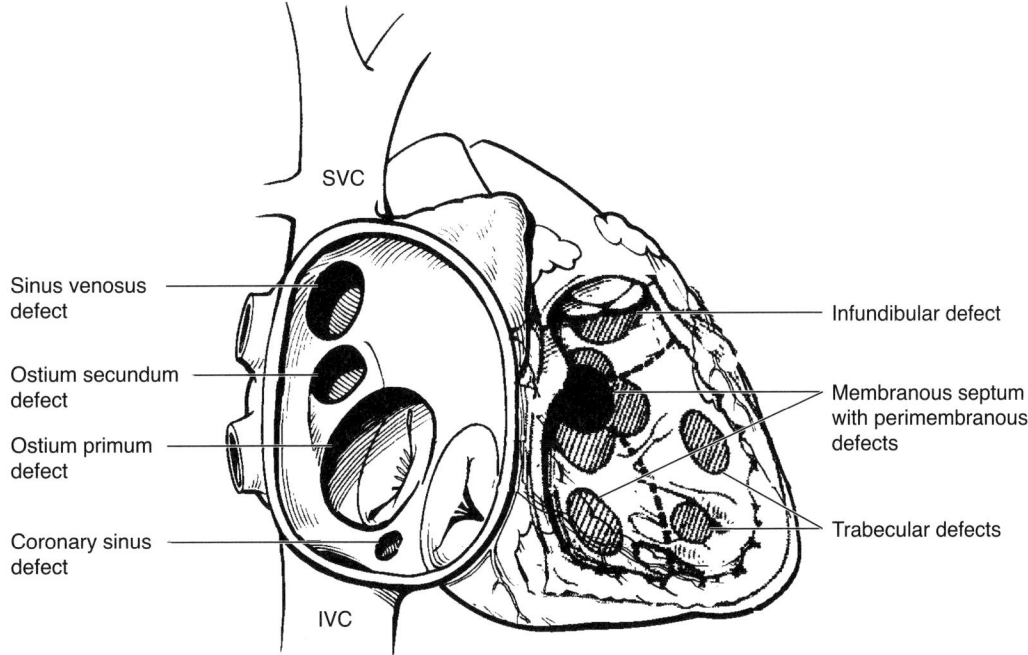

Figure 12.14 Schematic illustration of different types of atrial-septal defect and ventricular-septal defect which account for 40% of cases of congenital heart disease. (Reproduced with permission from Kambam, J. (ed) (1992) *Cardiac Anaesthesia for Infants and Children*. Mosby, St Louis, MO. p. 184.)

ventricle. Immunosuppressive therapy may be given preoperatively (cyclosporin) or intraoperatively (steroids), as required. As an immunosuppressed state is induced, meticulous attention to sterility must be maintained. Single lung transplantation may be undertaken with one-lung ventilation. These patients, however, already have end-stage respiratory failure, and CPB may become essential.

After CPB, weaning is similar to that for other cardiac operations. Isoprenaline is useful at this time to increase heart rate and contractility. Arrhythmias are common and may require pacing. Right heart failure may ensue if significant pulmonary vascular resistance is present, and may require inodilators, prostacyclin, inhaled nitric oxide or mechanical assist. Left heart failure may be secondary to poor myocardial protection or an inappropriately sized ventricle. Thoracic epidural analgesia may be used after lung transplantation.

HEART–LUNG TRANSPLANTATION

Heart–lung transplantation is more appropriate where significant pulmonary vascular resistance and right heart failure have developed (e.g. primary pulmonary hypertension, cystic fibrosis, Eisenmenger's syndrome) and has a 2-year survival rate of 60%. Anaesthesia is similar to that for cardiac transplantation. The trachea is divided and resutured to the donor trachea. This suture line may be assessed postoperatively by fibreoptic bronchoscopy. Bronchial artery anastomosis may be undertaken.

PATHOPHYSIOLOGY

The transplanted heart or lung responds differently to common stimuli. The lack of

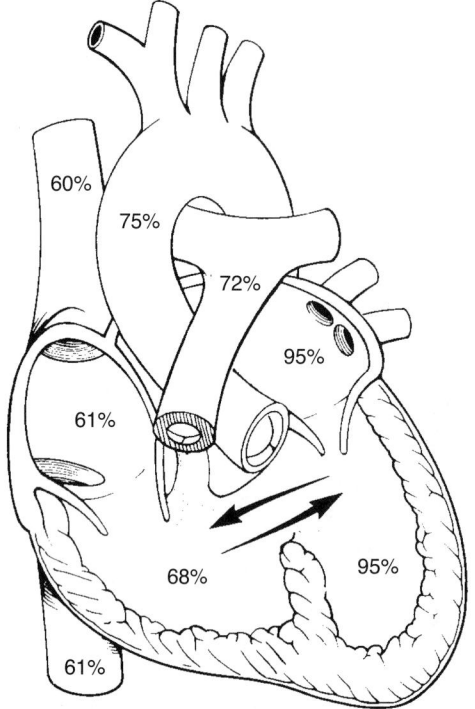

Figure 12.15 Tetralogy of Fallot (Sa_{O_2}%): pulmonary stenosis, overriding aorta ventricular septal defect and right ventricular hypertrophy. (Reproduced with permission from Kambam, J. (ed) (1992) *Cardiac Anaesthesia for Infants and Children*. Mosby, St Louis, MO. p. 222.)

cardiac innervation, the presence of immunosuppression and the risk of rejection, or accelerated coronary artery disease, should be borne in mind. Arrhythmias are common, and an elevated pulmonary vascular resistance may be found. Cardiac output increases with exercise in response to increased venous return initially, and then humoral stimuli. An increase in β-adrenoceptors makes the heart more sensitive to catecholamines

The transplanted lung lacks a lymphatic drainage and is unable to tolerate a fluid load. In addition to acute rejection and infection, lung function can be compromised in the long term by the appearance of obliterative bronchiolitis, the major cause of death.

OVERVIEW OF CONGENITAL HEART DISEASE

Congenital heart disease occurs in 8 of 1000 births (Table 12.9), with 50% of lesions accounted for by ventricular–septal defects (VSD), atrial–septal defects (ASD) (Figure 12.14) or patent ductus arteriosus (PDA). Associated conditions, such as Down's syndrome may be present. The most common complex congenital lesion is the Tetralogy of Fallot (Figure 12.15). Three separate characteristics of each lesion, and their response to changes in vascular resistance and volume loading, need to be assessed before anaesthesia.

SHUNTS

The persistence of a communication between the right and left circulation may allow blood to flow either from right to left (cyanosis), or from left to right (pulmonary plethora, right venticular hypertrophy and pulmonary hypertension). Common manoeuvres affect pulmonary and systemic vascular resistance and hence impedance to flow. This will alter the shunt flow characteristics. In a right-to-left shunt, the aim is to keep pulmonary vascular resistance to a minimum increasing pulmonary flow. In a left-to-right shunt, a low systemic vascular resistance encourages systemic flow, in preference to pulmonary flow. A left-to-right shunt may allow enough mixing of blood for cyanosis to occur. Additionally, as the pulmonary and right sided pressures increase, flow through the shunt may reverse giving rise to Eisenmenger's syndrome.

OBSTRUCTION TO FLOW

In some obstructive situations, mitral stenosis, aortic stenosis and a shunt may be critical to ensure an adequate cardiac output. If the only shunt is a PDA, efforts to keep it open may be necessary (prostaglandin E_1 infusion). Obstruction may also be dynamic, as in right ventricular outflow tract obstruc-

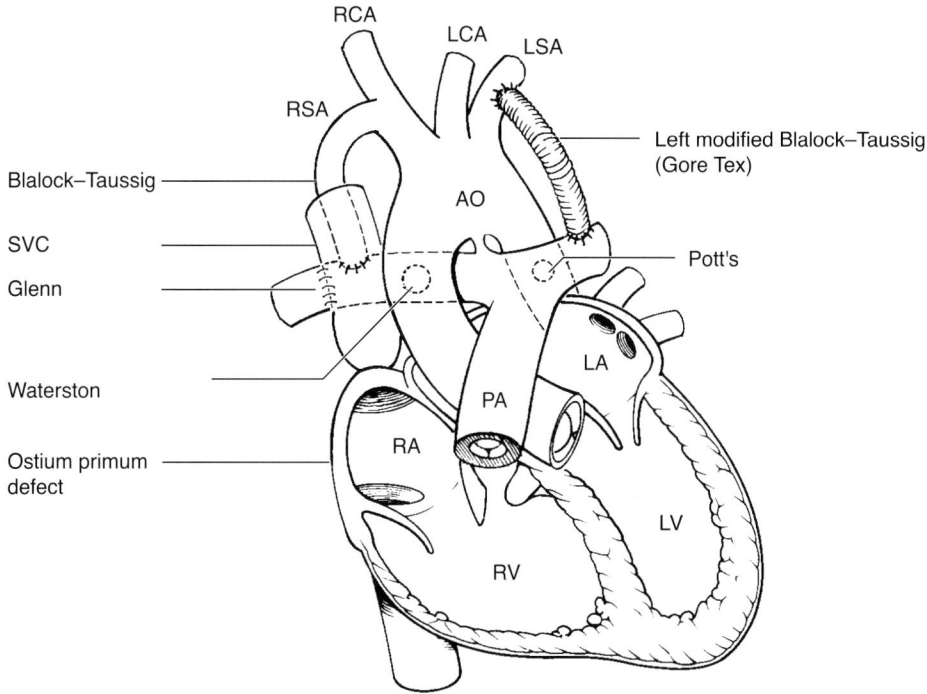

Figure 12.16 Palliative procedures to increase pulmonary blood flow. (Reproduced with permission from Kambam, J. (ed) (1992) *Cardiac Anaesthesia for Infants and Children*. Mosby, St Louis, MO. p. 126.)

tion in Tetralogy of Fallot, and may require treatment with β-blocking drugs.

VENTRICULAR STATUS

The myocardium is generally immature. If flow through the right or left ventricle has been bypassed, it may be unable to withstand correction of the circulation. A palliative operation (Figure 12.16), or appropriate timing of the operation, is then crucial to success.

The paediatric heart has little reserve and responds to stress such as hypoxia with a bradycardia (Table 12.10) or in the neonate, reverts to the fetal circulation (Figure 12.17). Premedication with atropine provides vagal inhibition and keeps the airway clear for a smooth, inhalational induction. Sedation with trimeprazine (3 mg kg^{-1}), or a benzodiazepine, may greatly assist by providing a calm child. Strenuous crying and struggling in the

Table 12.10 Significant characteristics of the paediatric, cardiac, surgical patient

---

Paediatric patient, not adult
Immature myocardium with limited reserve and reliance on heart rate
Return to fetal circulation in stress
Likelihood of pulmonary hypertension and cyanosis
Deep hypothermic circulatory arrest
Possibility of palliative surgery and definitive surgery when older

---

cyanotic, pulmonary hypertensive child may cause a hypercyanotic spell (Table 12.11). An inhalational induction is usually undertaken, although with ventricular dysfunction ketamine (i.m. or i.v.) or etomidate may be preferable. Minimal systemic disturbance requires appropriate management of pulmonary and systemic vascular resistances and volume status. Intraoperative echocardiography is

230 *Cardiac surgery*

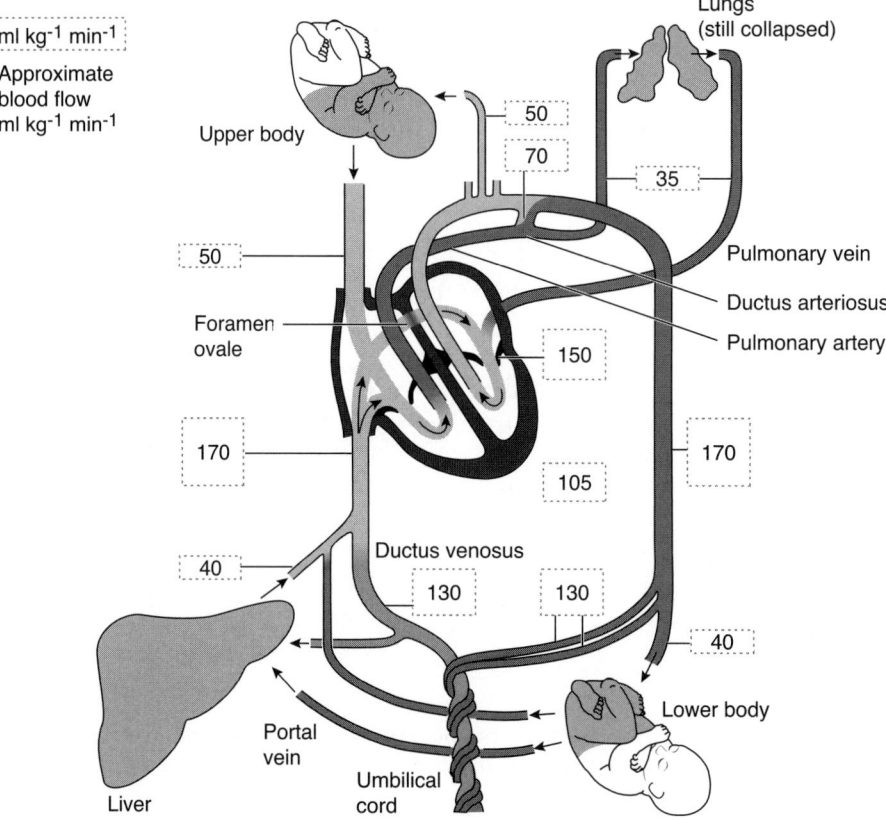

Figure 12.17 Fetal circulation. (Reproduced with permission from Despopoulos, A. and Silbernagl, S. (1991) *Colour Atlas of Physiology*, 4th edn, Thieme, Stuttgart, p. 191.)

Table 12.11 Factors influencing systemic vascular resistance and pulmonary vascular resistance in paediatric cardiac patients

	Systemic vascular resistance	Pulmonary vascular resistance
Increase	Sympathetic stimulation	Ventilatory: P_{O_2}, P_{CO_2}, pH, atelectasis, positive end-expiratory pressure, airway pressure
	α-agonists (adrenaline, noradrenaline, methoxamine)	Crying/struggling
	Squatting	
Decrease	Glyceryl trinitrate (GTN)	Prostacycline
	Sodium nitroprusside (SNP)	Inhaled NO
	Inodilators	Volatile anaesthetics
	Volatile anaesthetics	

extremely useful, providing early assessment of volume and ventricular status, and after surgery may reveal new defects that have been unmasked by correction of the primary lesion.

The priming fluid of the cardiopulmonary bypass circuit is a significant proportion of the blood volume, and the use of blood and plasma avoids undue haemodilution.

Postoperative problems may result from unmasked lesions, right ventricular failure with pulmonary hypertension and ventricular failure. As with adult cardiac anaesthesia, the best results are obtained with comprehensive preoperative assessment, surgical technical expertise and obsessive intraoperative and postoperative management.

FURTHER READING

Braunwald, E. (ed) (1992) *Heart Disease*, 4th edn, Saunders, Philadelphia.

Hensley, F. A. (ed) (1995) *The Practice of Cardiac Anaesthesia*. Little Brown, Boston, USA.

Kambam, J. (ed) (1994) *Cardiac Anesthesia for Infants and Children*. Mosby, New York.

Kaplan, J. A. (ed) (1993) *Cardiac Anaesthesia*. Saunders Philadelphia.

Prys-Roberts, C. and Biebuyck, J. F. (eds) *Current Opinion in Anaesthesiology*. Current Science, London.

VASCULAR SURGERY

J. P. Desborough

Postoperative cardiac morbidity and overall mortality are greater following vascular surgery than any other type of non-cardiac surgery. Many patients are elderly and have coexisting medical disorders. In particular, the cardiovascular and respiratory systems are likely to be affected. Most patients with peripheral vascular disease have generalized atherosclerosis; more than 70% have coronary artery disease. Much of the perioperative morbidity following vascular surgery is related to cardiovascular complications. In patients with stable, controlled angina, the risk of a perioperative myocardial infarction is 3–10% and the risk of death from cardiac causes is between 1 and 5%.

Careful preoperative assessment is the key feature of the management of patients presenting for vascular surgery. The aims of assessment are to determine the extent of co-existing cardiovascular and respiratory disease and to elicit factors which increase the risk of anaesthesia and surgery. If necessary, treatment can then be instituted to improve the physical state of the patient before surgery is undertaken.

RISK FACTORS

Certain clinical factors are associated with increased morbidity and mortality. Scoring systems have been compiled in an attempt to quantify the risk of perioperative complications. The Goldman index was proposed in 1977 to estimate the incidence of morbidity, or death, following major non-cardiac surgery. Nine risk factors, which could be elicited by clinical examination, ECG or chest radiograph, were assigned points in a scoring system. The most significant predictive features were clinical evidence of heart failure, recent myocardial infarction, arrhythmia and age greater than 70 years. (Table 7.2).

This scoring system has since been modified by other groups and the validity of its predictive power has been questioned. However, the major risk factors for non-cardiac surgery remain the same. These are previous myocardial infarction and current evidence of heart failure. One author has recently stated that the most important predictive factors for postoperative morbidity are clinical evidence of coronary artery disease and increased age.

CARDIOVASCULAR ASSESSMENT

All patients should be assessed by a history and physical examination, a 12-lead ECG and a chest radiograph. Current medication should be reviewed. An evaluation of the functional status of the patient should be made by assessing activity levels and exercise tolerance. Many patients with arterial disease affecting the lower limbs suffer from intermittent claudication or rest pain. It may be difficult in such cases to assess exercise tolerance accurately.

Evidence of myocardial ischaemia should be sought in the history taking. Risk factors for the development of ischaemic heart disease include smoking, diabetes and hypertension. Although hypertension is a frequent finding in patients with peripheral vascular disease, in itself it is not a useful predictor of perioperative morbidity. A history of angina pectoris should be noted and the severity and stability should be assessed. A history or ECG evidence of previous myocardial infarction is an important finding. In the 1970s, it was suggested that the risk of further perioperative infarction was as high as 30% for patients having surgery within 3 months of a myocardial infarction. More recent evidence from the early 1990s suggests that the risk is much lower; of the order of 5–10%. This may be related to improved care of patients in the perioperative period including optimization of medical therapy for coexisting diseases, the use of invasive monitoring of cardiovascular parameters, and close medical and nursing supervision after surgery.

Patients may have coronary artery disease, but be asymptomatic. More than half of patients with no history of ischaemic heart disease who undergo peripheral vascular surgery have significant coronary artery disease. Further tests can be performed to elicit the presence of ischaemic heart disease. In a 12-lead ECG, ST segment depression is indicative of subendocardial ischaemia, whereas ST segment elevation suggests transmural ischaemia or previous myocardial infarction. The presence of arrhythmias indicates the severity of the heart disease. A 24 h ambulatory ECG may detect episodes of silent ischaemia. Exercise ECG testing can be used to elicit angina or ECG changes indicative of myocardial ischaemia.

Other more sophisticated tests may be available at some institutions.

DIPYRIDAMOLE–THALLIUM IMAGING

Dipyridamole–thallium imaging is a chemical stress test which does not require the patient to exercise. Dipyridamole decreases the inactivation of the endogenous vasodilator adenosine, and also increases concentrations of c-AMP (cyclic adenosine monophosphate). This results in vasodilation of normal coronary arteries, whilst flow in diseased vessels is unchanged. It is infused intravenously, followed by an injection of the radioisotope thallium-201. Blood flow is diverted away from critically stenosed coronary vessels, so that the areas of myocardium supplied by these diseased arteries then have lower concentrations of the isotope on the thallium image.

ECHOCARDIOGRAPHY

Echocardiography is useful for assessing heart valve disease and left ventricular function. This can be a qualitative assessment of ventricular wall motion or can be combined with isotopic imaging. The ejection fraction, which is the ratio of stroke volume to ventricular end-diastolic volume can be measured. An ejection fraction less than 55% is regarded by some authors as an indication of increased operative risk. Values less than 35% have been associated with a high perioperative mortality. However, not all authors agree on a value, or indeed whether ejection fraction is useful as a predictor of perioperative myocardial events.

CORONARY ANGIOGRAPHY

In some centres, particularly in the USA, coronary angiography has been used to assess the severity of coronary artery disease in patients presenting for vascular surgery. If necessary, coronary revascularization can be performed before aortic or peripheral vascular reconstruction. Risk factors and cost implications are such that this is not undertaken routinely, but may be used for selected patients known to have significant coronary disease.

OPTIMIZATION

If a patient is identified as being at high risk of perioperative cardiac complications, their condition may require intensive medical therapy. Intensivists have noted that survivors of critical illness showed greater compensatory increases in tissue oxygen delivery than non-survivors. Improved cardiac output and delivery of oxygen have been used as goals in strategies developed to prevent multiple organ failure in severely ill patients. This concept has also been proposed for the management of high risk surgical patients. Cardiac output and O_2 delivery are measured using a thermodilution pulmonary artery catheter, and are then increased to a predetermined value: 600 ml min^{-1} m^{-2} is a commonly used target. This can be achieved using increased inspired oxygen, volume infusion to increase cardiac filling pressures, blood transfusion, inotropic drugs and vasodilators. Such preoperative management is termed 'optimization'. It requires additional resources in terms of invasive cardiovascular monitoring, medical supervision and high dependency nursing care. Some groups suggest that optimization of oxygen delivery may be beneficial in reducing postoperative mortality in certain high risk surgical patients. Patients over 70 years of age, those with limited cardiovascular reserve and with late stage vascular disease, are included in this group. At present, the goals are arbitrarily defined and the minimum increases in physiological parameters required to improve survival are not established. The availability of resources is a major limiting factor in the use of this technique.

RESPIRATORY SYSTEM

Chronic obstructive pulmonary disease is present in up to 50% of patients with peripheral vascular disease. In many subjects, this is associated with a long history of cigarette smoking. The aim of assessment is to identify chest disease so that respiratory function may be improved, if possible, to avoid postoperative complications such as atelectasis, pneumonia and ventilatory failure. A history should be taken, with specific enquiry about productive cough, wheezing and breathlessness. The patient must be examined for the presence of a chest infection or bronchospasm. The chest should be carefully auscultated and a chest radiograph inspected.

Simple, bedside respiratory function tests can be used to assess the severity of disease and the response to therapy. Peak expiratory flow rate can be measured with a peak flow meter. Values lower than about 100 l min^{-1} in adults indicate serious ventilatory impairment with an inability to cough effectively to clear secretions. A dry spirometer or vitalograph can measure forced vital capacity (FVC) and forced expired volume in one second (FEV$_1$). Restrictive lung diseases and loss of functional pulmonary tissue result in a decrease in FVC. Bronchospasm is associated with a decrease in FEV$_1$. Attempts should be made to reverse any bronchospastic elements, using bronchodilators, chest physiotherapy and antibiotics if appropriate. An arterial blood sample may be taken for estimation of arterial blood gases while the patient is breathing air. If the Pa_{O_2} is lower than 7.5 kPa and the Pa_{CO_2} greater than 7.5 kPa, a period of postoperative ventilation may be required, particularly after abdominal procedures. For patients with poor respiratory function having peripheral operations, regional anaesthetic techniques should be considered.

Patients should be counselled to avoid smoking before surgery. Blood levels of carboxyhaemoglobin (COHb) are increased in subjects who smoke, with values of 5–15% in heavy smokers. This equates to a decrease in O_2 carrying capacity equivalent to a loss of 2 g of haemoglobin. COHb has a short half-life of about 60 min. Cessation of smoking for

12–24 h before surgery will raise the O_2 carrying capacity of the blood as the concentration of COHb falls. However, the damage caused by decreased ciliary function and the risk of chest infection is not rapidly reversed.

OTHER SYSTEMS

Renal function should be assessed preoperatively by determination of circulating concentrations of creatinine, urea and electrolytes. The presence of renal impairment means that great care must be taken during the perioperative period to avoid factors which may further compromise kidney function. In patients with abdominal aortic disease involvement of the renal arteries can be determined by angiography.

Diabetes mellitus occurs in about 10% of patients with peripheral vascular disease. Cardiovascular disorders, neuropathies and renal dysfunction are common in longstanding diabetes. The stability of glycaemic control should be established before surgery. All patients, except those having the most minor surgery, will require an intravenous infusion of insulin with glucose. This should be started before surgery and continued until the patient resumes normal oral food intake. The aim of perioperative management is to maintain blood glucose values below 10 mmol l^{-1}. Good metabolic control may decrease the incidence of complications such as poor wound healing. Blood glucose concentrations should be monitored regularly with adjustment of the insulin infusion as necessary. Serum potassium values should also be checked. The anaesthetist must be aware of the possibility of autonomic neuropathy in diabetic patients. They may have symptoms of postural hypotension, which occurs from a lack of vasoconstriction, as a result of sympathetic nerve dysfunction. During anaesthesia, cardiac arrhythmias may occur. Haemodynamic disturbances are also possible, particularly with the onset of positive pressure ventilation. Delayed gastric emptying and impaired gut motility are features of autonomic neuropathy.

LABORATORY INVESTIGATIONS

Routine laboratory investigations are required before operation. These include a full blood count and estimation of urea and electrolyte concentrations. A coagulation screen is useful, particularly if patients have received anticoagulant therapy. Heparin infusions are often used in the treatment of critically ischaemic limbs.

ANAESTHETIC PROCEDURE

Monitoring of the cardiovascular system should begin before induction of anaesthesia with an ECG, measurement of arterial pressure and pulse oximetry. It is preferable to site invasive monitoring of arterial pressure before induction, if the patient has severe cardiac disease. Arterial surgery may involve rapid, large and continued blood loss. Cross-matched blood should be available before the patient is anaesthetized. Theatre staff should be instructed to weigh swabs and record blood loss in suction bottles. At least one large-bore intravenous cannula should be placed in a peripheral vein; two for aortic reconstructive procedures. Pressure infuser bags or a rapid infusion system must be available to allow fast transfusion of blood or blood substitutes. Fluid must be warmed.

The bladder should be catheterized so that urine output can be monitored. This is particularly important in patients with impaired renal function and in those operations where renal function may be compromised, for example with aortic cross-clamping close to the renal arteries. Urine output is a very good indicator of tissue perfusion. It should be maintained at at least 0.5 ml kg^{-1} h^{-1}.

Vascular surgery may take several hours. It is important to maintain normothermia if possible to avoid peripheral vasoconstriction. Nasopharyngeal or oesophageal probes can be used to monitor body temperature. Adjustment of the ambient temperature is an efficient method of keeping the patient warm. Various other devices may be used, including warming mattresses, heated overblankets, fluid warmers and warming of inspired gases with heat and moisture exchange filters. Positioning of the patient must be done carefully with protection of bony extremities and pressure points. If an arterial cannula and pressure monitor is used, the arm should be positioned so that arterial blood sampling is possible during surgery.

INTRAOPERATIVE MONITORING (Table 13.1)

The minimal standards of patient monitoring should be used in addition to vigilant clinical observations. An ECG with leads positioned to detect arrhythmias (lead II) and ST segment changes (V5) is essential. Observation of ST segment changes is useful for detection of myocardial ischaemia. Pulse oximetry and capnography are an essential part of monitoring. Ideally, arterial pressure should be directly measured by cannulation of a peripheral artery, usually the radial artery at the wrist. An arterial waveform can be displayed, together with a digital reading of systolic and diastolic pressure. Beat-to-beat monitoring of arterial pressure is useful in patients with cardiac disease and for surgery where profound changes in pressure may occur, for example with cross-clamping of the aorta or with sudden massive bleeding.

Table 13.1 Essential monitoring for major vascular surgery

ECG
Pulse oximetry
Direct arterial pressure
Central venous pressure
Inspired oxygen fraction (F_{IO_2})
Expired carbon dioxide fraction (F_{ECO_2})
Nasopharyngeal temperature
Urine output

Measurement of central venous pressure (CVP) is of value in patients having vascular surgery. This is usually done by a cannula placed percutaneously in the right internal jugular vein with the tip in the superior vena cava. The subclavian approach, or a long catheter placed from the ante-cubital fossa, may be preferable for procedures on the carotid artery. The reading indicates the filling pressure or preload of the right ventricle. It is a useful monitor of the intravascular volume status of the patient. The value of pulmonary artery catheters in the perioperative management of patients remains a controversial subject. These catheters are placed into the pulmonary artery percutaneously via a peripheral or central vein. The filling pressure of the left side of the heart can be monitored. This will be useful in circumstances where there is no close correlation between CVP and left sided filling pressure, for example in patients with poor left ventricular function, following myocardial infarction, or in cardiac failure. In addition, cardiac output can be determined by thermodilution and systemic and pulmonary haemodynamic parameters calculated. Therapeutic manoeuvres can be instituted to change these values to desired levels. However, it remains uncertain whether outcome is improved by the use of pulmonary artery catheters. The risks associated with insertion and use of these catheters are greater than with an internal jugular cannula. Complications include knotting of the catheter, cardiac arrhythmias, pulmonary infarction and haemoptysis.

A recent addition to cardiovascular monitoring is transoesophageal echocardiography (TOE). It has been used to estimate cardiac output but measurements have significant variability and do not correlate well with thermodilution methods. TOE can also be used to monitor ventricular wall motion abnormalities, which are a useful early indication of myocardial ischaemia. However, the technique requires continuous observation and considerable expertise for data evalu-

HEPARINIZATION

Heparin is used in vascular surgery to prevent clot formation while blood vessels are clamped. Its mechanism of action is to bind to antithrombin III and increase the reaction between antithrombin III and other activated clotting factors. The onset of effect is immediate. Heparinization can be monitored using a machine which determines activated clotting time, ACT. Ideally a baseline measurement should be taken; this is usually about 100–120 s. An intravenous dose of 5000 to 8000 units of heparin is given before cross clamping of vessels in vascular surgery. This dose should prolong the ACT into the range of 250–300 s. The ACT should be monitored during the course of the operation, so that additional top-up doses of heparin can be given if necessary.

After completion of the vascular anastomosis, the surgeon may request reversal of residual heparin activity by the administration of protamine. This may be unnecessary if adequate haemostasis has been achieved. A dose of 1 mg protamine per 100 units of heparin is required for full neutralization of the heparin effect. Consideration should be given to the half-life of heparin, which is approximately one hour. Ideally, reversal of residual heparin activity should be done in conjunction with measurement of ACT.

AORTIC RECONSTRUCTIVE SURGERY

Elective abdominal aortic aneurysm repair is commonly performed for aneurysms of 5 cm diameter or more. The aim is to avoid aortic rupture which has a very high mortality of about 80–90%; elective surgery has a mortality of 1–8%. Aneurysms of diameter less than 5 cm are generally managed conservatively, with yearly follow up and ultrasound assessment to detect any increase in size of the aneurysm.

ANAESTHETIC CONSIDERATIONS

A major consideration for the anaesthetist is the presence of pre-existing medical problems which must be fully evaluated before surgery. In addition there are potential problems relating to the operation itself. There may be massive haemorrhage requiring rapid transfusion. The anaesthetist should be aware of the haemodynamic consequences of aortic cross-clamping and the possibility of renal dysfunction and spinal cord damage.

BLOOD TRANSFUSION

Aortic aneurysm surgery often involves large blood losses. Homologous blood transfusion will be required in the vast majority of cases. The volume of transfusion required can be decreased if various blood conservation measures are undertaken. Preoperative collection and storage of the patient's own blood may be considered if donor blood is scarce. Iron supplementation may be required to restore the patient's haemoglobin before surgery. Intraoperatively, haemodilution by replacement of some of the blood losses with crystalloids or colloids may be considered. However, both these techniques cause anaemia, which is less easily tolerated in elderly patients with limited cardiovascular and respiratory reserve than in healthy young individuals. Intraoperative blood salvage can be used to decrease the volume of transfused blood. Various devices are available which collect, wash and return red cells to the patient. Blood from the surgical field is aspirated, mixed with a heparin solution and the cells are then washed free of plasma and debris. The heparin solution is removed, the red cells are concentrated to a haematocrit of about 60%, and can be reinfused. This process removes coagulation factors and platelets.

Any massive blood transfusion may lead to coagulation abnormalities. This results from haemodilution of the patient's blood with crystalloids and/or colloids and transfusion of red cells which are deficient in platelets and clotting factors. Coagulation should be monitored by regular laboratory assay and platelet counts. The results of these tests can be used as a guide to the necessity for transfusion of blood components.

HAEMODYNAMIC CONSEQUENCES OF AORTIC CROSS-CLAMPING

When the abdominal aorta is cross-clamped, the afterload or impedance of the heart increases so that stroke volume and cardiac output decline. Systemic vascular resistance increases. The venous return to the heart decreases, because the lower half of the body is excluded from the circulation, and perfusion pressures are low. Patients with poor cardiac function may not tolerate cross-clamping easily; the left ventricle may be strained severely by the increased afterload. In these patients, cardiac output decreases significantly with signs of myocardial ischaemia. Infusion of a vasodilator such as glyceryl trinitrate or sodium nitroprusside may be needed to lower the systemic vascular resistance.

During cross-clamping, filling pressures should be maintained above preoperative values by infusion of fluids. Blood and blood substitutes should be available to be given by rapid transfusion if necessary. When the cross clamp is removed, hypotension often occurs. There are several possible mechanisms for this. Brisk haemorrhage from the anastomotic site requires a further period of aortic clamping and surgical repair. Reactive hyperaemia and vasodilation may occur in distal vessels causing hypotension. A third cause of hypotension may be the adverse effect on the myocardium of metabolites which accumulate in poorly perfused, distal tissues during aortic cross-clamping. Hypotension can be avoided by careful attention to filling pressures during cross-clamping with maintenance of a value several cmH$_2$O above the starting value. Rapid volume infusion after removal of the cross-clamp should counteract any hypotension caused by reactive vasodilation.

RENAL FUNCTION

A small percentage (around 2%) of patients will develop acute renal failure following aortic aneurysm surgery. Renal function may be compromised as a result of hypovolaemia and hypotension, and massive blood transfusion. In addition, renal perfusion may be affected directly by cross-clamping at the level of renal arteries. Infrarenal cross clamping may also decrease renal perfusion by increased vascular resistance, turbulent flow and alterations in blood flow within the kidney.

The most easily measured parameter is urine output, but this does not predict the development of renal failure. However, renal impairment is unlikely if urine output is maintained at 0.5–1.0 ml kg^{-1} h^{-1}. Strenuous attempts must be made to avoid hypovolaemia, by monitoring of blood and fluid losses and measurement of filling pressures, and the maintenance of an adequate intravascular volume and cardiac output.

A number of pharmacological therapies have been advocated for renal protection during vascular surgery with aortic cross-clamping. Much of the evidence is based on animal studies and the results cannot be extrapolated to humans undergoing surgery where normovolaemia is usually maintained. The use of 'low-dose' dopamine has been advocated to protect against renal dysfunction. At doses of 0.5–2.5 μg kg^{-1} min^{-1}, dopamine stimulates dopaminergic receptors in the renal and mesenteric vasculature. Higher doses promote β-adrenergic effects, and α-adrenergic effects occur at doses greater than 5 μg kg^{-1} min^{-1}. The division of dosage is somewhat arbitrary as the effects of dopamine overlap, and there is much individual variation in response. Increased renal blood flow and urine output occur as a result of renal vasodilation and increases in cardiac output. This response is most pronounced in euvolaemic subjects. Although dopamine therapy may lead to an increased urine output, there is no documented evidence of a renal protective effect. A study of normovolaemic patients randomized to receive low-dose dopamine therapy following major vascular surgery showed no changes in urine output, creatinine clearance and creatinine concentrations. The use of dopamine is not without potential risk to the patient. Complications include tachycardia, myocardial ischaemia and infarction, and the development of gut ischaemia.

The use of diuretics to preserve renal function during vascular surgery has been advocated, but does not have a foundation in human studies. Mannitol in doses of 0.25–0.5 g kg^{-1}, and frusemide in doses up to 50 mg may be used if oliguria occurs. The best management is adequate fluid replacement to cover preoperative deficits, with meticulous attention to the maintenance of filling pressures and replacement of fluid and blood losses during surgery.

SPINAL CORD

A rare complication of aortic reconstructive surgery is damage to the blood supply to the spinal cord. It is more likely to occur during thoracoabdominal procedures than in operations on the abdominal aorta or aorto–iliac vessels. The incidence has been found to be much greater in surgery where aneurysms have ruptured, compared with elective procedures. The spinal cord is supplied by blood in a single anterior spinal artery and a pair of posterior arteries. There is much collateral input to these arteries from the vertebral artery, intercostal, lumbar and internal iliac arteries. The main supply to the anterior spinal artery and the distal part of the spinal cord is from a branch of an intercostal artery which arises between T8 and L2. This artery is sometimes called the radicular artery or the artery of Adamkiewicz.

Neurological consequences of ischaemic damage to the spinal cord include paraplegia and sensory losses. Various strategies have been proposed to avoid neurological deficits following thoracoabdominal aortic surgery. These include hypothermia, cardiopulmonary bypass, reattachment of intercostal and lumbar arteries, evoked potential monitoring, drainage of cerebrospinal fluid (CSF) and the use of drugs such as steroids and mannitol. Preoperative angiographic catheterization of intercostal and lumbar arteries may identify the level of the artery of Adamkiewicz. During surgery, intercostal arteries may then be reimplanted to preserve spinal artery flow below the level of the aortic cross-clamp.

ANAESTHETIC TECHNIQUE

Maintenance of haemodynamic stability and careful attention to patient monitoring are of greater importance than the choice of anaesthetic agents. For aortic surgery, general anaesthesia can be provided alone or combined with regional anaesthesia. General anaesthesia usually comprises a mixed opioid/volatile agent technique with neuromuscular blockade.

An anxiolytic premedication should be prescribed. Oral benzodiazepines such as temazepam are suitable to decrease anxiety without oversedation. Induction of anaesthesia should be slow to minimize cardiovascular effects such as hypotension. An intubating dose of neuromuscular blocking drug is used to facilitate tracheal intubation and ventilation of the lungs. Anaesthesia can be maintained with a volatile agent and an analgesic agent; morphine or fentanyl are suitable. During anaesthesia, arterial pressure, oxygenation and ventilation, urine output and patient temperature should be carefully monitored.

Regular arterial blood sampling should be done for estimation of acid–base status, plasma [K$^+$] and haemoglobin or haemocrit. Blood should be transfused to maintain a haemoglobin of at least 10 g dl^{-1}, or a haematocrit of 30%.

On completion of the procedure, if there is no surgical bleeding and the patient is physiologically stable and normothermic, neuromuscular blockade may be reversed and the patient extubated when awake. Supplemental oxygen should be given by face mask. Analgesia can be provided with opiates by intermittent, intravenous injection until analgesia is achieved, and then by continuous intravenous infusion, or by a patient-controlled device. If an epidural catheter is in place, analgesia is continued into the postoperative period. Ideally, patients should be carefully monitored in a high dependency facility. Observations of arterial pressure, oxygenation and urine output should continue at regular intervals. Immediate complications of aortic and peripheral vascular surgery include haemorrhage, hypotension and oliguria. Cardiovascular problems such as myocardial infarction, and renal failure usually occur later in the postoperative period.

PERIPHERAL VASCULAR SURGERY

Arterial disease is assessed initially by clinical examination. Non-invasive evaluation of arterial supply to the limbs is performed with Doppler ultrasound pressure measurements. An index of ankle systolic to brachial systolic blood pressure (ABI) can be derived. ABI is greater than 1.0 in healthy patients. Values decrease progressively with increasing severity of lower limb arterial disease. A patient with rest pain resulting from ischaemia, will have an ABI of about 0.25.

Anatomical evaluation of the location and extent of arterial disease is by arteriography. In the past, surgery has been the definitive treatment. Interventional radiological techniques may be used as an alternative. Percutaneous transluminal angioplasty (PTA) is most suitable for relieving obstruction caused by localized, short stenoses in proximal vessels, rather than multiple occlusions and those in distal vessels. Anaesthetists may be asked to provide sedation for patients having PTA. Intervention may also be required if complications arise, for example arterial dissection or haemorrhage. Surgical bypass of occlusive disease can be performed using a reversed autogenous saphenous vein graft or an *in situ* saphenous graft. If there are no suitable veins, graft materials such as Dacron® or Gore-Tex® may be used.

For peripheral arterial surgery on the lower limbs, regional anaesthetic techniques may be considered as an alternative to general anaesthesia. Procedures below the inguinal ligament such as femoropopliteal or femoro–distal tibial bypass grafts are very suitable for regional blockade with local anaesthetic agents. Spinal or epidural anaesthesia with blockade from T10 downwards are appropriate. It should be borne in mind that femoro–distal grafts may take many hours; thus an epidural local anaesthetic which can be topped up through a catheter may be more appropriate than a single-shot, spinal technique.

Preoperative assessment of the patient is essential; in particular, a check of the coagulation status should be included if regional anaesthesia is planned. The general principles of anaesthetic management and monitoring of cardiovascular parameters described earlier in this chapter also apply to peripheral arterial surgery. The patient may prefer to be sedated, particularly during long procedures. Supplemental oxygen should be given via a face mask, or nasal cannulae. The skin incisions and tunnelling for insertion of graft materials evoke the greatest responses in the cardiovascular system. Thereafter, anastomotic procedures may be lengthy, but are less stressful. There is always the potential for brisk haemorrhage which may require rapid transfusion.

Recent studies have shown that the type of

anaesthesia used for peripheral arterial surgery has little influence on the incidence of postoperative cardiovascular complications. Although most patients are theoretically at high risk of perioperative cardiac events, the risk of non-fatal myocardial infarction, or early death from cardiac causes, is around 2–6% with either general or regional anaesthesia. However, the type of anaesthesia may influence graft patency. There is some evidence that epidural regional anaesthesia may be of benefit in decreasing the risk of early graft failure. This improvement may be associated with enhanced fibrinolysis and requires further evaluation.

CAROTID ARTERY SURGERY

Carotid endarterectomy is performed to decrease the risk of stroke from emboli arising from atheromatous lesions in the carotid artery. Patients may already have suffered transient ischaemic episodes or have asymptomatic carotid bruits. The degree of carotid stenosis is determined by angiography. The aim of the operation is to remove atheromatous plaque leaving a smooth arterial wall. Multicentre trials have been performed to evaluate the role of carotid endarterectomy in the prevention of stroke. In patients with severe carotid artery stenosis (70–99%), the benefits of surgery outweigh the operative risks. For moderate stenosis (30–69%) results are unclear and further evaluation is required. In those patients with a mild degree of stenosis the risks of surgery outweigh the benefits.

PREOPERATIVE ASSESSMENT

Most patients presenting for carotid artery surgery are elderly, and as discussed earlier, many having coexisting medical disorders. There is a high incidence of cardiac disease, respiratory disorders related to smoking, and diabetes. These should be fully evaluated by history taking, clinical examination and investigations as described previously. A full neurological examination should be performed and recorded in the patients' notes. Systemic hypertension is very common in these patients. If controlled preoperatively, the risk of postoperative hypertension and stroke may be decreased. Routine medication should be continued on the day of surgery. In particular, antihypertensive therapy should not be stopped.

SURGICAL PROCEDURE

During surgery, the carotid artery in the neck is dissected out. After systemic heparinization, the artery is clamped on either side of the atheromatous plaque which is then removed through an arteriotomy. Oxygen delivery to the brain is compromised during carotid artery occlusion, although there will be some collateral flow via the circle of Willis and the vertebral arteries. Some surgeons use an intraluminal shunt as a bypass across the clamped vessel. The use of a shunt adds to the duration of surgery, and may increase the risk of embolization and arterial wall damage. The pressure in the carotid artery distal to the occluding clamp, called stump pressure, is generated from retrograde flow from contralateral vessels. It can be measured directly using pressure transducing equipment. A minimal acceptable stump pressure is around 50–60 mmHg; at this pressure surgeons who advocate the use of a shunt would consider one necessary to maintain brain perfusion. However, there is no correlation between signs of cerebral ischaemia, EEG changes and the stump pressure.

ANAESTHETIC CONSIDERATIONS

In the UK, most patients having carotid artery surgery receive general anaesthesia. This facilitates control of haemodynamic and respiratory parameters. Anaesthetists are much less familiar with providing regional anaesthesia for this operation. However, the advantage of a local or regional anaesthetic technique in a conscious patient is that changes in neurological status and hence a neurological deficit, will be detected very early. The effects of carotid occlusion on cerebral function may be readily assessed. The requirement is for blockade of the second and third cervical nerve roots by a cervical plexus block. Occasionally the fourth cervical root needs to be blocked. The use of cervical extradural anaesthesia for carotid artery surgery has been reported, although this technique should only be performed by experienced anaesthetists because of the potential for serious complications such as hypotension.

GENERAL ANAESTHESIA

The aims of general anaesthesia are haemodynamic stability with maintenance of oxygenation and ventilation. Monitoring of cardiovascular parameters is a priority, as many patients have severe atherosclerotic disease. Consideration of factors which affect cerebral perfusion is equally important, as cerebral blood flow will be compromised during clamping of the carotid artery.

CEREBRAL BLOOD FLOW

Cerebral blood flow is maintained by autoregulation at about 50 ml min^{-1} 100 g^{-1} brain tissue, over a wide range of perfusion pressures. Critical values are in the range of 18–24 ml min^{-1} 100 g^{-1}. Below these levels, blood flow may be too low to deliver sufficient oxygen for the brain's metabolic requirements ($CMRO_2$) and ischaemic damage may occur. Agents which decrease $CMRO_2$ may protect the brain from hypoxic damage in situations of cerebral ischaemia. Barbiturates are the only anaesthetic agents proven to have this effect; therefore, thiopentone may be of benefit in carotid endarterectomy. Midazolam decreases $CMRO_2$ and may be useful as an induction agent, but, it must be given cautiously to avoid hypotension. Many pharmaceutical compounds are being evaluated as potential neuroprotective agents. As yet, no drug has an established place in clinical practice for use in carotid artery surgery.

Other potential methods of protecting the brain include hypothermia and the avoidance of hyperglycaemia. Mild hypothermia (about 35°C) is achieved easily in theatre and may decrease cerebral metabolism sufficiently to be of benefit in carotid endarterectomy. More profound hypothermia is attainable only with cardiopulmonary bypass and is therefore of limited value. Hyperglycaemia has deleterious effects on the brain following global ischaemia; normoglycaemia should be maintained with regular blood glucose monitoring. This is particularly important with diabetic patients in whom metabolic control must be meticulous.

BRAIN MONITORING

There is no ideal monitoring system to warn of cerebral ischaemia during carotid artery surgery. Indeed, it is uncertain whether monitoring is useful because many systems lack a prognostic value. Stump pressure is the most commonly measured variable but it does not accurately predict neurological outcome. Cerebral function monitors and other automated EEG systems have been developed to overcome some of the complexities of EEG monitoring. However, skilled interpretation is still required, and unfortunately changes may indicate that neurological damage has already occurred.

Other methods of monitoring include xenon-133 clearance, transcranial Doppler ultrasound (TCD) and evoked potential monitoring. These are not used routinely. The radioisotope xenon-133 can be injected intra-arterially and subsequent scintillation counting over the brain indicates cerebral blood flow. Values below 18 ml min^{-1} 100 g^{-1} of brain tissue are regarded as critically low, although flow rates do not necessarily correlate with the appearance of neurological deficits. TCD can give an indication of cerebral blood flow, but only flow through the middle cerebral artery is usually measured. Monitoring of somatosensory evoked potentials has been shown to correlate with EEG findings of cerebral ischaemia during carotid endarterectomy. Unfortunately, neurological deficits may be detected only after emergence from general anaesthesia.

ANAESTHETIC TECHNIQUE

Anxiolytic premedication should be prescribed to attenuate pressor responses generated by stress and anxiety. Benzodiazepines are eminently suitable, for example temazepam orally 60–90 min before induction of anaesthesia.

Full monitoring of the patient should commence before induction of anaesthesia. Arterial pressure should be measured directly from a radial arterial cannula, and the trachea intubated to protect the airway. Induction and tracheal intubation should be performed carefully to avoid marked fluctuations in systemic arterial pressure. Hypotension may be deleterious to cerebral perfusion, and hypertension and tachycardia may precipitate myocardial ischaemia. Most anaesthetists institute mechanical ventilation of the lungs so that arterial carbon dioxide tension can be controlled; normocapnia should be maintained. The choice of anaesthetic agents is less critical than attention to the anaesthetic principles stated above. If necessary, lignocaine 1 mg kg^{-1} i.v., or fentanyl, can be given before laryngoscopy and intubation to avoid a surge in blood pressure. A suitable choice of anaesthesia would be induction with thiopentone, vecuronium or atracurium to facilitate tracheal intubation and ventilation of the lungs, and maintenance with isoflurane in an oxygen mixture with nitrous oxide or air. Fentanyl is a suitable opioid analgesic.

During surgery, normovolaemia should be maintained by infusion of fluids or blood if necessary. Fluctuations in arterial pressure may occur intraoperatively as a result of the patient's hypertensive disease or from manipulation of the carotid sinus nerve. Partial, or complete, baroreceptor denervation may abolish responses to carotid flow with subsequent reflex increases in heart rate and hypertension. The stimulus of improved flow after surgery may increase afferent stimulation leading to hypotension. Some surgeons use lignocaine infiltration to denervate the carotid baroreceptors, but this may result in hypertension.

Marked hypertension may be treated with specific antihypertensive agents, provided it has been ascertained that the level of anaesthesia is adequate. The combined α- and β-blocking drug labetalol, or the short-acting β-blocking drug, esmolol are suitable if tachycardia is also a problem. Sodium nitroprusside may be given by i.v. infusion. Treatment should be cautious to avoid hypotension. Hypotension may be treated with an α-adrenoceptor agonist such as methoxamine.

POSTOPERATIVE COMPLICATIONS

Cardiovascular and respiratory monitoring should continue for several hours after surgery. The most frequent, serious, postoperative complications are myocardial infarction (5–10%) and stroke (1–2%). One third of strokes occur peroperatively, one third in the first 24 h and the remainder occur later in the postoperative period. The appearance of a new neurological deficit on emergence from anaesthesia may necessitate an immediate return to theatre for re-operation.

Hypertension is a frequent occurrence following carotid artery surgery. It may occur as a result of pain, withdrawal of antihypertensive therapy, or interference with the innervation of the carotid sinus during surgery. Postoperative hypertension may also be an indication of a neurological deficit. After ensuring that analgesia is adequate, hypertension may be treated with an antihypertensive agent as described previously. Suitable drugs include sodium nitroprusside by i.v. infusion, or the combined α- and β-adrenoceptor antagonist, labetalol. A calcium channel blocker, such as nifedipine, is useful in the presence of myocardial ischaemia.

Hypotension may also occur and should be treated aggressively to avoid cerebral hypoperfusion. Hypovolaemia must be corrected by volume infusion before vasoconstrictor agents are used. If necessary, an α-adrenoceptor agonist such as methoxamine can be given. Ephedrine is also suitable, particularly if bradycardia is present.

Haemorrhage may occur postoperatively. Swelling in the neck can cause upper airway obstruction, necessitating prompt and effective management. Haematoma should be evacuated surgically. If it is necessary to re-anaesthetize the patient, intubation may be difficult. The anaesthetist should consider carefully whether the use of neuromuscular blocking drugs
is essential before securing the airway and intubating the trachea.

CONCLUSIONS

Patients for vascular surgery must be carefully reviewed before surgery to assess the severity of coexisting medical disease. Cardiovascular and respiratory disorders, diabetes and renal dysfunction are common. Vigilant monitoring of cardiovascular and ventilatory parameters during surgery is essential. The choice of anaesthetic technique and agents is less critical than a careful approach to induction and maintenance of anaesthesia. Monitoring of the patient should continue into the postoperative period.

FURTHER READING

Boote, R. H., Lewis, D. P., Zarich, S. W. *et al.* (1996) Cardiac outcome after peripheral vascular surgery. Comparison of general and regional anesthesia. *Anesthesiology*, **84**, 3–13.

Cunningham, A. J. (1994) Anaesthesia for abdominal and major vascular surgery, in *Anaesthesia* (eds W. S. Nimmo, D. J. Rowbotham and G. Smith.) Blackwell Scientific Publications, Oxford, pp. 1042–1076.

Garrioch, M. A. and Fitch, W. (1993) Anaesthesia for carotid artery surgery. *British Journal of Anaesthesia*, **71**, 569–579.

Juste, R. N. Lawson, A. D. and Soni, N. (1996) Minimising cardiac anaesthetic risk: the tortoise or the hare? *Anaesthesia*, **51**, 255–262.

Kaplan, J. A. (1991) *Vascular Anaesthesia*. Churchill Livingstone, Edinburgh.

NEUROSURGERY

R. Dwyer

Our understanding of cerebral physiology and pathophysiology has increased considerably in the last twenty years. This has led to a more rational approach to pharmacological management and to manipulation of physiological variables like arterial pressure and pulmonary ventilation. This chapter will summarize this information and point out areas where there is still uncertainty about management.

Anaesthetic considerations for neurosurgical patients differ from other types of surgery for a number of reasons.

- The presence of intracranial pathology alters patients' responses to drugs and procedures.
- Neurosurgery has unique requirements for optimization of operating conditions.
- The site of surgery puts neural tissue at risk.

CEREBRAL ANATOMY AND PHYSIOLOGY

The contents of the skull consist of brain tissue, blood and cerebrospinal fluid (CSF).

Brain tissue is made up of: neurons, excitable cells whose depolarization and repolarization is essential for central nervous system (CNS) function; and neuroglia, connective tissue cells, 10–50 times more numerous, which do not transmit nervous impulses but have other important functions.

Neurons are large cells with multiple connections to other neurons via dendrites and synapses. Synaptic connections have excitatory or inhibitory effects on a neuron, making it more or less likely to depolarize. Synaptic transmission in the CNS is mediated by over 40 neurotransmitters, excitatory and inhibitory.

Cell metabolic rate is high to provide energy to maintain ionic gradients, support cell homeostasis and neurotransmitter metabolism (40% of energy requirements) and to allow repolarization and depolarization (60%). Oxygen requirements are high; the brain is 2% of body weight but its oxygen consumption is 20% of the body total. Cerebral metabolic rate (CMR) may be defined by oxygen or glucose requirements ($CMRO_2$ or CMR_{glu}).

Oxygen extraction is similar to the rest of the body, and normal jugular venous oxygen saturation is 55–75%. Thus a large cerebral blood flow (CBF) is required. CBF varies considerably in different areas of the brain (grey matter > white); the normal global value is 50 ml 100 g^{-1} min^{-1}.

The energy substrate for brain cells is predominantly glucose, but reserves are limited and become exhausted in 3 min. Thus the brain is sensitive to hypoglycaemia which can lead to temporary or permanent dysfunction.

Substances such as trypan blue can penetrate all body tissues but do not enter the CNS. This is explained by the tight intercellular junctions in cerebral capillaries: 80 nm versus 650 nm elsewhere in the body.

Short Practice of Anaesthesia. Edited by M. Morgan and G. M. Hall. Published in 1997 by Chapman & Hall, London. ISBN 0 412 71890 1

This blocks entry of polar compounds such as water-soluble drugs or ions into the CNS. Highly lipid-soluble compounds such as anaesthetics are not affected.

CEREBROSPINAL FLUID

CSF is formed in the choroid plexuses of the lateral ventricles at a rate of 600 ml per 24 h. Total volume is 150 ml. It flows to the third ventricle and via the aqueduct of Sylvius to the fourth ventricle. It enters the subarachnoid space via three foramina. CSF is reabsorbed through arachnoid villi, principally in the superior sagittal venous sinus. CSF physically supports the brain and acts as a buffer to compensate for changes in intracranial pressure (ICP).

INTRACRANIAL PRESSURE

Normal ICP is 5–10 mmHg when supine. The skull is a rigid container and ICP is determined by the volume of intracranial contents (brain tissue, blood and CSF). Small increases in intracranial volume are accommodated by displacement of CSF through the foramen magnum, increased CSF absorption and venous compression. When compensatory mechanisms are exhausted further increases in intracranial volume increase ICP (Figure 14.1). On the steep part of this graph, small increases in intracranial volume cause large increases in ICP. This is why interventions causing small changes in intracerebral volume, e.g. thiopentone, have large effects on ICP. ICP consistently greater than 20 mmHg is considered pathological.

CEREBRAL BLOOD FLOW

Both decreases and increases in CBF may damage neural tissue. Decreased CBF (cerebral ischaemia) leads progressively to impaired cerebral function, loss of consciousness, impairment of structural integrity of brain cells, permanent brain damage and death. Increased CBF may be harmful because it increases cerebral blood volume (CBV) and ICP.

CBV changes with CBF, but the relation between the two is not constant. Nevertheless, when considering the factors which alter ICP it is often assumed the two are synonymous. CBF is readily increased or decreased by physiological and pharmacological manoeuvres unlike the other contents of the skull. This may cause problems for the anaesthetist if unwanted increases in ICP or decreases in CBF are induced. Alternatively, decreasing CBF may be therapeutically useful. CBF depends on blood pressure but CBF remains constant within the range 50–150 mmHg mean arterial pressure (MAP) due to the phenomenon of autoregulation (Figure 14.2).

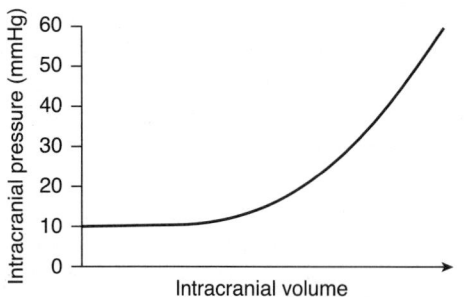

Figure 14.1 Increases in intracranial volume are compensated for initially, then intracranial pressure increases sharply.

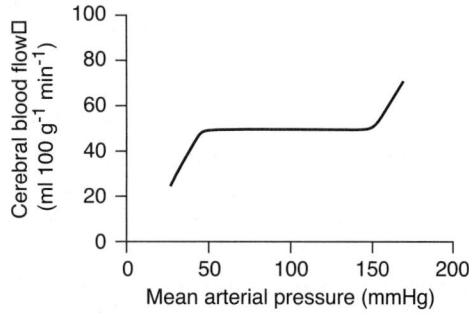

Figure 14.2 Autoregulation maintains cerebral blood flow constant while mean arterial pressure varies from 50 to 150 mmHg.

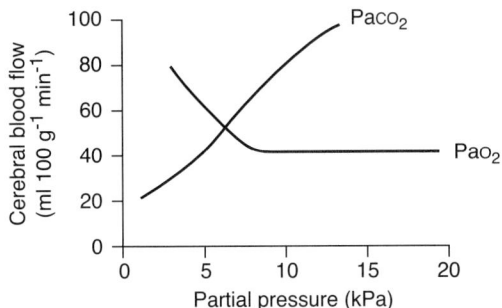

Figure 14.3 Cerebral blood flow changes linearly with $Pa{CO_2}$ within the physiological range. $Pa{O_2}$ influences cerebral blood flow only when very low.

Autoregulation is achieved: by the coupling of CBF to CMR; and by the intrinsic property of cerebrovascular smooth muscle to contract in response to increased intraluminal pressure. Factors that decrease CMR include decreased level of consciousness, decreased temperature and anaesthetic drugs. Other important influences on CBF are $Pa{CO_2}$, $Pa{O_2}$ and vasodilator drugs (Figure 14.3). These factors interact with each other, e.g. hyperventilation in a hypotensive patient can impair the usual vasodilator response to low blood pressure and cause decreased CBF and cerebral ischaemia.

Autoregulatory limits are shifted to the right by chronic hypertension. Hypotension may lead to cerebral ischaemia in hypertensive patients at blood pressures well tolerated in healthy patients. Autoregulation is impaired by acute conditions like head injury and cerebrovascular accident (stroke) and by chronic conditions like cerebrovascular disease and diabetes mellitus. Impaired autoregulation makes CBF more dependent on MAP; hypotension causes cerebral ischaemia and hypertension increases ICP. Patients with impaired autoregulation do not respond normally to the usual manoeuvres used to control ICP such as hyperventilation. There is extensive autonomic innervation of cerebral blood vessels, principally the larger vessels.

Sympathetic nervous system stimulation causes some cerebral vasoconstriction but less than that observed in other vascular beds. Cerebral vasoconstriction shifts autoregulatory limits to the right; normovolaemic hypotension is better tolerated than hypovolaemic hypotension.

PHARMACOLOGY

Anaesthetic drugs (except neuromuscular blocking drugs) are highly lipid soluble and cross the blood–brain barrier quickly. Most anaesthetic agents decrease CMR; an exception is ketamine which increases metabolic rate and CBF.

A number of anaesthetic agents can decrease CMR sufficiently to abolish cerebral electrical activity and produce a flat electroencephalogram (EEG) tracing. These include the intravenous induction agents thiopentone and propofol and potent inhaled anaesthetics such as isoflurane and desflurane.

Agents which decrease CMR tend to decrease CBF and ICP with some modifying factors. Volatile anaesthetic agents vasodilate cerebral vessels and increase CBF in a dose-related fashion. Flow-metabolism coupling is maintained but CBF is greater for a given value of CMR. The volatile agents have varying effects on CBF because of varying effects on CMR. Halothane depresses CMR less than isoflurane in equipotent concentrations so that CBF is greater with halothane. Isoflurane has a greater vasodilator effect in patients with low CMR (e.g. those with severe head injury), because its depressant effect on CMR is irrelevant. The cerebrovascular effects of sevoflurane and desflurane are broadly similar to isoflurane.

If anaesthetic agents (e.g. narcotics) decrease blood pressure, cerebral vasodilation follows as an autoregulatory response to maintain CBF. Increased ICP and decreased cerebral perfusion pressure (CPP) result. If MAP is maintained at baseline values, narcotics do not alter ICP as narcotics have no direct effect on CBF. Nitrous oxide (N_2O) increases CMR, CBF and ICP. CBF with nitrous oxide/isoflurane combined is greater than with isoflurane alone (in equipotent concentrations), i.e. nitrous oxide is a more potent vasodilator than isoflurane. The effect of nitrous oxide on CBF when used as sole agent can be prevented by the prior administration of a barbiturate or propofol, but not isoflurane.

CO_2 reactivity is retained during administration of isoflurane or nitrous oxide.

Thiopentone and propofol decrease CBF and ICP because they decrease CMR. Maximum effect from intravenous agents is achieved when an isoelectric EEG is achieved; further doses have no further effect on CMR and CBF. MAP must be maintained in order to maintain CPP. Etomidate may be a useful agent if hypotension is a problem; it decreases ICP but has less effect on MAP than the other agents.

Narcotics and benzodiazepines cause a small decrease in CMR and CBF related to a general decrease in arousal level. They have little specific effect on cellular metabolic rate or on ICP provided MAP is maintained. There is no difference between narcotics in their effect on ICP provided MAP is maintained. Non-depolarizing neuromuscular blocking drugs decrease ICP if a patient is agitated or straining. Suxamethonium has been considered to slightly increase ICP, but a recent study showed suxamethonium had no effect on ICP. Histamine released by neuromuscular blocking drugs increases CBF by cerebral vasodilation.

Vasodilator anti-hypertensive agents increase ICP. Agents like sodium nitroprusside, glyceryl trinitrate and nifedipine should be used cautiously in patients with increased ICP.

RAISED INTRACRANIAL PRESSURE

The normal ICP is 5–10 mmHg when supine, increased by coughing, Valsalva manoeuvre, head-down position, etc. Raised ICP occurs in neurosurgical patients due to increased volume of CSF (hydrocephalus), increased volume of blood (haematoma, malignant hypertension, CO_2 narcosis) or increased volume of brain tissue (brain tumour, cerebral oedema).

Clinical features of raised ICP include headaches, vomiting, papilloedema, cranial nerve signs and decreased level of consciousness. There may be characteristic changes on computed tomography (CT): decreased ventricular volume and loss of definition of the sulci on the surface of the brain.

ICP may be measured with a fluid-filled transducer system (like that used for arterial pressure monitoring) or by a fibreoptic transducer. The tip of the pressure monitoring system may lie in the extradural or subdural spaces, in the ventricles or in the brain substance.

ICP greater than 20 mmHg is considered pathological. The significance of increased ICP is two-fold: CPP decreases because of the well-known relationship CPP = MAP – ICP; and increased ICP causes cerebral distortion and herniation. Global increases in ICP lead to herniation through the foramen magnum ('coning') with brainstem ischaemia and death. Pressure can vary within the cranium. Localized increases in ICP lead to brain shifts, axonal disruption, pressure ischaemia and internal herniation.

Patients with raised ICP have decreased intracranial compliance (Figure 14.1). Small increases in intracranial blood volume cause marked increases in ICP. The principles of management are: to avoid further increases in ICP; to decrease ICP when it is dangerously elevated; and to maintain CPP.

This section discusses general principles of management for patients with increased ICP. Medical management aims to avoid increases in CBF (and by implication cerebral blood volume). Definitive treatment is also crucial, e.g. insertion of a shunt, drainage of a intracranial haematoma or treatment of malignant hypertension.

Sedation is avoided in non-ventilated patients; it depresses respiration causing hypoxia and hypercarbia and decreases the level of consciousness making assessment difficult.

Sedation is important in patients with raised ICP who are ventilated. Opiate and benzodiazepine combinations prevent coughing and straining without direct effects on MAP or CBF. Propofol is a cerebral vasoconstrictor and directly decreases ICP. Neuromuscular blocking drugs facilitate management when used intermittently, but prolong intensive care unit stay with long-term use. Mannitol is routine in the management of raised ICP. It increases plasma osmolality and draws water from areas of brain with an intact blood–brain barrier, thus decreasing ICP. It decreases CSF formation and it decreases blood viscosity; cerebral vasoconstriction follows as an autoregulatory response to maintain CBF constant. Frusemide 20 mg has a synergistic effect in prolonging the effect of mannitol. Using frusemide increases urinary loss of water and electrolytes, however.

Rapid administration of large doses of mannitol may decrease blood pressure because of smooth muscle relaxation in response to hyperosmolality. Mannitol may also cause hypernatraemia, hypokalaemia and dehydration. These problems can be minimized if mannitol is administered by infusion rather than as a bolus and by the use of smaller doses (0.25–1.0 g kg^{-1}). The dose of mannitol should be titrated against ICP and against plasma osmolality. Excessive plasma osmolality (>315 mOsm) should be avoided. Replacement of fluid losses maintains MAP, use of 0.9% sodium chloride solution or colloid, maintains plasma osmolality. Plasma osmolality is a more important determinant of brain interstitial oedema than colloid osmotic pressure. This differs from other tissues and is due to the blood–brain barrier.

Mannitol may enter brain tissue after long-term use, abolishing the osmotic gradient between brain and blood and leading to a rebound increase in ICP.

Steroids decrease cerebral oedema due to brain tumour with an onset of action of 12–24 h. Cerebral oedema after head injury does not respond and steroids do not have an established role in head injury at present; most studies show no benefit.

Hyperventilation decreases ICP by cerebral vasoconstriction. Routine use of hyperventilation in head injured patients, however, has been shown to worsen outcome. This is because: hypocapnoea decreases CBF causing cerebral ischaemia in some patients; the effect of hypocapnoea on CBF is transient because of adaptation of CSF pH to low $Paco_2$; and impaired CO_2 responsiveness is common after head injury and other CNS insults. However, hyperventilation may be useful as a short term method of controlling ICP.

Elevating the head 15–30° and maintaining the head in the midline decreases ICP by decreasing venous pressure. Tilting the patient head-down or coughing and straining increase ICP.

Occasionally barbiturate infusions may be used to control ICP. The dose of thiopentone infusion is titrated to control ICP or to achieve a flat EEG. If CMR is already low as in severe head injuries, agents which act by decreasing CMR have little effect in decreasing ICP.

Moderate hypothermia has begun to be used as a therapy to control ICP; its role is still uncertain but seems promising.

CSF drainage via an external ventricular drain may be used to decrease ICP. Excessive CSF drainage, however, can result in marked decreases in ICP leading to brain shifts and brain damage.

ANAESTHESIA IN PATIENTS WITH RAISED ICP

Voluntary hyperventilation before induction of anaesthesia helps control ICP before tracheal intubation. Thiopentone or propofol for induction of anaesthesia decrease ICP but overdosage causing hypotension decreases

CPP. A vasopressor may be used to maintain arterial pressure. Narcotics decrease requirements for other anaesthetic agents and obtund hypertensive responses. Non-depolarizing neuromuscular blocking drugs are the agents of choice unless there is a compelling reason to use suxamethonium to get rapid control of the airway.

Inhaled agents increase CBF; this is prevented by hyperventilation but it is difficult to control Pa_{CO_2} before tracheal intubation. Inhaled agents should be avoided before intubation in patients with critically raised ICP. Many anaesthetists will avoid inhaled agents until the dura is open when ICP is raised.

Intubation should take place after full muscle relaxation has been achieved. Sensory stimulation from intubation causes an increase in ICP (due to increased $CMRO_2$ and MAP) and further doses of intravenous induction agent before intubation will prevent this (e.g. thiopentone 100 mg). Alternatively a bolus of lignocaine obtunds ICP rises, with less depressant effect on MAP.

After intubation, anaesthesia is maintained by intravenous or inhalational agents, supplemented by narcotics. Propofol has theoretical advantages for neuroanaesthesia provided blood pressure is maintained, and is used widely. Isoflurane, sevoflurane and desflurane cause similar dose-related increases in CBF. Concentrations of these agents should be kept low and hyperventilation instituted if raised ICP is a possibility. The place of nitrous oxide has been controversial, but some practitioners will use it in concentrations up to 50% with hyperventilation. Narcotic supplementation decreases requirements for inhalational agents and propofol without directly affecting CBF or MAP. Muscle relaxation is maintained throughout surgery.

Insertion of head-pins increases MAP and ICP. This may be blocked by scalp infiltration with local anaesthetic, although this risks needlestick injury to the person holding the head. Alternatively thiopentone or lignocaine obtund increases in MAP and ICP. Initial dissection and wound suturing are the most painful parts of the operation and intracranial surgery is relatively pain-free. This makes depth of anaesthesia difficult to assess but sufficient anaesthetic must be given to prevent awareness.

Monitoring should include direct arterial pressure, ECG, oxygen saturation, end-tidal CO_2, temperature, nerve stimulator, urine output, blood loss, and direct observation of the brain. At the end of surgery a decision is made whether to waken the patient or to continue positive pressure ventilation This depends on the preoperative level of consciousness, events during surgery, the condition of the brain at the end of surgery, and the desirability of having the patient awake for neurological assessment.

It is important to know the effects of drugs on CBF and ICP, but these are not the only factors influencing the choice of drugs during neuroanaesthesia. If a particular agent is inicated for other reasons, undesirable effects on CBF or ICP can often be overcome by hyperventilation. A study comparing propofol, narcotic and inhalational anaesthesia showed no effect on outcome between these techniques despite varying effects on ICP. Nevertheless, there may be individual patients in whom the choice of agent alters neurological outcome.

HEAD INJURY

Head injury is the commonest cause of death after trauma. Residual brain damage in survivors leads to serious physical and neuropsychiatric disability.

Brain damage is caused by the primary insult at the time of impact and secondary insults which occur later due to the pathophysiological processes initiated by head injury. Management of head injury aims to minimize mortality and morbidity from the secondary insult.

Head injury damages brain tissue by direct trauma at the site of impact and on the oppo-

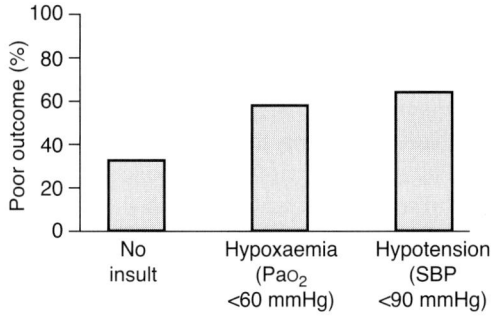

Figure 14.4 Poor outcome (death or severe disability) after head injury in patients who suffered no documented physiological insult, patients who were hypoxaemic and patients who were hypotensive. (Data from Miller *et al.* 1981)

site side of the brain ('contre-coup injury'). It also causes neuronal shearing injury by acceleration–deceleration forces. If these injuries are severe, breathing stops and the patient dies before receiving treatment.

Secondary brain damage occurs as a result of: arterial hypoxaemia; neuronal changes initiated by trauma; and cerebral ischaemia due to raised ICP or decreased MAP.

The main factors which predict poor outcome after severe head injury are: injury severity, age of the patient, hypoxaemia and hypotension (Figure 14.4). Poor outcome occurred in 30% of patients less than 20 years old versus 94% of patients aged 61–90 years in one study of severe head injury.

The injured brain is more sensitive to hypoxia and ischaemia. Documentation of hypoxaemia on admission increased poor outcome from 35% to 59% in one study (Figure 14.4). Hypoxaemia occurs commonly after head injury because of a number of factors: direct depression of the respiratory centre; airway obstruction; chest or airway trauma; and aspiration pneumonitis. Hypoxaemia is prevented by supplemental inhaled oxygen and early intubation and positive pressure ventilation.

Intubation is indicated in: severe head injury (Glasgow Coma Scale < 9), hypoxaemia (Sa_{O_2} < 95%), and before transport.

Maintenance of an adequate MAP and CPP improves outcome after head injury. MAP may be decreased due to vasomotor centre depression, blood loss or sedation. The brain is more sensitive to hypotension after head injury because: impaired autoregulation is common; CBF is usually decreased; injured neurons are more sensitive to hypoxia; and ICP may be increased. Secondary brain damage after head injury is largely caused by ischaemia. Autoregulation is often impaired after head injury and ICP increased so that a higher MAP is required. Data suggest that a CPP > 70 mmHg is required to optimize cerebral perfusion. The ideal arterial pressure varies between patients. Measurement of jugular venous oxygen saturation is a useful guide to the ideal CPP for individual patients. Arterial pressure is maintained by adequate fluid administration and, if necessary, by inotropic drugs.

Conversely many patients are hypertensive after head injury due to high levels of catecholamines. Hypertension is undesirable as it may increase CBF, increase intracerebral bleeding and worsen cerebral oedema by increased transudation of fluid. Arterial pressure may be elevated as a response to raised ICP ('Cushing reflex') and a high MAP may be necessary to prevent cerebral ischaemia in some patients.

Common practice is to treat arterial pressure consistently above 170–180 mmHg systolic. Labetolol does not directly affect ICP and is a useful agent. Vasodilators increase CBF and ICP. Arterial pressure limits are lower in children and higher in chronic hypertensive patients. Arterial pressure should be more tightly controlled in patients with rupture of the temporal lobe to prevent intracerebral haemorrhage.

Intracranial haematoma is a potentially treatable cause of secondary brain damage due to increased ICP. CT scanning is performed to exclude haematoma in patients with severe head injury and in patients who deteriorate neurologically. Intracerebral and sub-dural haematomas are associated with severe head injury; removal of the haematoma may or may not be beneficial depending on size and location. Extradural haematomas can occur without significant primary brain damage and outcome is excellent with early diagnosis and surgical drainage.

Most cases of raised ICP are due to cerebral oedema or contusion rather than haematoma. Management follows the principles described in the section on raised ICP.

The effect of hyperventilation has been discussed above. Routine use of hyperventilation in head injured patients worsens outcome. Hyperventilation should be reserved for short term control of ICP in a crisis, or with inhaled anaesthetics. Hypercapniea is associated with a worsened outcome and should be prevented; normocapniea is indicated in most patients.

Increased blood glucose worsens outcome after head injury (and after a variety of other cerebral insults). Hyperglycaemia exacerbates the intracellular acidosis that results from anaerobic metabolism after cellular hypoxia. Intracellular acidosis causes cell dysfunction and disruption and ultimately cell death. Therefore, blood glucose should be controlled after head injury, and glucose-containing fluids avoided.

In addition, glucose-containing fluids decrease plasma osmolality and increase cerebral oedema. Plasma osmolality, rather than colloid osmotic pressure, is the major factor governing movement of fluid into the brain as long as the blood–brain barrier is intact: 0.9% sodium chloride solution, or colloid solutions, are suitable fluids for maintenance and resuscitation.

Hypernatraemia is common after mannitol, and in patients who develop diabetes insipidus. Hypernatraemia can be treated with 0.45% sodium chloride solution. Rapid changes in serum sodium concentrations are dangerous because they cause rapid fluid shifts between brain and plasma. If abnormalities in serum sodium are of short duration they may be corrected relatively quickly, but if long standing they should be corrected more slowly at a rate of decrease of circulating sodium concentration of 0.5–1.0 mmol l^{-1} h^{-1}.

Intracranial pressure monitoring is used commonly in the management of severely head-injured patients. It guides treatment aimed at controlling ICP, allows monitoring of CPP and provides early warning of intracerebral haemorrhage. It is particularly important when patients are sedated and so not being assessed neurologically. The use of steroids, or barbiturates, is controversial in head injury. Most studies have shown no benefit from steroids, but interest has been reawakened by the improvement obtained with large doses of methylprednisolone in spinal cord injury. Barbiturates do not improve outcome if administered routinely to head-injured patients. However, in a small group with high ICP who were given barbiturates to achieve an isoelectric EEG, patients whose ICP was controlled had a better outcome than those who were not. There was no control group of patients and inotropes were needed to maintain MAP.

Moderate hypothermia probably improves outcome after severe head injury, but insufficent date are available as yet. Vigorous measures to prevent pyrexia are indicated after head injury.

CLINICAL MANAGEMENT OF HEAD INJURY

Many head-injured patients have other life-threatening injuries: 3% of patients with severe head injury have a fracture of their cervical spine. Chest, intra-abdominal and skeletal injuries are common.

Initial management of the head-injured patient involves provision of an adequate airway, assessment of level of consciousness (Glasgow Coma Scale, GCS), measurement of heart rate and arterial pressure, and auscultation of the chest. Patients with severe head injuries should be intubated, GCS < 9 is a common guideline, but patients with higher GCS scores may be intubated if they have other significant injuries or if they are to be transferred to the X-ray department or to another hospital.

The cervical spine is maintained in a neutral position for intubation. Intubation is facilitated by an intravenous induction agent and neuromuscular blocking drug to avoid large increases in ICP. Oral intubation is preferrable. The advantages of suxamethonium often outweigh any small increase in ICP it may cause and cricoid pressure should be used. Rapid control of the airway using suxamethonium prevents hypoxia and hypercarbia which are more damaging to patients than a small increase in ICP from suxamethonium. After intubation, the neck is immobilized in a hard collar and the patient assessed for other injuries. In a patient with a severe head injury, or who is deteriorating, mannitol is given and hyperventilation instituted pending CT scan. Mean arterial pressure and oxygen saturation should be stable before transfer to the radiology department for CT scan.

A regular dilemma is the patient with a head injury who requires prolonged anaesthesia for non-neurosurgical operations. Non-urgent surgery should be postponed to allow neurological assessment in the early stages after significant head injury. If surgery is urgent, ICP monitoring will provide early warning of intracerebral haematoma or cerebral oedema.

BRAIN TUMOUR

Primary brain tumours are benign (most commonly meningiomas, usually curable) or malignant. Malignant brain tumours do not metastasize outside the brain but are usually incurable because it is impossible to resect the entire tumour. Prognosis varies enormously depending on the histological type and rate of growth of the tumour.

Presenting symptoms include personality change, seizures, motor symptoms, headaches, vomiting and decreased level of consciousness. Most patients receive 2–3 weeks treatment with dexamethasone which provides a marked temporary improvement in symptoms. Surgery is ideally performed in this 'therapeutic window'. Patients occasionally require urgent surgery for tumour debulking or for drainage of hydrocephalus caused by tumours in the posterior fossa.

Preoperative assessment of neurological status provides a baseline for assessment after operation. Premedication is avoided in patients with impaired level of consciousness. Patients with brain tumours have decreased intracranial compliance and techniques appropriate for patients with raised ICP should be used (see above). Patients who are drowsy, or who have received mannitol, may be dehydrated. Patients are commonly taking phenytoin for seizures; dose requirements for the steroidal neuromuscular blocking drugs are increased.

The use of hyperventilation during general anaesthesia has been questioned. Hyperventilation was recently shown to cause ischaemia of brain tissue near retractors. Nevertheless, in patients with raised ICP, hyperventilation may be required to oppose the vasodilator effects of isoflurane. Short-term hyperventilation is a useful manoeuvre during episodes of acutely raised ICP. It also decreases brain bulk and improves surgical access.

Hyperventilation may be difficult in patients with respiratory disease. Ventilation with large tidal volumes, high inflation pressures and rapid respiratory rates may actually increase ICP by raising mean thoracic pressure. Choosing whether or not to hyperventilate requires an appraisal of the risks versus potential benefits. Measurement of end-tidal CO_2 as a guide to $Paco_2$ is not always reliable and arterial gas analysis should be performed to check the relationship.

Excessive pressure from brain retractors to expose the operative site may lead to ischaemic damage to areas of brain under the retractors. Measures to decrease 'retractor ischaemia' and improve surgical access to the operative site include decreasing brain bulk (mannitol, dexamethasone, head-up position, CSF drainage, propofol infusion), shorter surgery and maintaining adequate MAP.

Mannitol is commonly used to decrease brain bulk. Doses can be larger than those used for control of ICP: 0.5–1.0 g kg^{-1}.

Access to patients during neurosurgical procedures may be difficult and the endotracheal tube should be carefully secured and adequate intravenous access obtained before surgery starts. A urinary catheter is necessary before mannitol is administered. Direct measurement of arterial pressure allows rapid detection of changes in MAP and sampling of arterial blood. If central venous access is required it is commonly achieved via the antecubital fossa. This route does not need head-down tilt (increasing ICP) for insertion and avoids risks of obstruction to cerebral venous drainage.

Patients are extubated after operation unless the preoperative level of consciousness was impaired, or intraoperative complications have occurred. Emergence from anaesthesia and extubation should be as smooth as possible, avoiding coughing and straining on the tube. Smooth emergence decreases the risk of increased ICP and intracerebral haemorrhage. Early recovery facilitates neurological assessment. Pain is usually moderate, and NSAIDs and dihydrocodeine provide adequate analgesia.

STEREOTACTIC SURGERY

Stereotactic techniques are used for a variety of procedures, most commonly to biopsy a cerebral lesion without formal craniotomy. A special headframe is applied and CT scan performed to provide coordinates for the cerebral lesion relative to indicators on the

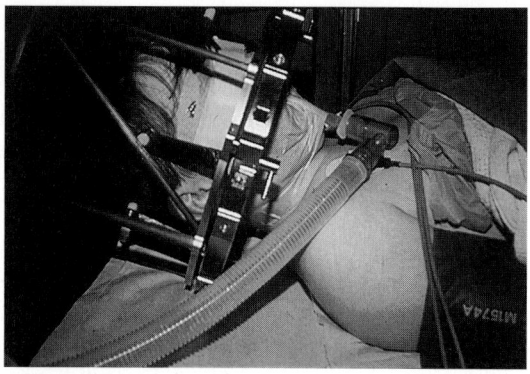

Figure 14.5 The metal headframe for stereotactic surgery makes direct laryngoscopy impossible.

headframe. The biopsy is taken via a small burrhole from the lesion as identified by the coordinates. The headframe is then removed.

Stereotactic biopsy may be performed under local or general anaesthesia. General anaesthesia presents problems because airway manipulation and laryngoscopy are impossible when the rigid headframe is in position (Figure 14.5). There is a choice between intubation before application of the headframe, or awake fibreoptic intubation after application of the headframe. Some centres insert a laryngeal mask with the headframe in place; there must be the ability to remove the headframe very quickly if airway difficulties arise.

POSTERIOR FOSSA/BRAIN STEM SURGERY

Most tumours in children and about 10% of tumours in adults arise in the posterior fossa below the tentorium cerebelli. Surgery in this area presents some specific problems for the anaesthetist.

Posterior fossa tumours often obstruct the flow of CSF causing hydrocephalus. Hydrocephalus may require drainage before definitive tumour surgery.

Surgical access to the posterior fossa requires positioning the patient prone or in the sitting position. The sitting position provides excellent operating conditions with good access to the posterior fossa and a slack brain. The sitting positioning carries a significant risk of air embolism and may make it difficult to maintain MAP. For these reasons the prone position is more commonly used.

The prone position has hazards also. The eyes and pressure points (face, chest, iliac crests, groins, knees, feet) must be protected and abdominal compression avoided. When the head is flexed there should be at least one fingerbreadth's distance between chin and sternum. Neck flexion during positioning may move the tip of the tracheal tube past the carina causing endobronchial intubation; tube position must be rechecked after positioning. Overflexion of the neck may lead to airway oedema due to venous obstruction. An armoured endotracheal tube is used and the tube securely fixed: displacement of the endotracheal tube intraoperatively could be fatal. This is more likely with an uncuffed tube in children. Circuit disconnection is also a risk.

The vasomotor centre and respiratory centre lie close to each other in the brain stem. Surgery in the posterior fossa may damage these structures. Intraoperatively this may be shown by unexplained changes in heart rate, arterial pressure or respiratory rate (if breathing spontaneously).

If these occur the surgeon should be informed immediately as this may be the only warning of damage to vital structures.

Most anaesthetists use positive pressure ventilation during posterior fossa surgery, relying on cardiovascular changes to warn of brain stem ischaemia. Occasionally spontaneous ventilation is used especially for surgery near the floor of the fourth ventricle where the respiratory centre is located. Spontaneous ventilation has the disadvantage of causing hypercapnoea. After posterior fossa surgery patients should be observed carefully for impairment of ventilatory control, or of the gag reflex.

AIR EMBOLISM

The sitting position makes the pressure negative in veins above the level of the heart and air may be entrained. Air embolism may occur via scalp veins, bony sinusoids, dural venous sinuses or from remote sources like venous catheters. Air embolism has been reported in 25–50% of all craniotomies performed in the sitting position. The volume of air entrained is often small and causes little upset, but larger volumes of air entering the circulation cause life-threatening hypotension and hypoxia. The effects of air embolism depend on the volume of air, the rate at which it enters the circulation and the general condition of the patient. Experiments in dogs suggest that volumes greater than 20 ml are potentially fatal.

A patent foramen ovale (or any other condition causing communication between the right and left sides of the heart) could allow a 'paradoxical embolus', an air embolus entering the systemic circulation. Air emboli in the cerebral circulation can cause neurological deficits.

There is controversy about screening patients for the presence of patent foramen ovale to prevent paradoxical air embolism. Some centres send all their patients undergoing surgery in the sitting position for echocardiography. If a patent foramen ovale exists, the prone position is used. Other centres point out that paradoxical air embolism can occur in patients without patent foramen ovale and that not all patients with patent foramen ovale get air embolism. These centres do not perform echocardiography before sitting-craniotomy.

Air collects in the heart and pulmonary artery causing obstruction to blood flow from the right side of the heart, hypotension and hypoxaemia. Pressures in the right side of the heart increase causing flow from the right to left atrium if the foramen ovale is patent. Management involves: prevention of further inflow of air; removal of air in the circulation; and supportive measures.

The surgical site is covered with wet packs and bone wax is applied to exposed skull vessels. The patient is ventilated with 100% O_2. Venous pressure is increased by placing the patient head-down or by jugular compression. Air is removed via a central venous catheter placed at induction. A multi-orifice catheter is the most efficient at removing air. If a single orifice catheter is used the ideal placement for the catheter tip is at the junction of the superior vena cava and the right atrium. Fluids, vasopressors and 100% oxygen are used to maintain the patients' general condition.

The left lateral, head-down position is said to move the air embolus from the pulmonary artery into the right ventricle and to improve pulmonary blood flow.

Adequate fluid administration and compression of the abdomen and extremities to reduce venous pooling (anti-gravity venous compression device, 'G suit') help maintain high venous pressures. This prevents air embolism and arterial hypotension. Nitrous oxide increases the size of air bubbles by diffusing into them and is usually avoided during surgery in the sitting position. Nevertheless one study showed that use of 50% nitrous oxide made no difference to clinical outcome with minor episodes of air embolism.

Early diagnosis of air embolism allows prompt institution of preventive measures, before the situation becomes critical. A number of monitors are useful in the diagnosis of air embolism. A precordial Doppler probe provides an audible monitor of normal smooth flow through the heart; as little as 1 ml of air is heard as a harsh grating sound.

End-tidal carbon dioxide tension is a relatively sensitive monitor of air embolism. A sharp decrease in end-tidal CO_2 tension, when ventilation has been unchanged, raises the possibility of air embolism. Pulmonary artery pressures increase during venous air embolism. Monitoring of end-tidal nitrogen by mass spectrometer allows detection of air entering the circulation.

Hypoxaemia, hypotension and the development of a precordial 'millwheel murmur' are relatively late changes. Adult respiratory distress syndrome (ARDS) may follow air embolism.

Air embolism can occur when the patient is horizontal, particularly in patients with low venous pressures like children. Air embolism has been reported during a wide range of operations including lumbar discectomy, varicose vein ligation and surgical procedures in the head and neck. A pneumocephalus is air trapped inside the skull during dural closure. This can increase ICP postoperatively. Diffusion of nitrous oxide into an air pocket may increase ICP also.

PAEDIATRIC SURGERY

Management of children undergoing neurosurgery follows the usual principles of paediatric anaesthesia. Poor access to the patient is a major concern especially as many patients are prone during surgery. Adequate monitoring and venous access are vital as blood loss may be large.

Hypothermia may be a problem in babies but is not usually a problem after one year of age; no body cavities are open and the body is covered by drapes. Body temperature may increase during surgery. This is prevented by exposing the child and decreasing environmental temperature. Intravenous glucose solutions should be avoided when there is a risk of cerebral ischaemia, but this must be balanced against the possibility of hypoglycaemia in smaller children.

PITUITARY SURGERY

Pituitary tumours present with endocrine disorders or with symptoms due to local compression, classically bi-temporal hemianopia.

Cushing's disease, acromegaly, diabetes insipidus and hypoadrenalism all have implications for anaesthetic management.

Transphenoidal resection under fluoroscopic control is the most common technique for pituitary resection. Surgery is performed in a head-up position. A throat pack prevents blood entering the hypopharynx. High doses of adrenaline solutions are injected into the submucosa for haemostasis which may cause hypertension and arrhythmias.

Measures to decrease brain bulk tend to retract the pituitary away from the surgeon and are not indicated unless ICP is increased. Postoperative replacement of glucocorticoids and sometimes ADH (antidiuretic hormone) are required.

CEREBRAL ANEURYSM

Defects in the muscularis layer of cerebral arteries develop into aneurysms. Aneurysmal rupture with subarachnoid haemorrhage (SAH) has catastrophic results; 50% die within 3 months and 25% have residual disability. Diagnosis is made on a history of headache and collapse, occurrence of neurological deficits, by CT scan and by angiography. Lumbar puncture is contraindicated if ICP is raised. Occasionally patients are diagnosed before rupture because of pressure symptoms or after screening of high-risk subjects.

SAH increases ICP causing headache and loss of consciousness. Smaller haemorrhages are followed by neurological recovery. Severity is graded 0–5, grade 5 implying deep coma.

Patients who survive subarachnoid haemorrhage are at risk of rebleeding (33% in 1 month) and of cerebral ischaemia from vasospasm. Vasospasm in cerebral vessels is thought to be due to release of vasoactive substances from red cells. Vasospasm is maximal 5–10 days after the initial bleed and has an incidence of 70% after SAH, half of whom are symptomatic. Early (<3 days) clipping of the aneurysm prevents rebleeding, decreases the incidence of vasospasm and allows aggressive management of vasospasm by induced hypertension.

Dehydration and electrolyte abnormalities (especially hyponatraemia) are common after SAH and can be prevented by infusion of 0.9% sodium chloride solution. Catecholamine values are increased after SAH, leading to hypertension, ECG abnormalities, cardiac dysfunction and neurogenic pulmonary oedema. Arterial pressure management before clipping of the aneurysm aims for normotension (120–150 mmHg systolic).

Nimodipine, a calcium antagonist, improves outcome after SAH. Initially used to treat vasospasm, it also acts as a cerebral protectant. No significant interaction with anaesthetic agents has been noted.

ANAESTHESIA

Induction of anaesthesia should avoid hypertension (which may rupture the aneurysm), hypotension (which may worsen cerebral ischaemia) and coughing and straining which increase ICP and MAP. Direct measurement of arterial pressure is indicated. An adequate depth of anaesthesia supplemented by narcotics provides cardiovascular stability at intubation. Volatile agents allow good control of the depth of anaesthesia, provided ICP is not raised. A dose of intravenous induction agent, β-blocking drug or lignocaine help control MAP and ICP at intubation.

In patients with recent bleeding, rapid changes in ICP could induce further bleeding by disrupting the clot. Mannitol to decrease brain bulk is given slowly (over 30 min), or is witheld until the dura is open. Hyperventilation decreases brain bulk, but causes vasoconstriction which is undesirable with vasospasm.

Maintaining a high CPP (>70 mmHg) during surgery prevents decreases in jugular venous oxygen saturation. Rupture of the aneurysm during dissection may be catastrophic; adequate intravenous access and rapid availability of blood are essential. Unfortunately control of haemorrhage from a ruptured aneurysm may require occlusion of a major cerebral vessel with the risk of cerebral ischaemia.

Temporary clips are commonly used to occlude vessels supplying the aneurysm. This may cause ischaemia in brain tissue supplied by the vessel; the temporary clip is applied for as short a time as possible. Maintaining a high blood pressure during this period maximizes collateral flow. Some centres administer a cerebral protectant, although no benefit has been shown from any agent to date. Induced hypotension is occasionally requested to decrease tension in the aneurysm, or to facilitate control of bleeding. Hypotension should be safe if MAP is maintained >50–60 mmHg except in sicker patients who commonly have impairment of autoregulatory mechanisms.

Mild hypothermia is increasingly used as a cerebral protectant during aneurysm surgery. It is discussed below in the section on cerebral protection. Increased temperature should be prevented when there is a risk of cerebral ischaemia.

Early wakening is desirable to allow neurological assessment and detection of intracerebral haematoma or vasospasm. If there have been intraoperative surgical problems, or if the brain is swollen, it may be necessary to continue sedation and ventilation postoperatively.

Vasospasm is a major concern postoperatively which can lead to transient, or permanent, neurological deficits and death. Vasospasm presents with confusion, decreased level of consciousness or focal neurological deficit. Prevention is by nimodipine and early surgery. Management aims to maintain perfusion of ischaemic areas. Hypervolaemia, haemodilution and hypertension are the mainstays of treatment. Volume loading (with monitoring of central venous or pulmonary artery pressures) and vasopressors are titrated to maintain a MAP that reverses neurological deficits, if possible. Excessive hypertension (>180 mmHg systolic) could, however, increase ICP and cerebral oedema especially in patients with impairment of autoregulation. The optimal haematocrit is 30%. Despite these measures vasospasm causes significant morbidity and mortality.

Arteriovenous malformations (AVM) present similar problems for the anaesthetist. Small AVMs may be resected surgically. Resection of large AVMs can cause torrential haemorrhage during surgery. Adjoining brain tissue can swell markedly after operation due to excess perfusion of adjoining tissue and local oedema ('normal perfusion pressure breakthrough'). Current practice is to embolize large AVMs under radiological control to decrease their size before surgery. This has led to a reduction in these complications

HYDROCEPHALUS

Hydrocephalus occurs due to congenital abnormality (Arnold–Chiari malformation) or due to intracranial pathology (haemorrhage, infection, tumour). Blockage of CSF flow increases ICP. Treatment is by drainage of CSF externally (external ventricular drain) or into the peritoneum (ventriculo–peritoneal shunt). Occasionally, drainage may be into the jugular vein or even the right atrium. The principles of anaesthetic management are the same as for any patient with raised ICP.

EPILEPSY SURGERY

Surgical excision of an epileptogenic focus is useful in patients with epilepsy resistant to conventional drug therapy. Electrophysiological mapping of brain structures may be required to allow excision of the epileptogenic focus while avoiding damage to essential structures. In some cases mapping must be carried out with the patient awake. These requirements pose a challenge for the anaesthetist.

General anaesthetic agents (volatile agents and intravenous induction agents) suppress cerebral electrical activity and are anticonvulsant. The anaesthetic technique should be based on narcotics and neuromuscular blocking drugs with nitrous oxide. Low concentrations of volatile agents, or low infusion rates of propofol, can be used to supplement these, but must be discontinued 15 min before electrophysiological mapping to avoid suppression of electrical activity.

Awake craniotomy is performed with local anaesthetic blocks to the nerves supplying the scalp, local infiltration and infusions of sedative agents. Sedation is required because of pain, and because these procedures are prolonged and uncomfortable. Sedation can be with a combination of narcotic and neuroleptic agent (droperidol), or with propofol. Both these techniques may cause airway obstruction and respiratory depression. Narcotics cause minimal interference with cerebral electrical activity, but are somewhat unpredictable as sedative agents. Propofol is easily titratable, but must be discontinued at least 15 min before recording of the EEG because of its anticonvulsant effect. Propofol is also capable of stimulating epileptiform activity on EEG.

NEURORADIOLOGY

An increasing number of anaesthetics are required in the X-ray department for diagnosis, or treatment, of neurosurgical conditions.

CT scan and cerebral angiography in small children and mentally handicapped patients require general anaesthesia. Anaesthesia for magnetic resonance imaging (MRI) poses specific problems. There is an increased requirement for general anaesthesia for MRI compared to CT scan because of the confined space, loud noise and longer duration of MRI. Ferrous equipment cannot come close to the MRI scanner and specialized equipment is needed for ventilation and monitoring. There

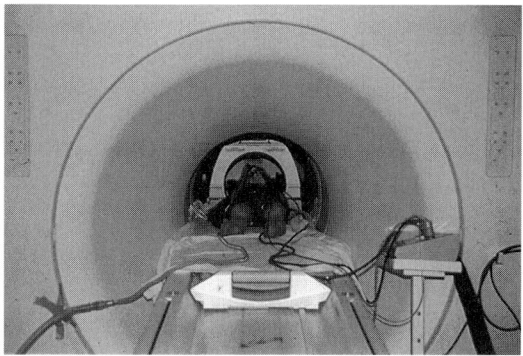

Figure 14.6 Access to patients in the MRI scanner is poor.

is no access to the airway while the patient is being scanned (Figure 14.6).

A number of different approaches to these problems have been described. Sedation with chloral hydrate, or with barbiturates, has been used, but our experience has been that sedation is time consuming, unreliable, may compromise the airway and causes delayed recovery. Propofol infusion has been used with and without the use of a laryngeal mask to maintain the airway. Our practice is to induce anaesthesia with propofol, insert a laryngeal mask airway and maintain anaesthesia with isoflurane. Patients with raised ICP receive an intravenous induction and positive pressure ventilation.

Extensions are used on breathing circuits and ventilator tubing. MRI-compatible monitors are available to record ECG, blood pressure and oxygen saturation. Sidestream end-tidal CO_2 analysers are used. All metal objects must be removed from the patient and from staff before entering the MRI suite to avoid injury from projectiles. Metal interferes with the quality of the images obtained – a reinforced tracheal tube degraded the quality of the images in one of our patients.

Interventional neuroradiology is an expanding area. Current indications are for embolization of AVMs and of cerebral aneurysms. These procedures can be performed under local anaesthesia allowing continuous assessment of neurological status. Vascular complications can occur, either hamorrhage or vessel occlusion. An anaesthetist must be available in case of deterioration in neurological status requiring intubation. Manipulation of ventilation and blood pressure can be useful therapeutically.

Many radiologists find that general anaesthesia provides better conditions. Light levels of anaesthesia are required with maintenance of the airway by a laryngeal mask airway or tracheal tube.

CEREBRAL ISCHAEMIA

Cerebral energy requirements are high but storage capacity for energy is limited. Neuronal function and viability requires oxygen and glucose; decreased supply has immediate effects.

Decreasing global cerebral blood flow (CBF) has graded effects on the brain (Table 14.1). Complete global ischaemia (i.e. cardiac arrest) causes a flat EEG within 30 s and cellular energy depletion within 2 min. Irreversible, ischaemic damage will occur unless blood flow is restored rapidly. Neurons are the most sensitive cells to ischaemia and the most sensitive areas are the cerebral cortex, the basal ganglia, the thalamus and hippocampus.

Severe ischaemia leads to rapid neuronal necrosis, but if ischaemia is incomplete neuronal necrosis may be delayed for hours or even days. Mechanisms initiated by ischaemia cause delayed neuronal necrosis despite restoration of perfusion. This delay provides an opportunity for therapeutic intervention to block the mechanisms causing neuronal necrosis.

Certain areas of the brain are more vulnerable to the effects of ischaemia than others: the concept of 'selective vulnerability'. These areas contain the highest concentrations of the excitatory neurotransmitter, glutamate. Glutamate concentrations increase during ischaemia and act on a number of receptors to promote calcium entry into the cell with lethal effects. The best known receptor is the *N*-methyl-D-aspartate (NMDA) receptor.

There is normally a calcium gradient of 10 000:1 between the exterior and interior of the cell. Calcium is essential for normal neuronal function, but Ca^{2+} enters the cell in inappropriate amounts during ischaemia. Entry of calcium into the cell occurs owing to excitatory neurotransmitters and the failure of normal energy-requiring homeostatic mechanisms. Intracellular calcium activates proteases and lipases which lyse cell structures and produce free radicals and fatty acids including arachidonic acid. Arachidonic acid leads to the production of prostaglandins and leukotrienes which mediate inflammatory responses in the brain.

Lactate formation due to anaerobic metabolism causes intracellular acidosis and impairs cellular homeostatic mechanisms. The amount of lactate formed during ischaemia is proportional to the blood glucose, which explains why outcome after ischaemic insult is worsened by an elevated blood glucose.

Focal ischaemia (e.g. temporary arterial clip) and incomplete global ischaemia (e.g. hypotension) differ from complete global ischaemia (e.g. cardiac arrest). Focal ischaemia causes localized dysfunction and neur-

Table 14.1 Effects of decreasing cerebral blood flow (CBF) on the brain

CBF	Effects
50 ml 100 g^{-1} min^{-1}	Normal cerebral function
22 ml 100 g^{-1} min^{-1}	EEG slowing, neurological dysfunction but cells viable
12 ml 100 g^{-1} min^{-1}	EEG flat, delayed cell death
<6ml 100 g^{-1} min^{-1}	EEG flat, rapid cell death

onal damage. However, focal ischaemia or incomplete global ischaemia cause considerably less permanent neurological damage than complete global ischaemia. In addition, cerebral protection is more effective in focal ischaemia than in global ischaemia. This finding is consistent with the graded effects of decreasing CBF shown above. Cerebral dysfunction occurs with low CBF, but permanent neuronal damage is prevented or delayed.

During focal ischaemia the central area supplied by the occluded vessel receives no perfusion and is likely to undergo infarction. However, there is a much larger surrounding area which receives a low blood flow via collateral vessels. This area of brain which is ischaemic, but still viable, is called the 'ischaemic penumbra'. The aim of therapy during periods of regional ischaemia is to maximize perfusion in this ischaemic area and to minimize the size of the central area receiving no perfusion. Maintenance of an adequate perfusion pressure is the most effective way of doing this. During incomplete global ischaemia the areas at risk of ischaemia are the 'boundary zones', the areas furthest from a major vessel.

Mechanisms of cerebral damage after ischaemia are complex and not fully understood. The description given above is a very much simplified version.

CEREBRAL PROTECTION

Cerebral ischaemia has devastating effects and a huge amount of research has been directed to prevent this. A wide range of therapeutic approaches has been used.

$CMRO_2$ reduction

Agents which decrease cerebral oxygen requirements should delay ischaemic damage. Barbiturates decrease CMR and have been shown to improve outcome after focal ischaemia. However, other agents (propofol, isoflurane) which decrease CMR are less effective than barbiturates, suggesting that additional mechanisms contribute to the beneficial effects of barbiturates. Isoflurane and propofol have been shown to have a cerebral protectant effect in specially designed studies, but it is not of a magnitude to be significant clinically.

Anaesthesia using any of the common agents protects against ischaemia compared to the awake state. This is related to a decreased level of arousal and a decreased autonomic response to ischaemia.

The unique effect of barbiturates as cerebral protectants is related to their action as sodium channel blockers, in addition to their effect in decreasing CMR. Maximum benefit from barbiturates is achieved with large doses (40 mg kg^{-1} thiopentone), which cause a decreased MAP and prolonged recovery. This has limited the usefulness of barbiturates in clinical practice.

Hypothermia

Hypothermia is presently the most effective method of cerebral protection. Hypothermia decreases CMR by lowering electrical activity and the energy requirements for maintenance of cell integrity. Deep hypothermia (18°C) has been used for periods of total circulatory arrest of up to 60 min. This severity of hypothermia causes complications and is impractical for regular use.

Moderate hypothermia (3°C below normal) improves neurological outcome after a wide variety of cerebral ischaemic insults. Hypothermia is beneficial in both global and focal ischaemia, even when induced after the ischaemic insult. These data come from animal studies. The only human studies to date showing benefit from hypothermia have been after head injury. Hypothermia has undesirable effects notably increasing myocardial ischaemia. Nevertheless, data from animal studies are so convincing that moderate hypothermia is widely used while the results of clinical studies are awaited.

Moderate hypothermia has a greater protective effect than is explained by its effect in decreasing CMR. Moderate hypothermia decreasing CMR by 15% has a markedly greater protective effect than deep isoflurane anaesthesia decreasing CMR by 50% at normothermia. Therefore, the effect of moderate hypothermia in improving outcome depends little on its depressant effect on CMR.

The mechanism of protection by hypothermia is probably multifactorial. Moderate hypothermia markedly decreases concentrations of the excitatory neurotransmitter, glutamate, after ischaemia. Inhibition of glutamate release is probably the most important mechanism responsible for benefit from moderate hypothermia.

The converse of benefit from hypothermia is that pyrexia worsens outcome after cerebral ischaemia. Pyrexia should be prevented and treated in patients at risk.

NORMOGLYCAEMIA

Increased blood glucose concentrations worsen outcome after global ischaemia and possibly after focal ischaemia. Even a glucose infusion, which does not increase blood glucose, worsens outcome after ischaemia. Glucose administration should be avoided in patients at risk. While no benefit in outcome has been shown from control of blood sugar by insulin, most authorities advocate maintenance of normoglycaemia. The threshold for damage from hyperglycaemia is not clearly defined; it may be 10 mmol l^{-1}, or it may be a graded effect from normal concentrations of blood glucose upwards.

PERFUSION PRESSURE

Maintenance of adequate CPP and CBF improves outcome after focal ischaemia. A small increase in regional CBF in the ischaemic penumbra may permit cell survival. The volume of the ischaemic penumbra may be large and survival of these cells greatly improves functional recovery. Hypertension, however, risks worsening cerebral oedema or causing haemorrhage.

HAEMODILUTION

Infarct volume after focal ischaemia is least when the haematocrit is 30%.

NORMOVENTILATION

Hypercapnia worsens systemic acidosis, may increase ICP or may cause a 'steal' phenomenon, diverting blood away from ischaemic areas. Hypocapnia decreases CBF. The 'inverse steal' mechanism proposed to divert blood to ischaemic areas has not been supported by experimental evidence. Normocapnia is recommended for patients with cerebral ischaemia.

ANTI-EXCITATORY AGENTS

A large number of agents which may interfere with the cascade of events following cerebral ischaemia have been investigated. A number with clinical potential will be discussed.

Calcium is intimately involved in the sequence of events causing permanent neuronal damage after cerebral ischaemia. Calcium antagonists improve outcome after SAH. Benefit has also been shown for nimodipine in subgroups of patients after head injury. However, SAH is the only widely accepted indication for calcium antagonists as cerebral protectants at present.

NMDA antagonists improve outcome after focal ischaemia, even when given after the ischaemic insult. They block the action of glutamate at the NMDA receptor, preventing excess calcium entry. NMDA antagonists also help prevent spontaneous depolarization of the neuron, decreasing energy requirements for repolarization. Other agents which block the effect of glutamate at different receptors are being investigated. No agent has yet been approved for clinical use.

FREE RADICAL SCAVENGERS

Methylprednisolone improves outcome if given in large doses within 8 h of spinal cord injury. Its mode of action is thought to be partly its effect as a free radical scavenger. Available evidence does not support the use of steroids after cerebral ischaemia. Tirilizad has been shown to be beneficial after subarachnoid haemorrhage but produced no benefit after cerebrovascular accident and worsened outcome after head injury. Superoxide dismutase has been shown to improve outcome after head injury. The role of these agents as cerebral protectants is still unclear and further clinical trials are required before they become widely used.

GLOBAL ISCHAEMIA

Complete global ischaemia is most commonly seen after cardiac arrest. Many studies have investigated methods of improving neurological outcome after cardiac arrest, but to date the only intervention of proven benefit has been the use of adrenaline during the period of cardiopulmonary resuscitation (adrenaline maintains CBF). Trials of the use of barbiturates have shown no benefit. Results with calcium antagonists have been inconsistent and do not justify use of these agents at present.

Maintenance of normal arterial pressure, oxygenation and CO_2 tension are the mainstays of management after global ischaemia. Cerebral oedema after global ischaemia indicates severe brain damage and ICP monitoring or mannitol are not usually indicated.

CNS MONITORING

The most sensitive monitor of CNS status is the awake patient. Global and regional ischaemia are readily detected when surgery is performed under local anaesthesia. Rapid return of consciousness after general anaesthesia allows early assessment and monitoring of level of consciousness. The Glasgow Coma Scale (Table 14.2) formalizes assessment of the level of consciousness. It is useful because it provides a shorthand index of level of consciousness and because it is an objective assessment, eliminating inter-observer variability.

Table 14.2 Glasgow Coma Scale

Observation		Score
Eyes open	Spontaneously	4
	To speech	3
	To pain	2
	None	1
Best motor response	Obeys commands	6
	Purposeful movement	5
	Localizes pain	4
	Flexion to pain	3
	Extension to pain	2
	None	1
Best verbal response	Oriented	5
	Confused	4
	Inappropriate words	3
	Incomprehensible sounds	2
	None	1

ICP measurement technique is described above. Measurement of ICP allows early detection of haematoma, optimization of CPP and rational management of raised ICP.

Jugular bulb venous oxygen saturation gives a measure of oxygen extraction from blood by the brain. The normal range is 55–75%. Decreases below 55% indicate cerebral ischaemia. Increases above 75% indicate hyperaemia. Changes in jugular venous bulb saturation must be interpreted in the light of changes in Pa_{O_2}, Pa_{CO_2}, MAP, temperature, drugs and ICP. Its most useful role is to guide therapy in patients with raised ICP.

Near-infrared spectroscopy monitors oxyhaemoglobin, deoxyhaemoglobin and cytochrome aa_3 in brain tissue using wavelengths which pass through the skull. It offers continuous, non-invasive measurement of brain oxygenation and has the potential to measure cerebral blood flow. Its most useful clinical application at present is during carotid endarterectomy or during induced hypotension.

Transcranial Doppler ultrasonography is a non-invasive method of measuring changes in CBF (e.g. during carotid endarterectomy) and of diagnosing vasospasm.

The electroencephalograph (EEG) monitors cerebral electrical activity. It diagnoses seizures or ischaemia (decreased high frequency activity progressing to absent electrical activity). The EEG in the operating theatre is usually monitored in two channels, electronically processed and displayed as the compressed spectral array. This facilitates interpretation of the EEG. EEG can detect cerebral ischaemia (e.g. carotid endarterectomy) and is a guide to depth of anaesthesia.

Somatosensory evoked potentials are elicited by stimulation of a nerve at a peripheral site (tibial nerve or median nerve) and the cortical response is monitored via scalp electrodes. The signal is small and must be averaged to distinguish it from background cerebral electrical activity. It provides a measure of cerebral function which is sensitive to cerebral ischaemia. It also monitors the integrity of sensory pathways in the spinal cord and brain stem and will detect ischaemia at these sites.

Motor evoked potentials (stimulation over the cranium) are more sensitive to ischaemia in the anterior part of the cord than somatosensory potentials.

NEUROSURGICAL INTENSIVE CARE

The management principles outlined above also apply in intensive care. Many head-injured patients never need neurosurgical intervention but outcome is improved enormously by appropriate management in the intensive care unit (ICU). Priorities in management in ICU are:

- maintaining CPP >70 mmHg and normal Pa_{CO_2} to maintain CBF;
- control of ICP (sedation, mannitol, head-up positioning, evacuation of intracerebral haematoma etc.);
- maintenance of normal Pa_{O_2};
- prevention of pyrexia;
- prevention of cerebral oedema (e.g. maintain plasma osmolality, treat hypertension);
- nutrition (enteral if possible), prophylaxis against stress ulceration;
- prevent and treat respiratory tract infection;
- early detection of intracranial pathology by monitoring of neurological status (Glasgow Coma Scale) and ICP.

FLUID MANAGEMENT

Fluid administration aims to maintain normal blood volume or, in certain patients (e.g. patients with vasospasm or low CPP) to expand circulating volume without causing pulmonary oedema. Fluids are chosen to avoid hyperglycaemia and maintain normal plasma [Na+]. Colloids are useful when plasma volume expansion is required.

Diabetes insipidus is common after head injury. It is diagnosed by large urinary output with low urine osmolality (<300 mOsm) in the presence of an abnormally high plasma osmolality. Diabetes insipidus is strongly suggested in patients with a high urinary output (>150 ml h^{-1}) and elevated plasma [Na+]: diuresis due to mannitol, or glucose, or rapid fluid infusion should be excluded. Management is by desmopressin 1 μg as required.

Sedation is an important part of ICP management. It also decreases anxiety and is essential in conscious patients requiring ventilation. The commonest agents are morphine/midazolam combinations and propofol. Propofol directly decreases ICP, is easily titratable and allows rapid recovery. However, it decreases MAP, cannot be used in small children and is expensive. Other agents which may be useful for sedation include haloperidol, dihydrocodeine and clonidine.

Neuromuscular blocking drugs are always used for endotracheal intubation and are indicated intermittently to facilitate sedation. They prevent movement and straining, but do not control MAP or ICP. They may mask seizures and permit awareness. Routine use of these drugs prolongs ICU stay in patients with head injury.

Seizures are common in neurosurgical patients and must be immediately treated and prevented. Seizures may impair oxygenation, increase CMR, and increase ICP. Thiopentone and benzodiazepines stop seizures, and phenytoin is the standard drug for prophylaxis.

Neurogenic pulmonary oedema may occur after a major intracerebral catastrophe such as severe head injury or SAH. It is characterized by pink, frothy, pulmonary secretions, hypoxia and diffuse pulmonary infiltrates. It is thought to be due to a surge in catecholamine output after stress. Management is supportive; pulmonary ventilation with positive end-expiratory pressure, high F_{IO_2} and removal of pulmonary oedema fluid in the airways by suction. The condition is usually relatively short-lived and resolves in 12–24 h.

TRANSFER

Transfer of neurosurgical patients to specialist units is often required. Inadequate care during transfer has a deleterious effect on outcome. Transfer of neurosurgical patients should only take place when adequate oxygenation can be guaranteed. Patients should usually be intubated and ventilated during transfer; even if oxygenation is adequate before transfer, deterioration may occur later. Cardiovascular stability must also be guaranteed; patients with unstable arterial pressure should only be transferred if they require specialized surgical intervention to stop bleeding. Patients must be accompanied by a person able to manage the airway and ventilation, usually an anaesthetist.

BRAIN DEATH (Chapter 45)

Patients without brain function may be kept alive indefinitely by pulmonary ventilation, i.v. fluids and inotropic drugs. Formal tests of brain stem function establish the diagnosis of brain death and allow discontinuation of therapy.

Reversible factors which could depress the level of consciousness must be excluded. These factors include drugs, metabolic or electrolyte abnormalities, hypotension, hypoxia and hypothermia. The cause of coma must be known. Tests of brain stem function may then be performed. These include:

- testing for motor response to painful stimulus in the cranial nerve distribution,
- pupillary responses,
- corneal reflex,
- caloric responses,
- dolls eye movements,
- cough and gag reflexes,
- ventilatory response to hypercapnia.

A positive response to any of these tests indicates that brain stem function is still present and the patient does not fulfil the criteria for brain stem death.

Regulations regarding the time of performing brain stem tests, and personnel who may perform tests, vary between different countries. Performance of an EEG to confirm absence of cerebral electrical activity is obligatory in the USA but not in the UK. Motor response to stimuli in the limbs may occur in brain dead patients due to spinal reflexes. This may cause confusion among family and staff, but does not indicate brain function and is compatible with a diagnosis of brain death.

When consent is given for the brain-dead patient to become an organ donor, optimization of the physiological condition of the donor improves outcome in organ recipients. Fluid administration, inotropic drugs and desmopressin may be required.

CONCLUSIONS

Many of the factors leading to neuronal damage have been identified but no 'magic bullet' has been found to prevent this damage. While advantages can be shown for different drugs, the choice of drugs is less important than the way they are used. The most important factors in achieving a successful outcome in neurosurgical anaesthesia are maintenance of oxygenation and arterial pressure, and an adequate depth of anaesthesia and working with a good surgeon.

FURTHER READING

Cucchiara, R. F. and Michenfelder, J. D. (eds) (1990) *Clinical Neuroanesthesia*. Churchill Livingstone, New York.

Drummond, J. C. and Shapiro, H. M. (1994) Cerebral physiology, in *Anesthesia* (ed. R. D. Miller) Churchill Livingstone, New York, pp. 689–730.

Miller, J. D., Butterworth, J. F., Gudeman, S. K. *et al.* (1981) Further experience in the management of head injury. *Journal of Neurosurgery*, **54**, 289–299.

Moss E., Dearden, N. M. and Berridge, J. C. (1995) Effects of changes in mean arterial pressure on SjO_2 during cerebral aneurysm surgery. *British Journal of Anaesthesia*, **75**, 527–530.

Sano, T., Drummond, J. C., Patel, P. M., Grafe, M. R., Watson, J. C. and Cole, D. J. (1992) A comparison of the cerebral protective effects of isoflurane and mild hypothermia in a model of incomplete forebrain ischaemia in the rat. *Anesthesiology*, **76**, 221–228.

Shapiro, H. M. and Drummond, J. C. (1994) Neurosurgical anaesthesia, in *Anesthesia* (ed. R. D. Miller) Churchill Livingstone, New York, pp. 1897–1946.

van Aken, H. ed. (1995) *Neuroanaesthetic practice*. BMJ Publishing Group, London.

Walters, F. J., Ingram, G. S. and Jenkinson, J. L. eds. (1994) *Anaesthesia and Intensive Care for the Neurosurgical Patient*. Blackwell Scientific Publications, London.

Young, W. L. and Pile-Spellman, J. (1994) Anaesthetic considerations for interventional neuroradiology. *Anesthesiology*, **80**, 427–456.

GENITOURINARY AND RENAL SURGERY

S.E. Hutchinson

Population changes have meant increasing numbers of elderly patients presenting for surgery. This is particularly marked in the speciality of urological surgery as many conditions, such as benign prostatic hypertrophy and bladder tumours, become more common with advancing age.

Surgery is now often carried out using minimally invasive techniques, which are advantageous for the patient and cost effective when performed on a day-stay basis. The anaesthetist is under considerable pressure to allow many elderly patients to return home a few hours after general anaesthesia. Providing a safe anaesthetic for these elderly patients requires knowledge of specific problems arising in this surgical speciality, and of the physiological changes occurring with age. This includes a reduction in renal function progressing, in some cases, to renal failure.

This chapter will cover specific anaesthetic techniques for the range of renal and genitourinary procedures, taking into account the physiological changes listed in Table 15.1 and their appropriate anaesthetic management.

ANAESTHESIA FOR GENITOURINARY SURGERY

Preoperative assessment must be appropriate to the age and overall medical condition of the patient, and the type of procedure planned.

A full history and examination should particularly note details of any previous anaesthetic records. Further investigations should include a recent chest X-ray, electrocardiogram (ECG) and routine blood tests. Where

Table 15.1 Physiological changes in the elderly

Cardiovascular	increased incidence of ischaemic heart disease
	increased incidence of hypertension
	reduction in cardiac output
	reduction in maximum heart rate
	reduction in vasomotor reflexes
Respiratory	reduction in vital capacity
	reduction in functional residual capacity to below closing volume
Renal	reduction in renal blood flow and glomerular filtration
	reduction in maximum concentrating ability
Haematological	increase in anaemia of varied aetiology
Metabolic	reduction in muscle mass
	reduction in basal metabolic rate
	reduction in capacity to retain heat

appropriate, these tests may extend to respiratory function tests, echocardiogram, or exercise ECG.

DAY-CASE SURGERY

Many urological procedures, such as check cystoscopy, are brief, cause minimal postoperative discomfort, and are ideally suited to day surgery. Flexible cystoscopy is often performed without anaesthesia. Patients requiring a general anaesthetic can only be considered for day surgery if their preoperative investigations have been satisfactorily carried out before admission. The results should be available and show the patient to conform to grades 1 or 2 of the classification laid down by the American Society of Anesthesiologists (ASA) (see Table 7.1).

- The duration of surgery should be less than 30 min.
- Adequate transport facilities and home support should be available.
- The degree of postoperative pain and analgesic requirements should be appropriate for early discharge.
- The choice of general anaesthetic or spinal blockade is open to the anaesthetist, however, regional blockade involves delay in return to full mobility, with a high incidence of urinary retention, and confers no benefit in minor surgery.
- No sedative premedication should be prescribed.
- Adequate monitoring and resuscitation equipment are essential.
- Induction agents should be given slowly and in smaller doses to elderly patients, bearing in mind the physiological changes with age.
- Anaesthesia may be maintained with inhalational agents or a total intravenous infusion.
- The patient may breathe spontaneously with, or without, the use of a laryngeal mask airway. Intubation and ventilation may be more appropriate for the patient, or the surgery.
- If elderly patients are slow to recover, or require more potent analgesia, they should remain in hospital overnight.

PENILE SURGERY

Most penile surgery is performed on children and young men. It is not within the remit of this chapter to discuss paediatric anaesthesia. Surgery for circumcision, or meatotomy, is satisfactorily performed with the patient breathing spontaneously. Limited regional blockade, given in addition to a general anaesthetic, provides good postoperative analgesia.

A caudal block gives excellent analgesia in small children, but has a high incidence of urinary retention, delays return to mobility in the older child, and is inappropriate for adults. A penile block is a very good alternative. Postoperative analgesia can be supplemented with NSAIDs and other simple analgesics.

Penile block

This gives excellent postoperative pain relief, avoiding motor and central sympathetic blockade and bladder disturbance. Some of the autonomic supply is unaffected, therefore erection may occur during surgery.

Anatomy

The somatic supply of the penis is from the second, third and fourth sacral nerve roots. The fibres run in the dorsal nerve of the penis (the terminal branch of the pudendal nerve). This nerve runs with the artery along the inferior ramus of the pubis, entering the fibrous tissue which surrounds the corpora cavernosa (Figure 15.1). This supplies the skin and glans of the penis. The autonomic supply arises from the inferior hypogastric plexus in the pelvis, some fibres accompanying these

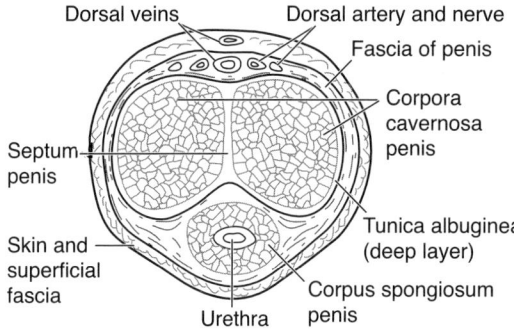

Figure 15.1 The anatomy of the penis in cross-section. (Reproduced with permission from Wildsmith, J.A. and Armitage, E.N. (1987) *The Principles and Practice of Regional Anaesthesia*. Churchill Livingstone, Edinburgh, p. 135.)

blood vessels to the corpora. The base and some of the ventral surface of the penis are innervated by cutaneous branches of the genitofemoral nerve.

Technique

A finger is placed under the pubic symphysis in the midline. A skin wheal is raised, then a small bore (23 G) needle is inserted vertically to a depth of 3–4 cm; 5–10 ml local anaesthetic is infiltrated onto the superior surface of the corpora cavernosa. Plain bupivacaine 0.25–0.5% is used. **Solutions containing adrenaline should never be used**. The whole area is very vascular and repeated aspirations avoid inadvertent intravascular injection.

A further 5 ml of solution should be placed subcutaneously in a ring around the base of the penis or as a single ventral injection. This blocks the branches of the genitofemoral nerve, reducing the failure rate to 4%. The technique and dose are modified for use in children.

TESTICULAR SURGERY

Males of all ages have minor surgery for epididymal cysts, hydroceles and sterilization, or more extensive surgery such as radical orchidectomy.

Vasectomy is frequently performed under local infiltration. Other procedures may be performed under regional blockade, such as spinal or epidural analgesia. This is particularly appropriate if the patient's condition makes a general anaesthetic hazardous (as in severe respiratory disease). The likely level of block required must be ascertained preoperatively. Most patients prefer to be asleep for penile and testicular surgery. A technique involving spontaneous ventilation is usually adopted. A field block can be performed targeting the ilio-inguinal, iliohypogastric and genitofemoral nerves. This gives extremely good post-operative pain relief particularly where the surgery involves the inguinal canal.

Torsion of the testes presents as an emergency and surgery should be performed as soon as possible. Pain is often severe, and can be assumed to reduce gastric emptying. Vomiting is a common occurrence after traction on the spermatic cord. A rapid sequence induction, with extubation in the lateral position, is therefore recommended.

TRANSURETHRAL ENDOSCOPIC PROCEDURES

The range of transurethral procedures now carried out through the endoscope is extensive. Before discussing these in detail it is appropriate to highlight the issues relating specifically to anaesthesia for transurethral surgery.

Spinal or general anaesthesic?

The choice of anaesthetic technique depends on the individual patient and the experience of the anaesthetist.

The place of spinal anaesthesia in patients with respiratory disease is well established. There is continuing discussion in recent literature on the merits of regional blockade in cardiovascular disease. The incidence of myocardial ischaemia increases in the postoperative period in elderly patients undergoing transurethral resection of the prostate. There is, however, no difference in morbidity between those having spinal or general anaesthetic techniques.

Cardiac output and mean arterial pressure changes are greatest immediately after induction of anaesthesia, and after institution of the regional block. Decreases in the heart rate are more pronounced in general anaesthetic patients in this period. A block that does not extend above T10 is consistent with the requirements for most transurethral surgery. At this level there is limited effect on the splanchnic bed, and vasodilation occurs mainly in the peripheral vessels. The potential risk of compromising the coronary circulation with sudden hypotension is therefore minimized. The positioning of the patient in lithotomy for transurethral surgery is thought to confer added benefit in maintaining systolic arterial pressure.

The use of regional anaesthesia avoids central nervous system depressants: a great advantage in the elderly.

The incidence of spinal headache is reduced with advancing age. Needle size is an important determinant, but the use of very fine needles in patients with ossification of spinal ligaments is of little benefit. The advent of 'atraumatic' spinal needles with pencil-points has decreased the incidence and severity of headache.

The details of performing a spinal block are dealt with elsewhere in this book. A safe technique must be used including appropriate monitoring, equipment and drugs for full resuscitation. Intravenous access must first be established. The extent of fluid preloading should be carefully considered. The cardiovascular system may not tolerate large increases and decreases in central venous pressure. Excessive fluid loading increases left ventricular end diastolic pressure inducing cardiac failure. Bolus doses of ephedrine counteract the hypotension caused by sympathetic blockade and maintain blood pressure by predominantly increasing heart rate, and so cardiac output, rather than by peripheral vasoconstriction. This is undesirable in patients with coexisting ischaemic heart disease, in whom, a combination of fluid and vasopressors is recommended (ephedrine can be administered by infusion). Several studies have used the α-agonist, metaraminol, as an alternative to ephedrine.

The lithotomy position

Transurethral surgery is performed in the lithotomy or Lloyd–Davis position. Asymmetrical, or excessively abducted, positions should be avoided to prevent straining the hip joints and pelvis, in a group of patients with a high incidence of osteoporosis. Padding minimizes pressure points on the lower leg avoiding venous thrombosis and possible neurological damage at bony prominences. The hands should be kept clear of metallic parts of the poles.

The Trendelenburg position further compromises the respiratory and cardiovascular function of the anaesthetized patient. Increased upward pressure on the diaphragm predisposes to reflux of gastric contents, and intubation should be considered, particularly in obese patients.

Estimation of blood loss

Significant blood loss is mainly confined to prostatic surgery, but may be seen in the transurethral resection of bladder tumours. Visual estimates of blood loss during endoscopic procedures are notoriously unreliable. Attempts have been made to quantify the loss by spectrophotometry of the drained irrigation fluid. This is time consuming and cumbersome, and has not gained widespread acceptance.

Clinical judgement, monitoring of the central venous pressure and estimation of the haematocrit must guide the anaesthetist to the need for volume replacement and transfusion.

Temperature loss

Maintenance of normal body temperature requires intact mechanisms to detect and respond to changes in environmental temperature. The elderly are less able to respond to these changes. There is a decrease in basal metabolic rate, reduced muscle mass, impaired autonomic function and an impaired ability to shiver.

All patients undergoing surgery are at risk of heat loss through evaporation and convection, and a reduction in the metabolic rate during general anaesthesia. This is exacerbated in endoscopic procedures by the use of irrigation fluids. Regional anaesthetic techniques prevent vasoconstriction in the lower body further increasing heat loss. Adverse effects following hypothermia include increased oxygen requirements and myocardial workload during the immediate postoperative period. There may also be a reduction in conscious level and delayed recovery from general anaesthesia. Preventative measures include the warming of intravenous and irrigation fluids, heated mattresses, and the humidification of inspired gases.

Antibiotic therapy

Urinary infection is common in the presence of outflow tract obstruction. Instrumentation of the urinary tract in the presence of infection leads to bacteraemia.

Prophylactic antibiotics are widely used when infection is known or suspected, before surgery. Aminoglycosides have been replaced increasingly by the third generation cephalosporins. Both these groups of antibiotics are predominantly excreted via the kidney, therefore care should be taken where there is any degree of renal failure. Up to 10% of patients with penicillin sensitivity will demonstrate a cross reaction to cephalosporins. Patients with prosthetic heart valves, pacemakers or valvular lesions should be given antibiotic prophylaxis for any transurethral procedure, even in the absence of documented infection. Guidelines are given in the *National Formulary* and are constantly updated. Current therapy uses a pre-induction combination of intravenous ampicillin and gentamicin, followed by postoperative oral amoxycillin. Substitution with vancomycin is recommended in patients with penicillin sensitivity.

MINOR TRANSURETHRAL PROCEDURES

This group includes cystoscopy, biopsy of bladder lesions, urethrotomy and bladder neck incision, and may be performed as day-case procedures. Patients catheterized for 24 h until bleeding has ceased may require inpatient stay.

Anaesthesia may be regional, or general, as appropriate. Postoperative pain relief is usually adequately provided by paracetamol-based analgesics or NSAIDS. Occasionally intramuscular opiates are required.

ENDOSCOPIC URETERIC SURGERY

This includes tumour biopsy, ureteric dilatation, or the positioning of stents. (Ureteric stones will be discussed in the next section.)

Instrumentation of the ureter often presents the surgeon with technical difficulties. Anaesthesia may be prolonged and radiological imaging may be needed.

Regional analgesia alone is rarely appropriate for this type of surgery. The block needs to extend well above the T10 level to provide adequate conditions for high ureteric instrumentation, which results in cardiovascular changes.

The surgeon may require cessation of breathing for radiological imaging, and a technique of intubation and ventilation is often advisable for all but the simplest of ureteric procedures. Removal of ureteric stents is often performed as a day case, and now increasingly with a flexible cystoscope under local anaesthesia. Pain relief following ureteric instrumentation must take into account the severity of spasm often occurring. The NSAID drugs are successfully used, but spasmolytic agents are sometimes required.

ENDOSCOPIC REMOVAL OF STONES

Many small stones are still removed transurethrally. While this is often a minor procedure, it may be prolonged with the use of copious amounts of irrigating fluid. Location and destruction of the stone is not easy, even with the use of the ultrasonic lithoclast and Dormier basket.

EXTRACORPOREAL LITHOTRIPSY

Extracorporeal shock wave lithotripsy is used to fragment renal, ureteric and bladder calculi. Externally generated shock waves are focused on the stones to cause the fragmentation. Early lithotripter machines relied on a capacitor charge across an electrode gap to generate the wave. This procedure presented the anaesthetist with many problems since the patient required general or regional anaesthesia sitting up in a bath of water. Some centres still use these powerful machines for hard stones. Second-generation lithotripters do not require patient immersion and are much less painful. Most stones are destroyed using this method.

General anaesthesia with spontaneous ventilation using an inhalational or total intravenous technique is rarely required. Most cases are satisfactorily carried out with sedation and small bolus doses of intravenous, short-acting opiates. Some centres advocate the use of local anaesthetic cream to the overlying skin surface, but this has not reduced the need for opiate analgesia. Surgery is usually performed as a day case, but two or more episodes may be needed to fragment the stone.

TRANSURETHRAL RESECTION OF BLADDER TUMOUR

The tumour may be a very small lesion, resected quickly under general or regional anaesthesia. Catheterization until bleeding has stopped makes inpatient stay likely for most of these cases.

At the other end of the spectrum are the large bladder tumours requiring extensive resection entailing time and considerable blood loss. The anaesthetist should be aware of the likely extent of surgery before choosing the method of anaesthesia, and be prepared for fluid and blood replacement.

Regional blockade, such as spinal analgesia, is very appropriate for these cases but consideration should be given to the patients medical and mental state. The surgeon's view may be hampered by straining and coughing. Therefore, quiet respiration through a clear airway is essential, avoiding any large swings in intrathoracic, and hence venous pressure, which may cause increased bleeding. Diathermy of the bladder wall close to the path of the obturator nerve (in the lateral pelvis), causes brisk leg jerks which are potentially hazardous during resection. For these reasons, intubation and ventilation is often the method of choice for the larger tumours. Absorption of irrigating fluid is unlikely to be a problem since large venous sinuses are not opened.

TRANSURETHRAL RESECTION OF THE PROSTATE (TURP)

This is a common operation, becoming more so as the elderly population increases. Choice of anaesthetic technique has already been discussed. Problems encountered by the anaesthetist during prostatic resection include:

- blood loss, sometimes substantial, but always difficult to quantify,
- heat loss causing hypothermia,
- positioning of the patient,
- absorption of irrigation fluid leading to TURP syndrome.

The first three problems have been covered already, but the last is an important cause of perioperative morbidity warranting full discussion.

TURP Syndrome

Reported incidence of this syndrome varies widely, but a mild form may be seen in up to 20% of resections: severe cases are limited to 1% patients.

Aetiology

During prostatic resection, a continuous flow of fluid through the resectoscope provides good visibility and allows for removal of resected prostatic fragments. The fluid currently used in the UK is a 1.5% solution of the amino acid glycine. Table 15.2 lists the properties of the ideal irrigation solution.

The average venous pressure in the prostatic fossa is 1.5 kPa. Venous sinuses of the prostate are opened during resection, and intravesical hydrostatic pressures above this level during intermittent filling cause irrigation fluid to enter the circulation. The rate of absorption is up to 30 ml min^{-1}, correlating with the extent and duration of the resection.

Table 15.2 Properties of the ideal endoscopic irrigating solution

Isotonic to prevent haemolysis
Non-electrolytic
Clear with good optical clarity
Easy to sterilize with long shelf life
Non-allergenic
Physiologically inactive
Easy and inexpensive to manufacture

Presentation

The awake patient will show signs of the syndrome at an earlier stage, with confusion or restlessness, often proceeding to convulsions and coma. Blood pressure is initially elevated, but hypotension supervenes.

ECG changes include bradycardia, T-wave inversion, and loss of P-waves. Mild dyspnoea occurs which may progress to cyanosis and respiratory distress.

Pathophysiology

Absorption of irrigating fluid causes a dilutional hyponatraemia and water intoxication. The glycine is osmotically active, so plasma osmolality does not immediately fall. Sodium concentrations below 120 mmol l^{-1} produce deranged tissue function, affecting nerve, heart, and muscle. Values below 100 mmol l^{-1} can lead to coma. The effects on the central nervous system are due to the hypervolaemia, causing cerebral oedema, and a rise in intracranial pressure. Glycine is metabolized in the liver to ammonia, which may produce encephalopathy. Fluid overload leads to cardiac failure with pulmonary oedema, cyanosis, and hypotension.

Prevention

Resection time should be limited to less than 1 h and surgical technique should involve good haemostasis and diathermy to the venous sinuses as soon as they are opened. The irrigation fluid should not be placed more than 60 cm above the patient to limit the hydrostatic pressure. Newer surgical techniques now use continuous irrigation with low pressure suction, to avoid over distention of the bladder.

Equipment has been developed which can detect fluid absorption immediately. Ethanol 1% is added to the irrigation fluid and expired breath analysis detects ethanol that has entered the circulation in the anaesthetized or awake patient. Computer technology represents this, several times a minute, as an accurate measurement of the volume of fluid absorbed. The operator can warn the surgeon, and resection can be stopped long before the syndrome develops.

Treatment

Early recognition of the signs of the developing syndrome is important.

Urgent measurement of the serum sodium concentration and central venous pressure monitoring will help in diagnosis and management. Termination of surgery limits further glycine absorption. Definitive treatment must then be supportive, with admission to the intensive care unit, and full invasive monitoring. The extent of the hyponatraemia will determine the need for positive pressure ventilation and inotropic support.

Active treatment with hypertonic saline is controversial, potentially increasing circulatory overload and cardiac failure. The rapid correction of plasma sodium concentration has been implicated in permanent neurological damage, and the suggested maximum rate of increase is 12 mmol l^{-1} per day. Others contest that rapid correction of circulating sodium to a mild hyponatraemia reduces the overall mortality.

Pacemakers and diathermy

In-dwelling pacemakers and diathermy are a potential hazard in any surgical procedure. The usual precaution of using bipolar diathermy is not possible in prostatic resections.

Interference with pacemaker function is rare with the more modern designs. The anaesthetist should determine the age and type of pacemaker, and diathermy plates should be placed as far away as possible. A magnet should be available so that it can be used in an emergency, if pacemaker function is affected.

Newer methods of performing TURP

Recent technological advances have enabled prostatic removal to be carried out using a laser probe through the endoscope. A suprapubic catheter is inserted before resection to enable a continuous flow of irrigation fluid, so improving visibility, and decreasing intravesical pressure. Laser time is in the region of 4 min, dramatically reducing overall operating time. This is a major advantage, as is lack of blood loss, and, since no venous sinuses are opened, avoidance of the TURP syndrome. The suprapubic catheter is replaced by an urethral catheter, which remains *in situ* for several weeks while the tissue oedema subsides. Postoperative pain can be severe for the first few hours, but patients are often able to return home 24–48 h later, with the catheter in place.

Precautions must be taken, as for all laser procedures, to protect the eyes of patients and staff in theatre.

The techniques of prostatic ablation with 'microwave thermocoagulation' or with the 'Vapotrode' are employed in some centres with great success. These techniques are relatively new, and while they confer major intraoperative benefits, their long-term outcomes are still being assessed.

RADIOLOGICAL PROCEDURES

Many urology procedures (particularly involving ureteric instrumentation) require the use of radiological screening. A suitable operating table allows for the positioning and function of an image intensifier, or for plain X-rays to be taken. The patient's position should be appropriate for the X-ray, and all radio-opaque objects moved from the field of vision.

The need for temporary cessation of ventilation, during imaging of the renal tract, means intubation and ventilation is most appropriate. Percutaneous procedures now commonly combine the skills of the radiologist and surgeon reducing the need for large, open operations. The patient is prone, semi-prone, or in the lateral position. Some procedures can be performed under local anaesthetic infiltration and intravenous sedation. Larger procedures, involving instrumentation of the renal pelvis and associated deep tissues, require a general anaesthetic.

MAJOR PELVIC SURGERY

This encompasses surgery for pelvic malignancy, such as cystectomies, (with the formation of conduits), radical prostatectomies, and total pelvic exenteration. Those patients with congenital and acquired bladder abnormalities may require repeated, complex, pelvic surgery. Such operations include bladder reconstruction, augmentation, or urinary diversion (through a conduit formed from bowel, appendix or fallopian tube). These major cases number few in the average hospital's urology lists, but they are a very important group which merits full discussion.

Genitourinary malignancy is seen in older patients, who are likely to be less fit. As well as intercurrent disease, they may be anaemic and cachectic. Often they will have required bowel preparation. These operations carry a significant morbidity and mortality, and the anaesthetist must be able to assess the patient and be involved with the surgeon in the decision to operate. Some patients are not able to withstand such major surgery, and alternative therapy may be more appropriate.

The operations are long, blood loss is significant, and the degree of monitoring must reflect all these factors. Invasive monitoring of the arterial and central venous pressure is necessary. It may be appropriate to insert a pulmonary artery catheter to monitor pulmonary capillary wedge pressure, and hence left ventricular function.

Many anaesthetists supplement general anaesthesia with a regional technique. Epidural analgesia can be continued into the postoperative period to give excellent pain relief. There is evidence to suggest that the sympathetic blockade and decrease in venous tone resulting from the epidural may increase the blood loss peroperatively.

Great care must be taken to measure and replace blood and fluid losses, correct haematocrit, electrolytes, acid–base balance and clotting. Body temperature should be monitored and maintained.

Postoperative care is crucial and should be within a high dependency or intensive care setting. Very extensive surgery may require a period of elective ventilation for hours, or even days, to allow physiological parameters to return to normal.

Major pelvic surgery may be carried out on patients with spina bifida and those with previous cord damage, to facilitate bladder emptying, and prevent urinary incontinence. In these patients the level of sensory loss must be established preoperatively. There is always the temptation to forego the use of analgesics if surgery is performed where the patient has no sensation. Surgical stimuli often extend above this level, and in addition, the presence of intact spinal reflexes makes the use of general anaesthesia plus adequate analgesia imperative in all, but the most minor, procedures.

OPEN PROCEDURES ON THE KIDNEY

Surgery is usually carried out with the patient in the lateral position, with the table 'broken' to maximize the area of visibility and access to the surgical site (Figure 15.2). Positioning can be difficult, and the anaesthetist must be involved in securing the patient, and checking that the limbs are in the anatomical position, well padded and supported to avoid nerve injury.

Intubation and ventilation is necessary and invasive monitoring may be needed. Breach of the pleura is not uncommon and a chest drain should be inserted at the end of the operation if a pneumothorax is a possibility. The anaesthetist should ensure that the lung

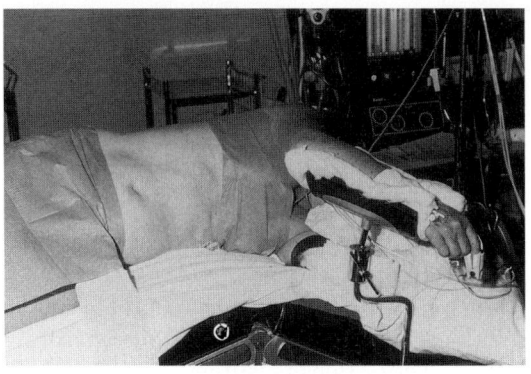

Figure 15.2 Lateral 'table-break' position for renal surgery.

is fully inflated as the pleura is closed. A postoperative chest X-ray should be performed. Very occasionally, resection of a huge mass, such as a polycystic kidney, may need a thoracoabdominal approach, and a double lumen endobronchial tube is required.

Postoperative analgesia must be tailored to cope with the level of pain and to encourage adequate coughing and chest movement. A high lumbar, or thoracic, epidural block gives excellent postoperative pain relief. Alternatives are interpleural or intercostal catheters to deliver boluses, or infusions, of local anaesthetic.

Patient-controlled analgesia with opiates is successful, but atelectasis and chest infections are common and exacerbated by sedation and hypoventilation. Chest physiotherapy and respiratory monitoring are important.

ANAESTHESIA IN THE PATIENT WITH RENAL FAILURE

End stage renal failure is defined as: creatinine clearance < 10 ml min^{-1} and plasma creatinine $> 500 \mu$mol l^{-1}. The incidence in the UK is about 140 per million per year. About 60 per million per year commence long-term renal replacement therapy. There are about 300 per million population with impaired renal function and annual mortality of 10%.

Isolated acute renal failure is uncommon as it is usually seen in conjunction with sepsis and multi-organ failure, or as a complication of another medical or surgical condition. Surgery, if urgent, is for the underlying primary condition. Mortality is high, and anaesthesia revolves around supporting cardiac and respiratory function. Surgery should be delayed if possible until the patient is dialysed and stable. The problems then approach those of end-stage renal failure (ESRF).

Safe anaesthesia for these patients demands a knowledge of the aetiology, pathophysiology, clinical manifestation, and medical management of ESRF.

CLINICAL PATHOPHYSIOLOGY

Table 15.3 lists the possible features associated with chronic renal failure, but several

Table 15.3 Clinical features of end-stage renal failure

Cardiovascular	hypertension
	ischaemic heart disease
	secondary valvular dysfunction
	congestive cardiac failure
	pericarditis
	endocarditis
Respiratory	infection
	dyspnoea due to acidosis and anaemia
	dyspnoea from cardiac failure and fluid overload
	pleural effusions
	pulmonary fibrosis
Haematological	anaemia (normochromic normocytic)
	platelet dysfunction
	prolonged bleeding time
Gastrointestinal	nausea and vomiting
	anorexia
	peptic ulceration
	reduced gastric emptying
Nervous system	autonomic neuropathy
	peripheral sensory and motor neuropathy
	myopathy

of these are of particular importance to the anaesthetist.

Anaemia

Haemoglobin is usually 5–10 g dl^{-1} in ESRF. This is as a result of several pathological processes.

- reduction in the production and release of erythrocytes from marrow,
- reduction in red cell life span, especially on haemodialysis,
- high incidence of peptic ulceration leading to chronic iron deficiency, and
- poor appetite resulting in deficiencies in vitamin B6, B12, and folate.

Haemoglobin values are higher in those with polycystic kidneys and patients maintained on continuous ambulatory peritoneal dialysis.

Biosynthetic erythropoietin is prescribed for those patients with haemoglobin < 8 g dl^{-1}, or who are symptomatic from their anaemia (angina and severe dyspnoea). This treatment is, however, expensive and adverse effects include vascular thrombosis and hypertension.

Compensations for anaemia

The physiological changes associated with anaemia are:

- elevated red cell 2,3-DPG concentrations (2,3 diphosphoglycerate), causing a right shift in the oxyhaemoglobin dissociation curve, and greater oxygen release to tissues, and
- an increase in cardiac output causing demands on the heart which may already be compromised by ischaemic changes.

Preoperative transfusion is recommended in all patients with ESRF and a haemoglobin < 5 g dl^{-1}, but may be necessary in those who are symptomatic with lesser degrees of anaemia.

Bleeding

Abnormalities of platelet function are thought to be the primary haemostatic defect. Deficiencies in platelet aggregation are not correlated with the severity of renal function, but improve on dialysis. Bleeding time is prolonged, but returns to normal with transfusion or erythropoietin.

Excessive bleeding after haemodialysis is treated with protamine. Poor haemostasis, not associated with heparin, has been successfully treated with desmopressin acetate.

Cardiovascular system

Cardiovascular disease is the main cause of death in ESRF. In the age group 25–45 years there is a three-fold increase in mortality compared to the patient with normal renal function. This is due to:

- hypertension,
- coronary artery disease,
- abnormal left ventricular function, and
- pericardial disease.

Although hypertension is an important cause of ESRF, approximately 80% of patients with ESRF from other causes will develop hypertension as a complication. This is related to an increase in systemic vascular resistance and salt and water loading. The resulting left ventricular hypertrophy increases myocardial oxygen demand. Many patients will be taking antihypertensive drugs, and these should be continued throughout the perioperative period. Angiotensin-converting enzyme inhibitors do not cause significant anaesthetic problems, but calcium channel inhibitors and β-adrenoceptor blockers exacerbate the cardiovascular depression caused by inhalational agents. Spontaneous ventilation techniques with inspired concentrations above 1 (one) minimum alveolar concentration (MAC) should be avoided.

Hypertensive patients often show exaggerated changes in arterial pressure and heart rate at induction of anaesthesia, laryngoscopy and intubation. Changes in the ST-segment and T-wave are seen on the ECG in response to marked increases and decreases of arterial pressure, and heart rate. These ECG changes are normally associated with myocardial ischaemia and everything should be done to avoid precipitating then. However, there is no evidence to suggest that, if transient, they cause any long-term effect on morbidity and mortality.

Since the advent of dialysis, pericardial disease is uncommon, but pericardial effusion is easily diagnosed with echocardiography and should always be excluded if the heart size suddenly increases.

Abnormal lipoprotein metabolism is seen in ESRF. Elevated cholesterol values and decrease in high density lipoprotein concentration are associated with coronary artery and peripheral vascular disease.

Low output cardiac failure is seen in 45% patients. In addition to ischaemic heart disease and hypertension, other mechanisms which may cause congestive failure are:

- volume overload, (a) extrinsic, failure of sodium and water excretion, (b) intrinsic, in aortic and mitral regurgitation,
- pressure overload, aortic stenosis.

Cardiac failure is a very high risk factor for general anaesthesia. Lowering of cardiac output with anaesthetic drugs induces a cycle of decreased arterial pressure, impaired myocardial blood flow and further depression of cardiac output.

Infective endocarditis is found in 2.5% of patients on haemodialysis and in up to 9% of patients with an infected vascular access sites. Mortality in these patients is extremely high.

Autonomic neuropathy occurs in diabetic patients and is therefore more common in ESRF. Impairment of sympathetic vasoconstriction and cardiac reflexes can lead to a marked fall in arterial pressure with intermittent positive pressure ventilation, exacerbated by hypovolaemia often found after dialysis.

Respiratory system

The presence of heart disease and the inability to excrete fluid loads makes patients susceptible to pulmonary oedema. Dyspnoea is often made worse by acidosis and anaemia. The cause of renal failure may be associated with respiratory pathology such as pulmonary fibrosis in rheumatoid arthritis and amyloidosis. Chest infections are common and associated with depression of the immune system.

Nervous system

Peripheral sensory neuropathy (predominantly of the lower limbs) is well recognized in ESRF and may progress to a motor neuropathy. The incidence is increased in patients with diabetes.

Uraemic patients often exhibit weakness which is due to myopathy rather than neuropathy, and may show an exaggerated response to neuromuscular blocking drugs. Other common symptoms such as twitches, cramps, restless legs and pruritus of unknown aetiology, are treated with quinine sulphate, with no anaesthetic implications.

Autonomic neuropathy is common in diabetic patients. The anaesthetist should be prepared for cardiovascular instability and take measures to minimize the effects.

Large shifts in fluid and electrolytes with dialysis have been known to cause fits and mental changes, but are rarely seen now. Severe uraemia causes drowsiness and an altered conscious level, which are reversed as treatment lowers urea and resolves the acidosis.

Gastrointestinal system

There is a high incidence of peptic ulceration in ESRF. Many patients are already taking histamine (H_2) receptor antagonist drugs. Continuation throughout surgery is important, since gastric acid secretion is often increased, and gastric emptying delayed, predisposing to oesophageal reflux and aspiration. Preoperative metoclopramide and pre-induction sodium citrate limit the risks during anaesthesia.

Calcium and phosphate

A fall in plasma calcium and a rise in plasma phosphate values are caused by the reduction in glomerular filtration. Acidosis permits the ionized calcium concentration to be preserved, so tetany is rare.

Defective vitamin D hydroxylation in the kidneys causes poor bone mineralization and reduced absorption of calcium from the gut. Reduced plasma calcium stimulates the production of parathyroid hormone, which raises calcium and lowers plasma phosphate. Prolonged stimulation of the parathyroid glands leads to hyperplasia and autonomous production of parathyroid hormone, often requiring parathyroidectomy. Many patients are prescribed calcium supplements. Hypocalcaemia combined with hypermagnesaemia (from excessive antacid consumption) potentiate the action of the non-depolarizing muscle relaxants.

Ectopic calcification occurs when the solubility for calcium phosphate is exceeded. This results in the formation of stones, exacerbation of atherosclerosis, and calcification in the conducting system of the heart, causing arrhythmias and conduction abnormalities.

Acid–base balance

Acidosis is due to the inability to excrete fixed-acid metabolites as the glomerular filtration rate falls. The compensatory mechanisms are:

- increased respiratory drive causing a fall in Pa_{CO_2},
- buffering with plasma bicarbonate,
- alkaline bone salts (raised urinary calcium) to buffer hydrogen ions, and
- increased production of ammonium ions in the kidney.

The anion gap, calculated as plasma sodium − (chloride + bicarbonate) increases as sulphate and phosphate are retained. Acidosis is renowned for potentiating the action of neuromuscular blocking drugs and is seen even with atracurium.

Potassium

As the glomerular filtration rate falls, potassium balance is maintained by increasing secretion in the distal tubule and reducing reabsorption. Faecal loss of potassium increases dramatically. As acidosis ensues with worsening renal function, the potassium moves from the intracellular to extracellular space. Plasma potassium is raised and there is an inability to cope with the normal dietary load. Fluids containing potassium must be avoided unless the plasma potassium concentration is known to be abnormally low. Hyperkalaemia causes well-known electrocardiographic changes:

- peaked T wave,
- wide QRS complex,
- decreased amplitude of P and R waves, and
- finally 'sine wave' ECG.

It should be treated before surgery (depending on severity and speed of correction necessary) by using:

- oral calcium resonium 30 g,
- rectal calcium resonium 30–60 g (appropriate if nil by mouth),
- 50% glucose 50 ml, plus soluble insulin 12 units, or
- 10% calcium gluconate 5–10 ml and 50 mmol bicarbonate.

DRUGS IN RENAL FAILURE

The influence of renal disease on the pharmacokinetics and the pharmacodynamics of anaesthetic drugs has been extensively investigated.

The most important problems relate to

increased elimination half-life and the effects of drugs on the cardiovascular system.

Drugs bind mainly to two proteins in plasma; α-1-acid glycoprotein and albumin. There is a small increase in the binding of mainly basic drugs to α-1-acid glycoprotein, but a significant decrease in the binding of acidic drugs to albumin. This is due to hypoalbuminaemia, seen in some renal diseases (as in nephrotic syndrome), and to alterations in the structure and affinity of the drug binding sites, caused by uraemia and changes in pH. As a result, the apparent volumes of drug distribution may be increased. This may be further altered by intravascular volume depletion after haemodialysis.

When the unbound fraction of many anaesthetic agents is increased, total drug clearance is either unaltered or increased. However, for those drugs and their metabolites which are eliminated through the kidney, there is a curvilinear relationship between the glomerular filtration rate and the drug's elimination half-life.

Premedicant drugs

Atropine and glycopyrrolate are about 50% eliminated by the kidney, however accumulation is unlikely since they are only given as a single dose. Hyoscine is not excreted renally. The elimination of phenothiazines and the shorter acting benzodiazepines is not influenced by renal failure.

Induction agents

With decreased plasma protein binding of all induction agents commonly used (thiopentone, propofol and etomidate) there is a higher, free-drug concentration reaching brain tissue. Assuming that brain sensitivity is unaltered, the patient requires a decreased rate of administration, rather than a reduced total dose of drug.

A slow induction minimizes the cardiovascular effects. Patients who are volume depleted, or severely uraemic, benefit from smaller doses, and the use of etomidate, instead of propofol or thiopentone, gives greater cardiovascular stability.

Neuromuscular blocking drugs

Renal dysfunction significantly affects the metabolism of some competitive neuromuscular blocking drugs (D-tubocurarine, gallamine, alcuronium and pancuronium) which are predominantly renally excreted. These drugs should never be used.

Atracurium is broken down by Hoffman degradation and ester hydrolysis and its elimination is unchanged in renal failure. Its effect can be prolonged by acidosis, but it is the drug of choice in renal dysfunction. Prolonged infusions result in an increase in the plasma concentration of the metabolite laudanosine. At very high values this causes convulsions in dogs. These are at significantly greater concentrations than recorded during anaesthesia in man.

Mivacurium is metabolized by plasma and tissue esterases. Plasma cholinesterase activity is reduced in renal failure, but the increase in duration of effect of mivacurium is minimal, and it is a suitable drug for use in ESRF.

Vecuronium is partially renally excreted and its effect, like that of the new agent, rocuronium, is prolonged in renal failure. It can be used, but will accumulate after multiple bolus doses or infusions.

Doxacurium and pipecuronium both exhibit reduced clearance in ESRF and there is no indication for their use.

Suxamethonium causes a rise in plasma potassium of about 0.5 mmol l^{-1} in normal patients. This increase may be far greater in those with uraemic neuropathy and suxamethonium should not be used if the potassium is above 5.5 mmol l^{-1}. The reduction in plasma cholinesterase activity does not prolong its action.

Opioid drugs

Most analgesic drugs are metabolized to inactive metabolites in the liver, which are then excreted in the urine in healthy patients. Only phenoperidine is excreted 50% unchanged and therefore should not be used.

The actions of fentanyl, alfentanil and sufentanil are unaltered in ESRF. The metabolites of morphine accumulate with poor renal function. One of these, morphine-6-glucuronide, is a potent analgesic, and is thought to be responsible for some of the prolonged clinical effects which have been reported. Morphine should be used with care, and not as a continuous infusion.

The action of pethidine is also altered, and one of its metabolites, norpethidine will accumulate. While this has only weak analgesic activity, it can cause excitatory phenomena and convulsions.

Inhalational agents

Isoflurane, halothane and enflurane have all been used successfully in renal failure. There have been reports of deterioration in renal function following enflurane, but the concentration of inorganic fluoride produced is usually well below that associated with renal toxicity.

Anticholinesterases

All these drugs are excreted by filtration and tubular secretion. There is therefore a significant reduction in their clearance, and repeat doses should not be given at reversal of neuromuscular blockade. It is wise always to use a peripheral nerve stimulator to monitor the degree of neuromuscular blockade.

SURGERY

Patients with ESRF present for surgery for a variety of conditions unrelated to their renal disease. However, there are certain surgical procedures which are performed frequently on this group of patients as listed below.

- Vascular access: fistula and graft formation, tunnelled central venous catheters.
- Peritoneal dialysis: insertion, revision and removal of catheters.
- Nephrectomy: polycystic, infected and transplanted kidneys.
- Vascular: limb revascularization and amputation.
- Eye surgery: cataracts and vitrectomy.
- Parathyroidectomy.

PREOPERATIVE ASSESSMENT

These patients have often had many surgical procedures before and much information can be obtained from the previous anaesthetic charts. It is very important to take a full history and perform a thorough examination of the cardiovascular and respiratory systems to elicit signs and symptoms of new, or worsening, disease.

Multi-organ dysfunction is common, but it is only worth postponing surgery if the overall condition can be improved, or further investigations are necessary. It is important to identify and quantify the presence of valvular lesions, hypertension, left ventricular hypertrophy and dilatation, ischaemic changes and coexisting pulmonary disease. A recent ECG, chest X-ray and echocardiogram will give a great deal of information. More invasive cardiovascular investigations will often have been done to provide a fuller picture. Antihypertensive medication should be continued throughout the perioperative period. The site of arteriovenous fistulae should be identified.

FLUID AND ELECTROLYTE STATUS

A history of the normal urine output of the patient is important. It should not be assumed that the patient with ESRF is anuric. Often the output is small and there is strict fluid restriction, which is important information for the anaesthetist. The margin for error is small and losses must be replaced very carefully perioperatively to avoid overhydration and pulmonary oedema. If the surgery potentially involves substantial blood loss, then a central venous catheter should be sited to accurately monitor intravascular volume.

The time of last dialysis, the weight removed, and the normal dry weight (compared with current weight) are all important factors in determining the preoperative degree of volume depletion or overload. It is best to avoid dialysis immediately before surgery since there are dramatic shifts of fluid and electrolytes between the intravascular and extravascular spaces.

Circulating potassium should be measured within the last 24 h and within 6 h of the last dialysis, and should be normal. For emergency surgery it is not always possible to achieve this optimal status, so it may be necessary to proceed and deal with problems as they arise.

PREMEDICATION

Most of these patients are acclimatized to the hospital and cope better without sedatives to delay recovery. A preoperative visit by a sympathetic anaesthetist prepared to explain procedures and allay fears is very important. If sedation is necessary a small dose of oral temazepam is far better than intramuscular opiates. The prescription of an H_2 receptor antagonist is advisable, given the night before and the morning of surgery. Metoclopramide and sodium citrate help reduce the risk of acid aspiration.

INTRAVENOUS CANNULATION

Arteriovenous fistulae should be identified, and the limb wrapped in gamgee to keep it warm and well protected. This limb should never be used for cannulation or arterial pressure measurements as damage to the fistula is possible.

The dorsum of the dominant hand is chosen; veins in the non-dominant arm should be preserved for future fistula formation, if required. If veins are scarce, the search should proceed from the hand proximally, to spare the larger veins. Indwelling dialysis catheters should be left untouched (unless in an emergency) to avoid the risk of infection.

INDUCTION

The following should be monitored from induction, throughout the anaesthetic:

- non-invasive arterial pressure,
- ECG,
- oxygen saturation, and
- expired carbon dioxide and inspired oxygen concentrations.

It may be necessary to monitor central venous and invasive arterial pressures, and in some circumstances, pulmonary capillary wedge pressure. All patients should be preoxygenated to avoid small, transient drops in oxygen saturation, which are undesirable in the presence of anaemia and ischaemic heart disease.

The induction agent chosen should be administered very slowly. This will minimize the cardiovascular effects, limiting the drop in arterial pressure. As explained earlier, there is a greater fraction of the drug in the unbound state, reaching brain tissue and other major organs. The overall induction dose is often unchanged, but induction time is greatly increased.

A rapid sequence induction is indicated if there is a history of reflux or symptomatic hiatus hernia. Serum potassium should be normal before suxamethonium is used.

Intubation and ventilation is recommended in all except the young and reasonably fit patient having a short procedure. The risk of aspiration must be considered, and if a technique is chosen using a laryngeal mask airway or face mask and inflation of the patients stomach is to be avoided; a very gentle and unhurried induction is necessary.

Lignocaine spray to the larynx is useful to attenuate the hypertensive response to intubation but **beware**, this renders the airway unprotected postoperatively in a patient with an increased chance of regurgitation. The benefit must outweigh the risk!

MAINTENANCE OF GENERAL ANAESTHESIA

The concentration of inhalational agent must be carefully titrated to avoid depression of the cardiovascular system and yet prevent awareness. A total intravenous technique using propofol can be useful for short operations. An inspired oxygen concentration of 50% should be given throughout anaesthesia, and if ventilated, normocapnia should be maintained. Atracurium is the neuromuscular blocking drug of choice, and reversal with anticholinesterase and anticholinergic drugs depends on the level of residual blockade. The elimination of both these groups of drugs is delayed in ESRF. Repeat doses should not be given.

REGIONAL ANAESTHETIC TECHNIQUES

Regional anaesthetic techniques offer many advantages. An epidural, or spinal, block may be appropriate for surgery on the lower limb and pelvis, but extensive regional blockade is hazardous because of possible profound hypotension.

Preloading the patient with large volumes of fluid intravenously is contraindicated where urine output is poor. Fluid overload and a decrease in haematocrit result. If a regional technique is adopted for abdominal surgery, central venous pressure measurement must be started before the block.

Some concern has been expressed over the increased bleeding time seen in ESRF, particularly after recent dialysis. Clotting should always be checked, but even when normal, the risk of an epidural haematoma will deter many anaesthetists.

Brachial plexus block is an excellent choice for the formation of an arteriovenous fistula. It can be used alone, or in conjunction with a general anaesthetic, giving good, postoperative pain relief. The axillary approach is safer, but provides a less predictable block for fistulae at the wrist (in the area supplied by the musculocutaneous nerve). Acidosis increases the spread of local anaesthetics away from the site of injection, shortening the duration of the block. The threshold for central nervous system and cardiovascular toxicity is also reduced in acidosis.

INTRAVENOUS FLUIDS

Fluid deficits from preoperative starvation, and recent dialysis should be replaced with 0.9% sodium chloride solution; Hartmanns solution should not be used. Operative loss, unless very small, should be replaced by blood. Depending on the level of anaemia colloid solutions can be given while monitoring the haematocrit. It is undesirable to raise the haemoglobin above $10 \, g \, dl^{-1}$ in most of these patients. Central venous pressure monitoring is desirable for large fluid losses, and in patients with compromised left ventricular function. Fluid management for renal transplantation is fully discussed elsewhere in this book (chapter 27).

POSTOPERATIVE MANAGEMENT

Patients should be extubated and transported to the recovery room in the lateral position. The left lateral position is preferred, but is contraindicated in the presence of a fistula in the left arm: the most common site.

Supplemental oxygen should be administered from the cessation of anaesthesia. A minimum inspired concentration of 40% should be given and this must be continued on the ward for 24 h in all but the young active patient with a normal haemoglobin concentration. In those patients with severe heart disease oxygen should be continued at 2 l min^{-1} for several days with measurement of saturations, especially at night. After major surgery, a period in a high dependency area is warranted.

Intramuscular injections are not contraindicated, but can cause exaggerated bruising. If opiate analgesia is required, patient-controlled analgesia has many advantages. The opiate of choice is fentanyl, although pethidine and morphine have been successfully used. Some protection against respiratory depression is conferred by the nature of the delivery system, and regular observations. NSAID analgesics are contraindicated in renal failure. Other simple analgesics can be used alone, or in combination with opiates.

FURTHER READING

Cranshaw, J. and Holland, D. (1996) Anaesthesia for patients with renal impairment. *British Journal of Hospital Medicine*, **55**, 171–175.

Critchley, L. A. H., Short, T. G. and Gin, T. (1994) Hypotension during subarachnoid anaesthesia. Haemodynamic analysis of three treatments. *British Journal of Anaesthesia*, **72**, 151–155.

Dobson, P. M. S., Caldicott, L. D., Gerrish, S. P., Cole, J. R. and Channer, K. S. (1994) Changes in haemodynamic variables during TURP. A comparison of general and spinal anaesthesia. *British Journal of Anaesthesia*, **72**, 267–272.

Edwards, N. D., Callaghan, L. C., White, T. and Reilly, C. S. (1995) Perioperative myocardial ischaemia in patients undergoing transurethral surgery. *British Journal of Anaesthesia*, **74**, 368–372.

Hanhe, R. G., Larsson, H. and Ribbe, T. (1995) Continuous monitoring of irrigation fluid absorption during transurethral surgery. *Anaesthesia*, **5**, 327–331.

Holland, D. E. and Old, S. (1992) Anaesthesia for patients with impaired renal function. *Current Anaesthesia and Critical Care*, **3**, 140–145.

Miyabe, M., Sonada, H. and Namiki, A. (1995) Effects of lithotomy position on arterial blood pressure after spinal anaesthesia. *Anaesthesia and Analgesia*, **81**, 96–98.

Reilly, C. S. (1993) Regional analgesia and myocardial ischaemia. *British Journal of Anaesthesia*, **71**, 467–468.

Ryall, D. M. and Dodds, C. (1992) Anaesthesia for urological surgery in the elderly. *Current Anaesthesia and Critical Care*, **3**, 200–205.

Swales, J. D. (1987) Dangers in treating hyponatraemia. *British Medical Journal*, **294**, 261–262.

HEPATOBILIARY AND PANCREATIC SURGERY 16

A. Holdcroft

The liver is the main metabolic organ in the body and is richly vascularized, receiving 25% of the cardiac output through a direct, high pressure connection with the aorta and also a low pressure portal system from the abdominal viscera. The hepatocytes are intimately in contact with the afferent blood supply and the cannaliculi which transport waste products through the biliary system. An anaesthetist should aim to identify any preoperative hepatobiliary dysfunction, to select appropriate anaesthetic drugs and techniques to prevent deterioration of liver function and to be aware of the effects of other procedures, such as surgery, on liver and biliary function.

ANATOMY

The liver is the largest organ in the body but is hidden by the rib cage and is not normally palpable. It is divided functionally into right and left lobes, both of equal size and each supplied by a branch of the portal vein. The portal vein drains the gastrointestinal tract and provides substrates for metabolism. Besides being the main metabolic organ in the body, it also stores glycogen, proteins and vitamins, detoxifies and excretes substances either into the blood stream or the bile.

Liver cells radiate from central veins which join to form the hepatic vein. Between the columns of liver cells are sinusoids which contain blood and whose walls are lined with phagocytic cells (Kupffer cells, part of the reticuloendothelial system). The functional unit is the acinus with entry from the portal tract (Figure 16.1) and exit through the hepatic venous system. Bile cannaliculi originate between hepatocytes with tight junctions sealing them. They drain into the larger bile ducts in the portal tract.

Bile is actively secreted by the hepatocytes, stored in the gall bladder and released into the duodenum. This opening at the ampulla of Vater can be visualized endoscopically and either the pancreatic or bile duct cannulated and contrast media injected (endoscopic retrograde cholangiopancreatography, ERCP). The endoscopy also allows relief of benign or malignant strictures by stenting, while sphincterotomy can relieve obstruction from impacted gall stones. Bile or pancreatic juice may be obtained for culture, cytology or chemical analysis.

BLOOD SUPPLY

Blood flow to the liver is supplied by both the hepatic artery and portal vein. The portal vein provides up to 70% of the total oxygen supply to the liver when fasting (Figure 16.2). Digestion will reduce the content of oxygen carried by portal venous blood. Liver blood flow is

Short Practice of Anaesthesia. Edited by M. Morgan and G. M. Hall. Published in 1997 by Chapman & Hall, London. ISBN 0 412 71890 1

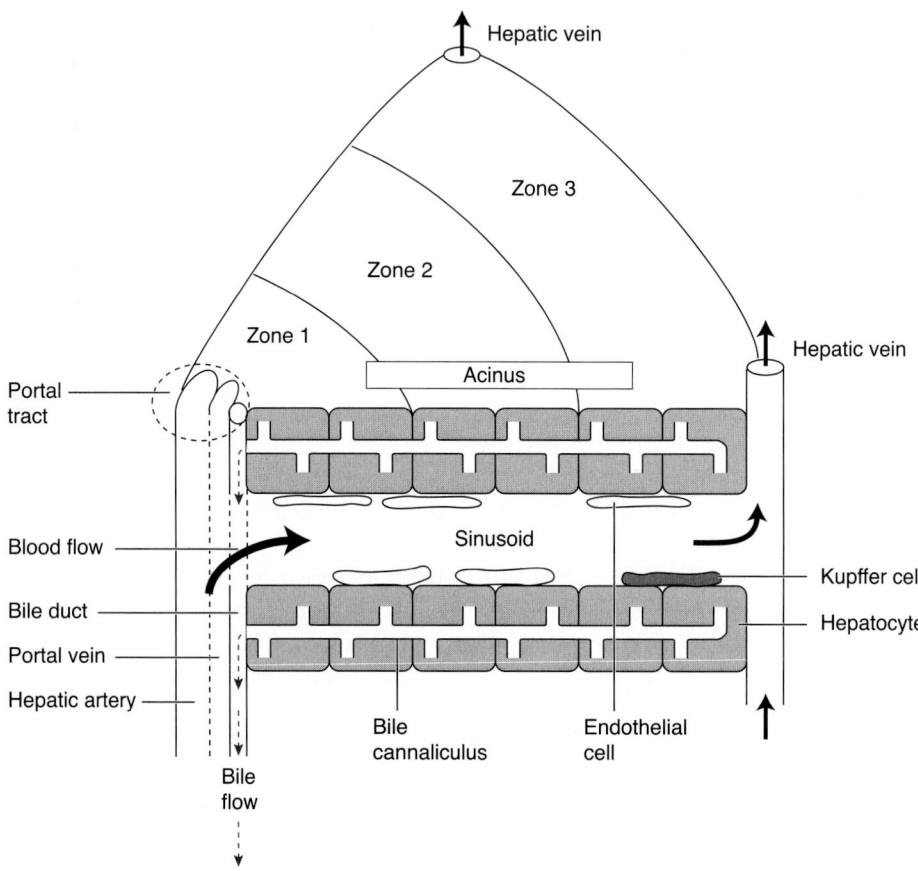

Figure 16.1 Blood supply of a liver acinus. The portal tract contains the terminal afferent vascular branches of the hepatic artery and portal vein, the bile ductules, the lymph vessels and nerves.

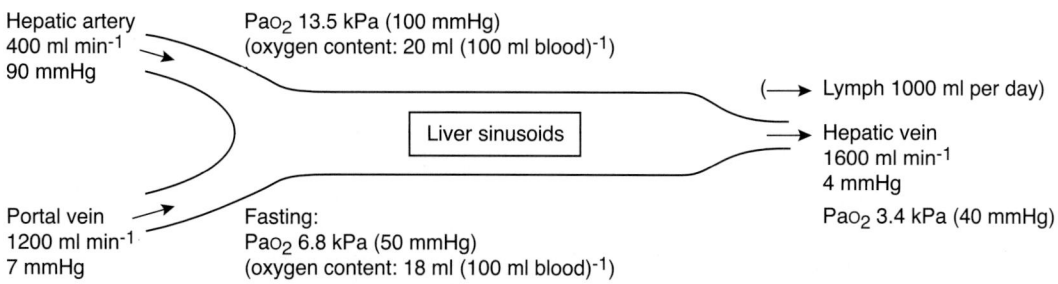

Figure 16.2 The blood supply of the liver. Pressures given as mean values.

therefore dependent on a low pressure system and the hepatic microcirculation is very sensitive to small increases in pressure in the hepatic venous outflow. Anaesthetic drugs and ventilation techniques reduce hepatic blood flow by reducing both portal venous blood flow and cardiac output so that hepatic artery flow also decreases and therefore cannot compensate by autoregulation for the decrease in portal flow.

Effect of surgery

Abdominal surgery can reduce liver blood flow more than the effect of anaesthetic drugs by surgical pressure on the portal system and the release of hormones, especially catecholamines, which cause hepatic artery vasoconstriction.

Effects of drugs

The effects of anaesthetic agents on liver blood flow can only therefore be studied without surgery using non-invasive methods. Dilatation of splanchnic vessels, such as occurs with isoflurane and desflurane, may partially improve the detrimental effects of surgery. No changes in hepatic blood flow were detected before surgery when fentanyl, 50 μg, was given epidurally.

Effects of ventilation

Blood flow may not be as important as oxygen supply. In humans, before surgery, hepatic blood flow and hepatic vein oxygen saturation were maintained with isoflurane and nitrous oxide anaesthesia despite significant reductions in cardiac output. When ventilation was maintained constant in anaes-

Table 16.1 Functions of the liver

Function	Major areas of activity	Examples
metabolic	carbohydrate	gluconeogenesis
	protein	deamination
		formation of urea
		synthesis of plasma proteins
		interconversions of amino acids
	fat	oxidation of fatty acids
		synthesis of lipoproteins, cholesterol and phospholipids
		conversion of proteins and carbohydrates into fats
	coagulation factors	fibrinogen
		vitamin K dependent: factors II, VII, IX, X and protein C
		non-vitamin K dependent except factor VIII
	toxins	drug metabolism and detoxification
storage	vitamins	
	iron	
	glycogen	
excretion	bilirubin and bile salts,	
	hormones	thyroxine
		steroid hormones: oestrogen, cortisol, aldosterone
blood reservoir of about 0.5 l phagocytosis	macrophages	remove bacteria from the blood

thetized animals, mild hypocapnia decreased hepatic artery blood flow, whereas hypercapnia caused a significant increase in cardiac output and portal vein blood flow.

FUNCTIONS OF THE LIVER

The functions of the liver are summarized in Table 16.1. The hepatocytes synthesize and store nutrients and metabolize substrates for energy and excretion. Bile production and excretion takes place in the reticuloendothelial cells and bile ducts.

METABOLIC FUNCTIONS IN THE ACINUS

The hepatocytes within an acinus are arranged in sheets of cells with functional zones (Figure 16.1). Zone 1 is adjacent to the afferent vessels with well oxygenated blood which has a high nutrient content from the gut and is used for gluconeogenesis. Zone 3 is the peripheral area adjacent to the efferent vein, and suffers most from injury whether viral, toxic or hypoxic. Zone 2 is intermediate and lies between.

BILE

Haemoglobin and haem proteins are broken down to liberate haem. Bilirubin is the end product of haem metabolism. Unconjugated bilirubin is lipid soluble and is transported in the plasma bound to albumin. The amount of drugs bound to albumin may therefore be influenced by increases in the concentration of unconjugated bilirubin. The latter is converted to a water soluble compound by conjugation; there is a deficiency of enzymes responsible for this process in Gilbert's syndrome and sometimes in neonates.

Bile acids are only synthesized in the liver. They are formed from cholesterol and are conjugated in the liver with amino acids. Conjugated bilirubin, bile salts, cholesterol, phospholipids, proteins, electrolytes and water are secreted by the liver cells into the bile cannaliculi. Water follows the osmotically active bile salts. Bile is released into the duodenum and that which reaches the colon is reduced by bacteria to urobilinogens.

The bile salts are absorbed in the terminal ileum and recirculated through the liver. They help to emulsify dietary fat and decreased secretion leads to steatorrhoea. Under these circumstances there is a failure to absorb the fat soluble vitamins: vitamin K (required for the production of clotting factors II (prothrombin), VII, IX, X and the fibrinolytic protein C); vitamin D and calcium, which in the long term can lead to osteomalacia; vitamin A; and vitamin E. Disturbance of bile flow at any level leads to cholestasis with jaundice, pruritis and steatorrhoea.

DRUG METABOLISM

Orally administered drugs are absorbed from the gastrointestinal tract to a greater or lesser extent, pass in the portal venous system to the liver and are metabolized to varying degrees before reaching the systemic circulation. This is first pass metabolism.

Many drugs cannot be excreted intact by the kidneys because they are highly lipid soluble. Their elimination depends on one or more processes to make them more polar and thus more water soluble for excretion by the kidneys. These are known as phase 1 or 2 biotransformations which are mainly inactivation processes. Phase 1 reactions tend to lead to the production of reactive metabolites, whereas phase 2 reactions produce more hydrophilic compounds ready for excretion. Many products of hepatic metabolism are eliminated by the kidneys. If the metabolites are biologically active there is a risk of hepatic or renal toxicity.

The main drug metabolizing enzyme systems for phase 1 processes are in the microsomal fraction of the liver where oxidation (that is, the loss of an electron), reduction and hydroxylation reactions can occur and cytochrome enzymes such as the haem P450 system are located. The drug metabolizing enzymes are present in greater amounts in zone 3 and enzyme induction also occurs here. Enzyme inducers such as barbiturates, other anticonvulsants and alcohol enhance drug metabolism and may increase the toxicity of drugs with toxic metabolites, e.g. the defluorination of fluorinated inhalational anaesthetics. Single doses of barbiturates do not cause enzyme induction. Alternative reactions include the conversion of alcohol to acetaldehyde by cytosolic enzymes and cleavage of the drug molecule by non-enzymatic reactions.

Phase 2 biotransformations involve conjugation of the drug or metabolite with other molecules. The enzymes for these reactions are present in high concentrations in the liver. However, there is evidence for the extra-hepatic glucuronidation of drugs such as midazolam, morphine and propofol, especially when liver enzyme function fails.

The hepatic porphyrias are characterized by abnormalities of haem biosynthesis. The enzyme δ-aminolaevulinic acid (ALA) synthase is increased so that an excess of ALA and subsequently porphyrins, are formed. The mechanism by which some drugs precipitate an acute attack of porphyria may involve an increase in ALA synthase activity. These drugs include barbiturates, benzodiazepines and NSAID analgesics.

There are large differences among patients in the ability to metabolize drugs or other compounds. This heterogeneity is largely the result of genetic factors. It can be considered that each patient has a unique liver enzyme profile which may not be constant but can be utilized to metabolize a wide range of compounds with the same enzyme systems.

TESTS OF LIVER FUNCTION

Normal values for liver enzyme and synthetic function are shown in Table 16.2. In chronic liver disease minimum alterations may be present. A variety of plasma proteins are synthesized. Albumin, although commonly measured, has a half-life of 22 days so it is not

Table 16.2 Normal values of liver function tests

	Normal value[a]	Comment
Tests for cholestasis		
Serum		
Bilirubin		
total	5–17 μmol l^{-1}	>20 μmol l^{-1} for jaundice
conjugated	<5 μmol l^{-1}	not normally present
Alkaline phosphatase	35–130 units l^{-1}	
Gamma-glutamyl		
transpeptidase (γ-GT)	10–48 units l^{-1}	
Urine		
Bilirubin	none	present in cholestasis
Tests for hepatocellular function		
Serum		
Transaminases		
aspartate (AST/SGOT)	5–40 units l^{-1}	also from heart, muscle
alanine (ALT/SGPT)	5–35 units l^{-1}	more specific to liver
Albumin	35–50 g l^{-1}	
Prothrombin time	12–16 s	
Urine		
Urobilinogen	+	increased in hepatocellular failure

[a] normal laboratory range may vary

reduced in acute liver failure. Fibrinogen (normal value 2–6 g l^{-1}), prothrombin (factor II), and acute phase proteins provide a more acute picture of loss of liver synthetic function.

Viral infections cause an early increase in transaminases and can be detected with specific viral antibody tests. Mitochondrial antibody is increased in primary biliary cirrhosis. Pre-hepatic disorders such as haemolysis and Gilbert's syndrome are manifest by increased conjugated bilirubin.

The diagnosis of liver cysts and tumours, and work up for definitive surgery includes ultrasound, CT scan and angiography.

EFFECTS OF DISORDERED LIVER FUNCTION

COAGULATION ABNORMALITIES

Qualitative or quantitative coagulation abnormalities are common as the result of a number of factors: reduced synthesis of blood clotting factors, both vitamin K and non-vitamin K dependent and fibrinogen; a reduced life of coagulation factors because of disseminated intravascular coagulation or variceal bleeding; and hypersplenism and reduced bone marrow function which cause thrombocytopenia.

Coagulation must be restored to the optimum condition preoperatively. Vitamin K can be given parenterally but if time is short, fresh-frozen plasma will provide factors II, V, VII, and IX, cryoprecipitate and fibrinogen. Preoperative intramuscular injections should be avoided in patients with impaired coagulation.

The safe limits for invasive procedures are: a prothrombin time of <17 s and platelets >80 × 10^{-9} l^{-1}.

CARDIOPULMONARY DISORDERS

Arteriovenous shunts can be cutaneous or intrapulmonary. They reduce the systemic and pulmonary vascular resistance and increase the heart rate, plasma volume and cardiac output leading to a hyperdynamic circulation. If severe, cardiac failure and hypoxaemia can result.

Pulmonary complications with arterial hypoxaemia are common and are of various aetiologies: intrapulmonary shunts; ventilation/perfusion mismatch; restrictive defects associated with ascites, hepatomegaly and pleural effusions; and alveolar diffusion defects. In addition, smoking is often associated with alcoholism and chronic obstructive airway disease can be present. Particular attention should be given to the careful use of theophylline derivatives in cirrhosis because their clearance is reduced and cardiac toxicity is potentially dangerous.

PORTAL HYPERTENSION

When there is portal venous obstruction, the pressure in the portal system will increase from the normal pressure range of about 4–9 mmHg. Above pressures of 20 mmHg, collateral vessels open. Compensatory mechanisms, which are not fully understood, develop to maintain liver blood flow. Vasodilatation occurs and the circulation becomes hyperdynamic. At a threshold portal vein pressure, the collateral circulation opens systemic connections at the following places: in the gastrointestinal tract epithelium when it changes from being protective to absorptive, that is at the cardia of the stomach and the anus (varices form in these areas); at the umbilicus where clinically a 'caput Medusae' is observed on the abdominal wall with blood flowing away from the umbilicus (these enlarged vessels can cause bleeding when the surgeon enters the abdomen); retroperitoneal structures in the splenic, renal and lumbar tissues. Splenomegaly is usually present as a result of which platelets will be sequestered and red blood cell survival reduced. There is an increased incidence of gastric ulceration in these patients and prophylactic gastric acid suppression is required.

Collateral blood flow from the portal system passes through the epidural space and dilated epidural veins may be traumatized. Epidural analgesia is contraindicated in portal hypertension because of the potential for blood vessel trauma and bleeding from a coagulopathy.

ASCITES

Ascites complicates cirrhosis because raised portal pressure increases lymph pressure. There is a reduction in serum albumin and hence in the plasma oncotic pressure and there is dilutional hyponatraemia (about 130 mmol l^{-1}) despite marked sodium retention.

Spironolactone, a potassium sparing diuretic, is the treatment of choice for this condition. Ascites should be drained slowly. If the abdomen is opened quickly, fluid will be lost rapidly. Pressure effects on the mesenteric vessels will diminish and vasodilation with loss of blood volume and hypotension quickly follows. Controlled drainage will prevent this, together with appropriate blood volume replacement. Ascites will also have pressure effects on the lungs and stomach. Preoperative drainage may help to relieve hypoxaemia. A rapid sequence induction of anaesthesia should be used with precautions against regurgitation of stomach contents.

RENAL FUNCTION

It must always be assumed that there is altered renal tubular function in cirrhosis. Water and sodium retention are the result of decreased glomerular filtration, increased renin–angiotensin activity and decreased antidiuretic hormone activity. The water retention is greater than sodium so the disorder manifests as hyponatraemia. Hyperaldosteronism and diuretic therapy enhance potassium loss and there is an associated alkalosis. Diuretic therapy may also precipitate hypovolaemia and oliguric renal failure which is reversible after diuretic withdrawal and fluid replacement.

Renal function may be disturbed during hepatobiliary surgery because of physiological disturbances which include massive haemorrhage and subsequent vasoconstriction and the need to clamp abdominal blood vessels such as the inferior vena cava during a hepatic resection, with consequent obstruction to the renal veins. In addition to these problems, the preoperative state of hepatic function will also affect renal function. Abnormalities of hepatic function in Wilson's disease and polycystic disease are also associated with renal disease. Renal toxicity from drugs such as aminoglycosides and NSAID analgesics increases in cirrhosis.

There is a direct correlation between the elevation of bilirubin concentration and the risk of acute tubular necrosis following surgery. Hypotension, sepsis and shock can complicate surgical intervention and can contribute to renal dysfunction. Renal failure can follow cholestasis because steatorrhoea allows the overgrowth of bacterial pathogens which produce toxic products. These effects can be reduced by prescribing oral bile salts (sodium taurocholate) to maintain normal bowel flora.

The hepatorenal syndrome describes oliguric renal failure associated with liver disease. In spite of a reduced systemic vascular resistance, intrarenal vascular resistances are increased. This is probably the consequence of the activation of systemic vasoactive factors and increased intrarenal vasoconstrictors such as leukotrienes, thromboxanes and endothelins. The balance between renal vasodilation with prostaglandins and kallikreins and vasoconstriction is lost. The differential diagnoses are hypovolaemia, causing prerenal uraemia, or acute tubular necrosis. Correcting fluid and haemodynamic abnormalities will differentiate hypovolaemia from other diagnoses of uraemia. Urine sodium is negligible (<10 mmol l^{-1}) in the hepatorenal syndrome whereas it increases in acute tubular necrosis. The hepatorenal syndrome is characterized by a high urine: plasma creatinine ratio.

EFFECTS ON DRUGS

Metabolism

When the liver can almost completely remove a drug in minutes by metabolism and biliary excretion that drug has a high extraction ratio (ER). If all the drug is extracted, then ER = 1. The extraction ratio depends on the concentration of the drug entering the liver and that extracted. It does not quantify the overall amount of drug removed. It is the clearance of the drug which measures the volume of blood from which the drug has been eliminated per unit time. If the extraction ratio is high and the intrinsic clearance is equivalent to hepatic blood flow then the drug will be almost entirely removed after entering the hepatic circulation. Drugs in this category are said to have flow-limited metabolism. These drugs include lignocaine, propofol, propranolol and opioids. The formation of lignocaine metabolites has been used as an assessment of liver function. Indocyanine green also has these characteristics and its clearance has been used to measure liver blood flow.

Poorly extracted drugs such as diazepam, thiopentone and warfarin are unaffected by changes in hepatic blood flow and their elimination is dependent on the capacity of the drug-metabolizing enzymes to remove them; clearance may be increased by enzyme induction and large changes in clearance may occur if variations in bound fraction of the drug occur. A drug that is capacity limited may be highly protein bound e.g. warfarin (binding sensitive) or have a low plasma binding, e.g. barbiturates. Some patients with liver disease have an altered end-organ sensitivity to benzodiazepines or barbiturates which, again,

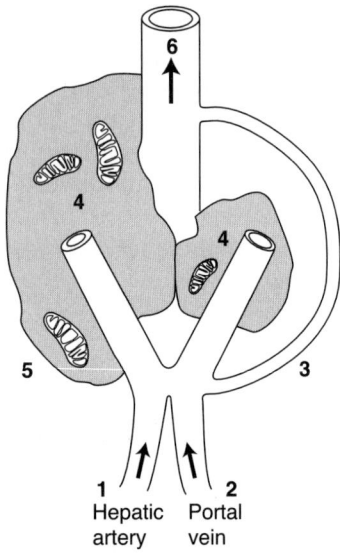

Figure 16.3 Liver disease and drugs. Changes in cardiac output, **1**, can affect blood flow to the liver, gut and other organs where drug absorption, excretion and site of action occur. These changes may be caused by liver cell failure, drugs or other diseases. Portal venous flow, **2**, carries drugs from the gastrointestinal tract. If this blood is shunted, **3**, bypass of the normal metabolic process occurs. Liver cell mass, **4**, can be reduced in the elderly or as part of the disease process. Enzyme synthesis or metabolic reactions can be increased or decreased, **5**, and this can alter drug binding to albumin or other liver proteins. Phase 1 is affected more than phase 2. Alterations in tissue and protein binding and retention of sodium and water change the volume of distribution. **6**, represents hepatic venous drainage.

makes it difficult to predict effect. The pharmacokinetics of drugs such as lorazepam and morphine appear to be relatively normal in patients with liver disease because they undergo glucuronidation, but the increased end-organ sensitivity increases their risk potential.

Drugs and hepatic disorders interact in various ways. These are summarized in Figure 16.3. If liver failure is severe, reductions in drug dosages are necessary to compensate for reductions in both liver and renal clearance.

Alcohol is a substance which can induce an acute increase in toxic metabolites from drugs under normal circumstances and also pancreatic and liver disease in the longer term. Chronic pancreatitis with acute episodes or liver cirrhosis are common complications of chronic alcohol use. There are a number of mechanisms proposed for alcoholic liver injury. Acetaldehyde, a metabolite, is extremely reactive and toxic. Fatty liver can develop as well as fibrosis. Acute alcohol hepatitis is rare.

The choice of anaesthetic agent is important because alterations in hepatic blood flow occur or metabolic products may be toxic and hepatocellular function can deteriorate as the result of anaesthesia and surgery. Isoflurane does not influence liver enzyme activity in contrast to halothane. Halothane reduces hepatic blood flow and inhibits phase 1 enzymes so that drugs such as fentanyl and lignocaine have a prolonged half-life.

Drug distribution

The volume of distribution of a drug is influenced by many factors including protein binding and the size of the fluid compartment. The greatest effect is seen on compounds which are normally highly protein bound and have a small volume of distribution, but effects can be unpredictable. Usually muscle relaxants which are not highly protein bound but are distributed in a large fluid compartment require a larger initial dose in hepatocellular failure. The synthetic opioids, fentanyl and sufentanil have virtually unchanged kinetics in hepatic failure, but alfentanil, with a volume of distribution about ten times less that of fentanyl, is more likely to be affected by an increase in the volume of distribution, such as occurs in ascites.

Recovery times after sedative drugs are prolonged in cirrhotic subjects. Propofol infusions have this effect. Benzodiazepines have an increased volume of distribution because of a decrease in protein available for binding and a decrease in drug clearance.

ANAESTHETIC MANAGEMENT

GENERAL MANAGEMENT OF ANAESTHETIC PROBLEMS

Precautions to prevent transmission of hepatitis are described in Chapter 34. In the presence of acute hepatitis, surgery should be delayed to avoid any further reduction of hepatic function by anaesthesia or surgery. Liver disease is frequently asymptomatic, but has widespread effects on various systems of the body. Table 16.3 summarizes the characteristics of liver and pancreatic disease which may be manifest on preoperative assessment.

The preoperative laboratory investigations which are required before major hepatobiliary surgery include: full blood count including

Table 16.3 Clinical signs and symptoms characteristic of liver and pancreatic disease

	Liver	Pancreas
History	Alcohol	Alcohol
	Smoking	Smoking
	Jaundice[a]	Jaundice
	Hepatitis	Pain
	Encephalopathy[a]	
Examination	Fever (hepatitis, septicaemia)	Fever (cholangitis)
	Cutaneous spider naevi clubbing palmar erythema	Poor nutrition
	Cardiovascular hyperdynamic	
	Bruising/ haemorrhage[a]	
	Fluid retention/ ascites[a]	
	Hypoxaemia/ cyanosis	
	Gynaecomastia	

[a]signs of portal hypertension

platelets; blood grouping and crossmatch; urea, creatinine and electrolytes; clotting screen; liver function tests; glucose; urine analysis; viral hepatitis screen; chest X-ray; electrocardiogram; and further lung function tests where appropriate (e.g. smokers, pulmonary complications) such as lung volumes, arterial blood gases and acid–base status. Hypovolaemia can also occur with sepsis in the perioperative patient. It is usual to treat preoperative infections with antibiotics intravenously and all surgery is covered by prophylactic antibiotics at induction of anaesthesia.

It is usual to pass a nasogastric tube for perioperative and postoperative stomach drainage.

RISK ASSESSMENT

Portal hypertension should be considered in all hepatobiliary cases even if cirrhosis or ascites is not present. The main causes of cirrhosis are alcohol and viral infections. The associated surgical risks are infection, bleeding, renal failure and hepatic failure and encephalopathy. Mortality significantly increases with the severity of liver damage (Chapter 27). Haemorrhage during surgery is the prime cause of mortality in severe disease. If liver resection is required the liver cell mass remaining may be inadequate. Renal and hepatic failure postoperatively are the major causes of mortality. Common operations for patients with cirrhosis include sclerotherapy for bleeding oesophageal varices, gynaecological surgery, general surgery, laparoscopy and inguinal hernia repair.

INDUCTION AND MAINTENANCE OF ANAESTHESIA

Maintenance of liver blood flow and oxygenation are major goals during hepatobiliary surgery. There are not many factors which increase blood supply. Severe hypoxia increases hepatic artery flow but will not pro-

Table 16.4 Causes of decreased hepatic blood flow

Sympathetic stimulation
Hypotension (reduced venous return/cardiac output) caused by
  haemorrhage
  cardiac depressant drugs
  regional anaesthesia, e.g. thoracic epidural analgesia
  IPPV and PEEP
Hypocapnia
Pressure effects caused by
  surgical retraction
  tumours
  ascites/laparoscopy

vide oxygenation. It is therefore important to minimize known causes of decreased hepatic blood flow. These are shown in Table 16.4.

These effects are minimized by maintaining cardiac output and hepatic perfusion pressure, normocarbia and by the appropriate choice of inhalational agent and fluid management. Isoflurane has been the volatile agent of choice because it has the least depressant effect on hepatic artery and portal vein flow when compared with halothane and enflurane. Isoflurane and sevoflurane maintain hepatic artery blood flow in the chronically instrumented dog and hepatic oxygen extraction does not change at <2 MAC. All inhalational anaesthetics reduce portal venous flow and their effects are reversible.

Pressure effects on the lungs from surgical retraction may require a positive end-expiratory pressure (PEEP) to maintain oxygenation. The increase in intrathoracic pressure will impede venous return and should only be used if indicated by a reduction in oxygen saturation. PEEP may also be useful in minimizing the risk of air embolism during dissection around the hepatic veins.

The choice of inhalational agent will depend on cardiovascular effects and drug metabolism. The proposed mechanism for liver injury following halothane anaesthesia is a drug metabolite acting as a hapten when covalently bound to a cell protein and inducing immunological liver injury. The drug metabolite is trifluoroacetate, which is also formed during the metabolism of enflurane and isoflurane. There is the potential for cross-sensitization to other halogenated anaesthetics such as desflurane. The degree of metabolism of these agents is much less than that of halothane so the risk potential for hepatotoxicity is minimized. Sevoflurane has a totally different structure based on hexafluoroisopropanol, such that the fluorine is liable to extensive metabolism and hexafluoroisopropanol is rapidly glucuronidated so that its capacity for toxic reactions is limited. Compared with halothane, 3% rather than 20% is metabolized, so that its potential for toxicity is much less.

Neuromuscular blocking drugs

Cholinesterase is synthesized in the liver. Suxamethonium and mivacurium are metabolized by this enzyme and will have a prolonged action in severe hepatic failure. Suxamethonium is not affected by alterations in volume of distribution and should be used when indicated for rapid sequence induction.

Onset of non-depolarizing drugs may be delayed and larger doses required because of an increase in the volume of distribution. Elimination of pancuronium and vecuronium are mainly hepatic and their duration of action can be prolonged. Atracurium is the preferred neuromuscular blocking drug in hepatic failure because it is destroyed by Hofmann elimination and so its duration of action is independant of liver function. The pharmacokinetics of its main metabolite, laudanosine, are also unchanged. Neuromuscular function should be monitored throughout the operative period and reversal also confirmed by the clinical sign of a head lift for >5 s. If postoperative ventilation is planned, these considerations may be less important.

MONITORING

Routine monitoring includes the ECG, oxygen saturation, end-tidal carbon dioxide concentration, ventilator alarms, inhalational agent concentration, core body temperature (e.g. oesophageal) and neuromuscular function.

For major hepatic and pancreatic surgery, continuous central venous pressure and invasive arterial pressure monitoring are required. Urine output should be measured half-hourly and arterial blood gases, pH, serum $[K^+]$, haematocrit and glucose hourly, unless values are abnormal and require more frequent monitoring. Careful assessment of blood loss from swabs, suction or other routes must be made at least half-hourly and a complete record of fluid replacement kept. A coagulation screen and platelet count should be performed when indicated either by preoperative abnormalities or by blood loss. Cardiac output must be maintained by reference to haemodynamic parameters, but its direct measurement is rarely indicated.

RENAL FUNCTION (Table 16.5)

Prevention of postoperative renal dysfunction begins preoperatively and continues during surgery. Hyponatraemia and hypokalaemia should be corrected before surgery if necessary. Correction of hyponatraemia with diuretics and/or dopamine will require haemodynamic monitoring.

Cardiac output must be maintained and adequate fluids administered. Continuous monitoring of cardiovascular function and urine output with invasive arterial and central venous lines is necessary and the ability to maintain cardiac output despite fast loss of blood. Good surgical technique can also help to meet these goals.

Half-hourly urine volume will monitor both renal function and, indirectly, cardiac output. The output should not decrease below 20–30 ml per 30 min. This is more than required in critical care to prevent renal failure, but much can happen to blood volume in

Table 16.5 Summary of methods for maintaining renal function[a]

Generally (to avoid renal drug toxicity)
  avoid NSAID and nephrotoxic antibiotics, e.g. aminoglycosides
Preoperatively (to reduce the occurrence of the hepatorenal syndrome)
  in obstructive jaundice give bile salts to normalize gut flora
  reduce hyperbilirubinaemia with drainage stent
Intraoperatively
  avoid hypotension and hypoxaemia
  maintain urine output
  avoid infection with prophylactic antiobiotics; it can precipitate sepsis and renal failure
  use fluids with monitoring of cardiovascular function, osmolality and serum electrolytes
  monitor haemotocrit to manage replacement of fluid and blood

[a]In future agents may be available to block endotoxins, thromboxanes and leukotrienes

half an hour during hepatobiliary surgery. If major blood loss occurs after a period of oliguria and is not fully corrected, a significant time of poor flow to the kidney may occur. If oliguria persists after filling pressures are adequate, a small dose of a diuretic such as frusemide, 2 mg, can be given intravenously. The dose can be increased incrementally if no response is observed. Dopamine, starting with a dose of 2–3 mg kg^{-1} min^{-1}, may be indicated, especially in older patients who may also require an inotropic effect. Patients with cirrhosis with a high cardiac output will not require dopamine. Inotropic support may be required following massive haemorrhage.

MAINTENANCE OF BODY TEMPERATURE

Heat loss can occur with prolonged surgery, infusion of cold fluids, reduced liver metabolism and a large area of surgical exposure. It also occurs during laparoscopic surgery because large flows of dry, cold gases are insufflated. Core temperature must be monitored. Passive methods of maintaining heat, such as drapes, wraps, and heat and moisture exchangers, can help to prevent evaporative, convective and radiant heat losses. These should be supplemented with active warming methods, with a warm environment around the patient (such as a warm operating theatre and/or warming blankets) and warmed infusions to allow maintenance of normal body temperature.

HAEMORRHAGE

Major haemorrhage is to be expected during hepatic and pancreatic surgery although the speed at which blood is lost during resections corresponds with the blood flow to the organ involved.

Facilities must be available for rapid pressurized infusion to maintain the cardiac output. Such blood infusors need wide bore tubing into the patient, and methods to warm the fluid to body temperature whatever the rate of infusion. When blood or fluids are pressurized, care must be taken not to let air enter the circulation. Autologous blood can be used except if there is infection or malignancy, which excludes many hepatic operations. Red blood cell suspensions are commonly available and colloid replacement is necessary. Human albumin solution is pasteurized and can be used in quantity. Synthetic colloids can be used initially to replace 1–2 l losses. Fresh frozen plasma may be necessary to replace clotting factors but it has a potential for viral transmission. Venous access is provided by large (13–8 G) peripheral lines in the upper body and a multiple lumen infusion line centrally in the internal jugular vein. Another large line is usually sited centrally for major transfusion.

Measurement of blood loss should be recorded in the operating theatre for both swab loss (weighing method, 1 g=1 ml) and suction loss (at 100 ml intervals). Clinically, central venous pressure measurements may not be helpful at times because of surgical traction. Continuous pulse rate, oxygen saturation and blood pressure monitoring are essential to detect early signs of shock with hypotension and tachycardia. An end-tidal carbon dioxide trace may show a reduction when cardiac output decreases. During major blood loss, continuous monitoring of the electrocardiogram and core body temperature are necessary to detect arrhythmias and hypothermia. Regular investigative procedures during haemorrhage include measurement of arterial blood gases and pH for adequacy of ventilation and the detection of metabolic acidosis, electrolytes such as potassium and ionized calcium and the haematocrit, platelet count and clotting screen for confirmation of the adequacy of blood replacement (see Chapter 41 for assessment of clotting abnormalities). In addition, cardiac output and pulmonary artery wedge pressures may also be required for assessment if cardiac function deteriorates.

Aprotonin has been shown to reduce the requirements of blood and blood products in liver transplantation, but its efficacy and risk of inducing morbidity or mortality as a result of excess clot formation has not been studied for major haemorrhage during surgery.

POSTOPERATIVE CARE

After prolonged major surgery and transfer from the operating theatre to a high dependancy or intensive care unit, continuous monitoring, especially of cardiovascular, respiratory and renal function, is required and maintenance of fluid balance. When a central venous pressure line has been inserted a chest X-ray should confirm its position and other abnormalities sought. Intensive therapy will be required if there has been massive haemorrhage during surgery, if postoperative ventilation is required or if there is cardiovascular instability.

Transient abnormalities of liver function are common after operation and associated with upper abdominal surgery, blood transfusion, sepsis and cardiovascular instability. When

Table 16.6 Causes of postoperative jaundice

Preoperative	Perioperative	Postoperative
Genetic (Gilbert's)[a]	Transfusion	Transfusion[c]
Viral hepatitis	Haematoma	Haematoma
Drugs	Haemolysis[a]	Haemolysis[a]
Alcohol	Sepsis[b]	Sepsis[b]
Previous anaesthetics	Hypovolaemia	Hypovolaemia
	Biliary surgery	Biliary surgery
	Hypoxia	Hypoxia
	Hypotension	Hypotension
	Anaesthetic agents[d]	Pancreatitis
		Non-anaesthetic drugs

[a]unconjugated
[b]fever
[c]viral studies for cytomegalovirus and other blood borne viral infections
[d]assay for antibody titre to trifluoroacetic acid if indicated

hepatic function is abnormal, signs of encephalopathy require early management.

Pain relief after upper abdominal surgery necessitates either thoracic epidural analgesia with low dose local anaesthetic and opioids or patient-controlled analgesia. Epidural opioids cause minimal changes in hepatic blood flow. Hypotension must be avoided when local anaesthetics are used. Adequate analgesia is required to allow good diaphragmatic excursion and coughing.

Causes of postoperative jaundice

These are listed in Table 16.6, and require full investigation and appropriate treatment.

ANAESTHETIC REQUIREMENTS IN SPECIFIC SURGICAL PROCEDURES

Surgery in patients with hepatobiliary disease may be coincidental or required to treat complications of the disease process.

OPEN CHOLECYSTECTOMY

An open cholecystectomy for uncomplicated gall stones has <1% mortality. This increases with sepsis, liver disease, emergency surgery and stones in the common bile duct. Laparoscopy can reduce postoperative morbidity but has perioperative morbidity (Chapter 28). Conversion from laparoscopic to open cholecystectomy occurs in about 5–10% of patients. The general condition of the patient and the need for rapid recovery will determine the choice of anaesthesia. Provision of anaesthesia requires attention to the following:

- assess abnormalities of liver function,
- in obstructive jaundice: treat clotting defects, prevent renal failure,
- choice of narcotics: biliary pressures increase with fentanyl (by 23%) and morphine (by 100%) from control; naloxone reverses these effects,
- blood loss, this is rare but may be concealed,
- vagal reflex stimulation can induce bradycardia,
- hazards of perioperative X-rays,
- prevent postoperative nausea and vomiting.

BILE DUCT OBSTRUCTION

Cholestasis is commonly caused by extrahepatic obstruction to the biliary system. Intrahepatic causes are from hepatocellular reasons such as hepatitis, infection, drugs and hormones. Mechanical obstruction in the biliary tract may present with pain in the right upper quadrant of the abdomen, classically in gall stone obstruction, but obstruction from carcinoma of the pancreas is usually painless. Fever may accompany both pathologies as a result of cholangitis. Extrahepatic obstruction can be relieved by stenting and this prevents most of the complications which follow hyperbilirubinaemia.

When obstructive jaundice presents as a result of malignancy, surgical excision is the only hope of long-term survival. High bile duct obstruction may require the formation of a hepaticodochojejunostomy. A low bile duct obstruction would require a pancreatectomy. Intestinal bypass surgery and pain control with percutaneous coeliac plexus blockade are palliative methods.

LIVER RESECTION

Elective

Metastatic deposits are the most common hepatic tumours, particularly from malignancies in the large bowel. A hepatoma may be associated with hepatitis B or C viral infection. Tumours of the biliary tract also occur and their removal may require both hepatic and biliary tract resection. Small tumours may be removed by wide local resection but most will require a number of liver segments to be removed. Air embolism can complicate dissection around the porta hepatis and can be minimized by avoiding nitrous oxide.

Occasionally, in order to provide adequate surgical access, a transthoracic approach may be used. Trauma may occur to the diaphragm and a chest drain should be inserted to maintain inflation, with a non-return valve to exclude air. Hepatic regeneration occurs at 50–110 g day^{-1}.

Emergency

Trauma to the liver may be blunt, leading to splits and tears from shearing forces, or direct, causing contusion and disruption. The main effects are injuries to the liver cells rather than to the major vessels. The possibility for other organ damage in the same area (spleen, intestines, lungs and kidneys) or other injury is very high. Emergency surgery is usually indicated and preparations to manage a full stomach must be made. In the majority of cases, a hepatic segmentectomy will be required and the patient should be transferred immediately to a specialized unit for this type of surgery. Ultrasound and angiography are usually necessary. Coagulopathy may accompany a large subcapsular haematoma, and major blood loss should be anticipated and prepared for before surgery, with red blood cells and blood products available.

The patient must be adequately resuscitated preoperatively. Blood loss, from direct sources and coagulopathies, is the main cause of mortality. After operation infections occur and packing the wound will increase the mortality from this cause. Appropriate antibiotics must be given intravenously.

SURGERY FOR PORTAL HYPERTENSION

Oesophageal varices are formed by the increase in flow through the gastric vein into the azygos veins when there is portal hypertension. The vessel walls are fragile so that bleeding occurs easily, especially if ulceration occurs. Prophylactic gastric acid suppression is routine. The bleeding presents either as haematemesis or melaena and blood loss can further reduce liver blood flow. Mortality from emergency surgery is high, at about 30%. It follows massive blood loss from acute bleeding, or encephalopathy, renal failure or coagulopathy after prolonged bleeding. It is therefore preferable to treat the condition electively. The long-term prognosis depends on the underlying liver function.

Management of variceal haemorrhage

Immediate treatment comprises resuscitation, monitoring and stopping the haemorrhage

Central venous access is required to replace and monitor blood loss which is not easily measured directly. When placing a central venous line, a coagulopathy may need to be treated first with fresh frozen plasma and platelets as indicated. Other fluids are also required, mainly colloids and blood; sodium containing solutions should be used with caution. Overtransfusion will increase portal pressure and increase bleeding. Central venous pressure must be closely monitored and if there is heart disease, the patient is elderly or haemodynamically unstable, a pulmonary artery catheter should be used to measure cardiac output. In addition a urinary catheter must be sited and urine output measured every hour on the ward or every half hour in the operating theatre. A nasogastric tube does not increase bleeding and may prevent aspiration, reduce the incidence of vomiting, allow some measure of blood loss and prevent blood from entering the intestines thus preventing encephalopathic deterioration.

Balloon tamponade is an effective, temporary measure to stop bleeding. Topical anaesthesia can be used to pass a Sengstacken–Blakemore tube orally while the patient is awake. The gastric balloon is used to exert compression for up to 24 h while other measures such as drugs to reduce portal pressure (vasopressin and somatostatin with their synthetic analogues, terlipressin and octreotide respectively), and surgical and endoscopic interventions are planned.

Endoscopy with banding or sclerotherapy is usually carried out under sedation. Close monitoring, however, will be necessary, and sometimes general anaesthesia is required if there is lack of patient cooperation. These procedures do not reduce portal hypertension. More definitive surgery is needed for this with either a portocaval shunt or transplantation. If bleeding is not controlled, transjugular intrahepatic portosystemic stent shunts are indicated. The complications with this intervention are similar to other shunt procedures which reduce portal pressure but can increase encephalopathy.

PANCREATECTOMY FOR CHRONIC PANCREATITIS

Pain is characteristic of chronic pancreatitis, which is a progressive inflammatory disease of the pancreas with deterioration of exocrine and endocrine functions. Pain usually appears within an hour after a meal and for this reason patients tend to reduce their oral intake and lose weight. Pain assessment is often difficult because patients can be addicted to alcohol, have unstable personalities and can also be addicted to narcotics.

Pancreatic resection provides pain relief by removing diseased tissue and reducing pancreatic duct pressure. The following operations have been performed to relieve pain and preserve function.

Pylorus preserving pancreaticoduodenectomy/partial pancreatectomy

This preserves gastric function and avoids the nutritional disturbances of a Whipple's procedure. If a partial pancreatectomy is indicated, pancreatic function is usually preserved as well. Three anastomoses are made following dissection and removal of tissues: the stomach with the ileum, the bile duct and the pancreatic duct into the end of the proximal stump.

Total pancreatectomy

This will necessitate insulin replacement in the postoperative period, unless disease progression has destroyed pancreatic function preoperatively, which is rare.

Distal pancreatectomy

This procedure does not involve the bile or pancreatic ducts. A splenectomy is usually required because of the blood supply to the region.

After operation patients with regular opioid usage before surgery will require about twice the normal opioid dosage together with more anxiolytics. Higher pain scores are to be expected but side effects will be fewer, except for sedation.

Table 16.7 Rare diseases of the hepatobiliary system and their expected complications

Diseases	Complications
Hydatid cysts (tapeworm cyst from dogs)	Anaphylaxis
Wilson's disease (copper deposition)	Renal and neurological dysfunction
Hepatic porphyria	Vomiting, abdominal pain, peripheral neuropathy (exacerbated by barbiturates, oestrogens and sulphonamides)

RARE CONDITIONS

Anaesthetists should be aware of rare diseases such as hydatid cysts, Wilson's disease and porphyria which can present with acute or chronic life-threatening complications. These are summarized in Table 16.7.

FURTHER READING

Frink, E. J., Morgan, S. E., Coetzee, A., Conzen, P. F. and Brown, B. R. (1992) The effects of sevoflurane, halothane, enflurane, and isoflurane on hepatic blood flow and oxygenation in chronically instrumentalised greyhound dogs. *Anesthesiology*, **76**, 85–90.

Gelman, S., Fowler, K. C., and Smith, L. R., (1984) Liver circulation and function during isoflurane and halothane anaesthesia. *Anesthesiology*, **61**, 726–730.

Goldfarb, G., Debaene, B., Ang, E. T., Roulot, D., Jolis, P. and Lebrec, D. (1990) Hepatic blood flow in humans during isoflurane–N_2O and halothane–N_2O anesthesia. *Anesthesia and Analgesia*, **71**, 349–353.

Kirsh, R., Robson, S. and Trey, C. (eds) (1995.) *Diagnosis and Management of Liver Disease*. Chapman & Hall Medical, London.

Sherlock, S. and Dooley, J. (1993) *Diseases of the Liver and Biliary System*, 9th edn Blackwell, Oxford.

Strunin, L. and Thomson, S. (eds) (1992) The liver and anaesthesia. *Baillière's Clinical Anaesthesiology*, **6** (4).

OPHTHALMIC SURGERY

A.P. Rubin

Anaesthesia for ophthalmic surgery encompasses both general and local techniques and involves patients from the neonate to the most elderly. Many of the elderly patients have coincidental medical problems, the most common being cardiorespiratory disease, diabetes mellitus and arthritis. Many of the procedures are suitable for day-case surgery, when established criteria for patient care should be followed.

INTRAOCULAR PRESSURE

Control of intraocular pressure is a vital aspect of anaesthesia for intraocular operations and it should be low or normal before surgical incision to minimize the risk of iris or lens prolapse, vitreous extrusion or choroidal haemorrhage.

The normal range of intraocular pressure is 8–16 mmHg with a value of 25 mmHg or higher being pathological and it may be measured by contact methods using the Perkins applanation tonometer or non-contact methods such as the pneumatic air puff technique. The applanation method uses the fact that the force needed to flatten part of the surface of the eye depends on the internal pressure. The pneumatic method uses a jet of air at constant pressure from a set distance to indent the cornea. The intraocular pressure is the balance between external forces, such as the extraocular muscle tone and the scleral rigidity on the one hand and the volume of the aqueous, vitreous and choroidal vasculature on the other hand. It is affected by the balance between the production and drainage of aqueous humour. The aqueous is produced actively by the ciliary process involving carbonic anhydrase and cytochrome oxidase, as well as by simple filtration through the anterior surface of the iris. The normal volume in the eye is only 0.3 ml. The aqueous humour flows out of the eye through the trabecular meshwork into the canal of Schlemm. From there it enters the orbital venous system and the jugular veins. Carbonic anhydrase inhibitors, such as acetazolamide, reduce aqueous production, whereas osmotic diuretics, such as mannitol, reduce vitreous volume; thus both lower intraocular pressure.

The patient's eye is at risk if the intraocular pressure exceeds the perfusion pressure of the vasculature of the optic nerve or choroidal systems and particular care must be taken if the patient has glaucoma and starts with an elevated pressure.

Intraocular pressure is thus of vital importance in intraocular operations and, to ensure safe surgery, measures should be taken to reduce it to a minimum. It is also essential to avoid a sudden increase in intraocular pressure, especially when the globe is surgically open, as that might precipitate iris or lens prolapse, loss of vitreous humour, or an expulsive haemorrhage which might threaten vision.

Short Practice of Anaesthesia. Edited by M. Morgan and G. M. Hall. Published in 1997 by Chapman & Hall, London. ISBN 0 412 71890 1

Much ophthalmic surgery is for the removal of cataract and intraocular lens insertion. The low pressure ensures that the posterior capsule of the lens, behind which is the vitreous face, remains concave and relaxed and is least likely to rupture. It also ensures maximum room behind the posterior surface of the cornea for the safe removal of the lens material and its replacement with the prosthetic lens. External pressure on the eye, which may result from surgical retractors or anaesthetic face masks, must be avoided.

Arterial blood pressure changes have little effect on intraocular pressure as there seems to be autoregulation over a wide range. The arterial blood pressure would have to be very low before there is any significant reduction in intraocular pressure. However, changes in venous pressure are rapidly transmitted to the vasculature of the eye and immediately affect the pressure. An increase in venous pressure will follow an obstructed airway, coughing, sneezing, straining, vomiting, a Valsalva manoeuvre, IPPV with PEEP, anything tight around the neck or the head-down position and will lead to an elevation of intraocular pressure. A marked increase in choroidal blood volume predisposes to choroidal haemorrhage.

A major determinant of intraocular pressure is arterial carbon dioxide tension. As it increases the choroidal vessels dilate, flow through them increases and the pressure rises and as it falls the converse follows. Thus control of ventilation of the lungs may be used to control intraocular pressure. Oxygen tension has little effect unless it is dramatically reduced, when the pressure will rise.

Drugs used in anaesthesia may affect intraocular pressure in a number of ways. They may act on the central nervous system and affect the control diencephalic centres, they may act via contraction or relaxation of the external ocular muscles including the recti, obliques and orbicularis oculi, or they may act via changes in cardiovascular or respiratory parameters.

In summary, it can be seen that smooth induction and maintenance of anaesthesia, avoiding laryngoscopy and tracheal intubation if the depth of anaesthesia is inadequate, a slight head-up tilt and smooth extubation and recovery are all desirable features to keep the pressure low. Local anaesthetic injections may cause an increase in pressure due to the volume injected into the relatively closed space around or behind the globe.

PREPARATION OF THE EYE

Many drugs that are used for ophthalmic reasons may influence the patient in other respects and influence anaesthesia. Drugs administered on the conjunctiva are rapidly absorbed either directly or, after passing through the nasolacrimal duct, from the nasal mucosa.

MYDRIATICS

The pupil is dilated by sympathomimetics and parasympatholytics. These are usually applied topically but are occasionally injected under the conjunctiva. Phenylephrine, an α_1-receptor agonist, may be used in 2.5, 5 and 10% concentrations. One drop of 10% phenylephrine contains 4000 µg, equivalent to about 60 µg kg^{-1} for an adult, whereas the intravenous dose is described as 1–10 µg kg^{-1}. There will be absorption and systemic effects may follow, including hypertension, headache, tachycardia and angina. Clearly the least amount should be used and combinations with anticholinergic mydriatics such as cyclopentolate are preferred. Adrenaline 5 µg ml^{-1} is often added to the irrigating fluid during cataract surgery to maintain maximal pupillary dilatation. There have not been any problems reported from this use.

Cyclopentolate and tropicamide are short acting parasympatholyics used to dilate the pupil and may result in other parasympatholytic signs such as tachycardia, flushing, dry mouth, dry skin, pyrexia, confusion or psychosis. They may cause an increase in pressure in closed-angle glaucoma or where the anterior chamber is shallow.

Mydricaine is a combination of atropine, adrenaline and procaine and is occasionally injected under the conjunctiva to improve and maintain pupillary dilatation. It has potent effects, causing tachycardia and occasionally arrhythmias and often increasing the blood pressure.

MIOTICS

These are cholinergics and include carbachol and pilocarpine applied topically and miochol which is injected directly into the anterior chamber. Bradycardia is a possible effect of systemic absorption.

DRUGS USED TO LOWER INTRAOCULAR PRESSURE

These include cholinergics, anticholinesterases, β-adrenoceptor blockers, carbonic anhydrase inhibitors and osmotic diuretics. Cholinergic agonists act by constricting the ciliary muscle and this helps to open the drainage channels in the trabecular meshwork that lead to the canal of Schlemm. Anticholinesterases, such as ecothiopate and isoflurophate, may lead to delayed hydrolysis of suxamethonium or mivacurium and prolonged apnoea. β-blockers act by reducing aqueous humour production; some, such as timolol, are non-cardioselective and may lead to bronchospasm in susceptible individuals and there is a risk of bradycardia or heart failure. Cardioselective agents like betaxolol may be preferred in susceptible patients. Carbonic anhydrase inhibitors, for example acetazolamide, reduce aqueous production and, after an initial increase, decrease choroidal blood flow. They may cause a diuresis and, if used for a prolonged period, acidosis, hypokalaemia and hyponatraemia. Acetazolamide is given in a dose of 500 mg slowly intravenously or orally as 250 mg q.d.s. or 500 mg slow release capsules. An osmotic diuretic such as mannitol may be given in a dose of up to 1 g kg^{-1} over about 30 min, but may cause dehydration and lead to an overdistended bladder. It is also toxic if it extravasates outside a vein. An alternative occasionally used is sucrose 50%, 1 g kg^{-1}, which has a more rapid effect, usually within 5 min.

ANTIBIOTICS

Aminoglycoside antibiotics might in theory prolong neuromuscular block, but this does not seem to be a practical problem in ophthalmology.

GENERAL ANAESTHESIA

Essential principles are that the operations are in the head and neck region, many performed with the aid of a microscope and that absolute immobility is usually required. Thus airway control is essential and laryngeal masks or tracheal tubes must be positioned correctly and fixed in a way that prevents them being dislodged. All monitoring devices must be in place and reliable and the patient positioned on the table with due protection of pressure points and, usually, the other eye. The most common procedure is cataract extraction and intraocular lens implantation, followed by glaucoma surgery such as trabeculectomy and corneal graft (keratoplasty). The following general points apply especially to these procedures and the specific points of other operations will be discussed later.

PREOPERATIVE ASSESSMENT

Preoperative assessment should be complete and the patient in optimal condition before surgery is undertaken. In particular, both diabetes and hypertension are common and should be controlled. Many will be receiving one or more drugs which might affect anaesthesia. Guidelines should be agreed so that relevant investigations are done and the results available.

An association of eye disease with other medical conditions is well established and care should be taken to look for metabolic and endocrine diseases and conditions affecting the neuromuscular system.

PREMEDICATION

Premedication is used less as many will be elderly and day-cases, but it will remain indicated for some children and particularly nervous adults. Opioids, which increase the incidence of nausea and vomiting and respiratory depression, are rarely needed. Prophylactic anti-emetics are often prescribed to prevent any risk to the eye associated with postoperative vomiting.

PREPARATION

The preparation of the anaesthetic equipment and the application of monitoring devices should follow the Association of Anaesthetists guidelines. Monitoring is particularly important as the anaesthetist does not have easy access to the airway, is usually positioned at the patient's side and the surgery may take place in a darkened operating theatre.

INDUCTION OF ANAESTHESIA

All intravenous induction agents, with the exception of ketamine, lower intraocular pressure, although it would appear that etomidate and propofol may lower it to a greater extent than thiopentone. Propofol is also the best agent if a laryngeal mask airway is to be inserted. Ketamine may have a small place for examination of the eye in children, but the increased intraocular pressure, nystagmus, blepharospasm and adventitious movements make it rather unsuitable. The choice of induction agent depends on age, physical status, the need for rapid recovery, cost and ultimately personal preference.

MUSCLE RELAXANTS AND AIRWAY CONTROL

Suxamethonium increases intraocular pressure rapidly, either by contracture of the extraocular muscles or by increasing choroidal blood flow and the increase lasts for up to 10 min. It should be avoided unless strongly indicated. All of the non-depolarizing agents may be used as they either have no significant effect or lower intraocular pressure. Atracurium and particularly vecuronium are especially popular due to their shorter duration of action, controllability of the depth of block and cardiovascular stability.

An adequate depth of anaesthesia should be achieved before a laryngeal mask or tracheal tube is passed. A small dose of opioid, for example 10 µg kg^{-1} alfentanil, may be used to obtund the pressor response to intubation in particularly high risk patients.

The use of the laryngeal mask airway is still controversial. The protagonists claim it works well, is safe and that it avoids the problem of difficult intubation. Also that it causes less increase in intraocular pressure and that the incidence of coughing or straining at the end is much reduced compared with the use of a tracheal tube. The antagonists remind one of the dangers of a less secure airway in a situation where there is restricted access to it during surgery, the risks of IPPV via the laryngeal mask and the risk of aspiration of gastric contents. A tracheal tube should be preferred to a laryngeal mask if the patient is obese, has a history of regurgitation and if the laryngeal mask cannot be placed correctly or does not provide a reasonable air-tight seal. The preferred tracheal tube is a 'south facing' pre-shaped 'Rae', which allows the connections and gas sampling connector to be well away from the face and does not need a catheter mount between it and the anaesthetic breathing system. It should be firmly fixed with adhesive tape so that it cannot be dislodged.

MAINTENANCE OF ANAESTHESIA

Maintenance of anaesthesia may be with inhalational agents, all of the currently available ones causing a decrease in intraocular pressure, or by continuous infusion of intravenous agents. Some allow spontaneous ventilation, although theoretically the likely increase in carbon dioxide tension would elevate the intraocular pressure and high concentrations of inhalational agents are more likely to lead to hypotension. More anaesthetists use controlled ventilation with normocarbia or even mild hypocarbia aided by the administration of muscle relaxants. Atracurium 0.5 mg kg^{-1} or vecuronium 0.1 mg kg^{-1} are the most widely used and an initial dose may be followed by increments or a continuous infusion if the surgery is expected to be prolonged. A nerve stimulator is desirable to monitor the level of neuromuscular block. It allows accurate control of depth of neuromuscular block to allow increments to be given at the appropriate time and a more accurate assessment of the level of recovery from the relaxant drug. The most important factor is a smooth anaesthetic without straining or coughing. Analgesics are not often required as most of the operations are not very stimulating and their use increases the incidence of postoperative nausea and vomiting. However, they may be indicated to obtund the pressor response to intubation or for extraocular and prolonged procedures.

RECOVERY

There are no adverse effects of normal doses of atropine or glycopyrrolate and neostigmine on intraocular pressure or pupil size. Extubation should be performed without excessive coughing, although as surgical incision and suturing techniques have improved the eye is usually safe. It is difficult in practice to prevent coughing unless the tube is removed at a deep level of anaesthesia which prolongs the recovery and adds to the risk. The newer inhalational agents such as desflurane or sevoflurane have lower blood-gas solubility coefficients and therefore ensure more rapid recovery and this may be an advantage in reducing the time until the patient regains their protective reflexes. The recovery is much smoother after a laryngeal mask has been used than after a tracheal tube and this is another reason for their growing popularity in ophthalmic anaesthesia.

Adequate facilities for the observation and monitoring of the patient must be provided until they are fit to return to the ward. Oxygen should be given and particular care taken to detect hypoxia, arrhythmias, hypotension, respiratory depression, or failure of adequate reversal of neuromuscular blockade

POSTOPERATIVE ANALGESIA

Most patients having intraocular operations require only simple analgesics such as paracetamol, but more complex and extraocular operations may produce pain requiring opioids. Attention should also be given to the prevention and treatment of postoperative nausea and vomiting which is more common in this latter group.

SMALL BABIES

Babies may require examination under anaesthesia or probing and syringing of their lacrimal ducts. These procedures are frequently done as day cases and although they may seem minor, the anaesthetic demands the full skills, facilities and equipment appropriate to this age group. Most will require a laryngeal mask airway or tracheal intubation as the lacrimal system communicates with the airway via the nasolacrimal duct. Babies may also present with lid problems, congenital cataracts or glaucoma, which may be operated on in any eye unit and occasionally with ocular or orbital tumours, which are usually referred to specialized units. The details of paediatric anaesthesia are outside the scope of this chapter, but basic principles apply, the airway must be secured and the oculocardiac reflex is more often encountered than in adults.

STRABISMUS SURGERY

Squint surgery is most commonly performed in children or young adults, but occasionally is required in older people. An association with a neuromuscular disease and the rare possibility of a malignant hyperthermia susceptibility should be considered. Squint surgery requires airway control and protection against the oculocardiac reflex, which is most often precipitated by traction on the external ocular muscles and is seen in about 90% of unpremedicated children. There is a very high incidence of pain, nausea and vomiting after strabismus surgery and many advocate the use of anti-emetics routinely for these patients.

OCULOCARDIAC REFLEX

This is a sinus bradycardia which may follow pressure on the eye, traction on the extraocular muscles or other manipulation of the eye. It is mediated via the ciliary ganglion along trigeminal afferents and the efferent loop is via the vagus nerves. It may be very dramatic, the rate being so slow that no complexes are seen on the monitor. Although the reflex tends to fatigue and vagal escape occurs, it must be rapidly identified and the stimulus immediately removed. A vagolytic such as atropine or glycopyrrolate must be given and in strabismus surgery many would advocate their prophylactic use, especially in children. Suitable doses would be atropine 0.02 mg kg^{-1} or glycopyrrolate 0.01 mg kg^{-1}. It is rare with surgery under regional block as the afferent input is blocked. However an increase in pressure associated with the injection of local anaesthetic may precipitate the reflex occasionally.

OTHER SPECIFIC OPHTHALMIC PROCEDURES

Dacrocystorhinostomy

The most common procedure on the lacrimal system is the dacrocystorhinostomy, where the lacrimal mucosa is linked to the nasal mucosa to correct a blockage. Bleeding is a problem and the nasal mucosa may be prepared with a vasoconstrictor such as cocaine or adrenaline. Deliberate hypotension may be requested although it is doubtful if it is necessary. A throat pack should be used to protect the lower airway from aspiration of blood.

Oculoplastic surgery

Oculoplastic operations on the lids are common and may be performed under local or general anaesthesia.

Orbital decompression and tumours

Orbital decompression operations may be required for exophthalmos in patients with thyroid overactivity or for tumours. These operations may be associated with considerable blood loss and may require fluid replacement. Hypotensive anaesthesia may be requested by the surgeon. Radiotherapy may be used in the treatment of tumours and in children will usually necessitate general anaesthesia. Special precautions are required to allow the anaesthetist to be outside the treatment area but to be able to observe the child and monitors and to return if necessary.

Retinal detachment surgery

Retinal detachment surgery may involve the injection of very insoluble gases such as sulphur hexafluoride to tamponade the retinal tear. These gases are therefore retained for several days. The importance for the anaesthetist is that if nitrous oxide, which is 117 times more soluble than sulphur hexafluoride is used, it will diffuse into the gas bubble enlarging it dramatically. This may compromise the retinal blood flow. When the nitrous oxide is discontinued it will diffuse out of the bubble and there may be a sudden decrease in intraocular pressure and the tamponade effect of the bubble will cease. The solution is to discontinue the nitrous oxide at least 20 min before the gas is injected and not to use nitrous oxide if it is within 5 days of a previous intravitreous air bubble or within 10 days of a sulphur hexafluoride injection.

EMERGENCY OPHTHALMIC SURGERY

A proportion of emergency patients will be children and most injuries do not involve intraocular structures. Most do not require immediate surgery and there is time for full assessment and preparation. Sometimes there are associated injuries which require urgent intervention and the eye injury should be considered in the choice of anaesthetic technique and drugs.

Patients with injuries that penetrate the globe may require urgent surgery and are likely to have a 'full stomach'. Therefore a technique of anaesthesia has to be employed to achieve early airway protection without causing further damage to the eye. Controversy surrounds the use of suxamethonium, which is known to cause an increase in intraocular pressure but is considered to be an essential feature of rapid sequence induction. There is little evidence that the transient elevation in pressure that follows suxamethonium is in fact detrimental to the eye and it is often forgotten that laryngoscopy and intubation under light anaesthesia will also increase the pressure significantly. Attempts that have been made to reduce the harmful effects of suxamethonium include a priming dose of suxamethonium or a non-depolarizing relaxant, or pre-treatment with diazepam or lignocaine, but these are not reliable. A review of 63 penetrating eye injuries failed to show any harmful effects of suxamethonium used following pre-treatment with a non-depolarizing relaxant.

If suxamethonium is to be avoided, the patient's trachea must be intubated after the use of non-depolarizing relaxants. Aspiration prophylaxis with antacid and H_2 receptor antagonist should be used. Techniques of priming with a preliminary use of a small dose of the relaxant drug have been described, but are also unreliable. A better method is to increase the intubating dose of relaxant, e.g. vecuronium 0.15–0.25 mg kg^{-1}, which reduces the onset time, or to use a relaxant with a slightly shorter onset time such as rocuronium 1.0–1.2 mg kg^{-1}, which will provide acceptable intubating conditions in the majority of patients 60 s after administration. Particular care would need to be taken if the patient's trachea is also predicted to be difficult to intubate or has other significant injuries and a careful plan should be drawn up weighing up the advantages and disadvantages of the possible choices.

Extubation should be carried out in a head-down lateral position with the operated eye uppermost to minimize the risk of aspiration of gastric contents.

REGIONAL ANAESTHESIA

There has been a dramatic increase in the use of local anaesthesia for intraocular surgery and estimates from the Royal College of Ophthalmologists suggest that it is used for over 70% of cataract operations. The predominantly elderly patients tolerate local anaesthesia very well and the frequency of intercurrent disease makes the avoidance of general anaesthesia more desirable. Most cataracts are performed on a day-case basis which is preferred by patients and justified on economic grounds.

The techniques are relatively simple and safe and should result in excellent operating conditions. Anaesthetists are more involved at the present time not only in a stand-by capacity to monitor, sedate and occasionally resuscitate, but to actually perform the blocks. With skilled administration of the blocks, the need for sedation is minimal and the systemic complications may be anticipated and prevented rather than crisis situations occurring which then need urgent treatment.

CONTRAINDICATIONS

Contraindications include cases in children, lack of cooperation, those with involuntary movements, an inability to lie fairly flat and relatively still, the rare situation of allergy to local anaesthetics and an informed preference for general anaesthesia. A relative contraindication would be a long eye (above 26 mm) where there may be a significant risk of globe perforation. Anticoagulation within the therapeutic range is not considered a contraindication as the risk of stopping anticoagulant drugs is greater than the risk of continuing their use.

PREOPERATIVE ASSESSMENT

Attention should be paid to the control of high blood pressure, heart failure or diabetes mellitus and the patient got into optimal condition. Protocols are required with the indications for investigations and unnecessary investigations which will not affect patient management should be discouraged. Preoperative starvation is unnecessary as failure of these blocks is very rare if sufficient time is allowed. Diabetic patients may therefore remain on their usual regimens which simplifies their management and allows for early discharge.

As for all local anaesthetic techniques full resuscitation equipment should be available and an indwelling intravenous cannula should be in place for the occasional administration of drugs for resuscitation, lowering of intraocular pressure, or for mild sedation. Effective preoperative counselling gives the patients confidence and reduces the need for sedation. If sedation is required, it should be judiciously selected, safe and must not be used to cover inadequate blocks. Very occasionally drugs such as midazolam 7 μg kg^{-1} and alfentanil 3 μg kg^{-1} may be used to allay anxiety, provide analgesia and to enhance not diminish cooperation; others might prefer an intravenous induction agent such as propofol in very low dosage. If sedative drugs are used, particular attention must be paid to monitoring of the airway, respiration and gas exchange, the desirability of maintaining verbal contact with the patient and safe recovery.

ANATOMY

The orbit is a quadrilateral pyramid with the apex posteriorly and the base to the front. The lateral wall passes posteriorly at an angle of 45° whereas the floor passes upwards at an angle of 5°. The medial wall and roof are vertical and horizontal respectively. The orbit contains the globe, orbital fat, extraocular muscles, conjunctiva, eyelids, nerves and blood vessels. The globe is normally about 22–24 mm long, but in myopic eyes may be as long as 30 mm. Longer eyes tend to have thinner sclerae. The globe is separated from the other orbital structures by the Tenon's fascia. The orbital fat is divided into a central (intracone) space and a peripheral (extracone) space by the muscle cone of the four recti muscles. However, the orbital fat is continuous and the muscle cone is not a complete barrier to local anaesthetic spread, so that solutions placed in the extracone space rapidly enter the intracone space and vice versa. All the nerves to the extraocular muscles, the ciliary ganglion, the branches of the ophthalmic division of the Vth nerve and the terminal branches of the VIIth nerve to the orbicularis oculi muscle may be blocked by injections into the orbital fat. The least vascular parts of the orbital fat are the inferotemporal, nasal and superotemporal and it is usual to make injections into some or all of these areas. The optic nerve enters the orbit through the optic foramen and passes anterolaterally to enter the globe at its rear surface a little to the medial side of the mid-point. It is covered by a dural cuff containing a prolongation of the subarachnoid space right up to the sclera.

TECHNIQUES

There are several techniques of regional anaesthesia for ophthalmic surgery:

- topical,
- subconjunctival injection,
- sub-Tenon's infiltration,
- retrobulbar and facial nerve blocks,
- combined retrobulbar/peribulbar block,
- peribulbar block.

Topical

Many cataract operations are performed under topical drops alone, using amethocaine, lignocaine or bupivacaine. The anaesthesia is satisfactory although the iris is not anaesthetized, but there is no akinesia of the globe. Oxybuprocaine (Benoxinate) 0.4%, although shorter acting, does not sting and is preferred to amethocaine before retrobulbar or peribulbar injections.

Subconjunctival injection

A small volume of local anaesthetic injected under the conjunctiva near the superior limbus will again produce good anaesthesia but has no effect on the motor nerves to the globe or periorbital structures.

Sub-Tenon's injection

An injection may be made deep to the Tenon's fascia layer which lies under the conjunctiva. It involves a small incision in the conjunctiva and Tenon's fascia usually in the inferonasal region and an injection of about 3 ml may be made via a blunt metal or plastic cannula. Anaesthesia is good and akinesia usually follows spread of the solution into the intracone space or along the muscle sheaths of the recti muscle.

Choice of solution

The blocks may be preceded by the injection of a dilute solution of lignocaine (0.2%) in balanced salt solution which does not sting on injection and the definitive solution may be warmed to body temperature before injection.

The traditional solution is an equal parts mixture of 2% lignocaine and 0.75% bupivacaine, giving rapid onset and long duration. High concentrations of local anaesthetic seem to be required to ensure adequate penetration and intense motor block. Adrenaline 5 µg ml^{-1} and hyaluronidase 7.5 units ml^{-1} are added freshly and while both seem to be beneficial in terms of quality and duration of block and reduction of pressure, many omit one or both. If a shorter duration is required, prilocaine is often preferred.

Retrobulbar and facial nerve blocks

This was the classical method and as the facial nerve endings may be blocked in the lids from within the orbit, a separate facial nerve block is rarely required. The retrobulbar injection remains very popular but is usually done on its own or combined with a nasal peribulbar injection.

Combined retrobulbar/peribulbar block

The eye must be looking straight ahead in the 'primary gaze' position. A retrobulbar injection is made from the inferotemporal region of the orbit and it is convenient to go through the conjunctiva which may be anaesthetized

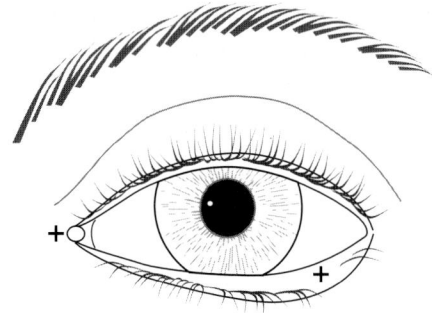

Figure 17.1 Left eye: sites for needle insertion.

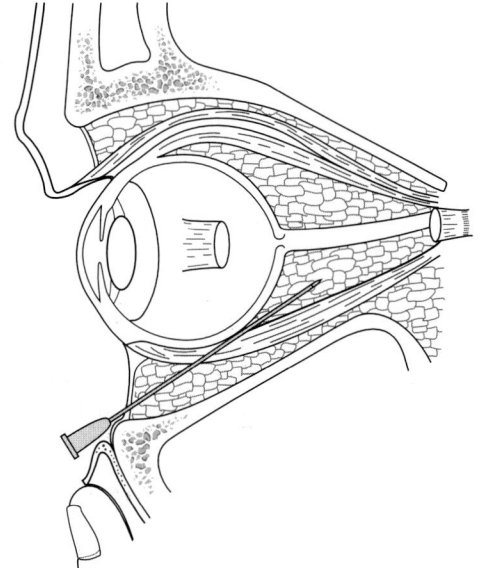

Figure 17.2 Retrobulbar injection.

with topical local anaesthetic drops rather than through the skin. A 25 G 2.5 cm needle is inserted half way between the line of the lateral edge of the iris and the lateral canthus avoiding conjunctival vessels (Figure 17.1).

The needle is then passed away from the globe, below it and then upwards and inwards until the needle is inserted to the full depth of 2.5 cm. This will usually allow the needle tip to enter the cone behind the hind surface of the globe (Figure 17.2).

The tip of the needle should not cross the line of the lateral edge of the iris so that it cannot reach the optic nerve. After careful aspiration, 2–5 ml of solution may be injected, monitoring any pressure rise, and stopping the injection if it rises excessively.

This injection should block all the relevant sensory nerves and the motor nerves to all the structures except perhaps the orbicularis oculi. When required, the orbicularis oculi is blocked by a nasal peribulbar injection, in which the 25 G 2.5 cm needle is inserted between the skin of the medial canthus and the caruncle and directed backwards for about 2 cm into the orbital fat (Figure 17.1). The feel of going through the medial orbital septum is often detected. About 5 ml of solution is injected and will spread into the medial orbital fat but also come forward above and below the medial orbital septum to fill the lids where it blocks the terminal branches of that part of the VIIth nerve that supplies the orbicularis oculi.

Peribulbar block

Traditionally the peribulbar block is performed with two injections through the skin, one inferotemporal and the other superonasal. More recently the technique has been modified so that all the injections are made through the conjunctiva and the superonasal injection has been superseded by the nasal one described above (Figure 17.3).

The inferotemporal injection is made in the line of the lateral edge of the iris about 2 mm from the sclera and the 25 g 2.5 cm needle is inserted away from and then below the globe. No attempt is made to go up or in towards the muscle cone and the needle need not go further than the equator of the eye. At least 5 ml of solution is usually injected assessing orbital pressure and stopping the injection if it increases excessively. More local anaesthetic is used than in a retrobulbar block, and 90% of patients will also require the nasal injection to complete the akinesia. This is performed as

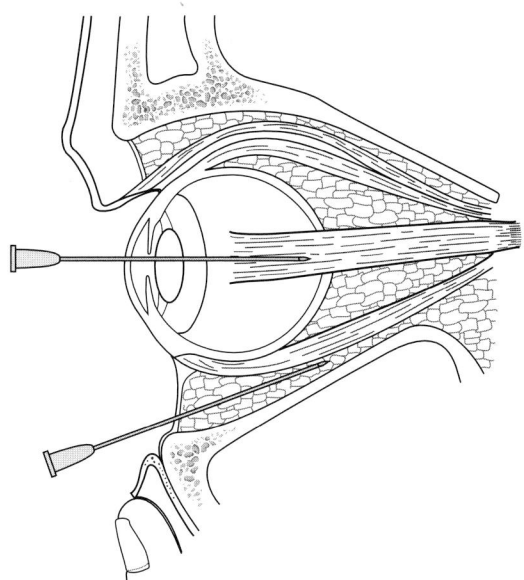

Figure 17.3 Right eye: peribulbar injections.

has been described for the combined retrobulbar/peribulbar injection inserting the needle medial to the caruncle and piercing the medial orbital septum before injecting 2–5 ml at a depth of about 2 cm (Figure 17.3). Indeed 25% of patients will require even more injections which should be chosen according to the deficiencies of the block. They may be inferotemporal, nasal, or superotemporal through the skin of the upper eyelid in order to achieve adequate akinesia. Thus up to 20 ml of solution may be required. More recently some are using a nasal injection of prilocaine only, using 6–8 ml and claiming good results.

Up to 30 min of a pressure device applied to the closed eye may be needed to allow for the absorption of the larger volumes of local anaesthetic and a return to normal or low pressure.

Assessment of the block

The block should ensure anaesthesia and motor block must be tested. Block of the levator palpebrae superioris is conformed by an inability to open the eye, of the orbicularis oculi by an inability to squeeze the lids and the external ocular muscles by a failure to move the globe in any direction.

CARE IN THE OPERATING THEATRE

The patient must be made as comfortable as possible and minimal monitoring should include oximetry, electrocardiography and blood pressure measurement. Oxygen is administered under the drapes which should be suspended off the patient's face. The patient requires someone to monitor them, reassure them and to explain some of the noises associated with modern cataract surgery. The patient should be encouraged to remain still and silent unless they have a problem.

COMPLICATIONS

Systemic toxicity

Complications may be due to systemic toxicity of the local anaesthetic or vasoconstrictor agents used. This may follow overdose or accidental intravenous injection. Allergic reactions to local anaesthetic or hyaluronidase may be seen very occasionally.

Bruising (Ecchymosis)

Ecchymosis is more likely if the injections are done through the skin, but may also follow transconjunctival injections.

Haemorrhage

Orbital (retrobulbar) haemorrhage is a serious complication that may occur in between 0.1% and 1.7% of patients. It is more likely to follow the use of longer needles as there are more large vessels in the posterior orbit. It is recognized by increasing proptosis, tight eyelids, periorbital and subconjunctival haemorrhage and a dramatic increase in intraorbital pressure. The operation may have to be postponed and orbital decompression may be required to prevent permanent loss of vision if the pressure causes occlusion of the central artery of the retina.

Globe penetration or perforation

The needle may enter the globe (penetration) or pass right through it (perforation). The risk is greater in myopic eyes which are longer and also have thinner sclerae and in those who have had previous retinal detachment surgery. The length of the globe is usually known from preoperative assessment for lens implantation. Detailed knowledge of the anatomy, an initially tangential approach and facing the bevel of the needle towards the globe all help to reduce the incidence. Diagnosis may be suggested by pain, sudden loss of vision, hypotonia of the globe, a poor red reflex or vitreous haemorrhage. It may follow both peribulbar and retrobulbar injections, but the incidence should not be more than about 1 in 15 000.

Amaurosis (loss of vision)

The blocks may lead to temporary loss of vision. This is more frequent after retrobulbar blocks due to more local anaesthetic reaching the optic nerve, but may be seen with peribulbar blocks as well. The patient should be reassured that, on the one hand, retention of vision does not imply failure of block and that on the other, loss of vision may be expected and is only temporary.

Optic nerve complications

There is a risk of direct damage to the optic nerve or injection or haemorrhage within the optic nerve sheath. Pressure on the optic nerve may also be a consequence of retrobulbar haemorrhage.

Central spread of local anaesthetic

Local anaesthetic may be injected into the optic nerve sheath which is a dural cuff communicating with the intracranial cavity. It is only likely if needles longer than 2.5 cm are used. The globe should be looking straight ahead during the blocks so that the optic nerve remains in its normal position behind the globe and does not rotate towards the needle. Symptoms include drowsiness, contralateral loss of vision, convulsions, or respiratory or cardiovascular depression. While it is likely to occur soon after the injection, its onset may be delayed, so the patient must be carefully monitored to detect early signs and to institute prompt treatment as required.

External ocular muscle palsies

Muscle palsies may rarely follow injection of high concentrations of local anaesthetic directly into a muscle, the medial rectus being the most common.

Subconjunctival oedema (chemosis)

Chemosis often follows orbital injections but is of little significance and usually disappears quickly with pressure.

FURTHER READING

Abbot, M. A. and Samuel, J. R. (1987) The control of intra-ocular pressure during the induction of anaesthesia for emergency eye surgery. A high-dose vecuronium technique. *Anaesthesia*, **42**, 1008–1012.

Cunningham, A. J. and Barry, P. (1986) Intraocular pressure – physiology and implications for anaesthetic management. *Canadian Anaesthetists Society Journal*, **33**, 195–208.

Davis, D. B. II and Mandel, M. R. (1986) Posterior peribulbar anesthesia: an alternative to retrobulbar anesthesia. *Journal of Cataract and Refractive Surgery*, **12**, 182–184.

Hamilton, R. C. (1995) Techniques of orbital regional anaesthesia. *British Journal of Anaesthesia*, **75**, 88–92.

Holden, R., Morsman, C. D. G., Butler, J., Clark, G. S., Hughes, D. S. and Bacon, P. J. (1991) Intraocular pressure changes using the laryngeal mask airway and tracheal tube. *Anaesthesia*, **46**, 922–924.

Hustead, R. F., Hamilton, R. C. and Loken, R. G. (1994) Periocular local anesthesia: medial orbital as an alternative to superior nasal injection. *Journal of Cataract and Refractive Surgery* **20**, 197–201.

Johnson, R. W. (1995) Anatomy for ophthalmic anaesthesia. *British Journal of Anaesthesia*, **75**, 80–87.

Johnson, R. W. and Forrest, F. C. (1994) *Local and General Anaesthesia for Ophthalmic Surgery*, Butterworth-Heinemann, Oxford.

Libonati, M. M., Leahy, J. L. and Ellison, N. (1985) The use of succinylcholine in open eye surgery. *Anesthesiology*, **62**, 637–640.

Rubin, A. P. (1995) Complications of local anaesthesia for ophthalmic surgery. *British Journal of Anaesthesia*, **75**, 93–96.

Smith, G. B., Hamilton, R. C. and Carr, C. A. (1995) *Ophthalmic Anaesthesia*, Edward Arnold, London.

Zide, B. M. Jelks, G. W. (1985) *Surgical Anatomy of the Orbit*, Raven Press, New York.

EAR, NOSE AND THROAT SURGERY 18

B. O'Donoghue

A minimally invasive approach had been established in ear, nose and throat (ENT) surgery since the early 1950s with the use of the operating microscope in ear surgery and for laryngeal surgery soon after. At the same time improvements in non-invasive anaesthetic monitoring and the availability of newly developed anaesthetic agents complemented these surgical techniques. The introduction of the fibreoptic laryngoscope in 1962 by Dr Peter Murphy, and of the laryngeal mask by Dr Archie Brain in 1983, enabled the development of a minimally invasive approach to airway control.

ANAESTHESIA FOR SURGERY OF THE PHARYNX, LARYNX AND TRACHEA

A thorough understanding of physiology and anatomy is a prerequisite for safe anaesthesia for upper airway surgery. The nerve supply to the larynx and pharynx is the IXth and Xth cranial nerves. Sensory innervation is provided primarily by the superior laryngeal nerve which arises from the inferior ganglion of the vagus. The upper branch innervates the mucosa of the lower pharynx, epiglottis and laryngeal vestibule. The lower branch, which passes under the surface of the pyriform fossa, innervates the arytenoepiglottic folds and posterior glottis. Below the vocal cords sensory innervation is provided by the recurrent laryngeal nerve, which also supplies motor neurones to all the intrinsic laryngeal muscles with the exception of the crico-thyroid and inferior pharyngeal constrictors, which are supplied by the superior laryngeal nerve.

TONSILLECTOMY AND ADENOIDECTOMY

The main indication for tonsillectomy and adenoidectomy is still recurrent tonsillitis, but a history of habitual snoring may also point out the need for surgery. Although surgery may be carried out at any age, it is most common in children between the ages of 4 and 6 years. After 8 years of age the postnasal space enlarges in proportion to the other pharyngeal structures and adenoidectomy is seldom indicated.

The aim of general anaesthesia is to provide an adequate depth to allow easy insertion of the mouth gag and prevent reflex tachycardia and hypertension. Inquiry about bleeding tendencies and recent aspirin ingestion should be made during the preoperative assessment, and a check made for loose teeth. Haemoglobin estimation should be carried out preoperatively if anaemia is suspected.

Increased vagal activity in children requires the preoperative administration of atropine or glycopyrrolate. Sedative medication is the subject of uncertainty and controversy. A proportion of children with large tonsils and adenoids suffer from intermittent upper airway obstruction during sleep, with resulting hypoxaemia, hypercapnia and swinging in-

Short Practice of Anaesthesia. Edited by M. Morgan and G. M. Hall. Published in 1997 by Chapman & Hall, London. ISBN 0 412 71890 1

trathoracic pressure. Pulmonary hypertension and cor pulmonale are recognized sequelae. Where obstructive sleep apnoea syndrome (OSAS) is suspected, preoperative sedative medication should be avoided. Otherwise there is no reason to withhold sedation.

Induction of anaesthesia is carried out via the inhalational or intravenous route, and is largely dependent on the child's cooperation. Gaseous induction in the presence of large tonsils and adenoids may be prolonged and difficult. Patients with OSAS usually have reduced hypoxic and hypercapnic ventilatory responses which are further decreased during inhalational induction. They will tolerate hypoxia and hypercapnia with little attempt to increase the respiratory rate or tidal volume. Early loss of upper airway muscle tone further exacerbates the hazards of the inhalational route of induction.

A depth of anaesthesia sufficient to insert an oropharyngeal airway will be attained more quickly with an intravenous induction agent. Propofol has several advantages. It maintains good muscle tone, reduces airway irritability, and may have analgesic and antiemetic properties. Induction is quick and smooth, whilst emergence and recovery are rapid with less risk of laryngeal spasm on extubation. In advanced OSAS ketamine offers the advantage of cardiovascular stability during induction.

Protection of the airway with an orotracheal tube in children and an oro- or nasotracheal tube in adults is required. Further protection is achieved by lowering the head and extending the neck, allowing blood to pool in the nasopharynx. A pre-shaped tracheal tube tightly strapped to the chin may accidentally enter the bronchus during neck extension, with resulting hypoventilation and lightening of anaesthesia. Increasingly the laryngeal mask airway (LMA) is used to secure the airway during adenotonsillectomy. Although surgical access may be more difficult, the LMA has the advantage of better airway protection during the immediate postoperative period. A smaller size LMA with a fully deflated cuff may be easier to insert when the tonsils are large.

Anaesthesia can be maintained by either volatile or i.v. agents, or a mixture of both. Stimulation due to positioning of the mouth gag may be associated with a rapid heart rate and hyperventilation if the depth of anaesthesia is inadequate. Tachycardia and hypertension may also be caused by hypercarbia, and in a child with OSAS, IPPV should be employed from the induction of anaesthesia.

Blood loss remains the main cause of morbidity and mortality. It is difficult to estimate, and therefore efforts should be made to weigh tonsillar swabs and measure the volume of blood in the suction bottle. The infusion of crystalloids 3–5 ml kg^{-1} h^{-1} not only increases vascular volume, but also induces a hypercoagulable state.

The tracheal tube is removed after both surgeon and anaesthetist are satisfied that the operating field is dry. After careful inspection with a laryngoscope for hidden blood clots, the child is placed in the lateral or semi-prone position with a pillow under the chest (tonsillar position), and the tube removed under deep general anaesthesia. Extubation when awake, although safer theoretically, may encourage coughing and postoperative bleeding.

A quiet recovery period is required. Intravenous opiates given during surgery will delay the time until postoperative analgesia is required, and prevent coughing and crying. Diclofenac (NSAID) is given almost routinely, but it is wiser to wait until bleeding has been controlled.

Tonsillectomy is now performed more frequently in a day-case surgery unit. Although postoperative bleeding is the most serious complication, persistent vomiting and inadequate fluid intake are the most common reasons for overnight admission. The incidence of nausea and vomiting can be as high as 70% during the first 24 h and it is important to administer anti-emetics prophylactically and not to force oral fluids.

Anaesthesia for tonsillectomy in adults is technically more difficult, carries a greater perioperative risk and requires prolonged postoperative analgesia. Very large tonsils may be the cause of chronic upper airway obstruction during sleep, with resulting hypoxaemia and nocturnal myocardial ischaemia. If OSAS is suspected, investigations should include a chest X-ray, overnight oximetry and a 24 h ECG. These patients are frequently very obese, have small lung volumes and desaturate very quickly. Hypoventilation occurs easily due to the reduced hypoxic and hypercapnic ventilatory drive so that IPPV is safer.

In the presence of a peritonsillar abscess, intubation may be required due to progressive upper airway obstruction. An abscess must be aspirated before the induction of anaesthesia. This relieves pain, reduces swelling and trismus, and prevents rupture of the abscess at the time of intubation. Intravenous antibiotic therapy and rehydration will improve the patient's general condition. Trismus in the patient with quinsy is due to muscular spasm and is relieved by induction of anaesthesia and the use of neuromuscular blocking drugs. The Mallampati score does not predict a difficult intubation in this situation. Stridor may complicate sublingual and submandibular cellulitis, and tracheostomy under local anaesthesia may be the safest way to protect the airway.

MANAGEMENT OF POST-TONSILLECTOMY HAEMORRHAGE

The incidence of post-tonsillectomy haemorrhage requiring surgical intervention is 0.3–0.6%. This complication usually occurs within 6 h of surgery and can be a daunting anaesthetic problem. The difficulties are caused by unsuspected hypovolaemia, a stomach full of blood and bleeding in the airway. The extent of blood loss may not be obvious and is often underestimated. Frequently the only indication of blood loss is a rising heart rate. The haemoglobin, haematocrit and coagulation status should be checked, and blood should be grouped and crossmatched. A large-bore venous cannula must be inserted immediately. Resuscitation with blood should be accomplished before the induction of anaesthesia, if at all possible. Anaesthesia is induced using a rapid sequence induction with the patient lying on their side. Competent help is necessary for the application of cricoid pressure and for continuous suction of blood from the pharynx. A slight head-down position will protect the trachea and glottis from the aspiration of blood. After induction of anaesthesia a gastric tube should be passed and the stomach contents washed out. Extubation is safest with the patient awake. If oozing persists, the possibilty of a bleeding diathesis should be considered, as a proportion of children with advanced OSAS have clotting abnormalities.

ANAESTHESIA FOR LARYNGOSCOPY AND MICROLARYNGOSCOPY

The common goal for endoscopic surgery of the airway is to provide the surgeon with a clear view, an immobile operating field and sufficient room in which to work. Anaesthesia has to be of sufficient depth to provide relaxation of the jaw, and to abolish the protective and autonomic reflexes from the larynx, pharynx and trachea. Rapid awakening and the return of all protective reflexes is required at the end of surgery.

Glycopyrrolate given preoperatively has a beneficial effect in drying secretions and protecting against vagal stimulation from the laryngeal stretch receptors. Topical lignocaine offers further protection against sympathetic stimulation, but its use in short cases is controversial because of the delay of the return of protective reflexes in the postoperative period.

The method of airway maintenance depends on the type of surgical procedure and the extent of the underlying pathology, which may range from a small nodule of the vocal cord to obstructing papillomatosis or a friable, extensive, supraglottic tumour. No single technique is appropriate for all cases and the anaesthetist should be familiar with several alternatives. Where signs and symptoms of upper airway obstruction are present, a detailed assessment of the anatomy should be carried out in conjunction with the surgeon.

Pre-oxygenation is prudent in all upper airway surgery, but is essential in cases where the airway is potentially compromised. An intravenous induction has to be given slowly, and neuromuscular blocking drugs can only be administered after the ability to ventilate the lungs has been established. Apnoea must not be allowed to occur until the airway has been secured. Anaesthesia can be maintained with inhalational agents, where a tracheal tube is being used, or intravenous methods in tubeless techniques. Ventilation is usually controlled; hypercarbia and resulting sympathetic overactivity may be the cause of tachycardia, arrhythmias and hypertension.

The technique of deep inhalational anaesthesia and spontaneous respiration is still in use, especially in removing foreign bodies from the airway. The high lipid solubility of halothane has the advantage of slow recovery, thus allowing the surgeon sufficient time to complete the procedure.

The apnoeic oxygenation technique refers to the insufflation of oxygen with a volatile anaesthetic, via a nasotracheal catheter, in a paralysed patient. The limitation of this method is the rate of rise of alveolar CO_2 and resultant hypoxaemia.

The posterior commissure or posterior one-third of the vocal cords are involved in only 5% of patients. Visualization with a small tracheal tube is usually adequate therefore, and direct laryngoscopy can frequently be carried out by this technique. The resistance to breathing is usually too great for spontaneous ventilation to be adequate.

A completely unobscured view can be obtained using one of the tubeless techniques. Ventilation using Venturi principles through an operating laryngoscope provides an unobstructed view and adequate ventilation. A Sanders injector, or a high frequency jet ventilator, delivers a jet of gas under high pressure within the lumen of an open-ended laryngoscope. Gas propulsion creates a negative pressure around the needle, and entrains ambient gas through the proximal end of the laryngoscope. The volume of gas leaving the distal end may be 20 times that of the jetting gas, and is at a lower pressure.

Tidal volume and peak inflation pressures depend on the driving pressure, needle length and diameter, and compliance of airways and chest wall. The best position of the needle tip for efficient gas exchange is at the middle third of the laryngoscope. Regulator pressures of 150–300 kPa are used in adults and 30–150 kPa is recommended in children. A needle of 12–14 G should be used in patients weighing 100 kg or over; 14–16 G in patients weighing 50–100 kg, and 16–18 G in patients weighing 50 kg or less. Jet ventilation should start at low driving pressures and be maintained at the lowest pressures giving chest expansion. It is contraindicated in patients with bullous emphysema and the jetted air must have a unobstructed exit at all times. General anaesthesia is usually maintained by intermittent, or continuous, infusion of an anaesthetic agent such as propofol, methohexitone or thiopentone with short-acting opioids. Full muscle relaxation will provide immobile vocal cords and maximal chest compliance.

In practice, following pre-oxygenation and i.v. or inhalational induction, the airway is secured with an LMA or tracheal tube. These are left in place until the surgeon has the laryngoscope positioned and larynx visualized, removed for the duration of surgery and reinserted to protect the airway during recovery. Signs of tachycardia or hypertension during microlaryngoscopy should be treated with deepening of anaesthesia before hypotensive agents are used.

The recent introduction of external high frequency oscillation using a Hyek curaisse oscillator has been found to provide adequate ventilation and oxygenation in patients undergoing microlaryngoscopic airway surgery. It generates both positive and negative pressure to maintain the respiratory cycle. The curaisse is applied to the chest and the oscillator is set initially at an inspiratory pressure of $-24\,\text{cmH}_2\text{O}$ and expiratory pressure of $+14\,\text{cmH}_2\text{O}$, and a frequency of 70 breaths per minute with an inspiratory/expiratory (I:E) ratio of 1:1. It is important to monitor transcutaneous CO_2 as the oscillator is an indirect pressure generator producing pressure changes in the curaisse rather than in the airway. The risk of aspiration is always present in a patient anaesthetized with an unprotected airway.

LASER SURGERY TO THE UPPER AIRWAY

Theory and applications

Lasers are intense sources of electromagnetic radiation. The word laser is an acronym for Light Amplification by Stimulated Emission of Radiation. The terms light and electromagnetic energy are used interchangeably in the scientific literature, although not all lasers are within the visible range. Monochromacity (very narrow range of wavelength) coherence (photons are in phase in space and time), and collimation (unidirectional beam with little divergence), are the characteristics of laser light.

Radiation is emitted or absorbed from an atom when electrons are transferred from one energy level to another. An atom moves from a higher to a lower energy state by **spontaneous** emission. Conversely when an atom is exposed to a specific amount of radiation it may absorb that energy and electrons are transiently raised to an excited energy state. If a photon is then incident upon an atom in the excited state, the atom can emit newly **absorbed** energy in addition to the existing amount of excited energy, by return of its electron to its lower level. Two emitted photons have the same energy level, frequency, phase and direction. The stimulating radiation has thus been **amplified**. The process of supplying high intensity energy is accomplished by an electrical discharge, another laser, or an intense light source.

Laser devices have three components: an active laser medium, an optical cavity and an energy source. Lasers are classified according to their active medium. The most important used in medicine are the CO_2, Nd-YAG, KTP, argon, krypton and the helium–neon laser. Most utilize light in the visible and infrared spectrum.

Absorption of the laser beam leads to tissue coagulation, water vaporization and cell destruction. Brief intermittent exposures allow controlled destruction of soft tissue, small blood vessel coagulation and heat dissipation. The CO_2 laser beam is absorbed strongly by water, blood and biological tissue; it has the shallowest penetration and reflection and scattering are negligible. Oedema formation is also minimal. It is particularly useful as a cutting tool in endoscopic excision of all obstructive lesions of the nasopharynx, oropharynx, larynx and trachea.

Nd-YAG and argon lasers are of shorter wavelength and are only very weakly absorbed by water. Scattering in the tissues is strong with back scattering of 20–40%. Nd-YAG provides the deepest penetration among medical lasers. Thermal effects will result in oedema formation in the postoperative period. The main advantage of the Nd-YAG is that it can be transmitted via optical fibres and hence its applications in tracheobronchial surgery. The argon laser exhibits considerable variability in its absorptive, scattering and reflective properties. It is especially suited for retinal photocoagulation and other ophthalmological procedures. The KTP has similar properties to the argon beam and is used in ophthalmology, and for resection of vascular tumours of the upper airways.

General safety considerations

Lasers used in medical practice do not cause ionization, are not carcinogenic and do not harm pregnant women.

If a laser beam is reflected by a shiny surface in an unintended direction, injury to patients and personnel can occur. The eye is the organ most susceptible to laser injury because of its high water and pigment content. The CO_2 laser beam primarily damages the cornea, whilst the Nd-YAG, argon and krypton are preferentially absorbed by the retina. Operating theatre personnel should wear protective glasses which absorb the radiation of the laser in use. Patients' eyes should be covered with moist cotton pads strapped with canvas tapes. Wet cloth towels should cover the surrounding surgical field to act as a heat sink. Surgical instruments ought to be of matt finish to avoid beam reflection. Above all, lasers should only be activated when pointing at the intended target and operated by personnel trained and accredited in safety techniques.

Anaesthetic hazards

Tracheal tube ignition and explosion, and unintended facial burns are the most common complications of the use of CO_2 lasers in the upper airways. The likelihood of tube ignition is determined by the type of tube, the energy of the laser beam, duration of exposure and composition of the gas mixture. The only non-combustible tubes are made of metal. The Norton tube is matt finished, convex and reflective with segmented coils which allow heat dissipation. To compensate for the gas escaping around the tube (it has no cuff), the fresh gas flow can be increased or ventilation established using a Venturi jet tracheal-tube coupler clamped onto the proximal end of the Norton tube. Metal tubes are relatively large and do not give an unobstructed view of the larynx. Their use is precluded therefore in paediatric surgery.

Polyvinyl chloride (PVC) tracheal tubes are more ignitable than red rubber tubes for a given gas mixture and laser beam energy. When comparing relative flammability red rubber tubes were the most flammable followed by silicone rubber, and then PVC. Tracheal tubes can be protected by wrapping with reflective metallic foil (aluminium or copper). Cuffs should be filled with isotonic saline and protected with wet cotton swabs. Metallic foil does not offer protection from damage caused by the Nd-YAG laser.

In an attempt to overcome the fire hazard a variety of commercially produced, laser-resistant, tracheal tubes have been developed. Most are made of silicone rubber, PVC or red rubber protected by metal loading, usually with an additional outer metal covering. For a tube to be resistant to laser penetration it should be able to withstand a beam of pulses of 5–25 W for a duration of 0.1–1.0 s.

In an attempt to increase visibility and reduce exposure of combustible material to the laser beam, silicone rubber catheters and small diameter metal tubes are inserted into the airway and ventilation accomplished by jetting a gas mixture. This form of ventilation does not depend on the Venturi principle. Pressures generated are directly transmitted to the lung and are more likely to result in barotrauma. A sufficiently long time must be allowed for expiration, and the exhalation route must be secured. Venturi jet ventilation through an operating laryngoscope provides an unobstructed view, avoidance of combustible material, and clearing of smoke generated by tissue coagulation. The Hyek oscillator can also be used to provide adequate and safe ventilation.

Various gas mixtures have been employed to reduce the risk of a fire. The anaesthetic vapours are not themselves combustible. Nitrous oxide, however, readily supports combustion and nitrogen or helium should be substituted as a diluting gas for oxygen. When using the Nd-YAG laser the inspired oxygen concentration needs to be maintained below 40% during firing. At this concentration, however, oxygen supports ignition and flammability of combustible apparatus: tubes and flexible endoscopes. In the absence of combustible material the use of oxygen and/or nitrous oxide is unrestricted. Dried carbonized particles may glow briefly, but without sequelae.

Management of airway fires

For an explosion to occur there must be a source of ignition (laser beam), a source of combustion (elastomeric tube), and a medium which supports combustion (oxygen or nitrous oxide). A laser-ignited explosion can cause thermal and chemical injury. The subglottic region, epiglottis and oropharynx are most likely to be affected. Inhalation of smoke may cause a chemical burn with bronchospasm, intra-alveolar fluid exudation and loss of surfactant.

Operating theatre staff should be well-rehearsed in the management of a sudden fire and drill protocols clearly displayed. **Immediate action**: the oxygen and nitrous oxide source should be discontinued immediately and the tracheal tube removed rapidly. The area should be flushed with cool saline or water. A new tracheal tube can be inserted, or ventilation may be maintained with a face-mask and 100% oxygen. Rigid bronchoscopy carried out soon after the incident will allow any debris to be cleared. **Further action**: IPPV, monitoring of pulmonary artery pressures and cardiac output with full intensive care unit support is usually indicated. Humidification is essential, and high-dose steroid and antibiotic therapy recommended. The progress of recovery can be monitored by repeated, flexible bronchoscopy.

ANAESTHESIA FOR MALIGNANT DISEASE OF THE UPPER AIRWAY

Upper airway malignancies frequently involve the larynx and pharynx. They may be treated by radiotherapy alone, or more frequently a combination of surgery with pre- or postoperative radiotherapy. Small tumours may be excised endoscopically using the laser, whilst large tumours may necessitate major soft tissue and organ excision with radical neck dissection and flap reconstruction. **Laryngectomy** with, or without, neck dissection of the lymphatic drainage involves total excision of the larynx with creation of an end-tracheal stoma in the base of the neck. The surgical approach is a wide horizontal neck incision at the lower level of the larynx. Following mobilization the larynx is separated from the tongue base and anterior pharynx superiorly, and inferiorly the trachea is divided and a stoma created. The surgical dissection is made in close proximity to the carotid arteries, internal jugular veins, and lower cranial nerves (IX, X, XI, XII).

Pharyngolaryngectomy involves total excision of the larynx, pharynx and oesophagus, with anastomosis of the mobilized stomach to the tongue base and residual pharynx. It can be carried out through a mid-sternal thoracotomy, or a wide neck incision with stomach mobilization through an upper abdominal incision.

ANAESTHETIC MANAGEMENT OF THE COMPROMISED AIRWAY

Preoperative assessment of a partially obstructed airway should be carried out in conjunction with the surgical team. Dyspnoea, tachypnoea, anxiety and restlessness, shortness of breath and stridor, tracheal tug and intercostal recession on inspiration may all be present in severe, upper airway obstruction. Inspiratory stridor is indicative of obstruction above the vocal cords, whilst expiratory stridor suggests obstruction at the subglottic or tracheal level. It is important to evaluate the airway carefully and systematically. A mixture of helium 79% and oxygen 21% will improve airflow and can be breathed by the patient during the investigative procedures.

Chest and neck X-rays and CT scans will indicate the size and location of the lesion. Solid tumours of the posterior pharyngeal/laryngeal wall are comparatively easier to manage during laryngoscopy with upward lift allowing visualization of the laryngeal inlet. Friable and vascular tumours located on the anterior wall of the pharynx or larynx can be a formidable challenge, even to the experienced anaesthetist. Fragments of tumour and haemorrhage may cause a complete upper airway obstruction. In subglottic lesions visualization of the glottis is easy, but tracheal intubation may be fraught with problems.

Whenever possible flexible endoscopy under topical anaesthesia should be carried out as a part of a planned procedure to assess the airway. It allows detailed examination of the anatomy and function of the upper airway during inspiratory and expiratory phases. Previous radiotherapy may cause airway displacement and compression due to tissue oedema and induration. The risk of major vessel or cranial nerve damage during surgery is also greater.

Each patient has to be assessed, and a strategy for the airway planned. A selection of various sizes of larygeal tubes and a means of transtracheal ventilation should be readily available. The surgical team should be scrubbed and prepared to proceed with emergency tracheostomy.

In patients with a severely compromised airway, awake tracheal intubation or elective tracheostomy under local anaesthetic are the only safe ways of securing the airway. To facilitate awake tracheal intubation topical anaesthesia with 4% lignocaine can be supplemented with a block of the superior laryngeal back of the vagus nerve. An injection of 2 ml of local anaesthetic 1 cm medially to the superior cornua of the hyoid bone produces a superior laryngeal nerve block.

Infiltration of local anaesthetic just posterior to the palatopharyngeal fold at its mid-point and 1 cm deep produces anaesthesia of the pharyngeal wall and paralysis of the tongue base. Care must be taken not to infiltrate the area supplied by the IXth nerve as the muscular hypotonia may render partial obstruction complete. Preoperative use of glycopyrrolate reduces secretions and the incidence of laryngeal spasm, and lessens the risk of vagal nerve stimulation during endoscopy. Sedative medication should be avoided and 100% oxygen must be given for 10 min.

Inhalational induction may be prolonged and depth of anaesthesia sufficient to perform laryngoscopy difficult to achieve. Furthermore, early loss of muscle tone predisposes to complete airway obstruction. Recently introduced sevoflurane, with its low solubility, offers rapid induction with an adequate depth of anaesthesia to perform a ventilation test and laryngoscopy.

Ketamine i.v. has been found not to be associated with a loss of airway patency, or with a decrease in airway muscle activity. In contrast, there is a marked loss of airway muscle activity with midazolam. Furthermore, ketamine produces analgesia and induces sleep with increasing dosage. **Apnoea must not be risked**, whichever route of induction is used. In patients with pre-existing, chronic upper airway obstruction withdrawal of the hypoxic stimulus during inhalational induction may lead to immediate apnoea. Neuromuscular blocking drugs can only be given after ventilation is assured.

After securing the airway, anaesthesia is maintained in a conventional way. Before the larynx is separated from the trachea, both the surgeon and anaesthetist should check the connections between the tracheostomy and ventilating circuits. The tracheal tube is then withdrawn slowly, and ventilation continued via the tracheostomy tube.

The anaesthetist should be aware that surgery of the neck carries a risk of sudden and large haemorrhage from a major vessel, and preparations for the administration of blood and clotting factors should be made in advance. Traction or compression near the carotid body may result in bradycardia and hypotension. Open neck veins create the possibility of air embolism, but the incidence is low. End-tidal CO_2 monitoring will show a sudden fall in expiratory CO_2, and a precordial Doppler examination will detect a characteristic murmur. Hypotension and ECG changes are late signs.

The airway management during pharyngolaryngectomy is similar to laryngectomy. The additional problems are those of preoperative malnutrition, the extent and duration of surgery with associated blood loss, and hypothermia. Intraoperative hypotension and arrhythmias may occur during oesophageal mobilization, and stomach or colon transposition.

Nutritional status should not be overlooked in the pre- and perioperative surgical and anaesthetic management of the cancer patient. Head and neck malignancies are commonly associated with concurrent nutritional deficiencies. There is a 40% incidence of undernutrition in head and neck cancer patients, and an 80% incidence in patients with tumours arising from, or involving, the upper gastrointestinal tract. Painful dysphagia, organic obstruction, anorexia, chronic alcohol abuse and advanced age predispose to an inadequate dietary intake, whilst tumour ulceration and necrosis, local infection and recurrent haemorrhage may cause increased protein loss. Anaemia, low albumin concentration and electrolyte imbalance cause low oncotic pressures perioperatively and may lead to impaired wound healing and increased susceptibility to infection. Enteral and parenteral nutritional support may be needed preoperatively.

Perioperative hypothermia leads to an increase in plasma catecholamine values and oxygen consumption. Both predispose to perioperative myocardial ischaemia. A new method of preventing hypothermia was recommended recently: the i.v. infusion of aminoacids which have thermogenic effects. This has to be used cautiously in patients with a compromised myocardium.

TRACHEOSTOMY AND EMERGENCY AIRWAY MANAGEMENT

Tracheostomy may be necessary for acute or chronic upper airway obstruction, loss of protective airway reflexes, prolonged unconsciousness and muscle weakness. Temporary tracheostomy may be indicated when tracheal intubation is not possible in certain head and neck procedures.

It should be carried out as a planned procedure under local or general anaesthesia. General anaesthesia can be given via a small tracheal tube, a rigid bronchoscope, face mask or laryngeal mask airway. Local anaesthetic is infiltrated progressively as the tissue layers are exposed. Transtracheal injection of lignocaine will minimize coughing and discomfort during tube placement. As soon as an airway is established intravenous sedation can be given.

Immediate complications of an inexpertly performed tracheostomy are loss of airway control, haemorrhage and malpositioning of the tube. The end-tidal CO_2 concentration must be checked, as breath sounds may be heard and the chest wall seen moving with ventilation, even with a tube misplaced in the anterior mediastinum. A chest X-ray should be obtained to verify correct tube placement and the absence of a pneumothorax or surgical emphysema. The most important late complication is tracheal stenosis at the cuff site or stoma. The use of high-volume, low-pressure cuffs, which are only inflated when necessary, reduces the risk of this complication.

Cricothyroid puncture using a 14 G intravenous cannula or cricothyrotomy at the third tracheal ring can be carried out in an emergency. Transtracheal ventilation with a Sanders injector, or flushing oxygen at the rate of

15 l min^{-1} with an intermittent rate of 6 to 8 breaths per min, can maintain adequate oxygenation until preparations for tracheostomy have been made.

Laryngeal spasm is an exaggerated and prolonged response of the protective, glottic-closure reflex to irritating stimuli such as blood, saliva or a foreign body. It is mediated by the superior laryngeal nerve, and can also be induced by instrumentation, or manipulation, in a lightly anaesthetized patient. The resulting hypoxaemia and hypercapnia reduce neuronal activity, and laryngospasm eventually ceases spontaneously. Sometimes reflex apnoea occurs in response to stimulation of the superior laryngeal nerve but more frequently vigorous see-saw chest movements follow laryngeal spasm. Markedly decreased intrapleural pressures, often as low as -50 to -80 cmH$_2$O, lead to the formation of interstitial pulmonary oedema. Hypoxaemia occurs within minutes, but pulmonary oedema can be delayed for several hours following relief of the obstruction. Pulmonary oedema is a well recognized complication of upper airway obstruction, commonly occuring in patients with large laryngeal tumours, or in children with acute epiglottitis.

Prevention of laryngeal spasm is an important concern in anaesthesia. Preoperative medication with an antisialogogue, and an adequate depth of anaesthesia before laryngoscopy, together with topical use of lignocaine, help to prevent spasm. Once spasm is fully established, the airway has to be cleared of any irritant materials, 100% oxygen applied through a closely fitting mask and a tracheal tube re-inserted.

FOREIGN BODY IN THE AIRWAY

The principles of anaesthesia for rigid laryngoscopy can be applied. Ventilation carries the risk of distal impaction of the foreign body, and therefore deep inhalational anaesthesia with spontaneous ventilation is used. Postoperatively, humidified oxygen, analgesia, dexamethasone and antibiotics will be required for 24–48 h.

SURGERY FOR SNORING

Obstructive sleep apnoea is frequently associated with anatomical abnormalities of the upper airway. Large tonsils and adenoids, nasal polyposis or poor activity of pharyngeal muscles predispose to intermittent upper airway obstruction during sleep. There is a generalized muscular hypotonia during all REM stages of sleep. If those anatomical abnormalities are added to already hypotonic pharyngeal and genioglossal muscles, complete airway obstruction may occur with resulting hypoxaemia and hypercapnia. Arousals with increased muscle tone are necessary to overcome the obstruction. Repetitive arousals with associated adrenergic discharges may lead to pulmonary and arterial hypertension. Hypoxic and hypercapnic ventilatory responses are reduced in these patients and their response to anaesthesia is unpredictable.

Sleep nasendoscopy

Sleep nasendoscopy refers to the fibreoptic endoscopic assessment of upper airway function under light general anaesthesia. The technique is used increasingly by ENT surgeons as a method of investigating the snoring patient. Anaesthesia can be hazardous, as patients may not infrequently have advanced OSAS, and the airway remains unprotected throughout the procedure. Midazolam is usually given until snoring commences and a small amount of propofol added, as necessary, to maintain sleep. The application of local anaesthetic to the nasal or pharyngeal mucosa is not advised, because it may modify reflex muscular tone and therefore intefere with the functional assessment. Anaesthetists are aware that the tongue base and lateral pharyngeal wall collapse in all anaesthetized patients. However observation that palatal flutter and epiglottic closure occur independently gives an indication to the surgeon of the site of snoring. It must be remembered, though, that during physiological sleep snoring does not always coincide with periods of maximum effort of breathing. Therefore, information obtained during sleep nasendoscopy can only be interpreted in conjunction with overnight polysomnography.

Anaesthesia for uvulopalatopharyngoplasty (UVPP)

The UVPP operation was designed to relieve loud snoring. There is a common misconception, however, that it can be used for the treatment of OSAS. Patients must be selected carefully and when OSAS is suspected, overnight polysomnography should be carried out and suitable treatment instituted. There is a danger that, with amputation of the palate, noisy OSA will be changed into a silent condition and any associated cardioneurological sequelae will deteriorate further. Thus, the vibrating palate in partial airway obstruction may serve the purpose of arousing the patient increasing muscle tone and limiting the period of upper airway obstruction. Theoretically, removal of this protective reflex may further exacerbate obstructive episodes during sleep. Use of CPAP may also be precluded when there is velopharyngeal insufficiency. Resection or stiffening of the soft palate is carried out with conventional surgery or with the CO_2 laser. Specific problems are peri- and postoperative airway management, use of sedation and postoperative analgesia.

The use of preoperative sedation is controversial. However, as already mentioned OSAS must be excluded before surgery is allowed to proceed and, therefore, in the simple snorer preoperative medication with its sedative effect need not be witheld. The antisialogogue effect of preoperative medication is useful in all types of pharyngeal surgery. The airway has to be secured and protected with an orotracheal tube, which has the advantage of depressing the tongue base giving better visualization of soft palate. The use of propofol and modern volatile agents ensures rapid recovery and return of pharyngeal reflexes. After careful inspection and suction of the pharynx and nasopharynx, the tracheal tube should be removed with the patient lying on their side. During the vulnerable period between extubation and awakening the airway may be protected with a laryngeal mask. Requirements for analgesia in the immediate postoperative period vary depending on surgical technique and skill. The pain is most severe on the third to the fifth postoperative day and may be exacerbated by infection and dehydration. In extensive palatal surgery i.v. opiates may be given via a continuous infusion supplemented by dexamethasone to minimize tissue oedema. Antibiotics are given prophylactically and if swallowing is painful i.v. fluid therapy may have to be continued. If i.v. analgesia is required the patient is best managed in a high dependency unit.

Laser palatoplasty can be carried out under local anaesthesia administered by the surgeon, though the postoperative pain is just as severe as after a conventional procedure. Regular paracetamol and diclofenac, with prophylactic antibiotic cover, should be started immediately after surgery and continued for 5 days.

ANAESTHESIA FOR EAR SURGERY

TYPES OF EAR SURGERY

Otitis media is a common disease of early childhood which may result in middle ear effusion, or chronic infection associated with perforation of the tympanic membrane, erosion of the ossicles or cholesteatoma. Surgery is required for persistent hearing loss and to eradicate chronic infection. Cholesteatomas cause local bone erosion resulting in spread into the mastoid bone, and in very advanced disease may cause facial paralysis, labyrinthitis with vertigo, or intracranial complications.

Myringotomy and drainage of fluid with insertion of a grommet to ventilate the middle ear is still the commonest of all surgical procedures, and is often performed with adenoidectomy and/or tonsillectomy. Tympanic membrane perforations are usually repaired in **myringoplasty** procedures using fascia taken from the outer surface of the temporalis muscle. The graft is placed on the undersurface of the eardrum remnant after opening the middle ear. The original 'onlay' technique is now rarely employed. **Tympanoplasty** involves grafting the tympanic membrane with, or without, reconstruction or replacement of the middle ear ossicles.

Mastoidectomy is undertaken to manage a wide spectrum of temporal bone pathology. Some operations involve the eradication of mastoid disease, for example chronic infection or cholesteatoma; in other instances the mastoid bone is removed to gain access to deeper structures, for example the labyrinth, facial nerve, endolymphatic sac or inner ear for cochlear implantation. Complete mastoid bone removal may be necessary in the treatment of malignant disease or for intracranial pathology.

Otosclerosis is an inherited disorder in which new bone formation occurs around the base of the stapes ossicle causing a conductive hearing loss. **Stapedectomy** involves a transcanal approach with removal of the stapes bone and replacement by a prosthesis. The inner ear is opened to allow insertion of the prosthesis. Occasionally inner ear fluid is lost which may result in postoperative nausea.

Inner ear disorders may cause severe attacks of vertigo and sensorineural hearing loss. The commonest of these conditions is Menière's disease, when there is an overload of fluid in the inner ear. This fluid is normally absorbed by the endolymphatic sac, and clearance can be enhanced by **sac decompression** via a mastoid approach and inserting a drain. Vertigo can be abolished by **labyrinthectomy**, though initially there are always severe vestibular symptoms with nausea and sometimes vomiting in the early postoperative period. Partial labyrinthectomy can be accomplished by a middle ear approach, whilst total labyrinthectomy is undertaken via a mastoidectomy. **Vestibular nerve section** is preferred when there is useful hearing, and can be performed by transmastoid, intradural or extradural, middle cranial fossa approaches.

Many skull-based tumours, such as acoustic neuroma and glomus jugulare tumours, are now removed jointly by ENT and neurosurgeons via oblique, lateral, transtemporal approaches. These approaches avoid significant brain retraction and facilitate cranial nerve identification and preservation.

ANAESTHESIA FOR EAR SURGERY

Most middle ear surgery is undertaken in young or middle-aged patients, and typically there are no associated or pre-existing systemic diseases. Safe and comfortable operating conditions can be provided by infiltration of local anaesthetic or administration of general anaesthesia. Local anaesthesia is popular and is commonly practised in other countries. However, in the UK general anaesthesia is the preferred technique for both patients and surgeons. The special requirements and considerations for both techniques are control of bleeding for microscopic surgery, absence of sudden movement, coughing or strained breathing, and careful positioning of the head and neck.

PREOPERATIVE ASSESSMENT

A medical history and examination with emphasis on cardiorespiratory status, cerebrovascular function and family bleeding tendencies should be taken. Neck auscultation to exclude a carotid bruit, reflecting underlying cerebrovascular insufficiency, should be carried out together with assessment of cervical mobility. Lateral rotation of the neck is necessary for all ear surgery, and the position of the head is altered frequently by the surgeon.

Whenever controlled hypotension is planned investigations should include assessment of cardiorespiratory reserve and oxygen-carrying capacity. A full blood count and ECG are essential in every patient, whilst Doppler echocardiography, chest and lateral neck X-rays, and blood biochemistry tests are undertaken if clinically indicated.

PREOPERATIVE MEDICATION

Undue anxiety may result in a tachycardia and an increased requirement for β-adrenergic blockade during surgery. Apart from commonly used anxiolytics, clonidine and β-blockings drugs may be used. There is no indication for opiates unless there is severe pre-existing pain.

Ear surgery is associated with a high incidence of postoperative nausea and vomiting, especially in ablative labyrinthine and vestibular nerve procedures. The aetiology of postoperative nausea and vomiting in ear surgery is multifactorial. Anti-emetic drugs blocking the chemoreceptor trigger zone and $5HT_3$-receptor antagonists are most effective when given before induction and in combination.

CHOICE OF ANAESTHETIC TECHNIQUE

Local anaesthesia with, or without, sedation can be undertaken satisfactorily. The preoperative assessment and intraoperative monitoring is no different to that required for general anaesthesia. The patient must be able to understand, communicate, and be fully cooperative.

Local anaesthesia of the sensory innervation of the ear involves infiltration of the anterior and posterior external meatal walls to block the following nerves: auriculo-temporal nerve supplying the outer external meatus; great auricular nerve supplying the medial-lower aspect of the auricle and part of the external meatus; and the auricular branch of the vagus supplying the concha and external meatus. This is usually carried out by the surgeon using a large fenestrated aural speculum, and by direct infiltration of the post-auricular sulcus. The addition of adrenaline produces vasoconstriction, reduces bleeding and delays absorption of the local anaesthetic. Sedation may be added by i.v. midazolam and/or propofol.

General anaesthesia for ear surgery requires particular attention to the maintenance of an unobstructed airway and provision of a bloodless field. The problems specifically related to ear surgery are: effect of nitrous oxide on middle ear pressure; postoperative nausea and vomiting; facial nerve monitoring and extremes of neck rotation.

An unobstructed airway and good ventilation from the beginning of induction until awakening is a prerequisite for good anaesthesia for ear surgery. Coughing and straining increase venous pressure, whilst hypoventilation results in CO_2 retention with its well-known physiological sequelae of tachycardia and vasodilation.

The airway should be secured with an orotracheal tube. To prevent kinking or compression when the neck is rotated a reinforced, armoured tube is preferred. The LMA is suitable for shorter procedures, and it is particularly useful in securing the airway during the recovery period. The tracheal tube can be exchanged for a LMA whilst the patient is deeply anaesthetized, and subsequently the LMA is tolerated well until full recovery. Lignocaine (4%) sprayed to the larynx and pharynx before intubation, or placement of the LMA, will assist further in avoiding coughing and preventing laryngeal spasm. Depending on the patient's cardiorespiratory status and duration of the procedure, breathing can be spontaneous or controlled. Spontaneous breathing offers the advantage of lower venous pressures whilst lighter planes of anaesthesia can be maintained during IPPV.

Otological surgery is carried almost exclusively using the operating microscope and small quantities of blood will obscure important anatomical structures. In addition, accumulation of blood in the middle ear during the postoperative period may **predispose** to infection.

The following principles must be observed before pharmacological control of blood pressure is undertaken.

- Venous pressure at the operating site is reduced by positioning the patient with a head-up tilt.
- Venous congestion is prevented by limiting head rotation, and ensuring smooth induction, maintenance and emergence of anaesthesia.
- Adequate ventilation is maintained to avoid hypercapnia and associated tachycardia and vasodilation.
- Adequate analgesia is provided to prevent adrenergic stimulation and resulting tachycardia and hypertension.

If a bloodless field is not achieved using conventional methods of smooth anaesthesia, posture and ventilation, controlled hypotension may be required. Before employing any hypotensive technique the risks and limitations of hypotension must be well understood. It is often thought that the risks are directly proportional to the degree of peroperative hypotension. It must be remembered, however, that if the mean arterial pressure provides adequate blood flow, a shortened duration of surgery may be safer. There must, of course, be a sensible balance between the degree of controlled hypotension and the quality of the surgical field which varies with each patient and the anaesthetist's experience. It must be emphasized that the quality of the surgical field is not only related to arterial pressure. In practice, pharmacological control of the heart rate to around 60 b.p.m. can be achieved with β-adrenergic or calcium channel blocking drugs. Peripheral vascular resistance can be lowered with α-adrenergic blockade, ganglionic blockade or drugs acting directly on vascular smooth muscle. Control of arterial pressure has to be extended into the recovery and postoperative period as sudden rises will predispose to haematoma formation with a consequent risk of infection and failure of the procedure. Smooth recovery is possible when analgesia is effective, ventilation unobstructed and adequate, and arterial pressure controlled, if necessary, to prevent rebound hypertension. Whenever controlled hypotension is used direct monitoring of the arterial pressure, and recording indices of organ perfusion are essential.

THE EFFECT OF NITROUS OXIDE ON MIDDLE EAR SURGERY

The early surgical technique of tympanoplasty and myringoplasty involved the onlay of a tissue graft onto the lateral aspect of the tympanic membrane. Excessive middle ear pressure after application of the graft tended to lift it outwards resulting in graft displacement. Presently an underlay graft technique is usually preferred. Excessive middle ear pressure will therefore only be important when the initial tympanic membrane perforation is large.

Nitrous oxide diffuses from capillary blood to a closed middle ear space. Expansion of gas is proportional to the duration of anaesthesia and the inspired fraction of nitrous oxide. After 2 h F_{IN_2O} of 0.5 will double the middle ear pressure, whilst an F_{IN_2O} of 0.7 will quadruple it. After discontinuation of nitrous oxide at the end of the procedure, the gas is rapidly reabsorbed and sustained, marked, negative middle ear pressures may develop, particularly if Eustachian tube function is abnormal. This low pressure may contribute to the transudation of fluid into the middle ear, or graft and prosthesis displacement. It is accepted practice to limit inspired nitrous oxide to 50%, or use an oxygen-in-air mixture, which avoids large fluctuations in intra- and postoperative middle ear pressure, thereby preventing graft displacement.

PATIENT POSITIONING

A head-up tilt is used to allow venous pooling into the dependent parts of the body and reduce venous pressure at the operating site. During prolonged ear surgery neuroskeletal injuries may occur and the ulnar and radial nerves are at risk, particularly if hypotension is used. Extreme neck rotation may cause compression of the internal and external jugular veins counteracting any measures taken to provide the bloodless field. Lateral rotation of the operating table with support of the patient is preferred, rather than extreme head rotation for adequate access. Arms should be placed in a neutral position, flexed and inwardly rotated to open the olecranon fossa to its maximum extent.

FACIAL NERVE PRESERVATION

Intraoperative monitoring of facial nerve function is used increasingly to reduce risks of surgical injury. Neuromuscular blockade should be discontinued, or reversed, before temporal bone drilling. Continuous infusion of neuromuscular blocking drugs at low doses slows the transmission in peripheral nerves, whilst activity in the cranial nerves is preserved. Hence the use of a relaxograph applied to a distal limb is helpful in maintaining the required level of muscle relaxation. In the spontaneously breathing patient the depth of anaesthesia should be sufficient to prevent any reflex movement, and this can be achieved using deep inhalational techniques or a combination of intravenous and inhalational anaesthesia. In a ventilated patient the degree of sympathetic stimulation is a guide to the depth of anaesthesia and it is essential to delay using sympathetic blocking drugs until sufficient anaesthesia has been reliably established. Use of perioperative EEG monitoring, although rarely practised, would be ideal.

POSTOPERATIVE NAUSEA AND VOMITING

Control of postoperative nausea and vomiting is essential, as retching increases venous and intracranial pressure and carries the risks of bleeding and surgical failure. Nausea and vomiting may occur after stapedectomy surgery, and are inevitable after labyrinthectomy and vestibular nerve section. In this group of patients preventative treatment is indicated. My preferred method is to give simultaneous chemoreceptor trigger zone and $5HT_3$-receptor blocking drugs commencing with induction and repeated at regular intervals for 48 h. If nausea prevents adequate fluid intake, intravenous therapy should be continued well into the postoperative period.

SPECIFIC ANAESTHETIC CONSIDERATIONS

Myringotomy and ventilation tube (grommet) insertion

This procedure is commonly performed in the UK for chronic middle ear effusions and hearing impairment, and is frequently carried out as a day-case procedure. In suitable adult patients it can be undertaken under local anaesthesia, and EMLA cream painted onto the eardrum is all that is usually required. In children and uncooperative adults, microscopic surgery can only be carried out satisfactorily under a general anaesthetic. Following induction with an intravenous or inhalational agent the airway can be maintained by an oropharyngeal airway or LMA. Paracetomol is adequate for postoperative analgesia, though rectal or oral NSAIDs are occasionally indicated.

Middle ear surgery

A bloodless field is important for all types of reconstructive middle ear surgery, but is a prerequisite for stapedectomy. Because surgery entails opening the inner ear, attempts to suction even small amounts of blood increase the risk of loss of inner ear fluid, resulting in postoperative dizziness and vomiting, and jeopardizing long-term hearing. Blood entering the vestibule may also compromise inner ear function.

During tympanoplasty, incision of the deep external canal skin or tympanic membrane may provoke refractory bradycardia due to intense vagal stimulation. Even when general anaesthesia is used it is important for the surgeon to infiltrate the external canal with a lignocaine and adrenaline mixture to prevent vagal stimulation.

Mastoidectomy

The duration of surgery varies depending on the precise nature of the procedure, the complexity of the anatomy and experience of the surgeon. When there is poor pneumatization of the temporal bone and the anatomy is compact, or when access to deeper structures is required, there is an increased likelihood of puncturing the sigmoid venous sinus with the possible risk of air embolism. The pressure in the venous sinuses is decreased in proportion to the degree of head elevation. It is important for the surgeon to inform the anaesthetist if there has been a puncture of the sinus. The open sinus should be sealed rapidly and the patient lowered immediately so that the wound is placed down below the heart level. The management of acute air embolism is discussed in Chapter 14.

Acoustic neuroma and skull base surgery

Although some of these procedures are entirely extradural, the anaesthetic considerations are those for neuroanaesthesia in a supine position. Lumbar and ventricular drains may be used to assist control of CSF volume and intracranial pressure. Invasive monitoring of arterial pressure should be carried out for about 48 h until the risk of complications has passed. Transmastoid, intracranial procedures require neurological monitoring in the early postoperative period which is best carried out in an intensive care unit. With large tumours and during prolonged surgery there is a recognized risk of non-specific disseminated intravascular coagulation due to thromboplastin activation. Coagulation studies should be carried out preoperatively and repeated intraoperatively if there are unexpected difficulties in obtaining a bloodless field.

ANAESTHESIA FOR NASAL SURGERY

Advances in tele-endoscopic technology have greatly increased the scope of the surgical management of chronic sinusitis and polypoidal disease of the nose. Increased awareness of the physiology of the upper airway during sleep has also lead to re-evaluation of the indications for surgical management of conditions affecting the nasal airway. The requirements of ideal anaesthesia for nasal surgery have changed dramatically during the last decade. A bloodless field, rapid awakening, pleasant recovery and postoperative course are expected and achievable with the use of recently introduced i.v. and inhalational anaesthetic agents and the LMA.

TYPES OF NASAL AND SINUS SURGERY

Corrective surgery to the septum is carried out to improve nasal airflow and ventilation of the sinuses. Nasal injuries are common and may result in displaced fractures. If not corrected within 10 days, permanent cosmetic deformity and nasal obstruction may result. Unilateral septal deviation causes hypertrophy of the contralateral inferior turbinate with further airway obstruction. Mucosal congestion may result in poor ventilation of the nasal sinuses and predispose to recurrent infections.

Septoplasty or **submucous resection** involve repositioning or resection of the cartilaginous or bony parts of the nasal septum. Inferior **turbinate reduction** is carried out by submucosal diathermy, partial excision using scissors or the KTP laser, or lateral outfracture. **Nasal polypectomy** can be undertaken using wire snares or forceps. However, dissection of their site of origin in the ethmoid sinus results in better clearance, and this is usually carried out endoscopically.

Endoscopes with angled lenses improve visualization of the anatomical structures of the lateral and superior walls of the nasal cavity and are now frequently used for access to the osteomeatal complex, diseases of the sphenoethmoid sinuses, and to open the maxillary antrum (antrostomy). Functional endoscopic sinus surgery has now largely superceded intranasal antrostomy and Caldwell–Luc procedures. More specialized surgery to the frontal sinuses, nasolacrimal duct and anterior skull base may also be carried out employing this technique. Postnasal space examination and biopsy can be carried out transorally using a Boyle–Davis tonsillectomy gag or transnasally using the endoscope.

Lateral rhinotomy was previously used for neoplastic conditions of the lateral nasal cavity. The anterior cranial fossa is the immediate superior relation to the ethmoid sinuses and nasal cavity. Management of malignant disease in this region frequently involves a limited craniotomy: **craniofacial resection**.

PREOPERATIVE ASSESSMENT AND INVESTIGATIONS

During the preoperative assessment attention should be given to the duration and severity of chronic nasal obstruction. Chronic nasal obstruction may trigger, and if not treated worsen, obstructive sleep apnoea with resulting pulmonary or arterial hypertension and myocardial ischaemia. If suspected, the patient should be fully investigated for this condition. In these patients nasal CPAP cannot be applied during the postoperative period, and if pre-existing OSAS is severe, a small peroperative tracheostomy tube may need to be inserted. This can be left in place for approximately 3 weeks until healing is complete, and nasal CPAP may be resumed.

Bronchial asthma and multiple allergies, in particular aspirin sensitivity, are commonly associated with polypoidal ethmoidal sinus disease. Topical anaesthesia may be preferred. Application of cocaine or lignocaine with adrenaline to the nasal mucosa usually provides acceptable analgesia and a relatively dry surgical field. Transient tachycardia resulting from the systemic effect of cocaine and adrenaline can be counteracted with i.v. calcium channel blocking drugs.

Anxiolysis is important as a slow heart rate is required throughout the perioperative period. Clonidine has been advocated as a suitable anxiolytic with additional α_2-agonist properties. However, it has a detrimental effect on the hypoxic ventilatory response and this must be considered in patients in whom large nasal packs will be placed postoperatively which may result in partial airway obstruction.

LOCAL PREPARATION OF THE NOSE

Anaesthesia for nasal surgery has to meet the requirements for endoscopic and microscopic procedures where the provision of a bloodless field is mandatory. The septum, inferior turbinates and polyps are very vascular structures and excessive bleeding will occur if effective preoperative vasoconstriction has not been achieved. Topical application of cocaine or lignocaine with adrenaline produces vasoconstriction and blocks the sphenopalatine ganglion which carries the vasodilator fibres to the nasal blood vessels. Cocaine readily penetrates the mucous membranes and is an effective topical anaesthetic with an intense vasoconstrictor action. It blocks the reuptake of noradrenaline at sympathetic nerve terminals and potentiates any sympathetic activity.

Arrythmias, hypertension and stimulation of the CNS may occur.

The *British National Formulary* recommends the use of cocaine in no more than 4% solution and a maximal dose of 1.5 mg kg^{-1}. It also advises against the concomitant use of adrenaline. Solutions and pastes of higher concentration reduce the time of onset and increase the duration of action. The addition of adrenaline significantly reduces the systemic absorption of cocaine during surgery. Despite theoretical benefits, there are reports of unusually rapid absorption when cocaine is combined with adrenaline, attributed to a decay in the adrenaline-induced vasoconstriction. Thus, the addition of adrenaline to cocaine is unpredictable, and may increase the risk of toxic effects which it is meant to reduce.

Lignocaine 4% with adrenaline 1:1000 is an alternative to provide vasoconstriction and decongestion. For instillation the head is positioned with full neck extension, and the septum and right and left turbinates are soaked in turn. The extended neck allows anaesthesia of the sphenopalatine ganglion in the lateral posterosuperior nasal quadrant.

ANAESTHETIC TECHNIQUES

Sensory innervation of the nasal mucosa is provided by the ophthalmic and maxillary divisions of the trigeminal nerve. Infiltration of the sphenopalatine ganglion, maxillary nerve and anterior ethmoidal nerve will provide analgesia of the frontal and maxillary sinuses. Topical analgesia of the nasal cavities is useful for surgery of the anterior septum, removal of polyps, turbinectomy and cauterization. To avoid the risks of coughing and laryngeal spasm, intravenous sedation should be started after local anaesthetic drugs have been absorbed.

General anaesthesia is better suited for longer operations and where the quality of the operating field is critical to the outcome. Propofol has an advantage as an induction agent: it depresses pharyngeal and laryngeal reflexes and facilitates quick insertion of an oropharyngeal airway or laryngeal mask. During surgery the airway is best protected with a cuffed tracheal tube, but in selected short cases where bleeding is not anticipated, the airway can be maintained with a LMA. Further airway protection is conventionally achieved by the insertion of a moist or greased gauze pack. Alternatively, a small-bore pharyngeal suction catheter can be placed alongside the tracheal tube or LMA and gentle suction applied intermittently. After the airway has been secured and protected, both nostrils are cleared of crust and secretions, gently wiped with saline-impregnated cotton buds, and cocaine or lignocaine with adrenaline applied as described above. A change from a tracheal tube to a laryngeal mask is recommended at the end of the procedure to maintain and protect the airway until the full return of pharyngeal reflexes.

The patient is positioned with a 15° head-up tilt and allowed to breathe spontaneously. The negative intrathoracic pressure during spontaneous ventilation assists venous return. Hypercapnia must be avoided due to its sympathomimetic and vasodilating effects. Patients with poor cardiorespiratory reserve, obesity, or suffering from OSAS require controlled ventilation.

To minimize bleeding during surgery the arterial pressure should be maintained at the preinduction value, or below. This should be readily achieved with an adequate depth of anaesthesia, controlled ventilation and good positioning. In some circumstances the arterial pressure may have to be lowered using a combination of β- and α-sympathetic blocking drugs.

Absence of coughing or sudden movement is of great importance in endoscopic nasal surgery where instruments are placed in close proximity to the optic nerve and anterior cranial fossa. Waking up must be very gentle as bouts of uncontrolled coughing or rises in arterial pressure may lead to a sudden and large haemorrhage, with the risk of accumulation of blood in the periorbital space causing increased orbital pressure and optic nerve damage.

In the past, restlessness during the recovery period after nasal surgery was accepted as inevitable. Large nasal packs contribute to increased upper airway resistance, and thiopentone may be responsible for restlessness which is frequently difficult to control. Modern practice using propofol, low solubility inhalational agents and protection of the airway with LMA ensure an uneventful postoperative recovery. Nasal surgery is not a painful procedure, and postoperative analgesia is easy to achieve with diclofenac or paracetomol.

DAY-CASE SURGERY

A minimally invasive approach and a pain-free postoperative course make nasal surgery well suited to day-case management. Turbinectomy and posterior septal surgery carry a higher risk of postoperative haemorrhage, and overnight stay is advised. A common postoperative complaint following nasal surgery is a sore throat, which is sometimes associated with uvular and pharyngeal abrasions following forceful insertion of the LMA, excessive packing or blind pharyngeal suction. This may prevent the patient from going home on the same day.

FURTHER READING

Brookes, G. B. (1982) Nutritional status in head and neck cancer: observations and implications. *Clinical Otolaryngology*, **8**, 211–220.

Department of Health. (1987) *Guidance on the Safe use of Lasers in Medical Practice*. HMSO, London.

Dodds, C. (1994) Sleep apnoea and anaesthesia, in: *Recent Advances in Anaesthesia and Analgesia*, (eds A. P. Adam and J. N. Cashma) Churchill Livingstone, Edinburgh, pp.179–197.

Hunton, J. and Oswal, V. H. (1988) Anaesthesia for carbon dioxide laser laryngeal surgery in infancy. *Anaesthesia*, **43**, 394–396.

Nair, I. and Bailey, B. M. (1995) Review of uses of the laryngeal mask in ENT anaesthesia. *Anaesthesia*, **50**, 898–900.

Ruttman, T. G., James, M. F. M. and Viljoen, J. E. (1996) Haemodilution induces a hypercoagulable state. *British Journal of Anaesthesia*, **76**, 412–414.

Walsh, G. R. and Navin, M. (1994) External high frequency oscillation ventilation. *Intensive Care in Britain* Greycoat Publishing, London.

PAEDIATRIC SURGERY

A. I. McEwan and A. E. Black

ANATOMY AND PHYSIOLOGY WITH ASSOCIATED ANAESTHETIC IMPLICATIONS

There exist significant differences in anatomy and physiology between the baby and the older child or adult that are relevant to the anaesthetist. A sound understanding of these differences is the basis of safe paediatric anaesthetic practice.

RESPIRATORY SYSTEM

The baby or young infant has a relatively large head with a protruding occiput and a short neck. Several factors conspire to make babies more difficult to intubate: the tongue is large and the larynx lies more anterior and cephalad at the level of C4 compared with C6 in the adult. The epiglottis is large, U shaped and floppy, and a laryngoscope with a straight blade is used to lift the epiglottis out of the way. The trachea is short making accurate, secure placement of the tracheal tube important. The trachea is lined with pseudostratified columnar epithelium which is only loosely connected to the underlying tissue. The narrowest point of the airway is at the cricoid cartilage and it is here that an oversized tracheal tube may cause trauma with subsequent oedema or subglottic stenosis. Resistance to gas flow is related to the fourth power of the radius and thus a small amount of oedema can cause a significant increase in resistance at this point.

The ribs are aligned horizontally and so the ability to increase lung volumes by an increase in the anterior–posterior distance by the 'bucket handle' effect is lost. Increases in ventilation must therefore be met almost exclusively by increases in respiratory rate. Oxygen consumption is 7–8 ml kg^{-1} min^{-1} which is 2–3 times that of the adult value, resulting in a higher respiratory rate of 30–40 breaths per minute. Muscle fatigue is also more likely in the neonate as the diaphragm consists of only 30% Type I muscle fibres (slow twitch, oxidative, fatigue resistant) compared with 55% at one year of age. Preterm babies have only 10% Type I fibres.

Functional residual capacity (FRC) is reduced because of the compliant chest wall and FRC is maintained primarily by the increased respiratory rate. Closing volumes encroach on tidal ventilation and ventilation perfusion ratios are poorly matched. Apnoea and anaesthesia both reduce FRC and thus impair oxygenation. Controlled ventilation is therefore nearly always employed during anaesthesia in babies and small infants, and high respiratory rates and positive end-expiratory pressure are useful in maintaining FRC.

Nasal air passages contribute up to 50% of total resistance to air flow. The insertion of a nasogastric tube may further increase airways resistance by 50%. Newborn babies have been described as 'obligate nose breathers' but it may be more accurate to say that they are

Short Practice of Anaesthesia. Edited by M. Morgan and G. M. Hall. Published in 1997 by Chapman & Hall, London. ISBN 0 412 71890 1

slow to convert to mouth breathing if nasal obstruction occurs.

Pulmonary surfactants are phospholipids produced by the Type 2 pneumocytes of the lung. The main surfactant produced is lecithin; production starts at about 22 weeks and increases during intrauterine development. The action of surfactant is to reduce surface tension in the alveoli preventing collapse and allowing easier re-expansion of collapsed alveoli. By measuring the lecithin/sphingomyelin ratio in the amniotic fluid of the mother the maturity of the fetal lungs can be gauged. The ratio increases from 1 at 32 weeks to 2 at 35 weeks and 4–6 at term. A lack of surfactant results in respiratory distress syndrome, and hypoxia, acidosis and hypothermia all inhibit production of pulmonary surfactant.

Ventilation is controlled primarily by the integration of signals from central and peripheral chemoreceptors and by mechanical receptors in the lung and chest wall. These mechanical receptors give rise to the Hering–Breuer and 'head' reflexes, and assume greater importance in the newborn baby than in the older child or adult. The ventilatory response to increased carbon dioxide tensions is less than in adults and further reduced by hypoxia. The response to hypoxia depends on the gestational age and on the general condition of the neonate. Healthy full-term babies over 2–3 weeks of age respond to hypoxia with an increase in ventilation, but preterm babies and full-term babies in the first week of life respond initially with increased ventilation followed by respiratory depression. If hypothermia is present hypoxia results in ventilatory depression.

Short periods of apnoea lasting up to 10 s, which are not associated with cyanosis or bradycardia, can occur in preterm and in some full-term babies. This is known as periodic breathing and poses no threat. However of greater concern is apnoea lasting longer than 20 s or associated with bradycardia or cyanosis. This type of apnoea may be central, obstructive, or a combination of the two, and indeed one may lead to another. These apnoeas maybe a result of sepsis, hypothermia, depressant drugs or may be simply related to prematurity.

Postoperative apnoea is more common in immature pre-term babies and occasionally may occur in full-term infants. Preterm infants of less than 60 weeks postconceptual age need to be monitored with an apnoea alarm for a minimum of 12 h postoperatively and full-term infants less than 45 weeks postconceptual age should also be monitored.

CIRCULATION

Fetal circulation and transitional circulation

Oxygenated blood from the placenta enters the umbilical vein, 50% of which bypasses the liver via the ductus venosus to enter the inferior vena cava (IVC). The well oxygenated blood from the IVC is directed from the right atrium through the foramen ovale into the left atrium and from there to the left ventricle and ascending aorta. This enables the well oxygenated blood to be preferentially distributed to the growing brain and to the coronary arteries. Less well oxygenated blood from the superior vena cava (SVC), and from the gut and liver, is directed from the right atrium to right ventricle and from here to the pulmonary arteries. Resistance to flow is high in the fetal lungs and only 10% of the cardiac output will pass through this high resistance circuit. The remainder of this poorly oxygenated blood passes through the patent ductus arteriosus (PDA) to the descending aorta and on to the lower body (Figure 19.1).

At birth the lungs are normally quickly expanded and fill with air. The pulmonary vascular resistance falls rapidly as a result of mechanical factors and because of an increase in the alveolar Po_2 and a fall in Pco_2. This results in a dramatic increase in flow to the pulmonary veins which increases the return to the left atrium and thus increases the left

Anatomy and physiology 339

creases perhaps as result of hypoxia, hypercapnia, acidosis or in cases of respiratory distress syndrome or diaphragmatic hernia. As pulmonary vascular resistance increases, flow through the ductus arteriosus may again revert to right to left creating a shunt that allows blood to bypass the lungs. This in turn creates worsening hypoxia, an increasing acidosis leading to yet higher pulmonary vascular resistance, and a downward spiral (Figure 19.2).

Neonatal circulation

The neonatal myocardium has only 30% contractile fibres and is relatively non-compliant.

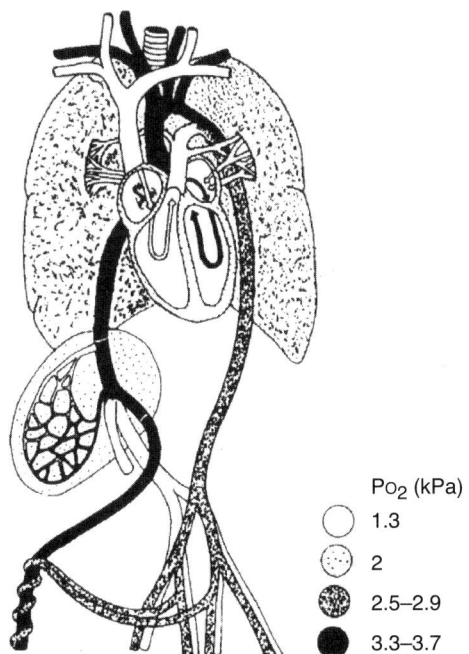

Figure 19.1 Fetal circulation. (Reproduced with permission from Davis, J.A. and Dobbing, J. (eds) (1981) Growth and development of the cardiovascular system, in *Scientific Foundations of Paediatrics*. 2nd edn. Heinemann Medical, London. p. 373.)

ventricular output. At the same time systemic vascular resistance increases, largely as a result of the loss of the low resistance circuit contained within the placenta. The overall effect is to increase pressures on the left side of the heart and reduce them on the right. This leads to closure of the septum over the foramen ovale and reversal of flow through the ductus arteriosus. In addition, the increased oxygen content of the blood passing through the ductus causes a prostaglandin-mediated constriction of the ductus. Permanent closure may take up to a week or occasionally longer. A similar period of time may be required to close the foramen ovale (Figure 19.2).

In the early neonatal period a transitional circulation may occur. This happens when pulmonary vascular resistance again in-

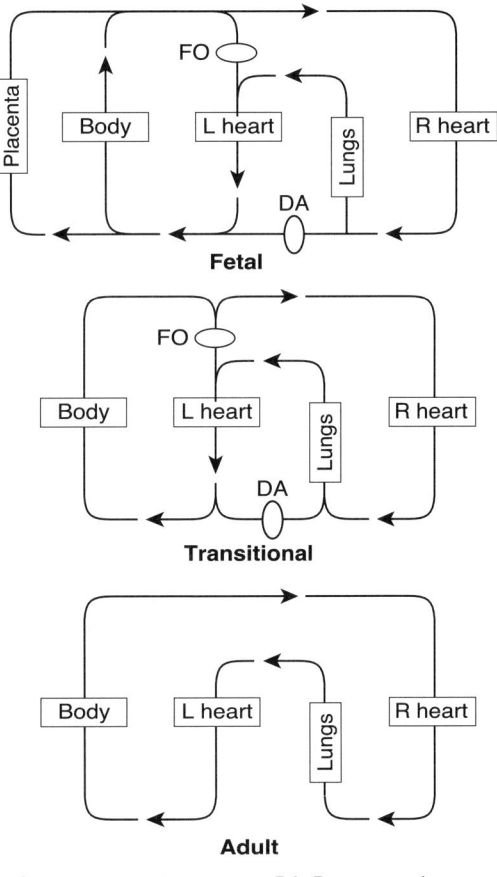

Figure 19.2 Changes in circulation after birth.

Stroke volume is fixed and cardiac output is therefore rate dependent and a bradycardia almost always causes a low output state. Systolic blood pressure is approximately 60 mmHg and the average heart rate is 120 b.p.m. Cardiac output is high reflecting the high metabolic rate. The circulating blood volume of a full-term baby in the immediate postnatal period varies widely depending on the placental transfusion at birth. The blood volume will, however, have stabilized by 48 h although the haematocrit will vary. The blood volume of a full-term baby is approximately 80–85 ml kg^{-1}, although in a preterm baby it may be as high as 100 ml kg^{-1}. By 6 weeks the value is 75 ml kg^{-1}. In the newborn baby, hypovolaemia causes a decrease in blood pressure and this fall appears to be directly related to the degree of hypovolaemia. The inability to compensate may be due to immaturity of the control of capacitance vessels. The haemoglobin value of 17 g dl^{-1} at birth falls over the next 4–8 weeks to 11 g dl^{-1}. This physiological anaemia of infancy is due to a low red cell production rate and a decreased survival time for red cells. The majority (80%) of haemoglobin at birth is HbF. This has a higher oxygen affinity than HbA with a p50 of 2.7 kPa compared with the adult value of 3.6 kPa. This high affinity is compensated for by the relatively high degree of acidosis, hypercapnia and hypoxia in the peripheral tissues. By three months the HbF has largely been replaced by HbA. In the pre-term baby the degree of physiological anaemia is greater.

TEMPERATURE REGULATION

Newborn babies are susceptible to hypothermia because of their large surface area to weight ratio, poor insulation because of reduced subcutaneous fat and inability to shiver. Heat is not only lost to the environment by radiation, conduction, convection and evaporation, but during anaesthesia core heat is also rapidly redistributed to the

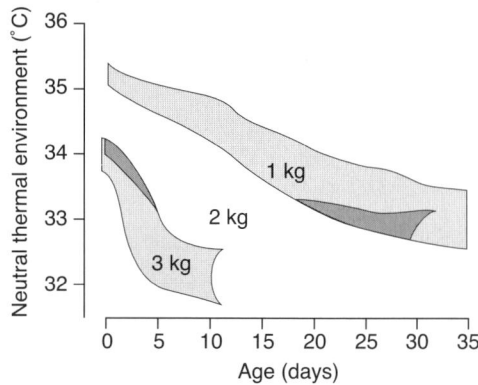

Figure 19.3 The changing neutral thermal environment for naked babies of differing birth weight and age. (Reproduced with permission from Hey, E.N. and Katz, G. (1970) The optimal thermal environment for naked babies. *Archives of Diseases of Childhood*, **45**, 328–34.)

periphery because of peripheral vasodilation. The response to cooling is an increase in heat production and this is achieved by non-shivering thermogenesis, by metabolism of brown fat and by peripheral vasoconstriction. Brown fat, which makes up 2–6% of body weight, surrounds the kidneys and adrenal glands and is present in the mediastinum as well as around the scapulae. Metabolism of the brown fat, which involves hydrolysis of triglycerides to glycerol, results in an increased oxygen consumption and heat production, and is mediated by noradrenaline released from sympathetic nerve endings in the fat. Increased oxygen and glucose consumption result in acidosis and may worsen any existing hypoxia. The temperature at which minimal metabolic demands are made on the baby is known as the neutral thermal environment. This is 36°C for the small, pre-term baby but lower for larger, full-term babies (Figure 19.3).

Measures to prevent cooling during surgery include measuring core temperature continuously, transfer to and from theatre in a heated incubator, a warmed theatre environment and minimal exposure. The head should be covered and the baby covered with a warmed blanket. A warm air mattress is used, and inspired gases are warmed and humidified. Intravenous fluids and cleaning solutions should be warmed.

METABOLISM AND COAGULATION

Hypoglycaemia is common in the sick, preterm or small newborn baby because of low carbohydrate reserves and immature gluconeogenesis. Infants of diabetic mothers may be particularly at risk. Blood glucose needs close monitoring in these infants and 10% glucose infusion 75–100 ml kg^{-1} per 24 h may be required to prevent levels falling below 2.2 mmol l^{-1}. Very low values need urgent treatment with 50% glucose 1–2 ml kg^{-1}. Neurological damage may occur in up to 50% of newborn babies with symptomatic hypoglycaemia.

Hyperglycaemia predisposing to cerebral haemorrhage, water and electrolyte loss in the urine, and exacerbation of hypoxic neurological damage may occur as a result of over zealous use of glucose containing intravenous fluids. Hypocalcaemia is common in pre-term or sick babies. Treatment is required if calcium levels fall below 1.5 mmol l^{-1}.

Coagulation factors are relatively normal at birth, although some vitamin K dependent factors may be deficient. Vitamin K 1 mg should be given to all neonates requiring surgery. Other coagulation abnormalities are common in sick newborn babies, particularly if they are pre-term and thrombocytopenia is a particular problem. Platelets, fresh frozen plasma, cryoprecipitate or specific factors may need to be given before surgery. Liver function is normal by three months of age.

FLUID BALANCE

Neonatal renal function is characterized by a low glomerular filtration rate as a result of high vascular resistance and limited tubular function. This results in a reduced ability to

Table 19.1 Maintenance fluid requirements after the first week of life

Weight (kg)	Rate (ml kg^{-1} h^{-1})	
Up to 10 kg	4 ml kg^{-1} h^{-1}	
10–20 kg	4 ml kg^{-1} h^{-1}	1st 10 kg+
	2 ml kg^{-1} h^{-1}	2nd 10 kg
20–30 kg	4 ml kg^{-1} h^{-1}	1st 10 kg+
	2 ml kg^{-1} h^{-1}	2nd 10 kg+
	1 ml kg^{-1} h^{-1}	last 10 kg

e.g. for a 15 kg child: 1st 10 kg 4 ml kg^{-1} h^{-1}= 40 ml h^{-1}
Next 5 kg 2 ml kg^{-1} h^{-1}=10 ml h^{-1}
Total=50 ml kg^{-1} h^{-1}

dilute or concentrate urine, and therefore increased difficulty in coping with a water or electrolyte load, or with dehydration. In addition, there is a tendency to hyponatraemia, acidosis and glycosuria.

At birth the total body water is high and the greater proportion is extracellular. In the first few days of life some of this water is excreted by the kidney and so in the absence of high losses, water requirements are low, 40 ml kg^{-1} per 24 h on day one increasing by 20 ml kg^{-1} per 24 h to a maximum of 120 ml kg^{-1} per 24 h. Preterm babies may require as much as 200 ml kg^{-1} per 24 h because of increased insensible losses. For older infants fluid requirements are summarized in Table 19.1. Maintenance fluid requirements can be met by use of 4% glucose with 0.18% saline.

During surgery blood and other losses are carefully assessed and replaced. Close attention to the haemodynamic state of the child, in conjunction with regular haematocrit determination, is usually the most reliable way of assessing blood and fluid loss. Third-space and evaporative losses during major surgery may be as high as 5–15 ml kg^{-1} h^{-1}. Maintenance fluids should continue and blood is replaced with fresh whole blood if possible, or a combination of red cells and human albumin solution or other colloids, if fresh whole blood is unavailable.

THE EYES AND RETINOPATHY OF PREMATURITY

Retinopathy of prematurity (ROP) (retrolental fibroplasia) describes a spectrum of retinal damage from early vasoconstriction, oedema and degeneration of the peripheral part of the retina (Stage 1) through to retinal detachment and blindness (Stage 4). Hyperoxia, once thought to be the only culprit, is now considered to be one of several risk factors which include sepsis, hypoxia, hyper and hypocapnia, blood transfusion, exposure to light and systemic illnesses.

ROP occurs most commonly in small preterm babies of less than 35 weeks of gestation and weighing less than 1500 g. A safe level of oxygenation is now thought to be 7–10 kPa or, if arterial saturation is monitored, a level of 90–95% should be safe.

PAIN

It is only recently that the long-held belief that newborn and small babies do not feel pain has given way to a realization that they do so. In addition to crying and grimacing, they respond with tachycardia, hypertension and raised intracranial pressure. Some suggest that adequate pain control may lead to increased surgical survival.

PHARMACOLOGY

GENERAL PRINCIPLES

The main differences between adult and paediatric pharmacology occur in very young children.

The larger, extracellular fluid volume in young children means that drugs such as depolarizing neuromuscular blocking drugs, which are distributed in the extracellular fluid need to be given in larger doses. Metabolism in neonates is unpredictable and they have a lower concentration of serum proteins. Drugs which bind to these proteins have an increased plasma concentration, and smaller doses are needed to achieve a given effect. The blood–brain barrier is immature, as are the renal, hepatic and nervous systems leading to unpredictable drug effects, and drugs with active metabolites may accumulate.

The presence of fewer receptors specific for drugs such as opiates is suggested as one of the reasons for increased sensitivity of babies to these drugs.

INHALATION AGENTS

Properties of an ideal agent for paediatric gaseous inductions include:

- safe, non-flammable, non-explosive,
- little effect on cardiorespiratory system,
- minimal toxicity,
- low incidence of side effects (airway irritation, nausea),
- rapid induction and recovery profile,
- high potency, i.e. low MAC,
- presence of some muscle relaxation or analgesic properties, and pleasant smell.

Increased alveolar ventilation in children results in a quicker uptake and elimination of inhalational agents, particularly with the less soluble agents such as sevoflurane. A higher percentage of the cardiac output is distributed to the vessel rich group, so that there is increased distribution to the brain, hastening induction. There is also lower tissue/blood and blood/gas solubilities in infants compared with adults, due in part to the higher water content and lower protein and fat concentration. The uptake of halothane, enflurane and isoflurane is inversely related to age. The rate of rise of alveolar to inspired partial pressures of the varying anaesthetic agents is inversely related to their blood solubility. MAC varies with age, decreasing at the extremes of age, it is low in the newborn and highest between 1 and 6 months (Figure 19.4).

Currently, halothane is the agent used most extensively in paediatric anaesthesia for gas-

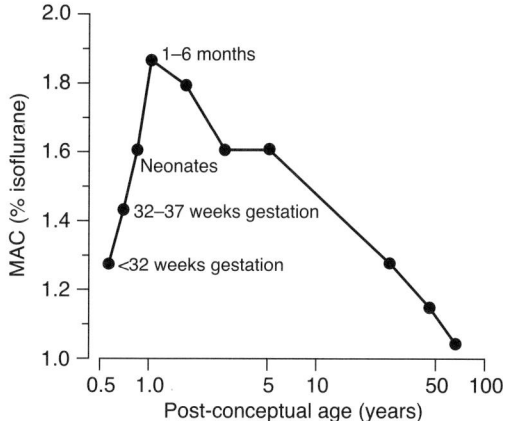

Figure 19.4 Changes of MAC values with age. (Reproduced with permission from Lerman, J. (1992) Pharmacology of inhalational anaesthetics in infants and children. *Paediatric Anaesthesia*, **2**, 191–203.)

eous induction. Halothane provides a smooth, gaseous induction and it is currently the drug of choice for any child with a potentially difficult airway. It causes dose-dependent depression of the myocardium and a bradycardia which result in a decrease in cardiac output; these effects may be partially offset by atropine. Arhythmias are also commoner with halothane, particularly ventricular ectopic beats and junctional rhythms. During halothane anaesthesia the myocardium has an increased sensitivity to exogenous catecholamines compared with isoflurane and sevoflurane. Although cases of halothane hepatitis have been reported in children, it is extremely rare and the risks of repeated halothane anaesthesia may be offset by its superior induction characteristics. It would be contraindicated, however, in any child who had had post-anaesthetic jaundice of unknown aetiology, and in children at risk from malignant hyperthemia, as would all other inhalational agents. Sevoflurane, which has recently been introduced, has good induction characteristics in children. It has a low blood gas solubility of 0.63, is pleasant smelling and non-irritant. Induction times are faster than with halothane and the side effect profile at induction is similar to halothane. During maintenance of anaesthesia in children there is a dose-dependent decrease in blood pressure with little effect on heart rate or systemic vascular resistance. The arrhythmia threshold with adrenaline is similar to that of isoflurane. Three to four per cent of sevoflurane is metabolized via the cytochrome P450 system and concern has been raised at the production of fluoride ions which are released in similar amounts to enflurane metabolism. Peak fluoride values occur about 30 min after anaesthesia, but concentrations are lower than those found in adults. The renal toxicity exhibited by methoxyflurane was probably related to free fluoride found in the renal microsomal metabolism system. Recent work has shown that the particular isoenzymes used to metabolize both sevoflurane and enflurane are predominantly hepatic and although the plasma concentrations of fluoride may rise the renal microsomal system is little involved. This may explain why renal damage has not been a problem with these two agents. Sevoflurane when used in circuits containing a soda lime absorber produces breakdown products including compounds A and B which are toxic in rats. The relevance of the products in either adults, or children, is unknown. Care should be taken when using sevoflurane at low flows with soda lime or baralyme.

Isoflurane is associated with an increased incidence of airway complications at induction such as cough, breath-holding and laryngospasm. However, slow, gentle inductions with isoflurane are possible with practice. Recovery is more rapid than with halothane and isoflurane reduces blood pressure predominantly by a decrease in systemic vascular resistance. Desflurane has the lowest blood gas solubility of 0.42, so it should have a rapid induction and recovery profile. Unfortunately studies in children have shown there is an unacceptably high incidence of complications including coughing, laryngospasm, decrease in oxygen saturation and excitement making it unsuitable for gaseous inductions in children. However, it is a good maintenance agent and provides muscle relaxation and a rapid recovery phase. Analgesic requirements seem to be higher following use of desflurane and delirium in recovery reached 50% in some studies.

Enflurane does not have specific advantages over other agents.

INDUCTION AGENTS

In general, larger induction doses of any agent are required in children because they have a greater central volume of distribution and distribution is more rapid, particularly to the vessel-rich group of organs. Also clearance is higher because of the increased metabolism.

Thiopentone (3–7 mg kg^{-1}) is the most commonly used i.v. agent. In neonates the dose may be smaller because they have lower values of plasma proteins. It is safe, painless, and has little cardiovascular or respiratory effect at these doses.

Propofol is also widely used and is licensed in the UK for children above three years of age. Propofol induction doses are 2.5–4.0 mg kg^{-1}. Onset is rapid and smooth, but it is associated with pain on injection in approximately 20% of patients, even after the addition of lignocaine, and apnoea rates of up to 80% have been reported in some studies. Propofol has been used by short-term infusion in children, particularly for sedation techniques, and in children in whom an inhalational agent is contraindicated.

Propofol use in intensive care, as a long-term sedative, has been discontinued. It was associated with several cases of untreatable cardiac failure in young children who required intensive care management, particularly of acute upper respiratory illness. The incidence of side effects such as nausea and vomiting does not seem to differ between thiopentone and propofol. The adult advantages of earlier, clearer recovery from anaesthesia with propofol are not apparent in young children. Propofol is associated with easier placement of the laryngeal mask airway possibly because of the high incidence of apnoea.

Ketamine is a useful drug in paediatric anaesthesia because it can be used i.v. (1–2 mg kg^{-1}) or i.m. (5–10 mg kg^{-1}). Additional advantages are that it is a good analgesic and will provide some amnesia. It is clear that older children can have the same dysphoric and hallucinogenic experiences that affect adults, but they appear to be less common in young children. It is used for many short, repeated, anaesthetics for procedures such as radiotherapy, laser and minor surgery.

NEUROMUSCULAR BLOCKING DRUGS

The role of suxamethonium has become controversial recently and its use has declined. However, it still has a place in paediatric anaesthesia. Babies require relatively larger doses (2–4 mg kg^{-1}) of suxamethonium, as they have a large, extracellular volume. It can be given i.m. if necessary. Plasma cholinesterase values may be lower, but this does not prolong the action of suxamethonium clinically. The use of atropine as premedication, especially in the younger patients, provides protection from bradycardia especially if a second dose of suxamethonium has to be used. Myalgic pain after suxamethonium is very uncommon in young children. Contraindications are the same as in adults, but particularly in children with muscular dystrophy.

Competitive neuromuscular blocking agents (NMB)

Newborn babies show an unpredictable response to these drugs. On the one hand sensitivity of the neuromuscular junction to NMB is increased, but in contrast there is an increase in the extracellular volume and volume of distribution which decrease the concentration of drug at the site of action. In practice, smaller doses are used and repeated, if necessary, depending on the response.

Tubocurarine is little used now, but in older children it is useful for long procedures requiring mild hypotension such as ear operations. Pancuronium is also long acting and is mainly used in cardiac anaesthesia where in combination with fentanyl it provides good cardiovascular stability. Atracurium is commonly used and it has a similar time of onset to that in adults. The ED_{50} varies with age, and is lowest in neonates. The Hoffmann elimination results is a predictable effect and the recovery profile is similar in different age groups. Vecuronium has a quicker onset of action with younger patients, but the duration of action is prolonged in newborn babies, and recovery slower than in children or adults. Mivacurium, a short acting drug, is rapidly metabolized by plasma cholinesterase and possibly other routes. Animal work suggests that lower doses are required in the youngest age groups presumably because of the immaturity of the neuromuscular system. In children, initial doses need to be high to provide predictable, rapid paralysis. Rocuronium has a more rapid onset in children than in adults and may be shorter acting.

LOCAL ANAESTHETICS

Local anaesthetic doses are lower in babies because of reduced protein binding, immature metabolism and increased sensitivity. Older infants and children will metabolize the drugs faster than babies and blood concentrations are lower. This is due in part to increased blood flow to the liver and other sites. However, peak plasma values are achieved earlier in the young, for example, following caudal anaesthesia, within 15 min as opposed to 30 min in the adult. Numerous schemes for calculating the maximum safe doses have been described and a simplified schedule is shown in Table 19.2.

Table 19.2 Safe maximum doses of local anaesthetics in children

Drug	Dose
Bupivacaine	2–3 mg kg^{-1}
	1.5 mg kg^{-1} (neonate)
Lignocaine (plain)	3 mg kg^{-1}
Lignocaine (with adrenaline)	7 mg kg^{-1}

OPIOIDS

Metabolism and clearance of opioids are unpredictable in babies, so that plasma concentrations are variable and side effects more likely. Of most concern when using opioids in babies, particularly those that were immature preterm babies or small-for-dates babies, is the risk of respiratory depression and apnoea. In this group of patients opioids should be used with great caution and always with close postoperative supervision including high dependency nursing and apnoea monitoring. Fortunately, for a large number of procedures in this group, simple analgesics with local infiltration are sufficient.

PREOPERATIVE PREPARATION

PREOPERATIVE EDUCATION

This can be achieved in many ways, direct discussion, play-therapy, videos and visits to the anaesthetic or recovery room. It is now usual for a parent to come with the child to the anaesthetic room. This is decided between the child, the parent and the anaesthetist. The final decision should be left to the anaesthetist as circumstances vary. It is important that there is a trained nurse present to support the parent and answer their questions on the way back to the ward. It is also becoming more common to ask parents to come to the recovery area.

PREOPERATIVE STARVATION

There is now evidence that shorter fasting times are safe in children of ASA status 1, 2 and 3, if there are no specific risk factors for a full stomach or for aspiration of gastric contents. Animal work has indicated that gastric volumes above 0.8 ml kg^{-1} and a pH less than 1.0 are associated with increased risk of lung damage should the gastric contents be accidentally aspirated. The exact relevance of these measurements to paediatric practice is unclear. Several large studies of paediatric anaesthetics have shown that clinically important pulmonary aspiration is very rare, of the order of 1 in 10 000, and that the majority of aspirations were associated with difficulties in intubation.

Those most at risk from either excessive or inadequate fasting are the smallest and sickest children. Breast-fed babies are not starved for more than 4 h before elective surgery as breast milk is very easily digestible. Older children should have no food for 6 h before operation, but can safely have clear fluids until 2–3 h before surgery as this does not affect either the average volume of gastric contents or pH. Patient and parental satisfaction is improved in children allowed more liberal fluids before operation.

Gastric emptying is prolonged after trauma and precautions should be taken to prevent aspiration.

PREOPERATIVE INVESTIGATIONS

There have been several large reviews of present practice and in healthy, elective patients over one year of age undergoing minor surgery no investigations are required. Laboratory tests are performed if clinically indicated. An accurate weight is essential. The anaesthetic implications of any particular syndrome should be reviewed before operation using specialist reference books.

SPECIFIC MEDICAL CONDITIONS

Sickle cell disease

Screening for haemoglobinopathies such as sickle cell disease or thalassaemia should be done in children in high-risk groups. Babies have high levels of fetal haemoglobin, HbF, and this decreases after birth and is replaced by the adult forms of haemoglobin by the age of 3–6 months. A sickle test in a young baby can give false negative results so, although this age group is actually protected by their high levels of HbF, the sickle test must be repeated later for correct identification.

The presence of sickle trait (HbAS and HbS levels <45%) is not associated with any additional morbidity and no other preoperative preparation is required. However, the management of a child with sickle cell disease must be discussed with a haematologist. It is uncommon now to undertake exchange transfusion in children if the surgery is minor, as the potential risks outweigh the benefits. If an exchange is necessary the aim is to decrease the HbS level from 85–95% to less than 30% and to increase the Hb to 10 g dl^{-1}. Patients should be kept warm and well hydrated and may need antibiotic prophylaxis.

Asthma

Mild asthma is common in children and usually poses no problem. Severe asthma needs careful assessment, investigation and planning. Elective surgery should not occur within one month of a severe attack. The preoperative condition is assessed and steroid and bronchodilator medication optimized, with additional doses given with premedication. In this small subgroup, the avoidance of histamine-releasing drugs, such as thiopentone, atracurium, tubocurarine or diclofenac, is wise as is the avoidance of unnecessary manipulation of the airway.

Sleep apnoea

Sleep apnoea may occur in children secondary to adenotonsillar hypertrophy. The history is of a normal respiratory pattern whilst awake, but severe snoring when asleep associated with periods of apnoea accompanied by marked oxygen desaturation. These children fail to thrive and may develop pulmonary hypertension and right heart failure. They may present for surgery unrelated to their airway and a careful history will identify those at risk. Postoperative monitoring is indicated and sedative drugs should be avoided. Nasal continuous positive airway pressure (CPAP) sometimes helps after operation.

Upper respiratory tract infection (URTI)

Children have very frequent URTIs (2–9 per year) and some children have nasal discharge most of the time. There is some evidence that anaesthesia undertaken during an URTI is associated with an increased risk of airway complications such as cough, laryngospasm, bronchospasm, oxygen desaturation and chest infection. The likelihood of these problems happening is increased if the trachea is intubated or the child is very young. An URTI is a relative contraindication to anaesthesia for purely elective surgery. The parents should be involved fully in the decision and should not be persuaded to proceed if they are concerned.

Child with a heart murmur

Many children are found to have a heart murmur on routine preoperative assessment, but the majority of these are innocent. However, it is important to exclude the very small number that may have haemodynamic consequences during anaesthesia. Thus, surgery should be postponed and the murmur investigated if the murmur is diastolic, pan systolic, late systolic or is associated with a thrill, or if the child is under one year of age, has signs or symptoms of cardiac disease or has evidence of left or right ventricular hypertrophy on ECG. Otherwise it is safe to proceed and have the child investigated at a later date. Antibiotics should be given if 'dirty' surgery such as genitourinary, bowel or dental surgery is undertaken.

Down's syndrome

Associated features may include cardiac abnormalities, difficulties with the airway associated with obstruction on induction, and atlantoaxial instability. Atlantoaxial instability, which increases with age, may be present in 12–18% of children. After tracheal intubation there is an increased incidence of stridor.

Muscular dystrophies

Muscular dystrophies have important anaesthetic implications. Respiratory function may be compromised and children are sensitive to sedative drugs and anaesthetics so that a period of postoperative ventilation may be required. Cardiomyopathy may occur and suxamethonium is contraindicated as it may cause severe hyperkalaemia and rhabdomyolysis. The relationship between the muscular dystrophies and malignant hyperthermia is unclear (Chapter 10).

Latex allergy

Latex allergy is increasingly recognized as a problem in paediatric patients. High-risk groups include children with spina bifida or major urological abnormalities. On exposure to any latex containing product an immune response ranging from simple urticaria to an extremely severe anaphylactic reaction may occur. The reactions are IgE mediated and patients will have positive skin and RAST (radio allergo sorbent test) tests to latex antigen. An anaesthetic plan for a sensitive child includes the scrupulous avoidance of any latex-containing equipment, and pretreatment with steroids, chlorpheniramine and ranitidine.

PREMEDICATION

This is important in some children, but optional in many, and the choice of drugs is wide. EMLA cream is useful to reduce the pain of injection if an intravenous induction is to be used. The use of EMLA in young babies is controversial, as they have lower levels of methionine reductase, which is required to metabolize methaemoglobin derived from the prilocaine in EMLA. Amethocaine provides topical anaesthesia more rapidly than EMLA.

Premedication is used to provide anxiolysis, sedation, analgesia and for drying secretions. Most premedication is given orally. Young infants do not usually require sedative premedication.

Trimeprazine, a sedative antihistamine, is given orally in a dose of 2 mg kg^{-1}. It is long acting and may delay discharge for day cases. Higher doses have been associated rarely with hypotensive episodes (grey baby syndrome).

Triclofos syrup, a chloral derivative, is widely used for premedication in a dose of 30–75 mg kg^{-1} (max. 1 g). Benzodiazepines such as temazepam (0.5–1.0 mg kg^{-1} orally) and midazolam, are all useful and well tolerated in children particularly those above 15 kg. Midazolam is particularly useful as it is short acting with a rapid onset. It can be given orally (0.5 mg kg^{-1}) or nasally (0.3 mg kg^{-1}), though many children find nasal administration unpleasant.

Atropine (20 μg kg^{-1}) can be given orally or i.m.; it is useful as a vagolytic and antisialogue. It is most often used in young babies.

Opiates such as morphine (0.1–0.2 mg kg^{-1}) i.m. are useful if a predictable degree of sedation is required such as before cardiac surgery. Although morphine can be given orally, the effect is less certain. Oral fentanyl has also been tried and is well tolerated.

ANAESTHETIC EQUIPMENT

FACEMASKS AND THE LARYNGEAL MASK AIRWAY (LMA)

Facemasks should have a low deadspace and also easily form an airtight seal around the mouth to provide effective CPAP or positive pressure ventilation. The older type Rendell–Baker mask provides the lowest dead space, but an airtight seal is more difficult to achieve. Newer masks are made from moulded plastic and provide a very effective seal. The laryngeal mask airway (LMA) is now commonly used in paediatric anaesthesia. It comes in four different sizes and the correct size and volume of air in the cuff are as follows:

Size 1	Up to 6.5 kg	Cuff volume 2–4 ml
Size 2	6.5–20 kg	Cuff volume 10 ml
Size 2.5	20–30 kg	Cuff volume 14 ml
Size 3	>30 kg	Cuff volume 25 ml

As in adults it does not protect the airway from regurgitated stomach contents and its use for positive pressure ventilation remains controversial. The LMA may be of particular use for patients with a difficult airway such as in the Pierre Robin syndrome. It has also been used successfully during neonatal resuscitation as an alternative to bag and mask ventilation.

LARYNGOSCOPES

Straight blade laryngoscopes are commonly used to intubate babies and small infants, because the technique involves placing the tip of the blade posterior to the epiglottis and lifting it, to expose the larynx. In bigger children a curved blade is more frequently used (Figure 19.5).

Anaesthetic equipment 349

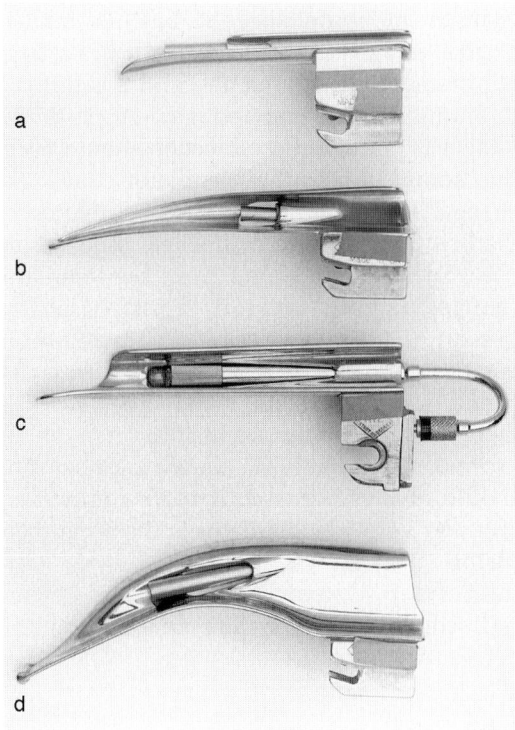

Figure 19.5 Various laryngoscope blades used in paediatric anaesthesia. (a) Miller; (b) Robertshaw; (c) Anderson Magill; (d) Macintosh.

Table 19.3 Oral tracheal tube sizes for neonates

Age	Weight (kg)	Tube size Internal diameter (mm)	Tube length (cm)
Newborn	0.7–1.0	2.5	7.0–7.5
Newborn	1.0–1.5	2.5	7.5–8.0
Newborn	1.5–2.0	3.0	8.0–8.5
Newborn	2.0–2.5	3.0	8.5–9.0
Newborn	2.5–3.0	3.0	9.0–10.0
Newborn	3.5	3.5	12
1 year old	10	4.0–4.5	13

Fixation of the tube is a matter of preference, as is the length to which the tube is cut, but secure fixation and accurate placement must be achieved.

TRACHEAL TUBES

Uncuffed tracheal tubes are used in young children and a small leak from around the tube is desirable. The correct tube size and approximate length are given in Table 19.3. For older children the **approximate** size for the tube is given by the formula: (age/4) + 4 = internal diameter (mm). The length of the tube placed orally is approximately three times the internal diameter in centimetres. These formulae can only be used as a rough guess, and positioning of the tracheal tube must be checked carefully to prevent endobronchial intubation.

Pre-formed tubes are available and these may be north or south facing. Uncuffed, reinforced, non-kinking tubes are also available and useful for surgery on the head and neck.

BREATHING SYSTEMS

The Mapleson classification of breathing systems is shown in Figure 4.6. The most commonly used systems in paediatric anaesthesia are the Mapleson D or Mapleson F. The coaxial version of Mapleson D is the Bain Circuit and used generally in bigger children. The Mapleson F, or Jackson–Rees modification of the Ayre's T-piece, is the system currently most suited to neonates and small infants. It can be used for spontaneous and controlled ventilation and is described as a partial rebreathing system. This is because at high fresh gas flows (FGF) there is no rebreathing of expired gas and end-tidal CO_2 concentration is dependent primarily on minute ventilation. As FGF is reduced partial rebreathing of expired gas begins to occur and this includes water vapour and heat. At low FGF the end-tidal CO_2 concentration depends less on the minute ventilation and more on the FGF. Recommended FGF varies between authors: e.g. 1000 ml + 100 ml kg^{-1} during controlled ventilation with a minimum of 3 l min^{-1}. For spontaneous ventilation a minimum of 4 l min^{-1} is appropriate.

Circle systems are not yet widely used in paediatric anaesthesia in the UK. The two most popular paediatric circle systems are the Ohio and Bloomquist systems.

VENTILATORS

Pressure generators have the advantage in paediatric anaesthesia of being able to compensate, to some extent, for a change in the leak around the tracheal tube. The ventilator used most commonly in operating theatres in the UK is the Penlon Nuffield 200 ventilator with the Newton modification (Figure 19.6). The Newton valve is simply a fixed orifice allowing a leak from the ventilator and converts this volume generator into a pressure generator. The Penlon can be used with both the Bain and the Ayre's T-piece and is simple to use, reliable, robust and inexpensive to buy. However, it is unable to compensate for changes in compliance, it has no built-in alarms, it is expensive to run as it has a large requirement for driving gas, and it is difficult to humidify the inspired gas. A particular danger is that if a disconnection should occur the sound from the ventilator does not change. In the same way, if an occlusion of the breathing system or tracheal tube should occur, neither the sound from the ventilator changes, nor the pressure registered on the pressure gauge. It is necessary, therefore, to use the ventilator in conjunction with a disconnection alarm and some other monitor that will detect an occlusion, such as an expired minute volume alarm. Capnography should always be used. A more comprehensive and versatile ventilator is the Servo ventilator. Most commonly used are the Servo B, C, and D although it is beyond the scope of this chapter to describe this ventilator in detail.

NEONATAL ANAESTHESIA

SPECIFIC CONDITIONS

Neonatal surgery is increasingly taking place in specialized centres and newborn babies needing surgery should be transferred to these centres for treatment. If antenatal diagnosis has been made the mother will frequently be transferred to an obstetric unit linked to a special centre. If the diagnosis is made after delivery, transfer will take place at this stage. The decision about how a baby is transferred is an important one and depends on the condition of the baby, the skill of local personnel and equipment available. Transfer of very sick babies is now frequently undertaken by a retrieval team sent by the receiving hospital that will have the necessary equipment and expertise.

Oesophageal atresia

Oesophageal atresia occurs in about 1:3000 live births. A tracheo-oesophageal fistula may

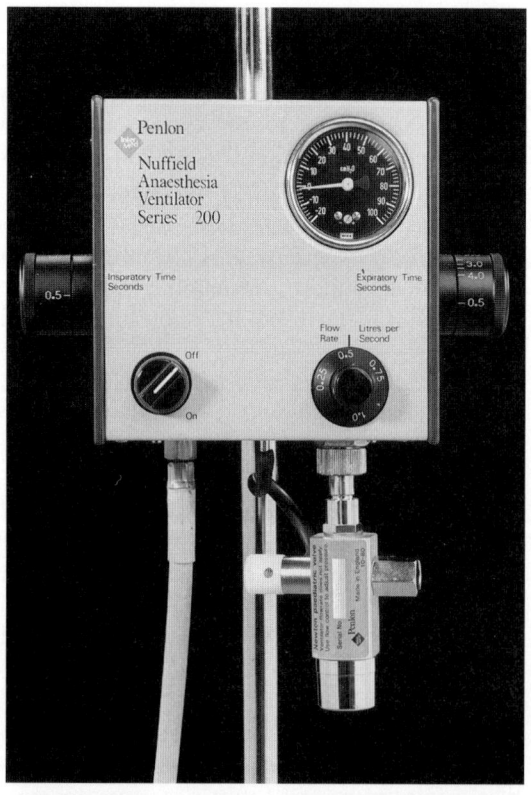

Figure 19.6 Photograph of Penlon Nuffield ventilator showing Newton valve attached.

also be present. Many different configurations of atresia and fistula exist, but the most common is that of oesophageal atresia with a fistula from the trachea to the distal oesophagus (Figure 19.7). The other much rarer types are shown in Figure 19.8. Antenatal diagnosis is now possible but if this has not occurred the diagnosis is made when a nasogastric tube cannot be passed into the stomach. Plain abdominal X-ray shows the nasogastric tube curled in the blind-ending oesophagus and, if a fistula is present, air will be seen in the stomach. Occasionally the diagnosis may be delayed and only made when the baby chokes on the first feed.

Oesophageal atresia is associated with prematurity and congenital heart disease. Cleft lip and palate may conspire with these features to make the intubation potentially difficult. Surgical outcome depends primarily on gestational age, birthweight and the severity of the associated conditions.

Surgical repair is either a primary, complete repair, or a staged procedure with a gastrostomy and ligation of the fistula, with later repair of the oesophagus. A double lumen Replogle tube should be positioned in the upper oesophageal pouch and left on gentle suction. Intensive respiratory care is required if pulmonary complications are present. Urgent ligation of the fistula is, however, usually required to prevent further soiling of the lungs, or to prevent gastric distension through the fistula if the patient is ventilated. An echocardiogram and cardiac assessment are useful.

Particular problems that may be encountered include:

- difficulties associated with prematurity, lung disease or congenital anomalies,
- difficult intubation,
- intubation of the fistula (rare), and
- surgical retraction of lung, decreasing ventilation.

Some centres still advocate awake intubation while others use an inhalational technique with a muscle relaxant. Hand ventilation is generally used so that changes in compliance can be detected. In addition to the usual clinical monitors a precordial stethoscope is useful. Fentanyl (2–3 $\mu g\ kg^{-1}$) can be given if extubation is anticipated together with the addition of low concentrations of volatile agent. Postoperative extubation is indicated if the baby is vigorous, there are no pulmonary complications, and the oesophageal anastamosis is not under tension. In 50% cases however, postoperative ventilation will be required when the oral tracheal tube should be replaced with a nasal tube.

Late complications include a diverticulum of the trachea, tracheomalacia, or oesophageal stricture. Overall mortality should now be very low.

Congenital diaphragmatic hernia

Congenital diaphragmatic hernia occurs in 1:4000 live births. It is associated with herniation of abdominal contents into the chest and hypoplastic lungs. The most common type (80%) involves herniation through the foramen of Bochdalek on the left side. Associated conditions include malrotation of the

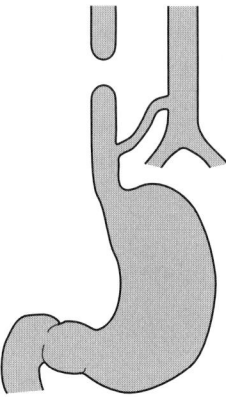

Figure 19.7 Most common form (85%) of oesophageal atresia with a fistula.

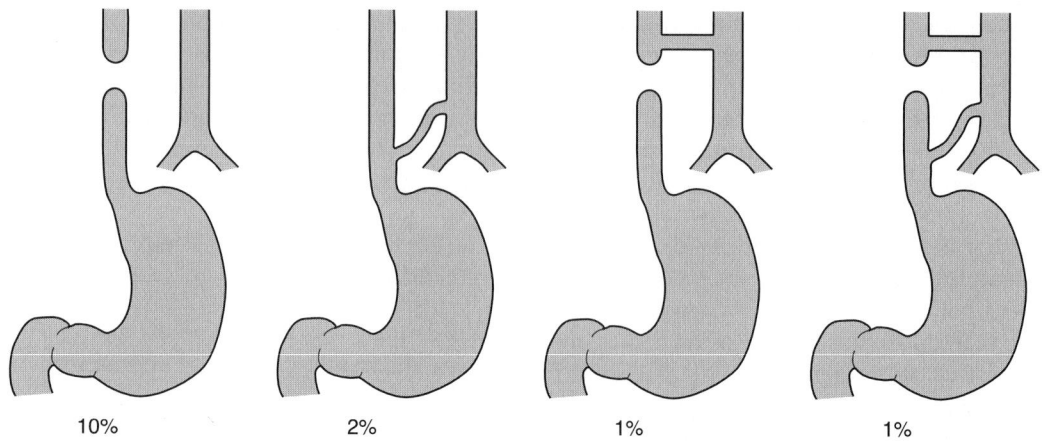

Figure 19.8 Other forms of oesophageal atresia.

gut and congenital heart disease. Less common are renal and neurological abnormalities. Antenatal diagnosis is now common which allows transfer of the mother to a centre with neonatal surgical services. The onset and severity of respiratory distress depends on the degree of pulmonary hypoplasia, as does the mortality. Respiratory distress, reduced breath sounds on the affected side of the chest along with bowel sounds audible over the chest, and a scaphoid abdomen, clearly point to the diagnosis. Chest X-ray reveals bowel in the chest, although this may be difficult to distinguish from congenital lobar emphysema. Mediastinal shift to the opposite side is progressive as the bowel fills with air. Pulmonary hypertension complicates the pulmonary hypoplasia.

Management is based on a period of ventilation so that the baby is presented for surgery in an optimal condition. Preoperative ventilation, with efforts to reduce pulmonary hypertension, has been shown to improve postoperative lung function and outcome. Invasive monitoring is required and cardiopulmonary stability is the aim. A nasogastric tube is passed to prevent further mediastinal shift and attempts are made to decrease pulmonary pressures with sedation (fentanyl), muscle paralysis, hyperventilation, minimal handling and the use of pulmonary vasodilators, the most specific of which is inhaled nitric oxide. Outcome with conventional treatment depends on the relationship between $Pa{CO_2}$ and the ventilation index (mean airway pressure and respiratory rate). A high $Pa{CO_2}$, despite high airway pressures and a fast respiratory rate, is associated with a high mortality. The use of extracorporeal membrane oxygenation (ECMO) is now being evaluated in this subgroup of patients and may improve mortality.

The movement of these sick patients to theatre should be done with minimal upset. Additional doses of neuromuscular blocking drug and fentanyl may be required before surgery and isoflurane, or other volatile agent, can be added with caution. Nitrous oxide should be avoided to prevent further distension of the abdominal contents.

Exomphalos and gastroschisis

Exomphalos and gastroschisis present similar anaesthetic problems but have different anatomy, embryological origins, associated conditions and incidence. Exomphalos is the herniation of abdominal contents into the umbilical cord. Gastroschisis is a defect in the abdominal wall lateral to the umbilical cord usually on the right side. Exomphalos is associated with other congenital abnormalities such as gastrointestinal, genitourinary and cardiac anomalies and with the Beckwith–Weideman syndrome (exomphalos, macroglossia and severe hypoglycaemia). Exomphalos occurs in 1:5000–1:10 000 live births whereas gastroschisis occurs less commonly (1:30 000) and is not associated with congenital abnormalities except prematurity.

The surgical options include primary closure, which is preferred if possible, a staged closure, or simply closure of the skin. The staged procedure is used when the abdominal contents cannot be returned to the abdomen, and a silo or pouch is fashioned to allow time for the abdominal contents to be accommodated in the abdomen. The main anaesthetic problems result from high intra-abdominal pressures which inhibit ventilation, and from heat, fluid and electrolyte loss from exposed viscera. In addition, hypoglycaemia is a potential problem. Preoperatively the patient needs resuscitation with crystalloid and colloid solutions. Plasma electrolytes and glucose need careful monitoring and correction. The exposed viscera are wrapped in sterile plastic to reduce heat and fluid loss and a nasogastric tube is passed to prevent gastric distension. A rapid sequence induction is performed, nitrous oxide is omitted and fentanyl in small doses with a volatile agent can be used. The decision about postoperative ventilation depends on the intra-abdominal pressure and the ease with which the baby is ventilated, as well as on the general condition.

Intestinal obstruction

There are various causes, but commonly duodenal atresia, malrotation, meconium ileus and duplication are encountered. As a result of vomiting there may be fluid and electrolyte abnormalities and there is a risk of aspiration both before and during anaesthesia. In addition, abdominal distension may compromise ventilation.

Fluid resuscitation should be complete before surgery and plasma electrolytes corrected. A nasogastric tube is passed to decompress the stomach and should be aspirated immediately before induction of anaesthesia. A rapid sequence induction with cricoid pressure is used. Large amounts of fluid may be required intraoperatively if necrotic bowel is present. Extubation is carried out in the lateral position when the neonate is awake and vigorous. Postoperative ventilation may be needed.

Congenital pyloric stenosis

Congenital pyloric stenosis is common and occurs in 1:300–1:400 live births. It is more common in first-born boys. Thickening of the circular muscle of the pylorus occurs which forms a tumour. The clinical presentation is with vomiting and a palpable tumour. The vomiting is sometimes projectile and occurs after feeding and, if undiagnosed, can cause marked dehydration and a hypochloraemic alkalosis.

Pyloromyotomy is not an emergency and it is important to correct the fluid and electrolyte abnormalities before surgery. The aim is a plasma sodium of 135 mmol l^{-1}, chloride 90 mmol l^{-1} and bicarbonate 24 mmol l^{-1}, and to have established a urine flow of 1–2 ml kg^{-1} h^{-1}. Fluid replacement is usually with 0.9% saline and maintenance fluid should be continued with 4% glucose 0.18% saline. Potassium may be needed in severe cases, but at a rate not exceeding 3 mmol kg^{-1} per day. A gastritis is sometimes present and 4 h gastric washouts are given with 0.9% saline through the nasogastric tube. Atropine may be prescribed as a premedication, but is often omitted as an intravenous cannula is present and it can be given i.v. if necessary. After aspirating the stomach, induction is either gaseous or iv. with cricoid pressure, suxamethonium and oral intubation followed by positive pressure ventilation. The surgery is usually quick and the patient is extubated awake in the lateral position. Postoperative analgesia is provided with bupivacaine infiltrated into the wound during surgery and feeding can commence 4–6 h after uncomplicated cases.

Necrotising enterocolitis

Necrotizing enterocolitis is primarily a disease of low birthweight infants. The predominant feature is intestinal mucosal damage following ischaemia of the bowel which may result in perforation, peritonitis and septic shock. Clinically there is abdominal distension, bloody diarrhoea, temperature instability, apnoea and lethargy. In addition, the baby may be shocked, acidotic and develop disseminated intravascular coagulation. Radiographically there may be intramural air in the bowel, or evidence of perforation with intraperitoneal air. Mortality is in the region of 30%. Indications for surgery include evidence of perforation, or intestinal gangrene, or portal venous air. Necrotic bowel is resected and an enterostomy is fashioned.

Aggressive management in the neonatal intensive care unit consists of fluid and blood replacement, antibiotics, a nasogastric tube to decompress bowel, mechanical ventilation, attempts to treat the coagulopathy, intravascular monitoring and possibly inotropic support. This management needs to be continued in theatre. Fentanyl, oxygen and air and a muscle relaxant can be used as the anaesthetic technique.

SPECIFIC ANAESTHETIC PROBLEMS IN CHILDREN

ACUTE AIRWAY OBSTRUCTION

The most common causes of acute airway problems in children are infections, such as laryngotracheobronchitis (croup), epiglottitis, or trauma from either an inhaled foreign body, or post-intubation, or after burns. Upper airway obstruction presents with stridor which, if inspiratory, usually suggests the pathology is above the thoracic inlet and if biphasic at or below the inlet.

A careful history may identify the likely aetiology, but frequently a laryngoscopy and bronchoscopy will be needed for diagnostic or therapeutic reasons.

CROUP

Croup is a common acute viral illness (frequently parainfluenza) affecting young children (<2 years), particularly in winter. The history is longer than that with epiglottitis and the child is comparatively well. Stridor is worst at night and there may be a cough. Management is essentially supportive with humidified air, maintenance of oral fluids and active management of the pyrexia. Only children with worsening symptoms require admission, further investigation, oxygen therapy, dexamethasone, nebulized adrenaline and occasionally intubation and management on the intensive care unit.

EPIGLOTTITIS

Epiglottitis is a haemophilus influenza infection and has become far less common with the advent of the HiB vaccine. It is a severe illness with rapid development of symptoms and major systemic upset. The child is unable to lie down, and cannot speak or swallow its saliva. There is no cough. Epiglottitis tends to affect slightly older children (>2 years). If the diagnosis is suspected the child must be managed quietly and gently avoiding interventions such as X-rays, blood tests or examination of the throat, any of which may cause acute total airway obstruction. The child is transferred to theatre where anaesthesia is induced and maintained with halothane in oxygen until deep enough for a direct laryngoscopy and intubation to secure the airway. A tracheostomy set must be readily available.

An oral tracheal tube is initially passed and if the situation is stable the anaesthetist can change this for a nasal tracheal tube as this will help management in the intensive care unit and is more comfortable for the child. Management consists of sedation, supportive therapy and antibiotic treatment until there is sufficient leak around the tracheal tube, or until the temperature has settled. The child is then extubated.

ASPIRATED FOREIGN BODY (AFB)

AFB may present as an acute respiratory problem, or more chronically, depending on the type of foreign body and the site at which it has lodged. A foreign body may lodge above or below the cords, and symptoms and signs will help in deciding the site. If the object is in the bronchus it may produce a ball valve effect and an X-ray will show hyperinflation on the affected side with mediastinal shift when expiratory and inspiratory film are compared. After atropine premedication, anaesthesia is induced with halothane in oxygen, and spontaneous respiration maintained until the anaesthetic level is deep enough to allow laryngoscopy. The airway is sprayed with topical lignocaine before passage of the bronchoscope. It is useful to maintain spontaneous respiration and avoid muscle paralysis, with inevitable ventilation, as this may push the foreign body further down the airway or, if expiration is partially obstructed, increase hyperinflation with the risk of pneumothorax. This procedure may take a long time and the airway can be damaged necessitating postoperative nebulized adrenaline and steroids.

PAIN MANAGEMENT IN CHILDREN

Children and babies feel pain and will mount a similar physiological response to pain as adults. It is sometimes more difficult in the very young to assess pain levels and hence the efficacy of analgesic methods. Monitoring and careful follow up are essential, and pain and sedation scales are available to help in this task. Analgesia is tailored to the requirements and physical status of the child, and the expertise and facilities available to the anaesthetist and postoperative care team. Pain management starts early and pre-emptive analgesia may be beneficial. The combination of an appropriate local anaesthetic technique with anaesthesia may be all that is required for pain relief after minor surgery. In addition, the use of simple analgesics such as paracetamol and diclofenac are surprisingly effective in children. Paracetamol in a dose of 12–15 mg kg^{-1} six hourly can be used in most children, including babies, and is given orally or as a suppository. Diclofenac is commonly used and it can be given orally or rectally in a dose of 1–3 mg kg^{-1} over 24 h.

Although sectionalized consent is not required in the UK it is good clinical practice to discuss with the family the available options for pain relief, especially if a local or regional block is to be used, or a suppository given.

REGIONAL ANAESTHETIC BLOCKS

Although few operative procedures can be undertaken exclusively with a local anaesthetic technique, these blocks are important adjuncts to general anaesthesia and postoperative pain relief. Contraindications to a local block include local or systemic sepsis, abnormalities of the blood clotting mechanism, allergy to local anaesthetic agents, the presence of a specific anatomical abnormality such as spina bifida, and patient or parent refusal.

Some blocks require large volumes of local anaesthetic agent and the maximum recommended doses must not be exceeded (Table 19.2).

Caudal block

This is one of the most common blocks for all age groups, and is useful for lower abdominal, perineal and leg surgery. The position of the sacral hiatus is shown in Figure 19.9. The

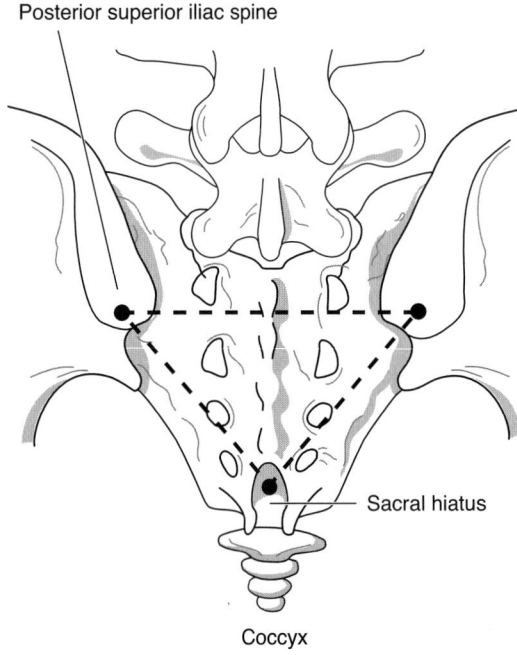

Figure 19.9 Anatomy of sacral hiatus. (Reproduced with permission from Steward, D.J. (1995) *Manual of Paediatric Anaesthesia*. Churchill Livingstone, New York.)

child is placed on its side with the neck and knees flexed. The sacral cornua are identified and a cannula or needle is inserted initially at an angle of 40° to the back, until the sacral coccygeal membrane is pierced. The angle of the cannula is moved more in line with the sacrum and advanced slowly (Figure 19.10). Once aspiration has confirmed no blood or CSF, the required dose of local anaesthetic is injected.

- Circumcision, hypospadias: L5–S5, bupivacaine 0.25% 0.5 ml kg^{-1}
- Hernia repair, orchidopexy: T9–S5, bupivacaine 0.25% 0.75–1 ml kg^{-1}

Children should be monitored during the procedure as a high incidence of ECG changes has been reported in very pre-term babies, although not in older groups. Cannulae are widely used now in preference to a needle to avoid the risk of an implantation dermoid,

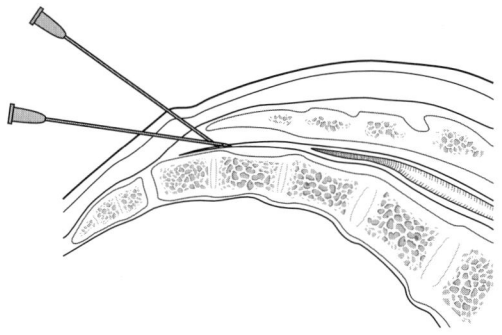

Figure 19.10 Position of needle while performing caudal block. (Reproduced with permission from Steward, D.J. (1995) *Manual of Paediatric Anaesthesia*. Churchill Livingstone, New York.)

and to allow placement of the local anaesthetic solution to a higher level without the increased risk of subarachnoid injection. Caudal catheters have been successfully placed in children and infants to high levels (thoracic) to provide analgesia.

Epidural

A Tuohy needle (19 G for child of less than 10 kg and 18 G above this weight) is inserted in the appropriate vertebral interspace and the epidural space identified with a loss of resistance technique. The use of saline and continuous pressure is associated with fewer complications. The space can be very superficial, less than 0.75 cm from the skin in infants and 1–2 cm in children. The catheter is then fed into the epidural space and fixed on the back. An aspiration test is done and an initial dose of 0.5 ml kg^{-1} of 0.25% plain bupivacaine injected. If used for postoperative analgesia an infusion of a lower concentration of bupivacaine is given, with or without opioid. The agents used include diamorphine, morphine and fentanyl. In children epidural opioid analgesia must not be used in patients treated as day-cases as postoperative monitoring is essential. Great care must be taken with small babies (less than 5 kg), and the availability of a 24 h pain service is essential before epidural analgesia can be used safely. The main side effects are itching, nausea and vomiting, urinary retention and, rarely, apnoea. Technical difficulties with the equipment may also occur. The possibility of these problems means that a risk–benefit analysis should be considered for every case. In one study the incidence of urinary retention in the 1–10-years-old group, who did not have peroperative urinary catheters was 50%. Nausea or vomiting occurred in 21% in the 5–10-years-old group, although it is reported to be less frequent in younger patients. Postoperative care includes monitoring of vital signs, sedation and pain scores, review of treatment by a dedicated pain control team, and assessment and treatment of side effects.

Spinal

This is popular in some centres for hernia repair in small babies, or quick, anorectal procedures, as it is thought to be associated with a lower incidence of postoperative complications such as apnoea. However, this is only true if no sedation is given during the procedure. A 22 or 24 G spinal needle is inserted into the subarachnoid space at the level of L3–4 or below, with the child held carefully in the position described for caudal blockade. Heavy bupivacaine is the agent of choice.

Ilioingual and iliohypogastric blocks
(Figure 19.11)

These are particularly useful for analgesia during, and after, unilateral hernia repair or orchidopexy. The needle is introduced at a point 1 cm medial to and just below the anterior superior iliac spine, as it is advanced the layers of external and internal oblique are felt as two separate 'pops'. If the aspiration test is negative, part of the local anaesthetic dose can then be injected; the remainder of the drug is then fanned out through the tissues as the needle is withdrawn. Direct application

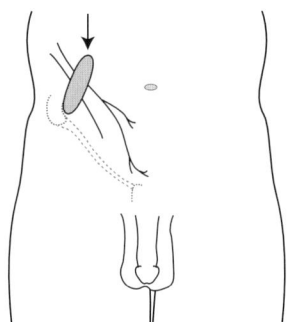

Figure 19.11 Area of infiltration of local anaesthetic for ilioinguinal block. (Reproduced with permission from Steward, D.J. (1995) *Manual of Paediatric Anaesthesia*. Churchill Livingstone, New York.)

of the local anaesthetic by the surgeon during the operation is a useful alternative, especially when the child is small and the small doses need to be very carefully placed. If, during an orchidopexy, an incision is made low in the scrotum additional direct infiltration is required.

Penile block

This provides useful analgesia for circumcision and distal hypospadias repair. Small volumes (0.5–3 ml) of plain bupivacaine (adrenaline must never be used) are required and are placed just below Bucks fascia which is identified by inserting a needle just below the symphysis pubis, in the midline, and advancing it slowly until it 'pops' through the fascia. Local haematoma formation is a potential risk.

Wound infiltration

Wound infiltration is a simple, effective method of providing analgesia if the wound is not too large. Bupivacaine 0.25% in a dose of 0.5 ml kg^{-1} is commonly used.

SYSTEMIC OPIATES

Opiates are extensively used. The main peroperative drugs are fentanyl, morphine and alfentanil. Postoperatively morphine can be administered i.m. by intermittent bolus, as i.v. infusions using either nurse- or patient-controlled mechanisms, or subcutaneously.

Infusion systems use a carefully programmed regimen that may involve a low level background infusion with the availability of an additional bolus of morphine as determined by the amount of pain present. This is chosen by either the patient, (useful in children above five years of age) or by the nurse. Additional safety features include a limit on the maximum dose and on the time between doses. Safety and efficacy are monitored with sedation scores and pain scales. Codeine phosphate is a very safe analgesic, particularly useful in the very young and in children in whom sedation should be avoided. It is given orally or i.m. Use of opiates is associated with potential side effects as previously discussed; babies are particularly sensitive to opiates and great care must be taken. In general, opiates are avoided if the baby weighs less than 5 kg, unless special circumstances apply.

RESUSCITATION

Cardiac arrest in infants and children, in contrast to adults, is often not a sudden event, but the result of a progressive deterioration in cardiorespiratory function. The causes of this deterioration are multiple but the final common pathway of cardiorespiratory failure is the same. Outcome is less good after cardiac arrest, mortality is high within 24 h and sur-

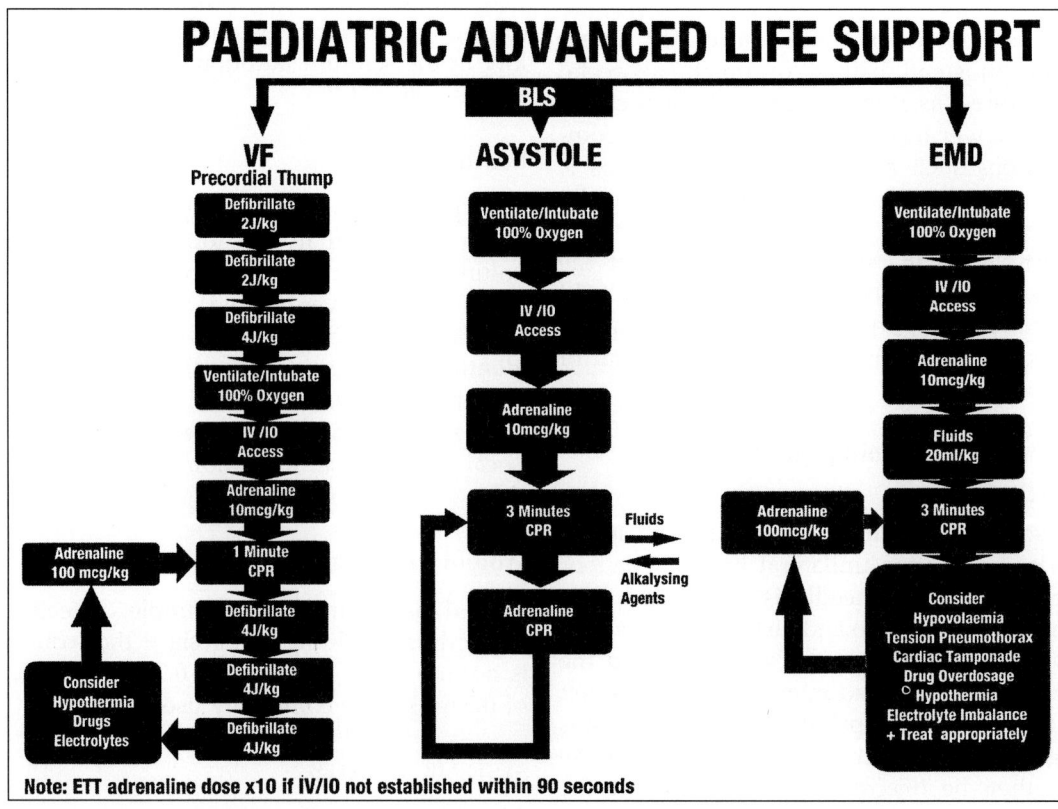

Figure 19.12 Resuscitation guidelines from the Resuscitation Council.

vivors have high morbidity. The outcome after a witnessed cardiac arrest is better, but if spontaneous circulation has not returned after 20 min the outlook is very bleak. The aim, therefore, must be to intervene at an early stage to prevent cardiac arrest from occurring, or once it has occurred, to act promptly. Outcome after respiratory arrest alone is much better. Management of cardiac arrest is outlined in Figure 19.12.

FURTHER READING

Arthur, D. S. and McNicol, L. R. (1986) Local anaesthetic techniques in paediatric surgery. *British Journal of Anaesthesia*, **58**, 760–778.

Berry, F. A. and Gregory, G. A. (1987) Do premature infants require anaesthesia for surgery? *Anaesthesiology*, **67**, 291–293.

Great Ormond Street Hospital for Children NHS Trust (1995) *Guidelines for Drug Administration*. Department of Anaesthesia and Acute Pain Service, Great Ormond Street Hospital, London.

Hatch, D., Sumner, E. and Hellmann, J. (1995) *The Surgical Neonate: Anaesthesia and Intensive Care*. Edward Arnold, London.

Lloyd-Thomas, A. R. and Howard, R. F. (1994) A pain service for children. *Paediatric Anaesthesia*, **4**, 3–15.

Steward, D. J. (1995) *Manual of Paediatric Anaesthesia*. Churchill Livingstone, New York.

Zideman, D., Bingham, R. Beattie, J. *et al.* (1994) Guidelines for Paediatric Life Support. A statement by the Paediatric Life Support Working Party of the European Resuscitation Council 1993. *Resuscitation*, **27**, 91–105.

DAY-CARE SURGERY

D. J. Wilkinson

Anaesthesia for day-case surgery has been taking place since January of 1842 when William Edward Clarke gave ether to a Miss Hobie in Rochester, New York so that a dentist, Elijah Pope, could remove one of her teeth. Much surgery before this had been performed on a day-case basis, but this was the first use of 'modern anaesthesia': day-case work has been increasing ever since. Much has been written over the last two decades on this subject but, like many areas of anaesthetic practice, it is still difficult to obtain a consensus view on even the basic principles of practice.

The patient has to be at the focus of all that takes place in day care. The ability to communicate clearly, to ensure that all involved understand the implications of day-stay care and then provide a high standard of care that continues out in the home, after the patient has left hospital, determines the quality of day-case care.

Day-care anaesthesia requires meticulous preparation, special facilities, extensive and often expensive equipment and drugs, highly qualified and motivated staff, considerable interdepartmental liaison both inside and outside the hospital and then careful audit, which must include a closing of the audit loop.

GUIDELINES, PROTOCOLS AND REPORTS

In 1985 the Royal College of Surgeons of England's Commission on the provision of surgical services, produced guidelines for day-case surgery which reflected the opinions of a multidisciplinary committee. The report tried to provide a policy for day work, some definitions of what this type of work was, an idea of the accommodation and facilities that are required, and then some thoughts on patient selection, anaesthetic considerations and postoperative care. This report initiated a reappraisal of day case surgery and was widely read. Unfortunately, its recommendations were often adopted as strict protocols and these were too prescriptive for modern practice.

The Value for Money Unit of the UK National Health Service Management Executive produced the 'Bevan report' in 1989. This document suggested that 'The expanded use of day surgery, especially where dedicated facilities exist or can be provided, may be one way to increase overall theatre utilisation and throughput at least cost. A limiting factor here is often the lack of day beds or infrastructure geared to this form of treatment.' The report, which became obligatory reading for all hospital managers, also highlights the lower cost of treating patients as day cases as opposed to inpatients. Hospital administrators began to take notice of day work but clinicians still continued to be uninterested, except for the few enthusiasts, like Burns in Southampton and Ogg in Cambridge, who for the most part were trying to influence their colleagues at a time when few were prepared to listen.

Short Practice of Anaesthesia. Edited by M. Morgan and G. M. Hall. Published in 1997 by Chapman & Hall, London. ISBN 0 412 71890 1

The other major breakthrough for day-case work in the UK was the introduction of propofol by ICI in the mid-1980s. This drug made this type of work so much easier; here was an induction and maintenance agent that was simple to use and from which the patients would emerge from anaesthesia feeling well, not vomiting, and wide awake. Even the worst sceptics of day work began to understand that patients could be treated for relatively major procedures, and yet still be able to go home on the same day. This was particularly ironic as the USA did not gain access to this new agent for several years further and yet surgeons in the USA were practising day-stay care in a manner far ahead of the UK.

The Audit Commission then reported on rates of day surgery practice within the UK. Their survey considered a 'basket' of 20 procedures which were particularly suited to day work and which could be used to compare performance between districts. They suggested that another half a million patients could be treated with very little increase in expenditure if District Health Authorities could improve standards of audit, provide specialized day facilities (or use current facilities more efficiently), improve the management of existing day facilities, and somehow stimulate some interest in this type of work by clinicians.

Paediatric day care was investigated in 1991 by the National Association for the Welfare of Children in Hospital (NAWCH) who published their findings as *Just for the Day*. This document sets very high standards for care and premises and bases much of this on what is now official Department of Health policy that children should be cared for in a separate environment to adults. This requires either a separate day facility or 'children-only days' in the main day centre. Purchasers now demand this in their contracts and this has proved very difficult for even the best units in the country to achieve. My personal view is that it is not necessary, provided that special facilities for children are available and that adequately trained nurses are employed, then any day unit can care for children safely and effectively, and can do so with adults on the same lists.

Most of the recommendations made by these reports had been published in the past by a wide variety of health care personnel from the UK, but their innovative ideas had been overlooked. As well as a myriad of papers reflecting the use of propofol in day-case work, a series of books were published at this time relating to day care in the UK, and the British Association of Day Surgery was inaugurated. This association expanded rapidly, attracting membership from all disciplines related to the specialty: surgical, anaesthetic, nursing and clerical, and thus doing much of what the Audit Commission had hoped might occur. The first European Congress on Ambulatory Surgery was held in Brussels in March of 1991 and delegates from all over Europe were joined by practitioners from North America. This meeting permitted an appreciation of the widely differing standards of day care across Europe and the need for some agreement on guidelines for care.

In 1992 The Royal College of Surgeons of England published an updated version of its 1985 report, which was a marked step forward from the original but did not embrace what I believe to be 'modern practice'. There is an acceptance of mixed medical and surgical facilities in the report, so that endoscopy, oncology and surgery are all potentially housed in the one unit. This does not provide the correct ambience for surgical day work. Surgical day cases are patients who are essentially well and they have different requirements to medical patients who are often quite unwell. There are statements such as, 'The elderly and the infirm will ordinarily be excluded. . . .'. This is again outdated practice; it is often the elderly that benefit the most from day-care surgery as they do not then become disorientated by an overnight stay in hospital. 'Even if accompanied, patients should not go home by public transport.' Why ever not? Patients go home from the wards by public transport and they are often a great deal less well than patients after day-case surgery. The report is a useful step forward but on the whole does not go far enough and is too conservative and didactic in its views. Perhaps its most useful aspect is the title itself: 'Guidelines' rather than a protocol. Most clinicians want guidelines to help them in their practice rather than prescriptive protocols which they are 'encouraged' to follow by the spectre of medicolegal problems.

The Audit Commission also produced another of its NHS Occasional Papers in conjunction with the Royal College of Surgeons report, entitled *All in a Day's Work*. This report showed that there was even greater potential for day cases and this was based on more accurate data collecting systems than had been available in the 1990 report. It highlighted the importance of purchasers and providers working together to provide the right facilities and standards of care for these day cases and then providing adequate audit of that work.

More documents have continued to be published to help those who are refining old, or creating new, day centres. NHS Estates have produced *Health Building Note (HBN) 52 Volume 1* entitled *Accommodation for Day Care: Day Surgery Unit*. This gives detailed plans on how to build a new unit, what facilities are required and what protocols can be adopted. Volume 2 has also been produced and deals with the setting up of endoscopy facilities. The third volume in this series details the requirements for medical investigation units. Volume 1 of HBN 52 is an immensely helpful document to all those trying to increase day care and has taken into account many of the North American experiences of this type of practice. In conjunction with this, NHS Estates have published a Nucleus Study Pack to aid those who are trying to design new units in a Nucleus hospital. It analyses day units using an interesting tool developed by University College, London, which looks at what they call spatial degree of integration! This essentially is the ease whereby patients can orientate themselves within a new building or room, and is based on line of sight analysis. The document is very slim and fantastically expensive.

In September of the same year (1993) the *Report of the Day Surgery Task Force* was published by the NHS Management Executive. This 'takes the form of a short report and a substantial "toolkit" which highlights current good and best practice taking place in the NHS in the development of high quality day surgery.' Again this is an excellent document for those involved in day work. It stresses the importance of total quality management and suggests methods whereby practitioners can collate data on their practice. The report stresses the importance of data collection being procedure-based and not just a set of numbers of cases treated. A target of 50% of all elective surgery to be performed as day-case work by the year 2000 has been set. This is realistic and can be achieved with relative ease. The Oxford Regional Health Authority produced another document in association with this entitled *Day Surgery – Your Help Pack*. This too is highly recommended reading. An update on the task force report has appeared which will set even higher, and yet still realistic, targets because of the huge increase in this type of practice that has occurred in the last 2 years.

The Association of Anaesthetists of Great Britain & Ireland had added its contribution to this growing volume of information with one of their booklets entitled *Day Case Surgery: The Anaesthetist's Role in Promoting High Quality Care*. This booklet, published in 1994, outlines selection of patients, documentation, staffing, anaesthesia, recovery, discharge, audit etc. as well as referring to contractual matters.

Further European Congresses in Ambulatory Surgery have now been followed by a World Congress which is set to be a regular event. Many countries are forming their own day surgery associations and this again promotes the concept and ethos of this type of work.

PREOPERATIVE PREPARATION

The most important factor in effective day surgery and anaesthesia is good preoperative preparation. Many patients are now requesting this type of care either from their general practitioners (GPs) or from the surgeons to whom they are referred. These patients must be given full information both written and verbal about the procedure they will undergo, what care they will need once they return home and the likelihood that they might have to stay in hospital postoperatively. Only then can they decide whether they wish to have the operation on a day-stay basis. Once that decision is made then they must have an appropriate assessment which will include their past medical history, current health status and social circumstances.

The preoperative screening that they undergo should be made by someone who is familiar with modern day surgical practice. This can be the patient's own GP, the surgical junior staff, the anaesthetist or a nurse. All that they will be doing is filling in a questionnaire which will identify areas of potential concern for the anaesthetist and surgeon. Each day surgery unit in the country has developed a version of this form and they are usually modifications of someone else's booklet. This has proved to be a very effective method of evolving care. There is no great mystique over what questions should be asked, every anaesthetist has a series of questions that they ask at every preoperative assessment; day surgery is no different. Each booklet creator has their own 'special' question that sorts the wheat from the chaff, but fitness for surgery and anaesthesia is self evident to any practising anaesthetist.

It used to be the case that only the super fit in their 20s and 30s having minor surface surgery could be considered for this type of care. The rules have now changed. Patients who are ASA grade II and III and even IV may be suitable for some day-stay procedures. The definitive question to ask is 'would their care be substantially different and safer as an inpatient?' If the answer is 'yes' then that is where they should go; if 'no' then day care is the place. There are no age barriers to day care. The very young and the very old are often most suited to day care as this prevents separation from their families. The mentally and physically handicapped should not be excluded from this service either, for exactly the same reasons.

Any chronic disease must be well or optimally controlled. Patients with insulin-dependent diabetes, hypertension, asthma, epilepsy and other cardiovascular and respiratory diseases need no longer be excluded. All such decisions should be based on the tenet of the most appropriate care in the most appropriate setting.

The most effective place to make these assessments of the patient is probably in a special clinic run in the day unit by the nursing and anaesthetic staff who will be subsequently involved in that patient's care. This is often difficult for logistical reasons, and so some form of compromise is needed. If the assessment occurs in the day unit then this gives the patient an opportunity to familiarize themselves with the unit and the staff and to see where their care will occur. Day-case care is particularly dependent on maintaining the patient's confidence and retaining their ability to feel in control of their situation and not become depersonalized. Everything should be patient focused, therefore, with how they feel at the forefront of everyone's mind and not what is 'the rule' or perhaps just convenient. Good information and an interested and sympathetic response to invited questions will do much to ensure that the patient then experiences a successful day stay in the future. It is also crucial to remember that many patients do not speak or read English as their first language and their needs must be met either with advocates, relatives or the use of language telephone lines. Even those for whom English is their first language may not be able to read or understand patient information leaflets, and this may cause considerable embarrassment, anxiety and resentment if it is not dealt with sympathetically.

Written information must confirm all the information that the patient has been given verbally, about fasting, medications, transport etc., as most patients cannot retain all this information during what, for them, is a particularly stressful time. Special emphasis must be made on the patient's social conditions, their housing, access to telephones, access to heating, cooking, and washing facilities and particularly who will care for them at home after the operation. Many units now produce special information sheets for the patient's escort who will take them home, as well as for their subsequent carer who may not be the same person.

Further information should be provided preoperatively about the operation itself, how the patient will feel afterwards and what care they will need at home. It is important that the patient can contact someone when they are at home to discuss symptoms or perceived problems. Some units have had considerable success in these circumstances with a mobile telephone which is carried by a senior nurse every night; the number of this telephone is on the information sheet. Other units rely on the on-call surgical team for out-of-hours consultation, but this team may have no knowledge of the procedure performed, nor can they readily access that information from a unit which is usually locked overnight. In the face of a major problem or just a lack of information the patient may then turn to their GP or to an Accident and Emergency (A & E) Department of their local hospital: this is not ideal.

It must be remembered that many patients will opt for day care because they do not wish to let their friends and family know they are having surgery. This may be for a variety of reasons and does not only apply to those who are undergoing procedures like termination of pregnancy. All such situations must be dealt with sympathetically and the patients wishes and beliefs respected.

Preoperative investigation of the patient should be limited to those indices that will significantly affect anaesthetic management. There is no place for the routine testing of anything unless there is a clinical indication; thus no one should have a routine haemoglobin test, chest X-ray or ECG. If the patient gives a history of respiratory or cardiovascular disease then those investigations should be performed, but not otherwise. All investigations should be made preoperatively and their results should be evaluated by an anaesthetist well in advance of the day of surgery. There is little point in arranging a patient's haemoglobin test three weeks in advance of surgery and then cancelling on the day of the procedure if the result is 8.3 g dl^{-1}. There is no value in routine urine testing at the time of admission on patients who are starved and dehydrated.

Consent forms should be completed and signed by the surgeon and patient in advance: this should help minimize delays on the day of surgery.

Rules regarding starvation are undergoing considerable re-evaluation; 6 h nil-by-mouth for food still seems to be a good rule, whereas 4 h for liquids is under considerable challenge. Each practitioner must weigh up in his or her own mind the risks and benefits for each patient in the light of their current health and the procedure they will undergo. The starving for 12 h of a patient undergoing the removal of a skin lesion under local anaesthetic infiltration is as ridiculous as letting a patient who will be managed with artificial ventilation via a laryngeal mask head-down for a laparoscopy, drink clear fluids up to an hour before the procedure. It is reasonable to let a patient drink a moderate volume of 'clear liquid' (defined as a solution that can be seen through when placed in a glass, i.e. apple juice, but not milk) up to 3 h before surgery. Some may wish to shorten that period even more.

Any patient taking regular medication should be encouraged to continue this on the morning or afternoon of surgery unless their is a specific reason not to do so (e.g. warfarin, insulin etc.). Specific instructions must be given in writing to the patient on these matters and this should be communicated to the referring GP as well.

Once a patient has been evaluated, screened and assessed as suitable for day care, then that information must be communicated to the community physicians, nurses and other allied professions who will be potentially involved in their subsequent care. This will allow time for feedback of potential contraindications to this treatment.

On the day of surgery the patient should arrive in the day unit at a specific time having been fully evaluated and investigated and with a background knowledge of what to expect. It should be exceptional for a procedure to be cancelled at this time unless there is a sudden onset of a new illness. It is vitally important that the whole day should reflect a confident and smooth process so that patient confidence and self-respect are maintained. There should be minimal disruption of clothing at all stages of the patient's care. The routine stripping of patients and their incarceration in ill-fitting hospital gowns is totally archaic and inappropriate for modern day-surgery. Glasses, hearing aids, teeth and the like should be retained unless there is a real medical/surgical reason why they cannot be.

Time must be allocated for the patient to express any concerns over the intended procedure with the nurse, anaesthetist or surgeon. The patient must be carefully identified by all personnel and sites of surgery should be clearly marked.

DRUGS

Once a patient has been selected for day surgery and fully prepared as described, then decisions must be made about their anaesthetic management. As in all aspects of anaesthetic care there are no absolute right and wrong ways of doing any procedure. Each anaesthetist must develop techniques which permit the patient to undergo their surgical procedure with the minimum of stress and the maximum of comfort. Analgesia is paramount and must be long lasting. Morbidity, such as nausea and vomiting, must be minimized.

The 'ideal technique' for day surgery will probably involve a blending of local anaesthesia with a varying degree of unconsciousness for all patients. Some will happily remain wide awake during local blockade and surgery, others will wish to be asleep.

Premedication is rarely useful in adults, but it is often necessary in children. The use of EMLA cream and benzodiazepines will minimize both intraoperative problems at induction and also postoperative problems at home later. To be fully effective, this EMLA cream may need to be given to the parents to apply to their children sufficiently in advance to be working by the time the child is admitted. Any adult who is particularly nervous may benefit from a short acting benzodiazepine like temazepam given orally, and this should not impair their subsequent discharge. Greater sedation from premedication may also be indicated for those who are mentally handicapped in whom reassurance and explanation may not be adequate to alleviate natural anxiety and fear.

The advantage of the use of preoperative non-steroidal anti-inflammatory drugs (NSAID) is popularly pursued by many, but is not conclusively proven. Rectal preparations may cause discomfort or offence, oral preparations in a dehydrated anxious patient may encourage renal or gastric side effects and parentral administration can be painful.

Other NSAID like piroxicam, which are formulated as a tablet to suck and is readily absorbed in the mouth, are not licensed for perioperative use. Each practitioner must develop a practice which benefits the patient and which is safe and rational based on published work and peer experience.

Sedation can be provided by the shorter acting benzodiazepines such as midazolam, which may or may not require reversal with flumazenil, or from the standard intravenous induction agents methohexitone, propofol and etomidate. These sedatives can be used as single doses, which may then be augmented by inhalational agents, or alternatively they can be given as continuous infusions.

Patient-controlled sedation, using propofol, during regional techniques has proved very effective in many units and permits the patient to decide the level of sedation best suited to them.

Full general anaesthesia will utilize the same induction agents as listed above. Propofol is now the drug of choice for day-case work, but methohexitone and thiopentone were the only drugs available to the North American pioneers of day-case work who had achieved a rate of day surgery above 50% of all elective surgery before propofol had been introduced! The use of small doses of midazolam (2.5 mg) before either a barbiturate or propofol significantly reduces the dosage of these agents required for anaesthesia. This concept of co-induction has proved popular in many units and does not influence recovery times.

Following or, more often, before the use of these induction agents I believe that there is still a major role for short-acting opioids like fentanyl and alfentanil. Many workers have suggested that their side effects of nausea and vomiting outweigh their usefulness as analgesics. This must be decided by the individual in their own practice, but effective analgesia must be paramount in all cases and should not be sacrificed for potential lack of nausea.

Anti-emetics should be given early at induction. All have side effects and none are always effective. Metoclopramide and prochlorperazine are old favourites whose value has been questioned. Cyclizine is probably more effective but can make patients drowsy later. Ondansetron certainly works, but is expensive as a routine drug and may be best saved as an 'escape' anti-emetic when others have failed. After operation small doses (3–6 mg) of ephedrine are remarkably effective in the treatment and prevention of postural hypotension which in turn leads to nausea. Propofol is undoubtedly a potent anti-emetic. I do not believe in the abandonment of nitrous oxide to prevent these symptoms.

The inhalational agents can be utilized according to the preference of each practitioner. Despite the plethora of scientific papers on this subject, the emergence times from these agents play little part in the final recovery of patients and their use and mode of administration should be according to local preferences. Closed circuit anaesthesia is appropriate on cost grounds for the most recently introduced agents like desflurane and sevoflurane.

The choice of airway control should be determined by the proposed surgery and the health of the patient. A face mask held by hand or with a harness is satisfactory for many procedures, although such a technique may impede completion of all the charts and forms that the anaesthetist is expected to fill in even the most brief of surgical operations. The laryngeal mask airway (LMA) has revolutionized airway control and is eminently suitable for day practice. It can be used for patients who are breathing spontaneously and those whose lungs are ventilated with or without muscle relaxants, but in the latter group careful consideration of lung and chest wall compliance and the positioning of the patient must be taken into consideration.

Tracheal intubation is not a contraindication to day surgery in any age group and may be safely performed where indicated. I intubate every patient that I paralyse and ventilate: this is a personal preference. Placement of the tube can be achieved after the use of a narcotic and propofol induction, but it is more usual to use a muscle relaxant. Suxamethonium is a useful agent for short procedures and the possibility of postoperative myalgia should not cause it to be discarded for day work. The patient can be warned of this side effect and, if indicated, it is a very useful drug. Mivacurium is a useful alternative for short procedures, but its duration of action in recommended dosages may prove to be particularly evanescent and higher doses may provoke the release of histamine as shown by wheals on the arm used for injection; this does not usually cause systemic effects.

Atracurium probably still remains the most commonly used agent for neuromuscular blockade for day surgery where it can be used in very low dosage with great efficacy. Other longer acting relaxants, like vecuronium and pancuronium, may have a place for prolonged surgery and the newer introduced agents like rocuronium may prove effective also.

Analgesia must always be provided. This may take the form of opioids or NSAID as discussed previously and should involve the use of long-acting local anaesthetics whenever possible. Bupivacaine should be infiltrated into incisions or applied to nerve trunks. Lignocaine and prilocaine may be used intravenously or may be appropriate for epidural or subarachnoid administration if appropriate formulations are available. Many countries have 'heavy lignocaine' available which permits spinal anaesthesia that is short in duration and allows patients to achieve rapid ambulation and safe discharge. Special care must be taken after central neural blockade to ensure that full proprioception has returned and that postural hypotension is not present. Retention of urine must also be borne in mind as a possible complication.

It is not helpful to try to develop 'pure techniques' which rely solely on narcotics or NSAIDs or local anaesthetics, as a blend of all three will usually provide the best perioperative conditions for the patient, the anaesthetist and the surgeon.

Newer anaesthetic agents and 'ancillary drugs', are being introduced regularly; each must be carefully evaluated to determine its place in day-stay practice. Each is usually heralded by their manufacturer as the new panacea for all day-surgery cases; then after a period of time it finds an appropriate niche in this type of anaesthesia.

When anaesthesia is complete the patient is moved into the operating theatre. Full monitoring is maintained and augmented where appropriate throughout surgery. Once the surgical procedure is finished the patient is transferred to recovery.

POSTOPERATIVE CARE

Day-care surgery and anaesthesia require meticulous attention to detail. As the patient will leave the day unit and travel home within a few hours, it is what might be regarded by the medical staff as the 'little things' that will make the biggest difference to them. They should be clean, dry and warm as they move through to recovery, not still covered in skin preparation, lying on a wet canvas and without a blanket. Do they feel nauseated, is the induction of anaesthesia site bruised? 'Minor morbidity' takes on major significance for the day-stay patient and yet is simple to prevent, and once these techniques become ingrained for day-work they also produce lasting benefits for inpatients.

In the recovery area each patient must be cared for by specifically trained nurses on a one-to-one basis until they are fully conscious. Full monitoring is maintained as before and once awake the patient is questioned on their level of comfort. As soon as they feel able to walk, they are escorted to a secondary recovery or 'step-down' area to complete their recovery. In this latter zone they can rest in reclining chairs until they wish to dress themselves and increase their mobility. Relatives or friends can join the patient at any stage of the recovery process at the discretion of the medical and nursing staff.

All patients must be seen during their postoperative course by the surgeon and anaesthetist who have been involved in their care. This will allow an explanation of what exactly has been done and what they can now expect as well as outlining future plans, if any, for their care. Once this has taken place, the majority of patients attending for day surgery can be discharged by the nursing staff who are able to follow simple discharge criteria protocols. The patients receive all appropriate medication, including analgesics, often in two formulations: a small number of tablets for severe to moderate pain (say DF118), and a larger number of less potent drugs (such as mefenamic acid or paracetamol).

Patients are also given detailed instructions, identical to those they received preoperatively, which outline the 'do's' and 'don'ts' of their immediate and late postoperative management. Patients are then allowed to go home with an escort, provided assurance has been given that they have someone to care for them that night.

The GPs involved can be informed by fax with a complete discharge summary of their patient's treatment before the patient leaves for home. For those without a fax, a telephone message to the practice and a message that the patient is about to be discharged has a similar effect. The practitioner has already been alerted to their patient's proposed treatment on that day by the preoperative request for medical and social information. The GPs are thus able to plan effective postoperative care for their patients based on up-to-the-minute information in conjunction with their own knowledge of the health and social background of the patient.

AFTER-CARE

Until the patient next attends for outpatient review by the surgeon they are cared for by their own practitioners, the community nursing services, and usually their immediate family. I believe that day centres must augment this care and provide a postoperative after-care service. The Audit Commission has published an audit questionnaire which is appropriate for patients to complete at home. This published work is a good starting format for each centre to use to develop their own audit. Failure to act in this way must jeopardize any success that a day centre is trying to achieve. Surgeons, anaesthetists and nurses should not think that they have done a good job in sending the patient home unless they can demonstrate that the following days spent at home were comfortable and incident free, and that a burden of care has not been placed on community medical or nursing services.

Day-stay care can provide the highest quality care that is available for patients today, provided it is done well. It can also provide some of the worst possible care if patients are sent home to suffer needlessly when local anaesthetics and potent narcotic analgesics have worn off. Most, if not all patients, go home relatively comfortable and relatively free from side effects (otherwise they would have to be admitted). The next 24 h are crucial and determine the standard of care that is achieved. Over the last decade we have addressed most of the urgent problems in the hospital care of day cases and it will be the next decade which will see anaesthetists facing and solving the postoperative problems described by patient audit when effective analysis of their experiences is obtained and then acted upon.

FUTURE DEVELOPMENT

Day-stay surgery will increase; all aspects will undergo change and development. Surgeons will increase the complexity and duration of their day-stay practice as new techniques of non-invasive surgery expand the range of procedures which can be attempted. Anaesthetists will continue to improve postoperative morbidity using newer and less toxic agents. Epidural and subarachnoid anaesthesia will expand in frequency and scope in this country as it has in the USA. Hotel facilities will be built close to hospitals to extend the possibilities of day care. Community and domiciliary nursing will extend its remit in these fields to cater for patient needs, much as can be seen in the USA with surgeons performing day-stay thyroidectomy and hysterectomy as well as routine cholecystectomy.

It is to be anticipated that many more new centres will evolve over the coming decades. Day surgery is not a static process, but one which is constantly evolving in new directions. All involved in this type of work must be prepared to adopt a flexible approach and to constantly re-evaluate their practice in the light of new developments.

FURTHER READING

Association of Anaesthetists of Great Britain & Ireland. (1994) *Day Case Surgery: the Anaesthetist's Role in Promoting High Quality Care.* AAGBI, London.

National Association for the Welfare of Children in Hospital. (1991) *Just for the day.* Caring for children in the Health Services. NAWCH, London.

National Health Service Management Executive. (1993) *Day Surgery: Report by the Day Surgery Task Force.* Health Publications Unit, Heywood, UK.

Twersky, R. S. (1995) *The Ambulatory Anesthesia Handbook.* Mosby, St Louis.

Wetchler, B. V. (1985) *Anesthesia for Ambulatory Surgery*, 2nd edn. Lippincott, Philadelphia.

Whitwam, J. G. (1994) *Day Case Anaesthesia and Sedation.* Blackwell Scientific Publications, Oxford.

DENTAL SURGERY

A. Chan and P. J. Flynn

Dental anaesthesia has always been considered to be in a different category from anaesthesia for other forms of surgery because of the historical involvement of the dental profession in its origin. It was an American dentist, Horace Wells, who noted the analgesic effects of nitrous oxide at a demonstration of its effects by a travelling chemist, G. Q. Colton, in 1844. In a spirit of inquiry, Wells persuaded Colton to administer the gas to him for extraction of a wisdom tooth. Shortly after, another dentist William Morton, demonstrated the successful use of ether for general surgery at Harvard. In England, the first anaesthetic was given by a dentist, James Robinson, who acted as both surgeon and anaesthetist in 1846. The dental profession has a unique association with anaesthesia, and anaesthesia developed in dental surgeries to a large extent in isolation from hospital practice. For many years the administration of a general anaesthetic was considered well within the competence of any medical or dental practitioner, but with the establishment of the UK National Health Service in 1948 anaesthesia was recognized as a speciality in its own right and acknowledged to be a postgraduate skill. Dental schools, however, continued to teach practical anaesthesia to undergraduates, but by the 1960s there was increasing concern regarding their training and about the anaesthetic techniques in use in the dentist's surgery. From 1965 onwards consecutive working parties set up by government and national bodies attempted to produce policies governing practice and postgraduate training in dental anaesthesia. However, no action was taken to implement the recommendations of these committees until the publication in 1990 of the Report of the Expert Working Party convened under the chairmanship of David Poswillo. A major recommendation of this report was that the same general standards would apply with respect to personnel, premises and equipment, irrespective of where a general anaesthetic was administered. While a 'no detriment' clause to cover dentists and non-specialist doctors already engaged in giving general anaesthetics was also included, it was stated that all general anaesthetics should be administered by accredited anaesthetists. The Poswillo report was accepted in full by the Department of Health and produced a considerable change in attitudes toward dental anaesthesia, especially with regard to monitoring equipment. A greater appreciation of the specialist knowledge and skills required in dental anaesthesia, coupled with the increased range and availability of physiological monitoring, has seen a reduction in the number of dental practices prepared to offer general anaesthesia with the service now concentrated in fewer, better equipped surgeries.

Short Practice of Anaesthesia. Edited by M. Morgan and G. M. Hall. Published in 1997 by Chapman & Hall, London. ISBN 0 412 71890 1

OUTPATIENT GENERAL ANAESTHESIA

INDICATIONS

Most dental procedures can be performed under local anaesthesia. There are, however, circumstances in which the use of general anaesthesia is indicated. The traditional 'chair' dental anaesthetic involved only a brief period of unconsciousness, so that painful carious teeth could be extracted. More recently the remit has been widened to include orthodontic extractions, conservative treatment and minor oral surgery. Procedures lasting up to about an hour are now considered suitable for the dental surgery, or a day-care centre. Accepted indications for general anaesthesia are as follows.

Dental procedures in young children

It may not be possible to obtain the cooperation of small children with dental treatment, especially when multiple extractions are required. Conservative treatment may be managed with the help of inhalational sedation, but on occasions general anaesthesia may be required.

Acute infection

Due to altered pH of the tissues, local anaesthesia is often unsuccessful in patients with dental infections. In addition, local injections may also spread the infection. General anaesthesia overcomes these problems; however, extra care must be taken if there is associated tissue oedema because of trismus and potential airway problems.

Adverse reactions to local anaesthesia

Patients with a genuine history of allergy to local anaesthetics, such as skin reactions or angioneurotic oedema, should have general anaesthesia.

Failure of local anaesthesia

Rarely local anaesthesia may be ineffective despite adequate dosage and apparently accurate placement. This may be due to aberrant anatomy, since the problem has been found in patients who have undergone previous surgery to the mandible.

Mentally or physically disabled patients

These patients may not be able to cooperate sufficiently to allow extractions, or conservative treatment, under local anaesthesia.

Very nervous adults

Some extremely nervous patients may request general anaesthesia. Most of these patients can be successfully treated under local anaesthesia by sympathetic and experienced dentists with the help of appropriate sedative techniques. However, in some cases the phobia may be so intense that a general anaesthetic becomes unavoidable.

Minor oral surgery

Extraction of impacted third molars is one of the most common surgical operations in fit young adults. Many easier extractions can be managed under local anaesthesia and sedation. For day-case extraction it is important to ascertain that the duration and difficulty of the surgery will not cause prolonged recovery, or severe postoperative pain and swelling.

CONTRAINDICATIONS

The majority of dental anaesthetics are given in dental surgeries or community clinics outside hospital. Only ASA Class I or II patients should be anaesthetized in such surroundings, and similar guidelines should be applied to dental outpatient or hospital day-stay units if they are remote from the main hospital block. Hospital admission is mandatory for patients with unstable or serious cardiovascular, respiratory or other medical disorders. Similarly, patients with oral sepsis who may present difficult airway problems because of severe trismus or oedema of the floor of the mouth or pharynx, must be admitted to hospital. Disabled patients with cardiovascular, respiratory or airway problems should also be treated as inpatients.

PATIENT ASSESSMENT

Health questionnaires are widely used to provide an initial screening of fitness. Many dental practices rely on dental staff, or the general practitioner, to complete these questionnaires and will give an appointment for general anaesthesia based on the result. It is, however, essential that the anaesthetist verifies the history with the patient. One should never be in such a hurry that a talk to the patient (or parent) is omitted. In hospital, junior medical, or dental, staff may be responsible for patient assessment. Although it is universally agreed that ASA I and II patients are fit for general anaesthesia in the dental chair, caution may be needed if using ASA grading by anaesthetic colleagues as there is evidence of difficulty in differentiating between Classes II and III. In addition, the system does not take into account age, obesity, extent of surgery proposed and specific anaesthetic problems. Each patient must be assessed on an individual basis by the person giving the anaesthetic.

Patients who invariably present the anaesthetist with a difficult decision are children with the common cold. Increased irritability and hyper-reactivity of the airway may lead to life-threatening hypoxia, and there is an increased incidence of intra- and postoperative respiratory complications for up to 6 weeks after a respiratory tract infection in children. It has been recommended that children with symptoms of a moderate to severe respiratory tract infection presenting for elective surgery should have the anaesthetic postponed for 6 weeks. However, this may be difficult if there is dental pain. If the infection appears to be mild with a non-productive cough, and the procedure is short enough for mask anaesthesia, then it is reasonable to proceed. Indications for postponing the procedure include an age of less than one year, nasal congestion, rhinorrhoea, a productive cough, signs of wheezing and the need for intubation. The role of the laryngeal mask in this situation remains to be clarified. Each case should be assessed on its merits and considerable judgement is required, as there are no definitive criteria on which to base the clinical decision.

When the history is unremarkable and the proposed procedure brief, it is still usual to omit a physical examination of the patient, especially children, unless the history suggests it. It is difficult to defend this practice when such an examination customarily precedes the administration of general anaesthesia for other surgical procedures. It would appear that auscultation of the chest together with recording of the heart rate, arterial pressure and weight should become a minimum acceptable practice for all patients. The nasal and oral airway, and the condition of the teeth should be assessed. A haemoglobin estimation should be performed on all patients of Afro-Carribean and Mediterranean descent, and a sickle or thalassaemia test performed as indicated. Studies have shown that approximately 10% of patients considered fit for outpatient anaesthesia have abnormal blood and urine results. A haemoglobin estimation and urinalysis should be considered the minimal tests in any patient presenting for anaesthesia. It has been suggested that an ECG should only be performed if indicated by the history. Children with undiagnosed heart murmurs should be referred for a cardiological opinion.

PREPARATION OF THE PATIENT

The preparation of the patient is no different from that of other patients undergoing general anaesthesia. Ideally, every patient must be seen by the anaesthetist beforehand, so that each party may have a chance to ask questions and be reassured. In the case of children the procedure should be explained to them in simple terms. Older children should be offered the choice of an intravenous or inhalational induction. The need for preoperative fasting must be emphasized. For elective procedures no solid food is allowed for 6 h but, although still controversial, it has recently been recommended that clear liquids be permitted for up to 2 h before anaesthesia. Studies in adults and children allowed freely available, clear liquids until 2 h before the scheduled time of anaesthesia found gastric contents to be similar to those who had endured a longer fast. Potential benefits include reduced thirst, better perioperative experience, improved compliance and less risk of hypoglycaemia.

A valid consent for the procedure must be obtained. This may need to include the method of pain relief, if a drug is to be administered per rectum, and it may be advisable to discuss pain relief at this stage. The consent for a child must be signed by the parent or legal guardian. The patient's escort is not required to be a relative, but must be at least 18 years of age.

TECHNIQUE OF ANAESTHESIA

In general, age and the extent of surgery determine the anaesthetic technique. Inhalational induction is commonly used in young children and may be offered to older children and adults if requested. It is usual to encourage a parent to hold the child's hand during induction. Small children may be anaesthetized sitting in the parent's lap. Induction should commence with high flows of nitrous oxide and at least 30% oxygen delivered by cupping the hand around the end of the circuit. Halothane may gradually be introduced increasing the concentration in a stepwise fashion by 0.5% every 3–4 breaths. As consciousness is lost a nasal mask may be placed over the face. Older children and adults will usually accept a mask from the beginning of induction. Adequate surgical anaesthesia is suggested by regular respiration and sufficient relaxation of the jaw to allow the dental prop to be inserted. Adults and older children usually prefer intravenous induction. In day-stay anaesthesia the most widely used induction agent is propofol in a dose of 2–3 mg kg^{-1}. Once surgical anaesthesia has been achieved, a pack consisting of folds of a length of gauze about 8 cm wide must be placed over the back of the tongue to isolate the operation site and prevent the aspiration of blood or dental debris. The vulnerable area, where leakage of blood and debris is likely, occurs where the edges of the pack meet the buccal walls. Care should be taken to ascertain that the airway is unobstructed by the pack as evidenced by the regular movement of the rebreathing bag and the patient's respiration. Anaesthesia may be maintained via the nasal mask with halothane, or other volatile agent if preferred. Throughout the procedure the airway must be maintained by holding the mandible upwards and forwards by supporting the angle of the jaw. During extraction of posterior teeth from the lower jaw it may be particularly difficult to counteract the downward pressure exerted by the dentist, although the experienced operator will support the jaw. For multiple extractions, once surgery on one side has been completed, a piece of the pack should be placed over the sockets over which is then placed the prop. The integrity of the barrier produced by the pack should be checked before extraction is performed on the other side. Where easy surgery is anticipated anaesthesia may be withdrawn before extraction of the penultimate tooth and 100% oxygen administered. At the end of the procedure fresh dental packs should be placed over the sockets with a length protruding from the mouth, and without obstructing the airway. The patient should be nursed in the recovery position until consciousness is regained. Most procedures are accomplished in less than 5 min and spontaneous respiration with inhalational agents is usual. For more prolonged procedures with intubation, a controlled ventilation technique may be considered.

Choice of drugs

Halothane remains a popular agent for inhalational induction. Enflurane and isoflurane offer the advantages of lower solubility of the gas in blood, with a more rapid onset and recovery, and a lower incidence of arrhythmias. In practice, it may be difficult to achieve sufficient depth of anaesthesia in young children with the maximum concentrations permitted by the enflurane vaporizer. Induction with isoflurane has been found to produce an unacceptably high incidence of coughing, breath holding and laryngospasm. Both agents, however, are widely used for maintenance of anaesthesia following intravenous induction. Of the newer volatile agents desflurane appears to have similar effects on the paediatric airway to isoflurane, but a more rapid recovery. Preliminary experiences with sevoflurane have found it to be acceptable at high concentrations and as non-irritant as halothane in paediatric patients and to produce a more rapid return to consciousness.

Intravenous induction offers the advantages of more rapid onset, less salivation, fewer arrhythmias and less atmospheric pollution. Although for many years the intravenous agent of choice was methohexitone, this has been replaced by propofol, which offers the advantages of rapid induction with minimum involuntary movements, diminished airway reactivity, rapid recovery and a very low incidence of nausea and vomiting. However, it causes more respiratory depression than methohexitone which may be considered a drawback if the anaesthetic is to be maintained by inhalational agents. Bradycardia and hypotension associated with propofol have been cited as reasons for preferring methohexitone. In intubated patients use of suxamethonium results in a high incidence of postoperative muscle pain despite various preventative strategies. For those experienced in the technique, blind nasal intubation avoids the use of suxamethonium, and nasal intubation has also been successfully achieved using only alfentanil and propofol. In addition, non-depolarizing neuromuscular blocking drugs such as atracurium, vecuronium, rocuronium and mivacurium are all satisfactory for outpatient, dental procedures.

CONTROL OF THE AIRWAY

In no other field of anaesthesia is the interaction between the anaesthetist and surgeon so vital. Dental anaesthesia breaks one of the fundamental rules of safe practice in that the patient is not intubated, despite the fact that the airway is shared with the surgeon. However, dentists have always been educated to share the responsibility for maintaining the airway during general anaesthesia. A calculated risk is taken by the anaesthetist, in that the skill and speed of the surgeon, support of the jaw and effective packing balance the potential problems of intubation. In 1965 it was noted that for 50% of patients the operating time was less than 1 min, and in no patient was it longer than 5 min. At present there may be less concern about speed, but a greater desire to effect a definitive result and avoid repeated anaesthetics. Extraction of 12 or more teeth in small children is not uncommon, and older children may require orthodontic extraction in all four quadrants. Intubation is now routinely practised in outpatient anaesthesia, and it is incumbent on the anaesthetist to consider whether it is indicated for each anaesthetic, although it is preferable to avoid it in outpatients below 6 years of age. If intubation is used, the tube is usually inserted by the nasal route, and a pharyngeal pack is always placed even in the presence of a cuffed tube.

An alternative method of airway control is offered by the laryngeal mask, which has been found to decrease the incidence of hypoxaemia during dental anaesthesia, when compared with the nasal mask. A dental pack should always be used since the evidence that the laryngeal mask produces an adequate seal around the laryngeal area during dental surgery is not conclusive. Dye studies have suggested that the cuff forms an effective barrier preventing aspiration from the oropharynx. A further modification in its design has resulted in the availability of a mask with an armoured tube which is narrower than the standard mask and thus takes up less room in the mouth. The reinforced laryngeal mask is available in four sizes and consists of a mask sealed to an armoured, narrow-bore tube with an internal diameter about 2–2.5 mm smaller and a length 10–15 mm longer, than the standard mask. The main disadvantage of this model is that it is too floppy to permit the usual method of insertion. A gloved index finger is needed to position the mask in the pharynx, keeping the finger as close as possible to the junction between the tube and the mask. A Magill's forceps may also be useful to place the mask, or it may be inserted under direct vision using a laryngoscope. It should be noted that the reinforced laryngeal mask is unsuitable for prolonged spontaneous respiration due to the increased resistance of the tube. There is no doubt that the laryngeal mask is an immensely useful addition to the armamentarium of the dental anaesthetist. Exactly where it stands in relation to the nasal mask and to intubation remains to be defined. A recent study of the reinforced laryngeal mask during third molar extractions found satisfactory airway maintenance and surgical access in procedures lasting up to 20 min. It is perhaps reasonable to assume that it cannot provide the degree of safety, in terms of maintenance and protection of the airway, offered by a tracheal tube.

The ideal airway requirements for dental surgery are the provision of a stable unobstructed airway, protection of the lungs from aspiration, minimal interference with the surgical field and a low complication rate. Neither the nasal mask, laryngeal mask, nor tracheal tube meets all of these requirements, although in theory the combination of tracheal intubation and an oropharyngeal pack is still probably the safest. Conventional anaesthetic wisdom dictates that a tracheal tube is mandatory where the airway is shared, but it is generally agreed that in carefully selected dental patients the need for intubation may be obviated. The decision of which method of airway control to choose can be difficult in some cases, nevertheless safety of the patient is paramount.

POSTURE

Although posture plays an important role in both respiratory and circulatory efficiency, it should be appreciated that no position offers a guarantee of safety for either respiratory or circulatory function. In dental anaesthesia the choice of posture lies between the traditional bolt upright sitting position at one extreme, and fully supine at the other. For many years a debate raged furiously about the merits and risks of the sitting as opposed to the supine position. Those in favour of the upright position argued that it provided easier maintenance of the airway, more efficient respiratory exchange and less risk of airway contamination. Those opposed cited the risk of unrecognized hypotension leading to cerebral ischaemia. The upright position facilitates airway maintenance since the effect of gravity directs the relaxed tongue into the floor of the mouth, rather than posteriorly into the obstructive position against the posterior pharyngeal wall in the supine position.

Vital capacity is some 15% less in the supine than in the upright posture. This difference is due partly to alterations in lung blood volume, and partly to the impairment of diaphragmatic movement imposed by the abdominal contents. It is well known that at low lung volumes, the phenomenon of airway closure may lead to some degree of hypoxaemia because of the continued perfusion with mixed venous blood of the non-ventilated areas of the lung. Low lung volume is a feature of both increasing age and the supine posture, in which it is approximately 1 l less than in the upright position. Thus, the upright posture may have an important overall respiratory advantage particularly in the elderly, and probably the obese.

The question of which position provides the better airway protection from aspiration is more difficult to resolve. McCormick studied four different postures for dental anaesthesia and found a higher incidence of blood soiling of the pharynx with patients in the supine position, although the results did not reach statistical significance. Scott found that 25% of patients anaesthetized in the sitting position showed evidence of aspiration of radio-opaque oil injected at the side of the pack, whereas only 2% maintained supine with 30° of head-down tilt inhaled the oil. In a similar study in children Love found that aspiration in the upright position was only prevented if the patient was maintained bolt upright without any head retraction, which is difficult to prevent during surgery. In patients maintained horizontal with a 5–15° head-down tilt, material tended to pool in the palatal and pharyngeal areas, but some inhalation occurred in 20% children. Airway protection during dental anaesthesia with the nasal mask depends primarily upon efficient packing and suction. Failure to achieve proper packing and suction is probably the most common cause of difficulty, and even catastrophe. Although efficient packing can be achieved in any posture, it is claimed that it is easier in the sitting position. Anaesthetic factors which increase the risk of inhalation of debris are hypoxaemia, coughing, struggling and mouth breathing. Those associated with the surgery are prolonged operating time, multiple extractions and excessive haemorrhage. Newer airway adjuncts such as the larnygeal mask may prevent the problems related to anaesthesia, but elective intubation should be considered where the duration of surgery, or number of extractions, poses a significant risk of airway contamination.

The supine position offers the advantages of a lower incidence of fainting, no postural effect if hypotension occurs and better visualization of the patient's respiration. In addition, it is a better position should resuscitation be required and it is easier to move the patient laterally for recovery, or if vomiting occurs. Reports concerning deaths in dental anaesthesia have consistently failed to detect any differences in mortality between the upright, reclining and supine positions. Each posture has its advantages and disadvantages, but none can be considered safe under all circumstances.

MONITORING

Traditional chair dental anaesthetics are very brief, but things can go wrong very rapidly. Pulse oximetry, electrocardiography and non-invasive blood pressure measurement should be applied to all patients, although arterial pressure measurement is often omitted in children where the procedure is not expected to exceed 5 min. It should be noted that some adult pulse oximeter finger probes give misleading values when used on children. Monitoring should also include capnography in all intubated cases and where the laryngeal mask is used. Measurement of expired volumes and airway pressure is necessary if the lungs are artificially ventilated. Ideally, monitors should be attached before the induction of anaesthesia, although this may be impossible in the very uncooperative child.

Monitoring should be continued at least until the patient regains consciousness and longer if clinically indicated.

RECOVERY

Mortality reports have found that 30–60% of all deaths in dental anaesthesia occurred in the recovery period. It is essential to observe the patient closely until they are fully awake. Whatever posture has been used for the procedure, the lateral horizontal position should be adopted as soon as possible. A 30% incidence of hypoxaemia has been found in patients recovering from dental anaesthesia, which is increased following intubation, intravenous induction and the use of neuromuscular blocking drugs. Pulse oximetry should be continued and supplemental oxygen administered until consciousness is regained. Even with oxygen supplementation the reported incidence of hypoxaemia is about 20%, suggesting unrecognized airway obstruction. It is mandatory that the patient is supervized by a suitably trained individual, either the anaesthetist or experienced general nurses, until consciousness is regained. Dental nurses are not trained to manage the unconscious patient, although they may supervize late recovery provided they have undergone appropriate instruction. The anaesthetist must not leave the premises until the last patient has been discharged. Recovery of street fitness, as shown by the ability to walk a straight line unaided, may take about 30 min. The speed of recovery depends on a number of factors of which duration and depth of the anaesthetic are probably the more important ones. Bleeding should have ceased and there should be no significant pain or nausea and vomiting. Packs must be positioned in such a way as to encourage maximum haemostasis and no obstruction. Patients must be escorted home by an adult. Written postoperative instructions should be given stressing the avoidance of driving, operating machinery, cooking, caring for young children, signing important documents and consuming alcohol for the remainder of the day. Advice about dental care and whom to contact in an emergency should also be given.

PAIN RELIEF

In the past little attention was given to postoperative analgesia in the belief that most patients would have the cause of the pain removed. In addition, concern that the use of opioid analgesics was likely to prolong recovery and decrease patient throughput discouraged any form of pain relief. Ideally, methods of analgesia should be discussed with the patient beforehand. Fear markedly decreases the tolerance to pain, and reassurance can go a long way to alleviate it and render it more manageable. Pre-emptive analgesia has much to recommend it. Local anaesthetic infiltration, or nerve blocks, should be performed before the surgical procedure. This offers the advantage of a reduced anaesthetic requirement and a lower incidence of cardiac arrhythmias, in addition to effective analgesia without major side-effects. The non-steroidal anti-inflammatory drugs, especially when used pre-emptively, have been shown to produce good postoperative pain relief without prolonging recovery from anaesthesia in both adults and children. A serious medicolegal issue has arisen in relation to the rectal administration of drugs and it is mandatory to seek consent if this route of administration is to be used. Combinations of analgesic drugs and local anaesthesia may be given whenever feasible. Opioids are widely used as part of the anaesthetic technique for extraction of third molars. Delayed recovery is not a problem, but there is some increase in postoperative nausea and vomiting. Dexamethasone has been shown to reduce the postoperative inflammatory response following third molar extraction, and hence the swelling and pain and probably should be more widely used. In addition, local anaesthesia with bupivacaine has been found to provide effective analgesia for such surgery.

COMPLICATIONS OF DENTAL ANAESTHESIA

The main complications associated with dental anaesthesia are usually respiratory or cardiovascular in nature.

Respiratory complications

Airway obstruction

The most common problem in dental anaesthesia is airway obstruction. This may be due to inadequate support of the jaw allowing the tongue to fall back. In most cases manipulation of the mandible will correct matters. Despite careful assessment, an inability to maintain a clear nasal airway may only occur when the patient is fully anaesthetized and the mouth is closed. Large adenoids and tonsils may be responsible. Insertion of a well lubricated, nasopharyngeal airway may solve the problem, but it is wise not to persist if this does not pass easily through the nose. The laryngeal mask may be used otherwise. A combination of airway obstruction and light anaesthesia is often followed by laryngospasm. As its name implies spasm of the laryngeal adductors occurs with further obstruction to air flow, and inspiratory stridor results. If this situation arises, manipulation of the mandible to keep the mouth open and airway clear is helpful. It is also worthwhile to deepen anaesthesia carefully with halothane in 100% oxygen and gentle positive pressure. As the situation improves the stridor disappears. It is important to differentiate this from complete laryngeal spasm, where the patient is silent in the presence of violent respiratory efforts. Persistent worsening of the airway obstruction, as shown by decreasing oxygen saturation and bradycardia, necessitates the use of atropine followed by suxamethonium and intubation. This is rarely required if the problem is recognized and remedied at an early stage.

Respiratory depression and apnoea

Apnoea may be due to breath holding under light anaesthesia, but a more common cause is failure to reduce the concentration of volatile agent once anaesthesia has been induced. Apnoea is an almost invariable side-effect of intravenous induction. As with respiratory depression, ventilation should be assisted until respiration resumes.

Contamination of the airway

Aspiration of blood and debris is an ever-present risk with dental anaesthesia. High powered suction must be available at all times. It is essential to realize that the oropharyngeal pack is only a relative, and not an absolute, barrier. Clearly the more teeth to be extracted, the more bleeding is likely and the greater risk of overwhelming the pack. It has been suggested that the semi-recumbent and sitting position allows the pack to act more like a barrier, which it is, rather than expecting it to behave as a seal, which it cannot be. Nevertheless, airway contamination has occurred in all positions and it may be that the amount of surgery, and therefore bleeding, is a determining factor. Patients undergoing multiple extractions require careful assessment. If the surgery can be accomplished rapidly, the laryngeal mask combined with a dental pack may provide adequate protection. The pack may need to be changed if it becomes soaked and inefficient. Suturing of multiple extraction sites should be considered. Where there is any major risk of airway contamination the combination of intubation and packing should be used.

Cardiovascular complications

Hypotension

A number of factors may result in hypotension in the dental patient. Dental patients are often nervous and and prone to faint. Fainting can only occur in the conscious patient and is much more common if the patient is in the upright position. Pallor, low pulse volume and bradycardia are the usual manifestations, and adoption of the supine position and atropine, if indicated will usually resolve the problem. It is certainly possible for a faint to coincide with induction and occasionally it has been indistinguishable from the onset of anaesthesia. In the nervous patient the time of greatest risk is probably following venepuncture. Thus, it is wise to leave a short interval between insertion of the cannula and induction of anaesthesia. The incidence of fainting is very low if the supine or semi-recumbent position is used. An important cause of hypotension in association with induction is anaphylaxis and this may be the first indication of the event. Most intravenous anaesthetic agents depress arterial pressure by 10% or more and this is usually counteracted by the stimulus of surgery. Studies during methohexitone anaesthesia found that the arterial pressure achieved preoperative or higher values during dental surgery, whether the patient was supine or erect. All the presently available volatile anaesthetics may cause a decrease in arterial pressure, but it usually attains preoperative or higher values once surgery commences. A rare cause of hypoension is vagal stimulation occurring in response to surgery, instead of the more usual sympathetic reaction. Ideally, all patients undergoing dental anaesthesia should have their arterial pressure monitored, however brief the procedure, and especially if a posture other than supine is used.

Arrhythmias

There is a 30–70% incidence of cardiac arrhythmias during dental anaesthesia with halothane. This has been ascribed to the effects of catecholamines, released in response to stimulation of the trigeminal nerve during surgery, on a myocardium rendered sensitive by halothane. The arrhythmias vary from nodal rhythm to multifocal ventricular ectopics with runs of ventricular tachycardia. Their clinical significance has yet to be ascertained. The vast majority of patients appear to come to no harm, but the possibility remains that the arrhythmias may be responsible for some of the deaths associated with sudden cardiovascular collapse. The incidence of arrhythmias is much reduced following intravenous induction and during enflurane, isoflurane, sevoflurane and desflurane anaesthesia. In addition, total intravenous anaesthesia, and the use of neuromuscular blocking drugs and controlled ventilation are associated with very few arrhythmias. The incidence of arrhythmias may also be decreased by preoperative buccal infiltration, or nerve block, with non-adrenaline-containing local anaesthetic. Many anaesthetists induce with halothane and maintain the anaesthetic with enflurane or isoflurane. If frequent, or multifocal, ventricular ectopics occur during halothane anaesthesia, surgery should cease, retention of carbon dioxide should be obviated by attention to the airway and ventilation, and a change to enflurane or isoflurane made if further surgery is needed. In the face of continuing arrhythmias local anaesthetic blockade to the remaining teeth should be considered. Intravenous β-blocking drugs and lignocaine have been found to be effective in abolishing intractable ventricular arrhythmias. The patient should not be moved until sinus rhythm has been re-established.

POLLUTION

Government reports in the late 1970s reflected widespread concern about the contamination of the operating theatre environment with anaesthetic gases and vapours. Pollution during dental anaesthesia is a significant problem. The level of contamination of the atmosphere with halothane during general anaesthesia for outpatients undergoing dental extractions was found to be far in excess of that recorded in surgical operating theatres. Cole and colleagues found that scavenging reduced levels of nitrous oxide by 80–90%, but concentrations were still approximately 12 times recommended levels in surgeries with no air conditioning. Pollution in dental anaesthesia derives from three main sources: mask leakage, mouth breathing and the expiratory valve. Scavenging from an expiratory valve positioned on the nasal mask increases the bulk of the apparatus. A modified parallel Lack breathing system has been described in which the expiratory valve is remote from the mask and is suitable for scavenging. The position of the expiratory valve in the Bain circuit also allows for easy scavenging and the Bain circuit is widely used for this reason. Intubation is associated with less pollution than the nasal mask, and recent work suggests this is also true when the laryngeal mask is used in dentistry. It must be acknowledged that when gaseous induction is carried out by traditional methods, the prevention of pollution is virtually impossible. To reduce the concentration of anaesthetic gases in the dental surgery Cole has recommended some form of room ventilation to provide at least 10 air changes per hour, routine scavenging of the exhaust valve, effective suction systems which should be exhausted outside the building and frequent equipment checks for leaks.

DENTAL SEDATION

Sedation has been defined as a technique in which the use of a drug or drugs produces a state of depression of the central nervous system enabling treatment to be carried out, but during which verbal contact with the patient is maintained throughout the period of sedation. The drugs and techniques used should carry a margin of safety wide enough to render unintended loss of consciousness unlikely. Any technique which exceeds this definition, and where contact with the patient is lost, may be regarded as general anaesthesia with all its attendant consequences and responsibilities. Anaesthetists are not often directly involved with sedation in dental practice, except in a teaching or an advisory capacity. The two main forms of sedation used in outpatient dentistry are classified according to their routes of administration. Sedation with nitrous oxide is known as relative analgesia, although the term inhalational sedation is preferable since local anaesthesia is required for all but the most minor procedures. In this technique a specially designed machine limits the maximum concentration of nitrous oxide to 70% and a hypoxic guard cuts the flow off, if the oxygen supply fails. Patients should be made comfortable breathing 100% oxygen for a few minutes and nitrous oxide should be introduced in 5% increments every 2–3 min. Patients should be warned of the likely paraesthesia of the face and extremities. Concentrations of 25–35% nitrous oxide are adequate for many patients and 50–70% carries the risk of the excitement stage or light anaesthesia. If the patient cannot maintain an open mouth or verbal contact is lost, the concentration must reduced. The rapid elimination of nitrous oxide results in a flexible and safe technique, and it is the only method of sedation recommended in children.

Intravenous sedative techniques owe their origin to the work of Niels Jorgensen who, in 1946, introduced the use of dilute mixtures of pentobarbitone, pethidine and hyoscine to produce sedation. The long induction and exceedingly long recovery lead to a search for more appropriate drugs, and in 1965 Drummond-Jackson claimed that using small increments of methohexitone it was possible to achieve a state of 'ultralight anaesthesia' without associated loss of airway control. However, subsequent investigators found it was extremely difficult to achieve this state without on occasions producing surgical anaesthesia. The introduction of diazepam in 1968 was rapidly followed by its application for sedation in dentistry. Wide interindividual variation in response was noted and Verrill attempted to titrate the level of sedation by using the drooping of the eyelid as a suitable end-point. Despite dose-related respiratory depression, brief impairment of laryngeal reflexes and prolonged recovery due to an active metabolite, diazepam had a sufficiently wide sedation to anaesthesia ratio to make it the most popular intravenous sedative until the advent of midazolam in early 1980. Midazolam was found to produce greater anterograde amnesia and a more rapid recovery than diazepam. It should be noted that midazolam is more than twice as potent as diazepam and that it takes effect more slowly. The initial recommended dose is 0.07 mg kg^{-1}, but patients' sensitivities vary and it is best to use a 1 mg per ml dilution and titrate the dose to an adequate level of sedation as indicated by drowsiness, slurred speech, delayed verbal response and past-pointing. It has been suggested that ptosis is indicative of a relative overdose. It is rarely necessary to use more than 10 mg. Adequate local anaesthesia will be required for conservative treatment or extraction. A number of studies have investigated combinations of midazolam with analgesics such as pentazocine and nalbuphine. The drugs potentiate each other and severe respiratory depression has been reported.

A more promising technique may be the use of patient-controlled sedation. Patient-controlled intravenous therapy, initially introduced for analgesia, was first adapted for controlled anxiolysis using diazepam, and more recently for perioperative sedation using either midazolam or propofol. Zacharias *et al.* used patient-controlled sedation during third molar extractions and found the technique satisfactory. The difficulty with all sedation is that it fails occasionally. If an anaesthetist is present, and the surgery is equipped for general anaesthesia, there is no difficulty in inducing deep sedation or general anaesthesia. If not the temptation to increase the dose, or embark on polypharmacy, should be resisted and an appointment made for a day that allows the option of general anaesthesia. The performance of dentistry under sedation requires a degree of skill which only comes with practice. It must be stressed that patients should be assessed and prepared for sedation in the same way as they would be for general anaesthesia, and the criteria for fitness are similar to those used in outpatient dental anaesthesia.

INPATIENT GENERAL ANAESTHESIA

Most dental surgery can be accomplished on an outpatient basis. The indications for inpatient treatment are usually the medical condition of the patient, or the duration of the surgery and/or the amount of postoperative pain. Sometimes infection with trismus and swelling of oral tissues produces an inability to fully open the mouth. Any suggestion of limited mouth opening requires full preparation for the difficult airway. Most patients can be managed with a dose of intravenous induction agent sufficient to allow an attempt to ventilate the lungs by mask. If this is possible, anaesthesia can be deepened to allow a rapid extraction, or the trachea may be intubated following administration of a neuromuscular blocking drug. An alternative is to use an inhalational induction. If the airway is clearly difficult to manage, awake intubation using the fibreoptic endoscope is indicated. For any other than the most rapid procedures intubation will be required, and this is usually via the nose to avoid encroaching on the surgeon's field. A pack is mandatory because of known ability of blood to track past the cuff of the tracheal tube. Bleeding from the nose may be provoked by the passage of the tube and has occasionally overwhelmed the pack and caused asphyxia. In children under six years old, an oral tube is recommended because of the presence of relatively enlarged adenoid tissue. Care must be taken to protect the eyes and to ensure that the headtowel does not cause disconnection or obstruction to respiration. Preformed, nasal, tracheal tubes may be an advantage, although they may require to be softened in warm water to lessen the risk of trauma to the mucosa.

Most patients are allowed to breath spontaneously, although the use of IPPV allows a lighter plane of anaesthesia, and decreases the incidence of arrhythmias. Local anaesthesia with bupivacaine provides good pain relief in patients undergoing extraction of third molars and dexamethasone lessens postoperative swelling and decreases the demand for analgesia. In general, ASA III and IV patients who require dental surgery should be admitted to hospital. Patients about to undergo cardiac surgery need to be made dentally fit preoperatively; this may require surgery under general anaesthesia. Attention must paid to the patient's cardiorespiratory state and drug regimen. Advice should be sought from the medical team with responsibility for the patient about the precise nature of the cardiac lesion, and for recommendations about their anticoagulant therapy and prophylactic antibiotics. The mortality rate for inpatients undergoing dental anaesthesia is significantly higher than that of outpatients, which is presumably related to the greater incidence of airway difficulties and serious medical disease in this group.

EQUIPMENT IN THE DENTAL SURGERY

Dental anaesthesia has been traditionally carried out in a chair in the upright position. However, after the 1950s unexplained deaths during dental anaesthesia were suggested to result from unrecognized hypotension in the sitting position, and were believed to be avoidable by adopting the supine position. In recent years many centres have adopted the semi- or fully recumbent position.

In general, dental chairs fall into two categories: the conventional chairs which are designed primarily for the upright or reclining posture; and the contoured chairs which are designed primarily for low seated dentistry. The conventional chair is designed to give the maximum range of mobility and is, therefore, particularly suitable for most general anaesthetic purposes. The disadvantage of this type of chair is that when used in the horizontal position the support afforded to the patient is not optimal for prolonged procedures. In the horizontal position it offers poor arm and back support.

There are a wide variety of contoured chairs available which are particularly suited for low seated dentistry. These chairs, however, present the anaesthetist with certain difficulties in the unintubated patient, since the solid one piece head-rest is non-adjustable, hinders manual support of the mandible, and renders the use of the twin tube nasal mask more difficult.

Almost all modern chairs are electrically operated. It is important that the mechanism which lowers the patient from upright to horizontal is rapid in action and has an overriding manual control. It should be borne in mind that the well-upholstered dental chair may provide too elastic a surface for cardiac compression to be effective.

For many years nitrous oxide was the mainstay of dental anaesthesia, while reliance was placed on more potent agents to produce anaesthesia for general surgery. For nitrous oxide to be effective in the more difficult patient an element of hypoxia was used. This led to the development of specific apparatus which claimed to allow breath by breath control of concentrations of oxygen and nitrous oxide, the so called 'on demand' anaesthetic machines. The most popular were the Walton and the McKesson machines. The popularity of intermittent flow machines resulted from their presumed economy, control of oxygen concentration at low values and the supply of gases at a positive pressure sufficient to overcome partial nasal obstruction. The essential requirement of an intermittent flow machine is that the mixture concentration should be controlled accurately despite large changes in flow rate produced by the patient. By 1960s the use of oxygen restriction fell out of favour and adequate anaesthesia required the use of inhalational or intravenous adjuvants such as halothane and methohexitone. In addition, considerable doubt was expressed as to the accuracy of the intermittent flow machines, and modern dental anaesthetic machines are not dissimilar to those used in other branches of surgery. The anaesthetic equipment and facilities which should be available in a dental outpatient surgery include a basic, continuous flow, anaesthetic machine with an oxygen fail-safe device and inability to provide less than 30% oxygen, an oxygen analyser, temperature compensated vaporizers, a suitable range of masks, valves, laryngoscopes, tracheal tubes, scavenging and suction apparatus.

The practice of dental surgery also necessitated the development of instruments to keep the mouth open. There exist a multitude of mouth props and the two commonly used designs are the Devonshire and the McKesson. The McKesson mouth prop is particularly useful in partially edentulous patients. Props should have a tether in case of dislodgement, often a short length of fine chain. Gags are nowadays only occasionally used, because of the risk of damaging the teeth and lips with them.

A variety of nasal masks are in use which include the following:

- The McKesson mask which has a spring-loaded expiratory valve with twin narrow-bore supply tubes for use with 'on demand' machines. The narrow bore and length of the twin tubing renders the resistance to inspiration undesirably high when the flow rate exceeds the minute volume of the patient.
- The Goldman nasal mask, although described as wide-bore has an inlet diameter of only about 1.4 cm. It incorporates an integral Heidbrink valve and was designed for use with the continuous flow machine.
- Clear plastic nasal masks are now available suitable for use in dental sedation or anaesthesia.

RESUSCITATION EQUIPMENT

Cardiac arrest can occur in the dental surgery, hence, it should be fully equipped to cope with such an emergency. Minimal equipment includes a means of inflating the lungs with 100% oxygen, pharyngeal airways, a full set of tracheal tubes, laryngoscopes and a cricothyrotomy set. An electrocardiograph, a defibrillator and a full set of resuscitation drugs with equipment for intravenous infusion should be available. Protocols for advanced life support and other emergencies such as anaphylaxis and malignant hyperthermia must be available and kept up to date. All persons working in the anaesthetic area must be familiar with the commonly used anaesthetic and resuscitation equipment and with the emergency drug tray, the contents of which should be checked daily. There should be a clear understanding of how to summon emergency assistance. The General Dental Council and the Poswillo report recommend that a simulated resuscitation is practised on a regular basis in every dental surgery. Clearly, this should also apply whenever general anaesthesia is administered without rapid availability of the cardiac arrest team.

THE FUTURE

It has at last been accepted that a dental anaesthetic is little different from that administered for other surgical procedures and the same standards of expertise and care must apply. Dental anaesthesia has evolved a long way from its initial, lowly status, and developments in airway management and anaesthetic agents offer further advances. With improvements in dental health and more patient care under local anaesthesia and sedation, it is likely that the number of patients requiring general anaesthesia will diminish and it will be feasible for these to be managed by accredited anaesthetists as proposed by the Poswillo report.

FURTHER READING

Brimacombe, J. and Berry, A. (1995) The laryngeal mask airway for dental surgery – a review. *Australian Dental Journal*, **40**, 10–14.

Cole, P. V. (1981) The problem of pollution in the dental surgery. *South African Association of Dentistry Digest*, **4**, 210–216.

Department of Health (1991) *Report of an Expert Working Party on General Anaesthesia, Sedation and Resuscitation in Dentistry*. Department of Health, Dental Division, London.

Dresner, M. and Soni, N. (1989) Preoperative assessment. *Current Opinion in Anaesthesiology*, **2**, 701–708.

Green, R. A. and Coplans, M. P. (1973) *Anaesthesia and Analgesia in Dentistry*. H. K. Lewis, London.

Haynes, S. R. and Lawler, P. G. P. (1995) An assessment of the consistency of ASA physical status classification allocation. *Anaesthesia*, **50**, 195–199.

Love, S. H. S. (1968) The complications of dental anaesthesia. *British Journal of Anaesthesia*, **40**, 188–196.

Phillips, S., Daborn, A. K. and Hatch, D. J. (1994) Preoperative fasting for paediatric anaesthesia. *British Journal of Anaesthesia*, **73**, 529–536.

Van der Walt, J. (1995) Anaesthesia in children with viral respiratory tract infections. Clinical Review. *Paediatric Anaesthesia*, **5**, 257–262.

Zacharias, M., Hunter, K. M. and Luyk, N. H. (1994) Patient-controlled sedation using midazolam. *British Journal of Oral & Maxillofacial Surgery*, **32**, 168–173.

PLASTIC SURGERY 22

C. E. Blogg

The mysteries associated with anaesthesia for plastic surgery come mainly from lack of familiarity, rather than the problems posed by the specialty itself. The general principles of anaesthesia apply to all fields of surgery, but with different emphasis. Patients who present for plastic surgery may be of all ages from newborn to elderly. The majority of the surgery is superficial, involving only skin or mucosa, but surgery includes bone, muscle and deeper layers when complex ablation and reconstructive surgery is performed. As the skin extends from head to toe, so plastic surgery may involve any part of the surface of the body. Overlap of interests occurs, for instance breasts may be reconstructed at the same time as performing a mastectomy. For plastic surgeons and other specialists to work together generally benefits the patient and all concerned.

The lesion and surgery are usually limited to skin and superficial structures. Major body cavities are rarely entered, so the results of surgery are highly visible. Plastic surgeons dissect lightly and accurately, and the anaesthetists can expect the tissues to be handled more gently than is usual with other specialties. Anatomical symmetry becomes important, blood loss should be minimized and in many cases pain can be avoided by use of local anaesthetic for infiltration, or regional block techniques. Plastic surgeons tend to use instruments delicately and treat tissues with respect.

GENERAL PRINCIPLES

MULTIPLE PROCEDURES

Several stages (e.g. delayed flaps, expansion techniques, reconstructions) may be necessary for completion of plastic surgery and so repetition gives the opportunity of enhancing an anaesthetic technique and building rapport with the patient; there are also the slight risks of repeated anaesthesia. With cosmetic surgery, the patient's dissatisfaction with body image may persist, resulting in a need for yet more surgery. In other cases, e.g. pressure sores, the causative factors continue.

MULTIPLE SITES

Plastic surgery often involves operating on several sites. For example, skin grafts are commonly taken from a limb and applied to the trunk or another limb. Free flaps have to be removed from one site and moved to another. The use of regional or local anaesthesia for multiple sites may be restricted to avoid the total dose reaching toxic levels.

TISSUE PERFUSION VERSUS BLOOD LOSS

There is potential conflict, for the anaesthetist, in trying to reduce blood loss to facilitate accuracy and speed of dissection and yet optimize perfusion. Striving for a 'totally

Short Practice of Anaesthesia. Edited by M. Morgan and G. M. Hall. Published in 1997 by Chapman & Hall, London. ISBN 0 412 71890 1

bloodless field' may be mistaken if viability of flaps is threatened.

BLOOD LOSS

Blood loss may be increased by:

- increased cardiac output (hypertension, tachycardia, pain and increased endogenous catecholamines);
- increased capillary blood flow (hypercapnia, pyrexia);
- increased venous pressure (gravity, partial venous occlusion, raised intrathoracic pressure, over transfusion);
- reduced clotting (anticoagulants, NSAIDs, steroid therapy and rarities such as a disseminated intravascular coagulopathy, incompatible blood transfusion);
- rebound hypertension after induced hypotension; and
- capillary fragility, (von Willebrand's disease, chronic steroid therapy, advanced age, etc.).

Conversely, blood loss can be reduced or minimized by:

- decreasing cardiac output (β-blockers, cardiodepressant induction agents, hypovolaemia, intermittent positive pressure ventilation);
- prevention of arterial flow (tourniquet, arterial ligation, bypass/shunt procedures);
- local vasoconstriction (adrenaline infiltration, cooling);
- reduced peripheral vascular resistance (nitroprusside, glyceryl trinitrate, hydralazine, adenosine, trimetaphan, ganglion blocking drugs, calcium channel blocker, regional block);
- enhanced venous outflow (gravity, reduced mean intrathoracic pressure, regional block);
- haemodilution (acute normovolaemic autologous blood donation then transfusion); and
- blood salvage (re-use of collected surgical blood loss).

PERFUSION

Perfusion, or flow of blood, depends on the pressure differential ($P_a - P_b$) and is related to radius (r) and length (L) of the vessel and viscosity (η) of the blood. If blood is assumed to behave as a Newtonian fluid (possessing constant viscosity) and the vessel is rigid, flow is expressed by the Poiseuille–Hagan formula:

$$\text{Flow} = \frac{(P_a - P_b)\pi r^4}{8\eta L}$$

Thus, small changes in radius will result in a large change in flow as it depends on the fourth power of the radius. If the pressure gradient is increased by maintaining the arterial pressure whilst the peripheral resistance is reduced, perfusion will be optimized. Viscosity of blood is closely related to haematocrit in larger vessels, but blood does not behave as a typical Newtonian fluid in small vessels (less than 1.5 mm diameter). Viscosity increases dramatically if the haematocrit is greater than 40% and declines with dilution. Oxygen transport decreases as haematocrit falls such that the ideal haematocrit for optimum perfusion, without impairing oxygen transport, is about 30–40%; cerebral oxygen delivery is also optimized at that range.

Perfusion can be impaired by venous outflow obstruction. Tissues become engorged, hypoxic then ischaemic and oedematous. If the venous outflow cannot easily be restored, application of leeches to draw off the retained venous blood can buy time whilst new venous channels develop.

Perfusion is not a simple product of shear stress applied to extensible tubes containing blood of varying viscosities since precapillary sphincters can be open or closed, diverting blood from, or shunting it into, the capillaries.

Demonstration of good effluent flow from a tissue flap can mislead and does not ensure that perfusion is equally distributed in the tissue. Optimum perfusion results from maintaining a high cardiac output, vasodilatation and a large pulse pressure and is indicated by a narrow differential ($< 2°C$) between core and skin temperature, urine output > 30 ml h^{-1} and clinical observation, e.g. rapid return of pink colour on blanching tissues. Mechanical methods of assessing perfusion are presently mainly at the experimental stage.

RED CELLS

If there is no flow, red cells form parallel clumps and platelets deposit at anastomotic sites. As flow progressively increases, rouleaux are formed, red cells become evenly distributed and then aligned axially. At high flows, the cells deform and preferentially flow in a narrower central stream. Rouleaux formations can variously be broken up by low-molecular-weight dextran, dilution and, probably, by increasing flow.

BLOOD LOSS

Skin is highly vascular. Blood loss from relatively small areas can be massive, e.g. in scalp surgery. Intraoperative bleeding may so hinder dissection that surgical progress may be impossible, e.g. craniofacial reconstruction. Postoperative bleeding under grafts may separate the graft from its bed and threaten its viability. In some circumstances, e.g. during palatal surgery, excessive bleeding may endanger the airway.

REDUCTION IN BLOOD LOSS

Active reduction in intraoperative bleeding begins preoperatively. Relief of anxiety is important. Pre-existing hypertension requires treatment. For major procedures, screening for clotting abnormalities is wise especially if there is a personal or family history of excessive bruising or bleeding. Patients should be warned to discontinue platelet function-inhibiting NSAIDs at least 10 days preoperatively. Debate continues about the potential value of preoperative or intraoperative NSAIDs in improving flap survival. None the less preoperative subcutaneous heparin is recommended for the prevention of deep vein thrombosis if postoperative immobility is likely.

Avoidance of cardiostimulatory agents (ketamine, pancuronium) and use of induction agents (propofol, etomidate), relaxants with minimal cardiovascular effects (atracurium, vecuronium) and adequate doses of opioids (fentanyl, alfentanil) should reduce adverse cardiovascular changes at induction of anaesthesia.

Reduction of the tachycardia and hypertensive response to tracheal intubation can be achieved by premedication (β-adrenoceptor blockers, (metoprolol, timolol) or calcium channel blocking agents, (nifedipine), α_2-agonists (clonidine), lignocaine, butyrophenones, (droperidol), etc.). Alternatively lignocaine, esmolol or large doses of opioids given intravenously immediately before intubation will obtund the response.

Induction of anaesthesia should be smooth, without hiccuping, coughing or straining by the patient otherwise venous hypertension and increased venous bleeding result. Venous bleeding can be reduced by ensuring that the operative site is uppermost. Adequate postoperative analgesia reduces restlessness and the changes in position which can result in arterial or venous obstruction and threaten viability of flaps.

Plastic surgery anaesthesia lends itself to the use of the laryngeal mask airway. Its insertion is probably associated with reduced hypertensive responses, less coughing on emergence from anaesthesia and might result in less postoperative bleeding compared to conventional use of tracheal intubation.

AUTOLOGOUS TRANSFUSION

Preoperative removal and storage of the patient's blood ensures that blood lost at surgery has a lower haematocrit. If 1 l of blood is lost with a low haematocrit (25%), 200 ml of red cells less is lost compared to the loss of the same volume of blood with a haematocrit of 45%. Total red cell loss is reduced since autologous replacement can restore blood volume when bleeding has stopped.

Excessive reduction in red cell mass may result in their redistribution and ischaemia in, for instance, the cardiac subendocardium and presumably, in transposed plastic surgical flaps. Oxygen transport remains adequate, despite reduction in circulating haemoglobin, if oxygen is added to inspired gases, normovolaemia is maintained and the haematocrit remains above 30%. This can be achieved by preoperative donation, acute normovolaemic haemodilution, or blood salvage. Crossmatching incompatibilities and transmission of donor infections are avoided. Reliance on the blood donor population is almost eliminated. Further benefits include virtual elimination of the allo-immunization to cellular and plasma protein antigens. Allergic, febrile or haemolytic reactions are reduced. Recurrence-free survival rates in cancer patients may be improved.

Preoperative blood donation

Preoperative donation of one unit of blood (450 ml) should be limited to patients who weigh more than 50 kg and be reduced proportionately for those with smaller body mass. Predonation haemoglobin values greater than 11 g dl^{-1} are necessary to avoid excessive anaemia. Larger volumes of fresh blood can be retrieved if replaced by the patient's previously-stored blood being transfused at the time of donation. Donations can be made at 3-day intervals and the last should be not less than 72 h before surgery. Anaemia can be reduced by oral iron supplements. However, despite the apparent attractions of autologous blood transfusion, the evidence for cost-effectiveness is sketchy.

Acute normovolaemic haemodilution

At the time of surgery, blood can be stored, taken in continuity from an arterial or central venous cannula and replaced simultaneously by an equal volume of colloid. The blood is then kept warm in the operating theatre and transfused when necessary. In some Jehovah's Witnesses this technique may avoid problems encountered when blood transfusion is refused.

Blood salvage

Collection of the patient's own blood spilled at surgery and transfusion has become practicable with cell-saving devices. Red cell survival varies with the technique used, but ranges from 40 to 60% survival for at least 24 days. However, plastic surgical procedures rarely warrant the costs involved.

CONTROLLED HYPOTENSION

Positive benefits for the patient, adequate training of the anaesthetist and a skilled, practiced surgeon are all prerequisites for controlled induced hypotension. History of stroke, transient ischaemic attacks, anaemia, postural hypotension, myocardial ischaemia and conduction defects all contraindicate profound hypotension (systolic pressure ≤ 60 mmHg). Preoperative investigations should include chest X-ray, record of ECG, measurement of creatinine, or urea and electrolytes to ensure that cardiac and renal function are normal.

Preparation includes premedication over the 24 h preoperation with calcium channel blocking agents (e.g. nifedipine 10 mg t.d.s.) or β-adrenoceptor blockers (e.g. propranolol 10–40 mg t.d.s.). Thymoxamine has also been recommended. Four-hourly ward blood pressure and heart rate measurements will indicate whether premedication is effective by reduction of blood pressure and heart rate. Use of β-adrenoceptor blocking agents reduces the increase in heart rate response commonly seen in young patients when induced hypotension is attempted. The symptoms and effects of anxiety may also be reduced. Droperidol premedication (5 mg i.m.) usefully combines amnesogenic, sedative and α-adrenoceptor blocking actions. Oral clonidine, an α2-receptor agonist, is likely to result in easier achievement of hypotension and reduces the doses necessary of hypnotic, hypotensive and sedative agents, but its effects may be antagonized by α-adrenoceptor blockers.

Intraoperative induced hypotension is most easily achieved by giving 2–5% isoflurane which, uniquely of the volatile agents causes vasodilatation in muscle as well as skin. Short-acting agents such as sodium nitroprusside, glyceryl trinitrate or trimetaphan can be titrated by intravenous infusion against arterial pressure directly measured by intra-arterial cannulation, but have the disadvantages of tachyphylaxis, potential toxicity, rebound hypertension and the difficulty in supervision of a potent infused vasodilator. If the right atrial filling pressure (CVP) is maintained whilst the peripheral vascular resistance is reduced, invasive arterial monitoring in the healthy young patient is rarely necessary. Profound hypotension (< 60 mmHg systolic) is rarely justified if attention is paid to other details of management. Systolic pressures reduced to 100 mmHg measured at the height of the brain appear to be safe and adequate to reduce blood loss.

Induction of anaesthesia should be smooth without coughing, straining or stimulation of the cardiovascular system. Propofol usefully results in decreased cardiac output and reduction in laryngeal reflexes. Use of tubocurarine to produce hypotension by histamine release is unreliable, whereas atracurium or vecuronium, given by bolus or infusion, have minimal adverse effects. Liberal use of opioids reduces or eliminates the cardiovascular consequences of otherwise painful surgical stimulation.

Regional blockade (lumbar or caudal epidural, or spinal block), results in a decrease in systemic arterial pressure, improved regional blood flow and enhanced venous drainage, in addition to producing good analgesia. However, regional blockade of widely separated anatomical sites is not feasible. Flaps separated from their parent blood supply are necessarily already sympathectomized.

Hydralazine, in small increments (2–4 mg) can be used as the sole agent to induce hypotension or, in smaller doses, with β-adrenoceptor blockers to reduce the tachycardia which may prevent adequate reduction in bleeding. Newer agents (e.g. adenosine) or clonidine have potential. The mainstays of induced hypotension remain the use of posture and avoidance of adverse factors whilst careful monitoring is continued.

OPERATIVE PROCEDURES

CONGENITAL ABNORMALITIES

Congenital lesions require correction if they are unsightly, interfere with the development of normal function, or (in rare instances, e.g. some giant hairy naevuses) if it is advisable to remove the lesion as early in the child's life as possible to prevent subsequent malignant change. Because healing with minimal scarring is enhanced in the baby and young infant, surgery is increasingly carried out on progressively younger children. The timing of surgery may be critical to achieve function, e.g. hand syndactyly should be corrected before hand grasp is required. Walking begins at about one year of age and syndactyly of the feet should therefore be corrected by then. It is important that associated cardiac abnormalities which could influence the conduct of anaesthesia are not missed at the preoperative visit.

Cleft palate and lip

Surgeons in most centres in the UK prefer to repair cleft lips at 3 months of age and cleft palates at around 6 months of age. In some units, cleft lips are repaired just after birth to help the bonding process between child and mother, achieve a cosmetic result before the child leaves hospital, and because healing is enhanced and scarring minimized. Early surgical management of cleft lip carries the possibility that other congenital abnormalities may not be apparent.

The ease with which a facemask can achieve an adequate airtight fit must be assessed. Children with some upper airway syndromes (e.g. Treacher–Collins and Pierre-Robin syndromes) may present extreme difficulty in intubation due to a combination of micrognathia and cleft palate. Intubation may be so difficult that techniques such as passing a Seldinger wire through the trachea and through the larynx into the mouth and then railroading a tube into the trachea may be necessary.

Cor pulmonale secondary to airway obstruction caused by glossoptosis may occur and can be relieved preoperatively by fixation of the tongue with a stitch to the mandible.

Premedication for cleft lip repair consists only of intramuscular atropine 0.02 mg kg^{-1}. Coughing on secretions is reduced and placement of the tongue gag during the operation is made easier. Opioid-induced respiratory depression should be avoided in small children with congenital abnormalities of the upper respiratory tract, since gaseous induction of anaesthesia is usual and obtunding ventilation in the presence of airway abnormality increases the risk of obstruction. Promethazine 2 mg kg^{-1} orally can be added for the 6-month-old infant or older, to produce sedation, reduction in secretions and perhaps some amnesia. Thiopentone 20 mg kg^{-1} rectally is used by some. Midazolam solution has recently been introduced for oral use (0.5 mg kg^{-1}) or 0.3 mg kg^{-1} nasally and usually results in a contented and playful child. Intranasal ketamine 6 mg kg^{-1} has also been successfully used in children.

Electrocardiographic and pulse oximetry monitoring are required before induction of anaesthesia. Gaseous induction with nitrous oxide, oxygen, then halothane is usual and preferable to intravenous induction and likely loss of control of the airway. An intravenous cannula is then placed and (having demonstrated that ventilation with a face mask and bag system is adequate), a neuromuscular blocking drug (suxamethonium 1.5 mg kg^{-1} or vecuronium 0.01 mg kg^{-1} or atracurium 0.5 mg kg^{-1}) is given. Fentanyl (1–2 µg kg^{-1} before laryngoscopy) reduces the hypertensive and tachycardiac response. An armoured flexometallic latex tube is useful as it can be bent under the gag without kinking. RAE tubes are also favoured. It is important to monitor breath sounds on the left side of the chest with a precordial stethoscope throughout the procedure so that if accidental intubation of the right main bronchus occurs it will be immediately detected and corrected. Manual ventilation allows the 'educated' hand of the anaesthetist to detect any changes in compliance or disconnections instantly.

C-section laryngoscope blades have been designed, e.g. Bryce-Smith Oxford blade, to 'bridge' the gap in the lip and palate and provide a clear view of the larynx when the child has a distorted upper airway. Heat loss is minimized intraoperatively by the use of a condenser-humidifier in the breathing system, covering the baby in warmed covers and the use of the heat reflecting outer layer as well as raising the ambient temperature in the operating theatre. Lignocaine and adrenaline is infiltrated to separate tissue layers, provide local anaesthesia and reduce bleeding. Topical cocaine or adrenaline also reduces blood loss during palatal surgery. Infra-orbital nerve block for cleft lip repair may spare the infant from the need for opioid analgesia and the potential for respiratory depression. Analgesia is achieved without disortion of the operative field. The depth of anaesthesia required is minimal and manual ventilation with nitrous oxide and 0.5–1.0% halothane is usually sufficient. Long-acting neuromuscular blocking drugs are rarely necessary if the surgeon is swift.

The general principles of paediatric anaesthesia apply, thus maintenance intravenous fluids are given. When blood losses reach 10–15% of the estimated blood volume, colloid and then, if necessary, blood should be given. Blood loss is, however, difficult to estimate since the throat pack absorbs much of the haemorrhage. The use of a trap in the suction tubing and encouragement of the surgeon to use the sucker in preference to swabs gives the anaesthetist some forewarning of undue blood loss.

Facilities for re-intubation should be at hand when the patient is awakened on the operating table until there is no problem of airway obstruction or stridor. Following cleft palate repair, babies may still position the tongue into the place of the gap in the palate and so obstruct their airway. A tongue stitch placed before the end of surgery enables the tongue to be pulled forward postoperatively to keep the airway clear. Paracetamol suppositories (60–120 mg) help to achieve analgesia in the early postoperative period. Feeding is usually possible within 2 h of the operation.

Further surgery may sometimes involve the use of an Abbé flap in which a section of lower lip is rotated and joined to the upper lip. Nasal airways help to maintain an adequate airway under difficult circumstances. Division of an Abbé flap is ideally carried out under local anaesthesia because of the difficulty of re-intubating a patient whose lips are joined together. When general anaesthesia **is** necessary, then a left-hand laryngoscope may give access if the flap obscures the view on the right side of the mouth.

Hypospadias

Hypospadias occurs in approximately 1 in 300 boy babies. Repair may be carried out by paediatric and urological surgeons as well as plastic surgeons and is commonly done in two stages. Correction begins at around one year of age with the second stage 6 months later.

The usual principles of paediatric anaesthesia apply. If postoperative analgesia is inadequate the child is likely to be restless, bleed into the operation site and require re-operation. Because of the potential for haematoma formation with penile block, caudal block is usually preferred and provides good analgesia into the postoperative period. Bupivacaine 0.25% 0.5 ml kg^{-1} without adrenaline is used. Pre-emptive lumbar epidural analgesia with bupivacaine and morphine is also effective and provides more stable cardiovascular variables, reduced anaesthetic requirements and better postoperative analgesia than intramuscular morphine or subpubic block alone. Postoperative caudal block is as effective after surgery as pre-emptive caudal analgesia.

Syndactyly

Fusion of components of hands or feet may be confined to one limb or even involve all four limbs. Other congenital abnormalities may be associated. The principal problem to be faced is of venous access. Also, if more than one limb is operated on, it becomes difficult to produce bilateral regional anaesthesia without the risk of achieving toxic levels of local anaesthetic.

Bat ears

Of the children who present for this surgery, 10% are acutely distressed and remain dissatisfied with the outcome. None the less, there is often strong pressure from the parents for the operation to be carried out. New surgical techniques, e.g. use of an endoscope, may encourage surgeons and patients to undergo the operation.

The laryngeal mask airway spares the children the morbidity of tracheal intubation. Local infiltration of lignocaine with adrenaline results in minimal postoperative pain. A peculiarity of this procedure carried out under general anaesthesia is also the high incidence (48%) of postoperative vomiting, which does not occur if the surgery is carried out under local anaesthesia alone by blocking the great auricular, auriculotemporal and small occipital nerves. Avoidance of packing of the external auditory meatus and concha significantly reduces postoperative nausea and vomiting. Transdermal hyoscine and low dose droperidol (20 μ kg^{-1} i.v.) are also effective.

SKIN GRAFTS

Skin grafting involves removal of skin from its blood supply and laying the skin onto a vascular bed. Skin grafts are commonly taken from the thigh, where the anterior aspect can be blocked by a femoral nerve block and laterally by block of the lateral femoral cutaneous nerve, or the medial aspect by an obturator nerve block. There is an increasing preference by surgeons to take skin grafts from inconspicuous areas such as the buttocks, which cannot be as readily blocked by a peripheral nerve block. Analgesia for split thickness skin grafts can be produced (without general anaesthesia) simply by placing EMLA cream on the donor site.

When malignant excision sites are to be grafted, it is usual for the graft to be taken from the opposite limb. Regional perivascular block in limbs where lymph nodes may be involved by malignancy or infection is discouraged.

SKIN FLAPS

When full thickness skin cover is required, rotation of skin flaps with an intact blood supply is used. Perfusion and viability of the flap is affected by smoking, endogenous catecholamines, reduced perfusion pressure, pain, cold and venous obstruction resulting from inappropriate positioning. It is debatable whether anticoagulation with heparin or warfarin improves survival.

SKIN EXPANSION

Saline-filled plastic bags can be inserted under normal skin adjacent to areas which require skin cover or are to be used to construct a free flap and then progressively inflated by transcutaneous injections of saline over a period of weeks to achieve maximal increase in skin cells. The expanded skin can then be rotated into the skin deficit. Insertion of the expander is usually straightforward. However, removal of the expander several months later when it has been increased considerably in size can pose problems especially if close to the airway or elsewhere in the head and neck. Preoperative emptying of the expander may be necessary.

COSMETIC SURGERY UNDER GENERAL ANAESTHESIA

Breast operations

Breast augmentation usually consists of placing a silicone or saline-containing bag below the skin of the breast under local anaesthesia (or more commonly in the UK with a general anaesthetic). Symmetry is essential and the anaesthetist's aesthetic powers of observation may be tested. A small incision is used and access to bleeding points and haemostasis can be difficult. Advances in technology have resulted in endoscopic breast augmentation and increasingly bizarre access points, e.g. transumbilical.

Breast reduction is commonly associated with large blood loss, especially if both breasts are operated on simultaneously by two surgeons, with but a common diathermy. Venous access may be impeded and the use of a foot or ankle vein may be necessary. Some surgeons prefer considerable head-up tilt to ensure that the ptosis of the breast is satisfactory and to reduce bleeding. To maintain blood pressure can be problematical in some circumstances, but a tourniquet and infiltration of lignocaine with 1 in 1 000 000 adrenaline will reduce blood loss.

Liposuction and tumescent anaesthesia

Liposuction consists of inserting under the skin metal tubes with a side hole and attached to a powerful suction system. Fat, which is near liquid at body temperature, is then sucked out. General anaesthesia is commonly used in the UK.

In the USA 'tumescent' anaesthesia is used for liposuction and other similar superficial procedures in the surgeon's 'office'. Very large volumes of dilute lignocaine with adrenaline are used. Among the claims made for this technique are that bleeding is reduced and peak blood levels of lignocaine are less than the toxic level. Absorption of lignocaine and adrenaline is less rapid and the anaesthesia and vasoconstriction (with the resulting reduction of blood loss) are longer lasting than with general anaesthesia or conventional concentrations of lignocaine or adrenaline. Prolific urine output may require indwelling bladder catherization or frequent trips to micturate.

Despite doses of lignocaine up to 34.4 mg kg^{-1} of pH adjusted drug (in combination with 1 in 1 000 000 adrenaline) being used, which are far in excess of the usually accepted toxic dose, few adverse effects have been noted. Use of diazepam premedication conveniently allows enterohepatic re-circulation of diazepam to raise the threshold for seizures at the time when peak blood levels of lignocaine are reached, 10 h or so after infiltration.

Rhinoplasty

The nose is obviously highly vascular, and the ease and success of rhinoplasty is influenced by the amount of bleeding. The anaesthetist can reduce the bleeding by the use of cocaine paste or solution sprayed to the nasal mucosa before or after induction of anaesthesia. Prior lavage with 8.4% sodium bicarbonate solution will remove nasal mucus and enhance the local analgesic effect of the cocaine. The surgeon usually infiltrates the surgical field with lignocaine and adrenaline to produce local vasoconstriction. The ECG should be closely monitored as arrhythmias may result. Modest head-up tilt further helps to reduce bleeding, none the less, significant blood loss complicates 3% of procedures. Since the nasal air passage is obstructed at the end of the procedure by nasal packs, it is prudent to place an oral Guedel airway before extubation, until the patient is fully awake. Regular gastroprokinetic agents (metoclopramide 10 mg i.m. or orally 8 hourly) appear to reduce the problem of swallowed blood causing emesis.

MICROVASCULAR SURGERY

The use of microsurgical techniques to join blood vessels, nerves, tendons and other small structures, complete with vascular pedicles, with and without nerve supply, has developed from salvage procedures following trauma. For reconstructive procedures the intentions are to restore function and achieve a good cosmetic result in one operation. Commonly-used free flap donor sites are groin, latissimus dorsi, transferred rectus abdominous muscle and, when bone grafts are needed, a composite rib graft.

Free flaps

During the raising of the free flap, reduction in bleeding can be achieved by modest induced hypotension. However, during the anastomotic phase of the procedure, a hyperdynamic circulation is required.

The survival of free flaps is enhanced by:

- maintenance of a hyperdynamic circulating blood volume,

- preventing vasosconstriction,
- reduction of venous obstruction,
- maintenance of body temperature and core/skin gradient < 2°C,
- adequate analgesia, reduction in 'stress response' to pain and immobility,
- haemodilution to reduce viscosity and improve perfusion,
- reduction in clotting and platelet aggregation,
- avoidance of cold, shivering, hypotension, haemoconcentration, hypovolaemia, pain, hypocapnia and vomiting, and
- prevention of adverse pressure effects.

Premedication and preparation should not be rushed. Nifedipine 20 mg b.d. in a long-acting preparation may contribute to reduction in vasoconstriction. Oral α_2-agonists may also find a place in vasodilatation, sedation and reduction in analgesia requirements.

For induction, large doses of opioids with droperidol, neuromuscular block, controlled ventilation and the use of isoflurane to promote vasodilatation combine to form the simplest technique. Fluid loading with a litre of crystalloid solution at induction contributes to achieving a hyperdynamic circulation. Thereafter the central venous pressure should be kept elevated by appropriate use of colloid and crystalloid solutions. Regional analgesia aids perfusion by sympathetic block of the area, arteriolar dilatation and enhancing venous outflow and providing analgesia and local immobility. Maintenance of anaesthesia using controlled ventilation and a circle system ensures that normocarbia, heat and humidity can be maintained.

Monitoring of central venous pressure, core/skin temperatures, urine output, fluid balance, oxygen saturation and expired carbon dioxide is required. Automated non-invasive blood pressure monitoring is sufficient in the majority of patients but, if access to the limbs is restricted, invasive intravascular monitoring of arterial pressure is needed. Neuropathy, oedema and compartment syndrome can, very rarely, follow prolonged use of an automatic arterial pressure monitoring device. A direct acting vasodilator (nitroprusside, glyceryl trinitrate (GTN), hydralazine, etc) can be used if flap perfusion is impaired. Survival of flaps may be improved by perioperative administration of nifedipine and anti-thrombotic therapy with NSAIDs, local heparin or infusion of Dextran. Dexamethasone has been used before separation of the flap to reduce intracellular oedema. Intravenous regional guanethidine block may enhance survival of flaps in limbs.

Viability of the flap is difficult to monitor. Clinical observation of capillary refill and colour or sensation of warmth are crude measures but appear to be almost as reliable as invasive monitoring such as transcutaneous measurement of pH or oxygen. Miniature flow probes may lead to a false sense of well-being since this may simply indicate a shunt phenomenon. Where access to the transposed tissue is difficult, implanted monitoring such as electrical impedance plethysmography or Doppler flowmeters may be useful. Blood levels of plasma endothelin-1 are related to mean arterial pressure, since it is released by vascular endothelium, binds to vascular smooth muscle cells and produces prolonged vasoconstriction. It could be speculated that endothelin-1 levels in plasma may predict flap survival.

Careful positioning with adequate padding to protect pressure points during these prolonged procedures is vital. Heat and moisture exchangers, a circle breathing system with carbon dioxide absorber help to conserve heat and permit economies in fresh gas flow. Ambient temperature must be 22°C or higher if effective warm air heating blankets are not available. If nitrous oxide is used for maintenance of anaesthesia, the tracheal cuff should be inflated with the same gas mixture to prevent over-distension. Eyes require careful protection. Anti-embolism stockings and sequential compression stockings reduce the risk of deep vein thromboses. Prolonged administration of propofol or isoflurane appears to cause no elevation in the sensitive marker of liver dysfunction, hepatic glutathione-s-transferase.

CRANIOFACIAL RECONSTRUCTION

Urgent treatment will be needed if there is: raised intracranial pressure; deterioration in function, e.g. auditory or visual loss; physiological impairment if, for instance, the deformity interferes with breathing, causes obstructive sleep apnoea or inhibits feeding. Adenotonsillectomy should be electively performed before major craniofacial surgery if tonsils or adenoids cause airway obstruction. Non-urgent surgery is needed for socio-emotional factors (for instance, to alleviate disfigurement and the psychological impact on the patient).

Craniofacial reconstruction falls into two broad groups: congenital defects in children, and abnormalities in adults secondary to trauma. The two principal problems are first airway access and potential difficulty in intubation and second, likelihood of massive blood loss.

Preoperative evaluation should include careful examination of the airway and evaluation of all available X-rays and scan films. Kink-resistant tracheal tubes are used. Difficulty in intubation may be overcome by the use of fibre-optic laryngoscopes, wire and catheter techniques, placement of a mini-tracheostomy or cricothyrotomy, or intubation through a laryngeal mask airway. Elective or emergency tracheostomy may become necessary. Liaison with the surgeon is important preoperatively since it may be necessary to change the tube from the oral to the nasal routes (or vice versa) for frontal advancement.

Blood loss may be considerable, particularly whilst bony dissection is in progress; it can be reduced by induced hypotension and posture. Fluid preloading is prudent. Heart rate changes and variation of systolic pressure with ventilation best indicate volume status in small children. For intracranial procedures, it may be necessary to reduce cerebral bulk and cerebral oedema by the use of hyperosmotic intravenous solutions, diuretics, posture and modest hypocapnia. Drainage of cerebrospinal fluid and systemic corticosteroids may be necessary.

Heat conservation is vital and the use of warm air blankets, heated humidifiers in the respiratory system, elevation of ambient temperature and the use of reflective plastic sheeting all help to maintain body temperature. Anti-embolism stockings should be used and sequential compressive pneumatic stockings help to reduce the potential for deep venous thrombosis in the legs. Particular attention to protecting pressure points is necessary.

Postoperative care is directed to maintenance of the airway, fluid balance and replacement of blood loss. Early close observation of the level of consciousness and the use of scanning should detect postoperative intracranial problems such as intracerebral bleeding.

COSMETIC SURGERY UNDER LOCAL ANAESTHESIA

Many minor procedures are necessarily superficial and can be carried out under local anaesthesia with or without sedation. If intravenous sedation is planned, the patient should be prepared as for general anaesthesia by appropriate starvation and a gastroprokinetic agent and H_2-receptor blockers to reduce acid secretion. Preoperative oral medication with temazepam, a short-acting anxiolytic benzodiazepine, or non-sedative agents, e.g. timolol, can be used to reduce anxiety. Preoperative psychological support and rapport will reduce the pharmacological needs. Fear of the initial injection of local anaesthetic can be greatly improved by early application of EMLA cream.

In general, it is not recommended that the

surgeon be both operator and 'sedator'. The common practice in the USA is for a nurse anaesthetist, trained in the techniques and resuscitation procedures, to monitor and administer the sedation. The surgeon may try to direct the anaesthesia whilst carrying out the surgery and create a conflict of interests.

Monitoring for intravenous sedation for procedures under local anaesthesia should include monitoring of ECG, pulse oximetry with pulse display and blood pressure measurement. Resuscitation facilities should include the means to give oxygen under pressure, suction apparatus and all the equipment necessary for intubation of the trachea. Monitoring should extend into the recovery period until the patient is able to leave.

INTRAVENOUS SEDATION TECHNIQUES

There are numerous techniques, using a wide variety of agents, to satisfy the need for a combination of analgesia, anxiolysis, amnesia, sedation and euphoria. The depth of sedation to be achieved ranges from 'conscious sedation' in which verbal contact is maintained and this is produced by the use of a single agent, e.g. nitrous oxide, propofol or midazolam, through monitored anaesthesia care (MAC) which requires the airway maintenance (and rescue) skills of an anaesthetist, achieved with a cocktail of drugs by which verbal contact is lost.

Midazolam, cautiously given intravenously in 0.5 mg increments for an adult, forms the basis of many of these requirements. Deep sedation is combined with sufficient analgesia to render the patient unresponsive and perhaps requiring mechanical assistance to maintain a patent airway, supplemental oxygen and, often, reversal of benzodiazepine actions with flumazenil. Alfentanil 0.25–0.5 mg i.v. given immediately before a brief painful manoeuvre reduces the discomfort to the patient without subsequent ill-effects. Droperidol (0.25–0.5 mg i.v. bolus doses) combines amnesia, sedation, dissociation, anti-emesis and vasodilation from alpha adrenergic block. Nitrous oxide in oxygen (50%) provides sedation with euphoria, some analgesia, and because of its low blood/gas solubility, is rapidly taken up or eliminated.

Propofol in small doses (10–20 mg boluses i.v.) or by infusion provides elevation of mood and anxiolysis with sedation. Effective patient-controlled anxiolytic systems using diazepam or propofol have been described. Early administration of midazolam and droperidol produces amnesia and then allows 'fine-tuning' with increments of propofol and alfentanil to produce sedation and analgesia as necessary. It is wise to give supplemental oxygen via facemask or nasal catheters and to confirm adequate oxygenation by pulse oximetry. For monitored anaesthesia care or deep sedation, premedication 1 h before surgery with a relatively short-acting oral benzodiazepine (midazolam 0.5–0.75 mg kg^{-1}, or temazepam 10–20 mg) reduces the doses of other drugs and helps the patient to make the transition from the awake state to sedation. Other agents, e.g. clonidine, have a multiplicity of actions (potentiation of sedation, analgesia and vasodilation) and are increasingly used to reduce the doses needed of other drugs and 'smooth' the course of the sedation. Providing a benzodiazepine has already established amnesia, ketamine in 10 mg boluses i.v. adds good analgesia to the cocktail, without significant respiratory depression.

Recovery can be hastened from benzodiazepine sedation by the use of flumazenil intravenously, but it is costly and the duration of action may be shorter than that of the benzodiazepine. Doxapram (1 mg kg^{-1}) can be used to stimulate the respiratory chemoreceptors and provoke adequate ventilation. Naloxone is best avoided as analgesia wears off very rapidly and quality of return of consciousness is better if achieved more slowly. Intravenous sedation has little place in paediatric practice and is applicable at the earliest to sensible 10-year-olds.

LOCAL ANAESTHESIA IN PLASTIC SURGERY

The use of local anaesthesia includes:

- topical (EMLA cream, lignocaine sprays, local installation)
- local infiltration
- peripheral nerve blocks
- field blocks
- regional blocks (spinal or epidural).

Details of appropriate blocks are found elsewhere, but it is a feature of plastic surgery that most surgeons choose to infiltrate the wound site with a combination of local anaesthetic and vasoconstrictor. It helps if the skin incisions are marked with an indelible pen before infiltration distorts the tissues.

Liaison with the surgeon before the use of local anaesthetics is important to ensure that near-toxic levels of local anaesthetic agents have not been given by the anaesthetist before the surgeon administers another dose sufficient to produce a reaction. Local anaesthesia is also useful in the postoperative period. After prolonged procedures, patients appreciate repeat of the local anaesthetic block when it begins to wear off. Retrograde injection of bupivacaine through wound drains may produce useful analgesia.

The use of spinal or epidural blockade for day-case procedures is controversial. Urinary catheterization may be necessary to empty the bladder. The loss of motor power may delay the discharge of the patient. However, the use of lignocaine, rather than bupivacaine, ensures a more rapid recovery. Improvements in spinal needles have resulted in an acceptably low rate of post-spinal puncture headache and extend the range of procedures which can be carried out under spinal blockade for outpatients.

TUMESCENT ANAESTHESIA

Tumescent anaesthesia has become popular. Large volumes of very dilute local anaesthetic solutions are injected into the operative site. This appears to be particularly valuable in highly vascular areas such as the scalp and also before liposuction.

FURTHER READING

Buckley, R. C., Davidson, S. F. and Das, S. K. (1993) Effects of ketorolac tromethamine (Toradol^R) on a functional model of microvascular thrombosis. *British Journal of Plastic Surgery*, **46**, 296–299.

Davies, K. H. (1976) Guanethidine sympathetic blockade: its value in re-implantation surgery. *Lancet*, **i**, 876–877.

Klein, J. A. (1990) The tumescent technique. Anesthesia and modified lipsuction technique. *Dermatologic Clinics*, **8**, 425–437.

Murray, J. M., Phillips, A. S. and Fee, J. P. H. (1994) Comparison of the effects of isoflurane and propofol on hepatic glutathione-S-transferase concentrations during and after prolonged anaesthesia. *British Journal of Anaesthesia*, **72**, 599–601.

Owall, A., Gordon, E., Lagerkranser, M., Lindquist, C., Rudehill, A. and Sollevi A. (1987) Clinical experience with adenosine for controlled hypotension during cerebral aneurysm surgery. *Anesthesia and Analgesia*, **66**, 229–34.

Pal, S., Khazanchi, R. K. D. and Moudgil, K. (1991) An experimental study on the effect of nifedipine on ischaemic skin flap survival in rats. *British Journal of Plastic Surgery*, **44**, 299–301.

Ridings, P., Gault, D. and Khan, L. (1994) Reduction in postoperative vomiting after surgical correction of prominent ears. *British Journal of Anaesthesia*, **72**, 592–293.

Robins, D. W. (1983) The anaesthetic management of patients undergoing free flap transfer. *British Journal of Plastic Surgery*, **36**, 231–234.

Salemark, L. International survey of current microvascular practices in free tissue transfer and replantation surgery. *Microsurgery*, **12**, 308–311.

Tuominen, H. P., Svartling, N. E., Tikkanen, I. T. et al. (1995) Perioperative plasma endothelin-1 concentrations and vasoconstriction during prolonged plastic surgery procedures. *British Journal of Anaesthesia*, **74**, 661–666.

Uppington, J. W. and Goat, V. A. (1987) Anaesthesia for major craniofacial surgery: a report of 23 cases in children under four years of age. *Annals of the Royal College of Surgeons of England*, **69**, 175–178.

Ure, R. W., Dwyer, S. J., Blogg, C. E. and White, A. P. (1991) Patient-controlled anxiolysis with propofol. *British Journal of Anaesthesia*, **67**, 657–658.

ANAESTHESIA FOR RADIOLOGY

C. J. Peden

The world of diagnostic imaging is advancing rapidly. The idea that the magnetic resonance phenomenon could be used to produce images was suggested in 1973 by Paul Lauterbur; now over 20 years later magnetic resonance imaging (MRI) has given us an enormously powerful diagnostic tool. Other techniques such as positron emission tomography (PET) and magnetic resonance spectroscopy are providing valuable research information particularly about the physiology and biochemistry of the brain. In everyday clinical practice the quality of images produced and the speed of imaging of the new generation of computerized tomography scanners has increased markedly.

In this new world of imaging, the roles of surgery, anaesthesia and radiology are becoming blurred. Surgeons have already started to operate within magnetic resonance scanners; imaging is used to guide location of the lesion. Neurosurgeons use MRI preoperatively to localize precisely tumours and to plan surgical access. Interventional neuroradiology treats central nervous system disease using endovascular access to deliver therapeutic agents such as drugs and devices for embolization. For all these procedures the patient must remain motionless. Not all patients will require general anaesthesia, but the anaesthetist still has an important role to play in providing sedation and monitored care.

WORKING IN THE RADIOLOGY DEPARTMENT

In many radiology departments the anaesthetist is an infrequent visitor. The department is often distant from the operating theatres and other high dependency areas where anaesthetists are usually to be found. He or she may, therefore, have to work in an isolated and unfamiliar environment. If anaesthesia is performed infrequently the equipment may be old, not regularly serviced and not of the standard used in the rest of the hospital. Normal monitoring standards should be applied and if adequate monitoring is not available anaesthesia should be delayed.

Piped medical gases may not be supplied, so the presence of adequate numbers of oxygen cylinders must be checked before the start of the procedure. Radiology personnel may be unaware of the problems facing the anaesthetist and are unlikely to be trained to provide anaesthetic assistance; the presence of a skilled anaesthetic assistant is essential. Space may be limited by bulky equipment and access to, or movement around, the patient may be difficult. Access to the patient may also be limited by radiation exposure hazards to the anaesthetist. Anaesthetic equipment may need to be kept distant from the patient because of magnetic field hazards. Lighting may be poor and the environment may be significantly colder than an operating

Short Practice of Anaesthesia. Edited by M. Morgan and G. M. Hall. Published in 1997 by Chapman & Hall, London. ISBN 0 412 71890 1

Table 23.1 Potential problems for the anaesthetist in the radiology department

Site distant from operating theatres and high dependency areas
Radiology personnel untrained in the management of anaesthetized patients
Equipment may be old and not regularly serviced
Piped medical gases not supplied
Cold, dark environment
Radiation hazards
Magnetic field hazards
Access to patient difficult
Non-tilting X-ray tables
Use of intravenous contrast media
No recovery facility

theatre. It is usually not possible to increase the temperature, even for small babies, as the function of computer equipment depends on the maintenance of a low environmental temperature. In addition, recovery facilities may not be available; patients must be fully awake before they are transported to recovery facilities elsewhere in the hospital. As in any environment where anaesthesia is performed a tipping trolley, suction equipment and full resuscitation and defibrillation facilities must be provided and carefully checked before the induction of anaesthesia. The problems facing the anaesthetist working in the radiology department are summarized in Table 23.1.

Most diagnostic radiological procedures are not painful but the patient must remain motionless during the examination. The newest computed tomography (CT) systems can generate images very rapidly and MRI is getting faster: however, some of the more complex MRI examinations may still take up to 20 min for one scan and up to 1 h for the whole examination. Both MRI and CT produce images composed of multiple data acquisitions; particularly in MRI movement of the patient (at any point during the acquisitions that make up one scan) will result in faulty spatial allocation of signal and so degrade the quality of the final image by the production of movement artefacts. Patients who need sedation or general anaesthesia to undergo radiological procedures are therefore small children, mentally disabled adults, and confused or unconscious patients. The latter group may be recently admitted trauma patients who require invasive monitoring and active treatment such as blood transfusion, cardiovascular support and cervical spine immobilization, or patients transferred from the intensive care unit whose supportive therapy must continue during transfer and examination. Management of these patients is difficult, but should aim to provide the same standard of care as elsewhere in the hospital and keep the time spent in the radiology suite to a minimum. Some patients, both adult and paediatric, may be managed with sedation.

SPECIFIC PROBLEMS

RADIATION HAZARDS TO ANAESTHETISTS

Anaesthetists working in operating theatres have a very low exposure to radiation even when orthopaedic screening and chest X-rays are being performed. However, exposure can reach significant levels during other procedures such as cardiac catheterization, or certain neuroradiological procedures. These are prolonged examinations during which invasive manoeuvres (which are not without risk) are performed: the anaesthetist may be loathe to move too far away from the patient, particularly if they are sedated rather than anaesthetized. Distance from the patient during the time of radiation exposure is an important safety factor as radiation scatter decreases with increasing distance from the source, based on the inverse square law.

There are two important factors in providing all personnel with adequate protection from occupational radiation exposure. The first is quality control. It is up to the department of radiology to ensure that equipment is regularly serviced and checked on a daily basis and that techniques such as short bursts of fluoroscopic time are always used. The second factor is personnel protection. 'Lead' aprons (tin amalgam) must be a minimum of 0.5 mm lead-equivalent thick, the sternum should not be exposed and the wraparound variety should be used in preference to the type with open sides. An apron with obvious cracks or tears in it should not be used. During procedures such as cardiac catheterization, staff should protect the thyroid with a collar and special protective eye glasses with side shields should be available and worn. The anaesthetist should always distance themselves as far as possible from the radiation source during imaging. Anaesthetists who work frequently in areas of high exposure should be issued with standard radiation film badges to monitor their exposure and to educate them about their degree of exposure. Pregnant anaesthetists should avoid involvement in radiological procedures; their maximum monthly permissible dose of radiation is one tenth of the whole body dose allowed for occupational exposure to non-pregnant personnel.

CONTRAST MEDIA

A particular hazard for the patient in the radiology department is contrast media, although not all diagnostic procedures require contrast media. Approximately 5% of radiological studies in the USA are complicated by reactions to contrast media, with a death rate of 0.9 per 100 000 reactors. All contrast media, except that used for MRI, contain iodine. The incidence of severe non-fatal reactions is decreasing with newer non-ionic low-osmolality contrast media, but there is no difference in the death rate. The cost of the newer agents precludes their routine use for all patients.

There are no reported cases of severe adverse reactions to contrast media during anaesthesia, but the presence of an anaesthetist may be requested for an awake patient who is at high risk of having a reaction. Reaction is more likely in patients with a history of previous reaction, cardiac disease, other allergies or atopic diseases, with increasing dose of iodine, and with a bolus dose of contrast. High-risk studies include cerebral and coronary angiography, excretory urography and cholangiography.

All contrast media are hypertonic to plasma and haemodynamic changes may result from the administration of these hyperosmotic solutions; most patients have an initial brief hypertensive response followed by mild hypotension. Central venous, right ventricular and pulmonary artery pressures increase as does cardiac output, a potentially dangerous effect in patients who have a history of cardiac failure. The increase in plasma osmolarity causes a diuresis which eventually reverses the increase in blood volume and may lead to hypovolaemia.

It is the properties of contrast media that are useful for imaging purposes, high-density and stability of iodine-organic binding, which cause reactions in all patients. The severity of the reaction depends on the patient's cardiovascular status and the concentration of contrast medium given. Some patients also have idiosyncratic reactions. The first symptoms occurring in patients about to have a serious anaphylactoid reaction are nausea, vomiting and urticaria caused by histamine release. Hypotension and arrhythmias occur as the first clinical sign in about 10% of fatal reactions. Severe reactions then progress to anaphylactoid shock; this may take up to 8 h to develop after the initial symptoms and so patients must be closely monitored in hospital after any signs of a reaction.

There are several underlying mechanisms proposed for the anaphylactoid reactions induced by contrast media. These include histamine release, complement activation, antibody–antigen reaction, direct cardiac toxicity and disruption of the blood–brain barrier. Most reactions to contrast media can be treated by radiologists, so anaesthetists will only be called to severe reactions. The first line drug is adrenaline: methylxanthines, steroids and anticholinergics can be used as appropriate and according to local treatment protocols. Adrenaline not only causes bronchodilation and increases cardiac output, but also decreases histamine release by increasing concentrations of c-AMP (cyclic adenosine monophosphate) in mast cells and basophils.

Prevention is better than cure and the risk-versus-benefit ratio of the procedure should be considered in patients who are at high risk of having a reaction. Pre-testing is controversial and has been known to trigger a genuine reaction. Pretreatment with steroids and antihistamines orally, commencing at least 18 h before the examination, has been shown to reduce the incidence of reactions in at-risk patients. Anaesthetists can contribute to general safety for all patients by ensuring that indwelling intravenous access is used, that resuscitation equipment meets current standards and is regularly checked and that the radiology personnel are familiar with its use. Monitoring of all patients undergoing contrast studies may aid the early detection of a developing reaction.

SEDATION

Not all patients require general anaesthesia to undergo a radiological procedure: babies may sleep through relatively long examinations if the study is performed after a feed and they are well wrapped up to keep them warm. Adults may need sedation and analgesia to tolerate long invasive radiological procedures, but sedation is most widely used for children undergoing CT or MRI. Up to 80% of toddlers are sedated for CT and even more for MRI; complications are not widely reported but those that do occur can be severe and include respiratory arrest and death. A survey of the practice of sedation of children for CT in the USA showed that in less than 2% of cases is an anaesthetist present when children are sedated; in approximately 50% of cases the sedation was prescribed by the radiologist and commonly the sole form of monitoring was visual inspection from the control room. These figures caused concern in the USA and prompted an editorial in *Radiology* recognizing that current practice failed to meet the recommendations of the American Academy of Paediatrics guidelines for sedation of children. The situation may not be as bad in the UK, but we do not know; guidelines have been issued here by a joint working party of the Royal College of Anaesthetists and the Royal College of Radiologists.

Basic guidelines are essential as the use of intravenous anaesthetic agents in non-anaesthetic hands is potentially dangerous, as is the synergistic action of the benzodiazepines with opioids.

There are many different sedation regimens that have been used for children. High dose chloral hydrate (50–100 mg kg^{-1}) is still commonly used, although it is less effective in children over 4 years; at this dose it has the potential to cause respiratory depression and loss of the airway. Midazolam is used intravenously and nasally. Anaesthetic agents are used for sedation although some of the doses described (thiopentone 7 mg kg^{-1}) suggest that general anaesthesia is the more likely result. Propofol, given as a loading dose followed by an infusion, is the current favourite agent for sedation. The use of propofol again prompted an editorial in *Radiology*, entitled *Sedating pediatric patients: Is propofol a panacea*, to remind radiologists that propofol is only licensed for use by persons 'trained in the administration of general anaesthesia and not involved in the conduct of the diagnostic procedure'. In the hands of anaesthetists propofol is a good agent for sedation, because of its rapid recovery characteristics. When compared with thiopentone it was found to be more cost-effective, as nursing time in recovery was reduced. Cost-effectiveness of a drug matters in imaging departments; rapid and predictable onset and offset are important as CT and MRI imaging time is limited and expensive.

Sedating children can be difficult and unpredictable; the advantages of general anaesthesia are that it has a more rapid and controlled onset and immobility is guaranteed. If sedation fails, the child will lose its imaging slot for that day and have to return for general anaesthesia: this is inefficient use of resources. Sick children may be better managed with general anaesthesia; certainly if there is any question of raised intracranial pressure then sedation is inappropriate and potentially dangerous. An anaesthetist administering sedation should enquire whether the patient has received any oral contrast medium. Patients should not be given oral contrast medium and then sedation, as oral contrast medium is hypertonic and can cause pneumonitis and pulmonary oedema if aspirated.

The presence of an anaesthetist with sole responsibility for sedated patients would be ideal, but is not always practical. Far too many patients are given sedation for an anaesthetist to always be present, although the concept of monitored anaesthesia care is becoming increasingly popular. The American Society of Anesthesiologists has defined monitored anaesthesia care as 'instances in which an anesthesiologist has been called upon to provide specific anesthesia services to a particular patient undergoing a planned procedure, in connection with which a patient receives local anaesthesia or, in some case, no anesthesia at all. In such cases the anesthesiologist is providing specific services to the patient and is in control of the patients non-surgical medical care, including the responsibility of monitoring the patient's vital signs and is available to administer anesthetics or provide other medical care as appropriate'.

Even if anaesthetists cannot always be present in the radiology department they have an important role to play in the education of their colleagues in using sedative drugs safely and in resuscitation training to prevent mishap if problems should occur. Strict protocols for patient selection, preparation and monitoring should be used in all radiology departments where sedation is given: preselection procedures may identify high-risk patients where more skilled help may be needed.

Recommendations for safe sedation are that all patients should have continuous venous access via an intravenous cannula and be continuously monitored with a pulse oximeter, ECG and blood pressure; resuscitation equipment, suction and oxygen must be available and the patient should be on a tipping trolley (not always feasible for radiological studies). Staff involved in sedation should have recently certified evidence of training in cardiopulmonary resuscitation. It is important that every unit where sedation is practiced should be self-sufficient in drugs, equipment and staff to manage the initial phase of critical situations before more experienced help arrives and if the worst should happen it should be easy to transfer the patient to an intensive care area.

ANAESTHESIA

All patients should be seen, fully assessed and have had appropriate investigations performed before the induction of anaesthesia. Children and mentally disabled or extremely anxious adults may attend as day cases and day-case management should be applied; the same discharge criteria should be applied as are used in the rest of the hospital. Emergency patients must be stabilized before transfer to the radiology department.

When planning anaesthesia or sedation for radiological procedures, the length of procedure, accessibility of the airway, underlying medical condition and the need for rapid recovery must be considered and the most appropriate agents used. In the majority of cases the procedure will not be painful and the use of potent long-acting opioids is inappropriate. Total intravenous anaesthesia may be ideal due to its rapid recovery characteristics and low incidence of nausea and vomiting: it is worth remembering when planning anaesthesia (or sedation) for MRI that infusion pumps will malfunction above a certain level of magnetic field strength.

The airway should be secured in whichever way is suitable for that patient and for the procedure. It is generally inappropriate, even if it is possible, to hold the patients airway during a radiological procedure as the anaesthetist is then forced to remain close to the radiation source. The laryngeal mask appears to offer the ideal alternative for the patient who does not need tracheal intubation. However, the laryngeal mask should be used with caution: a recent case report of aspiration during a radiological examination in a patient whose airway was secured with a laryngeal mask questioned its safety when access to the airway is remote and the patient is not on a tipping table.

COMPUTED TOMOGRAPHY (CT)

Tomograms are reconstructed by computer from narrow beams of X-rays rotated 180° around the area under examination; cross-sectional images of any part of the body can be obtained. Although MRI has superseded CT for the elective examination of the central nervous system, spinal cord and many orthopaedic conditions, CT remains at present the main radiographic tool for examination of structures within the body cavities and for emergency examinations of the central nervous system and spinal cord.

Young children may require sedation or general anaesthesia to undergo CT scan as immobility is essential for high quality diagnostic images (Figure 23.1). Another significant group of patients who require CT scans are trauma patients who may undergo CT of the head, cervical spine, thorax or abdomen to assess injury. These patients must be stabilized before being moved to the radiology suite. The trachea of any trauma patient with a depressed conscious level must be intub-

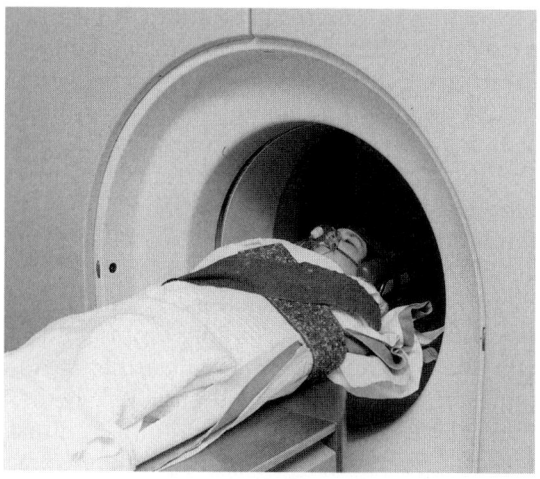

Figure 23.1 A sedated child in a CT scanner. Note that the patient is strapped into place and the head firmly fixed by pads to stop movement. Oxygen is being given, the child is fully monitored (although the monitoring is not visible in this photograph) and the child can be easily observed within the scanner.

ated and their lungs ventilated before the examination as they will be supine on a couch that does not tilt, with their head strapped into place. Intubation should be performed with a rapid sequence induction, cricoid pressure and unstable cervical spine precautions taken. Anaesthesia should be maintained appropriately for a head injured patient.

Before any patient is anaesthetized in the CT suite, or transferred to the CT suite from elsewhere in the hospital, all equipment must be checked and adequate supplies of oxygen and essential drugs ensured. The anaesthetist requires a dedicated assistant who will be present throughout the whole examination. It is safest to induce anaesthesia on a tipping trolley, secure the patients airway and then transfer to the CT couch for the examination. The airway of the anaesthetized patient must be secured with either a laryngeal mask (if appropriate) or a tracheal tube.

The patient is visible in the scanner and the anaesthetist can remain in the room wearing X-ray protection, or view the patient and

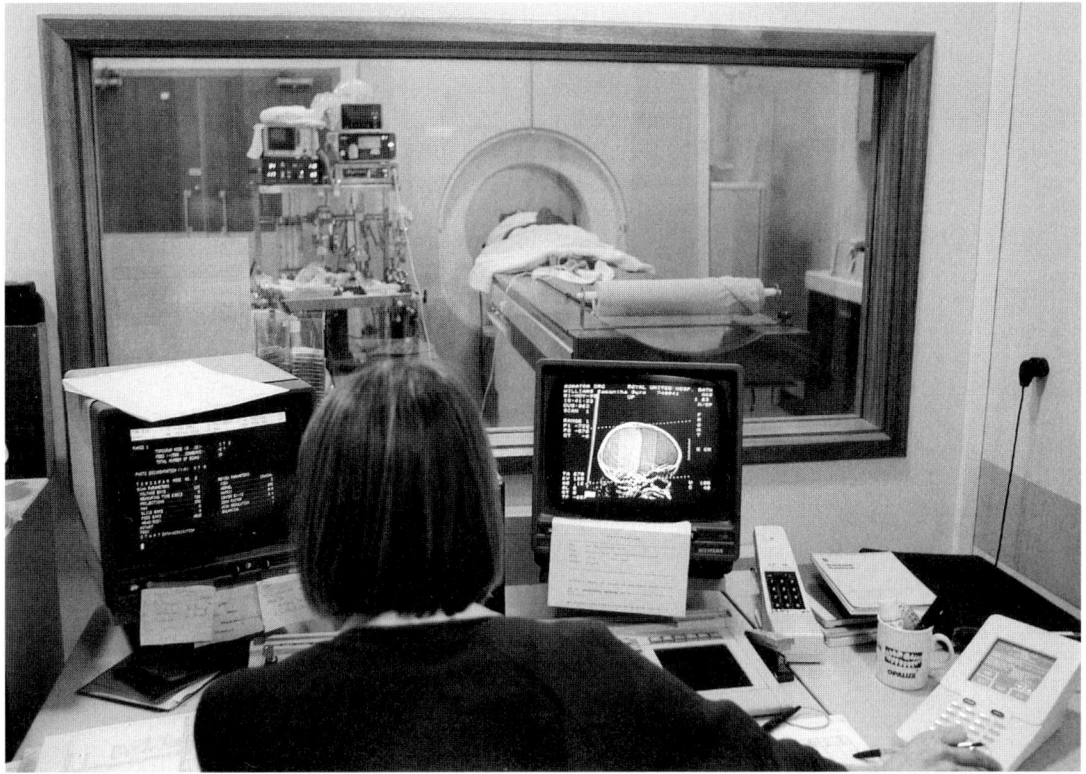

Figure 23.2 A sedated child within a CT scanner; the child and all the monitoring can be viewed through the window of the control room, or the anaesthetist can remain in the CT room wearing X-ray protection.

monitors from the control room (Figure 23.2). The CT scanner does not interfere with monitoring equipment, and the presence of monitoring equipment does not degrade CT scans. The scans are short and can be interrupted to check on the patient if necessary. The patient couch moves during the examination and ventilation tubing and intravenous lines should be secured and of adequate length. Interruption of ventilation may be requested to improve image quality particularly when examining the thorax and abdomen; changing the ventilation pattern to frequent small tidal volume breaths may be adequate. If ventilation is discontinued briefly, the anaesthetist must ensure that the patient's lungs are re-ventilated as soon as possible. Anaesthesia can be maintained with volatile agents or with total intravenous anaesthesia; the most appropriate anaesthetic for that patient should be used.

EMISSION COMPUTED TOMOGRAPHY

Emission tomography measures physiological function; it uses radiopharmaceuticals directed specifically at certain regions of the body. The photons emitted from these radionuclides are detected by scintillation crystals or arrays of solid state detector material which move around the patient, or surround the patient, to collect data from multiple angles. There are two types of emission tomography; photon emission and positron emission. Photon emission uses gamma ray emitters such as ^{123}I, ^{201}Tl and ^{99m}Tc. Positron emission tomography (PET) involves the use of radionuclides that emit two γ-rays after the annihilation of a positron with an electron; these travel in opposite directions and events are only registered when two opposing detectors are excited simultaneously. PET has been used to observe functional brain activity and regional cerebral blood flow, as well as alterations in myocardial metabolism associated with ischaemia. At present PET is mainly a research technique and anaesthesia is unlikely to be needed; considerations will be similar to those for CT.

INTERVENTIONAL NEURORADIOLOGY

Interventional neuroradiology is an expanding specialty. It is a mixture of neurosurgery and neuroradiology; its purpose is to treat central nervous system disease using endovascular access to deliver therapeutic agents such as drugs and devices to cause embolization. Most neuroradiological procedures involve the placement of special catheters into the arterial circulation of the head, neck or spinal cord; this is usually done by a transfemoral approach. A microcatheter is introduced into the cerebral circulation and through this drugs, embolic agents and balloons can be placed. More and more procedures can be performed without the need for craniotomy. Despite the fact that not all patients require general anaesthesia, the anaesthetist has an important role to play in providing sedation and monitored anaesthesia care, and to reduce the occurrence of morbidity and mortality during these high-risk procedures. Immediate intervention may be required if a disaster, such as intracranial haemorrhage, should occur.

ANAESTHETIC PRACTICE

Most adults are sedated; adults who cannot cooperate and small children, require general anaesthesia. As always the patient should be seen before the procedure and the anaesthetist should take a history and perform an examination. Points of particular relevance are previous experience of angiography, a history of contrast reaction, coagulation disorders and any neck, back or joint disorders which would make lying still for several hours very difficult. Premedication with an anxiolytic may be helpful. Nimodipine or nifedipine premedication given orally for prevention or treatment of cerebral ischaemia and reduction of the incidence of vessel spasm during catheter passage should be considered.

Many of these procedures can be carried out under conscious sedation. The aim is to provide pain relief, anxiolysis and immobility for patient comfort, which can be easily reversed when neurological testing needs to be performed. Sclerotherapy and chemotherapy are painful; the majority of other procedures are not, but traction on or distention of the cerebral arteries causes burning and discomfort from long periods of lying still is a significant problem. These procedures are psychologically very stressful for the patient with a risk of serious stroke or death. One anaesthetic technique which has been successfully used is neuroleptanaesthesia (fentanyl and droperidol) in conjunction with a propofol infusion titrated to give an unconscious patient with a patent airway. Supplemental oxygen is essential for all patients. The overall aim of monitored anaesthesia care in this setting is the ability to lighten and deepen sedation, keep the patient motionless and manipulate the blood pressure to minimize the effects of the intracranial interventions.

General anaesthesia with tracheal intubation is required for all patients who cannot cooperate and remain still, and for aneurysm ablation, sclerotherapy and certain types of chemotherapy. Patients may also need general anaesthesia for certain digital subtraction angiography techniques, where extensive multilevel angiography cannot tolerate even the smallest degree of patient movement; the radiologist may request apnoea during imaging, frequent very low tidal volume breaths may be tried. If apnoea is used, it is essential to remember to reconnect patient to the ventilator at the end of the procedure.

EQUIPMENT AND PATIENT SET-UP

The anaesthetic machine used should be able to give carbon dioxide for deliberate hypercapnia. The anaesthetist should have easy access to a telephone, as neurosurgical help may be needed urgently. A dedicated spotlight for notes and drug administration should be present as the lights may be dimmed for radiological purposes. Before starting these very long procedures, it is essential that the patient is comfortable. Each patient may be having multiple treatments and so great care should be taken to ensure continued patient acceptance. Two intravenous lines should be inserted and to maximize the distance between the anaesthetist and the fluoroscopy unit, extensions should be used. A three-way tap can be placed near the patient for continuous infusions and on the other line a three-way tap near the anaesthetist can be used for bolus drug administration.

MONITORING

Monitoring should include direct arterial blood pressure; transducers can be placed at three different sites. The pressure in the femoral artery introducer can be monitored, a second pressure is taken from the carotid or vertebral artery to detect thrombus formation or vascular spasm at the catheter tip and the pressure at the tip of the microcatheter can be measured for use during intracranial arteriovenous malformation embolization and for measuring stump pressures during balloon occlusions. A five-lead ECG is needed, a pulse oximeter should be placed on the toe of the leg receiving the femoral artery catheter, and the patient's temperature should be monitored. Supplemental oxygen should be given and a catheter attached to measure $P_{E'CO_2}$. The patient may require a bladder catheter depending on the predicted length of the procedure. All lines must have sufficient slack to advance the patient towards the image intensifier. If a CVP or a pulmonary artery catheter are needed, available fluoroscopy should be used to place these lines.

To monitor the central nervous system (CNS) during these procedures the ideal is to have the patient lightly sedated so that they can communicate and the CNS can be continuously evaluated; adjuncts which can be used and which are more important during general anaesthesia are the electroencephalogram, somatosensory and motor evoked potentials, transcranial Doppler ultrasound and ^{133}Xe cerebral blood flow monitoring.

MAGNETIC RESONANCE IMAGING (MRI)

Magnetic resonance imaging is now the imaging modality of choice for the diagnosis of many neurological and orthopaedic conditions. There are several thousand MRI installations in the USA and the number in the UK is increasing rapidly. As the number of examinations and applications increases so does the need for anaesthetic presence, to provide sedation and general anaesthesia and to manage critically ill patients in this challenging environment. MRI does not use ionizing radiation to generate images; instead information is generated from the spin of magnetically susceptible nuclei in a high magnetic field. If anaesthetists are to work safely in the MRI environment they should have a basic understanding of the principles of MRI.

BASIC PRINCIPLES OF MRI

MRI can use any nucleus which has a spin. MRI uses the proton nucleus; magnetic resonance spectroscopy can use the phosphorus, hydrogen, fluorine and carbon nuclei to produce biochemical information. Body water contains approximately $100 M\ ^1H$ and this high concentration provides the signal used to produce images.

When the proton nuclei are placed in a high magnetic field they align themselves with that magnetic field, behaving rather like small bar magnets; they continue to spin and at the same time their axis of rotation moves around the axis of the magnetic field (imagine this axis as a line running through the patient longitudinally from head to toe). Each nucleus has a characteristic frequency of spin at a given magnetic field strength; this is termed the resonant frequency. When these nuclei are subjected to a second magnetic field (the exciting field) oscillating at the resonant frequency of the proton nuclei and orientated at right angles to the initial static magnetic field, the nuclei flip away from their longitudinal alignment into another at right angles to their original alignment. When the second exciting field is turned off the nuclei return to their original alignment; as they do so their spinning magnetic fields induce current in a stationary wire. This current has a decaying sinusoidal waveform whose frequency is at the resonant frequency of the proton nucleus.

Images are produced by confining the exciting magnetic field to discrete slices of body tissue and by further transient magnetic fields called gradients, the data collection process can assign the signal from different parts of the body slice studied to the appropriate part of the pixel matrix on the screen or film. The intensity of signal in any given pixel depends on the density of water protons in the region, the delay between excitation of the proton nuclei and collection of the signal and the time allowed for the nuclei to recover before another excitation pulse is applied. T_1 and T_2 are the terms used to describe these sequence manipulations. The collection sequences can be manipulated to emphasize certain pathological conditions, e.g. oedema surrounding an intracranial tumour. For a detailed description of the principles of MRI the reader is referred to one of the major textbooks.

PRACTICAL ASPECTS

There are several problems facing the anaesthetist working in this challenging environment: principally these are the high magnetic field with associated risks of ferromagnetic attraction, an inability to see or get to the patient, lack of space to work in and malfunction of monitoring equipment. These problems are discussed in more detail in the relevant sections. MRI is developing and changing very fast and the advent of low field 'open' MRI systems will reduce some of the problems: the patient can be seen, access to them will be easier and the environment will be less claustrophobic. However, this type of scanner is likely to be suitable only for certain types of investigation and at present very few are available worldwide.

The magnetic field

The anaesthetist must work in a high magnetic field, which should be considered to be permanently on. It is very expensive to shut down the field and not without risk. If the field is suddenly shut down the cryogens, such as helium, on which all superconducting magnets are based may 'boil off' in an explosive event known as a quench. Dilution of the environment with the cryogen may cause hypoxia or asphyxia and the condensing vapour can cause cryogenic burns. Therefore, never assume that in case of emergency the field can be turned off.

Magnetic field strength is measured in Tesla (T). One Tesla is equal to 10 000 Gauss (G). The earth's magnetic field at the surface is of the order of 0.5–2.0 G. Clinical magnetic resonance imaging systems in the UK operate between 0.05 T and 2.0 T, that is 500 to 20 000 times the earth's surface magnetic field. The anaesthetist should know the extent of the magnetic field he or she is working in. A useful measure is the 5 G line; this is the field strength at which pacemakers will dysfunction, electrical equipment may start to malfunction and magnetic tape such as that on credit cards will be erased. The extent of the magnetic field depends not only on the field strength of the magnet but also on the type of magnetic field shielding in use. In general the more recent the system the better the shielding; but beware even with well-shielded systems the magnetic field increases rapidly as you get close to the magnet bore.

Ferromagnetic attraction

At a field strength of approximately 50 G the attractive force on ferromagnetic objects becomes significant and an object such as an oxygen cylinder can become a dangerous projectile accelerating into the magnet bore: 'the missile effect'! If someone is pinned to the magnet by a ferromagnetic object then the magnet may need to be quenched to extract them.

All MRI units operate certain patient and personnel exclusions because of the risks of ferromagnetic attraction and everybody entering the unit should complete a screening questionnaire. Pacemakers, automatic defibrillators, infusion pumps and neurostimulators may malfunction at very low field strengths and patients with these devices should not be allowed anywhere near the magnetic field. Many implanted prosthetic devices are non-ferromagnetic. Objects of unknown content, such as surgical clips, can be tested by suspending with thread from the magnet bore, or with a hand held magnet. Some ferromagnetic items pose little threat to the patient as they are firmly anchored, such as joint prostheses. There are some items where any movement would be critical, such as intracerebral aneurysm clips (as little fibrosis occurs in vessels in the central nervous system) or intraocular metallic fragments and patients with these *in situ* must not be placed in the magnetic field unless their nonmagnetic content is known unequivocally. The newer types of heart valves are not ferromagnetic and flow changes or heating do not seem to cause problems. There are extensive reviews of the magnetic susceptibilities of biomedical implants available and no patient should be taken near an MRI system if there is any query about the safety of any prosthetic device, implant or surgical clip, as disasters have occurred. Plain X-rays can be used to search for metal fragments if there is concern about their presence.

Biological effects of high magnetic fields

Large numbers of studies carried out to date suggest that there are no hazards of occupational exposure to high magnetic fields. Nevertheless, clinical MRI has only been in use for just over 10 years and caution is certainly advised to high-risk personnel such as women in the first trimester of pregnancy. Although there are no limits on total MRI exposure, local exposure levels are controlled. During MRI the patient is exposed to three different types of electromagnetic radiation; the static magnetic field, the gradient magnetic fields and the radiofrequency electromagnetic fields. Field strength for clinical use has an upper limit of 2.0 T, gradient varying magnetic fields must be kept at less than $3\,T\,s^{-1}$ and radiofrequency must be limited to $2\,W\,kg^{-1}$ over 1 g of tissue and $0.1\,W\,kg^{-1}$ averaged over the whole body

Other MRI problems

Gradient noise

The gradient magnetic fields produce a loud thumping or tapping which can be very disconcerting for the awake patient and may necessitate deeper levels of sedation or anaesthesia than might otherwise be required. Hearing loss has occurred. Magnet-compatible earplugs can be used.

Contrast media

The agents used for MRI differ significantly from conventional contrast media. The most

Table 23.2 Monitoring in a magnetic resonance system

Problems	Solutions
Static magnetic field means monitoring equipment must be kept away from the magnet	Use specifically designed compatible monitoring equipment when possible
Radiofrequency and gradient magnetic fields induce currents in leads and probes causing interference with monitoring degradation of images burns	Remove all magnetic components from probes or use plastic/disposable probes Keep leads short and do not form loops Position probes away from the area being imaged
Introduction of stray radiofrequency current by leads acting as aerials causes degradation of images	Remove probes and leads when not in use Use fibreoptic cables when possible

commonly used agent for MRI is gadopentate dimeglumine (Gd-DTPA. Magnevist) which has a high therapeutic ratio and a low incidence of side effects (2.4%) when compared with iodinated contrast agents. There is a reported incidence of severe hypertension and anaphylactoid reactions of about 1 in 100 000.

MONITORING IN THE MRI ENVIRONMENT

The changing gradient magnetic fields used for image localization, and the radiofrequency currents used to excite the proton nuclei, can induce currents and heating in monitoring leads, which cause interference with monitoring and have resulted in burns. Monitoring equipment and leads can also act as aerials which breach the radiofrequency screen surrounding the magnet and introduce stray radiofrequency currents which cause degradation of the magnetic resonance images.

There have been many changes in the field of monitoring in the MRI environment. When I began working with MRI in 1989 there was no specifically designed equipment available and so all the original papers about anaesthesia and MRI discuss modifying equipment. Now MRI compatible monitoring equipment can be purchased. However, it is very expensive and the anaesthetist must understand the problems of using monitoring with MRI in order to avoid the pitfalls that can still occur. The problems and some of the solutions are summarized in Table 23.2. Problems of breaching radiofrequency screens around magnets are less significant now, as current practice is to build the radiofrequency screens into the walls of the magnet room. The introduction of stray radiofrequency electromagnetic radiation by leads acting as aerials is then not a problem if all the anaesthetic equipment is inside the magnet room. If the anaesthetic equipment and monitoring is outside the room and leads are run through the radiofrequency screen, then the potential for problems still exists. Mains power supplies can also carry interference through the radiofrequency screen and monitoring equipment should use an adequately filtered and isolated power source or be run by batteries. Batteries are strongly ferromagnetic and battery powered monitoring equipment must be very firmly secured within the magnetic field.

Specific monitors

ECG

Voltage is induced as blood, a conducting medium, flows through the magnetic field. Changes are maximal when the blood flow is at 90° to the magnetic field and are seen as ST and T wave abnormalities, which should not cause concern. Artefacts produced by the gradient and radiofrequency fields can be interpreted as complexes resulting in an elevated heart rate. All electrodes and leads should be non-magnetic to avoid current induction. The beam of a standard cathode ray oscilloscope ECG display will be pulled off-centre by the powerful magnetic field: this problem can be overcome by using an ECG with a liquid crystal display. Many manufacturers now supply an ECG with the MRI system but this is usually meant to be used for timing imaging sequences with the heart beat (gating). Another ECG system may be required for monitoring purposes.

Pulse oximetry

Pulse oximetry provides information on adequacy of oxygenation as well as heart rate and cardiac output, but it has proved to be the most difficult monitor to use within magnetic resonance systems. When modified standard systems have been used, currents and heating have been induced in the cable resulting in interference which is aggravated by poor signal due to patient movement or to poor probe placement. More seriously, patient injuries, especially burns, have been particularly associated with the use of pulse oximeters in MRI. The use of fibreoptic monitoring systems solves these problems as there is no electrical or conductive material in which current and heating can be induced or transmitted. With MRI compatible equipment now available, patient injury from an adapted pulse oximeter would be difficult to defend.

Blood pressure

Non-invasive blood pressure monitoring is relatively straightforward to use. A system can be kept at the edge of the magnetic field and used with extended cables and nylon connections. If invasive pressure monitoring is required and the transducer leads will need to breach the radiofrequency screen, the leads should be passed through radiofrequency filters installed in conjunction with advice from the hospital medical physics department and the MRI system manufacturers.

Stethoscopes

Precordial and oesophageal stethoscopes seem appealing as basic monitors especially for neonates and infants undergoing MRI. However, long lengths of tubing are required and the noise produced by the changing gradient fields, which can be quite considerable, may obscure heart and breath sounds.

Capnography

Capnography is a very useful MRI monitor. It does not produce interference and can be used as a ventilation disconnect alarm. It can also be used to monitor respiration in sedated patients by taping the narrow-bore tubing close to the mouth or nose. Long lengths of tubing are required and there is an increased lag and alarm time. This is an important monitor that can be used, without risk to the patient and without causing image interference, if no specialized MRI monitoring equipment is available.

ANAESTHESIA IN THE MAGNETIC FIELD

Although new MRI systems are becoming much faster, one image can still take as long as 20 min to acquire and the whole examination may last over 1 h. Young children and confused or mentally disabled adults may require general anaesthesia to achieve this. Unconscious patients will need airway protection and controlled ventilation. The narrow magnet bore makes many patients feel claustrophobic; reassurance, counselling and prone positioning should overcome this. Only in rare cases should sedation or general anaesthesia be used for adults.

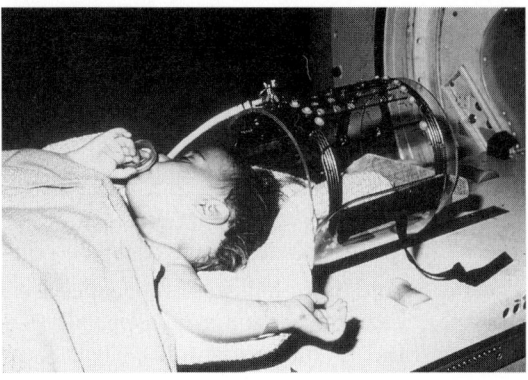

Figure 23.3 A sedated toddler about to be placed within an MRI head coil for imaging of the brain. The child will then go into the magnet bore and will not be visible or easily accessible. MRI head coils may make placement of connections and tubing difficult in the anaesthetized patient: use of a south or north facing tracheal tube eases this problem.

If an anaesthetized patient goes head first into the magnet then the airway is completely inaccessible and should be secured. For examination of the brain or cervical spine a head coil is placed around the patients head or neck (Figure 23.3). There may be insufficient space for a standard tracheal tube and catheter mount, a RAE type tube is ideal. All connections must be plastic. The laryngeal mask is also widely used for MRI and a mask with no ferromagnetic components is now specifically made for MRI. The individual anaesthetist must weigh the risks of using the laryngeal mask in this environment (difficult access to the patient, inability to see the patient, non-tipping table, the time required to detect an airway problem and then extract the patient from the magnet) against its advantages.

The major problem facing the anaesthetist setting up an anaesthetic service for MRI is where to site the anaesthetic machine. The best option in my opinion is to site the machine within the magnet field close to the magnet bore. This eliminates the need for extra long breathing systems and allows the anaesthetist to remain close to the patient. MRI compatible anaesthetic machines with MRI compatible ventilators are now made by most of the major manufacturers (Figure 23.4). A cheaper option, perhaps for occasional use, is to use a firmly secured wall mounted back bar if an anaesthetic machine is not required. The output of vaporizers within the field may vary slightly with position; output should be checked with the anaesthetic machine in its normal position. Anaesthetic machines must be run from piped medical gases as changing cylinders within the magnetic field can be extremely dangerous.

The anaesthetic machine can be sited at the edge of, or outside the magnetic field. Long lengths of breathing system tubing are required, with a large compressible volume and an increased risk of disconnection (Figure 23.5). Zorab (1995) has written a very practical review on providing a general anaesthesia service for MRI. He takes the opposite view to this author, i.e. the anaesthetic machine is better sited out of the MRI room.

The anaesthetized patient can breathe spontaneously or their lungs can be ventilated by hand. Ventilators used within the field must be MRI compatible; several commercial MRI

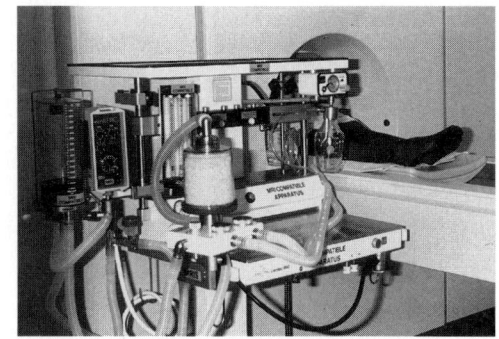

Figure 23.4 A patient within a 1.0 T magnet. In an adult having a brain scan only the legs are visible, the rest of the patient is within the magnet bore. An MRI-compatible anaesthetic machine and ventilator are sited next to the magnet bore within the magnetic field.

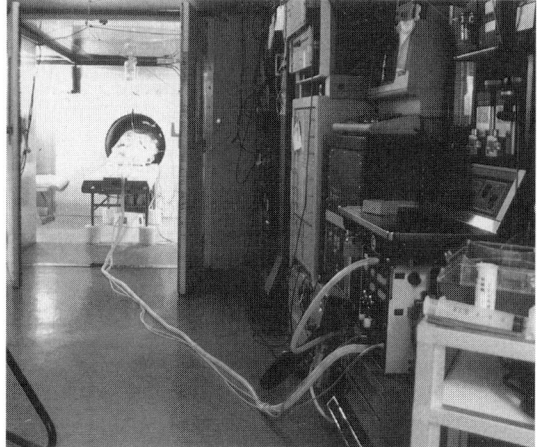

Figure 23.5 A patient from an intensive care unit being studied within a 1.6 T magnet research system. The anaesthetic machine and monitoring equipment are sited at the edge of the magnetic field. Note the long lengths of ventilator tubing required.

ventiltors are now available. A ventilator available in most hospitals is the Nuffield Penlon 200 (Penlon Abingdon, UK). It is valveless and only a small and insignificant part of its casing is ferromagnetic. With the addition of a Newton paediatric valve it can be used safely to ventilate babies as well as adults in the magnet. Breathing systems should be light weight, have no metal components and a low expiratory resistance and internal compliance. Suitable systems include the Bain, Lack and Ayre's T-piece. Anaesthesia can be maintained with a volatile agent or intravenously. The motor of infusion pumps may start to malfunction at field strengths of 30–50 G and extended infusion lines are required.

Specific problem groups of patients

Critically ill patients

As the scope of MRI expands there is likely to be an increasing demand to image critically ill patients. It is certainly possible to examine these patients with MRI but it needs planning and plenty of time made available in the MRI schedule. Ventilation has already been described. The main problems are presented by the number of lines and infusion pumps the patient may be attached to. These should be detached from the patient unless absolutely essential. Those infusions that must be continued need extensions of adequate length to keep the pumps outside the 30 G line as discussed above.

There is a theoretical risk of microshock being induced by the passage of conducting fluid such as 0.9% saline, through central venous or pulmonary artery catheters in contact with heart muscle in critically ill patients, or by the induction of current in intravascular pacing wires. This possibility has been investigated in a sheep heart model and there appears to be little risk to patients with a central venous catheter. Pulmonary artery catheters and intravascular pacing catheters should be disconnected from all electrical connections before the patient enters the magnet bore; pacing wires are unsafe and must be disconnected and taped separately with an insulating material if they must remain in place during a magnetic resonance examination.

Babies and infants

Maintenance of body temperature is critical in sick children, but the MRI environment is cold and air-conditioned to ensure optimal function of gradient coils and computer systems. Small children lose body heat rapidly in such a cold environment. The child's temperature can be measured during the examination using a rectal temperature probe passed to a monitor through a radiofrequency filter. Examination time should be kept to a minimum. Small children should be wrapped well and their heads covered. They should be returned immediately, at the end of the examination, to a warm environment or to a transport incubator.

RESUSCITATION

If you are unfortunate enough to have to resuscitate a patient who is in the magnet, remove them immediately from the magnet bore and as far out of the field as possible. If the arrest team are called they must be inspected for magnetic items before entering the field. Defibrillator and laryngoscope batteries are magnetic. Plastic laryngoscopes are available (e.g. Penlon, UK) and the standard batteries can be replaced by a single lithium battery, with an aluminium spacer: the whole unit can then be safely taken into the field. Resuscitation bags must have no magnetic parts.

PLANNING

Ideally an anaesthetist should be involved at the planning stage of an MRI unit. Piped medical gases are essential and the installation of isolated filtered a.c. power circuit and radiofrequency filters will minimize interference from monitoring equipment. Purchase of an MRI compatible anaesthetic machine and ventilator and fibreoptic monitoring systems will reduce potential anaesthetic problems. Space for resuscitation, induction and recovery from anaesthesia will enhance patient safety and increase patient throughput. Anaesthesia in an MRI unit should not be undertaken lightly; before working in an MRI unit the anaesthetist should have an awareness of the potential problems posed by MRI. The anaesthetist has a valuable role to play in increasing patient safety as well as facilitating optimal image acquisition in this exciting and uniquely challenging environment.

FURTHER READING

Goldberg, M. (1984) Systemic reactions to intravascular contrast media: a guide for the anaesthesiologist. *Anesthesiology*, **60**, 46–56.

Henderson, K. H., Lu, J. K., Strauss, T. K. J. et al. (1994) Radiation exposure of anesthesiologists. *Journal of Clinical Anesthesiology*, **6**, 37–41.

Holshouser, B. A., Hinshaw, D. B. and Shellock, F. G. (1993) Sedation, anesthesia, and physiologic monitoring during MR imaging: evaluation of procedures and equipment. *Journal of Magnetic Resonance Imaging*, **3**, 553–558.

Menon, D. K., Peden, C. J., Hall, A. S., Sargentoni, J. and Whitwam, J. G. (1992) Magnetic resonance for the anaesthetist. Part I: physical principles, applications, safety aspects. *Anaesthesia*, **47**, 240–255.

Patteson, S. K. and Chesney, J. T. (1992). Anesthetic management for magnetic resonance imaging: problems and solutions. *Anesthesia and Analgesia*, **74**, 121–128.

Peden, C. J., Menon, D. K., Hall, A. S., Sargentoni, J. and Whitwam, J. G. (1992). Magnetic resonance for the anaesthetist. Part II: anaesthesia and monitoring in MR units. *Anaesthesia*, **47**, 508–517.

Report of a Joint Working Party of the Royal College of Anaesthetists and the Royal College of Radiologists (1992) *Sedation and Anaesthesia in Radiology*. Royal Colleges, London.

Sury, M. R. J., Johnstone, G. and Bingham, R. M. (1992) Anaesthesia for magnetic resonance imaging of children. *Pediatric Anaesthesia*, **2**, 61–68.

Tobin, J. R., Spurrier, E. A. and Wetzel, R. C. (1992) Anaesthesia for critically ill children during magnetic resonance imaging. *British Journal of Anaesthesia*, **69**, 482–486.

Young, W. L. and Pile-Spellman, J. (1994) Anesthetic considerations for interventional neuroradiology. *Anesthesiology*, **80**, 427–456.

Zorab, J. S. M. (1995) A general anaesthesia service for Magnetic Resonance Imaging. *European Journal of Anaesthesiology*, **12**, 387–395.

ENDOCRINE SURGERY   24

R. A. Mason

This chapter describes a variety of endocrine diseases which, if untreated, may adversely influence the course of anaesthesia, or in which surgery is the definitive treatment. For anaesthesia and surgery to be undertaken safely, the anaesthetist must have a thorough knowledge of the effects of under- or overactivity of the particular gland, the diagnosis and treatment of the disease, and problems that might be encountered during surgery. The account of each condition is not intended to be exhaustive, but simply to include information that is pertinent to anaesthesia and surgery.

When discussing intraoperative management, the author has deliberately avoided giving detailed anaesthetic 'recipes', and has merely outlined principles that might guide the choice of drugs or techniques. It is now accepted that the safety of anaesthesia for patients with endocrine diseases rarely depends on the use of particular drugs, but on a detailed knowledge of the pathophysiology and pharmacology, on careful preparation of the patient for surgery, and on the thoughtful use of perioperative monitoring.

On the subject of monitoring, in order to prevent repetition, it is assumed that minimal standards of monitoring are normally undertaken. A specific monitor may be mentioned in order to highlight a particular problem, or because it is used in addition to basic monitoring.

THYROID

The thyroid gland is situated in the neck, deep to the strap muscles, and consists of two symmetrical, pear-shaped lobes joined by an isthmus, which lies anterior to the trachea at the level of the second to fourth rings. Local structures of particular relevance are the external branch of the superior laryngeal nerve, which descends close to the superior thyroid vessels to supply the cricothyroid muscle and the recurrent laryngeal nerve, which ascends in the tracheo-oesophageal groove in proximity to the inferior thyroid artery and provides the motor supply to all the intrinsic muscles of the larynx, apart from the cricothyroid. Although damage to these nerves is rare, they are potentially at risk when the adjacent vessels are being secured, particularly during thyroid re-exploration, or when the anatomy is distorted by a large goitre.

The gland synthesizes and secretes two types of hormone; iodine containing hormones, tri-iodothyronine (T_3) and thyroxine (T_4), and a polypeptide hormone, calcitonin. Calcitonin, in conjunction with parathyroid hormone, regulates serum calcium levels; the thyroid hormones control metabolic activity, growth and the development of the nervous system. Histologically, the functional unit of the thyroid is the follicle, an irregular, spheroidal structure consisting of an outer layer of epithelial cells resting on a basement

Short Practice of Anaesthesia. Edited by M. Morgan and G. M. Hall. Published in 1997 by Chapman & Hall, London. ISBN 0 412 71890 1

membrane, and a central part which contains iodinated thyroglobulin, the inactive, storage form of thyroxine. Iodine is absorbed from the gut, where it is reduced to iodide and enters the circulation. Iodide is subsequently concentrated by the thyroid epithelial cells, which oxidize it into iodine. Iodine binds with tyrosine residues to form mono-iodotyrosine and di-iodotyrosine. Coupling of these occurs to form either thyroxine (T_4) or tri-iodothyronine (T_3), both of which become bound to thyroglobulin, a glycolated protein which is synthesized in the lumen of the epithelial cell and secreted into the cavity. When thyroid hormones are required, small droplets of colloid re-enter the epithelial cell to fuse with lysosomes and proteolytic enzymes act to release T_4 (and some T_3), both of which enter the circulation. The majority of circulating hormone is in the form of T_4, but in the peripheral tissues it is converted into the biologically active form T_3, which is responsible for most of its effects.

Release of thyroxine is controlled by thyroid stimulating hormone (TSH) from the anterior pituitary, which in turn is controlled by thyroid releasing hormone (TRH) from the hypothalamus and by feedback inhibition of T_4 and T_3. TRH is manufactured in cell bodies in the hypothalamus and travels down the axon to the median eminence of the pituitary. It enters the circulation through a capillary plexus, passes into long portal veins and leaves from a second capillary plexus in the anterior pituitary, to act on target cells. These cells respond to the relevant releasing or inhibiting hormones, by increasing or decreasing the output of thyroid stimulating hormone.

THYROID ENLARGEMENT, WITH OR WITHOUT HYPERTHYROIDISM

Pathophysiology

Goitre is a general term for swelling of the thyroid gland. Goitres may be toxic or non-toxic and enlargement may be diffuse, multinodular or solitary. The commonest causes of hyperthyroidism are diffuse, toxic goitre (Grave's disease) and toxic, multinodular goitre. Other pathologies responsible for thyroid swelling include non-toxic, diffuse and multinodular goitres and carcinoma of the thyroid.

In thyrotoxicosis, there is an increase in size and number of thyroid epithelial cells and acceleration of their work rate, so that excess hormones are produced. The extensive influence exerted by these hormones at a cellular level means that in states of over- and under-production there are profound effects on a wide range of tissues. Thyroid hormones stimulate oxygen consumption and heat production; protein synthesis including that of specific enzyme proteins; carbohydrate and lipid metabolism; transport of aminoacids, carbohydrate and electrolytes into cells; influence neurotransmitters and their receptors; control cell growth and maturation. In addition, they affect the metabolism of specific drugs.

Activation of the adrenergic nervous system can account for many of the symptoms and signs of thyrotoxicosis. However, thyroid hormones do not actually increase plasma catecholamine levels, but may act on the density of adrenergic receptors and the sensitivity of tissues to catecholamines.

Surgery

Anaesthesia may be required for operations on the thyroid gland itself, or occasionally a patient with undiagnosed thyrotoxicosis may present for incidental emergency or elective surgery. Surgery is most commonly required for non-functioning thyroid nodules. Whilst thyrotoxicosis is mainly treated with either drugs or radioiodine, subtotal thyroidectomy may be indicated for large goitres producing symptoms of compression and for those patients who decline radioiodine treatment. During surgery, sufficient thyroid tissue should be left on each side to prevent subsequent hypothyroidism.

Clinical

A thyroid swelling in the neck, which sometimes extends retrosternally, is the usual presentation. The patient may be euthyroid or thyrotoxic. Signs and symptoms of classical thyrotoxicosis include weight loss, increased appetite, sweating, heat intolerance, nervousness, irritability, fine tremor, fatigue, tachycardia, goitre and exophthalmos. Older patients may develop atrial fibrillation and congestive cardiac failure. Clinically obvious myopathy is infrequent, but there is some degree of EMG abnormality in 90% of patients. If the thyroid is greatly enlarged it may cause compression and/or deviation of the trachea. If the tracheal diameter is reduced by more than 50% the patient will develop stridor, which may be positional, or may occur only on exercise.

On biochemical investigation, TSH levels are decreased and total or free thyroxine levels are high. T_3 thyrotoxicosis may occasionally occur, in which a low TSH level is accompanied by a high T_3 level, but normal total or free T_4 levels.

Preparation

Thyrotoxicosis must first be controlled, preferably using antithyroid drugs. When surgery has been undertaken in the absence of adequate control, perioperative complications have included tachycardia, atrial fibrillation, a hypermetabolic state resembling malignant hyperthermia, pulmonary oedema and thyroid storm.

Carbimazole, 30–45 mg daily, should be given until the patient is euthyroid. It interferes with thyroid synthesis by inhibiting organification of iodide and coupling of iodothyronines, but takes 6–8 weeks to produce adequate control. Since treatment with carbimazole sometimes increases the size and vascularity of the gland, it may be stopped 10 days before surgery and potassium iodide given, to inhibit temporarily the release of thyroid hormones and reduce gland vascularity. If the patient is troubled by tremor, anxiety and palpitations, β-adrenoceptor blockers can be started at the time of initial diagnosis. Propranolol, 30–60 mg 8 hourly, blocks the peripheral actions of thyroid hormone and also stops the deiodination of T_4 to T_3. Sometimes patients with mild thyrotoxicosis are prepared for surgery using β-blockers alone, with potassium iodide added for the final 10 days. However, since propranolol only blocks the peripheral effects of the thyroid hormones rather than their output from the gland, there is a small risk of precipitating a thyroid crisis, should the propranolol be omitted accidentally.

The sleeping pulse-rate gives a good clinical indication of the adequacy or otherwise of control on admission for surgery. Indirect laryngoscopy is undertaken in the ENT department to check for abnormalities of vocal cord movement before operation, for both clinical and medicolegal reasons. Routine chest X-ray with thoracic inlet views will demonstrate any retrosternal extension of the thyroid. If a large goitre is accompanied by respiratory symptoms suggestive of tracheal compression, such as breathlessness on exertion or positional stridor, or if there is superior vena caval or thoracic outlet obstruction, a CT scan is essential. This will show the exact site and dimensions of any constriction, and in the case of carcinoma, identify malignant invasion of the trachea. If there is stridor and critical airway narrowing, the patient should be prepared for an awake fibreoptic intubation.

For the thyrotoxic patient receiving propranolol, care should be taken that no dose is omitted in the perioperative period. A sedative premedication is usual.

Intraoperative

Since access to the patient is limited, monitoring should be carefully sited and a three-way tap and extensions to the intravenous infusion prepared. Rarely, severe tracheal narrowing results in stridor, in which case fibreoptic intubation should be undertaken before the patient is anaesthetized, since in the event of airway difficulty, the presence of the goitre prevents an emergency tracheostomy being performed.

An armoured orotracheal tube should be firmly fixed in place and care should be taken to protect the eyes, particularly if exophthalmos is present. Although nowadays it is usual to use intermittent positive pressure ventilation (IPPV) to prevent coughing and straining, only partial neuromuscular blockade should be maintained during thyroid dissection, in case the surgeon needs to identify the nerve supply using a nerve stimulator. The patient should be positioned with the head on a ring or horseshoe and with a sandbag under the shoulders, but hyperextension of the neck in elderly people is inadvisable. The table may be placed with a slight head-up tilt to reduce venous pressure, but care should be taken to prevent an air embolus. If possible, the anaesthetist should check the movement of the vocal cords at the end of surgery.

Postoperative

Permanent damage to the innervation of the vocal cords is rare. However, in the case of difficult and prolonged surgery, temporary partial paralyses may occur secondary to tissue oedema. The external branch of the superior laryngeal nerve supplies the cricothyroid muscle, a tensor of the vocal cords and damage results in hoarseness. The recurrent laryngeal nerve supplies the remainder of the motor supply to the larynx. Unilateral damage produces an immobile vocal cord that lies close to the midline and at a slightly lower level than the normal vocal cord, which can usually compensate. However, if partial or complete paralyses of both cords occur, there may be immediate postoperative problems, since both cords flap together. If the nerve supply to the abductors is damaged, airway obstruction secondary to glottic closure occurs immediately, in which case re-intubation should be performed followed by tracheostomy. If the vocal cords are partly paralysed in abduction, aspiration can occur.

Tracheal collapse is an extremely rare complication of surgery on a large, longstanding goitre that has softened the tracheal cartilage. Elective tracheostomy may be required.

Haemorrhage can occur in the first 24 h, usually as a result of failure to secure one of the thyroid vessels deep to the strap muscles. Bleeding into a confined space initially causes local pressure on veins, resulting in laryngeal and subglottic oedema. On the ward the patient presents with wound swelling, pallor and respiratory difficulty, whilst severe stridor may herald respiratory arrest, hypoxaemia and cardiac arrest. Prompt removal of clips and cutting of the sutures securing the strap muscles, should release the clot and control the immediate crisis. However, stridor may still be present because laryngeal oedema will take time to resolve and in a dire emergency urgent tracheal intubation or cricothyroidotomy may be required. The patient must be returned to the operating theatre as soon as possible to explore the wound and control the bleeding vessel. Tracheal intubation may be more difficult than normal because of the presence of laryngeal oedema and a range of tube sizes will be needed.

Thyroid crisis (or storm) is a term given to the abrupt onset of symptoms of a severe hypermetabolic state occurring in a patient with thyrotoxicosis. It is often precipitated by acute illness, surgery or trauma, usually if the disease is uncontrolled, or if treatment before surgery has been undertaken with β-blockers and potassium iodide alone. Thyroid storm is a clinical rather than a biochemical diagnosis. In the postoperative period it may present with hyperthermia, tachycardia, agitation, nausea, vomiting, abdominal pain, diarrhoea, jaundice, hepatomegaly, infection or the sudden onset of confusion or mania.

Treatment is urgent and should not await laboratory confirmation of thyrotoxicosis, since fatalities have occurred. Management includes administration of antithyroid drugs, therapy to control systemic effects of the crisis and identification and treatment of the precipitating factor. Carbimazole, 60–120 mg, or propylthiouracil, 600–1200 mg, is given orally or by nasogastric tube to inhibit new hormone synthesis and the drug will start to act within an hour. Potassium or sodium iodide immediately inhibits further release of thyroid hormone, but should not be given until at least 1 h after the antithyroid drug, to prevent the crisis worsening. Propranolol orally, 20–80 mg 6 hourly, or intravenously, 1–5 mg 6 hourly, blocks the peripheral effects of T_3, but should be given with caution in the presence of atrial fibrillation, since digoxin will be required. In the short term an esmolol infusion may be used. Hydrocortisone, 100 mg given 6 hourly, inhibits the peripheral conversion of T_4 to T_3. Active cooling will reduce metabolic demands and in cases of severe decompensation, IPPV and muscle paralysis may be required. Sources of infection should be sought, although antibiotics may be given empirically. Fluid, electrolyte and glucose replacement will be required and heart failure should be treated, if present.

Hypocalcaemia following thyroid surgery may be transient, or permanent. Symptoms of hypocalcaemia, which mainly result from increased excitability of muscle, include paraesthesiae, numbness, muscle cramps and tetany. Chvostek's sign of facial muscle twitching is elicited by tapping the facial nerve in front of the earlobe, below the zygomatic arch. Trousseau's sign is carpal spasm produced by inflating a sphygmomanometer above systolic arterial pressure. Myocardial contractility is decreased by hypocalcaemia and prolonged QT interval occurs on the ECG. Initially, calcium gluconate 10–20 ml should be given, which will increase the ionized calcium by 0.5–1.5 mmol l^{-1}.

HYPOTHYROIDISM

Pathophysiology

Hypothyroidism may be primary, or secondary to pituitary or hypothalamic disease. Autoimmune thyroiditis is the commonest primary cause, followed by the sequelae of surgical or radioiodine treatment of thyrotoxicosis. The disease is associated with deposition of a mucinous substance, a combination of salts, mucopolysaccharide and protein, that gives an abnormal puffiness of the skin and thickening of the subcutaneous tissues. Hypothyroidism is associated with a reduction in oxygen consumption and body heat production. Blood flow to skin surfaces is reduced and redirected to maintain core temperature, so that the patient is in a state of chronic vasoconstriction. There is a decreased end-organ response to catecholamines, reduced blood volume, cardiac output and pulse rate. In the absence of thyroid hormone, metabolism of certain drugs may be greatly impaired. If hypothyroidism remains untreated, an additional challenge such as an acute infection may precipitate myxoedema coma. This is a decompensatory state in which mental deterioration and impaired thermoregulation are imposed on the features described below. It may present in the immediate postoperative period, usually affects elderly patients and may be fatal.

Surgery

Patients with incidental hypothyroidism may present for operation, or alternatively emergency surgery may be inadvertently undertaken in hypothyroid patients. Elective surgery should be delayed in all but those with mild disease.

Clinical

Hypothyroidism produces a range of symptoms and signs, from mild to severe, affecting all systems of the body. Characteristic features include a pale, cool skin, husky voice, loss of the outer part of the eyebrows, weight gain and cold intolerance. There is a low metabolic rate, with a delay in the relaxation phases of reflexes. Cardiovascular complications include ischaemic heart disease, bradycardia, pericardial effusion, mild hypertension and cardiac failure. Neurological complications such as carpal tunnel syndrome, polyneuritis, myopathy and cerebellar syndrome may occur. The ECG is of low voltage with flattened or inverted T waves, prolonged QT interval and sinus bradycardia. In severe disease there is lethargy, hypothermia and respiratory depression, progressing to myxoedema coma. Chest X-ray may show mild cardiac enlargement or the presence of a pericardial effusion. There is a mild normocytic anaemia due to decreased red cell production and the white cell response to infection is depressed. Hyponatraemia may occur. Biochemical investigation shows an an increased TSH and decreased T_4 and sometimes T_3.

Treatment

Hypothyroidism should be treated cautiously, particularly in the elderly or those with cardiac disease, because of the danger of increasing cardiac workload in the presence of impaired coronary artery reserve. Oral l-thyroxine, 100–200 μg daily, or if heart disease is present, 25 μg daily, increasing at 3- to 4-weekly intervals, should be given. The only indication for intravenous thyroid replacement is in patients with myxoedema coma, or for those with severe hypothyroidism in whom urgent surgery is required, in which case management in a high dependency area is advisable. A single dose of lyothyronine sodium, 50 μg, should be given slowly, followed by 25 μg 8 hourly, using ECG control. Myxoedema coma may necessitate IPPV and invasive monitoring with a pulmonary artery catheter. Additional treatment includes gradual correction of hypothermia, antibiotics, hydrocortisone 100 mg 6 hourly and intravenous fluids, which should contain some dextrose. The patient's condition should start to improve within 24–48 h of initial treatment.

Intraoperative

Impaired drug metabolism means that hypothyroid individuals show extreme sensitivity to anaesthetic agents, narcotics and analgesics; therefore all drugs should be given with extreme caution. The combination of poor myocardial function, vasoconstriction and reduced blood volume, results in pronounced susceptibility to myocardial depressants and vasodilators. Severe hypotension, or even cardiac arrest, has been reported after induction of anaesthesia in unsuspected cases. Careful cardiovascular monitoring is needed because of minimal cardiac reserve. An impaired response to hypercapnoea, hypoventilation and reduced respiratory muscle strength means that ventilation should be controlled during all but brief procedures. Small doses of neuromuscular blockers should be used and if a nerve stimulator shows that return of function is incomplete, postoperative IPPV should be considered. Core temperature should be monitored and a warming blanket and blood warmer used.

Postoperative

Hypothyroidism can be unsuspected until after surgery, when the first indication may be delay in recovery from anaesthesia, hypothermia, or respiratory failure. Myxoedematous infiltration of the tongue and vocal cords can predispose to obstructive symptoms during sleep, particularly when analgesics or sedatives are used. Myxoedema coma may be precipitated by anaesthesia, or by any acute illness such as pneumonia.

PARATHYROID

HYPERPARATHYROIDISM

Pathophysiology

Four brownish yellow parathyroid glands are embedded in the posterolateral surfaces of the thyroid lobes and secrete parathyroid hormone (PTH), which is involved in calcium homeostasis. Its main actions are on bone, kidney and the gastrointestinal tract. Parathyroid hormone stimulates the activity of osteocytes and osteoclasts and, by increasing the rate of bone resorption, increases ionized plasma calcium and lowers plasma phosphate levels. In the kidney, its effect is to increase tubular resorption of calcium and decrease that of phosphate. Secretion of PTH is stimulated by a decrease in plasma calcium. Hypercalcaemia occurs when the amount of calcium released into the circulation exceeds the capacity of the renal excretion mechanism.

There are two types of hypercalcaemia of particular relevance to anaesthetists; hypercalcaemia associated with primary (and sometimes secondary) hyperparathyroidism, for which parathyroid surgery is needed, and hypercalcaemia associated with malignancy. Control of the latter becomes important when general anaesthesia is required for investigative procedures, such as gland or bronchial biopsy.

Primary hyperparathyroidism may be due to parathyroid adenoma (84%), parathyroid hyperplasia (15%) or parathyroid carcinoma (1%). Acute hypercalcaemia of malignancy is often more severe and the management of this is discussed below.

Surgery

Parathyroidectomy is the treatment for primary hyperparathyroidism and sometimes for the secondary form if it happens to be associated with parathyroid hyperplasia. In the latter condition, after parathyroidectomy, small amounts of parathyroid tissue may be transplanted into another site, such as the forearm, to facilitate access in the event of further hyperplasia occurring.

Clinical

There are a number of symptoms and signs common to all hypercalcaemias, regardless of aetiology. However, some may provide clues to the primary cause; for example, features such as renal stones, joint manifestations and peptic ulceration tend to be associated with hyperparathyroidism, whereas a sudden onset of dehydration, renal insufficiency and mental changes is more characteristic of the hypercalcaemia of malignancy.

General clinical features of hypercalcaemia can be divided broadly into neuromuscular, renal and gastrointestinal. Decreased tone in skeletal and intestinal muscle produces general muscle weakness, apathy, nausea, vomiting, constipation and abdominal pain. There may be signs of dehydration, with thirst, polyuria, polydipsia, renal insufficiency and mental confusion. Skeletal X-rays a show generalized decrease in bone density, bone cysts and subcortical bone resorption. A combination of hypercalcaemia (normal corrected Ca 2.20–2.55 mmol l^{-1}) and increased parathormone level is diagnostic of hyperparathyroidism.

Preparation

Symptoms usually start to occur when the plasma calcium levels exceeds 3.2 mmol l^{-1}, at which stage anorexia, vomiting and dehydration are prominent features. Dehydration is treated with fluid and electrolytes, giving 2–4 l per day for 48 h, alone or in combination with loop diuretics. This will enhance renal calcium excretion and lower plasma calcium levels by about 0.5 mmol l^{-1}. However, treatment with saline beyond this period carries the risk of electrolyte imbalance and cardiac failure. Some surgeons give 1-α-hydroxy-cholecalciferol 2–3 days before surgery. Methylene blue 5 mg kg^{-1} diluted in dextrose saline 500 ml may be given 1 h preoperatively to stain the parathyroids a greenish-blue colour.

Intraoperative

The management of parathyroidectomy is similar to that described for thyroidectomy. If methylene blue is accidentally infused rapidly in the anaesthetic room the patient may appear cyanosed.

Postoperative

Although the risk of haemorrhage and recurrent laryngeal nerve damage exists, it is much less than that associated with thyroidectomy. Plasma calcium starts to decrease at 4–12 h and reaches its lowest by 48–72 h. If it decreases below 1.6 mmol l^{-1} neuromuscular or cardiac irritability may occur, with tetany or a positive Trousseau's or Chvostek's sign. Treatment is with calcium gluconate 10% 20–30 ml.

HYPERCALCAEMIA SECONDARY TO MALIGNANT DISEASE

Pathophysiology

Severe hypercalcaemia may be associated with malignant disease, particularly carcinoma of the lung, head and neck, oesophagus, breast, renal cell and haematological malignancies. There are thought to be two main mechanisms contributing to the hypercalcaemia; the first humoral, the second local osteolysis due to metastases to bone. Hypercalcaemia may occur in the absence of bony metastases and there is evidence to suggest that the humoral mediator is a peptide, parathyroid hormone related protein, which is responsible for osteoclastic bone resorption.

Surgery

Anaesthesia may be required for surgery or investigative procedures in the presence of hypercalcaemia and the medical management is usually solely for the purpose of preparing the patient for diagnostic surgery.

Clinical

A characteristically sudden onset with profound dehydration, confusion and renal insufficiency. With severe hypercalaemia, bradyarrhythmias, bundle branch block, complete heart block and cardiac arrest may occur.

Treatment

Severe hypercalcaemia requires urgent treatment. Therapy may be divided into emergency and chronic. In acute hypercalcaemia, short term treatment with crystalloids should be given as above. For urgent lowering of calcium, calcitonin acts within hours, with a duration 2–3 days. However, its action is weak when compared with antiresorptive agents such as plicamycin, etidronate and pamidronate, whose onset is 24–48 h. However, the decision to use these latter drugs should be made with care, since in advanced stages of malignancy, hypercalcaemia may provide a kinder mode of death.

ADRENAL

The adrenal glands, situated above each kidney, consist of two embryologically distinct endocrine organs; the adrenal medulla and the adrenal cortex. The central, vascular, adrenal medulla is of ectodermal origin and contains chromaffin cells that manufacture and secrete the catecholamines, adrenaline, noradrenaline and dopamine. Chromaffin cells can manufacture a number of other peptides hormones, including enkephalins, somatostatin, neurotensin and substance P. The medulla receives a dual blood supply, from the medullary arteries and from the corticomedullary veins which carry cortisol-rich blood from the cortex. The adrenaline secreting cells are situated closest to the cortex, since they require high levels of cortisol to convert noradrenaline into adrenaline.

The surrounding adrenal cortex is of mesodermal origin and consists of three zones: an outer zona glomerulosa that secretes aldosterone (100 μg per 24 h), which is responsible for sodium balance and extracellular fluid control; the zona fasciculata which secretes mostly glucocorticoids (cortisol 16–20 mg per 24 h and corticosterone 4 mg per 24 h) and is responsible for carbohydrate, fat and protein metabolism; an inner zona reticularis, which secretes mainly androgens. All of the hormones are derived originally from the precursor, cholesterol. Aldosterone output is regulated by angiotensin II from the renin-angiotensin system and partly by an increase in plasma [K$^+$], with some support from adrenocorticotrophic hormone (ACTH). Glucocorticoids and androgens are controlled by ACTH from the anterior pituitary, which in turn is controlled by corticotrophin releasing hormone and antidiuretic hormone secreted into the hypophyseal portal system. The main regulators of ACTH output are cortisol, circadian rhythm, corticotrophin releasing hormone and stress.

PHAEOCHROMOCYTOMA

Pathophysiology

Phaeochromocytomas are rare catecholamine-secreting tumours of chromaffin cells; they are usually situated in the adrenal medulla, but may arise anywhere in the sympathetic chain. Ten per cent are extra-adrenal, but most of these lie within the abdominal cavity. They may be associated with a variety of syndromes, such as the multiple endocrine neoplasias, neurofibromatosis and von Hippel–Lindau disease. Intermittent secretion of catecholamines by the tumour produces paroxysmal episodes of hypertension, occurring spontaneously, or in response to a variety of stimuli. They may be associated with a variety of symptoms such as headache, sweating and palpitations, which can last anything from a few minutes up to an hour. The products mainly responsible for the symptoms are noradrenaline and adrenaline and to a lesser extent dopamine. However, the medulla contains a number of other vasoconstrictor peptides, whose role in the production of symptoms has not yet been defined. Secretion of these by phaeochromocytomas may account for the failure adrenoceptor blockade to completely control hypertensive crises. If adrenaline constitutes at least 20% of the total plasma catecholamine secreted, the tumour is likely to be in the adrenal, because high concentrations of cortisol from the cortex are required for synthesis of adrenaline from noradrenaline. In addition, larger tumours are usually noradrenaline secreting because they tend to outstrip the blood supply from the cortex.

The continuous secretion of a high level of catecholamines exerts a significant effect on the cardiovascular system and patients with predominantly noradrenaline secreting tumours are in a chronic state of vasoconstriction and hypovolaemia. In some individuals with longstanding disease this may result in a secondary cardiomyopathy. In addition, persistently increased catecholamine levels produce down-regulation of receptors, so that the receptors become less sensitive than normal to their effects.

Surgery

Anaesthesia may be required for elective excision of phaeochromocytoma, or previously undiagnosed patients may present with an unexpected cardiovascular crisis during surgery for an unrelated condition, or in labour. Surgical removal of the tumour is the only curative therapy, but before this is undertaken, pharmacological treatment is essential to prevent potentially fatal crises which may be associated with anaesthesia, radiological investigation, or handling of the tumour during surgery. The mortality from surgery has been reduced dramatically in the last 30 years, mainly as a result of drug treatment before surgery, but also because of improvements in monitoring and intensive care. However, phaeochromocytoma presenting during pregnancy still carries a high maternal and perinatal mortality. If the condition is diagnosed in early pregnancy, drug control followed by excision in the second trimester has been recommended. In later pregnancy, removal may be combined with Caesarean section. However, many tumours do not present until labour, when the signs and symptoms may be mistaken for those of pregnancy-induced hypertension.

Clinical

Episodes of headache, sweating and palpitations are the commonest presenting symptoms and in one series, the majority of patients had two or more of these complaints. Other common symptoms are pallor, nausea and vomiting, tremor, weakness, loin pain and dyspnoea. Paroxysmal hypertension may be superimposed on normotension, but in about 50% of patients the blood pressure is persistently elevated. During attacks patients may feel intensely unwell and have a feeling of impending doom. Chronic secretion of catecholamines may be associated with a cardiomyopathy, which resolves after tumour resection. Acute crises may be spontaneous, or provoked by exercise, bending, anaesthesia, tumour palpation or radiological procedures. Intraoperative presenting features of undiagnosed tumours include severe hypertension or hypotension with tachyarrhythmias, acute pulmonary oedema, myocardial depression and cardiogenic shock.

Preparation

The most important aspects of preparation from the anaesthetic point of view are diagnosis and localization of the tumour, together with careful pharmacological adrenoceptor blockade allowing gradual re-expansion of blood volume.

Although traditionally initial screening of suspects is undertaken by estimation of 24-hour urinary metabolites (HMMA, hydroxymethyl mandelic acid), measurements of plasma and urinary catecholamines are more sensitive and specific and are not subject to interference by dietary constituents or drugs. In the presence of equivocal results, suppression tests (using clonidine or pentolinium) may be useful, but provocation tests are hazardous and should not be undertaken. However, if in the presence of hypertension the plasma catecholamine levels are only slightly elevated, the diagnosis is unlikely. This is because chronic catecholamine secretion reduces the sensitivity of the receptors to their effects, and at least twice normal levels are required to produce hypertension. Impaired glucose tolerance may occur, particularly with the small, adrenaline secreting tumours.

A CT scan will identify most adrenal tumours, particularly if they are greater than 1 cm in diameter. MRI scans may assist in differentiation of tumours or in visualizing metastases. Radioisotope meta-iodobenzylguanidine (mIBG) imaging is helpful for locating extra-adrenal tumours or metastases; mIBG is similar in structure to noradrenaline and is taken up and concentrated in storage granules of chromaffin tissue. However, about 10% of tumours do not take up the radionuclide.

Elective surgery should only be undertaken after careful pharmacological preparation. In fact, once the diagnosis has been made, adrenoceptor blocking should be started immediately, since any crisis could produce serious, or even fatal complications. Phenoxybenzamine, a noncompetitive, mixed α_1/α_2-

antagonist, is still the mainstay of treatment and preparation should take place gradually over 10–14 days to allow cautious re-expansion of the blood volume. This is particularly important if there is evidence of cardiomyopathy or myocardial ischaemia. Oral phenoxybenzamine 10 mg twice daily initially, should be increased gradually until hypertension is controlled. Between 80 and 200 mg daily may be required. If a tachycardia develops, then a β-blocker, propranolol 40–80 mg daily, should be added. Beta blockers should never be given first, since they may precipitate a hypertensive crisis. Although the use of prazosin, a selective α_1-receptor antagonist, has been suggested as an alternative, in practice it has been found to give unsatisfactory control of hypertension and inadequate protection from catecholamine surges. This is because it is a competitive antagonist and can be displaced from its receptor site by excess circulating catecholamines, it is short acting and α_2-receptors are left unblocked. Labetalol, a mixed α- and β-blocker, has also been used. However, it is not recommended since it is a relatively weak blocker and its β-blocking effects exceed its α-effects, such that occasionally paradoxical severe hypertension has been reported. It also interferes with catecholamine estimation. Should more urgent blockade be required, an intravenous phenoxybenzamine regimen can be given, starting with an infusion of 1 mg kg^{-1}, increasing to 1.5 mg kg^{-1} on the second day, and 2 mg kg^{-1} on the third day. However, this is not recommended as routine preparation, but if urgency demands, it should be performed under strict medical supervision. During blockade there is an expansion of blood volume and decrease in haematocrit. Criteria for adequacy of blockade include control of hypertension through the 24 h, control of major symptoms and freedom from ischaemic changes on ECG. The anaesthetist should take an interest in the adequacy of preparation so that he/she is not presented in the anaesthetic room with a patient whose blood pressure is inadequately controlled. A sedative premedication and oral phenoxybenzamine and propranolol should be given on the morning of operation.

Intraoperative

During surgery, the aim is to provide conditions in which catecholamine release by the tumour, or the effect of any catecholamines released, is kept to a minimum. If the patient is hypertensive on arrival in the operating theatre, it suggests that blockade has been inadequate and surgery should be postponed. Problems during surgery, even in the apparently well-controlled patient, include severe hypertension during handling of the tumour, tachyarrhythmias, severe hypotension, and protracted hypoglycaemia following tumour removal.

A wide variety of drugs and techniques has been recommended. However, it is now accepted that adequacy of preoperative adrenoceptor blockade is of most importance in determining outcome, together with close monitoring of arterial and central venous pressures. Direct arterial monitoring should begin in the anaesthetic room and induction should be cautious, avoiding the use of suxamethonium, if possible. A combination of extradural anaesthesia with general anaesthesia can be used, but should vasopressors be required, higher than normal doses may be needed. A variety of drugs have been employed to treat intraoperative hypertension; these include phentolamine, sodium nitroprusside and GTN. Although propranolol, 1–2 mg, has traditionally been used for the treatment of tachycardia, a recent alternative is the short acting β-blocker, esmolol. A loading dose of 500 µg kg^{-1} given over 1 min is followed by an infusion of 300 µg kg^{-1} min^{-1} to maintain a pulse rate at 90–110 b.p.m. Hypotension may occur after ligation of the main veins from the tumour. Sudden reduction in catecholamine output from the tumour is in part responsible, but hypovolaemia may contribute. Patients with adrenoceptor blockade are extremely sensitive to changes in blood volume. Rapid infusion whilst monitoring the CVP will usually correct the hypotension. If it fails to do so, the use of phenylephrine or dopamine by infusion has been suggested.

Postoperative

Intensive monitoring in a high dependency area should continue in the postoperative period. Plasma glucose should be monitored, since protracted hypoglycaemia may occur. In addition it takes several days for the sensitivity of adrenoceptors to be restored to normal.

ADRENOCORTICAL INSUFFICIENCY

Pathophysiology

The three main causes of primary adrenocortical insufficiency (Addison's disease) are autoimmune (65–84%), infection and metastatic disease. Clinically apparent disease occurs only after a 90% loss of adrenocortical tissue. Secondary adrenal insufficiency results from a deficiency of ACTH secretion and usually as a result of a tumour of the pituitary or hypothalamus. Acute adrenocortical insufficiency may follow sudden withdrawal of corticosteroid therapy.

Surgery

Patients with unsuspected adrenal insufficiency may occasionally present for incidental surgery. Alternatively, patients receiving corticosteroids, or those who have received them within the previous 12 months, may have inadequate adrenal reserve to meet the demands of perioperative stress. Adrenal failure may also occur after trans-sphenoidal pituitary surgery or following the treatment of Cushing's syndrome.

Clinical

Addison's disease is more common in women than in men. Patients with chronic disease have weight loss, weakness, infertility, fatigue, emotional instability, abdominal pain, diarrhoea, hyperpigmentation of the skin and mucous membranes and intractable hiccups. Only in the later stages will the characteristic metabolic changes of hyponatraemia, hyperkalaemia, hypoglycaemia, hypercalcaemia and increased blood urea be seen. Acute cardiovascular collapse has been reported under a wide range of circumstances, in the casualty department, in the perioperative period and during pregnancy. Nausea, vomiting, severe hypotension are predominant features of the acute disease.

Treatment

In the acute situation, blood should be taken for plasma cortisol and ACTH determinations, after which therapy should be started without delay. If further investigations are likely to be required, dexamethasone, which does not interfere with plasma cortisol estimations, should be substituted for hydrocortisone. Hydrocortisone, 100 mg i.v., is given immediately and continued 6-hourly. Intravenous fluid in the form of saline, is followed by dextrose in the event of hypoglycaemia and any source of infection should be treated. For chronic glucocorticoid replacement therapy oral hydrocortisone, 20 mg in the morning and 10 mg in the evening is usual, although sometimes patients prefer 10 mg three times daily. For primary hypoadrenalism, fludrocortisone, 100–200 μg daily, should be added.

CORTICOSTEROID THERAPY AND SURGERY

Adrenal atrophy is detected 5 days after the onset of glucocorticoid therapy, if it has been administered in doses above the physiological level. If therapy is continued for more than a few weeks, it may take up to a year for the function of the hypophyseal-pituitary-adrenal axis to return completely to normal. Within this year, patients exposed to stress may have inadequate adrenal reserve and may require steroid supplements in the perioperative period. Ideally, in order to gauge the need for this, a patient's response to stress should be assessed with an ACTH stimulation test before operation. A dose of synthetic ACTH, 250 μg, is given i.v. and a blood sample for plasma cortisol is taken 30 min later. A level greater than 500 nmol l^{-1} indicates adequate adrenal function. In practice, testing is rarely done and steroid supplements are given empirically.

Traditionally, major surgical stress has been treated with hydrocortisone, 100 mg 6 hourly, but better knowledge of hypophyseal-pituitary-adrenal function and the levels of cortisol output from the adrenals suggest that this dosage is higher than is necessary. Replacement glucocorticoid therapy in the absence of adrenal function is hydrocortisone, 30 mg per 24 h. In normal patients in the perioperative period the increase in cortisol output occurs at the start of the operation. During major surgical stress it may increase to 150 mg per 24 h, although the maximum possible output from normal adrenals is almost double this level. In minor surgery the cortisol output reaches only 50 mg per 24 h. Even under major surgical stress, it has returned to normal by 48 h.

There is no advantage to be gained from giving more steroid than is necessary; on the contrary, the adverse effects on wound healing and immune function are detrimental to the patient. These considerations have led recent workers to propose that lower doses be given, based on the known glucocorticoid production rate and the magnitude of stress. For minor surgery, they suggest the equivalent of hydrocortisone 25 mg for the day of surgery and no additions unless complications occur; for moderate surgery, the equivalent of 50–75 mg 24 h^{-1} for 1–2 days and a return to normal dosages on day 2; for major surgical stress, the equivalent of hydrocortisone 100–150 mg 24 h^{-1} for 2–3 days. Thus, for those who are taking a maintenance dose of glucocorticoid, if the dose already exceeds the estimated stress requirement, additional drug will not be needed.

Equivalent dosages for a given glucocorticoid effect are: hydrocortisone 100 mg; cortisone 125 mg; prednisolone 25 mg; prednisone 25 mg; methylprednisone 20 mg; betamethasone 4 mg; triamcinolone 20 mg; or dexamethasone 4 mg.

PRIMARY ALDOSTERONISM (CONN'S SYNDROME)

Pathophysiology

Excess aldosterone production may be caused by an adrenal adenoma, adrenal hyperplasia or a carcinoma. Aldosterone is a mineralocorticoid secreted by the zona glomerulosa of the adrenal cortex. It promotes sodium reabsorption and potassium exchange, mainly in the renal tubules, but to a lesser extent in the intestine and salivary and sweat glands. The final stage of aldosterone secretion is controlled by the renin–angiotensin system, activation of which occurs in response to sodium or water depletion.

Surgery

Surgical resection of the tumour is usual.

Clinical

The main features are hypertension, hypokalaemia and alkalosis. Symptoms, should they occur, are usually secondary to the hypokalaemia and may include muscle weakness, polyuria, polydipsia and tetany. Urinary potassium is high, despite a low total body potassium and serum sodium may be in the upper range of normal, or be slightly elevated. Plasma renin levels are low and plasma aldosterone is elevated.

Preparation

A potassium infusion is required to correct depletion of stores. Hypertension should be controlled preoperatively; an aldosterone antagonist should be included, since this improves both the hypertension and potassium loss.

Intraoperative

Hypertensive peaks on induction of anaesthesia should be avoided if possible. The potassium infusion needs to be continued during surgery and normocapniea should be maintained to prevent potassium returning to the cells. An initial period of IPPV may be required in the postoperative period to counteract the respiratory acidosis that may occur at this time.

Postoperative

Provided the other adrenal is intact, steroid replacement should not be required. Following tumour removal, reversal of the electrolyte abnormalities occur earlier than correction of the hypertension.

CUSHING'S SYNDROME

Cushing's syndrome is the general term for a clinical disorder resulting from excess circulating glucocorticoid. The syndrome may be endogenous, secondary to increased secretion of cortisol or ACTH, or iatrogenic, from administration of either glucocorticoids or ACTH. Currently, Cushing's syndrome is classified into ACTH-dependent and ACTH-independent forms.

Pathophysiology

ACTH-dependent disease accounts for about 75–85% of cases of endogenous Cushing's syndrome and usually results from excess pituitary secretion of ACTH (formerly known as Cushing's disease). However, certain tumours, particularly those from lung, pancreas or kidney, may be a source of ectopic ACTH production. Relatively few cases of Cushing's syndrome are adrenal in origin (< 15%) and these consist of adrenal cortical adenomas or carcinomas. However, for the anaesthetist, features of Cushing's syndrome are most commonly seen as a result of therapeutic administration of glucocorticoids.

Surgery

In general, surgery is indicated in all types of endogenous Cushing's syndrome. It is important, therefore, to establish the exact diagnosis and the location of the lesion responsible. In the case of pituitary tumours, trans-sphenoidal pituitary microsurgery has become the treatment of choice and has an initial success rate of 95%. Adrenal adenoma or carcinoma is usually treated by unilateral or bilateral adrenalectomy.

Clinical

Cushing's syndrome is a multisystem disorder, resulting in profound long-term effects on the patient's physiology. In florid cases, the most striking external characteristics are moon face, plethora, central obesity with thin extremities, a dorsal hump and purple striae. Other clinical features include; weakness, thin skin, easy bruising, hypertension, menstrual disorders, hirsutism, impotence, proximal muscle atrophy, oedema, mental disorders, a diabetic glucose tolerance test (GTT), backache and acne. Fractures occur readily, secondary to decreased bone density, wound healing is poor and there is an increased incidence of infections. Advanced disease may be associated with severe left ventricular hypertrophy. Biochemical abnormalities include hypokalaemic alkalosis, sodium and water retention, hyperglycaemia, lack of diurnal variation in plasma cortisol with its failure to decrease at night and increased urinary free cortisol.

Thus, in a suspected case, the first step is to confirm the diagnosis of the syndrome by measurement of 24-hour urinary free cortisol and/or hydroxysteroid secretion, together with an overnight dexamethasone suppression test. If these tests are normal, Cushing's syndrome is excluded. If they are positive, the next step is to investigate the cause. Details are beyond the scope of this text, but the tests are divided into biochemical ones that examine feedback of the hypothalamic-pituitary-adrenal axis (including basal plasma ACTH and corticotrophin releasing hormone levels) and radiological imaging studies to identify pituitary, adrenal or ectopic lesions.

Preparation

For any patient with Cushing's syndrome in whom surgery is proposed, biochemical and cardiovascular evaluation and treatment are important. Initial examination may reveal hypertension with or without cardiac failure. Patients may require correction of hypokalaemia, reduced potassium stores and alterations in intravascular fluid volumes. After potassium replacement, treatment with spironolactone, an aldosterone antagonist, will stop further potassium loss. In florid cases, it has been suggested that perioperative mortality is reduced by drug treatment before surgery. Metyrapone, an 11-β-hydroxylase inhibitor which acts principally on the adrenal cortex, may be used.

Intraoperative

Anaesthesia may be required for pituitary microsurgery, bilateral or unilateral adrenalectomy, or for incidental surgery. Regardless of the surgery, gentle positioning is needed to avoid fractures of osteoporotic bone. Minimal trauma or friction to the fragile skin causes ecchymoses, so that patient transfer and application of monitoring or adhesive tape should be performed with care. The approach to bilateral adrenalectomy may involve removal of the 11th and 12th ribs and there is a significant incidence of pneumothorax. Haemorrhage may be a problem during either pituitary or adrenal surgery, therefore in the presence of cardiac disease, intravascular volumes should be carefully controlled. The presence of a myopathy means that neuromuscular blockers should be given cautiously and monitored closely. Spinal epidural lipomatosis, in which abnormal fat deposition occurs in the epidural space, may be sufficient to cause compression of the cauda equina. Anaesthetists should be aware of this complication if epidural anaesthesia is contemplated. Skeletal muscle weakness may contribute to postoperative respiratory inadequacy, therefore after major surgery, IPPV should be considered.

Postoperative

Packing of the nose after trans-sphenoidal hypophysectomy may predispose to airway obstruction and the insertion of suction catheters into each nostril before packing may prevent this. Glucocorticoid replacement (hydrocortisone, 20–30 mg daily, 20 mg in the morning and 10 mg in the evening) is required after removal of a pituitary adenoma or unilateral adrenalectomy, because the hypophyseal-pituitary-adrenal control has been suppressed by high glucocorticoid secretion. However, recovery of function may subsequently occur. After bilateral adrenalectomy, since lifetime replacement of both gluco- and mineralocorticoid will be needed, fludrocortisone 100 μg daily should be added. Blood pressure, body weight, serum electrolytes and plasma renin activity should be checked in the postoperative period.

Recovery may be prolonged by poor wound healing and sensitivity to infection. A significant mortality has been reported after major surgery, usually related to infection, thromboembolic problems or cardiovascular disease.

PITUITARY

The anterior pituitary secretes at least six hormones: growth hormone, prolactin, thyroid stimulating hormone, adrenocorticotrophic hormone, follicle-stimulating hormone and luteinizing hormone. The posterior pituitary secretes antidiuretic hormone (ADH or vasopressin) and oxytocin. The problems of ACTH-dependent Cushing's syndrome have been considered in the previous section.

ACROMEGALY

Pathophysiology

A clinical syndrome produced by a growth-hormone secreting pituitary tumour, usually an adenoma of the eosinophil cells of the pituitary, situated within the sella turcica. Growth hormone stimulates the secretion of insulin-like growth factor, somatomedin C, from the liver and it is the effects of both of these hormones that produce the syndrome of acromegaly.

Surgery

Trans-sphenoidal hypophysectomy is the surgical treatment of choice.

Clinical

Symptoms arise from a combination of hormonal effects, bulk effects from enlargement of organs and associated problems. The head, tongue, lips, jaw, hands and feet are enlarged; facial features are coarse and there is deepening and huskiness of the voice. Other features include profuse perspiration and seborrhoea, kyphoscoliosis, muscular weakness, arthralgias, skin tags, nerve entrapment syndromes, hypertension, acromegalic heart disease, goitre, diabetes mellitus, diabetes insipidus, hypercalcaemia and visual field and cranial nerve defects. Increased daytime somnolence and sleep apnoea have been described and both are more likely to occur in active disease, although treatment does not necessarily cure the problem. Extrathoracic airway obstruction occurs in 30–50% of acromegalics; upper airway obstruction is particularly common in men and results in nocturnal hypoxaemia.

Preparation

For the anaesthetist, assessment of airway and intubation problems are vital. Difficulties can occur both in tracheal intubation and in airway maintenance on a mask, so that awake fibreoptic intubation may need to be discussed with the patient. Hypertension, ischaemic heart disease, ventricular arrhythmias and diabetes, if not already treated, should be controlled. Octreotide, a somatostatin analogue, may be given before surgery.

Intraoperative

Four types of perioperative airway problem have been described during anaesthesia: difficulty in achieving an airtight fit with the mask; difficulty in visualizing the larynx on laryngoscopy, often because of massive hypertrophy of the pharyngeal mucosa; difficulty in passing a tracheal tube as a result of mucosal thickening, glottic stenosis, fixation or palsy of the vocal cords, or chondrocalcinosis of the larynx; and postoperative airway obstruction. If there are serious doubts about the ability to maintain an airway once the patient is asleep, awake fibreoptic intubation should be undertaken first. If this is not thought to be necessary, it should be ascertained that mask ventilation can be performed easily before a muscle relaxant is given. The patient's fingers may be too large to fit an oximeter probe.

Postoperative

Careful postoperative observation is required, since a variety of airway and cardiovascular problems have been reported. Central depression of respiration may be compounded by the residual effects of anaesthetic drugs and result in severe postoperative hypoxaemia, hypercarbia or respiratory arrest. Sudden deaths, which sometimes occur on return to the ward, may be explicable by a combination of these factors and respiratory obstruction. Acute pulmonary oedema, secondary to the relief of upper airway obstruction has also been described. Packing of the nose after the nasal approach to hypophysectomy may predispose to obstruction and insertion of suction catheters into each nostril before packing may prevent this.

DIABETES INSIPIDUS

Pathophysiology

Antidiuretic hormone (ADH or vasopressin) is a peptide synthesized in the supra-optic and paraventricular nuclei of the hypothalamus. It is packaged in granules and transported down the axon of the neuroendocrine cell to the nerve terminals in the posterior pituitary. It conserves body water and regulates the tonicity of body fluids, but also has a vasocontrictor action. The secretion of ADH is controlled by two main mechanisms. Plasma osmolality is the most important of these, acting via osmoreceptors in the hypothalamus, which rapidly respond to changes in osmolality. An increase in osmolality stimulates ADH secretion and a decrease suppresses it. Blood volume and blood pressure respond less sensitively, via baroreceptors in the left atrium, Purkinje tissue, aortic arch and carotid sinus; ADH output is stimulated by a decrease of 5–10% in blood volume or blood pressure. Antidiuretic hormone acts on the kidney via AMP. It causes reabsorption of sodium chloride in the ascending limb of the loop of Henle and increases the permeability of the collecting ducts to water and urea. A deficiency of ADH results in the syndrome of diabetes insipidus, in which large volumes of hypotonic urine are excreted.

Causes

Diabetes insipidus occurs either as a result of posterior pituitary failure, or secondary to a wide variety of other neurogenic conditions, including head injury, cerebral tumours, multiple sclerosis and brain death. It may occur temporarily or permanently following pituitary or hypothalamic surgery.

Clinical

Polydipsia and polyuria occur, with a urine volume of up to 24 l in 24 h, resulting in hypovolaemia and hypernatraemia. Urine osmolality is low (50–100 mosmol kg^{-1}) and there is increased plasma osmolality (normal 275–295 mosmol kg^{-1}).

Treatment

Treat the cause, if possible. Medical replacement therapy with either vasopressin, or desmopressin 0.5–2 µg intravenously or 10–20 µg b.d. nasally. Treatment should be guided by the urine output and plasma osmolality levels. Intravenous fluids may be required if the plasma osmolality is >290 mosmol kg^{-1}.

PANCREAS

The endocrine parts of the pancreas are the islets of Langerhans, collections of cells scattered throughout the organ and richly supplied with blood. They have no connection with the pancreatic ducts, but distribute their hormones directly into the blood stream. There are thought to be four basic types of cell; A cells, some of which secrete glucagon, β cells which secrete insulin, D cells which secrete somatostatin and F (or PP) cells which secrete pancreatic polypeptide. A number of other substances have been identified in the pancreas, including vasoactive intestinal peptide (VIP), gastric inhibitory peptide (GIP), 5-hydroxytryptamine (5-HT) and substance P. A variety of endocrine tumours originate in the pancreas, most of which are rare. They include insulinoma, gastrinoma, vipoma and glucagonoma. Diabetes mellitus is described elsewhere.

INSULINOMA

Pathophysiology

Insulinoma are rare, insulin secreting tumours of the B cells of the pancreatic islets, most of which are benign and solitary. Malignancy occurs in up to 8%, and 10% are multiple. The condition produces hypoglycaemia together with inappropriate, rather than excess, secretion of insulin. Insulin output does not suppress normally in response to hypoglycaemia, or respond normally to hyperglycaemia. The associated hypoglycaemia is mainly due to suppression of hepatic glucose release, as opposed to increased peripheral uptake of glucose.

Surgery

Surgery is the treatment of choice and consists of either enucleation of the tumour or partial distal pancreatectomy.

Clinical

Episodic hypoglycaemia produces diplopia, blurred vision, sweating, hunger, palpitations, weakness, confusion, focal neurological deficits and grand mal seizures. Patients are often amnesic for these episodes. Symptoms frequently occur before breakfast or during vigorous exercise, pregnancy or postpartum. The disease mimics other conditions, and symptoms may suggest CNS lesions, hysteria, epilepsy, sympathetic overactivity, intoxication or behavioural problems. The diagnosis is suggested if the symptoms can be shown to be associated with hypoglycaemia, or can be provoked by fasting or exercise. It is confirmed by elevated fasting plasma insulin and C-peptide levels in the presence of hypoglycaemia.

Preparation

The main aim is to prevent hypoglycaemia by frequent small, high protein, low glucose meals. Diazoxide, 200–600 mg daily, suppresses insulin release from beta cells in 60% of cases. Somatostatin analogues may help.

Intraoperative

Anaesthetic problems include the risk of hypoglycaemia under anaesthesia, secondary to insulin release during handling of the tumour and the problems of maintaining control of blood glucose between 5.5–8.5 mmol l^{-1}. The approach to the intraoperative management of blood glucose remains controversial. In some units an 'artificial beta cell', an automated feedback system, is used, which analyses glucose levels and controls the rate of glucose (or glucose and insulin) administration. Others consider that sampling for blood sugar every 15 min and altering the rate of glucose administration manually, is adequate.

Postoperative

The problem of hypoglycaemia is replaced by that of persistent hyperglycaemia, which may continue for several days postoperatively.

VIPOMA

Pathophysiology

A rare tumour that secretes vasoactive intestinal peptide (VIP), which is a neurotransmitter in addition to being a hormone and is found in nerve fibres within the pancreas. VIP inhibits secretion of gastric acid and stimulates pancreatic exocrine secretion and flow of intestinal juices. It has vasodilator properties. About 90% of vipomas arise within the pancreas and 10% in neural tissue. They are usually of pancreatic origin in adults, but ganglioneuroblastomas are more common in children. About 50% are malignant.

Surgery

Surgical excision is the treatment of choice.

Clinical

Produces a syndrome of Watery Diarrhoea, Hypokalaemia and Achlorhydria (WDHA syndrome). The volume of stools is often greater than $3 \, l \, 24 \, h^{-1}$ and there is massive loss of fluid and electrolytes from the gut. Presenting symptoms are weight loss, dehydration, abdominal colic and flushing. Untreated patients have developed paralyses and mental changes.

Biochemical investigations show hypokalaemia, acidosis, hypercalcaemia, increased urea, a diabetic GTT, increased plasma VIP and increased plasma pancreatic hormone.

Preparation

Diarrhoea should be controlled with octreotide, a somatostatin analogue. Correction of fluid losses, in particular potassium, glucose and bicarbonate, will be required.

Intraoperative

VIP is a vasodilator and hypotension during handling of the tumour has been reported.

GASTROINTESTINAL

CARCINOID SYNDROME

Pathophysiology

Carcinoids are hormone-secreting gastrointestinal tumours of neuro-ectodermal origin, most commonly arising from the midgut, but sometimes from the fore- or hindgut. The hormones, which are peptides and amines, frequently have little clinical effect since they are rapidly inactivated in the blood and the liver. However, if significant amounts enter the systemic circulation, the classical clinical signs of carcinoid syndrome occur. In effect, most patients with the syndrome have liver metastases, except for those with tumours in which the portal circulation is bypassed. Thus, only a small proportion of patients will have carcinoid syndrome and are mainly those with tumours of midgut origin. Tumours involving the ileum or appendix are the most common and less than 18% of these produce the syndrome. The peptides and amines that have been found to be associated with carcinoids include serotonin, bradykinins and tachykinins (substance P, neurokinin A and neuropeptide K). Other vasoactive peptides such as histamine and prostaglandins may be involved, but their part in the syndrome has not yet been defined. Serotonin can cause diarrhoea, hypertension and tachycardia, mild hyperglycaemia, hypoproteinaemia and possibly flushing. Bradykinins can cause flushing, hypotension, bronchospasm and increased capillary permeability, resulting in oedema and loss of fluid and electrolytes from the vascular compartment. Tachykinins cause vasodilatation and possibly play a role in bronchospasm and fibrosis of the cardiac valves.

Surgery

Since the tumours are slow growing, surgery is worthwhile, even in the presence of liver metastases. There is evidence that symptoms are proportional to the amount of secreting tissue, therefore surgery is directed towards debulking of the primary tumour and sometimes removal of liver metastases. Cardiac valvular replacement may be needed.

Clinical

The commonest features of the syndrome, in order of frequency, are flushing, diarrhoea, abdominal pain, cardiac valvular lesions (tricuspid or pulmonary), wheezing and oedema. Urinary 5-hydroxyindole acetic acid levels are increased and blood glucose may be elevated. CT scan of the liver will show metastases and there will be abnormal liver function tests and hypoproteinaemia. Echocardiography will show whether or not there is involvement of the heart valves.

Preparation

It is important to distinguish between carcinoid disease and carcinoid syndrome, since serious anaesthetic problems only arise from within the group of patients with the syndrome. Carcinoid crises have also been reported during radiology and liver biopsy. For patients with the syndrome, octreotide, a somatostatin analogue, is now the key drug. Before surgery, the patient may be having symptomatic treatment or antiserotonin agents such as cyproheptadine or ketanserin. In the presence of severe symptoms, subcutaneous octreotide may already have been started. Routine therapy can be continued, but if octreotide is not already part of the regimen, this should be begun 24 h before surgery (octreotide 500 μg 8-hourly s.c.) and given with the premedication. Evidence of carcinoid heart disease should be sought and treated appropriately.

Intraoperative

In the prepared patient, intraoperative problems are rare, but a small number of patients with carcinoid syndrome have developed serious cardiovascular complications or bronchiospasm during anaesthesia. These may be due to secretion of hormones by the tumour provoked by mechanical, biochemical or pharmacological stimuli, but have been reported most frequently on induction and during tumour handling. Acute crises have also occurred during liver biopsy and bronchial biopsy under local anaesthesia. Although with such a rare disease it is not possible to do a controlled trial, a number of authors have verified the value of intravenous boluses of octreotide, 50–100 μg, in the treatment of carcinoid crises. Episodes of hypertension and tachycardia, particularly in the presence of increased peristalsis can be treated with methotrimeprazine, 2.5 mg. Avoidance of agents that provoke histamine release is advisable and either etomidate or propofol are recommended. Direct arterial and CVP monitoring is required, and if heart disease is present, a pulmonary artery catheter as well.

Postoperative

Close monitoring in an intensive care unit should continue into the postoperative period.

FURTHER READING

Hull, C. J. (1986) Phaeochromocytoma. Diagnosis, preoperative preparation and management. *British Journal of Anaesthesia*, **58**, 1453–1468.

Mason, R. A. (1994) *Anaesthesia Databook*, Churchill Livingstone, Edinburgh.

Murkin, J. M. (1982) Anesthesia and hypothyroidism: a review of thyroxine physiology, pharmacology, and anesthesia. *Anesthesia and Analgesia*, **61**, 371–383.

Ober, K. P. (1995) Endocrine emergencies. *Medical Clinics of North America*, **79**, No 1.

Roizen, M. F. (1990) Diseases of the endocrine system, in *Anesthesia and Uncommon Diseases*, 3rd edn. (eds J. Katz, J. Benumof and L. Kadis), Saunders, Philadelphia, pp. 245–292.

Salem, M., Tainsh, R. E., Bromberg, J., Loriaux, D. L. and Chernow, B. (1994) Perioperative glucocorticoid coverage. Reassessment 42 years after emergence of a problem. *Annals of Surgery*, **219**, 416–425.

Southwick, J. P. and Katz, J. (1979) Unusual airway difficulty in the acromegalic patient – indications for tracheostomy. *Anesthesiology*, **51**, 72–73.

Veall, G. R., Q., Peacock, J. E., Bax, N. D. S. and Reilly, C. S. (1994) Review of the anaesthetic management of 21 patients undergoing laparotomy for carcinoid syndrome. *British Journal of Anaesthesia*, **72**, 335–341.

TRAUMA AND ORTHOPAEDIC SURGERY

P. G. Edge and M. Fennelly

TRAUMA

Anaesthesia in patients with multiple injuries and severe blood loss remains a challenge for even the most experienced anaesthetist. From the outset it is important to have a clear understanding of the mechanism of injury and its diagnostic significance in order to anticipate complications and institute appropriate management.

Trauma is the commonest cause of death between the ages of 1 and 41 years. Since the 1960s, while deaths from cardiovascular and malignant disease have decreased, deaths from trauma have increased. Conventionally, deaths from trauma are described as falling into three groups. In the first group death ensues within minutes irrespective of any intervention. This group accounts for half of all trauma deaths. The third group accounts for about a fifth of the total and death occurs days or weeks after the initial injury; these deaths are due to infection or organ failure. In the second group, accounting for about a third of trauma deaths, patients die within one to two 'golden hours' if injuries are untreated, but may survive if management is prompt and effective. These deaths are due to progressive respiratory failure, circulatory insufficiency or raised intracranial pressure secondary to injury. As part of the critical care team, anaesthetists require the knowledge to assess acute trauma and anticipate its effect on the perioperative management of the patient. To this end the Advanced Trauma Life Support and Advanced Paediatric Life Support courses have been devised to provide schemes whereby all doctors involved in trauma work can evaluate and treat multiply injured patients. Although these courses have been criticized for their dogmatic approach, on the whole the underlying principles provide a practical approach to immediate assessment, diagnosis and management. The procedures constitute the 'ABC' of trauma care and identify life-threatening conditions: A for airway management with control of the cervical spine, B for breathing and ventilation, and C for circulation and haemorrhage control. No potential neurological injury takes priority over ABC. A complete review of diagnosis and management of trauma to each system is beyond the scope of this chapter. However, some of the anaesthetic problems and pitfalls will be discussed.

AIRWAY MANAGEMENT

Establishing a patent and protected airway is the essential factor in reducing mortality from trauma. All trauma patients must be considered to have a full stomach and therefore to be at risk from vomiting and aspiration. Early tracheal intubation of unconscious or semiconscious patients will relieve airway obstruction, protect the airway from aspiration and allow positive pressure ventilation when spontaneous ventilation is inadequate. Secondary brain damage from a head injury

Short Practice of Anaesthesia. Edited by M. Morgan and G. M. Hall. Published in 1997 by Chapman & Hall, London. ISBN 0 412 71890 1

is a common cause of morbidity and mortality. Adequate ventilation and oxygenation, prevention of hypercarbia, reduction of intracranial pressure and restoration of perfusion pressure improve outcome considerably. During intubation an assistant should stabilize the head and neck in a neutral position. Cervical spine injury should be assumed in all trauma patients until definitively excluded and an adequate cervical spine film interpreted by an expert. Sedatives or anaesthetic induction agents should be used with caution before tracheal intubation in patients who are cardiovascularly compromised and muscle relaxants should only be administered when the anaesthetist has confirmed that the lungs can be ventilated using a bag and mask.

It should be remembered that trauma to the soft tissues of the face and neck can lead to massive swelling and a conscious patient with an injury to the anterior neck or lower face may require early semi-elective tracheal intubation before the airway becomes obstructed and intubation impossible.

Any factor which precludes the passage of a tracheal tube in a patient who requires definitive airway management is an indication for the creation of a surgical airway. Fashioning a tracheostomy under emergency conditions is a time-consuming, difficult and bloody procedure, and for these reasons a surgical cricothyroidotomy can be life saving when emergency oxygenation is required. Even needle cricothyroidotomy and jet insufflation of the airway can provide adequate oxygenation, but for a limited period only (up to half an hour) owing to accumulation of carbon dioxide.

THORACIC INJURY

Chest injuries account for half the deaths in fatal trauma. Indications that the injury correlates with severe pulmonary or vascular damage are fractures of the first or second rib, a wide mediastinum, flail chest and massive haemothorax. Injuries below the sixth rib are most likely to indicate intra-abdominal and not intra-thoracic trauma.

Pulmonary injury

Early recognition of respiratory distress requires no more than recognition of abnormal ventilatory efforts. Ventilatory support is the most common reason for admitting patients to the intensive care unit. Rib fractures, while not in themselves life-threatening, require pain control to permit adequate lung expansion and clearance of secretions. Patients with multiple rib fractures and large flail segments, are at greatest risk of developing respiratory failure or pneumonia. Pulmonary contusion produces direct damage to the lung parenchyma with haemorrhage, atelectasis and significant shunting; when severe, pulmonary contusion requires ventilation with positive end-expiratory pressure to improve oxygenation.

Cardiac injury

The most common cardiac injuries are cardiac tamponade, myocardial contusion and rupture. The anaesthetist needs to be aware that cardiac arrythmias or angina may be the presenting feature of myocardial injury. There may be no cardiac iso-enzyme elevation as the injury is due to extravasation of blood rather than myofibril death and degeneration and this type of injury does not carry the long-term disability of myocardial infarction. Ventricular fibrillation is probably the most frequent arrhythmia that occurs at the scene of an accident and causes death in many patients before reaching hospital. Inappropriate tachycardia is the most common arrhythmia in myocardial contusion. Frequent multifocal premature ventricular contractions and atrial fibrillation may also occur and ST segment changes and right bundle branch block are also seen. Atrial fibrillation is associated with pulmonary injury. If impaired perfusion occurs as a result, the arrhythmia will require treatment, as with arrhythmias of any cause. The risk of an arrhythmia occurring may be reduced by maintaining normal electrolyte balance. Supraventricular tachycardia may lead to impaired cardiac output because of poor ventricular filling with heart rates over 140 b.p.m. In these cases cardioversion may be necessary.

It is important to realize that the damage present when the patient is first seen may only be the tip of the iceberg and as cellular swelling, capillary leakage and fluid accumulation compromise tissue oxygenation, so symptoms progress. Angina due to myocardial contusion is classically unresponsive to nitrates.

ABDOMINAL INJURY

Intra-abdominal trauma frequently passes unrecognized and may result in late and avoidable death after injury. Physical examination that elicits positive signs of guarding or peritonism, particularly in the presence of injury to the abdominal wall, is the most reliable sign of significant injury. However, significant intra-abdominal injury is not precluded by a negative examination. Blunt injury causes 90% of abdominal trauma and the solid organs, the liver and spleen are most commonly injured. Injuries to hollow viscera often present insidiously. Large volumes of blood can accumulate in the abdominal cavity without obvious increase in girth and the anaesthetist needs to be aware of occult losses. Diagnostic peritoneal lavage is the quickest and most accurate means of diagnosing significant intra-abdominal haemorrhage.

PELVIC INJURY

The large pelvic bones have an extensive blood supply and the inner walls of the pelvis contain major arteries and veins. As a result, disruption of the bony pelvic ring can lead to life-threatening blood loss. Replacement requirements are frequently substantial and transfusion in excess of 5 l is not uncommon for this injury alone. Bleeding may remain resistant to treatment until the fracture is stabilized or the injured vessels are occluded by therapeutic embolization. Bladder and urethral injuries, and anorectal injuries are associated with pelvic fractures and must be suspected in all patients with this type of injury. Associated anorectal injury is a source of overwhelming sepsis. Neurological lesions associated with pelvic fractures involve the lumbosacral trunk and, in fractures of the sacrum, isolated sacral nerve damage.

TRAUMA TO THE EXTREMITIES

Limb injury is rarely life-threatening unless associated with uncontrolled haemorrhage. It may be permanently disabling if inappropriately treated. In addition the potential complications of long bone fractures increase the risk of multiple organ failure in patients with major trauma. Early definitive management including operative fracture fixation reduces these risks considerably.

Injuries to the extremities become limb-threatening when they are associated with ischaemia. This may result from vascular injuries *per se*, dislocation of major joints causing traction on blood vessels, compartment syndromes with localized neuromuscular ischaemia and crush injuries producing a mass of devitalized tissue. Compartment syndrome is a complication of closed fractures. Simple immobilization of a fractured or dislocated limb contributes significantly to relieving the pain of the injury.

ANAESTHESIA FOR TRAUMA SURGERY

MONITORING AND INTRAVENOUS FLUID REPLACEMENT

Patients who require emergency surgery for the management of major injuries require two large bore venous catheters; the flow of liquid is proportional to the 4th power of the radius of the catheter (Poisseuille's law) and therefore catheters should be at least 14 G or larger. Introducer sheaths for pulmonary artery catheters in a central vein are particularly useful. However, it is important to remember that a 14 G, 5 cm cannula in a peripheral vein will pass fluids twice as fast as a 16 G, 20 cm cannula in a central vein.

Pressurizing the bags of intravenous fluid facilitates rapid infusion. In addition to hand-inflated pressure bags, a number of automated devices are available that can deliver a litre of warmed fluid in under one minute. However, rapid infusion of blood under pressure through too small a cannula may lead to haemolysis.

The preferred site for measuring central venous pressure is the internal jugular vein. If thoracic injury is unilateral, use of the ipsilateral internal jugular vein reduces the likelihood of bilateral pneumothorax. Central venous pressure may also be measured from a catheter passed via the femoral vein but this site carries a greater risk of introducing infection.

Pulmonary artery catheters have little place in the acute management of the trauma patient. They are associated with endocardial injury in up to 50% of patients and with endocarditis in up to 7%. A patient who urgently needs a laparotomy to arrest further blood loss cannot possibly benefit from an additional half hour delay while a pulmonary artery catheter is inserted. These lines are best inserted in the postoperative period, when the information derived can be of most value in directing the future course of therapy. In many units less invasive methods of monitoring the cardiovascular system are being used, such as transoesophageal echocardiography.

Urine output is a direct measure of organ perfusion and in patients with normal renal function may be as useful as any pressure measurement. Therefore placement of a urinary catheter is mandatory. Five out of every 100 pelvic fractures are complicated by damage to the urinary tract. Suspicion should be aroused by radiographic confirmation of a fracture associated with perineal bruising or the presence of blood at the tip of the penis. Catheterization carries the risk of converting a partial tear of the urethra into a complete one with the added risk of introducing infection. The services of a urologist may be required in placement of a catheter.

It is important to remember that the goals of cardiovascular resuscitation are tissue perfusion and oxygen delivery and attempts to treat inadequate preload by increasing contractility with inotropic agents are likely to lead to further decrease in perfusion. The key to the treatment of hypovolaemia is aggressive intravenous fluid therapy. The subject of which type of fluid to use, crystalloid or colloid, remains controversial. Crystalloid infusion requires 2–4 times more volume to achieve the same haemodynamic effects; colloids do not cause more pulmonary oedema than crystalloids when pulmonary capillaries are damaged and analysis of controlled trials suggests that there is no difference in survival based on fluid choice alone. More importantly, survival in critically ill patients is associated with a haematocrit of around 33% even though oxygen delivery is constant to haematocrits as low as 22%. Most trauma victims are young and tolerate severe acute anaemia provided intravascular volume is supported. However, haematocrits of around 10% lead to increases in arterial lactate levels and are associated with mortality of around 70%. Haemodynamic stability will result from restoration of blood volume by the anaesthetist and control of bleeding by the surgeon.

TEMPERATURE CONTROL

Hypothermia is a frequent complication of trauma and all trauma patients should have their core temperature measured. Temperature loss may be due to exposure at the time of the initial injury and is exacerbated by removal of clothing for examination in inadequately heated accident and emergency departments. Resuscitation with cold intravenous fluids, surgery with open body cavities and prolonged anaesthesia compound the problem. Low core temperature predisposes to acidosis, coagulopathy, myocardial dysfunction and arrhythmias. Below 34°C the body is unable to generate sufficient heat to restore normal body temperature and active rewarming methods are necessary.

Warming blankets under the patient are rarely beneficial, as the surface area of the body in contact with it is inadequate. A warm operating theatre, warmed infusions and humidified anaesthetic gasses all contribute to maintaining body temperature. Where feasible, the newer warm-air circulation devices are a more effective method of reducing heat loss.

ADMINISTRATION OF ANAESTHESIA

Induction

There is no ideal anaesthetic agent or technique for the trauma patient. General anaesthesia is usually required for patients with multiple injuries; although regional anaesthesia may be useful in isolated limb injuries and is conducive to good postoperative analgesia. Techniques associated with major sympathetic nervous system blockade such as spinal or epidural blockade are contraindicated in the presence of hypovolaemia.

A rapid-sequence induction technique with muscle relaxation and oral tracheal intubation is the method of choice in most acute trauma. Preoxygenation to denitrogenate the functional residual capacity of the lungs is achieved by allowing the patient to breathe oxygen for 3–5 min via a close-fitting mask.

An induction dose of an intravenous anaesthetic drug is injected and as the patient loses consciousness, cricoid pressure (Sellick's manoeuvre) is applied. Suxamethonium is administered and the trachea is intubated with cricoid pressure maintained until the cuff has been inflated.

All the currently available anaesthetic agents have side effects which may prove detrimental to the patient with major injuries. The drug of choice will depend on the preference of the individual anaesthetist and prevailing clinical circumstances.

In unstable patients who require immediate surgery, the use of high dose opioid anaesthesia may be the method of choice. Fentanyl at a dose of 50–100 µg kg^{-1} may be used as the sole agent in conjunction with an amnesic dose of a benzodiazepine.

Muscle relaxants

Pancuronium causes an increase in heart rate, blood pressure and cardiac output as a result of its vagolytic action and will antagonize fentanyl-induced bradycardia. These effects may be of benefit in hypovolaemic patients. Vecuronium has minimal cardiovascular effects and like pancuronium, has little potential for histamine release. Both drugs provide suitable muscle relaxation for surgery.

Maintenance of anaesthesia

All the volatile anaesthetic agents in common use exacerbate hypotension in the presence of hypovolaemia. To minimize this it is usual to titrate the concentration against its effects. If unacceptable hypotension occurs with even very low doses of volatile anaesthetics it may be necessary to change to a high dose opioid technique. Nitrous oxide has little effect on cardiovascular parameters even in the presence of hypovolaemia. It should not be used until adequacy of oxygenation has been confirmed by blood gas analysis. Because of the ease with which it diffuses into cavities it should not be used in cases where there may be pneumothorax, open skull fractures or trauma to the gut.

Analgesia

Trauma patients are in particular need of adequate pain control. Continuous intravenous infusions of opioids contribute to the sedation required for many patients to tolerate the presence of a tracheal tube and mechanical ventilation of the lungs as well as providing good analgesia. In these circumstances respiratory depression is not an issue. In patients who do not require postoperative ventilation opioid infusions must be adjusted to allow adequate analgesia but without the risk of respiratory depression.

Supplementary techniques that have proved successful include intrathecal or epidural opioids, intrapleurally administered local anaesthetics and the full spectrum of regional and isolated nerve blocks, as well as intermittent infusion of opioids by patient controlled analgesia.

SPECIAL CONSIDERATIONS

PAEDIATRIC TRAUMA

Trauma is the leading cause of death in children between the ages of 1 and 19 years. Half of all these deaths are due to road traffic accidents. The traumatized child requires the same system of assessment and management priorities as the adult trauma patient but is less able to contribute to that management. Young children are unable to localize pain and may deny any symptoms.

The smaller and younger the child, the more difficult it is to secure the airway and achieve vascular access. Appropriate equipment and personnel experienced in paediatric management must be available to receive the injured child and a specially equipped area with weighing scales, overhead heater and suitable monitoring facilities. After achieving the ABC of trauma care further problems are treated according to clinical priorities. Although principles of paediatric management are dealt with elsewhere in this book, certain maxims of paediatric trauma may be usefully referred to at this point.

- Intrinsic cardiac dysfunction is rare in children and poor cardiac output is invariably due to hypoxia or hypovolaemia. Bradycardia in a shocked child is caused by hypoxia and acidosis and is a pre-terminal sign. Similarly, children's cardiovascular systems tolerate hypovolaemia remarkably well initially and hypotension is a late sign. If measured decreases in blood pressure are not rapidly reversed death may follow rapidly. A formula for calculating systolic blood pressure is $80 + (2 \times$ age in years). Hypoglycaemia may give a clinical picture similar to compensated shock and, particularly in small children, may coexist. Hypoglycaemia must always be excluded by blood glucose estimation.
- Intraosseous infusion is an important technique for gaining vascular access in life-threatening situations. Specially designed trochars are available which make this a rapid and safe technique. Infusion sites are usually the proximal tibia but the distal tibia and distal femur may also be used. Fractured bones should be avoided. Blood transfusions and all drugs can be injected through intraosseous needles. The greatest disadvantage is the need to infuse under pressure.
- Children have very elastic ribs which rarely fracture. A normal chest X-ray does not exclude major damage to and disruption of intrathoracic viscera. Because of the mobility of the ribs there is a high incidence of pulmonary contusion. Diaphragmatic rupture is also a more common injury in children, usually following blunt abdominal trauma.
- Gastric distension with air may severely compromise ventilatory efforts. It occurs as a result of air swallowing during crying and during bag and mask resuscitation. Early passage of a gastric tube should be considered particularly if anaesthesia is required.
- The bones of children are more pliant than bones of adults and are capable of returning to their normal shape after considerable deformation. If this limit is exceeded,

greenstick fracture and then complete fracture occurs. It follows that considerable forces must be applied to produce fractures in children and this can result in the degree of associated soft tissue damage being underestimated. Blood loss associated with long bone and pelvic fractures is proportionately greater in children. Although the injury itself is usually obvious the magnitude of associated blood loss is difficult to estimate. In patients with multiple trauma sites it is easy to underestimate the contribution of a single fracture to overall blood loss and attention must be paid to this in children who fail to respond to apparently appropriate therapy.

FAT EMBOLUS

Fractures of the pelvis and of the long bones, particularly the femur, are occasionally complicated by embolization of fat particles. The pathology of this condition is unclear. Originally thought to be due to particles of bone marrow fat escaping into the circulation from fracture sites, abnormal lipid metabolism has also been suggested as a cause. It is rare in children who have relatively less fatty bone marrow than adults. It occurs 2 or 3 days after injury and presents as a deterioration in the patient's general condition. Lung manifestations are the most common and constitute the major threat to life. Signs and symptoms include dyspnoea, cyanosis and frothy sputum containing fat globules. Chest X-rays show mottling of the lung fields. Blood gas analysis shows low arterial partial pressure of oxygen (in spite of high inspired oxygen concentration) due to ventilation/perfusion mismatch.

There is often a slight pyrexia, a petechial rash appears on the skin around the shoulders, neck and axillae. Conjunctival petechiae may occur and fundoscopy reveals fat emboli in the retinal vessels. Cerebral changes are probably secondary to hypoxia and may lead to an aggressive, confused or comatose patient. Coma and convulsions may occur and deep coma carries a poor prognosis. Renal involvement may occur with impaired renal function and the presence of fat droplets in the urine.

Therapy is maintained at respiratory support and the patient may need to be managed on an intensive care unit if there is major metabolic disturbance. The role of steroids is controversial; they may have a place in early management but are thought to be detrimental after the first 24 h. Heparin therapy has not been demonstrated to be effective. Prognosis is usually good and full recovery should be expected.

VOLKMANN'S ISCHAEMIC CONTRACTURE

This painful condition usually occurs as a complication of supracondylar fractures where the brachial artery may be vulnerable. The artery may be damaged directly when it is trapped by the fracture, or indirectly by compression due to swelling. As a result of ischaemia, the forearm muscles become oedematous increasing the interstitial pressure and exacerbating the problem. Eventually there is necrosis of the muscle which eventually becomes fibrosed and calcifies producing a fixed contracture deformity. There is a variable sensory loss usually involving the median nerve and paralysis of the ulnar nerve. The damage occurs over 12–24 h and is characterized by disproportionate pain on passive extension of the fingers. A palpable radial pulse does not exclude the diagnosis of ischaemia and early intervention to relieve the ischaemia is necessary. If signs are still apparent following reduction of the fracture further investigation is mandatory. Arteriography may reveal brachial artery spasm, which may be amenable to stellate ganglion block, or occlusion, when faciotomy and exploration of the artery are required.

HIP FRACTURES

Fractures of the femoral neck are a pre-mortal event. Patients over the age of 70 years who suffer this injury have a 50% mortality, from all causes, within 6 months. The injury commonly occurs as a result of a simple fall and is associated with a variable degree of pain. The incidence of fractures of the femoral neck increases with age, in later life it is three times more common in women where hormone-dependent osteoporosis and osteomalacia are contributory factors. Below the age of 60 years the fracture occurs more frequently in men, as a result of industrial trauma.

Fractures occur at two anatomical levels, intracapsular and extracapsular. Intracapsular fractures are prone to avascular necrosis. This is due to compromise of the blood supply to the femoral head as a result of either direct disruption of the blood vessels or compression of the blood vessels by intracapsular haematoma. Isolated intracapsular fractures are associated with minimal haemorrhage at the time of injury. In contrast, extracapsular fractures may be associated with significant blood loss and require preoperative fluid resuscitation.

In all cases, the aim of treatment is early internal fixation of the fracture and mobilization of the patient. The association of this injury with increasing age means that the cause of the initial fall must be sought. Cardiac arryhythmias, transient ischaemic attacks, electrolyte disturbances, occult chest or urinary tract infection may all cause falls in the elderly and factors such as these must identified and if possible treated before anaesthesia. However, protracted delay without active therapy is associated with a greater incidence of avascular necrosis and a significant increase in mortality and morbidity.

Surgical management of intracapsular fractures falls into three categories.

- Reduction and internal fixation. This is generally used for all fractures in younger patients and for fractures where there is minimal or no displacement of the femoral head.
- Primary replacement of the femoral head or hemiarthroplasty. This is carried out for fractures where there is significant dissociation at the fracture site in patients who are unlikely to have a long or very active life subsequently.
- Total hip replacement. This procedure affords the greatest chance of the patient returning to active life. It is also the procedure of choice in patients with rheumatoid arthritis who sustain a fracture.

Surgical management of extracapsular fractures requires reduction and internal fixation. Fixation is achieved with a nail and plate device following reduction of the fracture on an orthopaedic table.

Anaesthetic technique for urgent surgery for fractured neck of femur is determined by the patient's physiological status and the available anaesthetic experience. Although some studies have recommended a regional technique, either spinal or epidural anaesthesia, on the basis of a lower immediate mortality, after one month there is no difference in outcome between regional and general anaesthesia and mortality remains around 7% following surgery.

Access to patients on an elevated orthopaedic table is awkward and alert patients are often distressed by the need to lie still for long periods and the noise of surgical drills. In addition, securing the patients arms out of the surgical and radiographical field causes considerable discomfort and the lower half of the body is usually minimally draped which exacerbates intraoperative heat losses.

Regional anaesthesia for hip fractures

The problem of pain in the patient with a fractured femoral neck complicates suitable positioning for lumbar puncture or insertion of an epidural catheter. Spinal anaesthetics are usually sited more quickly than epidural catheters and onset of action and analgesia minimize the patient's discomfort. Hyperbaric bupivicaine solutions maintain the block best and before positioning on the operating table the patient can usually be turned fractured hip down without discomfort to augment blockade. Postdural puncture headache is rare in elderly patients even when larger bore spinal needles are used. Epidural anaesthesia has the advantage of being a continuous technique and may be topped up if surgery is unduly prolonged and to provide postoperative analgesia. It can be more difficult to site in the elderly patient who may have osteoarthritic changes in the lumbar spine. A volume of 10 ml bupivicaine (0.5%) usually ensures adequate spread of anaesthesia and density of neural blockade for surgery. With both techniques hypotension is likely to occur and may be profound unless measures are taken to prevent it.

General anaesthesia for hip fractures

The problem of prolonged gastric emptying must be borne in mind even when there has been an interval of 2 or 3 days between the accident and surgery, particularly as this will be aggravated by any opioid analgesia which may have been given. A rapid-sequence induction employing Sellick's manoeuvre should be used. There is no ideal induction agent but cognitive function has been shown to be better preserved in the immediate postoperative period and mobilization has been shown to occur earlier when propofol has been used in place of thiopentone. However, this difference was not apparent after one week and did not result in earlier discharge from hospital. Volatile agents may all cause significant hypotension and adequate analgesia to prevent marked swings of blood pressure in response to surgical stimulus are required.

General anaesthesia may be satisfactorily combined with a regional technique or with femoral nerve block or an inguinal perivascular lumbar plexus technique (3-in-1 block).

SPINAL INJURIES

The most common causes of spinal cord injury are road traffic accidents and sports injuries. Most patients are young men aged 15–35 years. Degenerative changes producing a narrowed spinal canal render elderly patients particularly vulnerable to significant injury from minor accidents.

The cervical spine is the region most susceptible to damage and hyperflexion and hyperextension are common. Instability occurs when the anterior or posterior supporting elements are disrupted. In adults, cervical spine injury most commonly involves the lower segments whereas in children the upper segments are more likely to be involved. A hangman's fracture is an unstable fracture of the pedicles of C2 with anterior movement on C3. It is important to remember that spinal cord damage may be present in the absence of radiographic evidence of bony injury.

Compression and rotation injuries affect the thoracolumbar region usually as a result of excessive forces applied to the posterior thoracic spine.

Disruption of nervous tissue, vasospasm and haemorrhage in the substance of the cord lead to ischaemia, oedema, release of amino acids and eventually infarction of the cord. Incomplete cord injuries produce a variety of defined neurological syndrome.

- Anterior cord syndrome. Motor function and pain sensation is lost below the lesion with preservation of proprioception and deep pressure sensation.
- Central cord syndrome. Upper limbs are affected to a greater degree than lower limbs with variable impairment of bladder and bowel function.
- Brown–Sequard syndrome results in ipsilateral hemiparesis and loss of proprioception in conjunction with contralateral loss of pain and temperature sensation.
- Lesions of the conus affect bowel and bladder function.

Anaesthetic considerations

Early involvement of the anaesthetist is of paramount importance in the management of the acutely injured patient, particularly when high cervical lesions are present. The increasing trend for early fixation and stabilization often results in the anaesthetist being presented with an unstable patient with a difficult airway. Early reduction of the fracture and decompression of the cord is mandatory in a neurologically deteriorating patient and early surgery facilitates management in the acute phase leading to earlier rehabilitation. It must never be forgotten that these patients may have accompanying intracranial, intrathoracic or abdominal injuries which should be excluded before definitive management of the spinal cord injury.

Airway management

If there is any doubt about the stability of the cervical spine an awake fibreoptic intubation by an experienced anaesthetist is now the preferred option. In the acute phase suxamethonium may be used safely, the problems of hyperkalaemia only developing after 48 h.

Ventilation

With lesions above C4 voluntary diaphragmatic movement is impossible. Lesions between C5 and C7 are associated with significant respiratory embarassment due to loss of intercostal and abdominal muscle function, and ineffective cough. Formal pulmonary function testing and blood gas analysis are essential preoperative investigations. Patients with significant thoracic injury are likely to have associated pulmonary contusion.

Cardiovascular problems

Spinal shock is a syndrome which develops within minutes of spinal cord injury and is characterized by flaccid paralysis below the level of the lesion and absent tendon and plantar reflexes. There is decreased systemic vascular resistance, increased venous capacitance, hypotension and bradycardia. The syndrome occurs with cord lesions above T5, which interrupt sympathetic outflow to the heart and unopposed parasympathetic tone. Parasympathetic efferent control of the heart rate, via the vagus, is unaffected. Bradyarrhythmias are associated with cervical, but not with thoracic or lumbar, lesions.

Maintaining spinal cord perfusion pressure is vital to prevent extension of the neurological injury; as autoregulation is lost, cord perfusion becomes pressure dependent. This may require the use of inotropes and anaesthetic manipulation especially in the perioperative phase. Direct arterial pressure monitoring and adequate venous access is imperative.

Patients with spinal shock have an unpredictable response to fluid challenge and, in the absence of sympathetic output to peripheral receptors, pulmonary oedema may develop rapidly during fluid resuscitation.

Temperature regulation

Normal thermoregulatory mechanisms are impaired in patients with spinal cord injury. Core temperature should be monitored and the patient kept warm particularly during the acute phase of injury and during surgery.

Gastrointestinal and urinary problems

A nasogastric tube may be required as ileus frequently occurs with spinal shock. In addition all patients with neurological deficit should be catheterized to avert potential distension of the bladder.

Positioning for surgery

Positioning patients with spinal cord damage requires great care and supervision by the surgeon. Movement may result in haemodynamic instability. Alignment of the spine must be maintained; for cervical injuries this is facilitated by the application of traction using skull tongs. When final positioning of the patient has been achieved, often in the prone position, the anaesthetist should confirm and secure the position of the tracheal tube and ensure adequacy of ventilation.

THE PATIENT WITH CHRONIC SPINAL INJURY

These patients commonly present for further stabilization of the spine, release of contractures, plastic surgery for pressure sores and genitourinary procedures. Autonomic hyperreflexia may occur in patients with lesions above T6 and is characterized by hypertension and cardiac arrhythmias due to excessive catecholamine release. It may be triggered by distension of the bladder or rectum or by surgical manipulation in inadequately anaesthetized patients. Treatment involves termination of the stimulus, increasing the depth of anaesthesia or raising the dermatomal level of a regional anaesthetic. If necessary the specific arrhythmia and hypertension should be treated. There is no clear advantage of one anaesthetic technique over another but these difficult patients definitely require an experienced anaesthetist. Temperature control remains an issue and careful positioning and padding are vital to prevent breakdown of vulnerable skin.

ELECTIVE ORTHOPAEDIC PROCEDURES

JOINT REPLACEMENT SURGERY

Elective joint replacement surgery has become an increasingly common procedure since the pioneering work of Charnley in the 1960s on the development of the total hip replacement. As a result of increased understanding of the biomechanical principles involved in the development of this prosthesis and the use of acrylic cement to transmit forces between metal and bone, this operation has become increasingly successful. Prostheses for other joints have been developed, in particular knee joints but also shoulder, elbow and other joints as well as customized prostheses for bone-tumour surgery.

Total hip replacement

This operation is normally carried out in the lateral decubitus position and many of the considerations for anaesthesia for fractured neck of femur surgery apply to hip replacement surgery. There is no single ideal technique. Blood loss is directly proportional to the patient's blood pressure, but while least blood loss occurs with deliberately hypotensive general anaesthesia, this may not be ideal in an increasingly elderly population. Postoperative complications have been found to be fewer with spinal anaesthesia. There is less blood loss with both spinal and epidural anaesthesia than with normotensive general anaesthesia. In addition, there is a lower incidence of postoperative deep vein thrombosis following the use of a regional technique. Although regional techniques are said to be associated with urinary retention, prostatism in elderly male patients and postoperative bed rest undoubtedly contribute to this complication. Certainly it occurs after both general and regional anaesthesia have been employed. As with anaesthesia for hip fractures, the technique used depends on a variety of factors, including the comfort and the preoperative mental state of the patient if a regional technique is to be used alone.

Total knee replacement

Knee replacement is carried out with the patient supine and has the advantage of being amenable to the application of a tourniquet which significantly reduces intraoperative blood loss. Occasionally, simultaneous bilateral knee replacement is carried out. This requires particular caution, firstly when tourniquets are inflated resulting in increased cardiac work and later when the cuffs are deflated; ideally cuffs should be deflated separately, about 20 min apart, to minimize metabolic upset. If a regional technique is used alone, it is not unusual for patients to complain of a dull aching in the region of the tourniquet cuff even though analgesia is adequate for surgery; the pain develops about 45 min after inflation of the cuff and gets progressively worse. The cause of this discomfort has not been elucidated. The same techniques and principles apply to anaesthesia for knee replacement surgery as to hip replacement.

Methyl methacrylate cement

The cement most commonly used in securing joint prostheses is a self-polymerizing acrylic compound, methyl methacrylate. It is supplied as a methyl methacrylate powder with a polymerization activator and an ampoule of liquid monomer which, when mixed produce a semi-solid which hardens over a matter of minutes. Being a polymerization reaction, it is exothermic and the temperature in large lumps of cement can reach over 100°C providing the potential for thermal injury to surrounding soft tissue. It acts as a space filler rather than as a glue and can withstand the compression that occurs between the bone and the prosthesis. Its mechanical strength is improved by eliminating air bubbles from the mixture. The addition of barium sulphate renders the cement radio-opaque and occasionally antibiotics such as gentamicin are included in the mixture, particularly if it is to be used in sites involving previous infection.

The sudden marked decreases in blood pressure sometimes associated with insertion of cement has been attributed to three factors:

- emboli being forced into the circulation by the pressure of inserting the prosthesis down the reamed medulla of the bone shaft;
- the release of vasoactive substances by the cement; or
- release of acrylic monomer into the blood stream.

The extent and duration of the hypotension are variable and all the proposed mechanisms may be involved. There may be an accompanying decrease in end-tidal carbon dioxide levels and oxygen desaturation can be resolved by increasing the inspired oxygen tension. These findings support the theory of embolic phenomena. In addition, cardiac arrest has been reported following insertion of cement down the femoral shaft. Postmortem examination in these cases has shown pulmonary bone marrow and fat emboli.

Thromboembolic prophylaxis

Pulmonary embolus is the most common fatal complication following surgery or trauma to the pelvis and lower limbs. Deep vein thrombosis occurs in 70% of patients undergoing hip arthroplasty and mortality due to pulmonary embolus may be as high as 1% in this group. Risk factors include increasing age and obesity, smoking, immobility and the presence of malignancy. The magnitude of the problem has resulted in the development of a variety of thromboembolic prophylactic regimens with no single scheme being demonstrably superior. Physical methods of promoting venous return, such as graduated compression stockings or intermittent compression leggings may be usefully combined with pharmacological methods of reducing coagulability. Low-molecular-weight heparin has been shown to reduce the incidence of deep vein thrombosis and pulmonary embolus without the excessive bleeding associated with low dose heparin and does not appear to increase the risk of bleeding when used with regional anaesthetic techniques.

Use of pneumatic tourniquets

Approximately 40% of orthopaedic procedures involve the use of a pneumatic tourniquet to reduce bleeding and improve the operative view. Although blood loss is markedly decreased, the use of a tourniquet is not free of metabolic and haemodynamic effects. The cuff of the tourniquet must be more than half the limb diameter in width and of sufficient length to encircle the limb one and a half times. It is applied to the proximal part of the limb as it is usually ineffective in preventing bleeding from vessels between the two bones in the distal part of the limb. It should be applied over padding which is free of wrinkles and other irregularities. Care must be taken to prevent skin preparation liquids seeping between the skin and cuff. The limb is exsanguinated prior to inflation of the cuff although in cases of infection or tumour exsanguination is contraindicated. The cuff is inflated with compressed air to a pressure approximately 100 mmHg above measured systolic pressure. Further inflation does not prevent bleeding from intramedullary blood vessels which is a particular problem in children.

The degree of metabolic disturbance is proportional to the duration of cuff inflation and is tolerated better by children than by adults. The duration of safe tourniquet inflation is unknown and recommendations vary from 60 min to 2 h. Electron microscopy after 2 h shows mitochondrial swelling, myelin degeneration and lysis of z-lines, (all of which are completely reversible) whereas after 1 h microscopy showed only depletion of sarcoplasmic glycogen granules. Overall injury is a function of inflation pressure and duration.

After inflating the tourniquet, tissue levels of oxygen decrease and carbon dioxide and lactate increase with a decrease in pH. On releasing the cuff the accumulated acid metabolites are buffered by plasma bicarbonate resulting in significant increases in Pa_{CO_2} and PE'_{CO_2} The maximum increase in PE'_{CO_2} is approximately 0.4 kPa after release of an upper limb tourniquet and may be as much as 1.2 kPa on releasing a lower limb cuff and is maximal within 3 min. Most of these changes can be compensated for by increasing minute volume for a few minutes before and several minutes after deflating the tourniquet cuff.

The use of pneumatic tourniquets in patients with sickle cell disease is controversial. On theoretical grounds vascular stasis, increasing acidosis and hypoxia might induce sickling but this has not been borne out by clinical experience when adequate oxygenation and hyperventilation has been maintained. Therefore the use of tourniquets is not necessarily an absolute contraindication in these patients, or in those with sickle cell trait, providing the necessary care is taken.

THE PATIENT WITH RHEUMATOID ARTHRITIS

Rheumatoid disease is a systemic connective tissue disorder in which arthritis is just one manifestation. It is three times more common in women than men and presents most commonly in the fourth decade of life. The childhood presentation, Still's disease, occurs most commonly between 2 and 4 years of age and in the same sex ratio as in adults. It is characterized by the production of rheumatoid factor, an antibody to an immunoglobulin, which, when deposited within the joint, stimulates the release of lysosomal enzymes. Fever, rash, joint swelling and redness, leucocytosis, anaemia and increased erythrocyte sedimentation rate are also features of the disorder. Severe cases may also develop splenomegaly and lymphadenitis. In both adults and children it classically involves multiple joints symmetrically: interphalangeal joints, metacarpophalangeal joints, the wrist, knees and ankles. Hence these patients usually present for release of joint contractures, repair of ruptured tendons or joint replacement surgery. Clinical features of rheumatoid arthritis are manifold but some are of particular importance to the anaesthetist. Certain features of the condition specifically affect airway management. These include the following.

- Atlantoaxial joint instability with erosion of the odontoid peg raises the possibility of cord compression, particularly with the neck in flexion. Clinical signs are frequently absent. A lateral view of the cervical spine in flexion and extension should be examined. A gap of 3 mm between the odontoid peg and posterior border of the anterior arch of the atlas indicates significant subluxation.
- Involvement of the temporomandibular joint may limit mouth opening. This is frequently a problem in Still's disease where it may be exacerbated by poor development of the mandible.
- Hoarseness of the voice may be an indication of cricoarytenoid involvement and limit size of the laryngeal inlet. This may predispose to airway obstruction.

Awake fibreoptic intubation using local anaesthesia may be the safest method of securing the airway should intubation be necessary.

Cardiac involvement is also a problem, occurring in one third of patients. It is more common in children and in men. Pericarditis with pericardial effusion may occur and significant tamponade has been reported. Pulmonary involvement is also more common in men. This may present as fibrosis with diffuse infiltration or as localized nodules within the lung, usually associated with a pleural effusion. Sternocostal and costovertebral joint disease reduce chest wall compliance and contributes to a restrictive lung defect.

Renal disease is common in these patients. Renal damage may be due to the disease itself or to drug therapy, particularly if gold or penicillamine have been used. In long standing illness, amyloid deposition may occur.

Regional techniques are particularly appropriate in this group of patients where feasible. Nerve blocks may be technically more difficult where anatomy is abnormal. In addition it may not be possible for the patient to remain immobile for the duration of the surgery and it is not unknown for the patient to need opioid analgesia for the pain in joints that are not being operated on. Positioning of the patient on the operating table must be particularly careful with deformed joints being supported and pressure points being well padded. Patients who have severe extra-articular involvement may require high dependency facilities for postoperative recovery.

ELECTIVE PAEDIATRIC SURGERY

Most elective paediatric surgery is performed for the correction of congenital anomalies which occcur as isolated orthopaedic findings or as part of a syndrome associated with other generalized physical and biochemical problems.

Talipes equinovarus

This condition affects 1 in 1000 live births. It is twice as common in boys and 10% of affected children have other congenital anomalies. Surgical correction may be undertaken as young as 3 to 4 months old. Although surgery is usually carried out under a tourniquet, bleeding sufficient to require transfusion may occur when the cuff is deflated and thus should be anticipated. Caudal epidural injection using bupivicaine 0.25% (0.5 ml kg^{-1}) provides satisfactory analgesia for surgery and the initial postoperative period. As corrective surgery involves predominantly soft tissue, prolonged postoperative analgesia is not usually required.

Congenital hip dislocation

Congenital dislocation of the hip is a condition in which the femoral head is displaced out of the acetabular socket. The condition occurs in 1 to 15 per 1000 live births, affecting girls seven times more frequently than boys. It may occur as an isolated abnormality or as part of a more generalized condition (e.g.

arthrogryposis); in 25% of cases both hips are affected. It is diagnosed by its characteristic appearance. In babies treatment consists of closed reduction by manipulation and subsequent splinting of the joint in abduction, but as the child gets older open reduction and osteotomy may be necessary. Providing the airway can be adequately managed with the child on the plaster frame, inhalational anaesthesia administered via a facemask is a suitable technique. Analgesic requirement after closed manipulation is usually minimal and an NSAID will usually suffice if analgesia is required at all.

Open reduction and osteotomy are associated with blood loss usually sufficient to require transfusion. Satisfactory analgesia may be provided by a caudal epidural injection of bupivicaine 0.25% using a volume of 0.5 ml kg^{-1}. This usually provides analgesia for a few hours after operation following which opioids will be required. Following open reduction a hip spica cast is usually applied which requires changing at intervals under general anaesthesia. This requires positioning the child on a spica table or frame and care must be taken to avoid accidental extubation during manipulation.

ELECTIVE SPINAL SURGERY

Surgical intervention is indicated for disc herniation, which may be acute or chronic, degenerative age-related changes, and in relation to connective tissue disorders and spondylolysthesis.

Cervical spine surgery

Both anterior and posterior approaches to the cervical spine are utilized for disc excisions and fusions, and for the resection of osteophytes. A transoral retropharyngeal approach is used to decompress and stabilize atlantoaxial subluxation which is pathognomic of rheumatoid arthritis.

Thoracic spine surgery

Patients with ankylosing spondylitis are particularly prone to fractures and may require correction of their kyphosis by multiple segmental osteotomies. Primary or metastatic tumours can lead to vertebral instability and neurological changes and may require thoracotomy for adequate stabilization. These procedures are often particularly haemorragic.

Spinal fusion

Fusion is performed for existing or potential instability and there are several techniques and instrumentations in current use. Spondylolysthesis requires fusion when the degree of forward slip of one vertebra on another is greater than 50%. In young, fit patients epidural catheters sited above the level of the fusion afford a very good intraoperative field and offer superb analgesia after operation.

Spinal cord decompression

Surgery for spinal stenosis involves decompression of the cord and nerve roots by laminectomy. Many of these patients are elderly and require careful anaesthetic evaluation and management. Discectomy is probably the most common spinal operation performed and a balanced anaesthetic facilitating a bloodless field is essential to its success.

Scoliosis surgery

Scoliosis is defined as a lateral and rotational deformity of the spine. The association between the resulting chest wall deformity and respiratory failure was recognized as early as the fifth century BC by Hippocrates. Increasingly complex surgical techniques and instrumentation are used to effect correction or halt the progression of deformity. Many of these patients are compromised by associated disease processes and anaesthesia for this

Table 25.1 Classification of scoliosis

Idiopathic	Infantile (<4 years old at onset)
	Juvenile (skeletal age 4–14 years)
	Adolescent (skeletal age >14 years)
Congenital	Due to vertebral abnormalities, e.g. spina bifida
Neuromuscular	Neuropathic
	Upper motor neurone – cerebral palsy, Friedreich's ataxia
	Lower motor neurone – polio
	Syringomyelia
	Myopathic, e.g. muscular dystrophy, myotonia
Scoliosis associated with neurofibromatosis	
Mesenchymal disorders	Congenital: Marfan's syndrome
	Acquired: Rheumatoid arthritis
Trauma	
Tumour	

type of surgery remains extremely challenging.

Idiopathic scoliosis accounts for 65% of cases, with a female preponderance and occurs at periods of maximum growth. The remaining 35% is secondary to congenital or acquired disease processes. Scoliosis may be classified as shown in Table 25.1.

The degree of curvature is measured by the Cobb angle on a radiograph. This is determined by drawing lines parallel to the superior border of the highest vertebra and inferior border of the lowest vertebral body of the curve. Perpendicular lines to these are then constructed and the cephalad (and caudad) angle at which they intersect is the Cobb angle. The greater the angle and associated problems, the more likely it is that surgical intervention will be required.

Preoperative assessment

Most patients with idiopathic scoliosis are normal, healthy children who have minimal associated pathology. Patients with syndromic scoliosis require careful evaluation and attention to accompanying pathology.

The most common problem in scoliotic patients is a restrictive ventilatory pattern associated with altered lung volumes, ventilation/perfusion defects and pulmonary vascular changes. Preoperative assessment of lung function is routine and these commonly show decreases in total lung capacity, vital capacity and functional residual capacity. Pulmonary impairment is significantly greater in patients with paralytic scoliosis due to the combination of reduced respiratory volumes and the increased inability to cough and clear secretions. The major abnormality in gas exchange is due to ventilation/perfusion mismatch and arterial blood gas analysis is desirable particularly in those patients who are unable to cooperate with formal lung function testing. As a result of earlier detection of scoliosis, very few patients now present with pulmonary hypertension as a secondary complication. Exercise tolerance is also a useful guide to pulmonary function. Patients whose lung function results are less than 30% of predicted values are at risk of postoperative respiratory insufficiency, particularly following thoracotomy. Children with cerebral palsy are prone to sleep apnoea and in these patients preoperative sleep studies are advisable.

There is a higher than normal incidence of cardiac anomalies in patients with scoliosis, 30% of whom have mitral valve prolapse. The association between cardiac disease and scoliosis is well documented and careful cardiac evaluation is indicated in patients with syndromes associated with cardiac dysfunction, e.g. cardiomyopathy in patients with Duchenne's muscular dystrophy. Echocardiography and cardiac catheterization studies should be assessed by a cardiologist where necessary.

Patients with neuromuscular dysfunction and developmental delay may have dysphagia, uncoordinated pharyngeal reflexes, reflux and hiatus hernia. After spinal surgery patients need to be nursed lying flat and the propensity for aspiration needs to be considered in any child who is at risk.

Existing neurological deficit should be documented preoperatively. Care should be taken to ensure that anticonvulsant medication is maintained within the therapeutic range throughout the perioperative period in patients who have seizures.

Surgical correction of scoliosis

When posterior fusion alone is inadequate to treat and control the scoliosis, corrective surgery may need to be carried out in two stages. This usually involves anterior release of the vertebral column by removing consecutive intervertebral discs, followed by posterior fusion of the vertebrae 7 to 14 days later. In the anterior approach a thoracoabdominal incision is used to expose the spine by retroperitoneal extension of the incision and detachment of the diaphragm.

For the posterior approach, positioning is important to reduce epidural venous pressure and minimize trauma to the brachial plexus and bony areas. Hooks are placed on the vertebral laminae at the upper and lower limit of the curve and the spine is distracted by moulded rods inserted between them.

In young children sequential plaster jackets may be applied to attempt correction. The child is placed on a Cottrell frame and a closely fitting plaster is applied to effect correction. General anaesthesia is invariably required for this procedure.

Anaesthesia for scoliosis surgery

Most of these patients fall into the paediatric and adolescent age groups and establishing a rapport with the patient and their often very anxious parents greatly aids their management. Adequate premedication is essential and with the advent of sevoflurane an inhalation induction may be employed in difficult children and adolescents with needle phobias. Intravenous access and placement of arterial and central venous catheters is often difficult due to deformity and contractures. A balanced anaesthetic technique using oxygen, nitrous oxide and volatile agents with adequate opioid supplementation is the usual technique unless the requirement for spinal cord monitoring restricts their use, as discussed elsewhere in this chapter. Moderate hypotension to a mean arterial pressure of 50–60 mmHg facilitates surgery and reduces blood loss; if necessary hypotensive agents such as labetalol or sodium nitroprusside may be used.

For the anterior approach epidural analgesia considerably aids blood pressure control and reduces postoperative morbidity. During posterior fusions blood loss may be considerable, particularly in patients whose scoliosis has a neuromuscular aetiology.

Postoperative care

All patients undergoing corrective spinal surgery should be nursed in a high dependency unit. Adequate analgesia is essential and epidural infusions of local anaesthetic and opioids are of enormous value in thoracotomy patients. Epidural catheters are also sited, where feasible, in patients undergoing posterior fusion. Patient controlled analgesic devices and standard opioid infusions also have a role. For patients with known respiratory compromise a period of postoperative ventilation may be necessary.

SPINAL CORD MONITORING

The consequences of postoperative paraplegia in young, fit patients undergoing spinal sur-

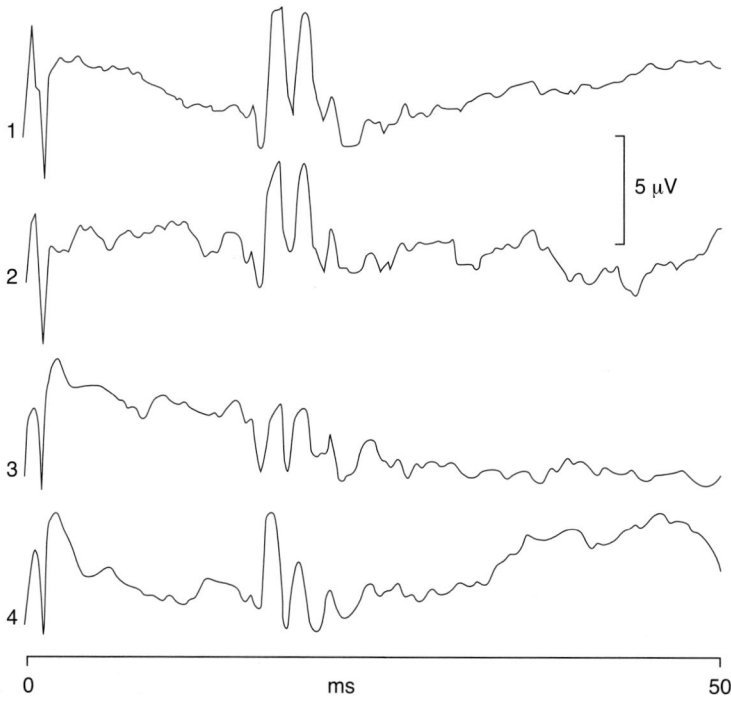

Figure 25.1 Spinal evoked potentials (SpEPs) recorded from the epidural space at C7 during surgery for correction of thoracic scoliosis: **1**, prior to correction; **2**, start of distraction; **3**, loss of amplitude of SpEP during distraction; **4**, recovery of amplitude of SpEP following reduction of distraction. There is no change in the latency of recorded SpEPs. The anaesthetic technique must have no effect on SpEPs.

gery are devastating. Today it is standard practice to institute some form of monitoring when performing any spinal operation that may be associated with high risk of neurological injury. The most primitive spinal cord monitoring is the wake-up test. This is only possible in cooperative patients and can be done no more than once or twice during the operation. The development of neurophysiological monitoring of the cord has depended on basic scientific observations of central nervous system electrical activity evoked by peripheral nerve stimulation. The scalp-recorded sensory evoked potential in response to peripheral nerve stimulation is still the most commonly used method. It is of particular value when surgery is performed on the cervical spine. However, nitrous oxide and the volatile anaesthetic agents supress the magnitude of the recording obtained. Epidural recording of spinal somatosensory evoked potential is now the gold standard in corrective spinal surgery and is more robust from an anaesthetic point of view. An example is shown in Figure 25.1. Monitoring of the motor evoked potential is justified by the small but significant incidence of anterior cord ischaemia occurring without any change in the sensory evoked potential.

Animal studies have shown the motor evoked potential to be an earlier predictor of impending cord damage. The development of a continuous intraoperative technique to monitor the motor tracts has been complicated by vulnerability to the anaesthetic and the need to stimulate central nervous tissue. Routinely administered anaesthetic agents completely obtund the evoked response elicited by magnetic stimulation and concern has been expressed about repeated transcranial electrical stimulation. Recently, a compound motor action potential has been elicited by direct spinal cord stimulation via an epidural electrode but this too is very sensitive to anaesthetic agents.

Although the anaesthetic contribution is central to intraoperative monitoring, operative decisions made on the basis of spinal cord monitoring remain the responsibility of the surgeon.

ANAESTHESIA FOR BONE TUMOUR SURGERY

Orthopaedic oncology involves the management of patients with primary tumours of bone, cartilage and related connective tissues as well as patients with other malignant disease that has metastasized to bone.

PRIMARY BONE TUMOURS

These most commonly occur between the ages of 5 and 25 years. Familiarity with the different types of tumour and an understanding of the planned operative procedure are integral parts of the preoperative evaluation. Chemotherapy, radiotherapy, or a combination of both are part of the preoperative management in many of these patients and consideration of the potential side effects is mandatory. Because treatment is multidisciplinary in the UK most of these patients are managed by tertiary referral hospitals.

METASTATIC BONE TUMOURS

These patients are usually over the age of 50 years. The primary tumours are most commonly carcinomas of the breast, prostate and lung and if metastases are present anywhere in the skeleton, the vertebral column is usually affected. Secondary bony deposits are commonly found in areas where haemopoietic marrow is present; the axial skeleton and proximal humerus and femur. Patients with metastatic bone disease are often offered palliative surgery, i.e. prophylactic fixation of long bones with intramedullary nails, or, in the vertebral column, stabilization to avert neurological deterioration.

SIDE EFFECTS OF CHEMOTHERAPY AND RADIOTHERAPY RELEVANT TO ANAESTHESIA

Side effects vary from minor inconvenience to life threatening.

- Myelosupression is common and may result in leucopenia, anaemia and thrombocytopenia. This type of surgery is inadvisable in patients whose white cell count is less than $4.0 \times 10^9 \, l^{-1}$, and recovery to a platelet count greater than $100 \times 10^9 \, l^{-1}$ is mandatory. The increased association between deep vein thrombosis and malignancy must not be overlooked.
- Cardiac abnormalities may manifest in the form of any arrhythmia. More rarely, cardiomyopathy may occur, particularly in susceptible patients receiving high doses of doxorubicin. In addition to routine cardiac investigations, in these patients an assessment of ejection fraction is desirable, in the form of either an echocardiogram or MUGA scan.
- Pulmonary fibrosis may occur following radiotherapy or chemotherapy with bleomycin, leading to a restrictive respiratory defect. Bone tumours frequently metastasize to the lungs.
- Nephrotoxicity is a hazard of chemotherapy with cis-platinum.
- Hepatotoxicity may occur. Preoperative liver function tests are essential and if abnormalities are found, coagulation tests should also be performed.
- Any biochemical abnormality may occur and monitoring of sodium, potassium, calcium and magnesium is routine.

SURGICAL PROCEDURES

Within the past two decades limb-sparing procedures have proved safe and effective alternatives to amputation for many patients with bony and soft tissue sarcomas. This advance has been further augmented by the development of new endoprosthetic devices and by progress in techniques of musculoskeletal reconstruction. Nonetheless, amputation still retains a role in high grade sarcomas and for recurrent tumours.

Disarticulation through both shoulder and hip joints are occasionally indicated and for more inaccessible or extensive tumours, forequarter or hindquarter amputation may be necessary. Standard hemipelvectomy is an amputation through the sacroiliac joint and symphysis pubis in which the entire hemipelvis and lower limb are removed. The indications for this operation are bony and soft tissue tumours of the pelvic girdle, proximal femur, groin and buttock.

INTRAOPERATIVE MANAGEMENT

This primarily centres around massive blood loss and transfusion, with attendant rapidly changing fluid shifts and the inevitable development of coagulopathy. Cannulae with as large a gauge as possible should be sited and all these patients require invasive arterial and central venous pressure monitoring. Hourly urine output measurement is also routine. A rapid infusion blood warming system should be available. Unfortunately, blood salvage systems are contraindicated in patients undergoing tumour surgery for fear of haematogenous dissemination of malignant cells.

In major reconstructive surgery large volumes of acrylic cement are often required, the problems of which have been discussed elsewhere in this chapter.

FURTHER READING

Alexander, R. H. and Proctor, H. J. (eds) (1993) *Advanced Trauma Life Support*, American College of Surgeons, Chicago, USA.

Conroy, J. M. and Dorman, B. H. (eds) (1994) *Anesthesia for Orthopedic Surgery*, Raven Press, NY, USA.

Katz, J., Benumof, J. L. and Kadis, L. B. (eds)(1990) *Anaesthesia and Uncommon Diseases*, 3rd edn, Saunders Philadelphia, USA.

Porter, S. S. (ed)(1995) *Anesthesia for Surgery of the Spine*, McGraw-Hill Inc., NY, USA.

ANAESTHESIA FOR THE THERMALLY INJURED PATIENT

L. Davis and T. L. A. Rylah

Improved survival of thermally injured patients has been accredited to the adoption of early tangential excision of the burn wound. Other reasons include improved control and treatment of infection; the use of cardiac, respiratory, and renal support in intensive care units; and more aggressive treatment by intensivists skilled in the early treatment of this injury. The percentage total body surface area (%TBSA) that results in death of half the victims up to the age of 45 years (LD_{50}) has risen to more than 70 over the past two decades. It can be seen that modern anaesthetic skills are needed to maximize these advances and an understanding of the pathophysiology of the thermal wound is essential for the anaesthetist.

The anaesthetist may encounter the burn victim during any stage of treatment. Initially the victim may present as a patient in need of fluid resuscitation or as an inhalation injury in the accident and emergency department. They may be asked to accompany the patient on transfer to a tertiary referral centre. The patient may need emergency surgery whilst undergoing resuscitation if any life-threatening major trauma has been sustained. Debridement of the wound and reconstructive surgery may entail many visits to the operating theatre. Thus the essence of burn care is communication and team work between all those involved in the care of these patients, especially the anaesthetist and the surgeon. This chapter will provide an insight into the changes that occur after a thermal injury and relate those changes to the anaesthetic management of these patients.

PATHOPHYSIOLOGICAL CHANGES

An injury is defined as a major burn when %TBSA > 20 or > 10 in a child under the age of 10 years or an adult over the age of 50 years. A full-thickness burn of 10% TBSA or any wound associated with an inhalation injury, major trauma or a chemical injury is also included in this definition. A burn involving the hands, feet, face or perineum is defined as major as it may have a significant impact upon function. If %TBSA ≥ 41, the injury is termed a severe burn.

The successful treatment of a burn relies upon the accurate assessment of the percentage body surface area that has been burned. A simple method for calculating this is the 'rule of nines'. This splits up the body into six parts and gives their percentages as shown in Table 26.1.

This rule does not apply to children, and a chart such as the Lund and Browder chart should be consulted. The size of a burn in a child can be assessed by using the palm of the child's hand as a guide, this approximating to one per cent TBSA and can be used as a

Short Practice of Anaesthesia. Edited by M. Morgan and G. M. Hall. Published in 1997 by Chapman & Hall, London. ISBN 0 412 71890 1

Table 26.1 The 'Rule of Nines'

Body sector	Percentage area
Head (including the neck)	9
Each upper extremity	9
Torso – front	18
Torso – back	18
Each lower extremity	18
Perineum	1
Total	100

template by being placed over the burned area.

The extent of the physiological changes is proportional to the size of the burn wound; a burn of over 20% TBSA will have a significant effect on the homeostatic mechanisms. There will be a loss of capillary integrity throughout the body which will result in a movement of plasma into the interstitial space and the burn wound. The finite plasma volume is expanded to a potentially infinite volume when this lost fluid is replaced during resuscitation. Thus oedema will form and gross swelling may occur all over the body. This may be particularly relevant if the airway has been involved or an inhalation injury has been sustained. The loss of capillary integrity over the whole body lasts for more than 8 h; after this time integrity is regained slowly so that at between 36 and 72 h after injury, fluid is lost only into the burn wound. Thus resuscitation regimens supply more fluid in the first 8 h and decrease the amounts proportionally over the next 18–24 h. The common regimens are summarized in Table 26.2. If the integrity is not regained after this time and large amounts of fluid are needed to maintain the plasma volume and organ perfusion, a resuscitation failure has occurred making the prognosis of the patient very poor.

Inhalation injury, glottic and sub-glottic burns may result in compromise of the airway and intubation and mechanical ventilation are recommended at the earliest possible time in these cases. Resuscitation fluids will exacerbate any oedema formation and increase this likelihood. Tracheostomy is associated with a higher mortality in patients with head and neck burns or inhalation due to the increased infection rates in these areas.

The cardiac output falls to a nadir in the first 2 h but will increase during resuscitation due to an increase in endogenous catecholamines, resulting in this returning to normal in 24 h and possibly doubling by about 36 h if resuscitation is successful. This catecholamine-induced hypermetabolic state will persist until the wound has been excised and skin coverage is complete. The core temperature is reset to 38.5°C and a 'normal' resting pulse rate of 110–120 b.p.m may mask the early signs of sepsis. An insulin resistant glycaemia may result from the increase in catecholamines and produce an osmotic diuresis. A high caloric intake will be needed to prevent muscle wasting and current practice is to start this within 24 h after injury. Parenteral nutrition may be required to supplement the enteral route.

These changes can affect the anaesthetic management and to simplify the strategies, treatment can be divided into three phases. The first phase is the resuscitation period when cardiovascular stabilization is established. This can be defined as the first 48 h after injury. Then follows the hypermetabolic phase when wound debridement and skin grafting promotes wound healing. Finally, after the wound has been closed comes the reconstructive phase when form and function are restored. Anaesthesia during the first phase is only recommended for small burns or life-saving surgical intervention. Thus the following discourse will concentrate mainly upon the second phase with reference to other phases where necessary.

OPERATIVE PROCEDURES

The likelihood of many operative procedures in a short period of time distinguishes these subjects from most other surgical patients.

Table 26.2 Common resuscitation regimens

	Muir and Barclay	Parkland	Hypertonic saline
Type of fluid	4.5% human albumin	Ringer's Lactate (Hartmann's)	0.9% saline+100 mmol sodium lactate per litre
Formula (ml of solution)	$\dfrac{\text{weight} \times \%TBSA}{2}$	$4 \times \text{weight} \times \%TBSA$	$0.3 \times \text{weight} \times \%TBSA$
Time period	per period	24 h	first hour
Distribution	3×4 hour periods 2×6 hour periods 1×12 hour period	Half in 8 h Quarter in 8 h Quarter in 8 h	Adjust to urine output and plasma sodium each hour

The members of the treatment team should show kindness and understanding at all times to the patients who are commonly frightened and in pain. The anaesthetist can play a major role in maintaining the patients confidence by supplying excellent pain relief and some continuity of care.

The surgical procedures can be divided into those performed early and those performed late.

EARLY PROCEDURES

Immediate excision and grafting

In otherwise fit and healthy patients with no other complicating factors and with injuries of up to 20% TBSA, excision of the wound can be performed immediately. This immediate excision will attenuate the burn response and convert the treatment into that of a patient with major trauma with an associated large blood loss.

Early excision should not be performed if the burn is larger than 20% TBSA or one with associated complications until resuscitation has been successful. This should occur at about 72 h after injury. However, there is increasing practice for the resection of the dead tissue to be performed during the resuscitation phase which in theory would shorten this period.

Escharotomy

This is a procedure classically performed without anaesthesia as dead tissue is analgesic and viable tissue has sensation. Escharotomy involves the incision of circumferential burns, usually full thickness, which are compromising either the circulation or the respiratory effort by constriction. However, as it is intensely painful to identify viable tissue in this manner, it is kinder to administer a general anaesthetic. This should make no difference to the outcome of the escharotomy but the risks of this procedure are greater during the resuscitation period.

Primary excision and grafting

This operation is commonly performed after resuscitation has been successful. Increased survival rates are associated with the removal of dead and non-viable tissue at the earliest opportunity by decreasing infection rates when compared to awaiting the separation of the eschar which may take in excess of 3 weeks.

A commonly accepted policy is to limit burn excision to about 20% TBSA per visit to the operating theatre, thereby reducing the stress response, blood and heat loss and allowing rotation of the donor sites. Alternatively, as it hastens recovery for all burn tissue to be excised at the earliest possible opportunity, it may be feasible to perform total burn excision with one visit to the operating theatre. This technique results in massive blood loss with resultant haemostatic problems, cardiovascular instability, massive heat loss and gross metabolic upset. It requires experienced critical care after operation and is very labour intensive. If this cannot be achieved, the patient will need to return to the operating theatre every 48 h (maximum). There is a case, therefore, for sedating these patients between operations and maintaining them on mechanical ventilation with adequate analgesia.

Dressing changes

These may be performed on a regular basis of every 2 days. The procedures are generally painful and distressing and should be carried out under general anaesthesia. The challenge to the anaesthetist is to develop a technique that interferes as little as possible with the patient's ongoing care and nutrition. Many variations have been used for this procedure including self administered Entonox (with or without an inhalation agent), ketamine and short acting anaesthetics such as alfentanil and propofol. To minimize the disruption to the patient these procedures could be performed as early as possible in the morning and in the burn unit room without transfer to the operating theatre, providing there is adequate monitoring.

LATE PROCEDURES

Reconstructive surgery

These procedures aim to restore form and function once full wound coverage has been obtained. Great efforts will have been made to prevent contractures, limit scarring and preserve function during the earlier treatment by the use of physiotherapy, pressure garments and splints. Nevertheless, in a large burn there is a high probability that contractures will develop. Anaesthesia for their release can pose problems, particularly if the contractures are on the neck or around the nose and mouth. The various reconstructive operations may span many years and it is important to plan well ahead.

Removal of eschar

If a patient has had a difficult resuscitation or has not been deemed fit for anaesthesia, the wound may be left to separate. This may take more than 2 weeks to occur. Anaesthesia may be required at this time to remove eschar that has not separated or to perform grafting. These patients are usually of the highest risk, often being elderly with concurrent illnesses. Blood loss may be massive.

COMMON ANAESTHETIC CHALLENGES

There are some areas where the anaesthetist is presented with particular challenges when dealing with the thermally injured patient both in the immediate and the long-term management.

THE AIRWAY

The burned patient is no different from a traumatized patient; the securing of a patent airway is vital and a tracheal tube may be required. Oedema may accumulate as a result of upper airway tissue damage or secondary to aggressive fluid resuscitation. If there is a clear history of upper airway damage or inhalation, the anaesthetist should assume there is a possibility that the airway will be jeopardized at a later time and intubation should be performed immediately. A tracheal tube may prove impossible to place correctly later, but an unnecessary tracheal tube can be removed without problems. Patients with inhalational injuries that need airway protection may also have burns to the face. These are likely to become infected and thus tracheostomy is not recommended as it can act as an entry point for mediastinitis and septicaemia and may contribute to a higher mortality rate.

Medium- and long-term problems for the anaesthetist are also common. Holding a face mask on a patient with facial burns may be difficult if the skin is covered with antibacterial cream and is greasy and slippery. There may be contractures on the face and neck, limiting mouth and neck movement making oral or nasal tracheal intubation difficult. For short procedures the laryngeal mask may prove invaluable but for longer operations or for those procedures where there is an expectation of special positioning the trachea should be intubated. It is in these circumstances that special techniques may need to be used. These include awake fibre-optic intubation and crico-thyroid puncture with retrograde cannulation. Inhalation induction with direct larygoscopy may be attempted but the airway is not guaranteed by this technique. It may be possible to release contractures under local anaesthesia before proceeding to induction of anaesthesia and more major reconstructive work. This possibility should be discussed with the surgeon.

INHALATION INJURY

Inhalation injury may occur with or without a thermal injury to the skin and may involve the upper airway or the lung parenchyma or both. Heat is responsible for only a small proportion of these injuries as the primary cause is exposure to the products of incomplete combustion. The diversity of these products has made it impossible so far to develop useful treatment strategies. Individuals exposed to the same toxic material at the same time may show great variance in their pathophysiological responses.

Many victims die at the scene due to hypoxia caused by cyanide, carbon monoxide or a low partial pressure of oxygen as the available oxygen is consumed. About half immediate thermal injury deaths are caused by carbon monoxide poisoning; burns alone accounting for only 20%. Other causes are cyanide and other toxin poisoning, pre-existing illnesses, coronary artery disease and acute alcoholism.

The victim may be unconscious or confused on presentation, making a history impossible to obtain first-hand. Patients may present with hoarseness or partial airway obstruction causing stridor, wheezing, supraclavicular and intercostal retraction or copious sputum which may be carbonaceous. A latent injury may be present with little or no symptoms but a strong positive history of exposure. These patients may deteriorate to full respiratory failure up to 48 h later. It is wise to observe these patients for changes during this period.

Diagnosis of an inhalation injury is sometimes very obvious but may have to be made by indirect evidence, i.e. second-hand accounts from fire-fighters or paramedical personnel. A history of exposure to smoke in an enclosed space, down a hole or being downwind of the incident will arouse a high degree of suspicion. Burned nasal hairs, carbonaceous sputum, soot in the nose and mouth, wheeze or voice change, and a burned face (including the cornea) are among the most common findings upon examination.

If a significant injury is suspected, the airway should be secured as soon as possible because resuscitation will result in swelling which may jeopardize the patency of the airways. Repeated indirect laryngoscopy may exacerbate the swelling and may pick up a partially obstructed airway at a time when it is difficult or impossible to intubate the trachea. Facial burns with no other signs or symptoms will not usually require intubation. Burns from the lips to the epiglottis will become oedematous with fluid resuscitation and intubation is recommended. If the oedema does not obstruct the airway when maximal (approximately 24 h after injury) and the airway is not thought to be at risk, the tracheal tube can be removed. If the airways below the epiglottis have sustained thermal injury or exposure to toxic or irritant substances, intubation, sedation, oxygen therapy and respiratory support will be necessary. It is humane to sedate and ventilate the lungs of these patients as they can be greatly distressed both physically and mentally. Blood gas analysis will reveal carbon monoxide or other poisoning and this should be treated by restoring optimum levels of oxygen transport.

If associated with a large burn, the lung will be assaulted further by the need for large amounts of fluids to resuscitate the victim. If the lung has also sustained a burn, this will further increase the fluid need. Respiratory support must be tailored to each patient to maintain oxygenation and carbon dioxide excretion. No mode of ventilatory support should be excluded but the effects of barotrauma must be borne in mind. Acid–base imbalance may be present and will need constant supervision and correction. Fibre-optic bronchoscopy may be used to assess the prognosis; burns to the airways after the third bronchial division carry a poor prognosis. It may also be used therapeutically to perform tracheobronchial toilet to remove epithelial sloughing. Steroids have not been shown to improve clinical response but increase infection and mortality rates in both inhalation injury and burns.

Carbon monoxide poisoning must be treated with high inspired oxygen concentrations and respiratory support. Any acid–base imbalance should be corrected. Hyperbaric oxygen treatment is seldom available and rarely results in any neurological recovery. Cyanide poisoning must be considered in patients slow to respond to treatment or with a persistent metabolic acidosis. Specific antidotes are available but may result in hypotension and excessive levels of methaemoglobin.

NUTRITION AND FLUID BALANCE

The post resuscitation phase is accompanied by a huge upsurge in the metabolic rate to the extent that in patients with a 50% TBSA burn it can double. This hypermetabolic phase lasts until there is effective wound closure. It is accompanied by an increase in oxygen consumption, carbon dioxide production, protein catabolism and a negative nitrogen balance. This hypercatabolism is mediated by a surge in endogenous catecholamines. A high caloric intake has to be maintained to minimize the catabolism of body mass and sometimes cannot be achieved by enteric means alone. This can cause problems for the anaesthetist as preoperative fasting must be kept to a minimum; dedicated parenteral nutrition lines cannot be used for induction and nasogastric feeding may be in progress. The nutritional requirements can be achieved by operating in the early morning and keeping to scheduled surgery times. The hypercatabolic state can also cause hyperglycaemia or an insulin-resistant diabetic state to occur which may complicate the anaesthetic care of these patients. An osmotic diuresis may dehydrate the patient; however, the good urine output may be mistaken for overhydration.

Wherever possible blood loss should be replaced with fresh whole blood as this will result in optimum coagulation and haemostasis. This is most important in children. Fresh frozen plasma and red-cell concentrate may be all that is available. Plasma volume may be replaced with human plasma protein fraction 4.5% or with Hetastarch 6% solution in 0.9% saline. An anaemic patient will benefit from preoperative transfusion so long as sufficient time is allowed for the transfused red cells to become fully competent in oxygen delivery by increasing their levels of 2,3-diphosphoglycerate.

MONITORING

All major burn patients should have a urinary catheter inserted to monitor and ensure adequate urine output (minimum of 0.5 ml kg^{-1} h^{-1} Hypovolaemia is difficult to detect in burned patients as they have a tachycardia even if adequate analgesia is given. In a patient who has satisfactory pain relief, a heart rate greater than 120 b.p.m. may signal the possibility of hypovolaemia. Other signs will include reduced capillary refill, a reduction in urine output and hypotension. Invasive monitoring will be of benefit. Central venous and/or a pulmonary artery catheter will give invaluable data on which to base fluid replacement when large losses are anticipated. The risk of infection is increased with the presence of these monitoring aids, so they must be removed as soon as the need for them has passed.

In all major burn excisions the blood pressure should be monitored with an arterial cannula as blood loss may be massive. It is often difficult to measure such loss but a rough guide would be 4% of the circulating volume per percentage body area excised. In areas where there is no underlying fascia such as the face, neck and buttocks this can be even more.

VENOUS ACCESS

It is essential that good venous access is assured and it is advisable that two large bore cannulae (14 G in an adult) are inserted before large excisions. Inhalational induction of anaesthesia may be necessary before cannulation in these patients, especially for children, as venous access can be difficult. Psychological support for these patients will improve the patient–anaesthetist relationship for the many future procedures. Cannulation sites are at a premium and should be selected first from any available peripheral sites, then to the central sites: groin, internal jugular and subclavian veins. If necessary, cannulation through a burned area is permissible but it is essential to keep this site meticulously clean. If there is a paucity of clean cannulation sites, grafting should be planned to create new sites for the future, as venous access through burned tissue will increase morbidity and mortality.

ANALGESIA

Pain is not solely dependent on a damaging insult to the body, but also on the anxiety, fear and depression that may be sequelae to the injury. Kind and thoughtful care from the burn unit staff will do much to allay these components of the patient's pain, having none of the disadvantages of pharmacological preparations. Nevertheless, there is a real need for alleviation of the physical pain of a burn which can be severe and protracted. Movement, physiotherapy and harvesting of donor skin all add to the patients' distress. Inadequate pain relief may contribute to the later development of post traumatic stress disorder in about half of major burn patients.

Intravenous administration of opioids is recommended to establish pain control as intramuscular routes are too unreliable and unpredictable. Ideally, a patient-controlled analgesia (PCA) device is the best option; it can be adapted to suit the wide variations in patients' requirements and it gives the patient some control and self determination which is important. PCA devices can be adapted for patients with disabilities and most children can be taught to use them. If PCA is not an option, some form of opioid infusion or nurse-controlled analgesia (NCA) is better than intermittent intramuscular boluses.

The opioid selected will vary according to the practice of each burn unit, the most commonly used being morphine although diamorphine, fentanyl and alfentanil are also used. Fentanyl and alfentanil may prove to have advantages over morphine in prolonged use, owing to the accumulative nature and possible renal effects of morphine. Long-term pethidine infusions should be avoided because of the potential accumulation of toxic metabolites. Once the acute phase has been passed, oral preparations such as Oramorph may be introduced, although it must be remembered that the bioavailability will be approximately halved when comparing enteral to intravenous administration. Slow release oral preparations such as MST are very acceptable in the long term.

Other analgesics for the burned patient include the simple analgesics such as paracetamol, co-proxamol, dihydrocodeine and NSAIDs such as diclofenac and ibuprofen. The use of NSAIDs should be limited to three days owing to their possible renal toxicity in these patients.

Local and regional anaesthesia techniques can be of use but are of limited application because the burn is classified as an infected wound and hence central neural blockade is contraindicated. In a well localized burn such as on the hand and forearm, a brachial plexus block may be performed. The transarterial technique in the axilla must not be used if reconstructive free-tissue transfer surgery is to be performed as this may later be blamed for poor perfusion to the flap.

Burn injuries also cause areas of hyperaesthesia and severe itching which is related to tissue healing and regeneration. This can sometimes be very severe and cause the patient much distress, but can be treated with small amounts of naloxone subcutaneously which will not intereferre with the analgesia already in progress. Alternatively, a partial agonist such as nalbuphine or buprenorphine may be used to good effect.

PAEDIATRIC BURNS

Children account for up to 40% of all burn admissions. A minor scald may develop life threatening sepsis in this age group. The child with burns, has specific problems in addition to the regular difficulties that a child would present to the anaesthetist.

The burned child exhibits a more severe physiological response to thermal trauma when compared to an adult. The increased core temperature may elicit febrile convulsions necessitating active cooling. Fluid requirements and nutritional needs are more accurately calculated if based on the body surface area rather than the weight of the child. It is even more essential that preoperative starvation is kept to a minimum as nutritional demand is high and there is a tendency for small children to become hypoglycaemic. Regular monitoring of blood sugar should help to avoid this. The use of dextrose solutions without saline can render the child dangerously hyponatraemic.

The difficulty of communication with a sick, frightened child is compounded when the child is not in the comforting surroundings of a paediatric ward and where he/she may well have had numerous previous general anaesthetics for grafting and dressing changes. It is important to gain the parents' and the child's confidence at an early stage. The parents can aid the anaesthetist in the smooth induction of a distressed child if they are willing and able.

Induction of anaesthesia should be as humane as possible with either the use of EMLA cream for venepuncture or inhalation induction and placement of intravenous cannulae once the child is unconscious. The technique of choice must ensure a swift recovery and a rapid return to feeding.

Ketamine has been used in children with a low incidence of postoperative hallucinations. This may be due to communication or perceptive differences in the child. The newer inhalational agents, desflurane and sevoflurane, show rapid recovery characteristics and may prove to be the agents of choice. Both enflurane and isoflurane have been used with good results.

Heat loss is a major problem with the high surface area to body weight ratio, thin skin and greater cardiac index. The core and peripheral temperature must be monitored and every effort made to ensure that heat loss is kept to a minimum. Smaller children can be operated upon under infrared heaters. The operating room should be kept sufficiently warm for the needs of the patient, and may be uncomfortable for the operating staff to work in. All fluids, including those used for antiseptic cleaning, should be warmed. Intraoperative monitoring will be a challenge in the thermally injured child where size complicates the issue.

Excellent pain relief is essential in children who may not be able to articulate their distress. Thus requirements may have to be measured objectively and a child-adapted visual analogue scale using smiling to frowning faces along a line can help the carers. Children of school age can be taught how to use a PCA, but younger children may need a nurse-controlled device or a constant infusion. Oral analgesia should be instituted as early as possible.

PHARMACOKINETICS AND PHARMACODYNAMICS

Many physiological factors contribute to the problems of drug metabolism in burned patients. These changes will become significant in a burn over 20% TBSA. Those factors that are known include: loss of vascular integrity; the release of vasoactive mediators and generalized vasodilation; a variable degree of renal failure; the intravascular release of haemoglobin and myoglobin leading to a loss of the renal tubular concentrating mechanisms; hypoperfusion of the liver leading to oedema and changes in the volume of distribution; a decrease in albumin which can be as much as 50% in a severe burn and an increase in α_1-glycoprotein (an acute phase reactive protein which binds many basic drugs) by a factor of two to three. Drugs that are primarily albumin bound such as diazepam will increase their potency whereas a drug bound to α_1-glycoprotein such as lignocaine or bupivacaine will decrease their potency. There will be an increase in cardiac output during the hypermetabolic phase which will increase organ perfusion resulting in a more rapid uptake and clearance of the drug. Drugs may interact with each other through enzyme induction or inhibition or through competition for protein binding places.

OPIOIDS

The requirement for opioids in severely burned patients is high and the intravenous route is the most reliable method of administration. There is a wide variation in the patient's requirements due to differences in pain tolerance and the factors discussed above; each treatment must be tailored to the patient's needs at that time. The amount of opioid needed is that which is enough to effect analgesia.

INDUCTION AGENTS

These patients are generally hypovolaemic and intravenous induction should be undertaken with great caution. The induction time will generally be short as there is a hyperdynamic circulation and low albumin concentrations will allow more free drug to be available. Propofol carries the obvious advantage that it allows rapid recovery but can cause precipitous drops in blood pressure. Care should be taken as propofol in combination with fentanyl can elicit an extreme bradycardia.

MUSCLE RELAXANTS

Animal studies have demonstrated a proliferation of acetylcholine receptors after a systemic burn. This is similar to a denervation or a disuse atrophy state; it is found in muscle where no nerve damage has occurred in freely moving animals. The appearance of these receptors depended on the severity of the burn; animals with 20% full-thickness burns showed increases in receptor numbers at 14 days and these had returned to control levels by 21 days. The animals which had 50% burns showed changes at day 10 which persisted until day 28 (and possibly longer). The underlying cause is not known but this phenomenon does explain the changed response of burned patients to depolarizing and non-depolarizing muscle relaxants.

Suxamethonium is the only depolarizing muscle relaxant available and it is contraindicated in major burns in all but the first 48 h. The reason for this is the exaggerated hyperkalaemic response which follows the administration of a depolarizing muscle relaxants. Increases in serum potassium to greater than 6 mmol l^{-1} have been observed in patients with burns as small as 8% TBSA. The consequences of a rapid and marked increase in the serum potassium concentration are ventricular arrhythmias and possibly death. The risk persists until there is complete skin coverage, although this sensitivity has been shown to be present for as long as 2 years after the burn.

The burn patient also shows a relative resistance to non-depolarizing muscle relaxants needing a 2–5 fold increase in drug dosage. This resistance is positively correlated to the size of the burn, and for atracurium the resistance is maximal at 15 to 40 days and has returned to normal after 100 days. No significant clinical resistance can be shown before one week after injury.

Plasma cholinesterase decreases following a burn, the magnitude and the rate of the fall being correlated with the size of the burn. Minimal levels of activity are reached 5–6 days after the injury and may be as low as 20% of pre-burn levels. In severely burned patients this can persist for 3–4 months after healing of the burn. The causes of this reduction in plasma cholinesterase activity are: decreased enzyme synthesis by the liver; a dilutional effect from resuscitation; increased catabolism; and trans-capillary loss. Complicated burns such as those with sepsis will show an even greater fall. Patients who are heterozygote or less commonly homozygote for an atypical cholinesterase gene would be very sensitive to a range of drugs which rely on ester hydrolysis for termination of action. As it is unlikely that suxamethonium will be used in these patients, the two most important drugs for the anaesthetist to be aware of are mivacurium and the ester local anaesthetic agents

ANAESTHESIA

No technique is regarded as the 'gold standard' and all anaesthetists will have their methods and drugs of choice. However, a number of general principles will apply in all cases.

LOCAL OR GENERAL ANAESTHESIA

The burned patient is regarded as an infected case, so there is no place for the central neural blockade as an anaesthetic technique in all but the most distal and minor of burns.

INDUCTION OF ANAESTHESIA

The burn patient is hypermetabolic with a hyperdynamic circulation. The patient is likely to desaturate quickly and must receive oxygen before induction. Generous doses of analgesic drugs will allow for a smooth balanced anaesthetic and should provide good postoperative pain relief. Propofol is suitable as an induction agent but should be used with caution. It is wise to administer a pre-emptive anti-emetic such as droperidol or ondansetron, with the induction of anaesthesia. Securing the tracheal tube can sometimes be a problem in facial burns and it may be necessary to suture the tube to the teeth.

TECHNIQUES TO FACILITATE SURGERY

Various techniques can be used to reduce blood loss in the primary excision and grafting phase. Subcutaneous infiltration of the wound and donor site with a weak solution of phenylephrine (15 mg in 1 l 0.9% saline) or swabs soaked in adrenaline (1 in 40 000) applied to the bleeding area will decrease blood loss. Alternatively, a synthetic vasopressin derivative, terlipressin, which has strong vasoconstictive properties but little systemic effects, may be used.

Hypotensive anaesthesia will allow easier surgery in the reconstructive phase by improving the operative field and will minimize the need for blood transfusion. However, free tissue transfer must not be jeopardized by hypovolaemia and poor blood flow. Vasodilatation must be accompanied by volume expansion allowing the dilated vessels to be easily handled. Once the infection risk has passed the use of regional blocks will improve blood flow to the receiving area and provide good analgesia.

MONITORING

Monitoring blood pressure, volume status and temperature have already been mentioned. Electrocardiography may require steel sutures or staples to be placed through burned tissue as adhesive electrodes will not adhere to the wound or the skin. Oesophageal electrodes or intracardiac electrodes on a pulmonary artery catheter are alternatives. The pulse oximeter probe may have to be positioned in an unorthodox place and the tongue, cheek nose and genitalia have all been used. Core and peripheral temperatures should be monitored, a falling peripheral temperature with a static core temperature indicates inadequate volume replacement.

POSTOPERATIVE CARE

Excellent analgesia is essential into the postoperative period; a relative perioperative overdose of opioid should not be antagonized but rather ventilation supported until there is a return of spontaneous breathing. Postoperative shivering will increase oxygen demand considerably and should be prevented by strict temperature maintainance rather than treated when it occurs. Heat is often lost during transfer from the operating table to the recovery room and care must be taken to minimize this. Warming blankets and warm air blowers are commonly used in the recovery room to restore temperature.

Cardiovascular instability during recovery may be due to concealed blood loss. Postoperative tests should be performed to estimate the blood loss and any derangement of the clotting system. Haemostasis is difficult to obtain and much blood can be lost into the copious bandaging. A consumptive coagulopathy may need to be treated with fresh frozen plasma and platelets.

SUMMARY

The burned patient presents the anaesthetist with many challenges. The airway may be difficult and cardiovascular instability may necessitate highly invasive monitoring. Analgesia is a key issue for patient welfare and drug handling can be unpredictable. Children will present a special challenge to all concerned. With good anaesthetic management it is possible to achieve a rapid recovery and attain resumption of enteral feeding within 2 h of a large burn excision.

The anaesthetist is an important member of the professional team who must support the patient both physically and psychologically through this major life trauma. Working in an environment where there will be failures, sometimes distressing, as well as successes, it is important that there is a feeling of mutual support between all the carers in order to provide the foundation for ongoing excellence in the burn unit.

FURTHER READING

Ellis, A. and Rylah, L. T. A. (1990). Transfer of the thermally injured patient. *British Journal of Hospital Medicine*, **44**, 206–208.
Frame, J. D. Taweepoke, P. Moieman, N. and

Rylah, L. T. A. (1990). Immediate fascial flap reconstruction of joints and use of Biobrane in the burned limb. *Burns*, **16**, 381–384.

Herndon, D. N. (ed) (1996) *Total Burn Care*, Saunders, London.

Hunt, J. L., Purdue, G. F. and Gunning, T. (1986) Is tracheostomy warranted in the burn patient? Indications and complications. *Journal of Burn Care and Rehabilitation*, **7**, 492–495.

Lund, C. C. and Browder, N. C. (1944) Estimation of areas of burns. *Surgery, Gynecology and Obstetrics*, **79**: 352–358.

Marathe, P. H., Haschke, R. H., Slattery, J. T., Zucker, J. R. and Pavlin, E. G. (1989) Acetylcholine receptor density and acetylcholinesterase activity in skeletal muscle of rats following thermal injury. *Anesthesiology*, **70**, 654–659.

Moran, K. T., O'Reilly, T. J. and Furman, W. R. (1988) A new algorithm for calculation of blood loss in excisional burn surgery. *American Surgery*, **54**, 207–210.

Rylah, L. T. A. (ed) (1992) *Critical Care of the Burned Patient*, Cambridge Univesity Press, Cambridge.

Yentis, S. M. (1990). Suxamethonium and hyperkalaemia. *Anaesthesia and Intensive Care*, **18**, 92–101.

TRANSPLANTATION OF LIVER AND KIDNEY

S. V. Mallett and T. Peachey

Organ transplantation is a field of medicine that has expanded enormously in the past two decades. Once considered a highly experimental procedure it is now established as a viable and successful treatment for patients with end-stage disease. Improvements in tissue typing, organ preservation, immunosuppression and surgical and anaesthetic techniques have led to greatly improved survival with an exponential increase in the number of centres performing transplants over the last ten years. However, with a limited number of cadaveric donors available, it is likely that this growth period has ended, and there is now an increasing trend towards looking critically at the economic effectiveness of transplantation. Careful scrutiny of selection criteria and outcome data are required to optimize the allocation of these precious resources and ensure the equitable and successful use of donor organs.

LIVER TRANSPLANTATION ANAESTHESIA

The first liver transplant was performed in 1963 by Thomas Starzl in Denver, USA, however it took another 20 years for this procedure to be recognized as an approved treatment for patients with end-stage liver disease. Orthotopic liver transplantation in most diagnostic groups now results in a one year survival in excess of 80%, and mortality in subsequent years is very low. In addition, the quality of life in long-term survivors is generally excellent. In the UK, liver transplantation is performed only in designated centres at the rate of approximately 700 transplants per year. Worldwide nearly 7000 liver transplants are performed each year.

Liver transplantation is one of the most challenging fields in anaesthetic practice. Liver transplant recipients may have severely deranged physiology as a result of their disease, together with impaired and unpredictable drug handling. The procedure itself can be complicated by massive blood loss, profound haemodynamic changes, pathological coagulopathies and numerous metabolic disturbances. Management of these complicated patients has contributed to the development of advanced, physiological monitoring and treatment, coagulation assessment, rapid infusion technology and temperature control systems. Many of these techniques are now used in other types of complex surgery.

INDICATIONS FOR LIVER TRANSPLANTATION

The major indications are as follows.

- Chronic end-stage liver disease with cirrhosis.
    Post hepatitis

- Alcoholic
- Cryptogenic
- Auto-immune
  - Chronic active hepatitis
  - Primary biliary cirrhosis
  - Primary sclerosing cholangitis
- Acute liver failure
  - Viral hepatitis
  - Drug induced (including halothane)
  - Poisoning (including paracetamol)
  - Miscellaneous.
- Metabolic disorders
  - Wilson's disease
  - α-antitrypsin deficiency
  - Tyrosinosis
  - Oxalosis
  - Haemochromatosis
  - Glycogen storage disease
- Malignant disease
- Budd–Chiari syndrome
- Re-transplantation
  - Primary graft dysfunction
  - Chronic rejection

The severity of liver disease at the time of transplantation can critically affect the probability of a successful outcome. In general, patients with end-stage liver disease (ESLD) are investigated and placed on the waiting list before the pre-terminal stage of their illness has been reached. Patients who are classified as Child's C (Table 27.1) at the time of operation have a significantly higher morbidity and mortality than those in Child's groups A and B. Waiting time varies but depends to a large extent on the recipient's blood group and body weight, and the availability of a suitably matched organ.

Patients with acute liver failure (ALF) meeting the criteria for transplantation, are registered with the UK transplant service as 'super urgent' and generally receive a graft within 24–48 h.

CONTRAINDICATIONS

As experience increases, and the results have improved the list of conditions that might prevent a patient being accepted for transplantation have decreased. Age is no longer considered a barrier, and a number of carefully selected patients over the age of 70 years have now been transplanted. Transplantation for hepatitis B infection and malignancy remains controversial, due to the high rate of recurrence of the original disease.

Currently the main contraindications as follows

- Widespread or extra-hepatic malignancy
- Sepsis outside the hepatobiliary system
- Severe cardiac or respiratory disease
- Active substance abuse
- Acquired immunodeficiency syndrome

Table 27.1 Modified Child's/Pugh risk grading

	Points		
	1	2	3
Encephalopathy	absent	mild	severe
Serum bilirubin ($\mu mol\ l^{-1}$)	<25	25–50	>50
Ascites	absent	good control	poor control
Albumin ($g\ l^{-1}$)	>35	30–35	<30
Prothrombin time prolongation (s)	1–4	4–6	>6

Equivalent Child's grading: Class A=5 or less, Class B=6–10, Class C=11–15 points

PATHOPHYSIOLOGY OF END-STAGE LIVER DISEASE

Patients presenting for liver transplantation do not all necessarily have grossly impaired liver function. Those with neoplasms or metabolic disease may have relatively normal function, and patients with cholestatic disease usually have quite well preserved hepatic synthetic function with little end-organ disease. However, patients with cirrhosis generally have severe, hepatocellular dysfunction and the classical, multi-system manifestations of ESLD.

Cardiovascular

ESLD is associated with a hyperdynamic circulation with a high cardiac output and low systemic vascular resistance, and reduced vascular sensitivity to catecholamines. Flow murmurs are common and some degree of functional mitral regurgitation may be present. There is an associated increase in plasma volume that may be up to 50% above normal. There is extensive arteriovenous shunting, resulting in a high mixed venous oxygen saturation (MV_{O_2}). Pathological oxygen supply dependency has been described in patients with cirrhosis. The cause of the vasodilation is incompletely understood, but is due in part to the production of, or inadequate clearance of, vasoactive substances by the failing liver (endotoxin, vasoactive polypeptide, nitric oxide). The magnitude of the haemodynamic changes is related to the severity of the liver disease, and becomes more severe as liver function deteriorates. These changes are reversible following successful liver transplantation. Patients with alcoholic cirrhosis and haemochromatosis may, in addition, have a cardiomyopathy. Atherosclerosis is less common in cirrhotic liver disease than in the general population, but coronary artery disease should not be overlooked and must always be fully investigated. Approximately 0.25–0.5% of patients with ESLD have significant pulmonary hypertension.

Portal hypertension

Life threatening gastrointestinal haemorrhage from oesophageal varices is of significant concern for patients on the transplant waiting list. Immediate treatment includes intravenous resuscitation and infusion of vasopressin or somatostatin and balloon tamponade. Following resuscitation, endoscopic sclerotherapy is the initial treatment of choice, but recurrence of bleeding occurs in one quarter of patients. Surgical portosystemic shunt may be considered but perioperative mortality may be as high as 25% when this is performed as an emergency. This surgery can increase the difficulty of a subsequent transplant procedure. The insertion of a transjugular intrahepatic portosytemic shunt (TIPS) is a relatively new, and far less invasive method of dealing with the complications of portal hypertension. TIPS results in a direct intrahepatic communication between the portal vein and hepatic veins causing decompression of the hepatic sinusoidal and mesenteric vascular beds. This technique is used in patients with recurrent, or life-threatening, variceal bleeds and also in some patients with intractable ascites.

Respiratory

Minor degrees of hypoxaemia are common in ESLD (30–50%) and many patients have a mild respiratory alkalosis due to compensatory tachypnoea. Ascites and pleural effusions result in atelectasis and ventilation–perfusion mismatch. Hypoxic pulmonary vasoconstriction is impaired. Pulmonary arteriovenous shunting can cause severe hypoxaemia, particularly when the patient is standing (orthodeoxia). Hypoxaemia can also be caused by massive dilation of pulmonary capillaries resulting in impaired transfer of oxygen to red cells in the centre of these abnormal vessels because of the increased diffusion distance ('diffusion disequilibrium'). Severe cases are labelled as having 'hepatopulmonary syndrome'. Low diffusing capacity for carbon monoxide has been found in 50% patients with chronic liver disease. Although there is evidence that intrapulmonary shunting reverses following liver transplantation, severe hypoxaemia ($Pa_{O_2} < 7$ kPa) is generally considered a contraindication to transplantation.

A small proportion of cirrhotic patients with portal hypertension also have portopulmonary shunts through mediastinal, paraoesophageal and ayzgous venous systems. These are not a significant cause of hypoxaemia as the saturation of portal venous blood is high (80–85%).

Some liver diseases may have specific pulmonary manifestations. Primary biliary cirrhosis is associated with both lymphocytic bronchitis and interstitial lung disease; autoimmune chronic active hepatitis is associated with pulmonary fibrosis.

Renal

Patients presenting for liver transplantation may have varying degrees of renal impairment. Hepatorenal syndrome is the term used to describe functional renal impairment due to advanced liver disease. It is characterized by a decreased renal blood flow, with reduced glomerular filtration rate and urine output in the absence of any renal histological abnormality. Free water excretion is impaired and there is dilutional hyponatraemia despite the occurrence of avid sodium retention. It appears to be caused by a physiological response to perceived vascular underfilling, perhaps due to the massive splanchnic vasodilatation that occurs with ESLD. There is activation of the renin–angiotensin system, enhanced sympathetic tone, increased ADH secretion and altered renal prostaglandin activity. The severity of the hyponatraemia is a good marker of the extent of altered haemodynamics in these patients. The development of actual hepatorenal failure heralds rapid deterioration of hepatic function and the need for urgent liver transplantation where appropriate. Pre-renal insufficiency is not uncommon due to the use of diuretics and the presence of tense ascites. It is essential to avoid nephrotoxic drugs (e.g NSAIDs) and to treat any infection aggressively in these patients to reduce the risk of acute tubular necrosis.

Central nervous system

Hepatic encephalopathy is a neuropsychiatric disorder associated with the accumulation of toxic substances (ammonia, γ-aminobutyric acid, short chain fatty acids) that are not cleared by the failing liver. There are also disturbances in the blood–brain barrier, changes in neurotransmitter concentrations and altered cerebral metabolism. It is important to appreciate that, although the basic mediators involved in the development of encephalopathy in acute and chronic liver disease are similar, there are some fundamental differences. In chronic disease, encephalopathy is usually associated with portosystemic shunting and has other obvious precipitating factors: gastrointestinal bleeding, protein loading, hypokalaemic alkalosis, sepsis. Cerebral oedema is rarely seen. In contrast, in acute liver failure 50–80% of patients develop cerebral oedema due to cytotoxic and vasogenic mechanisms. Brain stem herniation associated with a high intracranial pressure is the commonest cause of death in this group of patients. Many centres now use intracranial pressure monitoring in fulminant hepatic failure once the patient is placed on the superurgent waiting list for transplantation or is in grade 4 coma. If severe coagulopathy is present, there is also the potential for cerebral haemorrhage, especially if a sub-dural ICP monitor is used.

Hepatic encephalopathy grades are as follows.

1. Mild or episodic drowsiness
2. Increased drowsiness and confusion and disorientation
3. Very drowsy, frequently agitated and aggressive
4. Comatose, responds to deep pain.

Metabolic

Glucose

Hypoglycaemia is associated with acute liver failure or the pre-terminal stage of ESLD. In chronic liver disease hyperglycaemia with glucose intolerance is common and frank diabetes mellitus can occur especially in association with haemochromatosis and autoimmune chronic active hepatitis.

Electrolytes

- Hypokalaemia may result from diuretic therapy, respiratory alkalosis, secondary hyperaldosteronism and diarrhoea and vomiting.
- Hyponatraemia occurs frequently in patients with cirrhosis and ascites. It is usually dilutional and associated with increased ADH secretion, although sodium depletion from diuretics must be excluded. Corretion should always be undertaken slowly since rapid increases in sodium may cause central pontine myelinolysis. Hyponatraemia is usually treated with water restriction, reduced diuretic dosage and albumin infusions. Haemofiltration has been used before transplantation to correct refractory hyponatraemia.
- Hypomagnesaemia can result from increased excretion due to diureties. Alcoholic liver disease is often associated with severe total body depletion of magnesium which can predispose to the development of arrythmias such as atrial fibrillation.

Nutrition

Patients with ESLD are frequently malnourished with decreased muscle mass and low fat stores. This is due to decreased oral intake, malabsorbtion, abnormalities of hepatic synthesis and degradation of protein and substrates, and a catabolic state. Nutritional support is difficult because of the need to restrict dietary protein, and excessive use of glucose and fat can result in fatty changes in the liver and cholestasis. Branched chain amino acid solutions may enable protein intake to be increased to adequate levels.

Coagulation

Although coagulopathy is common in liver disease its nature and degree is variable and depends on both the underlying cause of the disease and its severity. Patients with mainly cholestatic disease (primary biliary cirrhosis or primary sclerosing cholangitis) generally have well preserved hepatic synthetic function and normal coagulation until very advanced stages of the disease. Patients with Budd–Chiari syndrome are usually hypercoagulable and may require anticoagulation therapy. Patients with chronic liver disease have a multifactorial cause of abnormal coagulation. Contributory factors include: malabsorption of vitamin K (leading to decreased synthesis of factors II, VII, IX and X and protein C and S), defective hepatic synthesis of all coagulation proteins except factor VIII, defective production and clearance of fibrinolytic inhibitors and activated coagulation factors, and hypersplenism resulting in thrombocytopenia and impaired platelet function. Also, in many patients with severe liver disease (Child's group C) a chronic low grade activation of the coagulation/fibrinolytic systems also occurs, perhaps due to endotoxaemia. Up to 30% of cirrhotic patients have evidence of accelerated fibrinolysis.

PREOPERATIVE PREPARATION

Patients are fully investigated before being placed on the transplant waiting list. Particular emphasis is placed on the cardiovascular system as this may limit patients' ability to withstand the haemodynamic stresses imposed by the procedure. If patients are on the waiting list for some months, it is important that they are reviewed again by the anaesthetic team as considerable deterioration in their overall status may have occurred.

Cardiac tests

All patients have a baseline 12-lead ECG, exercise ECG, echocardiogram and right heart catheter study. Echocardiography is useful for identifying valvular pathology, cardiomyopathy, ventricular dysfunction and reduction of ejection fraction. It may also give some indication as to whether pulmonary hypertension is present. If there is evidence of coronary artery disease on exercise testing, further studies such as thallium-dipyridamole scanning and even coronary angiography may be required. If there is overt coronary artery disease the patients may be referred for angioplasty or coronary bypass grafting before transplant if their liver disease is not yet end-stage. Patients with single vessel disease do not have an excess perioperative morbidity and mortality. Patients with mild to moderate pulmonary hypertension have been successfully transplanted although a difficult intraoperative course may be expected. However, severe pulmonary hypertension with right ventricular hypertrophy carries a high operative mortality and these patients may be considered for combined heart/lung/liver transplantation. Pulmonary vasodilators such as glyceryl trinitrate, prostacylcin and even nitric oxide are often ineffective in such patients. Echocardiography does not identify pulmonary hypertension unless it is severe, and a number of asymptomatic patients have been found to have unexpected pulmonary hypertension during surgery. It is for this reason that preoperative measurement of pulmonary artery pressure with a right heart catheter may be useful despite the low incidence of this problem.

Respiratory assessment

All patients have a chest radiograph, lung function studies and arterial blood gas analysis. Severe restrictive lung disease may not preclude transplantation, but a prolonged period of ventilatory support can be expected. Smokers are strongly advised to stop, and those patients with obstructive lung disease may require preoperative physiotherapy, antibiotics and bronchodilators. Large pleural effusions interfering with ventilation are drained. Severe hypoxaemia from whatever cause is considered a contraindication to transplantation.

Renal assessment

Liver disease is associated with lower concentrations of serum urea and creatinine and so it can be difficult to assess mild to moderate degrees of renal dysfunction. Creatinine clearance studies are used preoperatively to evaluate glomerular filtration rate. Renal failure is strongly correlated with an increased risk of postoperative sepsis and mortality; therefore renal protective measures (maintenance of intravascular filling pressures and adequate renal perfusion pressure together with low-dose dopamine) are of great importance perioperatively.

In our institution venovenous bypass is not used routinely except for patients with fulminant hepatic failure. In patients with severely compromised or deteriorating renal function, bypass is used to maintain renal perfusion pressure during the anhepatic phase.

Donor matching

Liver allografts, unlike renal transplants, do not require full tissue typing. Hyperacute rejection does not occur in liver transplantation. Improvements in preservation solutions have extended the maximum, cold ischaemia time for liver grafts up to 18–20 h, so liver transplantation can now be performed as a semi-elective procedure in daylight hours. However, the incidence of biliary strictures and graft dysfunction is increased with prolonged ischaemia, and this time is limited to less than 14 h where possible. Patients with acute liver failure who are deteriorating rapidly must be transplanted as soon as a graft becomes available. Grafts must ideally be blood-group compatible and of a suitable size for the recipient. In urgent cases it is possible to use a mismatched graft (ABO incompatible). Large grafts can be reduced in size for small recipients or only one lobe used, however this takes longer and is technically more complicated. Because there are so few paediatric donors, some centres now perform living-related liver transplants, grafting the left lobe of the donor into the child.

INTRAOPERATIVE MANAGEMENT

The surgical procedure

Liver transplantation is conveniently divided into three main stages: preanhepatic, anhepatic and postanhepatic, each has its own particular problems.

Stage 1: dissection

The abdomen is opened through a bilateral, subcostal incision extended up to the xiphoid and the liver and its vascular attachments (supra- and infrahepatic vena cava, portal vein and hepatic artery) and bile duct separated from surrounding tissues. In patients with portal hypertension there may be large variceal venous collaterals in the abdominal wall and mesentery which can result in heavy blood loss. Previous upper abdominal surgery, especially portocaval shunts, can also substantially increase bleeding in this stage.

Stage 2: anhepatic

The major vessels and bile duct are clamped and divided, and the native liver removed together with the retrohepatic inferior vena cava and hepatic veins. The donor liver is removed from ice and following suitable preparation on a back table is then placed in the recipient's hepatic fossa (beginning of warm ischaemia time). The suprahepatic vena cava, portal vein and infrahepatic vena cava are then anastomosed. When the last anastomosis is almost complete the liver is perfused with 500–1000 ml of human albumin solution through a cannula inserted into the portal vein through the incomplete anastomosis, flushing air and preservation solution from the liver through the incomplete infrahepatic caval anastomosis. Following completion of the anastomoses, caval flow is restored first by releasing the caval clamps (infra- then suprahepatic). This is followed by reperfusion of the grafted liver with portal venous blood.

The clamping of the vena cava and portal vein has obvious, and potentially serious, haemodynamic implications due to obstruction of venous return and may be managed with, or without, venovenous bypass (see below). During the anhepatic period, metabolic abnormalities may be severe and coagulation often deteriorates further due to exclusion of the liver.

Stage 3: after reperfusion

Immediately following reperfusion with portal blood there is often a period of haemodynamic instability and, occasionally, gross disturbances in coagulation. The extent and time course of these changes are variable, although in the majority of patients they are relatively short lived (< 10 min) and correct spontaneously, or with minimum intervention. In a few patients changes may be severe, requiring inotropic support for several hours. The rest of the procedure is usually uncomplicated. The hepatic artery is anastomosed followed by reconstruction of the biliary system (by duct to duct anastomosis or Roux-en-Y choledochojejunostomy depending on the recipient's anatomy). Finally, the donor gall bladder is removed before closure of the abdominal wound.

ANAESTHESIA

The primary responsibility of the anaesthetist during liver transplantation is to maintain physiological homeostasis and prevent, or at least limit, the progressive deterioration that would otherwise occur as a result of the numerous insults imposed by the procedure. To this end, techniques of anaesthesia, analgesia and muscle relaxation should be chosen to run with the minimum of intervention using continuous administration (by intravenous infusion or inhalation) where possible, so as not to detract from the task of maintaining physiological stability.

Premedication

If required, a short-acting oral benzodiazepine such as temazepam is ideal. Intramuscular premedication is contraindicated in the presence of coagulopathy.

Induction

Pre-oxygenation and a rapid sequence induction is usual and essential in patients with tense ascites or obtunded, neurological status. Both propofol and thiopentone are suitable induction agents. Suxamethonium can be used to facilitate tracheal intubation, any theoretical prolongation of its action due to low plasma pseudocholinesterase is not a practical issue.

Maintenance

The standard technique uses an air/oxygen mixture with isoflurane. Large tidal volumes and a slow respiratory rate with PEEP (5 cmH$_2$O) are used to minimize atelectasis, and the patient is ventilated to normocarbia. Nitrous oxide is avoided for a number of both practical and theoretical reasons. Bowel distension can be considerable during long procedures and may intefere with abdominal closure and prolong postoperative ileus. There also exists a risk of venous air embolism during the procedure. Bone marrow metabolism of vitamin B12 and folate is depressed after prolonged exposure and there is some evidence that nitrous oxide may reduce hepatic blood flow. Isoflurane maintains hepatic blood flow and oxygen delivery at higher values than either halothane or enflurane and also undergoes minimal metabolism. Preliminary data on desflurane indicate that it has no detrimental effect on hepatic blood flow and may be useful.

Sevoflurane has the potential for hepatotoxicity and its safety in end-stage liver disease has not been established. Fentanyl is used to provide analgesia since its clearance is minimally affected by liver disease and it provides cardiovascular stability. It is given as a bolus dose of 10–20 μg kg^{-1} followed by an infusion at 2–5 μg kg^{-1} h^{-1}. The possibility of drug washout due to massive blood replacement should be considered for any drug given by infusion. Atracurium is infused in normal doses for muscle relaxation as its metabolism (Hofmann elimination and ester hydrolysis) is not dependent on liver or renal function. Clearance of its metabolite, laudanosine, is partially dependent on liver function, but values do not reach those at which neurological stimulation is of concern. Vecuronium and pancuronium have a prolonged duration of action in patients with liver dysfunction and are avoided. Hepatobiliary clearance of rocuronium is 75%, so prolonged duration of blockade can be anticipated. Doxacurium is minimally affected by liver disease.

Vascular access

Dedicated, transfusion cannulae that provide the ability to rapidly transfuse large volumes of fluid (up to 1500 ml min^{-1}) are an essential part of a safe technique for liver transplantation. One 10 G cannulae is inserted by a Seldinger technique in the right jugular vein and a further two 10 G cannulae inserted in the left jugular vein if venovenous bypass is to be used. Subclavian catheterization is associated with a much higher incidence of local complications, especially in the presence of coagulopathy, and is generally avoided. Consideration should be given to this route in patients with raised intracranial pressure to prevent interference with cerebral venous drainage. Triple lumen central venous catheters and a peripheral venous cannula provide routes for infusions of drugs and maintenance fluids. Two arterial cannulae are inserted, one for monitoring and the other which is not heparinized for withdrawal of blood samples. An introducer sheath is placed for the insertion of a pulmonary artery flotation catheter (usually in the right internal jugular vein).

MONITORING AND MANAGEMENT

Cardiovascular and general monitoring

In view of the duration of surgery and the potential for rapid changes in haemodynamic status, monitoring of liver transplant recipients is intensive. The standard parameters include the following.

- ECG
- Direct arterial pressure
- Central venous pressure
- Core temperature
- Pulse oximetry
- Full airway gas analysis (O_2, CO_2, agent)
- Airway pressure and volume

With the exception of small children, a pulmonary artery floatation catheter (usually with mixed venous oximetry) is also inserted, and, full haemodynamic and oxygen transport parameters are calculated at regular intervals. Some institutions routinely use a right ventricular ejection fraction catheter, whilst others use rapid response catheters that give 'continuous' cardiac output determinations. In some centres pressure in the inferior vena cava is also measured which may give a better guide to volume status than either central venous pressure (CVP) or pulmonary artery wedge pressure (PAWP) whilst the inferior vena cava is clamped. This parameter may also give early warning of occlusion of the inferior vena cava in the immediate postoperative period.

Haemodynamic instability

There are many potential causes of haemodynamic instability during liver transplantation.

During the dissection phase intravascular depletion can result from surgical bleeding especially in the presence of a well-developed collateral circulation. Drainage and continued formation of ascites further contribute to vascular depletion. Hypotension may also result from surgical manipulation of the liver hilum and inferior vena cava interfering with venous return. Ionized hypocalcaemia from rapid infusion of citrated products can reduce myocardial contractility, as may severe acidosis. Patients undergoing liver transplantation for acute liver failure or for non-functional primary grafts may have significant haemodynamic instability from the outset and require inotropic support with adrenaline or noradrenaline.

During the anhepatic phase, haemodynamic changes depend on whether venovenous bypass is used. Most patients will tolerate cross-clamping of the vena cava provided they are normovolaemic or slightly hypervolaemic before clamping and have good collateral circulations. Following caval clamping the mean arterial pressure is usually well maintained by a compensatory increase in vascular resistance (which may double from baseline values) even though cardiac index falls by as much as 50%. Central venous pressure and PAWP fall with clamping of the vena cava whilst pressure in the inferior vena cava rises, often to within 30 mmHg of mean arterial pressure. Over transfusion should be avoided since right heart failure may occur with sudden volume loading on unclamping of the vena cava when normal venous return is restored. If the preoperative investigations have identified a limited cardiac reserve it is usual to bypass the caval cross-clamps with an extracorporeal circuit.

The most severe haemodynamic changes occur with reperfusion of the graft and are characterized by hypotension often associated with a profound fall in vascular resistance, high cardiac index and an increase in central venous and pulmonary artery pressures. There may be a degree of myocardial depression at this stage which further contributes to arterial hypotension. Occasionally, severe bradycardia or arrhythmias (including asystole) are also seen.

'Post-reperfusion syndrome' (a decrease in MAP of at least 30% from baseline for at least 1 min within 5 min of reperfusion) occurs in up to 30% cases. Interestingly, the incidence is much lower (8%) in patients in whom venovenous bypass has not been used. This may be attributable to the increased intravascular filling and higher vascular resistance before reperfusion in these patients. Reperfusion hypotension is probably caused by the sudden release of blood containing ischaemic metabolites and cytokines from the grafted liver and from the congested splanchnic circulation. Thorough flushing of the donor liver attenuates these changes but does not eliminate them. In the majority of patients the changes are transient and will at most require small doses of pressor agents. In a minority of cases, the haemodyamic changes persist and require continued use of vasopressor infusions. In some patients the increase in pulmonary artery pressures on reperfusion may also require treatment with vasodilators such as prostacyclin. Recently, some success has been found using nebulized prostacyclin to treat pulmonary hypertension. In addition to these changes, reperfusion can be complicated by profuse bleeding from a vascular anastomotic site or by pulmonary embolism of air or thrombi. Once the acute haemodynamic insult is over, the rest of the post-anhepatic phase is usually uncomplicated, although the vascular resistance frequently remains low for some hours into the postoperative period.

Metabolic function

Blood gas analysis together with the determination of sodium, potassium, ionized calcium, magnesium, glucose and haemoglobin values are performed at hourly intervals (more frequently during the anhepatic phase, if a specific abnormality is being treated, or if the patient becomes unstable). Progressive development of a metabolic acidosis is almost universal with an increase in circulating lactate. Severe acidosis due to hyperlactataemia developing in the anhepatic period, requires correction with sodium bicarbonate to keep the base deficit less than 10. Following reperfusion, acidosis corrects without treatment within a few hours if the graft function is good. Potassium changes are variable but hypokalaemia is not treated before reperfusion of the graft unless severe, as sudden hyperkalaemia may occur on reperfusion. Calcium supplementation (in 5 mmol increments) is usually required following transfusion of blood, or blood products, containing citrate. Hypomagnesaemia is also common and may increase the risk of arrhythmias especially in alcoholic patients and should be corrected with magnesium sulphate 20–40 mmol. Serial haemoglobin estimation is essential, as accurate measurement of blood loss is almost impossible. Glucose concentrations usually increase slowly due to blood transfusion, increased catecholamine secretion, administration of methylprednisolone and release of glucose when the graft liver is reperfused, and this hyperglycaemia may necessitate an insulin infusion. Severe hypoglycaemia may occur in patients with acute liver failure unless glucose infusions are administered.

Coagulation

Many changes may occur in the coagulation system in patients undergoing liver transplantation. In addition to pre-existing coagulation deficiencies, blood loss often leads to a dilutional coagulopathy. The anhepatic period results in complete failure to clear both activators and inhibitors of coagulation and fibrinolysis. Imbalances in these systems may lead to the development of a clinically significant fibrinolytic state. At reperfusion a 'pathological' coagulopathy can develop, the causes of which remain to be fully identified. Because of the complexity of the potential coagulation disorders, and the multiplicity of possible causes of non-surgical bleeding, it is essential to monitor coagulation serially throughout the procedure. Simple tests of clotting (PT, APTT, platelet count and fibrin degradation products) are inadequate for this purpose. They give little information about the quality of clot formation or of clinically significant fibrinolytic activity and do not provide a clear basis for direct replacement therapy. Whole blood clot analysis using the thromboelastograph or Sonoclot is used by many transplant centres for serial monitoring during transplantation, either in isolation or in combination with a battery of more sophisticated tests, and has proved of great value in guiding blood product and pharmacological therapy. A complete qualitative coagulation profile is provided by the thromboelastograph including information on clot formation rate (coagulation factor activity), speed and degree of clot strengthening (platelet number and function and fibrinogen availability), and clot stability (fibrinolysis). Administration of FFP, platelets and cryoprecipitate is guided by the thromboelastograph variables.

Pathological fibrinolysis developing towards the end of the anhepatic period or early in the post-anhepatic period may lead to significant blood loss from the operative site. This is usually a primary event associated with very high tissue plasminogen activator activity and low plasminogen activator inhibitor concentrations. It is more common in patients with advanced cirrhosis (Child's C) and in this group particularly, prophylactic administration of antifibrinolytic agents such as aprotinin or tranexamic acid can substantially reduce blood loss associated with fibrinolysis. A 'heparin-like' effect (as evidenced by an abnormal thromboelastograph trace which is normalized by the addition of heparin-cleaving enzymes *in vitro*) has also been described following reperfusion of the graft. Protamine sulphate (50–100 mg) may sometimes be effective in treating this condition.

Once liver function in the graft returns, the coagulation changes seen at reperfusion usually correct spontaneously; indeed the persistence of oozing from raw surfaces in the surgical field is often an early indication of poor graft function. Despite the problems with coagulopathy, thrombosis of the hepatic arterial anastomosis remains a constant danger and over zealous attempts to normalize coagulation are both unnecessary and potentially harmful.

Thermal balance

Unless active attempts are made to maintain core temperature, hypothermia is common during transplantation because of heat loss in presurgical preparation, evaporative heat loss occurring from the large exposed area of peritoneum and intestines during surgery, massive fluid replacement, the use of venovenous bypass and the placement of a cold donor graft.

Reperfusion of the grafted liver usually leads to a 1°C fall in temperature. Hypothermia (< 35°C) has a number of serious adverse effects including potentiation of coagulopathy, impairment of oxygen delivery, reduced renal concentrating ability and decreased splanchnic blood flow. Myocardial contractility and the response to inotropic agents is reduced and there is an increased likelihood of arhythmias. In addition, drug metabolism may be impaired. All intravenous fluids must be warmed, respiratory gases humidified and patient warming devices used. Warm-air convective warming blankets placed over the patient are particularly effective at maintaining core temperature.

Management of massive transfusion

Intraoperative blood loss varies considerably and depends on a number of factors including the nature of the liver disease, preoperative coagulation status, the presence or absence of portal hypertension, previous upper abdominal surgery, surgical technique and early graft function. Early transplants were frequently complicated by massive blood loss (losses in the range of 40–100 units were not uncommon). Improved surgical experience and a better understanding of coagulation disorders have led to a reduction in the average blood transfusion requirement, which is now 4–8 units of red cells. In some patients (generally those with less severe liver disease and no preoperative anaemia) it has been possible to perform liver transplants without transfusion of any banked blood, through the use of autologous blood transfusion and isovolaemic haemodilution. However, the possibilty of massive blood loss always exists, and it is prudent to have 20 units of blood available for every transplant. Blood loss is occasionally rapid and life threatening, so a rapid transfusion device should be available immediately. Such a device enables the transfusion of prewarmed fluid. For example, the Haemonetics RIS™ has a 2.5 l reservoir lined with a 170 μm filter for rapid mixing of blood and other fluids (saline, albumin solution and FFP) that can be infused at variable rates up to 1500 ml min^{-1} by means of a roller pump. It incorporates a heat exchange column, a 40 μm filter and air and overpressure alarms. In some patients loss of ascitic fluid is substantial and simple weighing of swabs gives a very inadequate quantification of actual blood loss. Therefore transfusion is guided by haemodynamic variables and determinations of haematocrit (maintained at 25–30%). Autotransfusion with cell salvage devices is used in many institutions and up to half the shed blood can be salvaged. However, a certain minimum blood loss must be exceeded before such systems become cost effective, and many of the more sophisticated systems need additional personnel to operate them.

Venovenous bypass

The use of venovenous bypass during the anhepatic phase of liver transplantation remains controversial. In some centres bypass is used for all liver transplant procedures in adults, whilst in others it is not used at all. Most centres have guidelines for the use of bypass in certain patients, however the potential benefits remain unproven and no properly randomized controlled study has been published.

The technique involves the extracorporeal circulation of venous blood from the venous system below the vena caval clamps to the central veins. Access to the inferior vena cava is achieved by surgical dissection of the femoral vein and direct cannulation using a 7 mm cannula. Blood may also be drained from the portal venous system, again by direct surgical cannulation. The pressure in the inferior vena cava during cross-clamping is usually in the range 30–50 mmHg and passive drainage of blood occurs along the bypass tubing to a centrifugal, non-occlusive pump. Blood is then pumped to the return cannula. Using two 10 G cannulae in the left internal jugular vein a flow rate of about 3000 ml min^{-1} can be achieved with return line pressures under 300 mmHg. If higher flow rates are required, which occurs when the portal vein has been cannulated, either direct cannulation of the axillary vein by cut-down or large percutaneous cardiopulmonary bypass cannulae can be used. Heparin-bonded tubing is used to prevent coagulation within the extracorporeal system. Systemic heparinization is not required.

The use of venovenous bypass is not without risks and several adverse factors and complications have been reported. The operation is always prolonged due to the requirement for surgical cut-down and subsequent closure. Cases of fatal pulmonary embolism have occurred resulting from thrombus either forming in the extracorporeal circuit or being translocated from the inferior vena cava to the right atrium. Blood clotting in the bypass system may occur if the flow rate is very low, and it is generally considered that at flow rates below 1 l min^{-1}, continuation of bypass is neither useful nor safe. Brachial plexus injury has been reported in association with the cut-down to the axillary vein and the need for additional percutaneous central venous cannulation carries its own risks.

There is no doubt that the use of venovenous bypass reduces inferior vena caval pressures (and portal venous pressures when the portal system is drained), increases renal perfusion pressure and maintains better cardiac output during caval cross-clamping, leading to improved haemodynamic stability and greater urine flow during the anhepatic phase. However, the potential benefits of a lower incidence of renal dysfunction, decreased surgical bleeding and lesser disturbance of gut permeability remain unproven. No effect on graft, or patient, survival has been demonstrated. It has been observed that post-reperfusion cardiovascular instability is more likely to occur in patients in whom venovenous bypass has been used.

In the authors' centre bypass is used in selected patients with either renal failure (established or impending) or cardiac disease (demonstrated either by echocardiogram or exercise ECG). Bypass is also used in patients with fulminant hepatic failure whose intracranial pressure may be raised and whose cerebral perfusion is critically dependent on haemodynamic stability throughout surgery.

IMMEDIATE POSTOPERATIVE CARE (48 h) AND COMPLICATIONS

After uncomplicated transplant operations, patients are usually extubated within 12 h and discharged from the intensive care unit in 24–36 h. Those patients that develop complications may stay in intensive care for a long time and can place enormous demands on resources. The major complications after operation are bleeding requiring re-operation, poor or absent graft function, sepsis, renal failure and vascular thrombosis with hepatic infarction.

Cardiovascular complications

The hyperdynamic circulatory state persists for some time and a high cardiac output and low vascular resistance is normal for the first 24 h. Severe hypotension with very low vascular resistance (< 200 dyne s cm^{-5}) requiring inotropic support is usually associated with marginal graft function. Later, hypertension may occur in 70% of patients after transplant and is related to cyclosporin and tacrolimus (FK506) administration. Occasionally, an unexplained hypodynamic circulatory state is seen with non-ischaemic dilated cardiomyopathy.

Fluids and electrolytes

Background maintenance fluids are administered in the form of 4% glucose in 0.18% sodium chrolide solution (1 ml kg^{-1} h^{-1}), and intravascular volume is maintained with colloid solutions if the haematocrit is above 30%, or blood if it is below 30%. Hypokalaemic alkalosis is common and potassium supplementation is usually required. If graft function is good, lactate values fall to normal (< 1.2 mmol l^{-1}) within 24 h. Mild to moderate hyperglycaemia is usual and may require insulin therapy. The combination of hypoglycaemia, hyperkalaemia, metabolic acidosis and deteriorating coagulation are suggestive of graft failure.

Bleeding and coagulation problems

After operation haematocrit is maintained at 30% to optimize hepatic arterial blood flow, using transfusion or venesection as required. Liver transplant patients generally have an increased International Normalized Ratio (INR) (around 2) and a low platelet count on arrival in the intensive care unit. Unless active bleeding occurs these variables are not corrected because of the risk of vascular thrombosis. Furthermore, administration of clotting factors masks changes in INR which are a useful index of graft function. With an adequately functioning graft INR becomes normal in 2–3 days, however thrombocytopenia may persist for a week or more. Up to 10% patients may have to return to theatre for postoperative haemorrhage, although a discrete bleeding site is identified in less than half these cases. Intra-abdominal bleeding is suggested by the need for continued red cell transfusion, drain loss with a high haematocrit, increasing IVC pressure and falling urine output. An underlying coagulopathy is often contributory, and in these circumstances efforts should be made to correct coagulation defects with FFP and platelets.

Analgesia

It is a well known, but poorly explained, fact that liver transplant patients have minimal narcotic analgesic requirements after operation and low dose infusions of fentanyl (0.5–1 $\mu g\ kg^{-1}\ h^{-1}$) or pethidine (0.1–0.3 mg $kg^{-1}\ h^{-1}$) are usually adequate. There are even some reports of patients completing their stay in the intensive care unit without receiving any narcotic analgesia at all! This is despite the large surgical incision, and contrasts sharply with other patients undergoing upper abdominal surgery. Postoperative analgesia with epidural opiates has been used in some carefully selected transplant patients with normal preoperative coagulation, but any possible advantage gained in this group of patients is unproven.

Infection

Infection is the most common cause of morbidity and mortality. Prophylactic antibiotics are administered at induction of anaesthesia and continued for 48 h after operation. Daily microbiological surveillance is performed routinely. Diagnosis of infection can be very difficult, as both rejection and liver infarction also result in pyrexia and an elevation of white cell count, however these conditions are associated with increased serum transaminase activity and deterioration in liver function. Sepsis can also cause hepatocellular liver dysfunction, although cholestatic changes are more common. Liver biopsy (percutaneous or transjugular) is required if rejection is suspected, and Doppler ultrasound or mesenteric angiography may be undertaken to exclude vascular thrombosis. Differentiation is vital, as graft rejection requires increased immunosuppression whilst infection may need a temporary reduction in therapy.

FULMINANT HEPATIC FAILURE

Acute liver failure accounts for approximately 10% of liver transplants. The nature of acute failure, characterized by rapid and relentless deterioration in liver function, differentiates it from other conditions in terms of the urgency with which transplantation must be performed and the need for highly specialized preoperative intensive care management. There is also a succession of difficult decisions involved, including identification of those patients that might recover without transplantation. Once a patient is placed on the 'super-urgent' waiting list for transplantation, constant regular review is required to assess whether the recipient's disease is too far advanced for recovery, even with a liver graft. The overall survival rate following transplantation for acute liver failure is around 50%, most of the mortality occurring perioperatively following which long-term survival is excellent.

CLASSIFICATION OF ACUTE LIVER FAILURE (ALF)

The condition is characterized by severe liver dysfunction, coagulopathy, hepatic encephalopathy and cerebral oedema in the absence of pre-existing liver disease. There are three groups.

- Hyperacute: encephalopathy arising within 7 days of the onset of jaundice, high incid-

ence of cerebral oedema, survival without transplant 36%.
- Acute: interval between jaundice and encephalopathy 8–28 days, high incidence of cerebral oedema, survival without transplant 7%.
- Subacute: interval greater than 4 weeks, low incidence of cerebral oedema, survival without transplant 14%.

MANAGEMENT

Patients with ALF who are deteriorating despite medical treatment should be transferred promptly to an institution that has experience of these patients and has the facility to perform emergency liver transplantation. Once grade 3 encephalopathy is reached, patients should be intubated to protect the airway. Those meeting the criteria for transplantation (Table 27.2) are registered urgently for a donor liver, which in the UK and USA is usually available within 48 h, although the urgency of the situation may necessitate ABO incompatible liver grafting.

SPECIFIC MANAGEMENT PROBLEMS

Cardiovascular instability

These patients frequently develop severe haemodynamic instability, with hypotension, high cardiac index (2–3 times normal) and low vascular resistance (often less than 200 dyne s cm^{-5}). Full haemodynamic monitoring using arterial, central venous and pulmonary artery catheters is established early to optimize cardiovascular function and oxygen delivery. Initially, hypotension may respond to intravascular volume expansion with colloid solutions such as albumin. Fresh-frozen plasma is not generally administered until the decision to proceed to transplant has been made, as clotting factor activity is one of the criteria used to assess the need for transplantation. The cause of the hypotension is usually profound arterial vasodilation and vasopressor support with noradrenaline to increase peripheral vascular resistance is almost always required. In many cases the patient will show progressive resistance to noradrenaline therapy and some may respond to adrenaline. Patients exhibiting noradrenaline resistance may show a response to angiotensin infusion. N-acetylcysteine has been reported to improve tissue perfusion and oxygen extraction in patients with ALF and may produce a small improvement in arterial pressure. Many patients with ALF demonstrate pathological oxygen supply dependency and combinations of noradrenaline or adrenaline with either prostacyclin or N-acetylcysteine appear to maintain or increase oxygen delivery and oxygen consumption; combination therapy may be more beneficial than vasopressors alone.

Table 27.2 Indications for liver transplantation in acute liver failure

Non-paracetamol related fulminant hepatic failure
  any three of
    age <10 or >40 years
    unfavourable aetiology (non-A non-B hepatitis, idiosyncratic drug reactions, halothane hepatitis and fulminant Wilson's disease)
    jaundice for >7 days before encephalopathy
    Prothrombin time >50 sec
    Plasma bilirubin >300 μmol l^{-1}
  or
    Prothrombin time >100 sec
Paracetamol-induced acute fulminant hepatic failure
  pH <7.30 (after volume resuscitation)
  or all of the following
    Plasma creatinine >300 μmol l^{-1}
    Grade 3 encephalopathy
    Prothrombin time >100 s

Using these criteria for acute liver failure not due to paracetamol 95% of fatal cases were identified, of those not meeting the criteria 82% survived. For those with paracetamol-induced liver failure 77% of fatal cases where identified and survival was 89% in those not meeting the criteria.

Renal failure

ALF is frequently complicated by acute renal failure. Renal replacement therapy is indicated if there is persistent hyperkalaemia, hyponatraemia, acidosis or fluid overload. Continuous methods of haemofiltration are essential (either continuous venovenous haemodialysis (CVVHD) or continuous arteriovenous haemodialysis (CAVHD), because of increased haemodynamic instability associated with intermittent haemodialysis. There is a trend in many units to use CVVHD, in preference, in these patients as arterial pressure may not be adequate to sustain CAVHD. There may be progressive acidosis due mainly to accumulation of lactate (circulating values may rise to 15 mmol l^{-1}) and large amounts of sodium bicarbonate may be required in association with haemofiltration, using lactate-free dialysis fluid, to maintain acid–base balance. CVVHD or CAVHD also facilitates the administration of blood and blood products. Some patients with ALF develop peripheral and pulmonary oedema and gas exchange may be severely compromised. Removal of large volumes of fluid (300–600 ml h^{-1}) may be needed to improve gas exchange and reduce cerebral oedema. Haemofiltration should be continued during the operation to facilitate management of the complex fluid and electrolyte balance in these patients.

Patients with ALF often become severely hypoglycaemic and blood glucose should be measured regularly; 50% glucose infusions are used to prevent hypoglycaemia.

Cerebral oedema

Brain stem herniation due to raised intracranial pressure (ICP) and cerebral oedema is the most common cause of death in ALF. Cerebral oedema is primarily of cytotoxic origin (accumulation of osmogenic metabolites) although vasogenic cerebral oedema (increased blood–brain barrier permeability) may occur at a late stage. Patients who are ventilated following the onset of grade 3 encephalopathy show few signs of raised ICP. Pupillary signs may be unreliable in these circumstances and when present, may indicate irreversible pathology. CT scans may demonstrate cerebral oedema; however, transferring such patients to radiology is hazardous and CT scanning may not show cerebral oedema even in the presence of a raised ICP. If the patient has evidence of a focal neurological abnormality, a scan is indicated to exclude intracranial haemorrhage. The only accurate method of monitoring ICP is to place an intracranial pressure transducer (see below). Care should be taken to avoid (or limit) factors that might further elevate ICP (neck vein compression, head turning, bronchial suction, fluid overload and seizures). Patients should be nursed with a 20° head-up tilt, and ventilated to achieve a $Pa\text{CO}_2$ of 3.5–4.0 kPa. Mannitol (0.5 g kg^{-1} i.v. bolus) is given if ICP remains above 25 mmHg for more than 5 min. Plasma osmolality must be measured and not allowed to rise above 320 mosmol kg^{-1}. If renal failure is present, dialysis should be used to remove mannitol and fluid. In cases of refractory intracranial hypertension maintenance of a cerebral perfusion pressure >50 mmHg becomes critical and vasopressor agents should be used if required. Infusions of thiopentone are sometimes given when patients no longer respond to mannitol. There are several non-invasive techniques that are currently being assessed as adjuvants, or alternatives, to ICP monitoring; these include transcranial Doppler ultrasonography, jugular oximetry and measurement of sensory evoked potentials.

Infection

Patients with liver failure are immune-deficient due to a variety of factors including Kupffer cell dysfunction, and overwhelming sepsis is the second most common cause of death in acute liver failure. In a high proportion of patients (30%), a pyrexia and raised white cell count will be absent and protocol-based cultures must be performed daily. The majority of infections are bacterial (both Gram negative and Gram positive organisms), but there is also a high incidence of systemic fungal infection (candida and aspergillus) and prophylactic antifungal therapy is routinely given.

ADDITIONAL SPECIAL PROCEDURES

Intracranial pressure monitoring

Direct measurement of ICP is the only technique which allows the early and accurate diagnosis of raised ICP, and objective measurement of the effectiveness of therapy. It also facilitates anaesthetic management during the perioperative period. Increases in ICP may occur during the procedure, particularly following reperfusion of the graft, and can take 24–48 h to return to normal following successful transplantation. ICP measurement may also identify patients in whom neurological recovery is unlikely, although recovery has been reported in some patients with ICP measurements in excess of 80 mmHg. ICP monitoring in patients with acute liver failure is not without risk because of the severe concurrent coagulopathy. Epidural catheters have the lowest risk of associated intracranial haemorrhage ($< 5\%$ compared with 20% for subdural or intraventricular devices). Epidural catheters also have the advantage that they can be inserted by experienced personnel without having to transfer the patient to an operating theatre. It is essential to correct coagulation deficits before placing ICP monitors. An international normalized ratio (INR) of 2 or less, a platelet count greater than 60 000 and a fibrinogen level of at least 1.5 g l^{-1} should be achieved before surgery. The coexistence of renal failure will require administration of blood products with concurrent removal of fluid by haemofiltration.

Plasmapheresis

High volume plasma exchange has been shown to reduce a raised ICP and improve haemodynamic stability for a short period (6–12 h) in some patients, when they have become unresponsive to more conventional therapy. It also ensures improved clotting function when FFP is given to replace removed plasma. Prothrombin time may be decreased from over 100 s to near normal when this technique is used.

Hepatectomy

Toxic substances released into the systemic circulation from areas of necrotic liver may contribute to the progressive haemodynamic and metabolic instability seen in acute liver failure. There have been several reports of an improvement in clinical state together with a reduction in ICP following hepatectomy. If a patient is rapidly deteriorating this is an option that may be considered when a donor liver has been identified but is not yet harvested.

Auxiliary liver transplantation

It is sometimes very difficult to predict in advance which patients with acute liver failure will eventually recover by spontaneous regeneration of the liver. In this situation transplantation eliminates the possibility of regeneration and commits the patient to immunosuppression for life. A few centres now use the alternative technique of auxiliary (heterotopic or partial orthotopic) liver transplantation in patients with acute liver failure. The complication rate is greater than for orthotopic transplants, but in some patients regeneration of their own liver occurs and later, following cessation of immunosupressive therapy, the auxiliary graft atrophies.

Bioartificial livers

Extracorporeal liver-assist devices are being developed in an attempt to provide a hepatic support system for patients with acute liver failure until the patient's own liver recovers function or a donor organ becomes available. Two devices are currently being evaluated, one using porcine hepatocytes and the other cultured human hepatocytes from hepatoblastomas. Both devices use cells cultured in the extracapillary space of a hollow fibre dialyser which is used to ultrafiltrate the patient's plasma. The patients are treated with *ex-vivo* perfusion through the bioartificial liver using a venovenous circuit. Preliminary results have shown these devices are capable of both removing toxins and providing some synthetic function (clotting factors, albumin), and that they can temporarily improve or stabilize the patient's condition.

RENAL TRANSPLANTATION ANAESTHESIA

The first human renal transplants were performed in the 1950s and were largely unsuccessful. The introduction of pharmacological immune suppression in the early 1960s first with azathioprine (a 6-mercaptopurine derivative) and then with azathioprine–prednisolone combinations greatly improved graft survival. Graft survival was further enhanced by the introduction of cyclosporin in 1978 by Calne. Renal transplantation is now a routine part of the management of end-stage renal disease and results in both improved quality of life for recipients and a decrease in healthcare costs. Approximately 1600 renal transplants are performed annually in the UK and over 5 000 patients are on the waiting list.

PREOPERATIVE PREPARATION

Intercurrent disease

A patient undergoing renal transplantation may present a formidable challenge to the anaesthetist and a thorough formal preoperative assessment is essential. The most common causes of end-stage renal disease are glomerulonephritis, essential hypertension and diabetes mellitus.

Cardiovascular complications

Patients whose renal disease is not caused by hypertension are usually hypertensive as a secondary phenomenon. It is unusual to see a patient with renal disease who is not hypertensive unless severe intravascular volume depletion is present. Most patients will be treated with β-adrenergic blocking drugs, and with either calcium channel blocking drugs, angiotensin converting enzyme (ACE) inhibitors or both. These drugs should be taken up to the time of premedication and consideration given to the management of hypertension after operation. There have been several reports of profound hypotension occurring following induction of anaesthesia in patients on ACE inhibitors, and the current recommendation is to omit the immediately preoperative dose. Coronary artery disease is much more common in patients with end-stage renal disease than in the general population. Hypertension, anaemia and chronic volume overload may lead to left ventricular hypertrophy and congestive cardiac failure. Atherosclerosis is rarely, if ever, confined to the coronary circulation and may, together with increased arterial calcification due to secondary hyperparathyroidism, lead to difficulties in the surgical procedure and an increased incidence of cardiovascular complications in the postoperative period. Hypertension should be adequately controlled preoperatively and patients with ischaemic heart disease may benefit from the infusion of glyceryl trinitrate during the perioperative period.

Gastrointestinal complications

Uraemic patients have delayed gastric emptying. There is an increased incidence of gastroduodenal ulceration and bleeding, and nausea and vomiting.

Metabolic factors

A significant proportion of end-stage renal disease is directly caused by diabetes and diabetes may be present incidentally. Up to 25% of transplant recipients in some centres may be diabetic. A glucose and insulin infusion should be started at the beginning of preperative starvation and continued through into the postoperative period. Many patients with end-stage renal disease exhibit relative insulin resistance, and infusion rates may be higher that expected. Potassium supplementation is usually not required. Development of hyperkalaemia and metabolic acidosis is universal and is controlled by dialysis. Plasma electrolytes should be measured immediately before operation. Lack of production of 1,25-dihydroxycholecalciferol in the failing kidney leads to phosphate retention and hypocalcaemia. This in turn causes secondary hyperparathyroidism and increases calcium resorbtion from bone. Osteoporosis and osteomalacia result and may be accompanied by metastatic calcification. Administration of 1,25-dihydroxycholecalciferol with dietary restriction of phosphate control these changes in many patients but in a minority sub-total parathyroidectomy is necessary. Increased sensitivity to non-depolarizing neuromuscular blocking drugs may occur in the presence of hypocalcaemia.

Haematological features

Anaemia is very common in end-stage renal disease but is often fully reversed by the administration of exogenous erythropoetin. It is multifactorial in origin. Lack of erythropoetin production by the kidney is compounded by secondary hyperparathyroidism which suppresses erythropoesis and increases red-cell turnover. Blood loss in dialysis systems contributes further and may exacerbate the iron deficiency caused by phosphate-binding drugs. Whilst patients with chronic anaemia compensate for, to some extent, for decreased oxygen availability by raising cardiac output, the margin of safety is greatly reduced and blood should be available for immediate intraoperative transfusion if bleeding occurs. A preoperative haemoglobin of 8 g dl^{-1} is acceptable in the renal transplant patient. Some anaesthetists will accept lower values, but the rapidly decreasing margin of safety must be recognized. In patients with pre-existing ischaemic heart disease or left ventricular hypertrophy, the ability of the cardiovascular system to maintain oxygen delivery may already be close to its limit.

Uraemia is associated with a mild coagulopathy caused by platelet dysfunction and decreased clotting factor activity, in particular factor VIII. Coagulation may be further impaired by residual heparinization from haemodialysis. Significant coagulopathy may develop rapidly if bleeding occurs during surgery. DDAVP (vasopressin analogue) 0.3 g kg^{-1} increases von Willebrand factor and improves platelet function in uraemic patients.

Neurological complications

Uraemic encephalopathy is rare, because of early diagnosis and appropriate commencement of dialysis. Dialysis disequilibrium syndrome may be seen after the first dialysis in patients presenting with previously undiagnosed end-stage renal disease and is characterized by nausea, vomiting, twitching, altered sensorium and, in severe cases, seizures.

Peripheral neuropathy occurs, and may be accompanied by autonomic neuropathy particularly in diabetic patients. The presence of advanced peripheral neuropathy specifically contraindicates the use of suxamethonium and all patients should be assessed for signs of autonomic neuropathy before anaesthesia.

Dialysis

Almost all patients presenting for renal transplantation will be on dialysis. Continuous ambulatory peritoneal dialysis may occur up to the time of surgery but peritoneal fluid should be emptied before induction of anaesthesia because of the increased intragastric pressure it may cause. Haemodialysis is usually conducted every two to three days and, unless the transplant recipient is suffering from volume overload or electrolyte imbalance, there is usually no need to schedule additional dialysis sessions before transplantation. Dialysis immediately before surgery carries an increased risk of residual heparinization.

Immediately after dialysis, patients are slightly volume depleted and their body weight should be compared to their normal 'dry' weight to assess their fluid balance before anaesthesia.

Premedication

Many patients presenting for renal transplantation require no premedication and this should be assessed on an individual basis. Diazepam is unsuitable in view of its decreased protein binding in renal failure. Midazolam is excreted at the same rate as in normal patients and temazepam is also suitable as a mild anxiolytic. The half-life of glycopyrrolate is greatly increased. Either morphine or pethidine can be given if a narcotic is required, but account should be taken of the total accumulated doses, as described later.

INTRAOPERATIVE MANAGEMENT

Anaesthesia

In the early days, many renal transplants were conducted under regional anaesthesia (continuous spinal), to avoid the greater risks of general anaesthesia. General anaesthesia is now much safer and, in view of the risks of coagulopathy and residual heparinization which may have catastrophic effects during the use of regional techniques, general anaesthesia is now preferred. Surgical access is greatly improved by the provision of muscle relaxation and the use of the head-down position. The nature of the surgical procedure requires a balanced anaesthetic technique with tracheal intubation and mechanical ventilation. For the induction agent neither thiopentone nor propofol nor etomidate is specifically contraindicated. Concentrations of thiopentone in the brain may be transiently higher than in patients with normal renal function since protein binding of the drug is reduced, but redistribution and clearance are unchanged. Because of the high incidence of intercurrent cardiac and vascular disease, and the possibility of fluid imbalance following recent dialysis, induction of anaesthesia should be conducted with caution and using adequate monitoring: (ECG pulse oximetry and automatic, repeated determination of arterial pressure). A large bore (14 G) venous cannula should be inserted before induction of anaesthesia. Isoflurane or desflurane are suitable agents for maintenance of anaesthesia because of their very low metabolism to free fluoride. Immunosupressive agents must be administered before reperfusion of the graft to prevent hyperacute rejection. Cyclosporin and/or anti-thymocyte globulin may have been administered peroperatively and methyl prednisolone is given shortly before reperfusion of the graft.

Surgical procedure

The donor kidney is usually transplanted into the contralateral iliac fossa of the recipient so that the renal vein lies laterally and does not cross over the artery. This ectopic extraperitoneal site facilitates the renal vascular anastomoses and ureteral implantation. Vascular anastomoses are dependent on the anatomy of the graft and recipient vessels, but are usually performed in the following order:

allograft renal vein to recipient's external iliac vein, allograft renal artery to the recipient's internal iliac artery (or if the graft has multiple arteries anastomoses are made to the external iliac artery). After the vascular clamps are released and the donor graft reperfused the ureter is implanted into the recipient's bladder.

DRUG METABOLISM

Neuromuscular blocking drugs

Suxamethonium will increase serum potassium by 0.2–0.5 mmol l^{-1} and so should be avoided in patients whose preoperative potassium concentration is >5 mmol l^{-1}. In patients with neuropathy (uraemic or diabetic), the rise in potassium concentration may be greater, and is unpredictable, but can be sufficient to induce cardiac arrhythmias or even asystole, so suxamethonium is contraindicated. Atracurium remains the neuromuscular blocking agent of choice as its elimination (Hofmann elimination and ester hydrolysis) is independent of renal function. Histamine release occurs in some patients following administration of atracurium which may contraindicate its use. Vecuronium or its newer derivative rocuronium may be used as alternatives. Both drugs are partially excreted by the kidney (10–15%) and may exhibit cumulative effects after repeated doses, so careful monitoring of neuromuscular blockade is mandatory. Cyclosporin augments the effects of neuromuscular blocking drugs and may prolong recovery time. Pipecuronium and doxacurium are both significantly dependent on renal excretion for elimination, and should be avoided.

Analgesics

Fentanyl is the opioid analgesic of choice as it has minimal haemodynamic effects and its pharmacokinetics are not significantly altered by renal dysfunction. Alfentanil, given by infusion, is also suitable. Pethidine is metabolized to norpethidine which is both neuroexcitatory and dependent on renal function for excretion; accumulation of this metabolite may cause convulsions. Norpethidine accumulation becomes significant at infusion rates greater than 1 mg kg^{-1} h^{-1} over a 24 h period. Both morphine and, to an even greater extent its active metabolite morphine-6-glucuronide, accumulate in renal failure, repeated doses, or infusions, of morphine-containing drugs may cause respiratory depression. Furthermore, reduced protein binding increases free morphine concentrations. Neither morphine nor pethidine are freely dialysable. Normal metabolism of these drugs in the postoperative period is dependent on early return of renal function in the graft.

Vascular access

Patients treated by haemodialysis will have a vascular access site, usually an arteriovenous fistula. Care must be taken to protect fistulae throughout surgery as these may be required for postoperative dialysis. Blood pressure cuffs should not be placed on a limb with a working fistula, and intravenous cannulae should never be inserted into a fistula. A 14 G peripheral cannula should be placed before induction of anaesthesia and a central venous catheter inserted before surgery. Direct arterial pressure measurement is generally not necessary and damage to peripheral arteries may prevent their subsequent use for establishing dialysis fistulae. In patients with severe ischaemic heart disease or demonstrated autonomic neuropathy a peripheral arterial cannula is inserted.

Fluid management

Most renal transplant programmes use set protocols for perioperative management of intravenous fluids to ensure optimal renal blood flow and adequate urine output. Probably one of the most important factors influencing immediate renal function (and avoidance of postoperative acute tubular necrosis) is the adequacy of perfusion of the transplanted kidney in the early period after reperfusion. The patient should be well hydrated before reperfusion of the graft. Central venous pressure should be maintained above 12 mmHg (allowing for head-down tilt if used) with either crystalloid or colloid solutions, and MAP should be at least 70 mmHg at the time of reperfusion. This value should be adjusted in patients with significant preoperative hypertension. Practice varies between centres, but most use low-dose dopamine throughout the procedure and give small doses of diuretics (frusemide 20–40 mg or bumetanide 1–2 mg) immediately before graft reperfusion. Some centres also administer mannitol (0.5–1.0 g kg^{-1}) as well, to promote a high urine flow in the early postoperative period.

IMMEDIATE POSTOPERATIVE CARE AND COMPLICATIONS

At the end of anaesthesia, special attention must be paid to the adequate antagonism of residual neuromuscular blockade. Close monitoring of haemodynamic variables is maintained for at least 24 h after operation usually in a high dependency unit or specialized renal transplant unit. Central venous pressure monitoring is continued and intravascular volume replacement reviewed regularly, taking the urine output, which may be very high, into account. Low-dose dopamine is usually continued and fluid lost in urine is replaced with a crystalloid solution, such as haemofiltration replacement fluid. Cardiac complications are a significant cause of postoperative morbidity and mortality, and hypertension should be carefully controlled as it may threaten both patient and graft survival, especially in diabetic patients. Hypotension and hypovolaemia will compromise the new graft and must be avoided. Postoperative analgesia is usually provided by PCA or infusions of pethidine, due care is taken if there is any doubt as to graft function. NSAIDs produce detrimental effects on renal blood flow by interfering with renal prostaglandin synthesis and are **absolutely contraindicated** following renal transplantation.

Complications related to the kidney graft

Acute tubular necrosis

This is more common following prolonged graft preservation times in excess of 24 h and following episodes of hypotension in the donor before organ harvesting. In many cases renal function will eventually recover, but these patients may require haemodialysis for up to 6 weeks after operation.

Graft rejection

Hyperacute rejection This starts within hours (sometimes minutes) of transplantation and is caused by preformed cytotoxic antibodies. It is irreversible and requires a transplant nephrectomy. With improved histocompatibility testing and crossmatching it is now rarely seen.

Acute rejection This is common in the first week following transplantation, but is usually reversible. Clinical signs include oliguria, pyrexia, hypertension and a swollen, tender allograft. The white blood cell count is usually elevated and circulating urea and creatinine rise. Rejection is treated by increased immunosuppresion, usually pulsed, high-dose methylprednisolone for three days. Increasing immunosuppression carries the risk of increased susceptibility to infection, and careful attention to infection screening is required. In addition, both cyclosporin and tacrolimus (FK506) are nephrotoxic, and high plasma concentrations may result in a deterioration in graft function so that circulating values must always be closely monitored.

Renal artery thrombosis

This is a rare complication that may be related to technical difficulty at the time of operation. It presents with acute anuria and severe hypertension. Management is usually by percutaneous transluminal angioplasty in the first instance, as surgical correction is associated with a high risk of graft loss. A renal vascular scan can be helpful to differentiate between acute tubular necrosis, graft rejection and renal artery thrombosis.

MANAGEMENT OF THE LIVING RELATED DONOR

Live related donation is a special circumstance in which the donor is voluntarily subjecting themselves to major surgery, and the small but definite risks this entails purely for altruistic reasons. It is essential for both ethical and legal reasons that the donor is properly counselled and that no coercion or undue pressure is involved. The moral issue is more complex with children; however, a number have donated to their identical twin.

The donor must have a full medical evaluation and be in good physical health without evidence of acute or chronic illness and with good bilateral renal function. Exclusion criteria include hypertension, significant coronary artery disease and diabetes mellitus. Upper abdominal surgery always carries a risk of pulmonary complications, therefore smoking is firmly discouraged and overweight patients should receive dietary advice.

Anaesthetic management

Hydration of the donor is started the night before surgery as maintenance of normal intravascular volume and urine output are essential to ensure good graft function. Light premedication such as oral temazepam is given if required.

Intraoperatively the main goals are to maintain haemodynamic stability and good renal perfusion. Full non-invasive monitoring is mandatory, but invasive pressure monitoring is not necessary. Live donor nephrectomies can be performed with the patient in the lateral 'flank' position or in the supine position which has less potential for cardiovascular instability. Intravenous crystalloid fluids are given (10–15 ml kg^{-1} h^{-1}) and low-dose dopamine is used routinely in some centres. Mannitol may be given to induce a diuresis and improve renal blood flow hence reducing cellular swelling. Blood transfusion is usually unnecessary, but is required occasionally. Significant haemorrhage occurs rarely both intra- and postoperatively.

Postoperative management

A chest X-ray is taken immediately after operation to exclude a pneumothorax. Unless adequately controlled, pain from the subcostal incision may be severe and cause diaphragmatic splinting with reduced basal ventilation and the concomitant risk of atelectasis. Epidural anaesthesia using an opiate/local anaesthetic mixture, or local anaesthetic alone, provides excellent analgesia, but the patient must be closely monitored for respiratory depression if opiates are used. The risk of serious postoperative complications such as bleeding requiring re-exploration, pulmonary emboli or chest infection is small (< 2%), but these patients should be closely supervised.

Although the well matched, live related donor offers the best likelihood of a successful transplant, some of these kidneys will be 'lost' due to rejection or recurrent recipient disease. The circumstances make the failure of a donated kidney particularly tragic for all concerned. In addition, the live donor is potentially putting their long-term health at increased risk. Cadaveric donation, when available, is usually preferred. Shortage of kidneys for transplantation is a worldwide problem, but has been alleviated to some extent by the increasing use of non-beating-heart donors.

CONCLUSIONS

Organ transplantation has become commonplace; it has taken nearly thirty years to achieve this spectacular success which has occurred as a result of major advances in the fields of immunosuppression, organ preservation, surgery and anaesthesia. Thomas Starzl, the surgeon who did so much to pioneer liver transplantation, once described his anaesthetic colleagues as 'warriors at the head of the table'. In effect he acknowledged the crucial role played by anaesthetists in the battle to preserve life in the face of end-stage disease and the numerous physiological insults presented by the transplant procedure. The experience gained from resolving the problems created by transplantation has done much to extend the field of anaesthesia. The application of these techniques and knowledge is now widely used to enable ever more complex surgical techniques to be undertaken and ensure the safer perioperative management of patients with organ dysfunction.

FURTHER READING

Lee, W. M. and Maddrey, W. C. (1995) Acute liver failure and transplanation: a symposium. *Liver Transplantation and Surgery*, **3**, 176–206.

McNair, A. N. B., Tibbs, C. J. and Williams, R. (1995) Recent advances in hepatology. *British Medical Journal*, **311**, 1351–1355.

Mallet, S. V. and Cox, D. J. A. (1992) Thromboelastography. *British Journal of Anaesthesia*, **69**, 307–313.

Mirenda, J. V. and Grissom, T. E. (1991) Anesthetic implications of the renin–angiotensin system and angiotensin converting enzyme inhibitors. *Anaesthesia and Analgesia*, **72**, 667–683.

O'Grady, J. G., Schalm, S and Williams, R. (1993) Acute liver failure: redefining the syndromes. *Lancet*, **342**, 273–275.

Rapaport, F. T. (1993) Present status of organ procurement and sharing: a summation of the second international congress of the society of organ sharing. *Transplant Proceedings*, **25**, 3311–3312.

Reiss, H. (ed) (1993) Hemostasis in liver transplantation. *Seminars in Thrombosis and Hemostasis*, **19**, 183–314.

Suthanthirian, M. and Strom, T. B. (1994) Renal transplantation. *New England Journal of Medicine*, **331**, 365–376.

Sutherland, F. R., Bloembergan, W., Mohamed, M., *et al.* (1992) Initial non-function in cadaveric renal transplantation. *Canadian Journal of Surgery*, **36**, 141–145.

Varty, K., Veitch, P. S., Morgan, J. D. T. *et al.* (1994) Response to organ shortage: kidney retrieval programme using non-beating-heart donors. *British Medical Journal*, **304**, 575–577.

LAPAROSCOPIC SURGERY

A. J. Cunningham and D. J. Kelly

Few developments have had as profound an effect on surgical practice as the recent 'explosion' in laparoscopic surgery. Such procedures, however, can hardly be described as being in their infancy. Endoscopy for rectal examination was first described by the Hippocrates-led Kos School around 460–375 BC. In 1910, Jacobaeus, a Professor of Medicine, described the application of endoscopy to inspect the peritoneum, pleura and pericardium. Since that time, gynaecologists have developed the instrumentation, operative principles, and techniques of laparoscopic surgery. Recently, reports of laparoscopic techniques have been described not only for cholecystectomy and gynaecological surgery, but also for a range of procedures including appendicectomy, inguinal hernia repair, nephrectomy, splenectomy, hemicolectomy and intrathoracic surgery.

Laparoscopy for diagnostic and therapeutic procedures offers specific patient advantages. The trauma of a large conventional incision is eliminated, without compromising the exposure of the operative field. Shorter hospital stay and decreased postoperative morbidity are strong arguments in favour of laparoscopic surgery. This realization has resulted in the concept of **'minimally invasive therapy'** with a general aim to 'minimize the trauma of any interventional process but still achieve a satisfactory therapeutic result'. In 1994, a UK report commissioned by the Department of Health to assess the implications of minimally invasive therapy for the National Health Service predicted that in 10 years 70–80% of surgical procedures would be performed endoscopically. The Working Party preferred the term 'minimal access surgery' to 'minimally invasive surgery', as the latter implied increased safety and minor procedures. Whilst minimal access surgery produces significantly less trauma than conventional approaches, it requires expensive technology and its adoption has major implications for patient services, operating room equipment, hospital design and surgical training.

THORACOSCOPY AND VIDEO-ASSISTED THORACIC SURGERY

Thoracoscopy gained popularity in the early 20th century, to divide adhesions and produce an artificial pneumothorax in the treatment of pulmonary tuberculosis. Its use declined rapidly, however, after the introduction of streptomycin in 1945. The advent of video-assisted thoracoscopes and the development of ancillary instruments has seen an increased interest in thoracoscopic surgery. Thoracoscopy and video-assisted thoracic surgery (VATS) are now regularly employed in the diagnosis and treatment of pleuropulmonary disease (Tables 28.1 and 28.2). Potential advantages include less postoperative pain, improved postoperative pulmonary function, a shortened hospital stay and operative time, and an earlier return to work.

Short Practice of Anaesthesia. Edited by M. Morgan and G. M. Hall. Published in 1997 by Chapman & Hall, London. ISBN 0 412 71890 1

Table 28.1 Thoracoscopy: clinical applications

Diagnostic	Pleural effusion
	Pneumothorax
	Blunt or penetrating chest trauma
	Solitary pulmonary nodules
	Staging pulmonary or pleural tumours
	Oesophageal perforations
Therapeutic	Pleural biopsy
	Pleural effusion drainage
	Pleurodesis
	Pleural adhesiolysis

Table 28.2 Video-assisted thoracic surgery

Lungs	Pneumonectomy
	Lobectomy
	Wedge, subsegmental, segmental resection
	Resection of pulmonary metastases
	Excision of blebs and bullae
Heart	Pericardiocentesis
	Pericardectomy
	Insertion of implantable cardioverter or defibrillator
Oesophagus	Oesophagectomy
	Repair oesophageal perforation
	Fundoplication
Mediastinum	Excision of tumours or cysts
Sympathetic nervous system	Transthoracic endoscopic sympathectomy
Vagus	Truncal vagotomy
Thoracic spine	Disc herniation
	Deformity correction
	Abscess drainage

The range of operative procedures falling within the realm of VATS continues to expand and now includes implantation of the cardioverter defibrillator device, oesophagectomy, excision of anterior and posterior mediastinal masses, transthoracic sympathectomy and management of thoracic spine deformities and disc herniations.

Thoracoscopy may be performed under local, regional or general anaesthesia. The choice is based on the patient's safety and comfort. Local anaesthetic infiltration of the thoracic wall and parietal pleura is the simplest method of providing anaesthesia. Intercostal nerve blocks or thoracic epidural anaesthesia at the appropriate level will provide better analgesia. During local or regional anaesthesia, partial collapse of the nondependent lung results when air enters the pleural cavity and this allows good visualization of the pleural cavity. Insufflation of gas into the hemithorax to enhance visualization can result in marked impairment of oxygenation, haemodynamic compromise or mediastinal shift. If the patient does not tolerate the procedure, or there is a need for conversion to an open thoracotomy, the awake patient in the lateral decubitus position presents difficulties to the anaesthetist.

General anaesthesia (GA) is appropriate for most modern thoracoscopies, given their duration and surgical complexity. Most VATS is performed under GA with one-lung ventilation (OLV) provided through a double lumen endobronchial tube sited in the left or right mainstem bronchus and verified bronchoscopically. A variety of GA techniques may be used for thorascopic procedures. The chosen technique must permit administration of 100% oxygen and result in early extubation without pain, haemodynamic compromise or arterial hypoxaemia. Frequently, anaesthesia is maintained using a combination of intravenous and inhalational agents. Thoracoscopic procedures are frequently similar to the corresponding open procedure in terms of length, duration of OLV, and the extent of resection. It is therefore prudent to adopt a similar monitoring strategy for thoracoscopic patients as one would for thoracotomy patients. An indwelling arterial catheter, continuous pulse oximetry and an end-tidal carbon dioxide monitor should be employed. Postoperative pain is managed by patient controlled narcotic analgesia, NSAIDs, or regional techniques. VATS-assisted siting of paravertebral catheters has been reported to assist post-thoracoscopic pain control.

The distribution of pulmonary blood flow and ventilation is influenced by the lateral decubitus position, and by the anaesthetized, paralysed, closed or open chest conditions. If the non-dependent lung is not ventilated, as during OLV, any blood flow to that lung constitutes shunt flow. Thus, OLV creates an obligatory right-to-left transpulmonary shunt through the non-ventilated non-dependent lung, which is not present during two-lung ventilation. Consequently, OLV results in a much larger alveolar–arterial oxygen tension difference and a greater risk of intraoperative hypoxia than two-lung ventilation. Factors operating to decrease blood flow to the non-dependent non-ventilated lung, and hence to minimize the risk of arterial hypoxaemia, include gravity, surgical interference with blood flow, and the extent of pre-existing disease in the non-dependent lung. The most important factor decreasing the size of the shunt is hypoxic pulmonary vasoconstriction which diverts blood flow towards ventilated lung segments, thereby improving ventilation (V) and perfusion (Q) matching.

The ventilated lung can usually eliminate sufficient carbon dioxide (CO_2) to compensate for the non-ventilated side, keeping the alveolar CO_2 tension to arterial CO_2 tension gradient small during OLV.

Creation of an artificial pneumothorax by CO_2 insufflation has been advocated to give complete non-dependent lung collapse and to optimize surgical conditions. However, significant haemodynamic compromise has been reported with such techniques. The extent to which the cardiac index (CI), mean arterial pressure (MAP) and left ventricular stroke work index (LVSWI) decrease is related to the CO_2 insufflation pressure exerted. Given the limited incision necessary for VATS, and hence the improved pulmonary function after operation, patients with severe pulmonary disease who were not previously considered for thoracotomy may be considered for VATS.

The VATS study group collected data from 40 North American institutions relating to 1800 thoracoscopic procedures in 1993. It was found that lung nodules (47.5%) and pleural effusions (19.4%) were the most frequent indications, and that almost 50% of the procedures performed were wedge resections. Conversion to a thoracotomy occurred in 24% of cases. Half of these conversions were to facilitate more extensive resection, but other indications included inability to locate the lesion, too large a lesion, a difficult surgical location, adhesions, bleeding, or a technical problem. Complications included prolonged air leak of more than 5 days (4.7%), bleeding necessitating transfusion (2.0%), postoperative pneumonia (1.9%), atelectasis (1.9%) and arrhythmia (1.6%).

LAPAROSCOPIC INTRA-ABDOMINAL PROCEDURES

Karl Langebuck performed the first open cholecystectomy in Berlin in 1882. Since then open cholecystectomy has become the 'gold standard' treatment for symptomatic gall bladder disease. Non-surgical approaches to treatment are associated with reduced morbidity and mortality, but are not curative. Laparoscopic cholecystectomy is a curative procedure with many advantages over the traditional surgical approach. (Table 28.3).

Audit of large series has, however, highlighted difficulties unique to, or more com-

Table 28.3 Laparoscopic cholecystectomy: comparison with traditional open cholecystectomy

---
Minimizes the abdominal incision
Preserves diaphragmatic function
Potential benefits
   Reduced adverse events
   Pulmonary function preserved
   Less postoperative ileus
   Early ambulation
Economic benefits
   Shorter hospital stay
   Early return to work and normal activities

Table 28.4 Laparoscopic intra-abdominal surgical procedures

Cholecystectomy
Vagotomy
Hiatus hernia repair
Diaphragmatic hernia repair
Appendicectomy
Colectomy
Inguinal hernia repair
Nephrectomy
Adrenalectomy

monly associated with, laparoscopic procedures. Minimal access surgery does not necessarily mean there is less risk associated with the therapeutic procedure: it merely indicates the surgical approach being taken. As with other surgical techniques, a learning curve exists and studies indicate that an inverse relationship exists between the number of procedures performed and the complication rate. Conversion to a laparotomy, which should not be considered a complication of laparoscopic cholecystectomy, averages 5% in most large series.

The current quest for procedures which can be performed endoscopically, coupled to improved surgical techniques and equipment, continues to expand the list of procedures performed in this manner. (Table 28.4). Proponents of the endoscopic approach claim that patients have decreased postoperative morbidity, a better cosmetic result, and can return home and to work earlier than after conventional surgery. Sceptics claim that the main reason for performing certain endoscopic-based procedures is that they are now possible and present a surgical challenge.

PHYSIOLOGICAL CHANGES AND COMPLICATIONS

Complications due to laparoscopic cholecystectomy may be broadly divided into those resulting from the surgical technique itself and those physiological derangements arising from creation of the pneumoperitoneum, systemic CO_2 absorption, venous gas embolism and patient positioning.

Trocar insertion

The first requirement for laparoscopy is the establishment of a pneumoperitoneum, to provide a clear view of the intra-abdominal structures and allow for the safe insertion of instruments. A Verres insufflation needle is usually introduced blindly into the peritoneal cavity periumbilically. This site has the shortest distance between the skin and the peritoneum, but the medial and lateral vessels are at risk of injury when the Verres needle or trocar are sited in this region. In addition, intra-abdominal structures may be damaged by 'blind' needle insertion. To avoid such injuries, a 'Hasson' minilaparotomy technique has been recommended by some for pneumoperitoneum creation.

Creation of a pneumoperitoneum

After placement of the Verres needle within the peritoneal cavity, a pneumoperitoneum is established by insufflating gas at low flow rates of $2-4$ l min^{-1} to a preset pressure level (usually of the order of 10–15 mmHg). Insufflation is continued until the abdomen is distended, hepatic dullness is lost and the upper abdomen has a tympanic percussion note: this usually requires 3–5 l of gas. At this point, the Verres needle is replaced by a trocar and sheath. The video laparoscope is then introduced through the sheath.

Extraperitoneal insufflation of CO_2 is a common complication of laparoscopy, occurring in 0.4–2.0% of cases. It may result in subcutaneous or retroperitoneal emphysema, thus prolonging or causing the abandonment of surgery.

Patient position

During laparoscopic surgery the patient is positioned so as to produce gravitational displacement of the abdominal viscera away from the surgical site. The Trendelenberg position is associated with a decreased functional residual capacity (FRC), decreased pulmonary compliance, increased intracranial pressure (ICP), increased pulmonary blood volume and pressure, and increased myocardial work and oxygen consumption. The cardiovascular and respiratory changes induced by the Trendelenburg and reverse-Trendelenburg positions may be influenced by the patient's intravascular volume, any associated cardiac disease, the degree of tilt employed, the anaesthetic drugs administered, and the ventilation technique. Other complications associated with anaesthesia in the Trendelenburg position include inadvertent right mainstem bronchial intubation and brachial plexus injury.

CO_2 homeostasis

Considerable CO_2 absorption can occur during laparoscopic procedures. The absorption of CO_2 from a closed cavity depends on its diffusibility and on the perfusion of the walls of the cavity, and not on the rate of gas insufflation. The pulmonary elimination of CO_2 during laparoscopic cholecystectomy appears to be biphasic: an initial brisk increase in elimination begins shortly after insufflation, followed by a more prolonged slower rate.

The increased $Paco_2$ results in haemodynamic alterations by causing vasodilation directly, and by stimulating the sympathetic nervous system (indirect effect). Hypercarbia can result in cardiac arrhythmias and pulmonary vasoconstriction, the latter may induce right ventricular failure. Elevation of $Paco_2$ is a major concern in those with raised ICP. Blood flow velocity through the middle cerebral artery, a marker for cerebral perfusion, increases up to 50% during laparoscopic cholecystectomy, presumably as a result of the increased $Paco_2$. Increasing the minute ventilation will help maintain a normal $Paco_2$ despite the increased CO_2 load. Thermocautery during CO_2 pneumoperitonea produces high levels of carbon monoxide intraperitoneally, but this does not appear to produce a significant change in haemodynamic function or oxygenation.

When a pressure gradient exists between the peritoneal cavity and the venous system, the insufflated gas may enter an open vein resulting in a gas embolism. Alternatively, gas may be insufflated directly into the systemic circulation when the Verres needle is introduced. The clinical effect depends on the volume of gas entrained, the rate of entrainment, the type of gas used for insufflation, and the patients intravascular volume status and overall condition. The signs of gas embolism are similar to those of venous air embolism. Often an acute decrease in the end-tidal CO_2 tension is the first sign. Treatment consists of discontinuing nitrous oxide, administering oxygen, releasing the pneumoperitoneum, and raising the CVP (by intravenous fluid administration and reversal of the head-up tilt). Inotropic support and aspiration of the gas via a central venous line may be required if the embolus is large.

The adverse effects associated with the creation of the CO_2 pneumoperitoneum have led to experimentation with other insufflation gases (nitrous oxide and helium) and with 'gasless' pneumoperitoneum techniques (an intraperitoneal mechanical device). To date none of these have replaced the use of the CO_2 pneumoperitoneum in routine clinical practice.

Pneumomediastinum and pneumothorax

Pneumothorax may complicate pneumoperitoneum and, if undetected, may be life threatening. It is most likely that gas passes from the abdominal to the thoracic cavity via a diaphragmatic defect. These defects or weak points occur at the Foramen of Bochdalek (the lumbocostal triangle), the outer crus or the oesophageal hiatus. In addition, congenital defects of the diaphragm (patent pleuroperitoneal canal) and the diaphragmatic hiati for the oesophagus and aorta can also allow gas to track from the peritoneal cavity into the mediastium. Excessively high intra-abdominal pressures during CO_2 insufflation may promote tracking of gas into the mediastinum. Alternatively, a pneumothorax may develop during a laparoscopic procedure independently of the pneumoperitoneum, due to a ruptured bleb or bulla.

Pneumothorax is an exceedingly rare complication of pneumoperitoneum. The majority tend to occur on the right side, and only occasionally do bilateral or tension pneumothoraces develop. A pneumothorax should be suspected whenever subcutaneous emphysema, increased airway pressure, haemodynamic compromise, oxygen desaturation, or unexplained hypoxaemia or hypercarbia develop, even if the characteristic physical signs are absent. If the patient is stable, a chest X-ray should be obtained to confirm the diagnosis. If a pneumothorax is recognized at the beginning or during the procedure, the abdomen should be deflated and a chest drain sited. The procedure may then be completed providing the patient remains stable. When the pneumothorax is detected towards the end of the procedure the surgery can be completed without therapeutic intervention, if the patient is stable. Once the abdomen is deflated, the CO_2 in the pleural cavity will be quickly reabsorbed, thereby obviating the need for a chest drain. In the presence of a tension pneumothorax, standard therapeutic measures should be instituted immediately including needle thoracotomy, deflation of the abdomen and insertion of a chest drain.

Cardiovascular effects

Although laparoscopic cholecystectomy is usually well tolerated, changes in cardiovascular performance may be caused by anaesthesia, patient positioning, mechanical and neuroendocrine effects of the pneumoperitoneum, and by hypercarbia. The extent of the haemodynamic changes is influenced by the intra-abdominal pressure attained, the amount of CO_2 absorbed, the patient's cardiovascular status and intravascular volume, the ventilatory technique, surgical conditions and the anaesthetic agents employed. The relative contributions of each of these variables to the overall haemodynamic change is difficult, if not impossible, to quantify.

There is a biphasic pattern to the cardiac index (CI) response to laparoscopic surgery, characterized by an early reduction (to approximately half of the awake value) followed by a gradual recovery over the 10 min following insufflation. The filling pressures of the heart, central venous pressure (CVP) and pulmonary capillary wedge pressure (PCWP), which are reduced by the induction of anaesthesia and the reverse Trendelenberg position, increase when CO_2 insufflation begins. Despite these changes in loading conditions left ventricular function, as determined by ejection fraction, is maintained in otherwise healthy patients. Such changes in left ventricular pre-load may have deleterious consequences in those with significant cardiovascular disease.

Calculated systemic vascular resistance (SVR) increases markedly, especially during the early phase of CO_2 insufflation, with partial restoration developing about 15 min after the creation of the pneumoperitoneum. The improvement in CI and reduction in SVR occur simultaneously. The rise in SVR may account, at least in part, for the increase in MAP observed during laparoscopy. Both mechanical (increased venous resistance and compression of the abdominal aorta) and humoral (alterations in catecholamines, prostaglandins, vasopressin and the renin-angiotensin system) factors could contribute to the increase in SVR. The increase in arterial pressure is associated with an increase in left ventricular wall stress. Pulmonary vascular resistance (PVR) also increases markedly during laparoscopy. Those with cardiac disease tend to show a similar pattern of change in CI, MAP, PVR and SVR to healthy patients, although there may be quantitative differences.

Cardiac output depends on venous return, myocardial contractility, and cardiac afterload. The initial reduction in CI is due to the direct myocardial depressant and the vasodilatory effect of general anaesthesia, coupled with the loss of sympathetic tone. The decreased venous return, and hence pre-load, that accompanies the reverse Trendelenburg position further decreases the CI and PCWP. The improvement in these parameters begins approximately 10 min after the start of insufflation and is probably due to a number of factors. The plasma concentration–time course profile of catecholamines and other humoral factors parallels that of changes in CI, MAP and SVR, suggesting a cause-and-effect relationship. The direct (vasodilatory) and indirect (sympathetic nervous system stimurcarbia also contribute to the haemodynamic changes seen during laparoscopy.

Acute hypotension, hypoxaemia and cardiovascular collapse have been described in association with laparoscopy. Postulated causes include: hypercarbia secondary to hypoventilation or CO_2 absorption, which may induce arrhythmias especially if the myocardium is sensitized by volatile anaesthetic agents; reflex increase of vagal tone as a result of excessive stretching of the peritoneum; compression of the inferior vena cava leading to decreased cardiac output; haemorrhage and venous gas embolism. Arrhythmias are common during laparoscopy and usually occur during or shortly after CO_2 insufflation. Bradyarrhythmias (A–V dissociation, nodal rhythm, sinus bradycardia) account for the majority of these and are not usually associated with significant falls in blood pressure.

Pneumoperitoneum and the reverse Trendelenburg position create a significant resistance to lower limb venous return resulting in decreased venous capacitance and outflow in most patients. Measures to reduce intraoperative stasis, such as compression stockings or pneumatic calf compression, may counteract this effect, thereby decreasing the risk of deep venous thrombosis.

Respiratory function

The division of abdominal musculature which accompanies open cholecystectomy produces incisional pain, diaphragmatic dysfunction, and impairment of ventilatory mechanics. The result is a restrictive pattern of pulmonary dysfunction after operation, with a shift from abdominal to rib cage breathing and a reduction in the vital capacity (FVC) and FRC. By avoiding the upper abdominal incision, laparoscopic surgery may reduce postoperative pulmonary complications.

The intraoperative pulmonary changes accompanying laparoscopic cholecystectomy are due to decreased lung compliance caused by upward displacement and splinting of the diaphragm during insufflation, and by changes in CO_2 homeostasis due to absorption of CO_2 from the peritoneal cavity. The increased arterial CO_2 tension that accompanies CO_2 insufflation is managed by increasing the minute ventilation. Preoperative evaluation with pulmonary function tests, which demonstrate forced expiratory volumes and diffusion defects less than 70 and 80% of predicted values, respectively, can identify patients at risk of developing hypercarbia and respiratory acidosis after CO_2-induced creation of a pneumoperitoneum.

After operation, the 20–40% reduction in FVC and forced expiratory volume in one second (FEV_1), is still considerably less than the 40–70% reduction which accompanies 'open' cholecystectomy. On the second postoperative day, the forced expiratory flow during 25–75% of the FVC breath (FEF 25–75%), an effort independent measurement, may be reduced almost twice as much following an open than after a laparoscopic cholecystectomy. In addition, the return to normal pulmonary function is approximately twice as fast following laparoscopic than following open cholecystectomy (5 versus 10–12 days). Nonetheless, 72 h after laparoscopic cholecystectomy pulmonary dysfunction persists with the FVC and FEV_1 at only 80% of preoperative values. The decrease in FRC after laparoscopic cholecystectomy is considerably less than that which accompanies open cholecystectomy. However, elderly patients, smokers and the obese are more likely to suffer greater reductions in FRC and sustain postoperative atelectasis regardless of the surgical approach.

In healthy subjects the pattern of change in lung function, after laparoscopic cholecystectomy, is qualitatively similar but of lesser magnitude than the change which accompanies open procedures. Adequate postoperative pain relief may improve pulmonary function after laparoscopic cholecystectomy. Towards this goal, thoracic epidural analgesia or patient controlled analgesia (PCA) can be of benefit.

ANAESTHETIC MANAGEMENT

Patient selection

Some surgeons consider laparoscopic surgery more suitable for higher risk patients than conventional approaches. Comparative studies of laparoscopic versus open procedures, in this patient population, have not been performed to date, so the anaesthetist must assess the risk/benefit ratio of the technique for each individual. Laparoscopic surgery should not be considered a suitable alternative in patients deemed unfit for the corresponding open procedure.

Preoperative assessment should include a detailed history and physical examination. Appropriate investigations should be performed, including a full blood count, urea and electrolytes, an electrocardiogram and a chest X-ray. Arterial blood gases, pulmonary function tests, further cardiological assessment and other investigations may be necessary. Premedication is prescribed according to the preference of the anaesthetist and the needs of the patient.

Monitoring

Monitoring should begin before induction with electrocardiography, non-invasive blood pressure and pulse oximetry. Peak inspiratory pressure and tidal volume should be measured. End-tidal CO_2 monitoring peroperatively is needed to monitor the adequacy of ventilation and to detect possible gas embolism. Controversy exists concerning the need for arterial cannulation to assess the effectiveness of oxygenation and ventilation after creation of a pneumoperitoneum. End-tidal CO_2 tension may differ considerably from Pa_{CO_2} during laparoscopic surgery because of V/Q mismatching. Erroneous clinical decisions can be reached if these two values are assumed to be equal, to change proportionately, or even to change in the same direction.

A study of 28 otherwise healthy patients undergoing elective laparoscopic cholecystectomy determined what increase in minute ventilation was required to maintain pre-insufflation Pa_{CO_2} and whether end-tidal CO_2 tension can be safely used as an index of Pa_{CO_2} and therefore, of the adequacy of ventilation during pneumoperitoneum. Increasing minute ventilation by 12–16% maintained the Pa_{CO_2} close to the pre-insufflation levels. End-tidal CO_2 tension was not a satisfactory index of Pa_{CO_2} if the latter exceeded 41 mmHg or if large volumes of CO_2 were insufflated. Otherwise, end-tidal CO_2 tension proved a reasonable approximation of Pa_{CO_2} in these patients, all of whom were free from cardiopulmonary disease

Placement of a urinary catheter and a nasogastric tube will minimize the risk of trauma to intra-abdominal contents at the time of trocar insertion and facilitate laparoscopic visualization. Hourly urine output measurement aids assessment of fluid balance. Intra-abdominal pressure should be monitored and not allowed to exceed 20 mmHg, both the rate of gas flow and the volume used should be noted. A praecordial or oesophageal stethoscope will aid detection of a venous gas embolus, although a Doppler ultrasound probe is more sensitive.

Anaesthetic technique

Although regional anaesthesia has been employed, general anaesthesia is the usual choice for upper abdominal laparoscopic surgery because of the discomfort caused by the pneumoperitoneum and the number of positional changes needed during the procedure. Tracheal intubation and mechanical ventilation are recommended, as several factors may induce hypercarbia, including depression of ventilation by anaesthetic agents, absorption of CO_2 from the peritoneal cavity, and impairment of ventilation by the pneumoperitoneum and initial Trendelenburg position.

A variety of agents can be used during laparoscopic surgery. The choice is guided by the personal preference of the anaesthetist and the general status of the patient. Usually a combined intravenous–inhalational anaesthetic technique is chosen. Despite the controversy surrounding its use, nitrous oxide has not been found to have a clinically significant effect on surgical conditions during laparoscopic cholecystectomy, nor on the incidence of postoperative emesis. Opioids and/or NSAIDs are usually given to reduce the stress response and provide analgesia. Intraperitoneal administration of 0.25% bupivacaine into the region of the gall bladder bed can provide effective pain relief following laparoscopic cholecystectomy. Postoperative nausea and vomiting are amongst the most common and distressing symptoms after laparoscopic surgery. Anti-emetic medication should therefore be administered prophylactically.

Adequate postoperative pain relief will help minimize patient discomfort, the stress response, and pulmonary dysfunction. The technique employed depends on the nature of the surgery, the patient's condition and the facilities available within the institution. The options available include PCA, regional techniques and oral, intramuscular or sublingual medications.

SUMMARY

The purpose of minimally invasive surgery is to achieve a satisfactory clinical result whilst avoiding the morbidity associated with more conventional approaches. Various authorities predict that in ten years 70–80% of surgical procedures will be performed endoscopically. This development will have major implications for hospital design and surgical training. Most intra-abdominal laparoscopic surgery is performed under GA to minimize patient discomfort and optimize visualization of structures.

Complications which accompany surgery are usually due to traumatic injuries associated with instrument insertion or the physiological changes which accompany anaesthesia, the creation of a pneumoperitoneum, CO_2 absorption and patient positioning. The relative contribution which each of the above makes is difficult to quantify. Laparoscopic cholecystectomy results in decreased CI and increased SVR, PVR and MAP in healthy patients. There are undoubted postoperative benefits in terms of better preservation of lung function and shorter convalescence.

FURTHER READING

Cunningham, A. J. and Brull, S. J. (1993) Laparoscopic cholecystectomy: anesthetic implications *Anesthesia and Analgesia*, **76**, 1120–1133.

Cunningham, A. J., Turner, J., Rosenbaum, S., Rafferty, T. *et al.* (1993) Transoesophageal echocardiographic assessment of haemodynamic function during laparoscopic cholecystectomy. *British Journal of Anaesthesia*, **70**, 621–625.

Horswell, J. L. (1993) Anaesthetic techniques for thoracoscopy. *Annals of Thoracic Survery*, **56**, 624–629.

Jones, D. R., Graeber, G. M., Tanguilig, G. G. et al. (1993). Effects of insufflation on hemodynamics during thoracoscopy. *Annals of Thoracic Surgery*, **55**, 1379–1382.

Joris, J. and Lamy, M. (1993) Neuroendocrine changes during pneumoperitoneum for laparoscopic cholecystectomy. *British Journal of Anaesthesia*, **70**, A33.

Joris, J., Noirot, D. P., Legrand, M. J. et al. (1993) Hemodynamic changes during laparoscopic cholecystectomy. *Anesthesia and Analgesia*, **76**, 1067–1071.

Putensen-Himmer, G., Putensen, C., Lammer, H. et al. (1992) Comparison of postoperative respiratory function after laparoscopy or laparotomy for cholecystectomy. *Anesthesiology*, **77**, 675–680.

Wahba, R. W. M., Béique, F. and Kleiman, S. J. (1995) Cardiopulmonary function and laparoscopic cholecystectomy. *Canadian Journal of Anaesthesia*, **42**, 51–63.

Wahba, R. W. M. and Mamazza, J. (1993) Ventilatory requirements during laparoscopic cholecystectomy. *Canadian Journal of Anaesthesia*, **40**, 206–210.

EPIDURAL AND SPINAL ANAESTHESIA 29

D. P. Dob and M. Morgan

Spinal and epidural anaesthesia are the two most common regional techniques used in anaesthesia. This chapter deals with the use of these techniques for operative surgery and does not consider their use in obstetric practice nor for acute or chronic pain relief.

ANATOMY

VERTEBRAE

There are seven cervical, twelve thoracic and five lumbar vertebrae. The sacrum consists of five fused vertebrae and the coccyx of four. The basic anatomy of all the vertebrae is the same and that of a typical lumbar vertebra is shown in Figure 29.1. Each consists of a body anteriorly and a vertebral arch which surrounds the vertebral canal containing the spinal cord and nerve roots. Arising from the posterolateral aspects of the bodies of the vertebrae are the pedicles, which meet the laminae, which lie posteriorly, at the origin of the transverse processes. Each lamina carries a superior and inferior articular process which bear the articular facets for articulation with adjacent laminae. The pedicles are notched near the junction with the transverse processes, the notches of adjacent pairs forming an intervertebral foramen through which the spinal nerves emerge.

A typical lumbar vertebra has a large body and the vertebral canal is triangular shaped with the apex posteriorly. The pedicles are thick and the transverse processes slender; the laminae are short and thick. The lumbar spines project horizontally backwards. Thoracic vertebrae have smaller bodies with long dorsal spines which overlap each other caudally, especially in the mid-thoracic region. In full flexion, the upper border of these spines may be inclined to an angle of 45–60° caudally. In the lower thoracic region the spines become more horizontal. The cervical vertebrae from C3 to C7 have small flat bodies and the vertebral canal is large. The transverse processes are short and from C1 to C6 are pierced by the foramen transversarium which transmits the vertebral artery. The cervical spines are short, often bifid and that of C7 is the most prominent in the vertebral column.

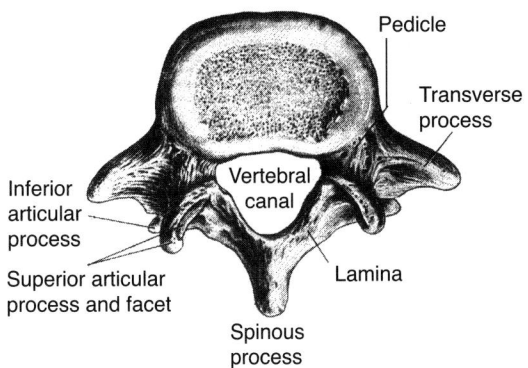

Figure 29.1 Superior view of the fifth lumbar vertebra with the large, kidney shaped body lying anteriorly. (Reproduced with permission from Gray's Anatomy, 37th edn.)

Short Practice of Anaesthesia. Edited by M. Morgan and G. M. Hall. Published in 1997 by Chapman & Hall, London. ISBN 0 412 71890 1

Ligaments

Between the bodies of adjacent vertebrae are the intervertebral discs. Running along the anterior aspect of the bodies of the vertebrae and intervertebral discs, from the foramen magnum to the coccyx is the broad, flat anterior longitudinal ligament, which does not come into relationship with the epidural space. A similar ligament, the posterior longitudinal runs along the posterior surfaces of the vertebral bodies and discs.

Joining adjacent laminae is the thick ligamentum flavum. The interspinous ligaments lie between the vertebral spines, while running along the tips of the spines is the supraspinous ligament.

The sacrum

The sacrum, which is wedge shaped with the base superiorly articulating with the fifth lumbar vertebra, consists of five fused vertebra. Its anterior aspect is concave and posterior convex. There are five large anterior sacral foraminae on each side and four posterior. The laminae of the fifth sacral vertebra fail to fuse, leaving a gap, the sacral hiatus, guarded by a rolled edge of bone, the sacral cornu. The apex of the sacrum articulates inferiorly with the coccyx. The sacral hiatus is closed by the sacrococcygeal ligament running from the sacral cornu to the back of the coccyx. The anatomy of the sacrum is variable and occasionally the sacral hiatus is absent.

MENINGES

The three meninges cover the brain and spinal cord. The innermost layer, the delicate piamater is applied directly to the brain and spinal cord. The outermost layer comprises the thick dura, which protects the neural tissue. In the skull, the dura consists of two layers, the outer endosteal layer which is applied directly to the skull and the inner meningeal layer. These two layers are tightly fused together, but split at certain sites to enclose the large intracranial venous sinuses. The arachnoid mater lines the dura and between it and the neural tissue is the sub-arachnoid space containing cerebrospinal fluid (CSF).

EPIDURAL SPACE

At the foramen magnum the two layers of dura are tightly fused together. The endosteal layer loses its identity, but the meningeal layer continues inferiorly as the spinal dura encasing the spinal cord and nerve roots. The epidural space (also known as extradural or peridural) lies between the spinal dura and the bones and ligaments that form the vertebral canal. The spinal cord usually terminates at the upper border of the second lumbar vertebra, although occasionally it may be higher or lower. (Figure 29.2) The dural sac normally terminates at the upper border of the third piece of the sacrum in adults and will contain nerves of the filum terminale and CSF. It may terminate at a lower level in children. The volume of the sacral component of the epidural space is about 20–25 ml in adults and besides the termination of the dural sac it contains the filum terminale which is a long extension of piamater, a venous plexus, sacral nerves and fat.

The boundaries of the epidural space are as follows.

- **Superiorly** the fusion of the two layers of dura at the foramen magnum; because of this fusion it follows that anything injected into the epidural space cannot directly enter the cranium.
- **Inferiorly** the sacral hiatus closed by the sacrococcygeal ligament.
- **Anteriorly** the posterior longitudinal ligament covering the posterior aspects of the vertebral bodies and intervertebral discs.
- **Laterally** the pedicles of the vertebrae and the intervertebral foramina.
- **Posteriorly** the laminae of the vertebrae and the ligamentum flavum.

Anatomy

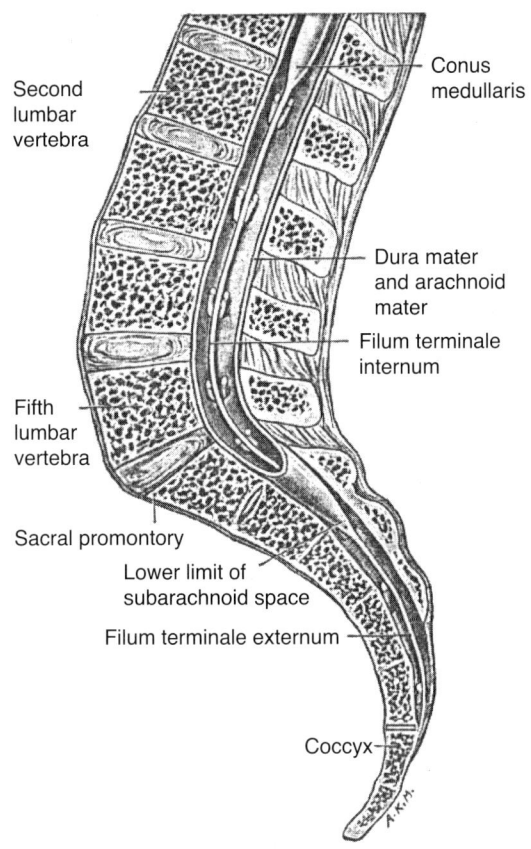

Figure 29.2 Median sagittal section of the lumbosacral part of the vertebral column. The spinal cord terminates at the upper border of the second lumbar vertebra while the dural sac ends at the upper border of the third piece of the sacrum. (Reproduced with permission from Gray's Anatomy, 37th edn.)

The epidural space can be entered anywhere along its length in the cervical, thoracic, lumbar or sacral regions.

NERVE ROOTS

The posterior (dorsal, sensory) and anterior (ventral, motor) nerve roots enter and leave the spinal cord respectively and fuse distal to the dorsal root ganglion in the vertebral canal before passing out of the appropriate intervertebral foramen. Due to the discrepancy between the length of the spinal cord (ending around L2) and the vertebral column, the nerve roots become more inclined vertically to reach their intervertebral foramina and those in the cauda equina pass vertically to their exit.

Each nerve root carries with it a prolongation of the dura which fuses with the nerve coverings just distal to the fusion of the nerve roots. These dural cuffs are lined by arachnoid and therefore contain pockets of CSF. If the nerve roots actually fuse within an intervertebral foramen, then there will also be CSF in this region. Arachnoid villi are found in the areas of the dural cuffs and are responsible for absorption of substances injected into the epidural space.

BLOOD SUPPLY OF THE SPINAL CORD

Arteries

The posterior spinal arteries, one on each side, arise from the posterior cerebellar arteries at the level of the foramen magnum. They descend along the length of the spinal cord and supply the posterior columns and dorsal horns. The anterior spinal artery extends along the length of the anterior median fissure of the spinal cord. It is made up of anastomosing branches of the vertebral, intercostal and iliac arteries and supplies the anterior horns of the spinal cord and the corticospinal tracts. Nutrient arteries which feed into the anterior spinal artery may be divided into three distinct areas:

- the cervical cord down to the level of the fourth thoracic vertebra which is supplied by vertebral, thyrocervical and costocervical arteries;
- the intermediate mid-thoracic cord which is supplied by the intercostal arteries; and
- the lumbosacral cord between T8 and L2 which is supplied by a single artery, the artery of Adamkiewicz.

There are no anastomoses between these arteries. Sensitivity to cord ischaemia increases from cephalad to caudad, the anterior region being most sensitive.

Veins

The epidural veins form a plexus in the anterolateral part of the epidural space on each side and drain the spinal cord and vertebral canal. The plexus communicates with the intracranial sinuses and with the inferior vena cava. Further tributaries drain into the azygos system and from there to the superior vena cava. There is therefore a venous network between the pelvis and the brain which can act as an alternative pathway to the caval system (vertebral venous plexus of Batson). As this system has no valves, any caval obstruction will lead to a large increase in the volume of blood in the epidural venous plexus. Obstruction may be caused by increased intrathoracic pressure, e.g. coughing, straining, Valsalva manoeuvre, or by caval compression by a large abdominal tumour, ascites or gravid uterus. Engorgement of these veins therefore results in a reduction in the volume of the epidural space and solutions injected under such circumstances may lead to an unexpectedly extensive spread.

Recent advances

Much recent research has utilized the techniques of magnetic resonance imaging, epiduroscopy and cryomicrotomy. The most important finding is that the contents of the epidural space are arranged in a repeating saw-tooth pattern between the vertebral bodies. Within the vertebral caval, the epidural contents are applied very closely to the vertebral walls.

Epiduroscopy has revealed the occasional existence of a dorsomedian raphé connecting the posterior aspect of the dura to the ligamentum flavum.

EPIDURAL ANAESTHESIA

EPIDURAL PRESSURES

In 1926, whilst measuring the CSF pressure in cadavers, Janzen frequently noticed the existence of a negative pressure after the needle had pierced the ligamentum flavum and before recording the positive CSF pressure following dural puncture. He noticed that this negative pressure was greater if the needle was blunt, if it had a side rather than an end hole and if the CSF pressure was low. He attributed these findings to the fact that having pierced the ligamentum flavum, the needle pushed the dura in front of it, thereby creating a negative pressure in a closed space, before it was eventually pierced, i.e. the negative pressure was an artefact. Other evidence has subsequently supported this theory.

Nevertheless, a number of other suggestions have been proposed to explain this phenomenon:

- transmission from the pleural cavity during respiration via the intervertebral foramina;
- the drag of the viscera, again via the intervertebral foramina;
- flexion of the spine increasing the volume of the epidural space; and
- growth of the vertebral column exceeding that of the spinal cord and dura.

LOCATION OF THE EPIDURAL SPACE

Performance of epidural anaesthesia requires the introduction of a needle, plus or minus a catheter, into the epidural space. There are two main methods of location.

Loss of resistance

This relies on the sudden change of resistance that occurs as the needle passes from the very tough ligamentum flavum, where it is virtually impossible to inject anything, into the epidural space where there is no resistance to injection. The loss of resistance is best appreciated by slowly, but continuously, advancing the needle whilst pressure is applied to the plunger of the syringe with the thumb. The syringe may be charged with either air or saline, both having their advocates. Saline has the advantage that it cannot be compressed so that false positives should be rare, but has the disadvantage that any fluid dripping from the needle after the syringe has been detached might be saline or CSF. The latter should feel warm if allowed to fall onto the exposed forearm and will test positive for sugar. If air has been used, then any fluid dripping from the needle must be CSF. Air, however, can be compressed so that more false positives can be expected; also the incidence of inadvertent dural puncture is higher.

Negative pressure

This depends on the existence of a negative pressure in the epidural space and this method of location is exemplified by the hanging drop method of Gutierrez. A drop of fluid is placed in the hub of the needle, which is advanced slowly and on entering the epidural space this fluid is sucked inwards.

Numerous methods and devices have been described in an attempt to aid location of the epidural space, all of which rely on one of these two basic principles. All serve to make what is basically a relatively simple procedure more complicated.

The majority of epidurals are performed in the lumbar region by the mid-line approach. The patient can be in the sitting or lateral position and the back fully flexed to make the space between vertebrae as wide as possible. Most are performed in the L2–3 or L3–4 interspace, the space being identified by a line joining the superiormost aspect of the iliac crest (Tuffier's line), which recent work has confirmed to cross the tip of the spinous process of L4. The importance of correct positioning cannot be overemphasized. The epidural space can be expected to be located 4–6 cm from the skin of the lumbar region in 70% of cases.

The paramedian approach is more frequently used in the thoracic region owing to the overlapping spinous processes. With the patient in the fully flexed position the needle is inserted 1 cm lateral to the superior aspect of the tip of a spinous process and advanced until it hits bone. This is the lamina of the vertebra below that whose spinous process was used as a landmark. The needle is then angulated about 10° from the horizontal so that the tip points to the mid-line and 'walked' in a cephalad direction off the lamina and into the ligamentum flavum. The needle is then advanced using the loss of resistance technique until it enters the epidural space.

Each method of using the epidural space has its advocates. The best method of locating it is that which works for the operator.

EQUIPMENT

Needles

As the usual technique relies on loss of resistance, then this is better appreciated the larger the needle. Also, to avoid inadvertent dural puncture after entering the epidural space, then the needle should preferably be blunt. There must obviously be a compromise between the degree of sharpness to permit reasonably easy passage through the tissues and the bluntness to prevent dural puncture.

By far the most common to be used for epidural anaesthesia is the Tuohy needle (Figure 29.3) which was originally described for intrathecal use. It is available in 16 and 18 G sizes for adults and is usually graduated in centimetres (Lee markings). The Huber tip of the needle is rounded and the thin walls allow passage of a catheter which emerges from the tip at an angle of 20°. There are smaller sizes for paediatric use.

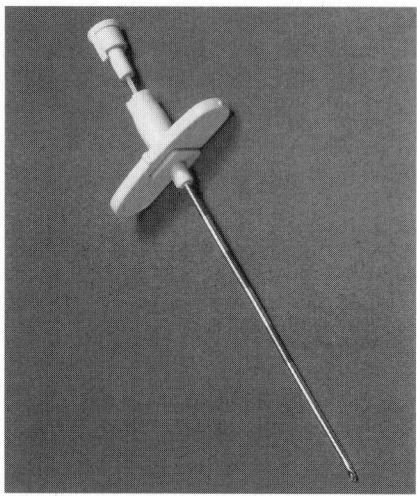

Figure 29.3 A modern Tuohy needle with Huber tip and flange. Note the centimetre markings (Lee markings) beginning, in this instance, 3 cm from the tip. The shaft of the needle is 8 cm long. (Reproduced by courtesy of Portex Ltd., UK.)

Epidural catheters

Several types are available. They are 90 cm long and radio-opaque. The tip may be rounded with side holes, reducing the possibility of dural puncture, or the hole may be at the tip of the catheter. (Recent evidence suggests more even spread of injected solution with the latter design.) A Luer hub may be fitted to the end of the catheter to which a 22 μm filter can be attached. Catheters usually bear markings at centimetre intervals from 5 to 20 cm (with 10 and 15 cm being identified), which, together with the Lee markings on the needle makes it possible to calculate the amount of catheter that has been left in the space when the needle has been removed. A typical catheter and filter are shown in Figure 29.4.

FACTORS INFLUENCING SPREAD OF
SOLUTIONS INJECTED

A number of factors can affect the spread of solutions injected into the epidural space and

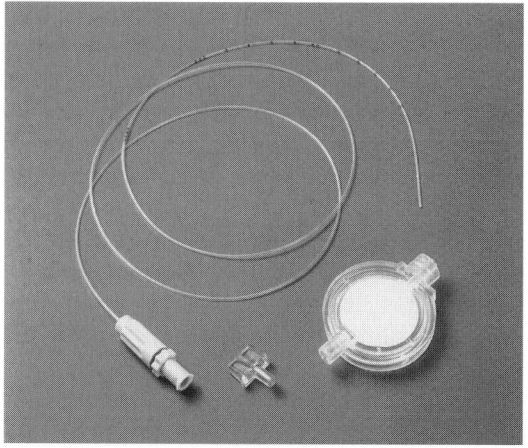

Figure 29.4 Typical epidural catheter and bacterial filter. Centimetre markings begin 5 cm from the tip and occur at 1 cm intervals to 15 cm. Double marks occur at 10 cm, triple at 15 cm and quadruple at 20 cm. (Reproduced by courtesy of Portex Ltd., UK.)

hence determine the ultimate height of the block.

Site of injection

The higher up the spinal column that the injection is made, then obviously the greater the height of the block, but the site of injection also influences the pattern of the block. Thus injection in the lumbar region always spreads more readily cephalad than it does caudad, whereas spread in the thoracic region is much more even. Spread after a caudal injection is much more erratic due to loss of solution through the large sacral foramina.

Volume of injectate

This determines the longitudinal spread of the solution. The concentration of local anaesthetic determines the speed of onset, intensity and duration of the block.

Age

From the age of 18 years, dose requirements decrease in a more or less linear fashion so that by the age of 80 years approximately half the volume of local anaesthetic is required to produce the same extent of block as at 18 years. This might be related to closure of intervertebral foramina by fibrous tissue with advancing age, blocking off an escape route for local anaesthetic from the epidural space.

Pregnancy, intra-abdominal tumours or ascites

As mentioned earlier, these conditions are associated with engorgement of the epidural plexus of veins and a consequent volume reduction of the epidural space. Injected solutions will therefore spread further.

Height

This correlates poorly with spread of injectate. The length of the vertebral column is a better marker, but still not particularly reliable.

Arteriosclerosis

Patients with arteriosclerosis require a lower dosage, but the reasons are not clear. These patients behave as if they are much older than their chronological age.

Gravity

Whether the block is performed in the sitting or lateral position has no clinically important effect on the eventual height of an epidural block.

SITES OF ACTION

The fate of local anaesthetic solutions injected into the epidural space and the sites at which they act are summarized in Figure 29.5. The main site is on the nerve roots in the epidural space, which involves diffusion of the drug through the meningeal coverings of the nerves. It must not be forgotten that significant amounts of drugs can be absorbed into the systemic circulation and a watch must always be maintained for toxic effects of local anaesthetics.

LOCAL ANAESTHETICS USED IN EPIDURAL ANAESTHESIA

Bupivacaine is by far the most common drug used epidurally in the UK although lignocaine is still used for operative surgery in some centres.

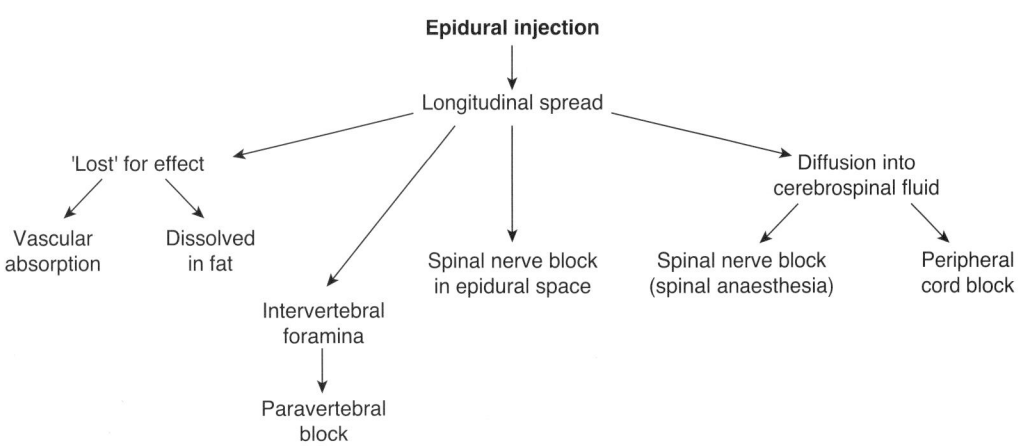

Figure 29.5 Fate of an epidural injection. (Modified from Bromage 1977, *Epidural Anaesthesia*. W.B. Saunders, Philadelphia.)

Bupivacaine

This is available as 0.25%, 0.5% and 0.75% solutions. It is the longest acting of the local anaesthetic agents, but in a concentration of 0.5% will only give effective anaesthesia for operative surgery for about 1.5–2.0 h, although postoperative pain relief may last for several hours. Muscle relaxation is superior with the 0.75% solution. The onset of action of bupivacaine is significantly slower than lignocaine and surgery may be delayed for 30 min after injection. Concern has been expressed about the cardiotoxicity of bupivacaine, especially the difficulty in achieving successful cardiac resuscitation. The 0.75% concentration is not licensed for use in pregnancy.

Lignocaine

For operative surgery, concentrations of 1.5 or 2.0% are used. The latency is about 10 min, but the duration is only around 1.0 h; this may be prolonged by the addition of adrenaline. Tachyphylaxis is a feature of repeat doses of lignocaine.

Prilocaine

This is the least toxic of the amide local anaesthetics. It may be used in concentrations of 2.0 or 3.0% for operative surgery. Its time of onset is similar to lignocaine, but it is of longer duration. Addition of adrenaline does not reduce the maximum plasma level obtained and hence is of little benefit. One of its metabolites, O-toluidine, causes methaemoglobinaemia and cyanosis will occur with doses greater than 600 mg.

Ropivacaine

This is the most recently introduced local anaesthetic and is not a racemic mixture like bupivacaine, but the (S)-enantiomer. It can be used in 0.5, 0.75 and 1.0% solutions and is still undergoing investigation. It is less cardiotoxic than bupivacaine.

Etidocaine

In a 1.0 or 1.5% solution, etidocaine produces good motor block which may outlast the duration of analgesia. It is very fat soluble and not currently available in the UK.

Adrenaline

Addition of adrenaline to bupivacaine and especially lignocaine, produces vasoconstriction, which results in a prolongation of the duration of action of these drugs and also reduces systemic absorption thereby increasing the maximum permissible dose. The optimum concentration is 1:200 000 (5 μg ml^{-1}).

Carbonated solutions

Using local anaesthetic as the carbonated salt results in an increase in the amount of un-ionized drug present. As it is only this form that can diffuse through tissue planes, this results in a decrease in onset time and denser block. These have found little favour in clinical practice.

Several other compounds have been given epidurally with good effect, e.g. ketamine, α_2-agonists, steroids and opioids, but they do not really have a place in operative surgery.

PHYSIOLOGICAL EFFECTS

For convenience these may be considered as the effects of blocking somatic nerve fibres and autonomic nerve fibres. The main site of action of the local anaesthetic is on the nerve roots within the epidural space.

Somatic nerve block

In order of sensitivity to local anaesthetic these nerve fibres consist of: unmyelinated C fibres subserving pain and temperature; A delta fibres also subserving pain and temperature; A gamma fibres, touch; A beta fibres, pressure; and Aα fibres, proprioception from muscle spindles and tendon end organs. Similarly, motor fibres are blocked in the order: unmyelinated C fibres (postganglionic sympathetic); gamma motor neurones to muscle spindles; and α-motor neurones to skeletal muscle.

The greater the concentration of local anaesthetic, the more types of fibre will be blocked. It is possible to choose a concentration that will block the smaller fibres whilst leaving the larger ones intact, i.e. differential nerve block. The block will always be densest at the site of injection. Assessment of the height of a block is usually done by assessing the response to a pin prick or to cold, e.g. with ethyl chloride. The block to temperature is, on average, two segments higher than to pin prick.

Autonomic block

Autonomic fibres leave the spinal cord in the thoracolumbar outflow (sympathetic) and sacral outflow (parasympathetic). The parasympathetic nerve supply to the gut is largely from the vagus nerve which is unaffected by epidural blockade. The 'physiological' effects of the latter are largely due to sympathetic blockade of preganglionic sympathetic fibres. These arise in the lateral horn of grey matter from T1 to L2 and pass in the ventral nerve roots into the mixed spinal nerve and then leave as white rami communicates to enter the sympathetic chain. These fibres are finely myelinated B fibres and are the most sensitive to local anaesthetics.

Cardiovascular effects

These result from a combination of sympathetic blockade and the effects of absorbed local anaesthetic and adrenaline on the cardiovascular system.

Blood pressure is the product of cardiac output and peripheral resistance. As sympathetic fibres are blocked, there is arteriolar vasodilatation and a reduction in systemic vascular resistance. Removal of sympathetic activity on the venous side results in an increase in venous capacity and a reduction in venous return and hence in cardiac output. There is thus a tendency for arterial blood pressure to fall. However, the body will attempt to maintain the blood pressure constant via the baroreceptor mechanism and there will be an increase in sympathetic activity above the level of the sympathetic block. The blood pressure is normally taken in the arm and thus only modest falls in blood pressure can be expected until the block increases to above T4 and the sympathetic fibres to the arm begin to be blocked. If the block reaches T1 and the cardiac sympathetic fibres (T1–T4) are blocked, then no compensatory mechanisms remain and control of blood pressure will have to depend on pharmacological means.

It should be stressed that if a block is confined to the thoracic region, e.g. T1–T6, then sympathetic activity below this level remains intact. Epidural block does not result in 'transection' of the spinal cord.

Local anaesthetics injected into the epidural space are absorbed into the systemic circulation. The amount absorbed usually has no important effect, but rapid absorption due to overdose or accidental intravascular injection can result in myocardial depression. Similarly, adrenaline injected with the local anaesthetic is absorbed and in the amount usually used, it is the β-effects that predominate. Thus an increase in heart rate and a reduction in systemic vascular resistance due to vasodilatation of muscle vessels results and a greater fall in blood pressure can be expected than with plain solutions.

The results of sympathetic blockade, however, will depend on a number of important factors.

- The degree of sympathetic activity that existed before the block: if this is high, e.g.

in hypertensive subjects, then a greater fall in blood pressure will result.
- Heart disease: these patients may not be able to compensate for changes in cardiovascular dynamics.
- The ability of the body to compensate for circulatory changes: this ability may be inhibited by concomitant use of vasoactive drugs such as β-blockers, calcium channel blockers, ACE inhibitors etc. Also depression of the vasomotor centre by sedative, opiod or anaesthetic drugs will inhibit the body's ability to compensate for changes in cardiovascular dynamics.
- Hypovolaemia: increased sympathetic activity results in an attempt to maintain venous return. Removal results in an increase in circulatory capacity with a profound decrease in venous return and cardiac output. Bonica and colleagues showed that in the presence of sympathetic blockade to T5, even a modest blood loss of 10 ml kg^{-1} resulted in a 41% decrease in mean arterial blood pressure and a 70% decrease in heart rate; two of five subjects had a cardiac arrest. Hypovolaemia is very poorly tolerated in the presence of extensive sympathetic blockade and it is mandatory that blood volume be maintained under these circumstances.

Respiratory effects

An epidural block to the level of T5 has virtually no effect on the mechanics of ventilation. A thoracic epidural used for pain relief after surgery will improve functional residual capacity and the patient's ability to cough.

Gastrointestinal effects

Block of sympathetic activity leaves unopposed vagal activity with the result that the gut is small and contracted, allowing easier surgical access. Sphincters are relaxed. Block of the sacral outflow (parasympathetic) from S2 to S4 results in bladder atony, whereas block of sympathetic activity to the bladder increases bladder sphincter tone.

Stress response

Abolition of the hormonal response to surgery will only result if all afferent input to the central nervous system (CNS) is blocked. This can be achieved for pelvic surgery provided the block extends to T5 thereby blocking the greater splanchnic nerve supply to the adrenals. The response cannot be prevented by epidural anaesthesia for upper abdominal surgery because there is no effect on vagal afferent activity. The stress response can be modified by utilizing the epidural for postoperative pain relief, but evidence that there is a long lasting benefit from this is scanty. The hypercoagulable state that exists after surgery is initiated by the stress response and this is limited by epidural analgesia, but evidence of a reduction in the incidence of pulmonary embolism is not strong.

Thermoregulation

The increase in skin blood flow due to epidural analgesia results in a redistribution of central heat to the peripheries. There is an increase in heat loss and attempts should be made to minimize this during surgery. No satisfactory explanation exists for the shivering that sometimes follows epidural anaesthesia.

INDICATIONS FOR EPIDURAL ANAESTHESIA

Before embarking on epidural anaesthesia for operative surgery it is essential to weigh up the advantages and disadvantages of the technique for each individual patient. Also to be taken into account is the fact that balanced general anaesthesia is an extremely effective and safe technique.

Epidural anaesthesia is an excellent choice for operations on the lower limb, particularly the hip, perineum, lower abdomen and pelvis. Intra-abdominal operations will require high concentrations of local anaesthetic to produce muscular relaxation. For upper abdominal surgery, considerable falls in blood pressure might occur. For vascular surgery of the lower limb, blood flow is improved as long as the sympathetic block is maintained, but there is no difference in outcome between regional and general anaesthesia. For intraperitoneal surgery, some form of sedation and possibly general anaesthesia will always be required and on purely humanitarian grounds should be provided during prolonged surgery on the extremities and those involved in cutting bone.

Epidural analgesia has distinct advantages for those procedures which necessitate the highest quality pain relief postoperatively, e.g. those with pulmonary disease. In patients with diabetes mellitus, the reduction in the stress response makes for easier control of blood sugar level after operation.

CONTRAINDICATIONS TO EPIDURAL ANAESTHESIA

Absolute

- Patient unwilling.
- Technical inexpertise.
- Failure to set up an intravenous infusion and lack of resuscitation equipment and drugs.
- Sepsis, local or systemic. Passage of the needle through an area of sepsis may result in infection being introduced into the epidural space and abscess formation. Epidural blood vessel puncture is one of the most common complications of epidural anaesthesia and in the presence of septicaemia subsequent bleeding may result in the development of an infected haematoma and an abscess.
- Known allergy to local anaesthetics.
- Uncontrolled haemorrhage due to the known possible disastrous consequences of extensive sympathetic block under such circumstances.
- Coagulopathy, due to either disease processes or full anticoagulant therapy because of the risk of persistent bleeding into the epidural space.

Prophylactic anticoagulation

This is now being practised extensively, usually in the form of miniheparin, in the hope of preventing deep vein thrombosis and subsequent pulmonary embolism. Little hard information is available as to the risk of epidural haematoma formation in the presence of prophylactic anticoagulant therapy. Such haematomas do occur spontaneously, but they have also been reported, albeit very rarely, in patients receiving this type of prophylaxis. The current thinking on this problem and the recommended course of action is summarized in Table 29.1.

Relative

Under some circumstances, special thought must be given before performing epidural

Table 29.1 Recommended safety precautions for performing spinal and epidural anaesthesia in the presence of anticoagulant therapy

Anticoagulant regimen	Safety precautions
Low dose unfractionated heparin	Before first dose or 4–6 h after last
Low molecular weight heparin	Before first dose or 12 h after last
Aspirin	Before first dose or 7–10 days after last. Bleeding time <10 min
Therapeutic anticoagulation	Block contraindicated
Intra-operative anticoagulation, e.g. cardiac surgery	Start 1 h before. If bloody tap, abandon surgery
Postoperative anticoagulation with heparin	Stop 1–2 h before removing catheter

anaesthesia. Thus, although there is no evidence that modern local anaesthetics cause permanent nerve damage, many neurological diseases (e.g. multiple sclerosis) are relapsing in nature and any deterioration might well be blamed on the regional block. In patients with spinal deformities, technical difficulties in performing the block may distress the patient. Potential massive haemorrhage (e.g. presence of placenta praevia) is also a relative contraindication. Extensive blocks are best avoided in those with fixed cardiac output states. It should also be noted that there is always a considerable delay in the S1 nerve root being blocked and to a lesser extent L5. This is purely due to the much larger size of S1 and operations involving this dermatome are probably best not done under epidural anaesthesia. The same consideration applies to spinal anaesthesia.

COMPLICATIONS OF EPIDURAL ANAESTHESIA

Technical problems

Technical problems involve failure to locate the epidural space and to pass the epidural catheter. This should not occur on more than 1% of occasions. Only about 25% of catheters actually travel in the direction intended and most curl up at the point of insertion. Occasionally a catheter passes out of an intervertebral foramen.

Blood vessel puncture

This is one of the commonest complications of epidural anaesthesia, particularly in obstetric practice. It may occur with the needle or, more often, the catheter. The latter must always be aspirated prior to any injection and all injections should be made slowly and stopped if there is any sign of toxicity. If a blood vessel is punctured, the most prudent action is to choose another interspace.

Accidental dural puncture

Inadvertent dural puncture with a Tuohy needle is usually obvious and another site should be chosen. There is a high incidence of post-dural-puncture headache under these circumstances which will require treatment (see below).

Accidental spinal anaesthesia

One of the major concerns in performing epidural anaesthesia is injection of an epidural dose intrathecally, which would usually be via the catheter. For this reason, most anaesthetists inject a test dose of 3 ml of lignocaine and observe the patient for signs of spinal block. Inclusion of adrenaline in the solution would indicate inadvertent intravenous injection because of the resultant, but transient, tachycardia.

If a large volume is injected intrathecally, a total spinal anaesthetic might result. Cephalad spread of the anaesthetic results in paralysis of the intercostal muscles and eventually the diaphragm with resultant apnoea. There is total sympathetic blockade with a profound fall in blood pressure. Intracranial spread is indicated by loss of consciousness and inability to maintain the airway. The first sign of an excessively high block are complaints of difficulty in breathing and whispering. Such a complication should never be fatal, treatment consisting of tracheal intubation and ventilation of the lungs with oxygen enriched air and maintenance of blood pressure with vasopressors, atropine and fluid therapy.

Subdural block

This results from injection of local anaesthetic between the dura and arachnoid, usually via a catheter; because of its position, CSF cannot be aspirated from the catheter. Although it is often said that the catheter migrates through the dura, this is not so as the latter is an extremely tough membrane; the catheter has been positioned there in the first place, the epidural needle having punctured the dura but not the arachnoid. Under these circumstances, injection of small volumes of local anaesthetic then produce unexpectedly and unpredictably extensive blockade. As the injected fluid tends to stay posteriorly, the sympathetic outflow tends to be spared and often there is little decrease in blood pressure.

Toxic reaction

Toxic reaction to local anaesthetics is always a possibility during epidural anaesthesia, so the patient must be closely observed for warning signs of such an event.

Neurological damage

This is a rare complication and occasionally might be permanent. It is always possible that the complication might be due to a pre-existing, undiagnosed neurological condition. When it occurs, the opinion of a neurologist must always be sought to exclude conditions unrelated to epidural anaesthesia. There is no evidence that neurological damage is more likely to occur after spinal than epidural anaesthesia. Problems might arise for a number of reasons:

- direct trauma to nerve roots or spinal cord by the needle or catheter;
- erroneous injection of incorrect and toxic solutions; e.g. ether, potassium;
- sepsis, with abscess formation;
- haematoma formation;
- VIth nerve palsy causing diplopia and resulting from a low CSF pressure as a result of dural puncture, usually with a large needle;
- introduction of foreign particulate material with resultant granuloma formation; or
- spinal artery thrombosis and spinal cord infarction, which results in permanent damage; the anterior spinal artery is most often affected. Conditions favouring this complication are the presence of arteriosclerosis, hypotension and adrenaline containing solutions.

A rapid diagnosis and treatment are essential in these cases in order to prevent damage.

CAUDAL EPIDURAL ANAESTHESIA

This involves passage of a needle, with or without a catheter, through the sacrococcygeal membrane into the caudal epidural space. It is extremely useful in children to provide intraoperative analgesia for procedures on the groin and penis. In adults it may also be used for similar procedures and for operations on the perineum.

The sacral hiatus is usually identified with the patient in the left lateral position. Strict attention must be paid to asepsis. The sacral cornu can be palpated as two tubercles above the coccyx; the hiatus forms the apex of an equilateral triangle, the base being a line joining the two posterior superior iliac spines. A short 20 or 22 G needle is then introduced through the sacrococcygeal membrane at an angle of 45°, when a distinct 'give' should be appreciated. The needle should then be directed more cranially at angle of approximately 20° and moved along the axis of the sacral canal for a short distance. Correct placement can be confirmed by injecting a small volume of air, which can be felt as crepitations over the sacrum if it is placed subcutaneously. Listening over the lower lumbar region with a stethoscope reveals a 'whoosh' if the needle is in the caudal canal. It is also possible to inadvertently place the needle in front of the sacrum or even in the rectum.

Following negative aspiration for blood and CSF, the local anaesthetic is injected; there should be no resistance. In adults, 20–30 ml 0.25% bupivacaine will usually give a block to L1. Because of the variable volume that can escape from the large sacral foramina, it is difficult to estimate reliably the volume needed and the technique is not used very often in adults; also, the large dose of local anaesthetic required means that toxic reactions are an ever present possibility.

Caudal blocks are much more valuable and extensively used in children. Great care must be taken to avoid accidental intravenous and intrathecal injection. In children under 30 kg, the dose of 0.25% plain bupivacaine is 0.5–1.0 ml kg^{-1}, the smaller volume being used for circumcisions and the larger for groin procedures. The total dose of bupivacaine should not exceed 2 mg kg^{-1}.

SPINAL ANAESTHESIA

The basic anatomy of spinal anaesthesia is as for epidurals. The resultant physiological effects are also the same, but appear faster with spinal anaesthesia, although there is no contribution to the cardiovascular effects from absorbed local anaesthetic due to the very small doses used. Spinal blockade also tends to be more dense than epidural and uneven blocks are much rarer. The main difference between the techniques results from the fact that for spinal anaesthesia, the local anaesthetic solution is injected into another fluid, the CSF.

EQUIPMENT

Spinal needles (Figure 29.6) are now designed to make as small a hole as possible in the dura in order to reduce to a minimum the incidence of post-dural puncture headache (PDPH). Inevitably there must be a balance between the size of the needle and the technical feasibility of introducing it into the CSF. Needles as small as 30 and 32 G have been used, but have been abandoned because of technical problems.

Recent needle design has concentrated on the tip of the needle and position of the distal orifice and a number are shown in Figure 29.6. Quincke type needles have a sharp tip, with an end orifice which cuts the dural

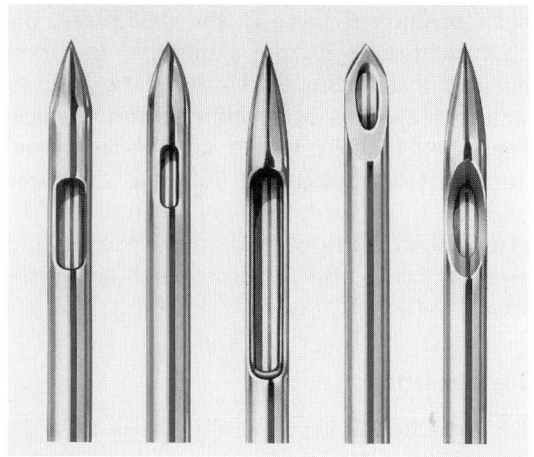

Figure 29.6 A selection of spinal needles. The two on the left are Whitacre needles while the one on the right is another example of a pencil point needle. The fourth from the left is a Quincke needle. In the centre is a Sprotte needle and note the length of the side aperture which might straddle the dura.

fibres. Use of fine needles (27–30 G) of this type do reduce the incidence of PDPH compared to 24 G needles, but are difficult to use. Whitacre and Sprotte needles have pencil points which part dural fibres rather than cutting them, so that the fibres close on removal of the needle. Numerous studies have shown a much lower incidence of PDPH with this type of needle. They are easier to use as the design allows a larger needle. The distal orifice is in the side of the needle about 2 mm from the tip. As this side orifice may be quite long, it is possible for it to straddle the dura so that some local anaesthetic is injected into the CSF and some into the epidural space. This might result in partial failure of a spinal block.

Spinal anaesthesia may be performed with the patient sitting or lying. The needle should be introduced in the mid-line in the L2/3 or L3/4 interspace (L4/5 being more difficult). If possible injection above this level should be avoided because of the danger of trauma to the spinal cord. As the needle is much finer than an epidural one, it is more difficult to 'feel' the layers, but a distinct 'click' is usually felt as the needle penetrates the dura. CSF will then emerge from the needle, but this may take some time when these are very fine. This can be aided by gentle suction with a syringe.

SPREAD OF SOLUTION

As spinal anaesthesia involves injection of one liquid into another, account must be taken of the baricity of the local anaesthetic compared to CSF and the subsequent posture of the patient.

Baricity

The specific gravity of CSF at 37°C is about 1.006. A local anaesthetic with the same specific gravity is isobaric with CSF, while if it is lower it is hypobaric. Thus, after injection a hypobaric solution will tend to rise and this can be aided by suitable posturing of the patient. However, hypobaric solutions have a reputation for relatively unpredictable spread in the CSF with a patchy block.

Solutions which are more dense than CSF will move downwards under the effect of gravity after injection and are known as hyperbaric. Local anaesthetics are rendered hyperbaric by addition of 8% dextrose and these are the most commonly used; e.g. 0.5% or 0.75% bupivacaine in 8% dextrose; 5% lignocaine in 8% dextrose. (Bupivacaine is by far the most commonly used in the UK). These hyperbaric solutions are much more controllable than hypobaric and isobaric.

Posture

Spread of solution depends largely on the use of posture after injection, the hyperbaric solution always following gravity. Thus low blocks (saddle block) can be obtained by injection in the sitting position and maintaining the patient sitting for at least 5 min. Unilateral blocks can be achieved by keeping the patient on the side after the injection. If the patient is kept horizontal after injection, the hyperbaric local anaesthetic follows the curves of the spine as described by Barker, but the block will only extend to the low thoracic region in a cephalad direction. Placing the patient head down, will result in a greater cephalad spread of the block.

Dose

The volume of hyperbaric solution injected should never exceed 3 ml. Increasing the concentration but maintaining the same volume has little effect on the spread of the block, but does increase the duration.

Barbotage

This is the technique of repeatedly injecting a small volume into the CSF and then aspirating and re-injecting. A greater spread is then obtained from a given volume, but the results are not predictable and the method is not recommended.

COMPLICATIONS OF SPINAL ANAESTHESIA

To all intents and purposes these are identical to epidural anaesthesia apart from the occurrence of PDPH. An incidence of transitory deafness to higher notes also occurs after spinal anaesthesia.

Post-dural-puncture headache

This headache is due to a low CSF pressure consequent upon leakage of CSF through the hole made in the dura. The incidence is directly related to the size of the needle used and is most common after inadvertent dural puncture with the large needles used for epidural anaesthesia. The headache can affect any part of the head, but is often occipital and frontal. It usually comes on very shortly after the event, but can be delayed for as long as three days. It can be severe and accompanied by photophobia, nausea, dizziness and occasionally diplopia. It has a marked postural component, becoming exacerbated on sitting or standing and relieved by lying down. The headache can be quite incapacitating, which is particularly undesirable in nursing mothers. The diagnosis is usually obvious, but occasionally such headaches have masked the presentation of much more serious pathology, e.g. intracranial tumours.

A large number of symptomatic treatments have been reported in the literature. The headache is due to low intracranial pressure consequent upon CSF leakage. Simple analgesics should never be withheld and lying down frequently relieves the worse symptoms. Some treatment aims at increasing CSF production with synthetic ACTH, while hydration with increased oral intake, or intravenously, is encouraged. Caffeine has been used as it is thought to produce cerebral vasoconstriction and is occasionally helpful. Infusion of saline into the epidural space has been claimed to help by decreasing the CSF leak. An abdominal binder is recommended by some. Although each of the various treatments has its advocates, none have been particularly successful.

By far the most effective method of treating PDPH is with an epidural blood patch. Up to 20 ml of autologous blood is injected into the epidural space under strict aseptic conditions, absence of any infection having been confirmed. The resultant clot seals the tear in the dura. The relief produced is remarkable and the patient can usually mobilize within 2 h; a repeat blood patch is occasionally necessary. Side effects of blood patching are backache and rigors, which are usually transient. Performing a blood patch usually has no effect on subsequent epidural anaesthesia, although occasionally limited and patchy blocks have been reported.

CONTINUOUS SPINAL ANAESTHESIA

This was originally done by passing a catheter into the subarachnoid space through a 15 G needle. The incidence of PDPH was around 30% and the technique was abandoned. More recently very fine 32 G microcatheters have been used, with a marked reduction in the frequency of PDPH. However, reports appeared of permanent nerve damage using these catheters and they were withdrawn. It is unlikely that the catheters were the cause of these problems, but rather the prolonged exposure of the cauda equina to high concentrations of local anaesthetic (usually 5% lignocaine) and dextrose. The technique has never found favour in the UK.

COMBINED SPINAL–EPIDURAL ANAESTHESIA

This technique was largely developed for use in Caesarean section. The epidural space is located in the usual way with a Tuohy needle. A spinal needle (nowadays usually a pencil point) is passed through the Tuohy needle into the subarachnoid space and the local anaesthetic injected into the CSF. The spinal needle is then withdrawn and a catheter inserted into the epidural space in the normal way. The technique has the advantage of a quick onset, dense spinal block combined with the option of extending the block via the epidural catheter, which can also be used for postoperative pain relief.

DIFFERENCES BETWEEN SPINAL AND EPIDURAL ANAESTHESIA

Although these techniques are largely similar, there are a number of differences:

- spinal blockade is more rapid in onset and can also be performed more rapidly;
- it is more difficult to control the height of a spinal block;
- hypotension can develop more rapidly in

spinal anaesthesia and too high a block can produce respiratory embarrassment;
- spinal block is denser and missed segments and unilateral blocks much rarer;
- PDPH is a feature of spinal anaesthesia; and
- because of the dose of local anaesthetics used, systemic toxicity is always a problem during epidural anaesthesia, but never during spinal.

CARE OF PATIENTS DURING SPINAL AND EPIDURAL ANAESTHESIA

The basic principles of care apply to patients undergoing surgery under epidural or spinal anaesthesia as with general anaesthesia. A fully equipped anaesthetic machine and resuscitation equipment must be present.

The principles of care are as follows.

- The patient should be prepared as for general anaesthesia, including fasting. No regional anaesthetic technique will ever be 100% successful for 100% patients and when failure does occur, the only recourse is to general anaesthesia.
- Informed consent must be obtained from the patient for the regional technique, even though it might be the intention to perform the block under general anaesthesia.
- The anaesthetist must remain with the patient throughout the entire operation, hand the patient over to the recovery room staff with instructions as to further care and must not leave the patient until they are satisfied with his/her condition.
- An intravenous infusion must be set up before commencing the block and a vasopressor of the anaesthetist's choice and atropine must be drawn-up ready for immediate use.
- It is always safer to perform spinal and epidural anaesthesia with the patient awake. Some patients will not tolerate this and some form of sedation will be necessary. Under these circumstances, the patient must be monitored by a properly trained person during performance of the block. Debate continues over the safety of doing the block in a fully anaesthetized patient, which is a common practice in the UK. Although theoretically this is not ideal, adverse reports have not been forthcoming.
- The procedure must be performed under full aseptic conditions, with the operator gowned, gloved and wearing a face mask and hat.
- During surgery, most patients will require some form of sedation or general anaesthesia. If sedated, great care should be taken to ensure a patent airway.
- Monitoring should be as for general anaesthesia.
- Blood pressure must be taken at regular intervals. Some degree of hypotension is an invariable accompaniment of spinal and epidural anaesthesia and it is up to the anaesthetist to decide the lowest level to be accepted. The best and most efficient treatment of hypotension is with a vasoconstrictor, either by intermittent injection or by infusion. However, the circulatory volume must be maintained at all times and fluid loading prior to the block is common place, although its effectiveness dubious. Vasopressors can be used prophylactically if necessary. Awake patients will often indicate significant hypotension by yawning or restlessness.
- Awake or sedated patients should be given oxygen via a facemask or nasal spectacles.

The importance of monitoring cannot be overemphasized and, for whatever reason, it must be stressed that cardiac arrests occur more frequently under spinal and epidural anaeshesia than under general anaesthesia.

FURTHER READING

Bromage, P. R. (1978) *Epidural Anaesthesia*. Saunders, Philadelphia.
Bonica, J. J., Kennedy, W. F., Akamatsu, T. J. and Gerbershagen, H. U. (1972) Circulatory effects of

peridural block: effects of acute blood loss. *Anesthesiology*, **36**, 219–227.

Liu, S., Carpenter, R. L. and Neal, J. M. (1995) Epidural anesthesia and analgesia: their role in postoperative outcome. *Anesthesiology*, **82**, 1474–1506.

Reynolds, F. (1993) Dural puncture and headache. *British Medical Journal*, **306**, 874–875.

Van Aken, H. (1993) New developments in epidural and spinal drugs administration. *Baillières Clinical Anaesthesiology*. Volume 7. Baillière Tindall, London.

PERIPHERAL NERVE BLOCKS 30

S. M. Geddes

GENERAL CONSIDERATIONS

THE PREOPERATIVE VISIT

The preoperative visit provides the opportunity for the anaesthetist to discuss the proposed anaesthetic technique with the patient. When a local anaesthetic technique is to be used, there are some special points to consider.

The anaesthetist must have a thorough understanding of the intended surgical procedure, in particular the innervation of the superficial and deep structures involved, the requirement for muscle relaxation, the likely duration of surgery and the potential for resort to a more extensive procedure. Consideration must be given as to whether surgery can be performed under a block alone or if sedation or general anaesthesia will also be required. If the duration of surgery might exceed that of the block, the anaesthetist should consider placing a catheter or the practicalities of repeating the block during the procedure.

The attitude of the patient to a local anaesthetic technique is extremely important. Most patients in the UK expect to be 'asleep' during surgery and, despite a calm and confident explanation, the prospect of being awake or only 'drowsy' during the performance of the block and the subsequent surgery is often met with misgiving. Unless a general anaesthetic will incur a substantial additional risk, there is nothing to be gained by coercing an unwilling patient to accept a local anaesthetic technique. It is also important to reassure the patient who prefers general anaesthesia that he has not rejected a technique which is overwhelmingly 'better' or 'safer'. In many cases the block can be performed, (with consent), under a general anaesthetic; however, it should be remembered that the unconscious patient can report neither pain on injection (indicating intraneural injection) nor the symptoms of systemic toxicity.

If the block is to be performed with the patient fully conscious or lightly sedated, it is essential to describe the phenomenon of paraesthesia or the sensations resulting from electrical peripheral nerve stimulation. If only light sedation is to be provided during surgery, the difference between anaesthesia and analgesia must also be explained. The patient should be warned when the block will persist into the postoperative period and when motor block will accompany the loss of sensation. Finally, the patient must be reassured that should the block prove inadequate, an alternative technique will be provided immediately.

CONTRAINDICATIONS TO A LOCAL ANAESTHETIC BLOCK

Apart from patient refusal and allergy to local anaesthetic agents there are two major contraindications.

Short Practice of Anaesthesia. Edited by M. Morgan and G. M. Hall. Published in 1997 by Chapman & Hall, London. ISBN 0 412 71890 1

There may be local soft tissue sepsis. Inserting a needle through such an area may introduce infection into previously healthy tissues and should be avoided. In addition, absorption from the inflamed tissues will be rapid and toxicity may ensue even when 'safe' doses are injected.

Second is the more difficult issue of coagulopathy. There is general agreement that when the patient has a major coagulopathy (therapeutic or pathological), local anaesthetic techniques should be avoided. The risks of central (spinal, epidural) block in patients receiving 'low-dose' subcutaneous heparin or aspirin have been widely debated and despite reports of large series of uncomplicated central block in patients receiving these drugs, this remains a controversial area. There is even less information about the incidence and consequences of haematomata after peripheral nerve block in patients receiving these drugs. However, there is a growing body of opinion that the risks in this second group have been overestimated, thus they should not routinely be denied the benefit of a peripheral nerve block. Anaesthetists should consider their experience with the proposed block, the anticipated ease of performing the block, whether pressure can be applied to any traumatized vessels and the potential benefits to the patient before recommending the technique. The block should be performed at a time when tissue heparin levels are low. This may mean manipulating the order of the operating list or the heparin regimen.

THE PEROPERATIVE PHASE

Environment

Monitoring and resuscitation equipment should be provided exactly as for general anaesthesia. An intravenous cannula is always placed before performing a block.

Asepsis

There is no reason not to use an aseptic technique. The skin should be cleaned with a chlorhexidine solution, which is then allowed to dry. Sterile gloves should be worn on all occasions and a gown and mask should be worn when a catheter is to be placed.

Drugs and doses

Recommended doses of the local anaesthetic drugs for peripheral nerve block are shown in Table 30.1. They are for an average patient having an unspecified block. Plasma and tissue concentrations following injection of local anaesthetic depend on many factors including absorption from the site of injection, distribution into the various tissue compartments and metabolism of the drug. For example, absorption is notably extensive following intercostal, brachial plexus and sciatic

Table 30.1 Maximal recommended doses of the local anaesthetic agents commonly available in the UK

Drug	Maximal recommended dose for peripheral nerve block	
	Plain solution	With adrenaline 1:200,000
Bupivacaine	2 mg kg^{-1} in any 4 h period	As for plain solution
Lignocaine	3 mg kg^{-1}	5 mg kg^{-1}
Prilocaine	5 mg kg^{-1}	

Table 30.2 Clinical features of local anaesthetic drugs

Drug	Equipotent concentration (%)	Relative duration of action
Bupivacaine	0.25	2–4
Lignocaine	1	1
Prilocaine	1	1–1.5

nerve blocks. It follows that the recommendations are not a licence to inject the 'maximum' dose with impunity. Conversely, in certain situations, they might be regarded as conservative.

In the descriptions of the blocks which follow, the volume and concentration of bupivacaine suitable for a healthy adult of average build are suggested. Judgement is required when applying these. As a general rule, bupivacaine 0.25% is suitable for minor nerve block, while 0.375%–0.5% is required for major trunks. Addition of adrenaline 1:200 000 is particularly recommended when moderate to large doses are injected into vascular areas. Solutions of lignocaine or prilocaine may be substituted and the equivalent potencies are in Table 30.2.

The latency, intensity and duration of a block depend on the accuracy of placement of solution, the diameter of the nerve to be blocked, the concentration and volume of the solution and the physicochemical properties of the drug, which are reflected in its clinical profile (Table 30.2). The relationship between these factors is complex, but as a general rule, latency is reduced and duration increased by increasing dose. Increasing volume (dose constant) improves the chance of successful block more than increasing concentration (dose constant).

Infusion techniques have been used to prolong brachial plexus block, paravertebral, intrapleural and intercostal block, psoas compartment block and block of the femoral and sciatic nerves. A wide variety of infusion regimens have been described, but, apart from brachial plexus anaesthesia, the doses are not so well established as for single shot techniques and so no recommendations are made. Repeated assessment and adjustment of infusion rate will be required.

Toxicity

There are two main mechanisms of systemic toxicity. The risk of intravascular injection is minimized by repeated aspiration during performance of the block. The conscious patient should be questioned about the early symptoms of central nervous system toxicity (tinnitus, dysphoria, circumoral or lingual dysaesthesia) while the block is performed. Major toxicity will present as excitatory symptoms such as muscle twitching or tremor and may progress to generalised seizure activity with secondary cardiovascular complications. Primary cardiovascular toxicity occurs at higher plasma concentrations and includes depression of contractility arrythmias and cardiac arrest. Toxicity due to absorption of a relative overdose from the perineural tissues may be more difficult to diagnose as the likely time of this complication is difficult to predict.

Vasoconstrictors

Addition of adrenaline to a local anaesthetic solution produces local vasoconstriction and decreases the peak plasma concentration, thus reducing the potential for toxicity. The duration of block will also be increased. Adrenaline should never be used when performing nerve blocks of the fingers, toes or penis. It should be used with caution in patients with cardiac disease, and the potential for interaction with sympathomimetic drugs should be remembered.

Locating the nerve

The traditional method is to seek paraesthesia. However, this implies that the nerve has at least been contacted by the needle and thus there is the potential for direct trauma or secondary damage resulting from oedema or haematoma formation. Despite this, there is no clear evidence that nerve damage commonly results from this technique, although neither is it vindicated.

Although no substitute for thorough knowledge of the anatomy, correct use of a peripheral nerve stimulator will increase the incidence of successful block in anaesthetized patients and it is also helpful in conscious or sedated patients. The needle is inserted deep to the skin and the output of the unit set to a level known to be adequate for nerve stimulation (usually 1 mA) before slowly advancing the needle. Having approximately located the nerve and elicited a response, the output of the unit is reduced stepwise to 0.5 mA or less and the change in response is used as a guide to redirect the tip of the needle so as to produce the strongest response at the lowest output. There is no evidence that the use of nerve stimulator reduces the risk of nerve damage.

Whichever technique is used, it is essential to be gentle and orientate the needle so that the bevel will part rather than transect fibres should the nerve fascicle be entered.

In the description of individual blocks, where it is recommended that paraesthesia is sought, it may be assumed that the use of a nerve stimulator is a suitable alternative technique.

Needles, cannulae and catheters

Disposable 22 G short-bevelled needles are suitable for most of the major nerve blocks described in this chapter. The short bevel produces a distinctive 'feel' as the needle passes through the tissues. This is best appreciated if the needle is held like a dart and is advanced with fine repeated 'bouncing' movements. The use of an 'immobile needle', where the syringe is connected to the needle via a primed extension set has the advantage that the needle is more easily manipulated and positioned if not directly attached to a syringe and that an assistant can perform aspiration, injection and change the syringe while the anaesthetist maintains the correct position of the needle. Insulated needles, where the current emanates only from the needle tip, are available for use with a peripheral nerve stimulator.

A catheter or Teflon cannula may be inserted so that repeated boluses or an infusion may used to prolong the block. When correct placement of the solution depends on localization of a fascial compartment, rather than an individual nerve, a standard 18 G Tuohy needle and epidural catheter may be used.

POSTOPERATIVE CARE

The anaesthetized, paralysed parts must be protected from injury until the block has regressed. When an infusion is used to extend the block, the anaesthetist must ensure that the nursing staff are competent in assessing the extent of the block and detecting the symptoms of local anaesthetic toxicity.

NERVE BLOCKS OF THE UPPER LIMB

These fall into three categories: the various techniques of brachial plexus anaesthesia, the peripheral nerve blocks which may be used to supplement a deficient plexus block or in combination as a sole technique for minor procedures and intravenous regional anaesthesia (IVRA).

BRACHIAL PLEXUS ANAESTHESIA

Formation of the brachial plexus

The brachial plexus provides the motor innervation and almost all of the sensory innervation of the upper limb (Figure 30.1). The anterior primary rami of C5–8 and T1 become the roots of the plexus as they emerge from the intervertebral foramina and there are also variable contributions to the plexus from the anterior rami of C4 and T2. Between scalenus anterior and medius, the roots combine to form the superior (upper C5, 6) middle (C7) and inferior (lower C8, T1) trunks which lie in a vertical plane and converge as they run caudally and laterally to cross the first rib beneath the clavicle. At the lateral border of the rib each trunk divides into anterior and posterior divisions. These form the lateral,

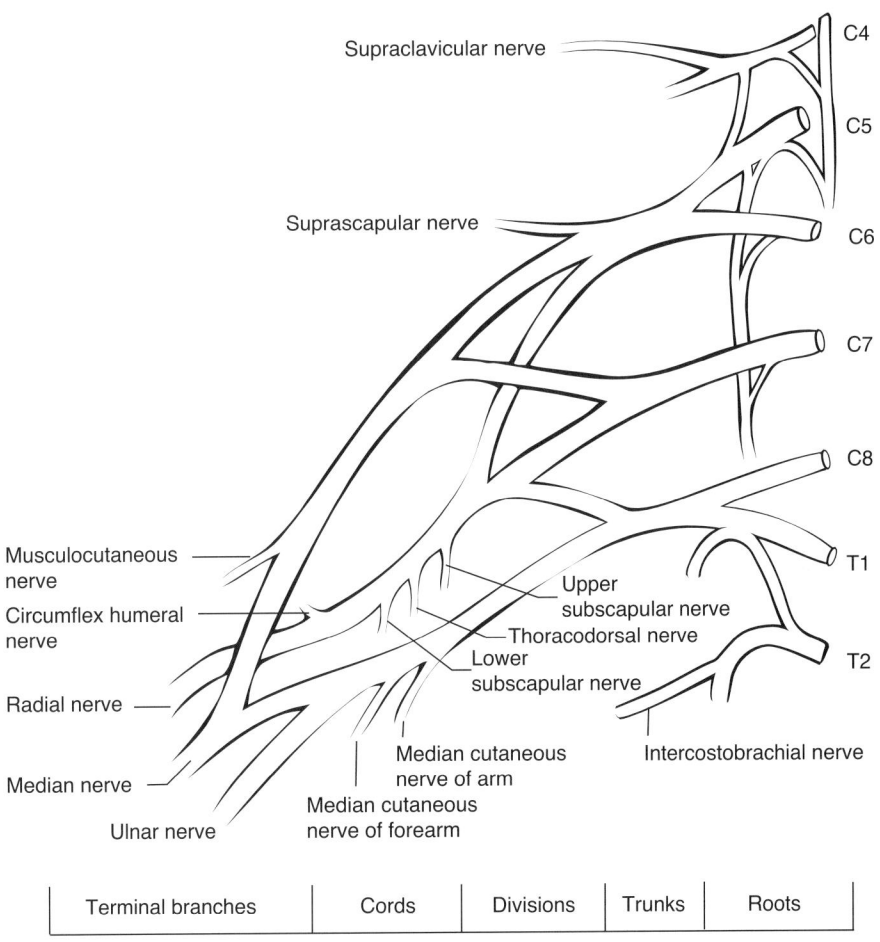

Figure 30.1 The brachial plexus. (Redrawn with permission from *Principles and Practice of Regional Anaesthesia* (eds J.A. Wildsmith, E.N. Armitage), Churchill Livingstone, Edinburgh, 1993.)

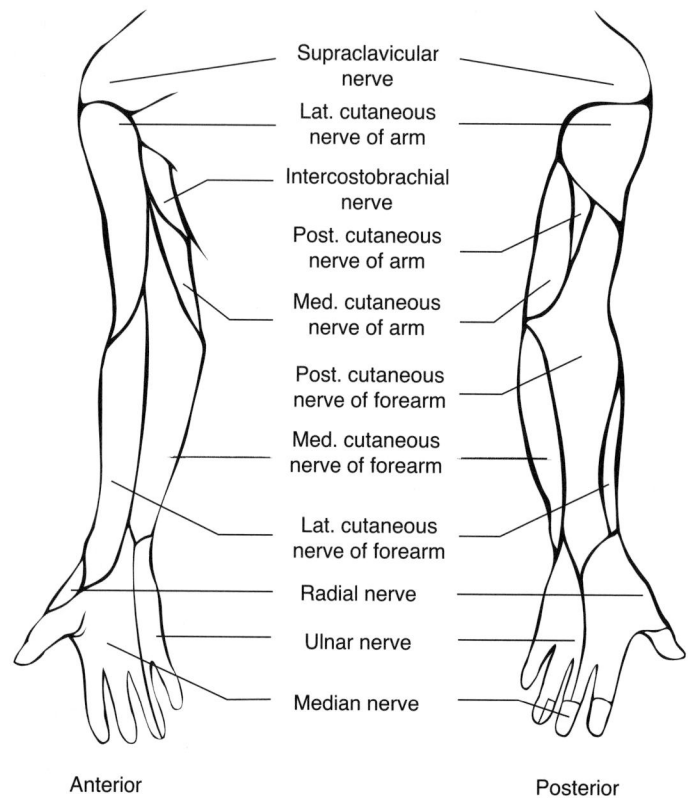

Figure 30.2 Distribution of cutaneous nerves arising from the brachial plexus.

medial and posterior cords which take up their named positions relative to the second part of the axillary artery.

Branches arise from the roots, trunks and cords. The distribution of the cutaneous nerves is shown in Figure 30.2. The terminal branches of the cords form the main nerves of the limb as they run with the axillary artery behind the lateral border of pectoralis minor. The posterior cord continues as the radial nerve, the ulnar nerve is the continuation of the medial cord and the large median nerve is formed from branches of the medial and lateral cords.

Detailed anatomy is given in the description of each technique, but there are two important general considerations. The first is proximity of the plexus, especially in the neck, to a number of important neural, vascular and other structures (most importantly the dome of the pleura); thus there is a substantial risk of unwanted conduction blockade, intravascular injection or pneumothorax when performing brachial plexus block.

The second is the fascial sheath which encloses the plexus throughout its course in the neck and axilla. Proximally, this compartment is continuous with the prevertebral fascia where it splits to envelope scalenus anterior and medius before fusing at their lateral margins. The subclavian vessels join the trunks of the plexus within the sheath in the root of the neck and the sheath continues around the neurovascular bundle to the distal limit of the axilla. Local anaesthetic solution deposited within this fascial compartment is contained in close proximity to the plexus thus maximizing the chance of a successful block. Compression of the sheath at its extremities prevents loss of local anaesthetic solution and may enhance spread within the sheath.

Brachial plexus block

The brachial plexus is accessible at many points in its course in the neck and axilla (Figure 30.3). Three popular techniques are described below. These differ not only in the likely distribution of the block, but also in the spectrum and risk of complications.

The intercostobrachial nerve (T2) runs from the thoracic wall, across the floor of the axilla and supplies the skin of the axilla and the medial aspect of the upper arm. A supplementary block of this nerve is required when a tourniquet is to be used in a conscious or sedated patient; 5–10 ml of solution are injected subcutaneously across the medial aspect of the arm at the lower border of the axilla.

Drugs and doses

In healthy adults of average build, injection of 30–35 ml bupivacaine 0.375–0.5% with adrenaline 1:200 000 will produce an adequate block via the subclavian perivascular approach, while 40–50 ml solution is required for axillary or interscalene block and thus the concentration of the solution may need to be

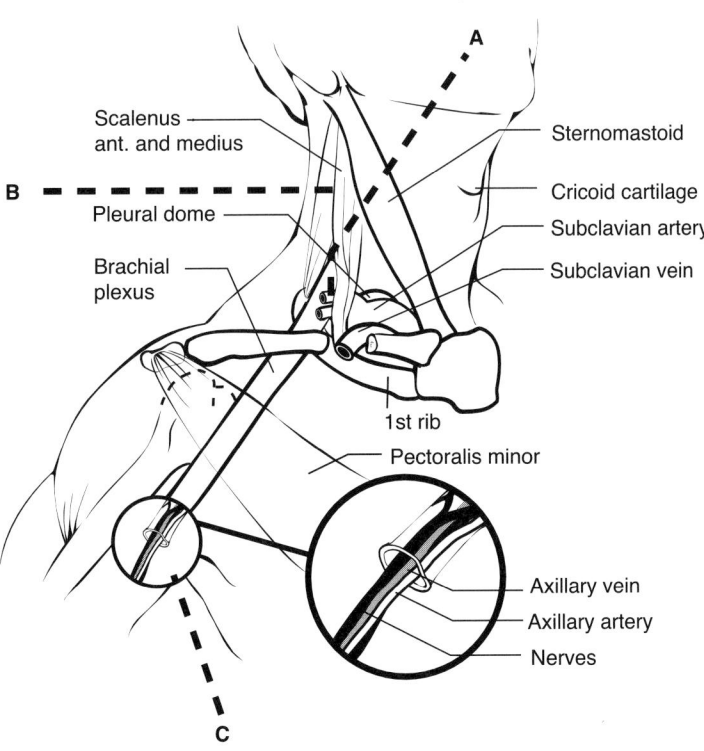

Figure 30.3 Injection points for brachial plexus block: (**A**), subclavian perivascular approach, (**B**), interscalene approach, (**C**), axillary approach.

reduced. It is important to retain some of the 'dosage allowance' so that supplementary peripheral nerve blocks may be performed if required.

Subclavian perivascular block

This is the most popular of the techniques which have been devised in order to retain the benefits of the extensive block resulting from introduction of local anaesthetic into the perineural sheath where the trunks lie close together, whilst minimizing the risk of pneumothorax. The arm and the radial aspects of the forearm and the hand, are reliably blocked (approximately 90% success). The inferior trunk (C8, T1) and thus the medial aspect of the arm and forearm are less reliably blocked (75–80%). Despite the relatively low risk of pneumothorax, this technique should not be used in day-case patients or those with severe respiratory disease.

Anatomy

As the trunks of the plexus approach the clavicle they are arranged in a vertical plane. They pass under the clavicle between the insertions of scalenus anterior and medius on the first rib. Here, the subclavian artery is anterior to the inferior trunk of the plexus and is within the fascial sheath. The dome of the pleura is immediately inferomedial to the plexus and lies against the inner margin of the rib.

Technique

The patient lies supine with his arm by his side and his head turned slightly away from the side to be blocked. A finger placed immediately lateral to the lateral border of sternocleidomastoid in the middle third of the neck lies on scalenus anterior. The finger is then rolled laterally into the interscalene groove. Scalenus anterior is tensed and thus the groove more easily located if the patient sustains a maximal inspiration. The groove is followed downwards until the pulsation of the subclavian artery is felt. In the event of difficulty, the patient is asked to turn his head towards the side to be blocked. This relaxes the tissues and allows the finger better access to the thoracic inlet. After the artery has been located the patient readopts the position described above. The needle is inserted immediately cephalad to the finger palpating the artery and is advanced directly caudally between the scalene muscles. A 'give' may be felt as the sheath is pierced. If the first rib is contacted before paraesthesiae in the hand or arm are elicited, the needle should be carefully redirected and walked along the line of the first rib. It should not be redirected posteromedially. If the subclavian artery is punctured the needle should be withdrawn and redirected posterolaterally.

Complications

Despite the fact that the angle of insertion of needle insertion is tangential to the pleura, the risk of pneumothorax remains. Proximal spread of the local anaesthetic solution may result in block of the stellate ganglion (resulting in Horner's syndrome), the recurrent laryngeal nerve (hoarseness) or the phrenic nerve. Unilateral phrenic nerve block is unlikely to cause serious respiratory embarrassment in the normal patient.

Interscalene block

This technique provides reliable block of the nerves arising from roots C5–C7 (90% success) and is the technique of choice for surgery to the shoulder, clavicle or upper arm. The medial border of the hand, forearm and arm and the deep structures innervated by the nerves arising from the inferior trunk will be less reliably blocked (40–60% success).

Anatomy

The roots and proximal sections of the trunks of the plexus run in the interscalene space above the dome of the pleura. Close relations are the vertebral artery and the dura (and thus the contents of the cervical spinal canal), the stellate ganglion and the phrenic and recurrent laryngeal nerves.

Technique

The interscalene groove is located as described above. The injection point is where the groove is crossed by a line drawn parallel to the clavicle from the cricoid cartilage, i.e. the level of the sixth cervical vertebra. The needle is inserted at 90° to the skin in all planes, i.e. medially, dorsally and caudally. This last is most important as it minimizes the risk of the needle passing between adjacent transverse processes and puncturing the vertebral artery or dura. Paraesthesia in the arm or forearm is sought at a depth of 2–3 cm. Paraesthesia in the shoulder is caused by stimulation of the supraclavicular nerve which lies outside the sheath. During injection the neck is compressed above the injection point to occlude the communication with the fascial space surrounding the cervical plexus thus favouring caudal spread although, despite this, cervical plexus block may occur.

Complications

The most serious potential complication is injection of local anaesthetic into the vertebral artery. The drug is carried directly to the cerebrum and a severe toxic reaction will occur following injection of only small doses. Similarly, local anaesthetic injected into the cervical epidural or subarachnoid space may cause bilateral phrenic nerve block or may spread cephalad to the brain stem. As with the subclavian perivascular approach, block of the stellate ganglion or the recurrent laryngeal or phrenic nerves may occur. Although the risk of pneumothorax is theoretically avoided, this has been reported and the possibility should be borne in mind.

Axillary block

This technique reliably blocks the medial aspects of the arm and forearm and of the median and ulnar distributions in the hand (90% success). Blocks of the musculocutaneous, circumflex and radial nerves are less certain (50–60%). The technique should be used where the supraclavicular landmarks cannot be easily palpated (e.g. the obese), patients in whom a pneumothorax or the other complications of supraclavicular block would be particularly serious and patients undergoing day-care surgery.

Technique

The patient lies supine with the arm externally rotated and abducted to 70–80° with the elbow flexed. The pulsation of the axillary artery is sought and traced as high in the axilla as possible. It may be easier to locate the pulse in the axilla with the arm in a lesser degree of abduction; the limb can then be repositioned before performing the block. The injection is made immediately above i.e. in a coronal plane anterior to, a finger placed on the artery. The needle is inserted at an angle of 20° to the skin, directed cephalad and parallel to the long axis of the arm. A distinct 'give' is often felt as the needle penetrates the sheath. During injection, compression is applied over the sheath distal to the injection point to enhance proximal spread.

Complications

The only common complication is inadvertent vascular puncture which should be detected by careful repeated aspiration.

Because of the low potential for complications with axillary block of the brachial plexus, there has been extensive investigation of measures which might increase the success rate of block of the posterolateral aspect of the limb. There are two problems: the musculocutaneous and circumflex nerves originate from the lateral cord high in the axilla (inadequate proximal spread) and the radial nerve may be inadequately blocked because it lies deep to the axillary artery (inadequate circumferential spread).

Measures to enhance proximal spread include digital compression of the sheath distal to the needle and having the arm in adduction during injection (thus a cannula rather than a needle must be used) so that the head of the humerus does not compress the sheath. Increasing the volume of injectate will enhance proximal spread but this approach is limited by the safe dose of local anaesthetic and other requirements of the block such as onset and intensity. Circumferential spread may be limited by the incomplete longitudinal septa which run within the axillary section of the sheath. A transarterial technique, where the axillary artery is deliberately punctured and solution deposited in the deep part of the sheath before withdrawal of the needle and injection superficial to the artery has theoretical advantages but is not reliably superior to the perivascular approach. Finally, axillary and interscalene blocks may be combined in order to provide satisfactory anaesthesia of the entire limb.

Continuous brachial plexus block

A cannula or catheter may be placed using any of the techniques described above, thus allowing the block to be extended by repeated injections or a continuous infusion. There is limited information about 'safe' regimens for continuous brachial plexus anaesthesia although infusion of 0.25 mg kg^{-1} h^{-1} of a solution of 0.25% bupicavine has been used without exceeding the currently accepted toxic plasma levels.

NERVE BLOCKS AT THE ELBOW AND WRIST

These maybe used to supplement brachial plexus anaesthesia or for minor surgery to the distal part of the limb. Bupivacaine 0.25% with adrenaline 1:200 000 is a suitable solution.

Lateral cutaneous nerve of the forearm

This is the terminal sensory branch of the musculocutaneous nerve. It perforates the deep fascia and enters the anterior compartment 1–2 cm proximal to the elbow joint and lateral to the biceps tendon, which separates it from the brachial artery. This block is often required as a supplement to axillary brachial plexus block.

Technique

The elbow is flexed 90° and the needle is inserted immediately lateral to the tendon of biceps, 1 cm proximal to the elbow joint and at right angles to the skin until the lateral condyle of the humerus is contacted. The needle is withdrawn 0.5 cm and 2 ml solution injected. The needle is then further withdrawn and redirected proximally. The process is repeated 3 or 4 times until the tip of the needle is 3 cm proximal to the point of its initial contact with bone.

Ulnar nerve

Two injections are required. The mixed palmar branch is blocked by an injection at the level of the styloid process of the ulna (Figure 30.4). The needle is introduced at right angles to the long axis of the forearm from the

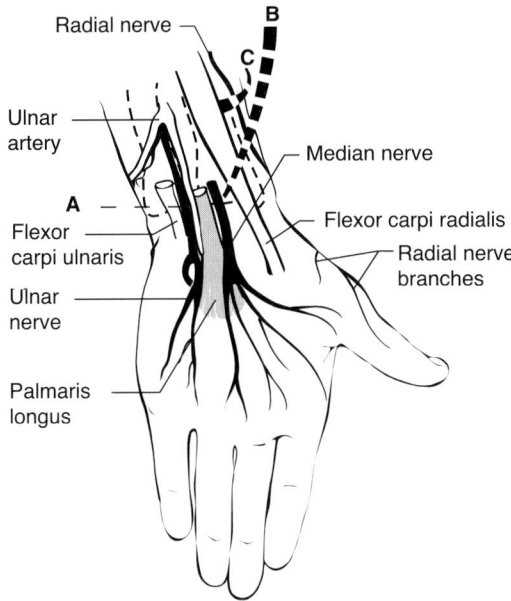

Figure 30.4 Nerve blocks at the wrist: (**A**), ulnar nerve, (**B**), median nerve, (**C**), radial nerve.

medial aspect of the wrist underneath the tendon of flexor carpi ulnaris. The nerve lies under the lateral border of the tendon and the ulnar artery is an immediate lateral relation. If paraesthesia is elicited 3 ml of solution is injected; if not 5 ml is injected. The dorsal branch is entirely sensory and is blocked by a subcutaneous track of solution deposited around the ulnar aspect of the wrist 2–3 cm proximal to the styloid process.

Median nerve

The median nerve lies immediately below or slightly lateral to the deep surface of the tendon of palmaris longus at the level of the proximal skin crease of the wrist (Figure 30.4). If palmaris longus is absent, the nerve is found in the mid-line of the wrist, medial to the tendon of flexor carpi radialis. The tendons will be more easily palpated if the wrist is flexed against resistance. The needle is inserted at right angles to the skin and paraesthesia is sought using small fanwise movements. 3 ml of solution is injected where paraesthesia is obtained. A 2 cm subcutaneous track of solution is then injected across the course of the nerve at the same level; this is to block the palmar branch of the median nerve which arises in the forearm.

Radial nerve

The radial nerve passes under the tendon of brachioradialis approximately 8 cm proximal to the wrist and runs subcutaneously on the dorsal surface of the forearm before dividing into its terminal sensory branches which supply the dorsum of the hand (Figure 30.4). A track of 5 ml of solution injected around the radial and dorsal aspects of the wrist will block these.

Digital nerve block

Solutions containing a vasoconstrictor should never be used for this block because of the real risk of severe ischaemia or gangrene.

Each finger has two palmar and two dorsal digital nerves. The needle is inserted on the dorsal aspect of the finger at the base of the proximal phalanx and directed towards the palmar surface. The needle is advanced until the point is just deep to the palmar skin and 0.5 ml solution is injected. It is then withdrawn until the point of the needle is just to the dorsal surface where a further 0.5 ml is injected. The process is repeated on the other side of the finger.

INTRAVENOUS REGIONAL ANAESTHESIA

This technique produces reliable, rapid-onset anaesthesia and muscle relaxation of the forearm and hand. However, it breaks the golden rule that local anaesthetic agents should not be injected into the circulation and thus there is the potential for serious complications resulting from systemic toxicity. Thorough understanding of the technique and meticulous attention to detail are required to ensure that these do not occur. Only clinicians who can recognize the symptoms of local anaesthetic toxicity and are competent in the management of circulatory collapse and convulsions should perform IVRA. When choosing to use this technique, the discomfort produced by the arterial tourniquet should not be underestimated. Prilocaine is the drug of choice because it is sequestered in the pulmonary tissue to a greater extent than any other local anaesthetic agent, thus the concentration of local anaesthetic in the blood perfusing the heart and brain is considerably lower than that in the pulmonary artery.

Technique

The patient's systemic arterial blood pressure is measured and noted. Two venous cannulae are inserted: in the hand of the arm to be blocked and in the opposite hand. A single-cuff orthopaedic tourniquet is applied to the arm to be blocked. The arm is elevated, exsanguinated and the cuff then inflated to apply a pressure of 100 mmHg above the systolic arterial pressure. The presence of an arterial pulse or venous congestion indicate that isolation of the limb is inadequate and the process should be repeated. The local anaesthetic solution (30–50 ml preservative-free 0.5% prilocaine) is injected slowly so as to minimize the risk that the intravenous pressure will exceed cuff occlusion pressure. Sensory and motor block develop within 15–20 min.

The clinician performing the block observes the patient for signs of systemic toxicity and monitors the cuff pressure during surgery. There is a risk that intravenous pressure may exceed cuff occlusion pressure during manipulation of the limb.

The drug will be fixed in the tissues at 20 min. Under no circumstances should the cuff be deflated before this. The cuff should be deflated step-wise and immediately re-inflated if signs of systemic toxicity are observed. Return of sensation is rapid following deflation.

The duration of the technique is limited by the patient's tolerance of tourniquet discomfort, at most 30 min in a stoical patient. A double cuff technique does not reliably reduce discomfort but introduces another potential source of error.

Complications

The risk of systemic toxicity is minimized by meticulous technique. This technique results in tissue ischaemia and is contraindicated in patients with sickle cell or peripheral vascular disease. It should also be avoided in patients with Paget's disease because of the potential for spread of solution via the venous channels within the bone.

NERVE BLOCKS OF THE THORAX AND ABDOMEN

Spinal and epidural anaesthesia are popular techniques which produce reliable, rapid-onset anaesthesia. However, a unilateral nerve block of the trunk may be the technique of choice when central neural blockade is contraindicated or technically difficult due to disease of the vertebral column and indeed may have other advantages.

The extent of a central block may be far greater than is required for surgery or postoperative analgesia and problems resulting from widespread sympathetic block, motor block and urinary retention may outweigh the benefits of the technique. With a unilateral technique the block can more easily be restricted to the relevant spinal segments and these problems can be avoided. These techniques are particularly suited for postoperative analgesia where a unilateral wound follows the line of a dermatome, e.g. a thoracotomy or a subcostal incision. However, the 'end point' is less well defined than for spinal or epidural analgesia and consequently the failure rate is higher. The spread of solution, and hence the extent of the block is less predictable and multiple injections are often required.

INNERVATION OF THE TRUNK: GENERAL PRINCIPLES AND EXCEPTIONS

The innervation of the skin and muscles of the trunk is by pairs of posterior and anterior rami of the spinal nerves arising from levels T2–L1. The nerves at the extremes of the range pursue somewhat different courses, but the typical anatomy is shown in Figure 30.5. The posterior rami arise immediately the spinal nerves emerge from the intervertebral foramina and pass posteriorly to supply the paravertebral tissues. The anterior rami T2 to T11 become the intercostal nerves, and that of T12 is the subcostal nerve. The anterior portions of the lower five intercostal nerves (T7 to T11) run in the anterior abdominal wall parallel to the ribs as do the subcostal nerve

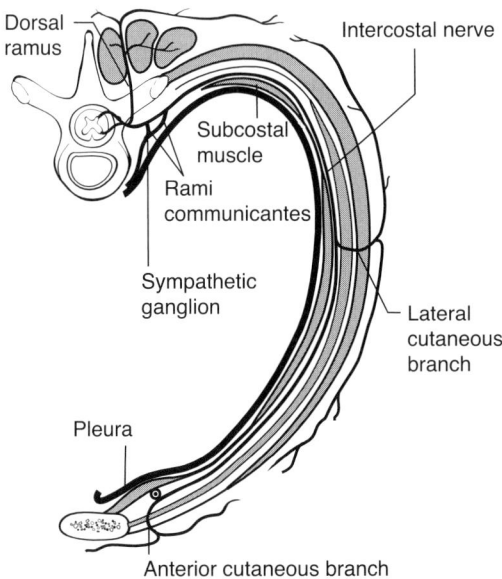

Figure 30.5 Course and relations of a typical thoracic spinal nerve. (Redrawn with permission from *Principles and Practice of Regional Anaesthesia* (eds J.A. Wildsmith, E.N. Armitage), Churchill Livingstone, Edinburgh, 1993.)

and the anterior ramus of L1. The corresponding dermatomal 'belts' also follow the line of the ribs and so, for example, the fibres arising at the level of T10 supply the skin at the level of the umbilicus.

The majority of the fibres in the anterior ramus of T1 join the brachial plexus, but there may be a small anterior cutaneous branch. The large lateral cutaneous branch of T2 (the intercostobrachial nerve) crosses the axilla to supply the skin over the medial aspect of the arm. A large part of the anterior primary ramus of T12 joins that of L1.

INTERCOSTAL NERVE BLOCK

Anatomy

The intercostal nerve may be blocked as it runs below the intercostal vessels in the subcostal groove on the inner surface of the caudal margin of the rib. Although accessible throughout its course the nerve is most easily blocked at the posterior angle of the rib where the subcostal space is relatively deep and is separated from the pleura by the subcostal muscles, thus minimizing the risk of pneumothorax (Figure 30.5). The lateral and anterior branches of the nerve will be blocked by this approach.

Technique

The patient's arm should be abducted and lie in a plane anterior to the shoulder so that the scapulae move laterally thus allowing access to the ribs. This can be achieved in the sitting, prone or lateral position. If the block is to be used to supplement general anaesthesia for thoracotomy, it is more easily performed after the anaesthetized patient has been positioned for surgery. This is a painful block and supplementary analgesia should be provided when the injection is made in a conscious patient.

The angle of the rib is palpated 8–10 cm from the mid-line and the overlying skin is tensed by pulling it cephalad. The needle is inserted at right angles to the skin so as to contact the lower margin of the rib and the depth is noted. The tension on the skin is then relaxed and the tip of the needle is walked caudally until it just slips under the rib. The patient is asked to hold his breath as the needle is inserted and the injection made. After aspiration (seeking air in addition to blood), 3–5 ml bupivacaine 0.25% with adrenaline 1:200 000 is injected. The block is repeated at adjacent costal levels to produce the desired extent of anaeshesia.

There is evidence that a large-volume injection (10–20 ml) will spread to up to four adjacent intercostal spaces. The route of spread is uncertain but is probably via the paravertebral and the subpleural spaces. (The subpleural space is between the pleura and the neck of the rib.) Whatever the mechanism, intercostal catheters, placed three to four spaces apart and directed medially, may be used to provide prolonged analgesia after thoracic or upper abdominal surgery.

Complications

Due to the vascularity of the intercostal space, systemic toxicity may ensue, even in the absence of vascular puncture. Adrenaline-containing solutions should be used. If an infusion technique is used, there is a risk of cumulative toxicity. Pneumothorax may present some hours after the block has been performed. The anaesthetist should ensure that the ward staff are alert to the possibility of these delayed complications.

PARAVERTEBRAL BLOCK

The paravertebral spaces are in communication via a common, fat-filled paramedian compartment which runs parallel to the vertebral column, thus three or four spinal levels may be blocked by a single injection. In contrast to intercostal block, the posterior rami of the spinal nerves, which supply the posterior ligaments, paravertebral musculature and overlying skin, are blocked.

Anatomy

In transverse section, the paravertebral space is roughly triangular (Figure 30.5). The borders are the pleura anterolaterally, the lateral surface of the vertebral body medially and the superior costotransverse ligament posteriorly. This ligament runs from the lower border of the transverse process to the upper border of the rib below. The spinal nerve enters the space through the intervertebral foramen, and divides into anterior and posterior rami. The anterior ramus sends and receives fibres from the sympathetic ganglion, which lies anteriorly, then passes laterally to run in the subcostal groove or in the abdominal wall.

Technique

With the patient sitting or in the lateral position with the side to be blocked uppermost, the spinal level corresponding to the middle of the area to be blocked is identified. In the lumbar region the transverse process lies at the level of the top of the corresponding spinous process; in the thoracic region it is found at the lower border of the spinous process of the vertebra above. The needle is then inserted 3–4 cm from the mid-line and at 90° to the skin until the transverse process is struck at a depth of 4–6 cm: distance and depth depend on the spinal level at which the block is performed. A saline-filled syringe with a free-running barrel is attached and the tip of the needle is walked off the transverse process until loss of resistance is encountered as it passes through the costotransverse ligament and enters the paravertebral space. Following aspiration for blood and air, injection of 15 ml bupivacaine 0.375–0.5% with adrenaline 1:200 000 will normally produce a block of three to four segments. If a more extensive block is required, a second injection will be more effective than increasing the volume injected at a single site. Solution may spread into intercostal spaces and the epidural space and occasionally minor contralateral block results. If a catheter is to be used, only a short segment should be inserted so as to minimize the risk of migration from the space.

Complications

There are many potential complications reflecting proximity to both the pleural cavity and the spinal canal. The common complications are moderate hypotension resulting from sympathetic block, vascular puncture, pleural puncture and pneumothorax. The incidence of these is comparable to that found following epidural or intercostal block. There is extensive absorption from this vascular area, thus adrenaline containing solutions should be used.

FIELD BLOCK FOR INGUINAL HERNIA REPAIR

This block may be used in combination with general anaesthesia or, in the frail patient, with intravenous sedation or analgesia. This technique is most successful when the tissues are strong and the sensation of piercing the musculofascial planes can be readily appreciated. Unfortunately, this is unlikely to be the case in the majority of adult patients presenting for this procedure.

Anatomy

The muscles and skin of the groin and adjacent areas are innervated by nerves arising from T12 and L1 (Figure 30.6). A large part of

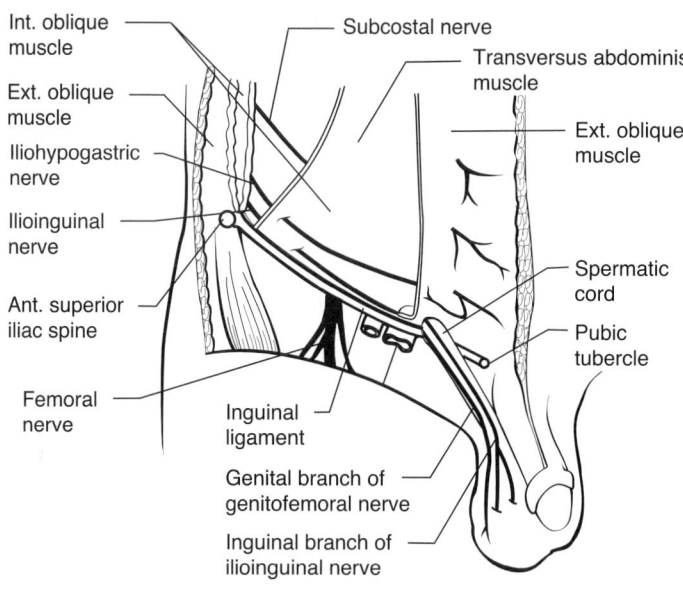

Figure 30.6 Course and relations of the nerves of the lower anterior abdominal wall and the inguinal regions. (Redrawn with permission from *Principles and Practice of Regional Anaesthesia* (eds J.A. Wildsmith, E.N. Armitage), Churchill Livingstone, Edinburgh, 1993.)

the anterior primary ramus of T12 (subcostal nerve) joins that of L1 before the latter divides into iliohypogastric and ilioinguinal nerves on quadratus lumborum. All three nerves run in the lateral abdominal wall between transversus abdominis and internal oblique. The subcostal and iliohypogastric nerves give off lateral cutaneous branches above the posterior superior iliac spine. In the anterior abdominal wall, the anterior cutaneous branch of T12 runs almost to the mid-line before piercing the rectus sheath. The iliohypogastric nerve pierces the internal oblique muscle 2 cm medial to the anterior superior iliac spine, and runs deep to the aponeurosis of external oblique before piercing this approximately 3 cm from the mid-line. The ilioinguinal nerve pierces internal oblique below the iliohypogastric nerve and then runs in the inguinal canal, supplying the structures running in the canal and the skin of the scrotum and root of the penis.

Technique

The iliohypogastric and ilioinguinal nerves may be blocked as they run above the anterior superior iliac spine. A needle is inserted 3 cm medial to the spine and directed so as to contact the inner surface of the ileum. If the musculofascial planes can be identified as they are pierced then 10 ml bupivacaine 0.5% with adrenaline 1:200 000 should be deposited in each layer; if not 10–15 ml solution is infiltrated as the needle is slowly withdrawn to the subcutaneous tissues. From the same point, the needle is reintroduced at 90° to the course of the nerves and a further 10 ml injected superficial and deep to the aponeurrosis of external oblique. The terminal fibres of the ipsilateral nerves and any fibres crossing the mid-line may be blocked by subcutaneous infiltration of 5–10 ml of bupivacaine 0.25% with adrenaline 1:200 000 in a line running superiorly from the pubic tubercle. Finally, if

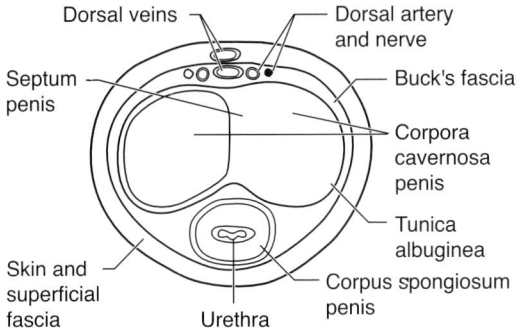

Figure 30.7 Transverse section of the penis. Redrawn with permission from *Principles and Practice of Regional Anaesthesia* (eds J.A. Wildsmith, E.N. Armitage), Churchill Livingstone, Edinburgh, 1993.)

this block is to be used as a sole technique, the surgeon must inject anaesthetic into the cord and the peritoneal sac at the deep linguinal ring to block visceral afferents.

Complications

A large volume of solution is required for this block and thus, even with careful aspiration, there is a risk of systemic toxicity. This may be minimized by using a more dilute solution for the subcutaneous infiltrations.

DORSAL NERVE BLOCK

Anatomy

The dorsal nerves of the penis (S2, 3, 4) run under the pubic arch, lateral to the dorsal arteries and the midline deep dorsal vein. These structures run within the loose fascial layer (Buck's fascia) which encompasses the corpora cavernosa and corpus spongiosum (see Figure 30.7). The terminal branches of these nerves pierce the fascia and supply the skin of the distal penis and the glans.

Technique

A fine needle is inserted in the midline, immediately inferior to the symphysis pubis and directed 15° laterally immediately the skin has been pierced. The needle is advanced until a 'give' is felt as Buck's fascia is pierced and 5 ml 0.25–0.5% bupivacaine without adrenaline is injected. The needle is withdrawn almost to the skin and redirected to repeat the block on the other side. Resistance to injection indicates that the fascial compartment has been filled and no further injection should be attempted.

Complications

Arterial compression and even gangrene may result if an excessive volume of solution is injected into the non-elastic fascial compartment. The dorsal veins of the penis are midline structures and may be punctured when performing bilateral injections from a single mid-line site.

NERVE BLOCKS OF THE LOWER LIMB

The arrangement of the nerve supply of the lower limb is less well-suited to the needs of the anaesthetist than that of the upper limb. The seven roots of the lumbosacral plexus arise over a relatively long portion of the vertebral column and the branches immediately separate and follow diverse routes rather than running together within a well-defined fascial sheath. Consequently, anaesthesia or the lower limb requires at least two injections (for the lumbar and sacral 'divisions') and a large dose of local anaesthetic solution. It is not surprising that many anaesthetists choose subarachnoid or epidural block when they wish to provide local anaesthesia for surgery to the leg. However, cases will arise where a lumbar plexus or peripheral block is the technique of choice. The arguments are essentially as advanced in

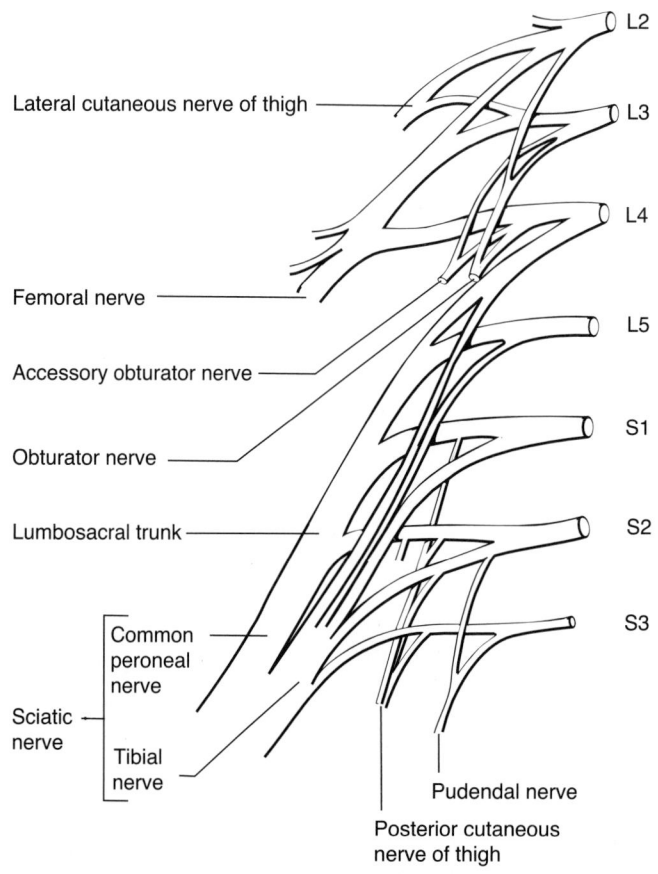

Figure 30.8 The lumbosacral plexus. (Redrawn with permission from *Principles and Practice of Regional Anaesthesia* (eds J.A. Wildsmith, E.N. Armitage), Churchill Livingstone, Edinburgh, 1993.)

favour of unilateral blocks of the trunk. In addition, many of the nerves of the limb follow a superficial course and may be used when the patient is receiving aspirin or 'low-dose' subcutaneous heparin, as pressure may be applied directly to the injection point should a vessel be punctured. Special consideration should be given to the use of solutions containing adrenaline in patients with peripheral vascular disease.

THE LUMBOSACRAL PLEXUS

This combined plexus is formed from the anterior primary rami of spinal nerves L2–S2. The lumbar portion provides cutaneous innervation to the anterior, medial and lateral surfaces of the thigh and the anterior and medial surfaces of the leg, and supplies the muscles producing flexion (L2, 3) and extension (L4, 5) at the hip and extension of the knee (L5, S1). A schematic diagram of the plexus is shown in Figure 30.8. The areas of cutaneous innervation by the terminal branches are shown in Figure 30.9.

At the lumbar level, the plexus forms within the substance of psoas major and runs caudally and lateral on quadratus lumborum. The lateral cutaneous nerve of thigh, the genitofemoral and the femoral nerves leave the

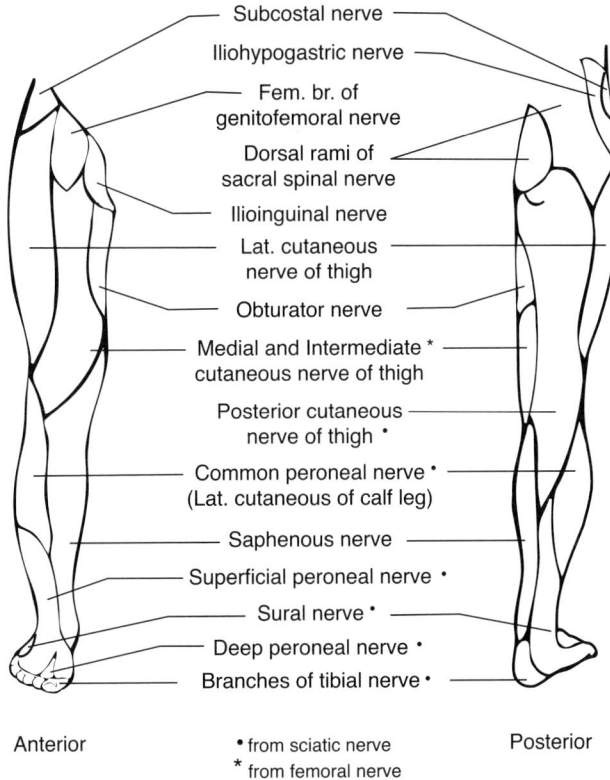

Figure 30.9 Distribution of the cutaneous branches of the lumbosacral plexus.

pelvis under the inguinal ligament and the obturator nerve leaves via the obturator foramen (Figure 30.10). The sacral portion of the plexus lies on piriformis muscle on the posterior wall of the pelvic cavity. The sciatic nerve and the posterior cutaneous nerve of the thigh leave the pelvis though the greater sciatic foramen. Detailed anatomy is given with the description of each block.

GENERAL COMMENTS

A peripheral nerve stimulator is recommended for all proximal blocks of the nerves of the lower limb.

Circumferential anaesthesia of the limb is required if an arterial tourniquet is used. Thus if a tourniquet must be placed on the thigh a block of the posterior cutaneous nerve of the thigh (sciatic nerve block) and of the femoral, lateral cutaneous nerve of the thigh and the obturator nerve (three-in-one block) are required. Surgery may be possible if an upper limb tourniquet is placed around the calf in which case blocks of the saphenous nerve at the knee and the branches of the sciatic nerve in the popliteal fossa are required.

BLOCKS OF THE LUMBAR PLEXUS

The nerves of the plexus may be blocked by an anterior or posterior approach. The posterior approaches result in more extensive block, but carries the risk of inadvertent epidural or intrathecal injection.

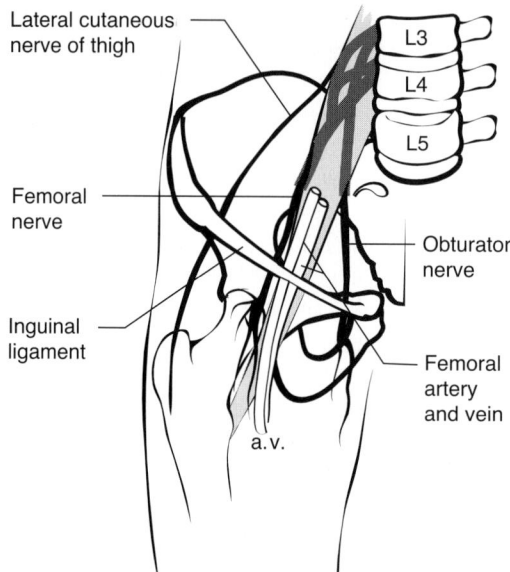

Figure 30.10 Course of the branches of the lumbar plexus.

Paravertebral block

Paravertebral block of the roots of the lumbar plexus is described above.

Psoas compartment block

Anatomy

The branches of the lumbar plexus emerge between quadratus lumborum and psoas major and run caudally in a fascial compartment (the psoas compartment) which arises from the investing fasciae of these muscles. The nerves lie relatively close together at the level of L4/5 (Figure 30.10) and may be blocked by a single injection of local anaesthetic solution spreading within the compartment.

Technique

The patient lies in the lateral position with the side to be blocked uppermost. A line joining the tips of the iliac crests is drawn and a point 3 cm caudal to this line and 5 cm lateral to the mid-line is identified: this point should lie over the transverse process of L5. A long 18 G Tuohy needle is advanced to contact the transverse process at a depth of 4–6 cm and a 'loss of resistance' type syringe charged with air is attached. The needle is walked cephalad and laterally off the transverse process until it contacts the dense fascia on the dorsal surface of quadratus lumborum. The needle is advanced through the muscle until loss of resistance to injection occurs as the tip of the needle enters the psoas compartment at approximately 10 cm deep to the skin; 10 ml of air are injected to open the potential space and 30 ml bupivacaine 0.375–0.5% with adrenaline 1:200 000 is injected. A catheter may be placed before withdrawing the needle.

Complications

Epidural and spinal injection have been reported.

A similar technique, using the transverse process of L3, has recently been described. The potential advantages are that as the process is longer than that of L5, the injection is made at greater distance from the midline thus reducing the risk of epidural or intrathecal injection and that the spaces between transverse processes are greater at this level, thus the needle passes more easily.

The 'three-in-one' block

The principle of this technique is that the branches of the lumbar plexus which lie deep to the fascia iliaca in the pelvis can be blocked by a single injection.

Anatomy

In the pelvis, the femoral nerve runs in the groove between iliacus and psoas major deep to the fascia iliaca before passing beneath the mid-point of the inguinal ligament, lateral to the femoral vessels. Here it lies within a sheath which arises in part from the fascia iliaca and is continuous with the subfascial compartment. The obturator nerve and the lateral cutaneous nerve of the thigh also run deep to the fascia iliaca before leaving the pelvis through the oburator foramen and beneath the lateral part of the inguinal ligament respectively. The lower border of the fascia iliaca is continuous with the posterior margin of the inguinal ligament, except where it lies posterior to the femoral vessels as these pass beneath the ligament. In the thigh, it blends with the fascia covering sartorius muscle.

Technique

The key to this block is accurate placement of local anaesthetic solution within the femoral nerve sheath. The main nerve trunk may divide immediately below or occasionally above the linguinal ligament and the use of a peripheral nerve stimulator is recommended. The pulsation of the femoral artery is located just below the linguinal ligament and the needle is inserted 1 cm lateral to this point, parallel to the course of the nerve and directed cephalad. The nerve is approximately 3 cm deep to the skin and a give may be felt as the needle pierces the fascia lata and the femoral sheath. If the nerve is not located, the needle should be redirected laterally. When the needle lies adjacent to the femoral nerve, 30 ml bupivacaine 0.375–0.5% with adrenaline 1:200 000 is injected while firm compression is applied distal to the injection site in order to promote proximal spread.

Fascia iliaca block

This technique aims to introduce local anaesthetic directly into the compartment deep to the fascia iliaca rather than via the sheath surrounding the femoral nerve; thus there is no need to locate this structure. An imaginary line joining the pubic tubercle and the anterior superior iliac spine is divided into thirds. The needle is inserted, at right angles to the skin, 1 cm below the junction of the outer and middle thirds. Two 'gives' will be felt as the needle pierces the fascia lata and then the fascia iliaca: 30 ml bupivacaine 0.375–0.5% with adrenaline 1:200 000 is injected while firm compression is applied distal to the injection site.

NERVE BLOCKS AT THE HIP

Femoral nerve

The technique is as for the 'three-in-one block' but only 10–15 ml of bupivacaine 0.25–0.375% with adrenaline 1:200 000 is required. While evidence of nerve stimulation is essential for the combined block, if this cannot be obtained and only femoral nerve block is required it is reasonable to inject 20 ml of solution fanwise across the likely course of the nerve.

Lateral cutaneous nerve of the thigh

This nerve enters the thigh beneath the inguinal ligament just medial to the anterior superior iliac spine and runs deep to the fascia lata before dividing. A needle is inserted at right angles to the skin 2 cm medial and distal to the anterior superior iliac spine. A 'give' will be felt as the fascia lata is pierced: 5 ml 0.25–0.375% bupivacaine with adrenaline 1:200 000 is injected. The needle is redirected so as to pass medially and laterally beneath the fascia lata and a further 5–10 ml solution is injected fanwise.

Obturator nerve

This block is difficult to perform and has little value as a sole technique. When anaesthesia of the small area of the medial aspect of the thigh is required the 'three-in-one' or fascia iliaca block can be used. When motor block of the adductors of the thigh is required central neural blockade is the most reliable technique.

Sciatic nerve

Anatomy

The sciatic nerve arises in the pelvis as the continuation of the sacral portion of the lumbosacral plexus. It enters the buttock with the posterior cutaneous nerve of the thigh via the greater sciatic foramen and runs deep to gluteus maximus. It follows a direct route, deep to the hamstrings towards the popliteal fossa where it divides into the common peroneal and tibial nerves. Occasionally this division occurs proximal to the popliteal fossa, but when this occurs these nerves run together to the knee.

The posterior and anterior approaches to the sciatic nerve are described. The use of a peripheral nerve stimulator is invaluable for both techniques.

Posterior approach

The patient lies on his side with the limb to be blocked uppermost. The hip is flexed to approximately 45° and the knee rests on the bed anterior to the lower limb; thus the pelvis is rotated slightly anteriorly. The posterior superior iliac spine and the tip of the greater trochanter are identified (Figure 30.11). The degree of flexion at the hips is adjusted so that the femur lies as a continuation of a line drawn between these two points. A second line is drawn from the tip of the greater trochanter to the coccyx. The point of insertion of the needle is where a perpendicular dropped from the mid-point of the first line crosses the second. A long needle is inserted at right angles to the skin in all planes and is advanced until a motor or sensory response in the foot is elicited (normally at a depth of 7–10 cm) or bone (the ischial spine) is encountered. If the nerve is not located the needle is withdrawn and redirected medially or laterally along the course of the coccygeal–trochanteric line: 20–25 ml bupivacaine 0.5% with adrenaline 1:200 000 is required. The posterior cutaneous nerve of the thigh will also be blocked.

Anterior approach

With the patient supine and the thigh fully externally rotated (so that the nerve may be located when it runs directly behind the femur), a line is drawn between the anterior superior iliac spine and the pubic tubercle. This line is divided into thirds and a perpendicular dropped from the junction of the middle and medial thirds. A 15 cm needle is inserted where this perpendicular crosses a second line, parallel to the first and arising from the tip of the greater trochanter, and is directed so as to contact the femur. The needle is then walked medially and advanced a further 5 cm. A technique where loss of resistance is obtained as the needle enters the posterior compartment has also been

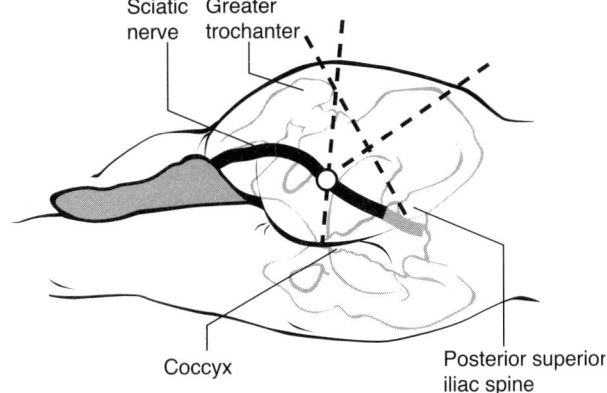

Figure 30.11 Landmarks for posterior approach to the sciatic nerve.

described. Bearing in mind the likely course of the nerve, motor or sensory response in the foot is sought and when obtained, 20–25 ml bupivacaine 0.5% with adrenaline 1:200 000 is injected.

NERVE BLOCKS AROUND THE KNEE

If surgery below the knee is proposed, these techniques avoid the loss of mobility resulting from sciatic or femoral nerve block.

Saphenous nerve block

The saphenous nerve lies on the medial aspect of the tibia, just below the knee joint. It can be blocked by subcutaneous infiltration of 10 ml bupivacaine 0.25% with adrenaline 1:200 000. The nerve runs with the greater saphenous vein, thus aspiration before injection is particularly important.

Nerve block in the popliteal fossa: common peroneal and tibial nerves

Anatomy

The common peroneal and tibial nerves are the terminal branches of the sciatic nerve and run together to the apex of the popliteal fossa.

Technique

The patient lies prone. The knee joint is flexed and the upper tendinous margins of the diamond-shaped poplitial fossa are palpated. The apex of the fossa is identified and the knee extended. If the popliteal artery can be palpated the needle should be inserted 1 cm lateral to this landmark and directed cephalad. If not, the needle is inserted at a point just lateral to the apex of the fossa. Paraesthesia or a muscular response in the dorsum of the foot (the tibial nerve) and in the lateral aspect of the calf (the common peroneal nerve) are sought separately from this point to the lateral border of the fossa and at a depth of up to 5 cm: 10–15 ml bupivacaine 0.25–0.375% with adrenaline 1:200 000 is injected at both points.

NERVE BLOCKS AT THE ANKLE

The lines of subcutaneous injection to block the deep peroneal, superficial peroneal and

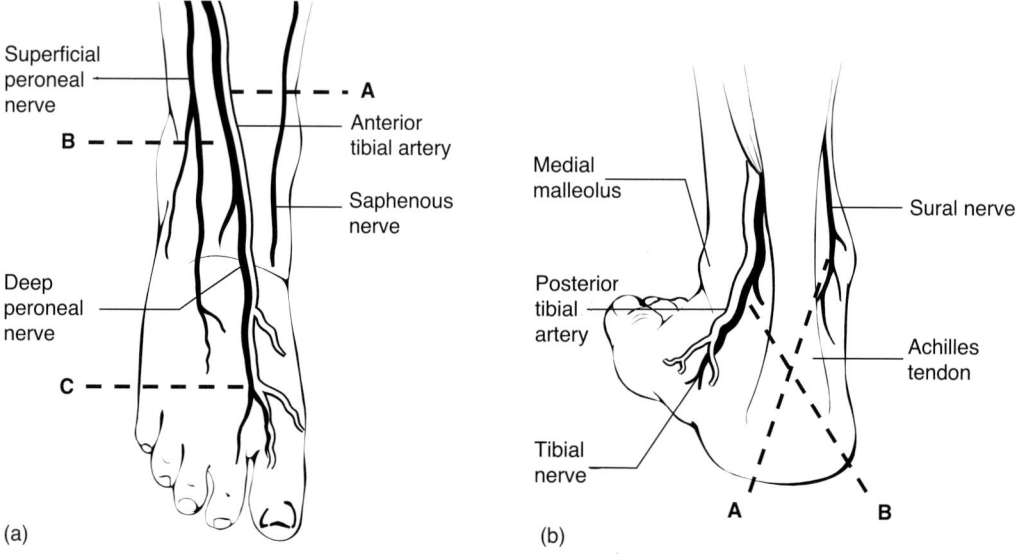

Figure 30.12 (a) Nerve blocks on the anterior aspect of the ankle: **A**, saphenous nerve; **B**, superficial peroneal nerve; **C**, deep peroneal nerve. (b) Nerve blocks on the posterior aspect of the ankle: **A**, sural nerve; **B**, tibial nerve.

saphenous nerves on the anterior aspect of the ankle and foot are illustrated in Figure 30.12. Up to 5 ml bupivicaine 0.25% solution with adrenaline 1:200 000 is required in each case. The tibial nerve is blocked behind the medial malleollus. The posterior tibial artery is palpated, the needle is inserted from the posterior aspect of the ankle, aimed towards the great toenail, and 5–10 ml solution is injected just superficial and posterior to the artery. The sural nerve is blocked by subcutaneous infiltration of 5–10 ml solution along a line from the border of the Achilles tendon to the lateral malleolus. Again, this is most easily performed if the needle is inserted on the posterior aspect of the ankle.

DIGITAL NERVE BLOCK

The technique is as for block of the digital nerves of the hand. The solution should not contain a vasoconstrictor.

IVRA OF THE LOWER LIMB

IVRA using a tourniquet placed on the thigh should not be used because of the large dose of local anaesthetic solution required and because the tourniquet pressures require to occlude the circulation are much greater than in the upper limb because of the substantial muscle bulk.

An 'upper limb' tourniquet may be placed at mid-calf level. Proximal placement will result in trauma to the superficial peroneal nerve. The technique is as described in the section on upper limb blocks. Tourniquet pressure should be at least 200 mmHg above systolic arterial pressure measured in the brachial artery. Suitable doses are as for IVRA of the upper limb.

NERVE BLOCKS OF THE HEAD AND NECK

This section describes commonly-used blocks of the superficial nerves of the head and neck.

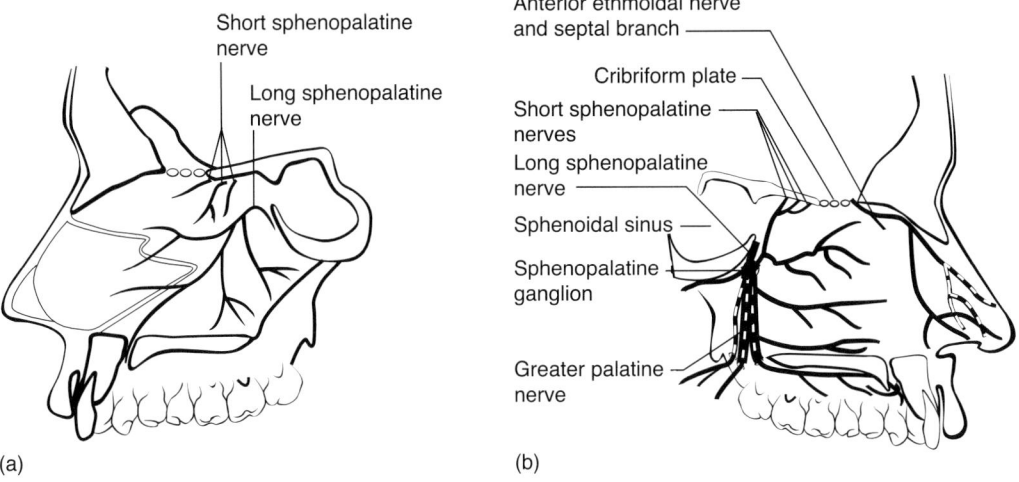

Figure 30.13 Innervation of the septal wall of the nasal cavity.

TOPICAL ANAESTHESIA FOR NASAL CAVITY SURGERY

This technique has the additional benefit of decreasing the vascularity of the nasal mucosa. Local anaesthetic solutions are readily absorbed and thus the recommended dose limit must be strictly observed.

Anatomy

The nasal mucosa is innervated by branches of the ophthalmic and maxillary divisions of the trigeminal nerve (Figure 30.13).

Technique

Three cotton-tipped pledgelets soaked in lignocaine 4% with adrenaline 1:200 000 or 5% cocaine without adrenaline (maximum topical dose of cocaine 1.5 mg kg^{-1}) are used for each nasal cavity. The first pledgelet is wedged in the vault of the nasal cavity anterior to the cibriform plate so as to block the anterior ethmoidal nerve proximal to the origin of its septal branch. The second and third pledgelets should be placed on the mucosa anterior to the sphenoidal sinus above and below the middle turbinate, i.e. above and below the sphenopalatine ganglion, thus the long and short sphenopalatine nerves and the greater palatine nerve will be blocked. The pledgelets should remain in place for at least 10 min. Any remaining solution should be instilled in to the nasal cavities. To complete the block the membranous septum and columella must be infiltrated.

OUTER SURFACE OF THE NOSE

This may be anaesthetized by a fan of subcutaneous infiltrations made from the tip of the nose. If it is essential that the tissues are not distorted, individual nerve blocks are performed; 1–2 ml bupivacaine 0.25% with adrenaline 1:200 000 is required in each case. The external nasal nerve is blocked at the junction of the bony and cartilaginous skeleton half way between the mid-line of the nose and the cheek, the infratrochlear nerve is blocked on the side of the nose just below the medial canthus of the eye and the infraorbital nerve is blocked immediately below the infra-

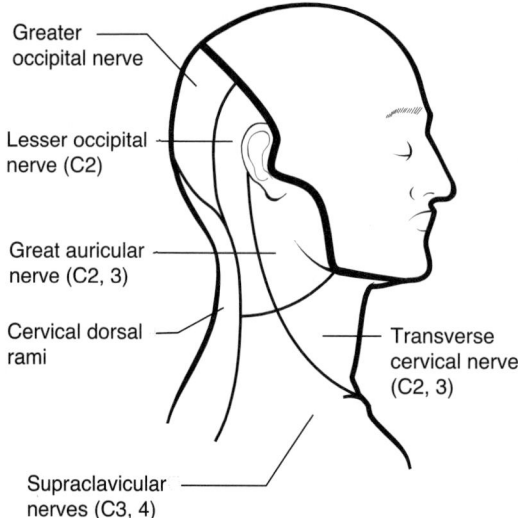

Figure 30.14 Distribution of the cutaneous branches of the cervical plexus.

orbital forearm. The needle should never be inserted into the foramen because of the risk of neural ischaemia.

SUPERFICIAL CERVICAL PLEXUS BLOCK

This block produces analgesia at the points of insertion of both internal jugular and subclavian venous catheters.

Anatomy

The cervical plexus is formed from the anterior rami of C1-C4 and lies deep to sternocleidomastoid. The superficial cutaneous branches of the plexus provide sensory innervation to an area which extends from the skin behind and below the ear (lesser occipital (C2) and greater auricular (C2,3) nerves), over the anterolateral surface of the neck (transverse cervical nerve (C2, 3)) and the skin overlying the shoulder as far as the manubriosternal joint (supraclavicular nerves (C3, 4)) (Figure 30.14).

Technique

The nerves are blocked as they pierce the deep fascia and curve around the middle third of the posterior border of sternocleidomastoid before running in the superficial tissues of the neck. The needle is inserted at the mid-point of the posterior border and is directed upwards and then downwards along the border while some 5–10 ml bupivacaine 0.25% with adrenaline 1:200 000 is injected in each direction. The external jugular vein crosses sternoclediomastoid at, or near, the injection point thus careful aspiration is required.

FURTHER READING

Brockway, M. S. and Wildsmith, J. A. W. (1990) Axillary brachial plexus block: method of choice? *British Journal of Anaesthesia*, **64**, 224–231.

Charlton, J. E. (1993) The management of regional anaesthesia, in *Principles and Practice of Regional Anaesthesia*, 2nd edn. (eds J. A. W. Wildsmith and E. N. Armitage), Churchill Livingstone, Edinburgh, pp. 47–75.

Covino R. G. (1989) General considerations, toxicity and complications of local anaesthesia, in *Anaesthesia*, 1st edn (eds W. S. Nimmo and G. Smith.) Blackwell Scientific, London, pp. 1101–1033.

Dalens, B., Vanneuville, G. and Tanguy, A. (1989) Comparison of the fascia iliaca compartment block with the 3-in-1 block in children. *Anesthesia and Analgesia*, **69**, 705–713.

Hanna, M. H., Peat, S. J. and D'Costa, F. (1993) Lumbar plexus block: an anatomical study. *Anaesthesia*, **48**, 675–678.

Lanz, E., Theiss, D. and Jankovic, D. (1983) The extent of blockade following various techniques of brachial plexus block. *Anesthesia and Analgesia*, **62**, 55–58.

Lönnqvist, P. A., MacKenzie, J., Soni, A. K. and Conacher, I. D. (1995) Paravertebral blockade. Failure rate and complications. *Anaesthesia*, **50**, 813–815.

Moore, D. C., Mulroy, M. F. and Thompson, G. E. (1994) Peripheral nerve damage and regional anaesthesia. *British Journal of Anaesthesia*, **73**, 435–436.

Neill, R. S. (1989) Head and neck, in *Anaesthesia*, 1st edn (eds W. S. Nimmo and G. Smith) Blackwell Scientific, London, pp. 1134–1145.

Winnie, A. P., Ramamurthy, S. and Durrani, Z. (1973) The inguinal paravascular technic of lumbar plexus anesthesia: the 3-in-1 block. *Anesthesia and Analgesia*, **52**, 989–996.

OBSTETRIC ANAESTHESIA AND ANALGESIA

M. H. Nathanson and D. G. Bogod

The obstetric anaesthetist, uniquely within anaesthetic practice, has the care of two patients in his or her hands. This burden of responsibility is increased by the fact that pregnancy is a physiological state, and the mother and her attendants understandably expect the outcome to be favourable and any interventions to be safe.

For the anaesthetist to perform to these high expectations, it is necessary to have a good understanding of how pregnancy and labour alter maternal physiology, and the ways in which these changes may impact upon, and be affected by, anaesthetic procedures. The anaesthetist does not work in isolation on the labour ward, and close communication with obstetric and midwifery colleagues is essential to ensure appropriate timing of interventions and to prevent crisis from becoming chaos.

Not only are anaesthetists expected to take an increasing part in obstetric management, they will also find their involvement extending to a greater proportion of the obstetric population. The use of epidural analgesia is increasing in the UK and other countries in the West, and the Caesarean section rate is rising inexorably, up to a quarter of all deliveries in some parts of the USA. In many maternity units, the anaesthetist is directly involved with more than half of the patients. Despite this increasing involvement, anaesthesia appears to be becoming safer as lessons from audits such as the UK Report on Confidential Enquiries into Maternal Deaths are learnt and applied in practice. Death, however, is a crude indicator of quality and safety and recent refinements in regional analgesia and anaesthesia demonstrate that anaesthetists are aware that there are still considerable improvements to be made.

This chapter aims to provide a solid grounding in the physiology and pathology of pregnancy, with particular reference to how these changes impact on anaesthesia. Pain relief in labour is discussed, emphasizing some of the recent advances in regional techniques. The alternative methods of anaesthesia for Caesarean section are presented, and the reasons for the increasing pre-eminence of spinal and epidural techniques discussed. Finally, we introduce the care of the sick obstetric patient, who can benefit greatly from anaesthetic skills learnt in the intensive care unit.

PHYSIOLOGICAL CHANGES DURING PREGNANCY

During the development of pregnancy physiological changes occur which affect nearly every organ of the body. These changes influence the interpretation of physical signs and symptoms, the results of diagnostic labora-

---

Short Practice of Anaesthesia. Edited by M. Morgan and G. M. Hall. Published in 1997 by Chapman & Hall, London. ISBN 0 412 71890 1

tory tests, the management of anaesthesia and analgesia, and the care of the complicated pregnancy and labour. A knowledge of these changes is, therefore, vital in providing safe anaesthetic care of the labouring woman.

RESPIRATORY SYSTEM

Ventilation increases from an early stage of pregnancy, mainly because of an increase in tidal volume. At term, minute volume is increased by about 50% compared with the non-pregnant state and the Pa_{CO_2} is approximately 4.05 kPa. This state of hyperventilation is thought to result from increased circulating progesterone and produces a concentration gradient down which carbon dioxide can pass from the fetal to the maternal circulation. Functional residual capacity (FRC) is reduced by 15–20% by the third trimester. Although closing volume remains the same, one-third of pregnant women have airway closure at term because of the reduction in FRC. The likelihood of airway closure increases in the supine and Trendelenburg positions and in women who smoke, who are obese or have skeletal abnormalities affecting the chest.

CARDIOVASCULAR SYSTEM

Cardiac output increases by 30–40% during early pregnancy but then decreases slowly and is just above normal at term. However, there is a further dramatic increase in cardiac output during labour. Heart rate is increased by 10–15 b.p.m. throughout pregnancy. Arterial blood pressure is decreased by 5–10 mmHg during pregnancy, despite the increase in cardiac output. The systemic vascular resistance is reduced due to lowered resistance in the uterine, renal and other vascular beds. Displacement of the diaphragm by the gravid uterus pushes the heart upwards leading to left axis deviation on the electrocardiogram. Ventricular ectopic beats, sinus tachycardia and paroxysmal supraventricular tachycardia may occur and, in the absence of organic heart disease, are not a significant hazard.

From the second trimester onwards the enlarging uterus causes progressively more significant aortocaval compression. Complete vena caval obstruction may occur in up to 90% of women at term when placed in the supine position. Although venous blood may be shunted to the superior vena cava by the azygous system and vertebral plexus, the reduced venous return in the supine position leads to maternal tachycardia, hypotension, faintness and pallor in 10% of women. This state is known as the supine hypotensive syndrome. Even in the absence of maternal arterial hypotension, the obstructed venous return from the pelvis combined with partial aortic compression causes a marked reduction in uteroplacental blood flow. During the second and third trimesters the supine position should be avoided if possible, but if necessary, manual displacement of the uterus to the left or lateral tilting of the body must be used.

HAEMATOLOGICAL CHANGES

Red cell volume increases by 20% and plasma volume increases by 40–50%. This discrepancy leads to the physiological anaemia of pregnancy, and at term the normal range of haemoglobin is 11.0–12.0 g dl^{-1}. Lower blood viscosity and a shift to the right of the oxygen–haemoglobin dissociation curve ensures an increased oxygen carrying capacity despite the dilutional anaemia. The white cell count may increase to 10×10^9 l^{-1} towards term, and the platelet count remains unchanged. Although the total amount of plasma proteins increase, the increase in plasma volume results in a fall in the total plasma protein and albumin concentration. Plasma fibrinogen concentration increases by 50% and there are increases in factors VII, VIII and X.

GASTROINTESTINAL AND HEPATIC CHANGES

Hormonal changes and direct pressure effects of the gravid uterus significantly alter gastrointestinal function. Progesterone reduces intestinal motility, absorption of food and the volume of intestinal secretions. Lower oesophageal sphincter tone is reduced from the end of the first trimester. Although it is often stated that gastric acid production is increased in pregnancy, there is no evidence for this and most studies point to a relative achlorhydria from the first trimester onwards. Pressure from the gravid uterus leads to rotation and upward displacement of the stomach. During labour, pain, anxiety and the use of anticholinergic agents and opioids slow gastric emptying. The duration of these changes is not known, but precautions against acid aspiration should be taken for at least 48 h after delivery.

Blood concentrations of aspartate transaminase, alkaline phosphatase and lactate dehydrogenase are increased during pregnancy. Serum bilirubin is unchanged and plasma cholinesterase activity is reduced by 20%. In practice the slower metabolism of suxamethonium is unimportant.

RENAL CHANGES

Renal plasma flow and the glomerular filtration rate are increased by 50% and the blood urea and creatinine concentrations are reduced by half. Glycosuria is common because of the reduced renal threshold for glucose. There is dilation of the renal calyces, collecting systems and ureters above the pelvis.

CENTRAL NERVOUS SYSTEM

The minimum alveolar concentration for inhaled anaesthetic agents is reduced by up to 40%. The requirement of local anaesthetic for epidural or subarachnoid blockade is reduced compared to the non-pregnant state. This latter change is commonly attributed to engorgement of the epidural venous plexuses reducing the volume of the epidural and subarachnoid spaces. However, there may also be a pharmacodynamic effect as a result of increased sensitivity of nerves to conduction blockade.

UTERINE PHYSIOLOGY

At term the uterine blood flow is about 700 ml min^{-1}. The maternal uteroplacental blood vessels have a continuous flow of blood throughout the cardiac cycle. Absence of flow, even during diastole, is abnormal. Uterine blood flow may decrease during periods of hypotension, for example after sympathetic blockade, or following the use of vasoconstrictors with primarily α-adrenoceptor agonist activity, such as phenylephrine. Ephedrine is the vasoconstrictor of choice during pregnancy. The most important factor in the transfer of drugs across the placenta is the movement of drugs by diffusion across the barrier separating the maternal and fetal circulations. Small lipid soluble molecules such as thiopentone cross readily. With normal induction–delivery intervals at Caesarean section, equilibration between the two circulations has not occurred and the concentration of thiopentone in the baby's blood at delivery is insufficient to lead to clinically important sedation. Similarly, the induction–delivery interval is usually too short for equilibration of inhaled anaesthetic agents. However, benzodiazepines given to the mother in labour will depress neurobehavioural function in the baby. Highly ionized molecules such as the non-depolarizing neuromuscular blocking agents do not readily cross the placenta. The degree of protein binding in the maternal circulation is important, as is the acid–base status of the fetus. An acidaemic fetus will 'trap' the ions of weak bases such as bupivacaine and pethidine, leading to accumulation of these drugs in the fetal tissues. The neonatal liver is able to metabolize amide local anaesthetics, but the elimination of pethidine and its metabolite norpethidine is prolonged.

ANALGESIA

For most women the pain during labour is moderate to severe. However, the degree of pain is variable and some women are able to deliver without any analgesia. Pain is worse in primiparae. Pain during the first stage of labour is caused by uterine contractions and cervical dilatation. Impulses are carried along visceral C-fibres that cross the base of the broad ligament and accompany the sympathetic nerves to the spinal cord. The pain is referred to the associated dermatomes: initially T11 and T12, and as the first stage progresses the adjacent dermatomes (T10 and L1) are involved. Backache may be severe and is often associated with an occipitoposterior fetal position. In the second stage, pressure from the descent of the presenting fetal part causes pelvic distension and stretching and tearing of the perineum. These structures have a somatic innervation from the pudendal nerves (S2–S4).

As well as the humanitarian importance of pain relief, effective analgesia in labour has physiological benefits for both mother and fetus. Maternal release of catecholamines is lowered, reducing the hypertensive response to contractions and lessening maternal metabolic acidosis. Hyperventilation during contractions that might otherwise lead to a detrimental shift to the left of the oxygen–haemoglobin dissociation curve is eliminated. Uterine blood flow may increase and a dysfunctional labour (uncoordinated uterine contractions) may become normal.

The woman (and her partner) who has attended childbirth classes will be better educated about the physiology of childbirth and the techniques of pain relief during labour. Techniques such as hypnosis, transcutaneous electrical nerve stimulation (TENS) and acupuncture have not been shown to be of use for the majority of women. Psychological conditioning or psychoprophylaxis aims to distract the mother from the pain by focusing her concentration on specific objects and breathing patterns. Pain scores may be reduced but requests for analgesia are similar to women not using the technique.

INHALATION ANALGESIA

The only inhalation analgesia currently licensed in the UK for obstetric use is 50% nitrous oxide in oxygen. This is usually given from a pre-mixed preparation known as Entonox and administered through a Tunstall (demand) valve. Entonox is most useful in the first stage of labour when it must be inhaled with each contraction. The mother must be instructed in its use, particularly the necessity to begin inhalations at the very beginning of the contraction as the onset time to analgesia is in the order of 45 s. Entonox will not produce a completely pain-free labour and one-third of women find it completely ineffective. Concerns regarding environmental pollution and chronic exposure to nitrous oxide may lead to this form of analgesia becoming less popular as effective scavenging is difficult to achieve. Use of low concentrations of volatile agents, for example isoflurane in oxygen are well described but little used.

SEDATIVES AND TRANQUILIZERS

Barbiturates and benzodiazepines are no longer used to sedate mothers because of the risk of neonatal depression. Furthermore, most mothers wish to be aware of the events at parturition and dislike the amnesia induced by these drugs. Diazepam is used, however, for control of eclamptic seizures.

OPIOIDS

Opioid drugs provide useful, if incomplete, analgesia. Their use necessarily involves a balance of unwanted maternal and fetal side-effects and effective analgesia. Pethidine causes nausea, vomiting and drowsiness in the mother. Pethidine may cause respiratory depression in the newborn baby and its metabolite norpethidine may depress neurobehavioural scores for 3 days after birth. In the UK intramuscular pethidine is licensed for use by unsupervised midwives. The peak effect occurs after 40 min and the duration of action is about 3 h. Pethidine provides some analgesia for about half of the women it is given to. Other opioid drugs produce equal analgesia, but may differ in their side-effects. Morphine is associated with an increased incidence of respiratory depression in the baby; synthetic opioids such as fentanyl and alfentanil produce a rapid onset of analgesia but placental transfer occurs early; and the antagonist–agonist drugs such as butorphanol and nalbuphine lead to maternal sedation. Patient-controlled analgesia using intravenous opioid drugs is useful when regional blockade is contraindicated and gives the mother a degree of control over her analgesia.

REGIONAL ANALGESIA

Regional analgesia provides the labouring mother with the most effective and reliable method of pain relief. Importantly the mother remains awake, alert and able to participate in the birth. Regional analgesia techniques include lumbar epidural blockade, caudal epidural blockade, paracervical and pudendal block and spinal (subarachnoid) anaesthesia.

CHOICE OF DRUGS FOR REGIONAL TECHNIQUES

Local anaesthetics

Bupivacaine is the most commonly used local anaesthetic agent in obstetric practice. It has a moderate speed of onset, produces relatively little motor block, provides good analgesia in low concentrations and has a long duration of action. A 0.5% solution produces good analgesia, but many mothers experience weakness of the legs. Bupivacaine 0.25% produces analgesia that is satisfactory, but not as complete as with bupivacaine 0.5%, and the incidence of motor block is reduced. Once an effective block is established it may be maintained with either repeated bolus injection of 0.25% solutions or a continuous infusion of 0.125% solution or weaker. Bupivacaine 0.75% is no longer recommended because of the high incidence of systemic toxicity following accidental intravascular injection. A hyperbaric solution of bupivacaine 0.5% in 8% dextrose is available for spinal blockade.

Lignocaine has a shorter duration of action than bupivacaine and is not suitable for providing continuous analgesia during labour. However, onset times are slightly shorter for lignocaine when compared to bupivacaine and 2.0% solutions of lignocaine may be combined with adrenaline 1:200 000 to establish a block suitable for Caesarean section. Alternatively lignocaine may be combined with bupivacaine to produce a block of rapid onset and long duration.

Prilocaine is not suitable for analgesia in labour because of the risk of methaemoglobinaemia in both mother and fetus. Etidocaine produces an unacceptably high incidence of motor blockade. 2-chloroprocaine is an ester local anaesthetic with a rapid onset and short duration of action. Its use has been linked with possible neurotoxicity. Ropivacaine has a similar profile to bupivacaine, but with less cardiotoxicity. Etidocaine and 2-chloroprocaine are not currently available in the UK; ropivacaine has recently been granted a license in the UK.

Opioids

The use of epidural opioids for obstetric analgesia has not been universally successful. Epidural morphine (up to 10 mg) produces only moderate analgesia. Fentanyl, 100–200 µg, produces analgesia within 10 min and will last for 60–140 min. The pain relief may be adequate in the first and second stages of labour (but not for instrumental or operative delivery). However, up to 50% of mothers will experience troublesome side-effects such as pruritus, nausea and vomiting, urinary retention or drowsiness. There is also significant risk of respiratory depression in the mother. The use of opioids alone may be an acceptable technique in mothers with contraindications to local anaesthetics such as aortic stenosis, or cyanotic congenital heart disease. Opioids given directly into the subarachnoid space may be of more use.

Adjuvant drugs

Adrenaline mixed with local anaesthetics in a concentration of 1:200 000 reduces absorption of the local anaesthetic, lengthens the duration of the block and may intensify the block. Such actions are useful when large volumes of local anaesthetic are being used to create a block for Caesarean section. Sodium bicarbonate may be added to local anaesthetic drugs to carbonate the drug and increase the speed of onset.

EPIDURAL ANALGESIA

The primary indication for epidural analgesia is pain. Other indications include maternal, fetal and obstetric reasons. Women with significant heart disease benefit from effective analgesia to prevent further stress being placed on the heart during contractions and expulsive efforts. However, a technique which induces sympathetic blockade should be used with caution if the heart condition precludes an increase in cardiac output to compensate for systemic vasodilatation, for example aortic stenosis. The avoidance of hyperventilation is beneficial to women with respiratory disease and the prevention of increases in intracranial pressure may benefit those with cerebral disease. Epidural analgesia reduces the increase in blood pressure during labour and is used in hypertensive mothers, particularly those with pregnancy induced hypertension, providing their coagulation and platelet function is normal. Fetal indications include prematurity, breech delivery and multiple birth. Obstetric indications include prolonged or dysfunctional labour and an increased likelihood of instrumental delivery or Caesarean section. The contraindications to epidural analgesia are maternal refusal, hypovolaemia, coagulation disorder, local sepsis, bacteraemia, spinal deformities and severe fetal distress. The technique should be used with caution in women with neurological disorders as a relapse may be attributed to the epidural analgesia. The relationship between the antiplatelet effect of aspirin and the likelihood of epidural haematoma is not clear. It is impractical to perform a bleeding time test before placement of an epidural catheter. An assessment of the likely risks and benefits must be made and the potential risks discussed with the mother. Finally, epidural analgesia must only be performed if there are sufficient trained staff (including anaesthetists, obstetricians and midwives) to care for the mother and if there are resuscitation facilities immediately available.

The effect of epidural analgesia on the mode of delivery is hotly debated. Although many studies have confirmed that the likelihood of an instrumental delivery is increased following epidural analgesia, many women receive such analgesia because of an obstetric indication which by itself increases the change of an instrumental delivery. Furthermore, mothers who choose epidural analgesia may have other differences compared to those who do not. Because of the effects of sensory and motor block on maternal expulsive efforts and pelvic floor musculature, it is accepted that the second stage of labour may be prolonged. Providing time is allowed for descent of the fetal head and there is no evidence for fetal distress, the incidence of instrumental delivery is probably no higher than in those women not receiving epidural analgesia. The status of the fetus must be carefully monitored during epidural analgesia especially while the block is being established.

PLACEMENT OF THE EPIDURAL CATHETER

The epidural catheter is usually placed when labour is established. Intravenous access must be ensured with a large-bore (16 G or larger) cannula. Historically it has been taught that fluid preloading with 500–1000 ml of crystalloid reduces the incidence of hypotension secondary to sympathetic blockade. However, recent work has failed to confirm reliable benefit from preloading. 1000 ml of crystalloid should be started and infused while the catheter is being positioned. Episodes of hypotension can be treated as necessary. The mother is placed in either the sitting or lateral decubitus position and the skin overlying the lumbar vertebra thoroughly disinfected and anaesthetized by infiltration with local anaesthetic. Identification of the epidural space is usually by the loss of resistance technique using either saline or air. The catheter is inserted through either the L2/3 or L3/4 interspace. No more than 4 cm of catheter should be left in the epidural space and a bacterial filter should be attached to the distal end of the catheter.

The position of the catheter must be checked to detect intravenous or intrathecal placement. Aspiration through the catheter is not a reliable test although it is recommended before each top-up as the catheter tip can migrate during use. A more reliable technique is the test dose of local anaesthetic. The composition of the test dose must be such that it can detect subarachnoid placement without causing a dangerously high block: 3 ml of either lignocaine 1.5% or bupivacaine 0.5% is usually used. The addition of adrenaline 15 µg (3 ml local anaesthetic with adrenaline 1:200 000) is recommended to aid detection of the catheter being placed intravascularly. The maternal heart rate must be continuously observed for at least 2 min and an increase of more than 20 b.p.m. is regarded as indicative of intravenous placement. However, false positives may occur, for example if a contraction occurs immediately after the injection. Adrenaline should not be used in mothers with hypertension or cardiovascular disease. Subdural catheterization (when the catheter tip lies between the dura and the arachnoid membrane) is frequently unrecognized and may lead to a dangerously high block unless the sensory level is measured regularly during labour. It can be differentiated from a normal block and a total spinal block on the basis of the associated clinical features described in Table 31.1.

TECHNIQUES OF EPIDURAL ANALGESIA

The most common technique for provision of analgesia during the first stage of labour following the establishment of an adequate block is intermittent injection (topping-up) of local anaesthetic. The block is established with 10 ml of bupivacaine 0.25% or 0.5%. Thereafter the block is maintained with intermittent injections of a low concentration of bupivacaine such as 0.25% or 0.125%. In most hospitals in the UK midwives are allowed to perform such top-ups according to a local protocol after the medical staff have confirmed the position of the catheter. The protocol should describe the volume and strength of agent to be used, the posture of the patient during administration and the details of blood pressure (every 5 min for 20 min) and other measurements required immediately following the top-up. The protocol may also include instructions for providing a block for the second stage of labour.

The use of continuous infusions or patient-controlled epidural analgesia is becoming more common. The advantages of infusion techniques are avoidance of pain before the next top-up, less work for midwifery staff and reduced episodes of hypotension and fetal heart rate abnormalities compared with bolus

Table 31.1 Clinical features of epidural block, subdural block and total spinal block

	Epidural block	Subdural block	Total spinal block
Onset time	Slow	Slow	Rapid
Spread	As expected	Higher than expected, sacral sparing	Higher than expected, sacral block
Nature of block	Segmental	Patchy	Dense
Motor block	Minimal	Minimal	Dense
Hypotension	Less than spinal, dependent on extent of block	Less than spinal, dependent on extent of block	Marked
Apnoea	Unlikely	Unlikely	Common
Conscious level	Normal	Normal	Depressed

Modified, with permission, from Glosten, B. Epidural and spinal anesthesia/analgesia, in *Obstetric Anesthesia: Principles and Practice* (ed D.H. Chestnut) pp. 353–78 (Table on page 371) published by Mosby-Year Book Inc, St Louis, 1994.

Table 31.2 Suggested technique for continuous epidural infusion of local anaesthetic and opioid to provide analgesia during labour

1. Exclude patients with contraindications and obtain informed consent
2. Ensure intravenous access with large bore cannula and start to infuse 1000 ml of crystalloid
3. Start fetal heart rate monitoring
4. Place patient in lateral decubitus or sitting position as preferred
5. Disinfect skin and infiltrate with local anaesthetic
6. Locate epidural space with loss-of-resistance technique
7. Thread catheter and leave no more than 4 cm in epidural space
8. After negative aspiration give test dose of 3 ml 1.5% lignocaine with 1:200 000 adrenaline
9. Measure maternal heart rate continuously and blood pressure after 2 min. Continue to measure blood pressure every 5 min for 20 min
10. If test dose negative after 5 min, give 10 ml 0.25% bupivacaine with 50 µg fentanyl (1 ml) in two divided doses
11. Prepare infusion of 10 ml 0.5% bupivacaine, 150 µg fentanyl (3 ml) and 47 ml 0.9% normal saline and start at 10 ml h^{-1} by syringe pump
12. Maintain sensory block between T10 and L1 by varying infusion rate between 5 and 15 ml h^{-1}
13. Continue regular sensory level, maternal blood pressure, and fetal heart rate measurements
14. Prescribe escape top-up (5 ml 0.25% bupivacaine) and instrumental delivery top-up (10 ml 0.5% bupivacaine)

dose top-ups. However, top-ups may still be required for break-through pain. Infusion protocols often use opioid drugs added to the local anaesthetic. The addition of opioids reduces the requirement for local anaesthetic drugs by up to 50% (usually a lower concentration is used) and may, therefore, allow retention of the ability to push in the second stage of labour and reduce the incidence of motor block. A suggested regimen for a continuous infusion technique is given in Table 31.2. These continuous infusions of local anaesthetic and opioid drugs have become known colloquially as 'mobile epidurals' as the mothers may remain able to walk and transfer to a chair. In addition there is a reduced need to catheterize the bladder. However, the use of opioid drugs in the epidural space introduces other side-effects. Patient-controlled epidural analgesia may allow the mother more control over her pain relief, but experience with this technique is still limited.

FAILURE OF EPIDURAL ANALGESIA

Most women experience complete analgesia throughout labour after establishment of an epidural block with local anaesthetic. Complete failure of the block is usually due to incorrect placement of the epidural catheter. Epidural analgesia may also fail if an inadequate dose of local anaesthetic is used or if the block is allowed to wear off before the next top-up is given.

Unilateral block may occur if the catheter advances anterior to the spinal cord and is trapped against the anterior aspect of the dura. Withdrawal of the catheter and further injection of local anaesthetic may help. A missed segment (an unblocked spinal segment often corresponding to a dermatome in the groin) is the most common failure of epidural analgesia (5%). Withdrawal of the catheter followed by administration of a stronger concentration of local anaesthetic with the unblocked groin in the dependent position is usually effective. For these partial blocks the use of a bolus dose of an opioid (for example, fentanyl 50–100 µg in 5–10 ml normal saline) may be helpful. If the block remains unsatisfactory the catheter should be re-sited. Backache in the presence of an otherwise satisfactory block is often due to a persistent occipitoposterior position of the fetal head and may be helped by a top-up with the mother in the sitting position.

COMPLICATIONS OF EPIDURAL ANALGESIA

The most common complication of epidural analgesia is maternal hypotension. The incidence can be reduced by adopting a position to minimize aortocaval compression. If hypotension occurs, the full lateral position should be used, oxygen given by face-mask, a further infusion of fluid started and, if necessary, a vasoconstrictor such as ephedrine given (3–6 mg bolus, intravenously).

During pregnancy and particularly during a contraction, the epidural veins are engorged. The risk of placement of the catheter in an epidural vein is consequently higher than in the non-obstetric population. A catheter that has entered a vein can be withdrawn until blood can no longer be aspirated and then a test dose cautiously given. If local anaesthetic is inadvertently given intravenously toxic reactions including generalized convulsions and cardiovascular collapse may occur. If the early signs of toxicity such as peri-oral paraesthesia, tinnitus and confusion are detected, measures must be taken to prevent progression to convulsions. Prophylactic anticonvulsants (for example diazepam 5 mg i.v. or p.r.) and oxygen by face-mask should be given. If fits occur the mother will require tracheal intubation and ventilation of the lungs. Toxicity may progress to cardiac arrest. Successful resuscitation of cardiac arrest in the mother at term requires left lateral uterine displacement by an assistant whilst external cardiac massage is performed. Emergency Caesarean section may be required before the mother can be resuscitated, and external cardiac massage may be needed for a prolonged period to allow the local anaesthetic to 'unbind' from the myocardium.

Dural puncture with the Tuohy needle is usually obvious. However, intrathecal placement of the catheter may go unrecognized and is the reason why a test dose is mandatory. Furthermore, migration of the catheter during labour may lead to intrathecal injection occurring at any time even after several uneventful top-ups. The result may be a total spinal block and is characterized by apnoea, profound hypotension and unconsciousness (see Table 31.1). Full resuscitative measures are indicated and Caesarean section may be necessary before full recovery can take place. Headache following accidental dural puncture is common in obstetric patients. The characteristic frontal or occipital headache is exacerbated by bright lights and the upright position and is relieved by lying flat. After dural puncture the catheter should be resited and all subsequent top-ups given by medical staff. Some authorities recommend that, if dural puncture occurs, the catheter should be deliberately passed into the intrathecal space and small spinal doses of local anaesthetic used for analgesia. If a headache occurs during labour, elective forceps delivery should be advised. After delivery, 1000 ml of normal saline should be infused down the resited catheter over 24 h. In addition, an intravenous infusion should be continued to keep the mother well hydrated. If the headache persists or causes increasing debility an epidural blood patch should be performed. Using full aseptic precautions 20 ml of autologous blood is placed into the epidural space over 1 min. Although the injection may be painful and can result in long-term backache, it is successful in relieving the headache in 90% of patients. The blood patch may be repeated once if the first attempt is not helpful.

Women receiving epidural analgesia may be at increased risk of developing persistent backache, although this has not been demonstrated by prospective studies. Although it has been suggested that the pain is due to adoption of abnormal postures during labour the exact aetiology and prognosis have yet to be determined. Permanent neurological damage is very rare following epidural analgesia. However, persistent distal paraesthesia or pain at the site of catheter insertion warrants further investigation for epidural abscesses or haematoma. Shivering is common following epidural analgesia with local anaesthetic drugs and if troublesome can be reduced by the addition of epidural fentanyl.

SPINAL ANAESTHESIA

Spinal anaesthesia is popular for instrumental vaginal deliveries and has also been used by continuous infusion to provide analgesia during the first stage of labour. Spinal anaesthesia is rapid to perform, has a high success rate and produces reliable analgesia. The saddle or low-spinal block provides analgesia to the vulva, vagina and perineum and may be used for low forceps, episiotomy or repair of tears: 1 ml hyperbaric local anaesthetic such as 0.5% bupivacaine is usually satisfactory; 1.5–2.0 ml hyperbaric solution produces a mid-spinal block up to the lower thoracic dermatomes and provides analgesia for intra-uterine manipulation, breech delivery and operative vaginal delivery. The mid-spinal block is also used for manual removal of the placenta. It should be remembered that there is a wide individual variation in the spinal level of block produced after introduction of local anaesthetic into the subarachnoid space. As well as ensuring that the block has reached the required level for the planned procedure it is essential to be aware of the possibility of an unexpectedly high block. Combined spinal/epidural techniques are now being used in some centres in the UK and USA to provide pain relief in labour.

SPINAL OPIOIDS

Small doses of opioids placed in the subarachnoid space reduce the possibility of significant transfer of drug to the fetus and produce more effective analgesia compared with epidural opioids. Morphine 0.25–1.5 mg produces good analgesia for the first and second stage of labour within 45 min. Fentanyl 25–50 μg produces analgesia after 5 min which lasts about 1 h. Morphine and fentanyl may be combined to produce analgesia of rapid onset and long duration. Like epidural opioids, spinal opioids avoid motor block and pharmacological sympathectomy in the mother. However, there is also a high incidence of side effects similar to those seen with epidural opioids.

CAUDAL ANALGESIA

Although caudal epidural analgesia has been used for many years it is unpopular because of the risk of the introducing needle passing through the mother's sacrum and rectum and into the fetal presenting part. Even small volumes of local anaesthetic injected directly into the fetus lead to toxicity and fetal death. Large volumes (10–20 ml) of local anaesthetic are needed by the caudal route to establish a block up to T10. The technique is usually rapid to perform and quickly establishes perineal anaesthesia for the second stage of labour, although there is a failure rate of around 10%. A finger placed in the mother's rectum during insertion of the needle will reduce the likelihood of transversing the rectum and entering the fetus.

PARACERVICAL BLOCK

An injection into the parametrium at the base of the broad ligament provides effective analgesia for the first stage of labour for up to 90% of women. It is performed by injecting local anaesthetic submucosally into the fornices either side of the vagina. Continuous fetal heart monitoring has shown that paracervical anaesthesia is associated with a high incidence of fetal bradycardia, as well as depressed neonates and even intrauterine death. This may be due to a direct action of local anaesthetics causing vasoconstriction of the uterine arteries in the broad ligament and so reducing uterine blood flow. As a result this method of analgesia is no longer recommended except in exceptional circumstances.

PUDENDAL NERVE BLOCK

The pudendal nerves are formed from the lower sacral roots (S2–S4) and supply the vaginal vault, perineum and the rectum and may be blocked as they pass through the pudendal canal on the lateral wall of the ischiorectal fossa posterior to the ischial spines: 10 ml of local anaesthetic is injected around each nerve using a 10 cm needle passed either transvaginally or transperineally. In addition the labia must be infiltrated to block the perineal branches of the ilio-inguinal and genito-femoral nerves. Because of the large volumes needed to complete the block a weak solution of local anaesthetic must be used. Pudendal nerve block should provide analgesia for outlet procedures in the second stages of labour. However, many women do not obtain full analgesia after pudendal nerve block and it is not a reliable technique for instrumental delivery. It does not provide effective analgesia for contractions in the first stage of labour or for high forceps deliveries.

LOCAL INFILTRATION

Local infiltration of local anaesthetic into the perineum provides satisfactory analgesia for episiotomy or repair of simple tears. More severe tears require a more extensive block. Under exceptional circumstances a Caesarean section can be performed with local infiltration; large volumes of dilute solutions of local anaesthetics combined with 1:400 000 adrenaline are injected by the surgeon into each layer before its incision.

GENERAL ANAESTHESIA FOR CAESAREAN SECTION

The proportion of mothers being delivered by Caesarean section depends on many factors both medical and cultural and varies widely from the UK and Europe (13%) to the USA (20–25%) and even higher elsewhere. General and regional anaesthetic techniques are used. The choice of technique depends on the degree of urgency, associated medical conditions and, most importantly, the mother's wishes. The number of women receiving general anaesthesia for Caesarean section in the UK is gradually falling. This probably represents an improvement in the training and skills of anaesthetists in providing regional anaesthesia and increasing acceptance of these techniques by mothers and their attendants.

The primary advantage of general anaesthesia for Caesarean section is the reliability and rapidity of onset of a state in which the operation can be performed. When delivery is truly an emergency, for example with persistent severe fetal bradycardia or cord prolapse, general anaesthesia can be induced within 3 min and the patient ready for surgery within 5 min. The triennial UK Report on Confidential Enquiries into Maternal Deaths indicates that many of the deaths directly due to anaesthesia are related to general anaesthesia. Although aspiration of gastric contents, failed intubation and unrecognized oesophageal intubation have become less common in recent reports, their continuing occurrence represents a depressing failure of care. The standard general anaesthetic technique involves pre-oxygenation, intravenous induction, rapid sequence tracheal intubation, balanced general anaesthesia with muscle relaxation and artificial ventilation of the lungs. Physiological and anatomical differences of the term mother and the presence of the fetus mandate some alterations to the anaesthetic technique compared with that used for the non-pregnant patient.

ASPIRATION OF GASTRIC CONTENTS

Aspiration of gastric contents is a catastrophic event during late pregnancy and labour and leads to the 'asthma-like' syndrome described by Mendelson. The risk of regurgitation and aspiration is increased because of delayed gastric emptying during labour, raised intragastric pressure and reduced lower oesophageal sphincter tone. Most labour wards operate a policy of withholding solid food to women in labour and restricting fluids to frequent but small amounts of water or tea. Other fluid requirements can be supplied by intravenous therapy. Although attempts can be made to empty the stomach with emetics or large-bore orogastric tubes, these techniques are extremely unpleasant for the mother and are not guaranteed to be completely effective. Pharmacological attempts to speed up the emptying of the stomach or increase the lower oesophageal sphincter tone are also unreliable because of the antagonistic action of other commonly used drugs such as the opioids and atropine. The H_2-antagonists such as ranitidine and the proton-pump inhibitor omeprazole will reduce both gastric volume and acidity. Premedication with ranitidine 150 mg, orally the night before surgery and again 1 h before induction is effective before elective surgery. The prophylactic use of H_2-antagonists during labour is usually restricted to high-risk pregnancies such as breech presentations and twins. Their value when given parenterally immediately before emergency Caesarean section is not proven. To further reduce the acidity of gastric contents oral antacids are administered before induction of anaesthesia. Particulate antacids such as magnesium trisilicate may actually contribute to lung damage if aspirated and a non-particulate antacid such as 30 ml 0.3 M sodium citrate should be used. Because many factors contribute to the increased risk of aspiration in pregnant women, it is not clear what the exact period of risk is. Most authorities assume that it starts from the second trimester of pregnancy. After delivery, the risk continues for at least 24 h and precautions probably be taken for the first 48 h after delivery. Any pregnant women with symptoms of gastro-oesophageal reflux should be considered at risk.

TRACHEAL INTUBATION

A balanced technique with tracheal intubation is considered the safest form of general anaesthesia. Correct positioning of a cuffed tracheal tube as soon as possible after loss of consciousness is essential to prevent aspiration of regurgitated gastric contents. Any

Table 31.3 Failed intubation drill

1. Call for help
2. Maintain cricoid pressure
3. Attempt IPPV with facemask and 100% oxygen until suxamethonium metabolized
4. If obstructed, try oropharyngeal airway, nasopharyngeal airway, LMA, or release of cricoid pressure
5. If still obstructed proceed to needle cricothyoidotomy and jet insufflate lungs
6. If oxygenation adequate decide if immediate Caesarean section is essential? (For severe fetal distress or maternal haemorrhage)
7. Yes – proceed with spontaneously breathing inhalational anaesthesia (e.g. halothane and 60% nitrous oxide in oxygen), maintain cricoid pressure. Prepare for greater than normal loss of blood
8. No – turn to left lateral position and allow to awaken
9. Consider regional technique or awake fibreoptic intubation

technique using spontaneous respiration without tracheal intubation is unacceptable. The laryngeal mask airway (LMA) does not form an effective seal around the larynx and may even direct regurgitated material from the oesophagus in to the laryngeal opening. However, the LMA may be helpful in establishing a patient following failed intubation.

The incidence of failed tracheal intubation is approximately eight times higher in obstetric than in non-obstetric practice. Ideally, difficult tracheal intubations should be detected prior to induction of anaesthesia and a careful evaluation of the upper airway for ease of intubation should be performed as part of the preoperative assessment. Unfortunately, all the currently popular bedside methods of predicting difficult intubation suffer from both low sensitivity and specificity. However, if intubation is predicted to be difficult, extra assistance may be requested, an awake fibreoptic intubation considered or a regional technique recommended. There are many possible reasons why intubation may be more difficult in pregnant women including large breasts preventing laryngoscope insertion, the presence of laryngeal oedema in patients with pre-eclampsia, full dentition in young women, cricoid pressure distorting the larynx and the fact that most anaesthetics for emergency Caesarean section are given by trainee anaesthetists (who may not allow enough time for onset of full muscle relaxation after suxamethonium). A failed intubation drill is essential and one suggested drill is described in Table 31.3. Patients do not die from failure to intubate the trachea, but from prolonged attempts to intubate and inadequate oxygenation. In the vast majority of cases, including most emergency Caesarean sections, there is sufficient time to allow the mother to regain consciousness and be intubated by more experienced personnel or for a regional technique to be used. If oxygenation can be maintained and the procedure must proceed, then cricoid pressure is maintained whilst the depth of anaesthesia is increased with inhalational agents in the spontaneously breathing patient.

INDUCTION OF ANAESTHESIA

Following premedication the patient is placed on the operating table with left lateral tilt. A large-bore intravenous cannula is inserted and an infusion of crystalloid fluid started. Full monitoring including ECG, non-invasive blood pressure and pulse oximetry is attached to the patient. All other equipment including capnograph, a selection of laryngoscopes and tracheal tubes, a laryngeal mask airway, stylets and gum elastic bougie and equipment for cricothyroid puncture and transtracheal jet ventilation are checked. The presence of a trained assistant able to apply cricoid pressure correctly is mandatory. Full pre-oxygenation with 3 min of 100% oxygen from a tight fitting face-mask and oxygen reservoir is important because of the reduced functional residual capacity and increased oxygen consumption at term. In a true emergency 3 or 4 vital capacity breaths of 100% oxygen is an acceptable alternative. Cricoid pressure is applied from the start of injection of the intravenous induction agent and continued until the airway is secured by a cuffed tube in the trachea. Thiopentone 4–5 mg kg^{-1} is the most commonly used induction agent. Etomidate may be used if there are concerns about cardiovascular stability and ketamine is the safest agent in patients who may be hypovolaemic or have acute asthma. Ketamine will depress the fetus and is contraindicated in patients with hypertension. The dose of induction agent used must ensure complete loss of consciousness in these patients, who have not received a sedative premedicant. To permit rapid tracheal intubation, suxamethonium 1.5 mg kg^{-1} is the muscle relaxant of choice following induction of anaesthesia. It is essential that correct placement of the tracheal tube is immediately confirmed by capnography.

MAINTENANCE OF GENERAL ANAESTHESIA

Anaesthesia is maintained with a balanced technique including muscle relaxation with an intermediate duration non-depolarizing neuromuscular blocking agent such as atracurium or vecuronium. The lungs are ventilated with nitrous oxide 50% in oxygen and a low dose of a volatile agent. Care should be taken to avoid hyperventilation which leads to vasoconstriction, reduced uterine blood flow and a leftward shift of the oxygen–haemoglobin dissociation curve. Higher inspired concentrations of oxygen may be of benefit in cases of severe fetal distress. Before the use of volatile agents in obstetric practice, there was a high incidence of either recall or vivid dreaming. The risk of recall can be dramatically reduced by the addition of low inspired concentrations of volatile agents without increasing bleeding secondary to uterine relaxation.

The minimum alveolar concentrations of the volatile agents are reduced in pregnancy and halothane 0.5% or enflurane 1.0% is sufficient. Higher concentrations should be used in the first few minutes to provide 'overpressure' and reduce the risk of awareness, and are also required if 100% oxygen is being used because of fetal distress. Following delivery of the baby and clamping of the umbilical cord, syntocinon 10 units is given intravenously and an opioid analgesic drug, for example morphine 10–15 mg, is given. Blood loss is usually about 500–1000 ml, but transfusion is rarely required. There is an 'auto-transfusion' of blood from the uterus at delivery and after administration of syntocinon.

REVERSAL AND RECOVERY

At the end of surgery, the anaesthetic agents are discontinued, neuromuscular blockade is reversed and the mother's trachea extubated when she has regained consciousness and her airway reflexes have returned. Extubation and immediate recovery should be in the lateral position and oxygen given until the mother is fully awake. Non-steroidal anti-inflammatory drugs (NSAIDs) are a useful supplement to opioid analgesics postoperatively. A diclofenac 100 mg suppository can be placed in the rectum before the end of surgery and diclofenac continued for 48 h. Specific contraindications to NSAIDs include a history of peptic ulceration, asthma, renal failure and pregnancy induced hypertension. An opioid such as morphine 10–15 mg intramuscularly, 3 hourly as required, should be prescribed. Alternatively a patient-controlled analgesia system to deliver morphine can be used.

REGIONAL ANAESTHESIA FOR CAESAREAN SECTION

The keen awareness of the risks of general anaesthesia in obstetric practice, highlighted by the triennial reports in the UK, have stimulated the refinement of regional anaesthetic techniques. In addition, maternal desire to be awake and for both parents to be present at the birth have encouraged anaesthetists to pursue these techniques further. The advantages of regional anaesthesia are the avoidance of the hazards of inhalation of gastric contents and failed intubation, the elimination of the problem of awareness, absence of respiratory depression in the baby, reduction of blood loss, and avoidance of the 'hangover' effects of general anaesthesia whilst the mother is establishing bonding and feeding. Disadvantages of regional anaesthesia are the time taken to establish the block, hypotension leading to a reduction of placental blood flow, pain or discomfort during surgery because of inadequate block and vomiting and shivering during surgery. Patient satisfaction with regional anaesthesia for Caesarean section is increased by a careful explanation preoperatively of the technique, its benefits and risks. This should include the possibility of headache after dural puncture, the use of general anaesthesia should the regional technique fail and reassurance that any pain will be treated. It should be emphasized that, although pain is unlikely, not all sensation will be lost. Visceral stimulation may occur with placement of high abdominal packs or delivery of the uterus onto the abdominal wall. Surgeons should be discouraged from either of these manoeuvres. The choice of regional techniques includes lumbar epidural, spinal and combined spinal–epidural anaesthesia. With these techniques it is essential to ensure that the block to cold sensation extends from T6 (preferably T4) to S5. Preparation of the patient is identical to that for general anaesthesia including oral antacids before the start of the anaesthetic. In addition, it is customary to infuse 1000 ml of crystalloid fluid before establishment of the block to reduce the incidence of hypotension. The benefit of such preloading remains unproven. The practitioner should be prepared to supplement intravenous fluids with ephedrine at the first sign of hypotension.

EPIDURAL ANAESTHESIA FOR CAESAREAN SECTION

Epidural anaesthesia may be used for emergency Caesarean section in women who already have a working epidural catheter *in situ*. It is also the technique of choice in some centres for elective surgery particularly if cardiovascular stability (achieved with careful small, incremental doses of local anaesthetic) is desirable such as in severe pregnancy induced hypertension, providing clotting is normal.

For elective Caesarean section, the epidural catheter is inserted in the usual manner and a test dose given to ensure correct placement. An initial bolus of 10 ml 0.5% bupivacaine or 2% lignocaine with 1:200 000 adrenaline is given in the supine wedged position. However, lignocaine may not provide anaesthesia of sufficient duration should surgery be prolonged. The sensory level is determined and then further local anaesthetic given on the basis of 1.5 ml for every unblocked dermatomal level below T6. The total volume of local anaesthetic required is very variable (15–45 ml). For emergency Caesarean section a rapid-onset block can be obtained by the use of a mixture made up as follows: 10 ml 0.5% bupivacaine with 1:200 000 adrenaline, 10 ml 2% lignocaine, 2 ml 8.4% sodium bicarbonate. Depending on the presence of a pre-existing level of block from the use of the catheter for analgesia, 15–22 ml of this mixture is given slowly over 5 min. A block suitable for Caesarean section will be obtained within 10–15 min. The mother must be maintained in a wedged position to prevent aorto-caval compression and she should breathe oxygen until after delivery of the baby. Breakthrough pain during the surgery can be treated with intravenous opioids such as fentanyl and persistent discomfort must be 'relieved' with general anaesthesia. Fentanyl 50–100 μg given epidurally before delivery does not appear to have an adverse effect on the baby. Following delivery and clamping of the umbilical cord, epidural fentanyl 100 μg or morphine 2–3 mg may be given for postoperative analgesia. Parenteral opioids should not be given within 6 h of epidural fentanyl or 12 h of morphine without careful assessment of the mother and use of respiratory monitoring. However, NSAIDs may be used and should be started at the end of surgery.

SPINAL ANAESTHESIA

Spinal anaesthesia is popular in many centres for both elective Caesarean section and emergency procedures because of the ease and rapid onset of the block. The success rate for spinal anaesthesia is high and an extensive block (to permit surgery) is easily obtained. Only small doses of local anaesthetic are used and there are no risks of toxicity. The incidence of post-dural puncture headache has been reduced with the introduction of smaller 'pencil-point' needles such as the Sprotte or Whitacre. A needle no larger than 25 G should be used. Hypotension is more common after spinal anaesthesia compared with epidural anaesthesia and this has led to concerns regarding the effect of spinal anaesthesia on placental and umbilical blood flow. Spinal anaesthesia is not a suitable technique for patients with cardiac disease or severe hypertension or in cases with severe fetal distress. Aorto-caval compression must be studiously avoided and hypotension treated urgently. Many practitioners add ephedrine 30 mg to the second one litre bag of crystalloid as prophylaxis against hypotension; 2.5–2.75 ml of hyperbaric ('heavy') 0.5% bupivacaine will produce an adequate block for most patients. However, spread of local anaesthetic after spinal administration is unpredictable even with the use of hyperbaric solutions. Preservative-free morphine 0.1–0.2 mg may be mixed with the local anaesthetic to provide postoperative analgesia.

COMBINED SPINAL–EPIDURAL ANAESTHESIA

To overcome the limitations associated with spinal and epidural techniques, they can be combined. A small dose of hyperbaric local anaesthetic is injected into the cerebrospinal fluid to provide a dense lumbosacral block. The extent of the block is determined and the block is then extended cranially with epidural administration of local anaesthetic to provide anaesthesia up to T6. The epidural catheter can also be used to give opioid drugs after delivery of the baby to provide postoperative analgesia. The spinal injection can be performed at one lumbar intervertebral space and the epidural catheter inserted at another space. Alternatively kits are now manufactured with modified Tuohy needles that permit passage of a spinal needle through the lumen into the subarachnoid space or through a tunnel welded to the side of the Tuohy needle. The spinal needle is then removed and a catheter threaded into the epidural space.

ANAESTHESIA FOR COMPLICATED PREGNANCY

HAEMORRHAGE

Haemorrhage is a major cause of death during pregnancy. Antepartum haemorrhage is usually due to placental abruption or placenta praevia. Abruption is often associated with development of disseminated intravascular coagulation (DIC). Postnatal haemorrhage, which may occur with conditions such as placenta accreta or uterine trauma, may necessitate anaesthesia for hysterectomy. The role of the anaesthetist in the management of severe haemorrhage includes resuscitation, correction of coagulopathies which may be dilutional or due to disseminated intravascular coagulation and provision of safe anaesthesia for Caesarean section or other surgery if necessary. The assistance of the transfusion laboratory staff and haematologists is essential. Ideally lost blood should be replaced with crossmatched whole blood. Group O Rhesus negative blood may be life-saving in severe haemorrhage before crossmatched blood is available. Clotting factor and platelet transfusions will be wasted if given during massive on-going haemorrhage and are best reserved until surgical haemostasis has been achieved. Because of the likelihood of continuing hypovolaemia and bleeding disorders, regional anaesthesia is usually contraindicated and general anaesthesia is induced with reduced doses of intravenous agents. Ketamine, 0.75–1.0 mg kg^{-1} i.v. may be preferred.

AMNIOTIC FLUID EMBOLUS

Amniotic fluid embolus is a rare, but frequently fatal, complication of pregnancy. The syndrome is caused by obstruction of the pulmonary vascular bed and activation of the coagulation cascade leading to DIC. It can occur during labour, especially when contractions are powerful and the membranes are intact, during or immediately after delivery and during Caesarean section. There is usually some degree of trauma to the uterus which permits the passage of amniotic fluid and fetal debris into the maternal circulation. Amniotic fluid embolus presents as acute dyspnoea, cyanosis, hypoxia and circulatory failure. A coagulopathy is detectable within an hour. The differential diagnosis includes other emboli (clot or air), pulmonary aspiration and eclampsia. The diagnosis is made by finding fetal debris in the maternal sputum, blood or lung tissue. Treatment is supportive, with correction of the coagulopathy.

PRETERM DELIVERY

Preterm delivery, which is defined as delivery before completion of the 37th week of gestation, is associated with high neonatal mortality and morbidity. Preterm labour is usually inhibited to allow increasing fetal maturity and for administration of glucocorticoids to the mother which accelerates formation of surfactant in the fetal lung. Epidural analgesia will assist safe vaginal delivery. Perineal relaxation and the use of outlet forceps reduces the likelihood of damage to the immature fetal skull from maternal expulsive efforts. β_2-receptor agonists such as ritodrine are frequently used to inhibit labour. Their use is associated with maternal tachycardia, arrhythmias, hypotension and pulmonary oedema which may complicate anaesthesia for eventual Caesarean section. Pulmonary oedema may be exacerbated by the use of excessively dilute β_2-agonist solutions. Although these agents should normally be diluted in 5% glucose, the solutions can be made more concentrated (ritodrine 3 mg ml^{-1}) if they are given using a syringe driver, so reducing the load of hypotonic fluid.

HYPERTENSIVE DISORDERS OF PREGNANCY

Along with pulmonary embolism, the hypertensive disorders of pregnancy are the leading cause of maternal mortality in the UK. These disorders may be subdivided into pregnancy induced hypertension (pre-eclampsia) and pre-existing chronic hypertension, although the one may be superimposed on the other. The diagnosis of pregnancy induced hypertension is based on the presence of hypertension and proteinuria. The hypertension is defined as an arterial blood pressure greater than 140/90 mmHg after the 20th week of gestation or an increase of at least 30 mmHg of systolic pressure or 15 mmHg diastolic above baseline antenatal booking clinic values. Proteinuria is defined as more than 0.3 g of urinary protein in 24 h.

Table 31.4 Clinical features of severe pregnancy-induced hypertension

Systolic blood pressure >160 mmHg, or diastolic >110 mmHg
Proteinuria >5 g 24 h^{-1}
Oliguria (urine output <400 ml per 24 h^{-1})
Abnormal liver function tests
Epigastric or right upper quadrant pain
Hepatic rupture (rare)
Thrombocytopenia
Coagulopathy
Headache
Visual disturbances
Hyperreflexia
Pulmonary oedema

Oedema may be present but is an unreliable sign. The hypertension is associated with a shift of fluids from the intravascular into the extravascular space and generalized vasoconstriction. Pregnancy induced hypertension is defined as severe if the arterial pressure is greater than 160/110 mmHg and proteinuria is 5 g or more in 24 h. There are a number of other clinical features associated with severe disease described in Table 31.4. The aetiology of pregnancy induced hypertension is unknown, although it probably has an immunological basis. There are abnormalities of placental implantation and function and of prostaglandin synthesis. It is more common in adolescents, primigravidae (especially when elderly) and in women with multiple pregnancies, diabetes or hydatidiform mole. There may be a genetic predisposition. The disease process can only be halted by delivery of the fetoplacental unit. The HELLP syndrome (**h**aemolysis, **e**levated **l**iver enzymes, **l**ow **p**latelets) may be a variant of severe pregnancy-induced hypertension or a separate condition.

Pregnancy-induced hypertension is managed by treating the symptoms and delivering the fetoplacental unit. The aim is to prevent progression to convulsions, control blood pressure, improve organ perfusion, correct coagulopathies and permit safe delivery. These measures need continuing for at least 48 h after delivery while the disease processes reverse. In the USA and South Africa, magnesium sulphate is used to prevent convulsions. Magnesium sulphate is gaining in popularity in the UK, where phenytoin is also used. The exact role of prophylactic anticonvulsants is not established. Magnesium sulphate is given as an intravenous loading dose of 40–80 mg kg^{-1} followed by an infusion of 1–2 g h^{-1}. The aim is to produce a blood level of 2–4 mmol l^{-1}. Toxicity causes muscular weakness and respiratory and cardiac arrest occur with severe toxicity. Phenytoin is given intravenously as a bolus of 15 mg kg^{-1} at a maximum rate of 50 mg min^{-1} with ECG monitoring followed by 100 mg three times daily.

Hypertension is usually treated with vasodilators. Despite peripheral oedema, these women are intravascularly depleted and diuretics are not indicated. Oral β-adrenoceptor antagonists (for example, atenolol), clonidine and α-methyl dopa are used to manage mild hypertension. Hydralazine and labetalol may be infused continuously for more severe disease and refractory hypertension can be managed with sodium nitroprusside. The aim is to maintain the diastolic pressure at less than 90 mmHg. Effective epidural analgesia may be sufficient to control blood pressure. Urine output should be measured hourly. Intravascular fluid depletion, particularly if associated with oliguria and renal failure, requires careful rehydration. Crystalloid is infused to maintain a urine output of at least 1 ml kg^{-1} h^{-1}, with small boluses of colloid such as 5% albumin being given if required. Monitoring of the central venous pressure is advisable during infusion of these fluids. Because of the likelihood of coagulopathy, a long line placed in the antecubital fossa may be safer than the internal jugular or subclavian route.

Analgesia and anaesthesia for Caesarean section for patients with pregnancy induced hypertension can be best provided by the epidural route. Epidural analgesia assists in control of blood pressure and can be extended for Caesarean section. Spinal anaesthesia is less appropriate for these patients as the fall in blood pressure may be dramatic and compromise uteroplacental blood flow. Carefully performed epidural anaesthesia with local anaesthetics may actually increase uteroplacental blood flow. Regional anaesthesia should be avoided in mothers with platelet counts of less than $100\,000 \times 10^9\, l^{-1}$ or clotting factor deficiencies. Oedema may cause difficulties in placement of intravenous cannulae and the epidural catheter. Preloading must be performed carefully to avoid pulmonary oedema.

General anaesthesia may be indicated, particularly if there is a coagulopathy or an eclamptic fit has occurred. Problems associated with the use of general anaesthesia include difficult intubation, marked pressor response to airway stimulation and increased haemorrhage. Intubation may be more difficult because of oedema of the tongue, epiglottis or other pharyngeal structures and bleeding following intubation. Equipment to deal with a failed or difficult intubation must be available and consideration given to awake fibreoptic intubation. Marked hypertension can occur both at intubation and extubation and may lead to pulmonary oedema or cerebral haemorrhage. An attempt must be made to attenuate this response. The choice of drugs which may be used includes short-acting opioids such as alfentanil 10 $\mu g\, kg^{-1}$, β-adrenoceptor antagonists such as esmolol (0.5–1.0 $mg\, kg^{-1}$), labetolol, sodium nitroprusside or trimetaphan infusions, or a bolus dose of lignocaine 1 $mg\, kg^{-1}$. Magnesium sulphate used to prevent or control seizures increases the maternal sensitivity to nondepolarizing neuromuscular blocking drugs. These drugs should be used with monitoring of neuromuscular function with a peripheral nerve stimulator.

ECLAMPSIA

Eclampsia occurs when convulsions complicate pregnancy-induced hypertension. Eclamptic fits can occur even when the blood pressure is only mildly raised. Seizures occurring in late pregnancy or labour should be regarded as eclamptic until proven otherwise. The differential diagnosis is epilepsy, cerebrovascular accident, water intoxication or local-anaesthetic toxicity. Seizures should be stopped with intravenous benzodiazepines and preparations made for delivery of the fetoplacental unit. The mother should be nursed in a quiet environment, with a clear airway maintained by tracheal intubation if necessary (with attenuation of the pressor response) and drug therapy given to control blood pressure and prevent further seizures. Magnesium sulphate is the agent of choice for seizure prophylaxis in these circumstances. Caesarean section should be performed under general anaesthesia and all eclamptic patients should be sedated and their lungs ventilated after operation. If after 6 h the mother is unresponsive or has localizing neurological signs a CT scan should be performed. Cerebral oedema may require intracranial pressure monitoring for optimum care. Before extubation the larynx should be inspected to exclude continuing laryngeal oedema.

MATERNAL HEART DISEASE

The changes of cardiovascular physiology during pregnancy and the stresses placed upon the heart during labour can cause cardiac decompensation and death in women with heart disease. The greatest risk is in women with right-to-left shunts, tight mitral stenosis with atrial fibrillation, coarctation of the aorta or recent myocardial infarction. Cardiac output increases by 30% during the first stage of labour and by 45% during the second stage. With each uterine contraction about 200 ml of blood is forced into the systemic circulation. After delivery of the placenta and contraction of the uterus the increase in blood volume may cause cardiac output to increase to 150% above pre-labour values. Girls with congenital heart disease and associated left-to-right shunts may develop pulmonary hypertension (Eisenmenger's syndrome) by the time they reach child-bearing age. Along with women with cyanotic congenital heart disease such as Fallot's tetralogy, they tolerate pregnancy very poorly. The systemic vasodilatation induced by pregnancy leads to an increase in the right-to-left shunt and worsening of the cyanosis. Further systemic vasodilatation as a result of epidural or spinal blockade with local anaesthetics may be fatal. Intrathecal opioids may provide safe analgesia and pudendal nerve block may suffice for instrumental delivery. Carefully balanced general anaesthesia is usually well tolerated. However, increases in pulmonary resistance, for example caused by hypoxia, must be avoided as they will also increase right-to-left shunt. Regional anaesthesia with local anaesthetics should also be avoided in patients with lesions which produce a fixed stroke volume such as significant aortic stenosis.

The majority of other heart valve disease in pregnancy will be either rheumatic valve disease or due to a floppy mitral valve. The most serious is mitral stenosis, especially if associated with atrial fibrillation. The increased cardiac output during pregnancy and labour leads to a higher diastolic flow rate across the mitral valve orifice. As a result the left atrial and pulmonary venous pressures are increased and pulmonary oedema can occur. Atrial fibrillation should be cardioverted if possible and open or closed mitral valvotomy may be lifesaving in severe stenosis. Continuous lumbar epidural analgesia with local anaesthetics is useful as it reduces the increase in cardiac output and the strain on the heart especially during contractions and maternal expulsive efforts. Epidural anaesthesia can also be used to provide safe anaesthesia for Caesarean section.

SUMMARY

The first part of this chapter examined the physiological changes that occur during pregnancy and labour. Mechanical alterations to the respiratory system in pregnancy, coupled with increased oxygen demand, mean that hypoxia can occur very rapidly and the anaesthetist must take this into account when planning general anaesthesia. Cardiovascular changes include a marked increase in cardiac output, especially during labour, and this can compromise patients with pre-existing heart disease. Aortocaval compression can cause hypotension in the supine position in the third trimester, and this can also interfere with placental perfusion. Although the alterations in gastric function in pregnancy, especially emptying rate and acid production, are often overemphasized, the process of labour has a deleterious effect which is worsened by treatment with opioids. Gastric reflux is a common problem from the first trimester and this can lead directly to the feared complication of Mendelson's syndrome.

Epidural analgesia remains the most effective method for relieving pain in labour, and recent attention has turned to reducing the degree of motor block, increasing the chance of vaginal delivery and minimizing complications such as hypotension. Many of these problems have been successfully addressed by the use of low concentrations of local anaesthetic used in conjunction with opioids, especially fentanyl. These mixtures can be delivered by bolus, but continuous infusions may have advantages. Patient-controlled epidural analgesia is very popular with women who want better control over their pain relief and combined spinal–epidural analgesia may have some advantages, particularly with respect to speed of onset of block.

The current trend towards regional anaesthesia for Caesarean section, driven by an increasing awareness of the hazards of general anaesthesia and by improved design of spinal needles, has been highlighted. Epidural anaesthesia remains the best option if an epidural is already in place and strategies for rapid attainment of a satisfactory block in the emergency situation are presented. Spinal anaesthesia is the method of choice for elective procedures, or when there is no epidural *in situ* for emergency Caesarean section. The importance of proper patient preparation before regional anaesthesia for Caesarean section has been emphasized; the anaesthetist must always be prepared to supplement the block, or even induce general anaesthesia, if necessary. There will always be indications for general anaesthesia and suitable techniques have been discussed, with emphasis on prevention of acid aspiration, the precautions that should be adopted to minimize the risk of failed intubation and the actions that should be taken if it arises.

Finally, some common emergencies have been dealt with. Haemorrhage remains one of the most frequently causes of maternal death, largely due to the early appearance of disseminated intravascular coagulation as a complicating factor. Early and accurate resuscitation is the key to success. Pregnancy-induced hypertension is common and in its severe forms is a significant threat to both mother and fetus. Anaesthetists, by virtue of their knowledge of invasive monitoring, fluid replacement and vasoactive drugs, are uniquely well-placed to manage these women and to treat the rare, but devastating, complication of eclampsia.

FURTHER READING

Bogod, D. G. (1994) The postpartum stomach – when is it safe? (Editorial). *Anaesthesia*, **49**, 1–2.

Chestnut, D. H. (ed) (1994) *Obstetric Anesthesia: Principles and Practice*, Mosby–Year Book Inc, St Louis.

Chestnut, D. H., Owen, C. L., Bates, J. N. *et al.* (1988) Continuous infusion epidural analgesia during labor: a randomized, double-blind, comparison of 0.0625% bupivacaine/0.0002% fentanyl versus 0.125% bupivacaine. *Anesthesiology*, **68**, 754–759.

Datta, S. (ed) (1991) *Anesthetic and Obstetric Management of High Risk Pregnancy*, Mosby–Year Book Inc, St Louis.

Department of Health *et al.* (1994) Report on Confidential Enquiries into Maternal Deaths in the United Kingdom 1988–1990, HMSO, London.

Felsby, S. and Juelsgaard, P. (1995) Combined spinal and epidural anaesthesia. *Anesthesia and Analgesia*, **80**, 821–826.

Mendelson, C. L. (1946) The aspiration of stomach contents into the lung during obstetric anesthesia. *American Journal of Obstetrics and Gynecology*, **52**, 191–204.

Moir, D. D. (1970) Anaesthesia for Caesarean Section: an evaluation of a method using low concentrations of halothane and 50 per cent oxygen. *British Journal of Anaesthesia*, **42**, 136–142.

Morgan, B. M. (1995) 'Walking' epidurals in labour (Editorial). *Anaesthesia*, **50**, 839–840.

Pearson, J. F. and Davies, P. (1974) The effect of continuous lumbar epidural analgesia upon fetal acid–base status during the first stage of labour. *Journal of Obstetrics and Gynaecology of the British Commonwealth*, **81**, 971–974.

Shnider, S. M., Abboud, T. K., Artal, R. *et al.* (1983) Maternal catecholamines decrease during labor after lumbar epidural anesthesia. *American Journal of Obstetrics and Gynecology*, **147**, 13–15.

ANAESTHESIA IN THE ELDERLY 32

C. Traynor

The number and proportion of elderly people is rising at an unprecedented rate both in developed and developing countries. Improved social conditions and preventative medicine are the main contributors to the achievement of a longer lifespan. Declining birth rates will result in an increase in proportion of the population aged over 65 years and, in particular, that proportion aged over 85 years. Half of all people over 65 years are predicted to need surgery during their life time. This has serious implications for those responsible for planning health care funding. There is increasing awareness among anaesthetists that the requirements of management of elderly patients are as different from the conventional, normal, adult population as is paediatric anaesthetic care. The elderly patient is distinguished by the biological consequences of ageing and age-related disease. Social conditions and lifestyle choices significantly contribute to disease in this population such that emphasis must be placed on medical state rather than chronological age. Many elderly patients present for surgery 'out of hours' needing rapid assessment often by relatively inexperienced anaesthetists. A thorough knowledge of the alterations in physiology, drug metabolism and perioperative requirements specific to their needs is mandatory.

PHYSIOLOGY

One of the hallmarks of ageing is heterogenicity, and the discrepancy between chronological age and functional or biological age can be very large indeed. However, the ageing process invariably affects all organ systems to the extent that the geriatric patient is physiologically quite different from a young adult. Of particular significance to anaesthetists are the changes in body composition, general metabolism and cardiorespiratory function. The most important end result of these changes is a diminished reserve capacity in all elderly patients.

Under non-stressful conditions, these changes may produce little functional impairment in the absence of disease. However, the ability to respond to the increased haemodynamic and metabolic demands of anaesthesia and surgery is greatly impaired.

CARDIOVASCULAR CHANGES

Structural changes in the vasculature with ageing result in increased stiffness of the aorta and systemic arteries. This contributes to the higher systolic arterial pressures, often with normal mean pressures, that tend to be the rule, rather than the exception, in elderly patients. The most important effect of ageing on the cardiovascular system is a reduction in maximal cardiac output. Cardiac performance

---

Short Practice of Anaesthesia. Edited by M. Morgan and G. M. Hall. Published in 1997 by Chapman & Hall, London. ISBN 0 412 71890 1

is affected by structural, functional, and central control deterioration. Changes in the heart include ventricular wall thickening, myocardial fibrosis and calcification of the valve edges. Heart murmurs have been found in more than half of patients aged over 75, but less than 10% have functional valvular disease. There is a significant loss of sinoatrial node pacemaker cells (80–90% are lost by age 75 years predisposing to ectopy). There is a decreased responsiveness to catecholamines leading to an increased tendency to rhythm disorders. Myocardial contraction and relaxation times are 20% longer. Because of the reduced ventricular compliance and lower maximal heart rate, the elderly increase cardiac output by increasing stroke volume, mainly by augmenting end-diastolic volume. Alterations in intravascular volume or venous capacitance, common with anaesthesia and surgery can, therefore, readily compromise the older patients' ability to maintain or increase cardiac output. Excessive intravenous fluid therapy may lead to congestive cardiac failure and pulmonary oedema, since the ageing patient has optimum cardiac function over a relatively narrow range of end-diastolic pressures.

Plasma concentrations of adrenaline and noradrenaline are 2–4 times higher in the elderly, but this difference is not clinically apparent because of reduced end-organ responsiveness to catecholamines. Autonomic reflexes essential to cardiovascular homeostasis are progressively diminished in the elderly including baroreflex vasoconstriction to cold and chronotropic responses to postural change.

RESPIRATORY PHYSIOLOGY

The elderly pulmonary system restricts the uptake of oxygen such that by age 70 years, the normal alveolar–arterial oxygen difference is 2.7 kPa.

The diaphragm and chest wall muscles decrease in strength and are more vulnerable to fatigue owing to loss of muscle fibres and infiltration with fat cells. Calcification around the articulations of the ribs results in decreased chest wall compliance. The work of breathing is increased by up to 20% for any given rate and depth. The surface area for gas exchange is reduced due to a decrease in the number of alveoli and an increase in the number of fenestrations between them. Elastic recoil is reduced due to a change in morphology of elastin. This loss of elastic recoil causes a fall in intrapulmonary tension gradients leading to increased airway closure at lower lung volumes, so that closing volume progressively encroaches on vital capacity. Residual volume rises owing to the increase in closing volume. These changes adversely affect the ventilation–perfusion ratio such that oxygenation can be readily compromised by perioperative events such as lying supine, alteration in diaphragmatic efficiency, drugs or fluid therapy (Figure 32.1).

Control of breathing is inefficient due to an age-related decrease in chemoreceptor function and reduced neuronal output from the medulla. The hypoxic ventilatory response is decreased by up to 30% even while awake, and a reduced hypercarbic drive of up to 50% with age, hampers CO_2 elimination so that respiratory acidosis can rapidly occur. Periodic breathing patterns are common, as is obstructive sleep apnoea which has a more pronounced effect on oxygenation and CO_2 retention even after transient episodes. The control of breathing is further compromised by the administration of volatile agents and opiates.

RENAL FUNCTION

There is a gradual loss of renal mass, primarily affecting the cortex, to about 70% of adult values. Renal perfusion declines to about 50% of maximal by age 80 years. The fall in glomerular filtration, estimated at about 1 ml min^{-1} for each year over 40 years of age, is not reflected by an increase in serum

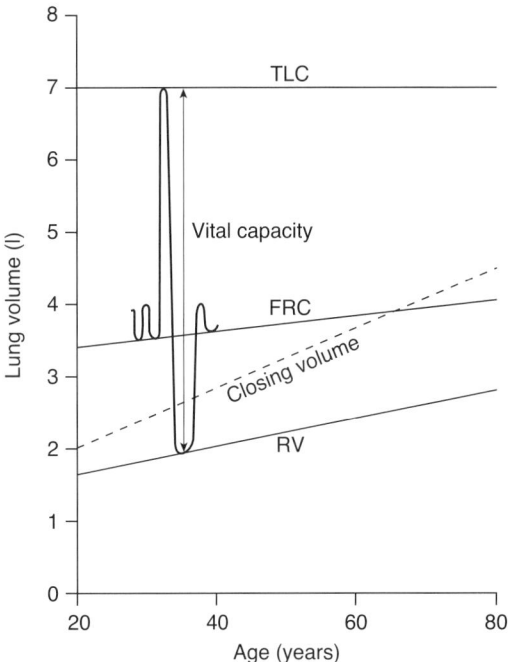

Figure 32.1 The effect of age on lung volume. (Reproduced with permission from Tockman, M.S. (1990) Aging of the respiratory system, in *Geriatric Surgery* (ed M.R. Kattic) Urban & Schwarzenberg, Baltimore, p. 77.)

creatinine because of the concomitant reduction in lean body mass and, therefore, creatinine load. Estimates of serum creatinine in the normal range may conceal impaired renal function and even modest rises are of much greater significance than in younger patients. Decreased glomerular filtration rate renders the patient more susceptible to acute renal failure in the event of ischaemic or nephrotoxic insult perioperatively. Renal functional reserve to withstand gross water and electrolyte imbalance is minimal. Maximal concentrating ability diminishes due to antidiuretic hormone resistance and reduced activity of the renin–aldosterone system leads to decreased reabsorption of sodium during sodium restriction. Maximal absorbtion rate for glucose is also decreased. The reduced capacity of the ageing kidney to maintain homeostasis is compounded by the prevalence (30%) of renal disease in this group of patients and has important implications for perioperative fluid management and drug therapy.

BODY COMPOSITION

Body weight tends to increase in middle adult life and then to decrease to values comparable with young adults after the age of 60 years. However, body composition changes progressively and irreversibly as part of the ageing process. The major changes are an increase in the proportion of adipose tissue relative to lean body mass, a decrease in total body water and a loss of bone mass. The increase in adipose tissue occurs centrally with loss of subcutaneous fat on the limbs and face. The reduction in total body water is mainly from the intracellular compartment due to a loss of cellular mass. Plasma volume is well maintained in fit, elderly patients although this may not be so in hospitalized, ill patients or those on certain medications. There is a gender difference in the change in body composition, women having a greater propensity to lay down adipose tissue and develop osteoporosis, while men have a more marked contraction of both intracellular and interstitial body water.

TEMPERATURE REGULATION

Thermoregulation is progressively impaired with old age. Extremes of heat and environmental cold can have very serious consequences and even lead to death.

The reduced ability to maintain thermal homeostasis in the elderly is multifactorial. All sensory systems are blunted and peripheral thermal perception may be reduced. Inactivity, loss of lean body mass and lack of nutrients in the diet may all contribute to diminished heat production. Thermoregulatory vasoconstrictor and shivering responses to cold are reduced and may require a lower triggering core temperature. Social factors, dementia, disease, drug therapy or injury may all exacerbate the poor response. Hypothermia, defined as a core temperature of < 35°C is a frequent occurrence during anaesthesia and surgery. One patient in three will develop a core temperature of < 35°C. General anaesthesia and regional anaesthesia inhibit thermoregulatory control, albeit by different mechanisms. Low ambient temperature in theatre, prolonged or major body cavity surgery, dry inspired gases and fluid therapy all contribute to a perioperative fall in temperature. Significant physiological changes occur with cooling and rewarming which may adversely affect outcome. The diminished cardiorespiratory reserve in older patients puts them at particular risk of emerging cold, hypoxic, acidotic and peripherally vasoconstricted from surgery. Hypothermia is associated with a fall in cardiac output and heart rate, and an increase in peripheral resistance. Hepatic and renal blood flow decrease significantly prolonging drug elimination. The duration of action of vecuronium, for example, is doubled at a core temperature of 34.5°C compared with 36.5°C. Haematocrit and blood viscosity are increased and blood coagulation is impaired. Respiratory rate and tidal volume fall and the ventilatory response to hypoxia is diminished. A cold-induced shift in the oxygen–haemoglobin dissociation curve to the left reduces tissue oxygen uptake. Shivering increases oxygen consumption by 400–500%. Elderly patients have a particularly limited ability to increase cardiac output and oxygen uptake to meet these demands. Arterial desaturation is common and tissue hypoxia may result in lactic acidosis. Even mild hypothermia has been shown to be associated with an increased incidence of early postoperative myocardial ischaemia. Wound healing is impaired. Protein degradation and nitrogen loss are increased by hypothermia which may contribute significantly to postoperative morbidity in older patients.

OTHER PHYSIOLOGICAL CHANGES

Liver mass is decreased by about 40% by age 80 years. Blood flow to and from the liver shows a corresponding decrease as liver mass decreases. This is important in the metabolism of several drugs normally cleared from the plasma in the 'first pass' through the liver. There is little qualitative change in hepatocellular enzymatic function with age. Routine liver function tests should be normal. Quantitative loss of hepatic tissue appears to be the most important factor in the age-related decrease in clearance of drugs requiring hepatic biotransformation.

The ability to metabolize a glucose load is progressively impaired with age so care must be taken in administering intravenous carbohydrates. Insulin secretion is not reduced and the probable cause is insulin antagonism, or changes in target-organ, receptor response. Changes in the ageing immune system are reflected in the increased incidence of autoantibodies and decreased cellular immunity; response to infection may be attenuated. Changes in the autonomic nervous system result in an increased incidence of postural hypotension with age, which may be compounded by some medications.

PHARMACOLOGY

There are fundamental differences in drug metabolism in elderly patients when compared with younger patients, some of which are as yet incompletely understood. Enormous physiological variability in this group can make successful and appropriate treatment a great challenge. In addition, elderly patients consume a disproportionate amount of varied and sometimes unfamiliar drugs, have an increased incidence of adverse drug reactions and a threefold increase in the incidence of unwanted side effects. Anaesthetic management can be profoundly affected by altered drug distribution and excretion, as a result of age-related changes in body composition and renal and hepatic function (Figure 32.2). Age-

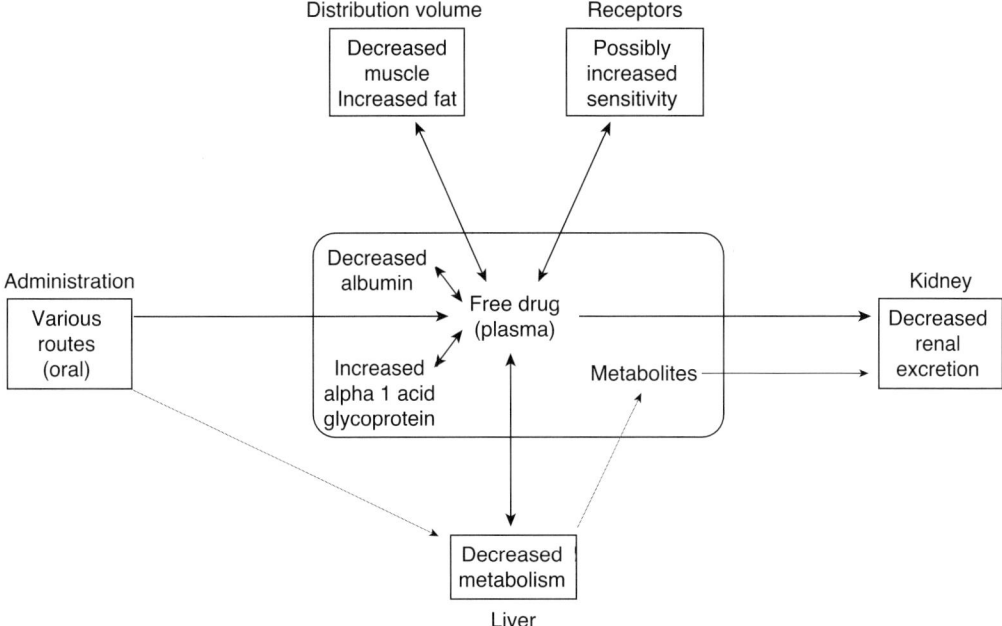

Figure 32.2 Summary of changes in pharmacokinetics and pharmacodynamics in the elderly. (Reproduced with permission from Mangat, P.S. and Jones, J.G. (1993) Post-operative pain control in the elderly. *Baillière's Clinical Anaesthesiology*, **7**, 171.

related changes in receptor and target site function affect the final pharmacological effect. The administration of anaesthetic drugs is compounded by the reduction in homeostatic reserve which counterbalances the effects of many drugs.

The increased proportion of body fat leads to a greater volume of distribution for lipid soluble drugs and acts as a reservoir, slowing elimination and prolonging plasma half-life. Plasma albumin declines slowly with age and may fall dramatically with illness while α_1-glycoprotein values rise with age. This can contribute to altered drug availability depending on the degree of protein binding. The initial volume of distribution for drugs is contracted resulting in a higher serum concentration for a given dose of drug. Reduced hepatic blood flow and greater variability in hepatic metabolism result in a longer plasma half-life for many drugs which undergo significant hepatic degradation. The fall in glomerular filtration rate decreases renal clearance of drugs by up to 50% even in the absence of disease. The resultant increase in plasma half-life of drugs, or metabolites, with low therapeutic ratio and high fractional renal clearance increases the risk of adverse reaction. Clinical evidence of increased sensitivity to certain drugs is not consistently explained by pharmacokinetics. Changes in receptor density, receptor affinity and age-related changes in the target tissue are among the factors thought to contribute to altered pharmacodynamics in the elderly. There appears to be a reduced β-adrenergic response in the myocardium, both inotropic and chronotropic responses are diminished. A differential reduction occurs in α-adrenoreceptor responsiveness, α_1-responsiveness is preserved but α_2-responsiveness diminished. There is evidence for a decline in cholinergic receptor sensitivity with age both centrally and peripherally, the ability of atropine to correct a bradycardia is attenuated. The precise mechanism of the clinical, increased sensitivity to benzodiazepines and opiates has not yet been fully elucidated. The relative effects of the above considerations on specific anaesthetic drugs are often complex and multifactorial.

Bearing in mind that different factors may be relevant to the metabolism of specific drugs within a particular group, the following broad generalizations can be made in regard to anaesthetic drugs. Absorbtion of drugs administered orally to the healthy patient is not affected by age. Intravenous induction agents are given at a lower dose and at a slower rate because of altered distribution, slower circulation time and attenuated autonomic response. In the presence of normal plasma cholinesterase concentration, the dose of succinylcholine is not altered by age. Non-depolarising neuromuscular blocking drugs are administered at a normal initial dose, but a lower maintenance dosage owing to altered pharmacokinetics. Minimal alveolar concentration for inhalational agents is decreased by about 80%, their volume of distribution increased, and elimination delayed. Agent specific data for MAC in the elderly is now available for inhalational agents. There is evidence to suggest that the data on cardiovascular effects of inhalational agents may not hold true for older and younger adults. Glycopyrolate is agreed to be the anticholinergic agent of choice since it does not cross the blood–brain barrier. Hyoscine and atropine can be associated with delirium and the anticholinergic syndrome due to altered central receptor sensitivity. Opioids are given in lower doses and have a prolonged duration of action due to combined pharmacokinetic and pharmacodynamic effects. Similarly, benzodiazepines have a prolonged half-life and increased sensitivity to their effects occurs. The combination of opiates and benzodiazepines together has a more pronounced effect on oxygenation and carbon dioxide retention and calls for caution.

COGNITIVE FUNCTION

Postoperative delirium is a common complication of surgery in elderly people. Its importance has been increasingly recognized not least because of increasing awareness of health costs, but also because it is associated with an increased mortality of 20–30%. It is associated with a three-fold increase in hospital stay, delayed functional recovery and increased morbidity from infection, falls, decubitus ulcers etc. after both elective and emergency surgery. Of particular importance to anaesthetists is its association with postoperative hypoxaemia and perioperative drug administration. Delirium is an organic brain syndrome which develops acutely and has a fluctuating course. It usually develops during the first four days after operation often at night firstly and may be agitated or withdrawn in type. It is characterized by disturbances of attention, memory, orientation, perception, psychomotor behaviour and sleep. The incidence is related to the type of surgery varying from 1–3% after cataract surgery to 60% after orthopaedic surgery.

The pathophysiology of delirium is not fully understood and is probably multifactorial. Changes in neurotransmitter function in the brain are suggested; in particular, cholinergic neurotransmission, and there is an association between postopertive delirium and anticholinergic drug activity. Preoperative factors predisposing to delirium include increasing age and multisystem disease, dementia and cerebrovascular disease, trauma, depression and alcohol or benzodiazepine abuse. Peroperatively, drug therapy and factors contributing to cerebral hypoxaemia such as hypotension, hypocarbia and hypothermia are important. Elderly patients are particularly susceptible to the central effects of anticholinergic medication: atropine eye drops have been associated with delirium after cataract surgery. Hyoscine is particularly deleriogenic and should be avoided. Glycopyrolate, which does not cross the blood–

brain barrier, is the drug of choice and its use has been shown to reduce the incidence of postoperative delirium compared with other anticholinergic drugs. Opiates and benzodiazepines are associated with delirium, but it is not clear if this is a direct association or secondary to respiratory depression. The most deleriogenic opiate is pethidine possibly because its active metabolite norpethidine has anticholinergic activity. Other drugs associated with delirium are H_2 receptor blockers (not dose or drug dependent), corticosteroids (dose related), digoxin and antibiotics.

After operation, hypoxaemia particularly on the second postoperative night is associated with, and implicated in, the decline in mental function after surgery. Chest and urinary tract infections, common after operation in this age group, may present with delirium. Dehydration, which may be difficult to detect, and hyponatraemia are also implicated. The management of postoperative delirium demands an early diagnosis and maintenance of a high index of suspicion in susceptible patients. There is evidence that meticulous medical care and nursing interventions can possibly influence the incidence and course of delirium. A vigorous search must be made for an underlying cause and this must be aggressively treated. Adequate analgesia is considered very important. Sedation must be used with caution. Benzodiazepine therapy may lead to further deterioration although its use is appropriate if there is associated alcohol or benzodiazepine withdrawal. Sedatives with anticholinergic side effects must be used with caution. Haloperidol is probably the drug of choice when agitation is a problem and has been found to be safe and effective. Chlorpromazine is also effective, but its adrenergic antagonist effect may lead to a significant drop in arterial pressure.

Dementia, or chronic brain failure, affects an increasing proportion of patients with advancing age. It comprises a group of about 70 diseases in which a very low proportion are truly reversible. Preoperative assessment and perioperative management and pain relief can be a great challenge in patients with dementia. It is important to recognize that the risk of postoperative delirium is increased in these patients and that both elective and emergency surgery have a much higher morbidity and mortality rate.

Attention should also be paid to the detection of depression in hospitalized, elderly patients which may lead to slowing of recovery and prolonged rehabilitation.

PERIOPERATIVE RISK AND OUTCOME

With intraoperative mortality now rare and improved facilities to prolong short-term survival, the standard time over which perioperative mortality is assessed is 30 days. Except in isolated cases, it is now often difficult to distinguish death from, or related to, anaesthesia *per se*, from that due to other causes. Current estimates of mortality in well prepared patients over 65 years are 5–10%, i.e. 3–5 times that for younger adults. There is no consistent evidence that the incidence of death is further increased with advancing age, certainly up to the age of 95 years.

Cardiac disease including myocardial infarction and congestive cardiac failure, respiratory disease and sepsis are the major causes of death in elderly patients. Three factors are consistently found to influence the mortality rates: the physical status of the patient, the urgency of the surgery and the site of surgery.

The American Society of Anesthesiologists Physical Status Classification Assessment correlates well with predicted mortality. Patients over 80 years of age are usually identified as Class II, even when defined fit and healthy. The incidence of multiple, concomitant diseases increases with age and 90% of patients over 80 will have pathological findings on examination.

Coronary artery disease, overt or subclinical, is common and is associated with increased risk of perioperative complications.

Previous myocardial infarction increases the risk of postoperative reinfarction, but the very high incidence previously reported has not been confirmed in recent studies. This is thought to be due to improved management of acute myocardial infarction with the advent of newer drugs, thrombolysis and early coronary artery surgery or angioplasty. Angina is known to increase risk in proportion to its severity. Unstable angina is considered a contraindication to non-cardiac surgery. Assessment and aggressive management is required. Silent myocardial ischaemia is associated with an adverse outcome including sudden cardiac death, myocardial infarction, acute left ventricular failure and life threatening arrhythmias. Recent evidence has shown an increased incidence, both in number and duration, of episodes of silent myocardial ischaemia following anaesthesia and surgery and a strong association with late postoperative hypoxaemia. Successful strategies to reduce the incidence are, as yet, not clear.

Severe hypertension is a contraindication to anaesthesia and surgery; 10% of treated, hypertensive patients and 50% of untreated or poorly controlled patients have been found to have silent myocardial ischaemia. Antihypertensive treatment should be continued before surgery, and treatment of mild to moderate hypertension has been shown to be associated with an improved outcome. The high prevalence of arrhythmias also increases the risk of cardiovascular complications. The effects of atrial fibrillation on ventricular filling can have serious consequences on cardiac output in the elderly patient. Isolated non-sustained ventricular ectopic beats are not associated with an adverse outcome.

The most common predictor of postoperative pulmonary complications is preoperative pulmonary disease. No single pulmonary function test has been found independently to be predictive of major pulmonary complications which occur in up to 40% of elderly patients. Malnutrition and low plasma albumin values increase the risk as does obesity, smoking, immobility and dementia. Surgery involving an abdominal wall incision impinges on diaphragmatic function and is associated with a two to threefold increase in the risk of postoperative atelectasis and pneumonia.

Urinary tract infection is the most common postoperative infection in this group of patients and is particularly associated with urinary catheterization of > 48 h. Respiratory and wound infections increase postoperative morbidity and mortality as a result of the diminished immune response to infection.

The incidence and number of coexisting diseases adversely affects outcome; the occurrence of cancer, diabetes and dementia are particularly significant.

Emergency surgery is associated with a 3–10 fold increase in mortality and a 20-fold increase in morbidity. The Confidential Enquiry into Peri-Operative Deaths (CEPOD) report highlighted this problem in the elderly. Factors deemed to be contributory included the 'out of hours' nature of the surgery with disproportionate junior personnel responsibility. Inadequate preparation and evaluation, and failure to apply knowledge, were also emphasized by this report. However, it is known that elderly people may present later in the course of a disease, necessitating more radical procedures. Diagnosis is often more difficult with obtunded classical signs. The surgical lesion may result in haemorrhage, acidosis or alterations in circulating volume, placing the patient in a higher ASA class. The emergency nature of the procedure often leaves little time to assess the patient and precludes optimization of their condition.

The site of surgery is an important predictor of risk and outcome. With the exception of fractured neck of femur, non-body-cavity surgery is associated with an excellent prognosis in most instances. Cataract surgery has a morbidity of 1–2% and prostate resection carries a low mortality of 1–3% whether it is performed transurethrally or as open prostatectomy.

Surgical entry into a major body cavity, whether elective or emergency, greatly increases morbidity and mortality in this group of patients. Major vascular, colonic, and intrathoracic surgery increase risk 10–20 times. The urgency of the surgery is particularly reflected in these procedures, one study of patients aged over 80 years showed an 8% 30-day mortality for elective aortic aneurysm repair compared with 78% mortality for ruptured aneurysm.

Consideration of the factors contributing to postoperative morbidity and mortality in elderly patients has led to the view that it is unwise to defer elective surgery on the basis of age alone. Forty per cent of patients have an uneventful recovery and a high proportion have minor morbidity and improved function. Undue delay or urgency are equally undesirable, and remain the subject of much debate particularly in relation to repair of fractured hips.

PREOPERATIVE ASSESSMENT

Elderly patients do not present themselves to the anaesthetist as a homogeneous group and preoperative evaluation may be complex. Emphasis must be placed not on chronological age, but on establishing the level of pre-existing disease and optimizing physiological function. The number and severity of coexisting medical problems is the strongest predictor of postoperative outcome. In the case of emergency surgery, the patient is at an increased risk and maximizing fitness in the time allowed is attempted.

A full history is important, though the interest and focus differs from what is classically taught. Past medical history, current problems and details of all drug therapy should be established. Information on daily living activities and nutrition help with functional assessment, as does social history. The incidence of medical problems highlights the need for a thorough individual preoperative assessment. It is imperative to bear in mind the blunting of physical signs in older patients and the sometimes atypical and insidious presentation of acute illness.

A thorough physical examination requires careful interpretation of the findings in older patients. Myocardial ischaemia may be silent, peripheral oedema may be caused by venous insufficiency and basal crepitations may not be pathological. Heart murmurs are commonly heard but their significance may be difficult to establish. Decreased skin elasticity may make the diagnosis of dehydration difficult. Slowness in movement or communication with old age means that extra time should be allocated for the preoperative visit. Pre-anaesthetic consultation with other specialities may be warranted.

Ancillary testing is based on the history and physical examination with, as a minimum, full blood count, serum electrolytes, creatinine and glucose, a 12-lead ECG and chest X-ray. Pulmonary function has been found to correlate best with forced expiratory volumes over the first second of expiration (FEV_1). Values of less than 2 l, or less than 75% of predicted value for age and gender, are associated with postoperative pulmonary complications. Full pulmonary function testing with arterial blood gas analysis is warranted only in specific situations, e.g. lung resection.

Almost half of all elderly patients have hypertension and treatment must be instigated, or reviewed, as appropriate. Particular attention should be paid to the ECG to detect previous myocardial infarction, arrhythmias and myocardial ischaemia. Circulating blood volume must be considered as volume depletion can have adverse effects on renal function during anaesthesia and postoperatively.

Cognitive function and mood should be documented. Elderly patients have specific fears and anxieties which may not be readily expressed. Time to discuss and allay anxieties should be allocated as in younger patients.

The need for premedication in elderly patients is questionable and care in the prescription of sedative and anticholinergic medication is required.

A full review of drug therapy is mandatory and, with the exception of oral hypoglycaemics and insulin, most essential medications are maintained until the day of surgery and restored as soon as possible thereafter. There is evidence that continuation of adrenergic or calcium channel blocking drugs during anaesthesia has a beneficial cardiovascular effect without increasing the hypotensive response to surgery. Psychotropic drugs need to be individually assessed with regard to an anaesthetic interaction. Regimens for insulin for the control of hyperglycaemia are planned and timed on an individual basis.

Finally, the choice of anaesthetic technique, regional or general, can be decided on discussion with the patient or relatives. Deep venous thrombosis prophylaxis must be considered and instituted as appropriate.

ANAESTHETIC MANAGEMENT

There is no ideal anaesthetic technique or agent for older patients. Regional anaesthesia is often preferred in patients with pulmonary disease or fractured femur. Local infiltration and nerve blocks, where applicable, will achieve minimal morbidity and mortality.

Successful anaesthetic management depends on an understanding of the reduced, functional reserve in older patients and the altered pharmacokinetics or pharmacodynamics of the various agents used. The presence of cardiovascular, pulmonary, renal or hepatic disease demands increased caution and vigilance with the choice of drug and dose. Age-related physiological changes call for increased care when handling elderly patients. Decreased lacrimation requires eye protection. Skin and subcutaneous tissue changes result in an increased tendency to bruising from tape and adhesives. The prevalence of osteoporosis and osteoarthritis requires gentle positioning and neutral head alignment if a risk of cervical arthritis is present. Visual or hearing deficits demand extra courtesy. Precautions must be taken to minimize heat loss and prevent hypothermia, particularly with prolonged or body-cavity surgery. Decreases in body temperature may occur inadvertently in the anaesthetic room during prolonged establishment of regional anaesthesia or intravenous cannulation. Suitable plans for heat conservation must be instituted. Loss of facial subcutaneous fat and poor dentition may make mask fitting difficult. Obtunded airway reflexes and decreased gastro-oesophageal sphincter tone increase the likelihood of silent regurgitation in elderly patients. Oropharyngeal secretions are diminished with age but mucus production is increased so that humidification of inspired gases is important.

Monitoring is dictated by the surgery and the condition of the patient. There is no evidence that routine monitoring with a pulmonary artery catheter is beneficial in elderly patients. Stable vital signs during anaesthesia and surgery result in less postoperative morbidity and mortality. Intraoperative arterial pressure monitoring and active correction of deviations may be beneficial for postoperative renal, mental and cardiac function. The margins for error are considerably narrowed in an elderly patient and complications are less well tolerated. Meticulous attention to fluid management and blood replacement is required. Preloading before regional anaesthesia has been questioned in elderly patients and the use of ephedrine may be preferred. Blood loss in excess of 10% of the calculated blood volume is poorly tolerated. A fall in haemoglobin concentration acceptable in a younger patient, may overwhelm the elderly patient's ability to maintain adequate oxygen delivery since maximal cardiac output is reduced. Temperature and acid–base monitoring, particularly after prolonged surgery, may identify the apparently healthy 'at risk' patient.

Monitoring of neuromuscular function is particularly relevant to older patients. Decreased elimination of non-depolarizing neuromuscular blocking drugs, exacerbated by hypothermia, can result in incomplete reversal of neuromuscular blockade. This may severely compromise respiratory reserve with resulting hypoxaemia. Planned postoperative ventilation and active warming to diminish shivering, and improve oxygenation, may be indicated.

REGIONAL ANAESTHESIA

There has been a rapid expansion in the use of regional anaesthetic techniques in recent years, both for the provision of surgical anaesthesia and for postoperative pain relief. While increased knowledge and expertise have undoubtedly benefited certain subgroups of surgical patients, data obtained from younger patients on management and risk–benefit analysis of spinal and epidural anaesthesia often need reappraisal when applied to elderly people.

Positioning for regional anaesthesia may be painful or unpleasant in an elderly patient. Access may be limited by arthritic changes in the spine, calcification of the ligaments or a confused, uncooperative patient. However, the infrequent occurrence of dural headache in older patients allows the use of larger gauge spinal needles. Technical difficulties prolong the time taken to achieve the block and increase the risk of exposure and hypothermia. Age *per se* is a poor predictor of the height of segmental block with plain, or hyperbaric, solutions for spinal anaesthesia. Similarly the spread and duration of blockade with moderate volumes of epidural local anaesthetic may be more unpredictable and the consequences of an extensive somatic and sympathetic blockade more serious. The hypotensive response correlates poorly with the height of the block, may be more profound, and may occur at a low segmental level of block. Subclinical dehydration is common in older patients and may compound the diminished cardiovascular compensatory mechanisms. The greater incidence of hypotension could increase the risk of anterior spinal artery thrombosis, if solutions with adrenaline are used.

The safety of regional anaesthesia in patients on aspirin or low-dose heparin has not been established. This is an important consideration in view of the increasing use of thrombosis prophylaxis in elderly patients.

Controlled, randomized trials suggest that regional and general anaesthesia are equally safe when administered to patients for whom either technique is suitable. The physiological and clinical benefits of regional anaesthesia are well established in patients with respiratory disease. The ventilatory response to hypoxia and hypercapnia is preserved and postoperative analgesia may be superior. A significant reduction in oxygen saturation may occur if benzodiazepine sedation is given and supplementary oxygen is mandatory. The benefits of regional anaesthesia in patients with cardiovascular disease is less clear. The potential risks of compromising the coronary circulation with sudden hypotension, or of precipitating congestive cardiac failure with fluid preloading, must be taken into account when choosing regional anaesthesia. The value of fluid preloading before spinal anaesthesia in the elderly has been questioned and the preferential use of vasoconstrictors has been advocated. The potential for producing a tachycardia with some vasoconstrictors is undesirable in patients with coronary artery disease. Regional anaesthesia causes vasodilation and the decrease in afterload may be beneficial in many cases. Increased lower limb blood flow and reduced blood viscosity may decrease thromboembolic complications. In patients having total hip replacement, interoperative blood loss is reduced by 50%, but postoperative blood loss is not related to anaesthetic technique. Overall blood loss during surgery for repair of fractured neck of femur is not affected by the choice of anaesthetic. Contrary to popular belief, investigation of cognitive and functional competence in elderly patients has not demonstrated any advantage of regional over general anaesthesia. Regional anaesthesia does not reduce the risk of hypothermia in older patients and temperature monitoring and management must be instituted.

Early postoperative mortality (less than 4 weeks) has been shown to be improved by the use of regional anaesthesia. The incidence of silent myocardial ischaemic episodes has been found to be reduced by the use of postoperative regional analgesia. However, long-term morbidity and mortality studies (up to 2 years) are disappointing; cumulative long term mortality has not been shown to be influenced by the anaesthetic technique. Regional nerve block, e.g. peribulbar or retrobulbar block for ophthalmic surgery, has important benefits for older people. The metabolic response to anaesthesia and surgery is prevented, fasting can be eliminated (which is particularly advantageous in diabetic patients) and mobilization is maintained.

POSTOPERATIVE MANAGEMENT

The postoperative period is recognized to be the most crucial time for elderly patients. The level of monitoring depends on the surgical procedure and concomitant diseases. However, in view of their limited physiological reserve, the special needs of this population must be addressed. Abdominal, and especially emergency abdominal, procedures are particularly hazardous and all elderly patients should be admitted to a high dependency unit after operation. The cold, acidotic, vasoconstricted, elderly patient is at great risk and may require re-anaesthetizing and ventilation to permit active rewarming. Hypothermia causes:

- shivering with increased oxygen consumption,
- exaggerated haemodynamic responses,
- increased ventilation,
- ventilation–perfusion mismatch,
- reduced hypoxic drive,
- delayed drug elimination.

This is associated with hypoxaemia, postoperative myocardial ischaemia and an increased incidence of wound infection. Studies have not supported the concept of diminished pain perception in elderly patients. Inadequate analgesia reduces the ability to cough and mobilize, and increases the incidence of respiratory problems. Tachycardia and hypertension increase the risk of serious cardiac problems. There is a reluctance, or inability, of some older patients to complain of pain and many medical staff fail adequately to prescribe analgesics for fear of overdosage. Increased awareness of the importance of the provision of good analgesia in the prevention of morbidity and mortality make it a great challenge. Pharmacokinetics and pharmacodynamics of the elderly demand that drug doses are decreased and treatment intervals prolonged. Medical problems such as renal insufficiency, gastrointestinal bleeding or respiratory insufficiency must be considered in addition to the available monitoring and nursing care. Full advantage must be taken of newer analgesic agents, better methods of delivery and combined therapies to reduce side effects. Achievement of pain relief at rest may be inadequate in elderly patients; functional analgesia on coughing or mobilization is vital. Treatment of postoperative pain using peripheral nerve blocks or the infiltration of local anaesthetics at the site of injury should be considered. Multimodal analgesia such as combinations of NSAIDs and opiates, or local anaesthetics and opiates can be used advantageously. Patient-controlled intravenous analgesia may require time and patience to demonstrate to an elderly patient, but allows for individual patient variability. The judicious use of intrathecal or epidural opiates and local anaesthetics can decrease unwanted sedation and improve mobilization. The advent of acute pain services in many hospi-

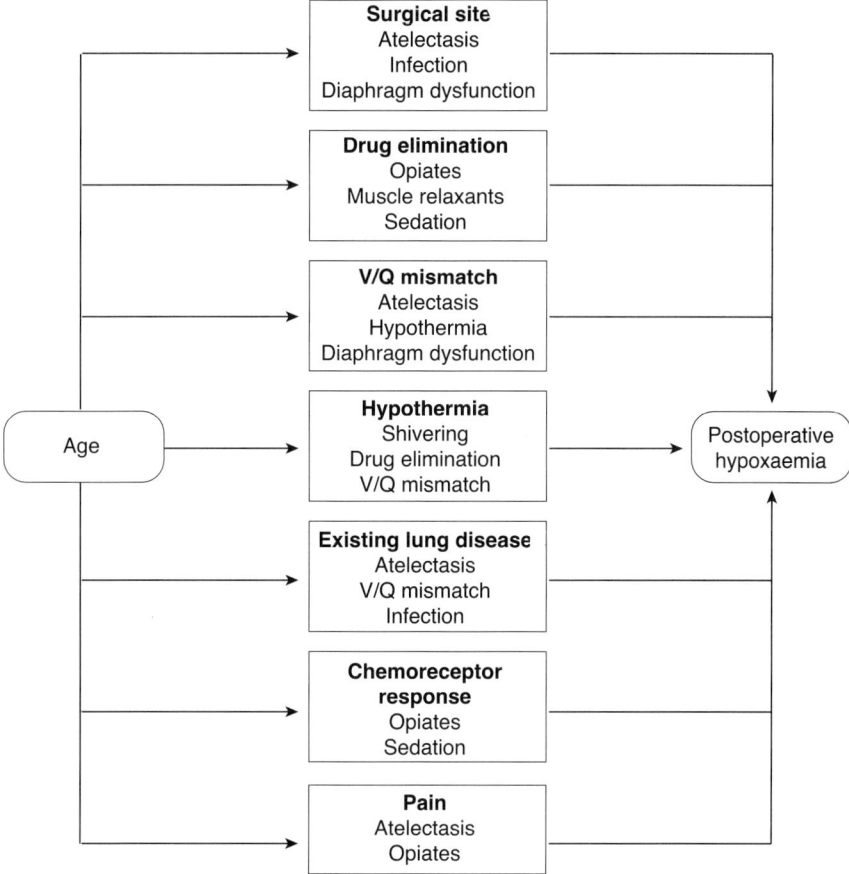

Figure 32.3 Factors contributing to postoperative hypoxaemia in elderly patients.

tals is of particular benefit to elderly patients. Absorption of intramuscular injections of analgesics is unpredictable, especially in obese, cold or muscle-wasted patients. The routine use of this method of analgesia has long been criticized, and it should be improved upon particularly in older patients.

Postoperative hypoxaemia is common, may be profound, and is often unrecognized. Early hypoxaemia can be acute and dramatic, but occurs while the patient is monitored and supervised, and therefore is treated or prevented. Late postoperative hypoxaemia tends to be nocturnal, particularly on the second and third postoperative nights, but may persist for up to five nights or more. Oxygen saturations of less than 85% are not uncommon and may reach 60% (Figure 32.3).

Diminished physiological reserve, an increased incidence of obstructive sleep apnoea, drugs (particularly opiates) and postoperative pain all contribute to an increased vulnerability to the occurrence of hypoxaemia and its consequences. Irregular respiratory rhythms and obstructive sleep apnoea are accompanied by increases in heart rate and arterial pressure which together with hypoxaemia may lead to myocardial ischaemia or impaired myocardial performance. Postoperative nocturnal hypoxaemia can cause confusion and is associated with delayed wound healing. Inappropriate treatment by sedation of the confusion resulting from unrecognized hypoxaemia, particularly in the late postoperative phase, worsens the hypoxaemia. Prolonged oxygen therapy for elderly patients has been recommended, particularly at night. Binasal catheter delivery is the method of choice, as $2\ l\ O_2\ min^{-1}$ delivery has been shown to be as effective as $4\ l\ O_2\ min^{-1}$ by face mask. It also has the advantage of being better tolerated by patients and less likely to be removed. Nasal CPAP has been used to overcome upper airway hypotonia.

Silent myocardial ischaemia is common in elderly patients and increases in incidence, severity and duration after surgery. The highest incidence is found on the third or fourth postoperative day, often not accompanied by haemodynamic changes. There is an established relation with postoperative hypoxaemia, although it can also occur during times of normal oxygen saturation values. Oxygen saturations < 85% and of greater than 5 min duration are particularly significant, and oxygen therapy may abolish associated S–T segment fluctuations. Tachycardia and hypertension may be contributing factors and attention to adequate pain relief and haemoglobin concentration is important. The relationship between episodes of myocardial ischaemia and death from myocardial infarction or arrythmia is not established. There is no direct evidence to date that reducing the frequency of silent myocardial ischaemia improves postoperative morbidity or mortality. However, it is not known whether repeated episodes, particularly in the presence of hypoxaemia may cause myocardial infarction or dysfunction. It is recommended that patients at risk are identified and the level of monitoring and oxygenation increased.

Renal function must be carefully monitored in elderly patients after operation. Changes in cognitive function, confusion, delirium or depression require a thorough search for a cause and appropriate treatment. Infection, especially urinary or respiratory, may not be classical in presentation. Deep venous thrombosis prevention must be considered and instituted where appropriate; low dose heparin may also reduce the incidence of silent myocardial ischaemia. Adverse sequelae after operation in elderly patients are exceptionally important in view of their limited physiological reserve.

CONCLUSIONS

Continually improving anaesthetic, surgical, and intensive care skills ensure than an increasingly elderly population will present for ever more complex surgery. The achievement of good results with low morbidity requires the highest possible standard of care throughout the perioperative period. The postoperative period is a particularly hazardous time for elderly patients. A diminished physiological reserve is most apparent when older patients are subjected to the stress of anaesthesia and surgery. This physiological phenomenon, together with an awareness of the altered pharmacodynamics in this age group, emphasizes the need to prevent postoperative problems. Many issues remain to be resolved. The wisdom of operating on patients classified as ASA grade 5 is frequently questioned. The long-term benefits of many standard practices for this population are often reviewed. Identification and prevention of postoperative problems is being actively researched. Anaesthesia for elderly patients and their care in intensive care units is now comparable in specialist knowledge to that for paediatric patients.

FURTHER READING

Djokovic, J. L. and Hedley-Whyte, J. (1979) Prediction of outcome of surgery and anaesthesia in patients over 80. *Journal of the American Medical Association*, **242**, 2301–2306.

Dodds, C. (1993) Anaesthesia and the geriatric patient. *Ballières Clinical Anaesthesiology*, **7**, 1.

Anon. (1989) Anaesthesia in old age (Editorial). *Anaesthesia* **44**, 337–378.

O'Keeffe S. T. and Ni Chonchubhair, A. (1994) Post-operative delirium in the elderly. *British Journal of Anaesthesia* **73**, 673–687.

Thomas, D. and Ritchie, C. S. (1995) Pre-operative assessment of older adults. *Journal of the American Geriatrics Society* **43**, 811–821.

Zenilman, M. E. and Roslyn J. J. (1994) Surgery in the elderly patient: I. *Surgical Clinics of North America*, **74**, 1.

ANAESTHESIA AND OBESITY 33

C. S. Reilly

It is not uncommon for the anaesthetist to be presented with an obese patient requiring anaesthesia. These patients have a high risk of per- and postoperative complications. The aim of this chapter is to help the anaesthetist to identify the preoperative problems potentially present, and to produce a structure for the anaesthetic and postoperative management which minimizes the risks inherent in this group of patients.

Obesity can be defined simply as having adipose tissue in excess of the normal range. The normal range in young men is 15–18% of total body weight and in young women it is 20–25%. The amount of body fat tends to increase with age. However, this may reflect the fact that the prevalence of obesity increases with age and may not reflect a physiological change. One definition of obesity is a total body fat content greater than 25% in men and greater than 30% in women. This definition, however, raises the question of how one measures, or estimates, body fat mass.

MEASUREMENT OF OBESITY

The simplest method of estimation is to use the relationship between weight and height. This relationship is the foundation for life insurance charts such as the Metropolitan Life Insurance Company charts. These tables, which relate mortality to weight, height and frame size, are used as an estimate of insurance risk. Mortality demonstrates a reasonable correlation with height and weight in these charts, but there is little scientific basis for the introduction of frame size. Based on survival data from a large population, these insurance charts suggest that increased risk of mortality occurs when an individual is greater than 20% heavier than the 'ideal' body weight. Obesity can therefore be defined as more than 20% heavier than ideal body weight. Such a definition can be extended to define morbid obesity as greater than 50% heavier than ideal body weight.

A measurement in much wider use is the height–weight index which is usually known as the body mass index (BMI). This measurement is obtained by dividing the weight in kilograms by the height in metres squared. This number has been used to grade the extent of obesity; a normal BMI is 20–25, grade I obesity or 'overweight' is 25–30, grade II obesity is > 30, severe or morbid obesity is > 35. This index is relatively easy to calculate and can be determined from a nomogram or from a table such as Table 33.1. The relation between body mass index and mortality from all causes has been described. The mortality ratio increases from 1.0 when body mass index is 20–25 to approach 2.0 when body mass index is 35, and increases steeply thereafter.

The major problems relating to anaesthesia and obese patients occur in the morbidly

---

Short Practice of Anaesthesia. Edited by M. Morgan and G. M. Hall. Published in 1997 by Chapman & Hall, London. ISBN 0 412 71890 1

Table 33.1 The relationship between height and body mass index (BMI=W/h^2) illustrated by approximate weight (kg) for a selection of values over a range of heights

Height		Weight (kg)			
ft:in	m	BMI=25	BMI=30	BMI=35	BMI=40
5:0	1.52	58	69	81	92
5:2	1.58	63	75	88	100
5:4	1.63	67	80	93	106
5:6	1.68	71	85	99	113
5:8	1.73	75	90	105	120
5:10	1.78	79	95	110	127
6:0	1.83	84	101	117	132
6:2	1.88	88	106	124	141

obese (BMI > 35). The problems and risk increase with increasing BMI.

PHYSIOLOGICAL CHANGES ASSOCIATED WITH OBESITY

CARDIOVASCULAR SYSTEM

Obesity produces significant physiological changes in the cardiovascular system and systemic cardiovascular disease is a common finding in obese patients. Although adipose tissue has a relatively low blood flow, in morbidly obese patients the cumulative adipose tissue blood flow constitutes a significant part of the cardiac output. There is an increase in intravascular volume and an increase in cardiac output to compensate for this. Systemic hypertension and left ventricular hypertrophy are common findings. Pulmonary hypertension is also a risk in this group of patients. Ischaemic heart disease and cardiac failure are common causes of death. Cardiac failure can occur even in the relatively young (< 30 years old) patient with morbid obesity.

RESPIRATION

Obesity has significant effects on respiratory function producing an inefficiency in ventilation. Oxygen demand and carbon dioxide production are increased because of the enhanced tissue metabolism and also by the increased energy expenditure that is required. There is, therefore, a potential imbalance between increased oxygen consumption and a decrease in oxygen availability.

The primary respiratory defect in the obese individual is a decrease in the functional residual capacity (FRC). This occurs as a result of a number of factors including decreased intercostal movement as a result of the increased weight of the chest wall which results in diaphragmatic breathing. The diaphragm, however, is splinted by the increased intra-abdominal mass. Of the components of FRC, it is the expiratory reserve volume which is reduced as a result of small airway closure. Because tidal volume is essentially unchanged, FRC encroaches on the closing volume within the normal range of tidal volume. This may, in turn, lead to further early closing of airways resulting in significant pulmonary shunt, which may in certain cases result in hypoxaemia although hypercapnoea is rare. However, in a small number of individuals progressive obesity can lead to the development of a raised $Pa\text{CO}_2$. This is known as the obesity hypoventilation syndrome, which is a form of Pickwickian syndrome. Obviously such individuals present considerable risk during their postoperative management. A possibility of the presence of obesity hypoventilation syndrome is justification for the preoperative measurement of arterial blood gases; the presence of hypoxaemia and hypercapnoea will indicate increasing risk. Obesity is associated with the development of obstructive sleep apnoea; patients can undergo periods of significant oxygen desaturation during sleep. This has important indications for the perioperative period where a relationship between desaturation and silent myocardial ischaemia has been demonstrated.

As described above, the FRC may encroach on the closing volume. It must be remembered that placing the patient in the supine position will cause a further decrease of around 20% in the FRC, and that a similar decrease of around 20% is probable during anaesthesia. This is likely to result in significant shunting and hypoxaemia and requires an increase in inspired oxygen concentration (F_{IO_2}).

Lung compliance will be decreased in obesity. This will be almost entirely due to a decreased compliance of the chest wall. The reduced compliance means that relatively high inflation pressures will be required to achieve an adequate tidal volume. It is not uncommon to use inflation pressures greater than 30 cmH$_2$O in these patients. There is also a relatively high incidence of asthma in obese patients.

GASTROINTESTINAL SYSTEM

Obese patients are at risk of passive regurgitation occuring during anaesthesia. Although there is a higher incidence of hiatus hernia in this group, oesophageal reflux is common in these individuals even in the absence of a demonstrable hiatus hernia. Obese patients are known to have a relatively high volume, low pH, gastric residue.

The combination of these factors, oesophageal reflux, raised intra-abdominal pressure and increased gastric residual volume, considerably increases the risk of regurgitation and aspiration pneumonitis. For this reason, anaesthesia should always be induced using a rapid sequence technique and the airway protected with a cuffed endotracheal tube.

ENDOCRINE ABNORMALITIES

Obesity is associated with abnormal carbohydrate metabolism and glucose intolerance. There is a relatively high incidence of diabetes mellitus in these patients. It is important that the blood glucose is checked preoperatively and there should be a low threshold of intervention for prescribing insulin in the perioperative period. This is particularly important in the postoperative period as the stress response results in a relative hyperglycaemia and a period of insulin resistance.

Fatty infiltration of the liver is a common finding in obese patients, but abnormal liver function tests are relatively rare, unless associated with excessive alcohol intake. Transient abnormalities of hepatic function have been noted following general anaesthesia in some individuals of normal body weight, and it is possible that obese patients have an increased likelihood of abnormal liver function tests after operation. Indeed, obesity is one of the factors associated with the rare complication (1:35 000) of halothane-associated hepatitis. This may be a reflection of the increased risk of reductive metabolism of halothane in patients with a large volume of distribution for the drug, and who have a greater risk of hypoxaemia in the postoperative period. Obese patients have a greater risk of thromboembolic disease in the perioperative period, with pulmonary embolism a major cause of death in this group. The amount of the endogenous anticoagulant antithrombin III in the circulation has been shown to be reduced in the morbidly obese.

DRUG METABOLISM

Judging the appropriate dose of a drug to use in the obese individual is difficult. Most drugs are given on a mg kg^{-1} basis, but this would potentially lead to overdosage in the obese patient and an increased incidence of adverse side effects. It is more appropriate in the obese patient that drugs are given on the basis of lean body mass rather than total body weight. Anaesthetic drugs are lipid soluble and the duration of action is more dependent on re-distribution than metabolism or excretion. In the obese patient there is a large volume of distribution at steady state and also a smaller increase in the initial volume of distribution resulting from the increased intravascular volume. These factors suggest that a larger induction dose may be required to produce the same response. However, in practice, at induction of anaesthesia there is only a small increase in the dose required above that which is calculated from the lean body mass, because the initial distribution of the drug by the cardiac output directs it to the areas of high blood flow including the brain. It is obvious that achieving a steady state concentration for maintenance of anaesthesia, with either an inhalational or intravenous agent, takes longer because of the increased volume of distribution. It might be anticipated that awakening at the end of surgery would be delayed because of the considerable amount of drug within the body. Despite this, there is no delay in the arousal of these patients and awakening occurs at a similar concentration to that in non-obese patients. However, at awakening the patient has a larger reservoir of drug within the body, which may be important in the development of halothane-associated hepatitis.

MANAGEMENT

The perioperative management of an obese patient undergoing anaesthesia and surgery is best dealt with under the headings of pre-, per- and postoperative management. However, there are a number of general considerations which should be addressed.

GENERAL CONSIDERATIONS

Movement of the patient

Movement of the morbidly obese patient to and from the operating theatre, and within the theatre, is a serious logistical problem which has to be considered before the operation. There are considerable practical problems in lifting, or turning, the morbidly obese patient in a way that minimizes the risk of accidental injury to either the patient, or the staff involved in lifting. It is important to minimize the number of times that the patient needs to be moved, and the most practical arrangement is to transfer directly from the patient's bed to the operating theatre table, and at the end of the operation transfer back to the bed. It is essential that an adequate number of staff trained in lifting techniques are available at the time the patient is to be moved or may require movement, for example to be placed in Trendelenburg position or the lateral position for surgery.

Access

Related to the above problems are the difficulties of access for both the anaesthetist and the surgeon. From the anaesthetic point of view, venous access, and access for additional monitoring such as CVP or arterial cannulae, may be made very difficult by the sheer size of the patient. Tracheal intubation and positioning of the patient for intubation can also cause problems. Size can also impede monitoring. It is often difficult to obtain a clear ECG trace and to ensure that the blood pressure cuff is of adequate size to give an accurate reading. The use of local analgesic techniques such as limb blocks, and epidural and spinal anaesthesia is attractive in these patients. However, the loss of landmarks can make these techniques very hard, if not impossible to perform, and may require different equipment, such as 15 cm Tuohy needles.

Coexistent disease

There is a relatively high incidence of coexistent disease and this must be remembered in the overall management of the patient. The plan for the anaesthetic in these patients must take account of problems such as ischaemic heart disease, hypertension, asthma and oesophageal reflux, which are all particularly common in these patients.

PREOPERATIVE MANAGEMENT

It is important that the patient is adequately prepared preoperatively for the procedure. Patients may present for surgery related to their obesity or may present for any procedure. The most common operation used to assist in weight loss is the vertical-banded gastroplasty. Jaw wiring and jejunoileal bypass are now rarely used. The aim of vertical-banded gastroplasty is to reduce the volume of the stomach, and therefore produce a feeling of fullness quickly and hence reduction in the amount eaten. The procedure involves a laparotomy with a vertical or subcostal incision and a set of staples are placed vertically along the stomach with a band placed round the outlet of this pouch which results in a stomach volume of 30–50 ml. The procedure takes around 1 h to perform. Because of the significant perioperative risks in this group of patients it is important that they are appropriately selected for this operation. In most centres a team involving a surgeon, a nurse, a dietician, a psychologist and an anaesthetist are involved in the selection and preparation of these patients.

Preoperative investigations should include a full blood count, plasma urea and electrolyte estimations, and a number of blood pressure measurements, ensuring that an adequate cuff size is used. In addition, because of the high incidence of cardiovascular and respiratory disease, preoperative assessment should include ECG, chest X-ray and pulmonary function tests. It is important that coexistent diseases in these patients are well treated preoperatively to minimize the risk of complications in the postoperative period. This is particularly important for the cardiovascular and respiratory systems. If the patient is a smoker they should be requested to stop several weeks before the operation.

As tracheal intubation is potentially difficult it is essential to make a full assessment of the airway at a preoperative visit. If considerable difficulty is anticipated, awake fibreoptic intubation should be considered and discussed with the patient.

Drug therapy

The patient should continue all preoperative drugs required for cardiovascular or respiratory disease up to and including the day of the operation. There is a higher risk of deep venous thrombosis and pulmonary embolism in these patients so it is important that anticoagulant therapy with heparin is started preoperatively and is continued in the postoperative period. There is a risk of failure of low-dose heparin regimens which has been shown to increase with increasing BMI. Monitoring of anticoagulant therapy with heparin to maintain a prothrombin time in the high-normal range is recommended.

Antacid therapy should be included as part of the premedication and the use of H2 receptor antagonists is appropriate. Sedative premedication should be used with caution, as in the larger patients the respiratory depressant effects of benzodiazepines may be significant. It is probably best to avoid the use of opioids preoperatively unless they are required for analgesia.

ANAESTHESIA

Anaesthesia should be induced on the operating table to minimize the need to move the patient. Before commencing anaesthesia, monitoring consisting of ECG, pulse oximetry and non-invasive blood pressure should be undertaken. Venous access with an infusion should be started. In obese patients, particularly those with coexistent cardiovascular disease, there is a strong argument for intra-arterial pressure monitoring which should be undertaken before anaesthesia.

It is necessary to undertake a rapid-sequence induction of anaesthesia in these patients. Tracheal intubation and assisted ventilation is required even for short procedures in obese patients. As described above, obese patients have a reduction in FRC particularly when in the supine position. Pre-oxygenation is, therefore, less effective in the obese patient than in a person of normal body weight. Indeed, it has been shown that, following 3 min pre-oxygenation, the time for oxygen saturation to fall to 90% was around 3 min in a group of patients with a mean body mass index of 46 compared with 10 min in patients with a mean body mass index of 24. In this study one patient desaturated to below 90% in less than 1 min.

In any morbidly obese patient there is the potential for difficulty in achieving tracheal intubation. Therefore, it is important in the preoperative evaluation to make a full assessment of the patient's airway. A particular problem is positioning of the head to allow access for intubation, as there is limited ability to flex and extend the neck because of size. A study has previously made use of neck size as a potential guide to difficulty in intubation. A number of studies have suggested that the incidence of difficulty in intubating the trachea in obese patients is no higher than in the general population. However, because of the combination of the potential for rapid desaturation and difficulty in maintaining an airway to achieve adequate ventilation of the lungs, a cautious approach is strongly recommend. In some centres particularly in the USA, awake, fibreoptic intubation is used as a matter of routine in the largest patients.

The choice of drugs for induction is largely dependent on the presence of coexistent disease. For example, moderate cardiovascular disease or asthma dictates the choice of intravenous agent to one which minimizes the potential changes in cardiovascular variables or with the lowest incidence of histamine release. As discussed above, the dosage required for an intravenous agent and suxamethonium during a rapid-sequence induction is difficult to determine. It is appropriate to have additional induction agent and suxamethonium drawn up in case they are needed. It is common practice to add a short-acting opioid to the induction sequence to minimize the stress response to intubation.

Anaesthesia is best maintained with nitrous oxide and a volatile agent and intermittent doses, or infusion, of a short-acting opioid. Isoflurane is probably the agent of choice for maintenance as it undergoes the smallest amount of metabolism in the body. These patients have a large fat mass in which the agent is sequestered and halothane is best avoided. Assisted ventilation of the lungs may be difficult in some patients because of high inflation pressures which may be beyond the capabilities of standard operating theatre ventilators. This is particularly the case for intra-abdominal operations where the patient is supine and may have a number of retractors in place. If difficulty is encountered in achieving adequate ventilation, it is important to remember that these patients have a relatively high incidence of asthma and the presence of bronchospasm should be actively sought and treated.

Monitoring

It is important that a high standard of monitoring is maintained in all obese patients, even for very short surgical procedures. It is obvious from the description above that these patients have a greater risk of adverse cardiovascular or respiratory events. Therefore, the anaesthetist must be continuously aware of not just abrupt changes but also trends suggesting a deterioration in any cardiovascular or respiratory variable. It is important that monitoring is established in the anaesthetic room before induction of anaesthesia. As a minimum this should consist of ECG, pulse oximetry and non-invasive blood pressure measurements. The accuracy of arterial pressure measurement using a non-invasive technique can be poor in these patients and it is essential that a blood pressure cuff of adequate size is used. Use of a cuff which is too small results in over-reading of arterial pressure, which may be misinterpreted as inadequate anaesthesia with increasing doses of volatile agents or opioids given to the patient and delayed recovery. In view of this problem early consideration should be given to intra-arterial pressure monitoring. A number of factors will contribute to this decision including the anticipated length of surgery, the patients preoperative cardiovascular status and the availability of an effective non-invasive method of arterial pressure measurement.

The use of other invasive monitoring inserted in the anaesthetic room must also be considered. In a patient whose obesity has resulted in cardiovascular complications such as pulmonary hypertension, left ventricular failure and severe hypertension, the use of an internal jugular catheter or pulmonary flotation catheter should be considered. It must be remembered that access for placing such a catheter may be difficult. The benefit of the increased monitoring must then be balanced against the potential risk of vascular trauma in the neck incurred while attempting to place a catheter. Following the induction of anaesthesia and endotracheal intubation, the monitoring must be extended to cover the respiratory system. At a minimum this includes end-tidal CO_2 and peak airway pressure measurement. These are essential to monitor the adequacy of ventilation of the lungs. In the anaesthetized morbidly obese patient inadequate ventilation is a common problem and the accurate diagnosis of the cause may be difficult. For example, a high peak airway pressure and raised end tidal CO_2 could be the result of hypoventilation due to the decreased compliance of the chest wall or, alternatively, could be due to some degree of bronchospasm. A number of modern monitoring systems include the facility of a pressure–volume loop which may be of assistance in differentiating these two causes. The inspired and expired concentrations of oxygen and volatile agent should also be monitored continuously. As discussed above, the accurate judging of drug dose may be difficult and so the degree of neuromuscular blockade should be monitored using a peripheral nerve stimulator. Because of the patient's size, obtaining an adequate response from the ulnar nerve may be difficult and the facial nerve may be used in preference.

Reversal and extubation

The problems to be overcome at this point of the anaesthetic are the re-establishment of adequate respiration, continuation of analgesia and prevention of aspiration. The factors that will influence adequacy of respiration include reversal of neuromuscular blockade, and the presence of opioids and inhalational anaesthetic agents. It is essential that neuromuscular blockade is adequately reversed with an anticholinesterase and the use of a peripheral nerve stimulator to measure the extent of blockade is essential. The time required to eliminate the volatile agent from the body may be prolonged because of the large reservoir of tissue with which the volatile agent equilibrates. It is important therefore, that the vaporizer is turned off promptly to allow adequate washout of the inhalational agent. The measurement of end-tidal concentrations of the inhalational agent is of great value during this period. Extubation should only be attempted when the patient is fully awake, with adequate reflexes and a stable respiratory pattern. Extubating the trachea when the patient is awake is one way of minimizing the risk of acid aspiration. In a patient of normal body size who is at risk of aspiration, the usual procedure is to extubate them on their side, head down. This would lead to several problems in obese patients. First, the problem of turning these patients and second, placing the patient in the head down position further compromises their respiratory reserve. An alternative is to transfer the patient to their bed asleep and then allow them to awaken in a sitting position before extubation. This is the author's practice with larger patients (BMI > 40).

There is a often a fine line between providing adequate analgesia for the patient at this time and preventing the respiratory depressant effects of opioids. It is important that all respiratory and cardiovascular monitoring is continued through the period of reversal. The patient should be kept in the operating theatre until the anaesthetist is completely satisfied that adequate respiration will be maintained during the period of transfer to the recovery room.

POSTOPERATIVE CARE

There are a number of problems which require specific attention in the postoperative management of the morbidly obese patient. These include provision of analgesia, ensuring adequate oxygenation and continued monitoring of the cardiovascular system.

Analgesia

It is essential in these patients that adequate analgesia is provided in the postoperative period as the consequences of inadequate, or excessive, analgesia carry a higher risk than in normal patients. As described earlier, the respiratory reserve in these patients is considerably reduced and is further decreased following anaesthesia and surgery. Poorly controlled analgesia, with either an excessive dose of opioid producing respiratory depression or inadequate pain relief making deep breaths or coughing painful, will result in hypoventilation, retention of secretions and hypoxaemia, and the increased likelihood of respiratory complications. In a recently reported series about 6% of patients had respiratory complications in the postoperative period (Table 33.2). The cardiovascular consequences of hypoxaemia or hypertension and tachycardia associated with pain, must also be considered. In the majority of patients intravenous opioids delivered by PCA, usually morphine with a bolus dose of 1 mg with a lockout period of 5 min, will provide adequate analgesia. If an epidural catheter has been placed for the operation, this is an excellent route for delivery of postoperative analgesia. However, from experience it is easy for these catheters to become displaced or pulled out when the patient is awake and moving, as there is excessive movement of the catheter where is emerges through the skin because of the increased tissue depth.

Table 33.2 Incidence of major complications in a study of 200 patients (mean BMI 46) undergoing vertical banded gastroplasty

	n	(%)
Major complications	31	15.5
Death from pulmonary embolus	1	0.5
Cardiovascular	14	7
Pulmonary embolus/deep vein thrombosis	7	3.5
Hypertension	5	2.5
Respiratory	12	6
Chest infection	11	5.5
Surgical	5	2.5

Based on Goulding and Hovell, 1995

Oxygenation

It is essential that these patients are given oxygen continuously over the first 24 h either by a mask or nasal prongs. It is also preferable that the level of oxygenation is monitored by continuous pulse oximetry in the first 24 h. There is good evidence, also, that these patients should have oxygen on the second and third night as they are at risk, particularly following laparotomy, of hypoxaemia overnight. A history of sleep apnoea also increases the risk at this time.

Monitoring

In view of the potential problems described above and the overall risk, it is preferable that these patients have cardiovascular and respiratory monitoring for at least the first 24 h. This is most satisfactorily conducted in a high dependency unit, if this is available. This allows continuous pulse oximetry, intraarterial pressure and ECG monitoring to be followed during the first 24 h. If there is no high dependency unit there is a good argument that these patients should be monitored in an intensive care unit overnight for the first postoperative night.

Intensive care and resuscitation

As a result of postoperative or surgical complications, or indeed as a *de novo* medical complication, some morbidly obese patients may require ventilation in an intensive therapy unit. A prolonged period (> 12 h) of postoperative ventilation carries a significant increase in morbidity and mortality. The decision to prolong ventilation in the postoperative period, or to intubate and ventilate the morbidly obese patient, must be taken with full consideration of the potential problems that will ensue. Postoperative ventilation increases the likelihood of nosocomial pneumonia in this group of patients in whom the risk of postoperative respiratory infection is already high. The need to reintubate and ventilate the morbidly obese patient, as a result of postoperative ventilatory failure, carries a high mortality. The lungs are difficult to ventilate and require a high airway pressure, which results in a significant fall in venous return and cardiac output, and an increased risk of a pneumothorax. Sepsis is likely in these patients. After any period of ventilation, weaning from the ventilator can be a difficult and prolonged process which may require an elective tracheostomy.

The ventilated obese patient is a major nursing problem, and is best managed on an airbed which reduces the incidence of pressure sores and skin infection, and aids turning.

Resuscitation

Resuscitation of morbidly obese patients following cardiovascular collapse is often unsuccessful. There are a number of factors which contribute to this difficulty. As described above, these patients become rapidly hypoxaemic during any period of apnoea. Venous access, airway management and tracheal intubation are all difficult making the delivery of drugs and oxygen slower. Because of their size it is hard to produce adequate pressures during cardiac compression and, moving them to a firm surface where cardiac compression is more effective may take time.

SUMMARY

When presented with a morbidly obese patient requiring anaesthesia there are a number of major considerations to be addressed.

- General points
    Difficulty of access and in moving patient
    Significant effects on cardiovascular and respiratory function
    Coexistent disease

- Preoperative assessment
    Assess cardiovascular and respiratory function
    Potentially difficult intubation
- Anaesthetic management
    Premedication including anticoagulant and H2 antagonist
    Rapid sequence induction
    High standard of monitoring throughout the entire anaesthetic procedure
    Awake extubation
- Postoperative care
    Analgesia - PCA
    Oxygen therapy

FURTHER READING

Berthoud, M. C., Peacock, J. E. and Reilly, C. S. (1991) Effectiveness of preoxygenation in morbidly obese patients. *British Journal of Anaesthesia* **67**, 464–466.

Bray, G. A. (1978) Definition, measurements, and classification of the syndrome of obesity. *International Journal of Obesity* **2**, 99–114.

Buckley, F. P., Robinson, N. B., Simonowitz, D. A. and Dellinger, E. P. (1983) Anaesthesia in the morbidly obese. A comparison of anaesthetic and analgesic regimens for upper abdominal surgery. *Anaesthesia* **38**, 840–851.

Goulding, S. T. and Hovell, B. C. (1995) Anaesthetic experience of vertical banded gastroplasty. *British Journal of Anaesthesia* **75**, 301–306.

Gray, D. S. (1989) Diagnosis and prevalence of obesity. *Medical Clinics of North America*, **73**, 1–14.

Mason, E. E., Renquist, K. E. and Jiang, D. (1992) Perioperative risks and safety of surgery for severe obesity. *American Journal of Clinical Nutrition* **55** (Suppl.), 573S–576S.

Sjostrom, L. V. (1992) Mortality of severely obese subjects. *American Journal of Clinical Nutrition* **55** (Suppl), 516S–523S.

Vaughan, R. W. (1982). Pulmonary and cardiovascular derangements in the obese patient, in *Anesthetics and the Obese Patient* (ed. B. R. Brown). Contemporary Anesthesia Practice Series, Davis, Philadelphia, pp. 19–39.

Wilson, A.T. and Reilly, C. S. (1993) Anaesthesia and the obese patient. *International Journal of Obesity* **17**, 427–435.

THE INFECTIOUS PATIENT 34

D. A. Zideman

Anaesthesia is a multidisciplinary specialty and anaesthetists therefore meet a wide range of medical conditions. Sometimes the conditions may be complex and the diseases and pathology relevant to each other. Quite often though, there may be a primary pathology that needs urgent surgical attention but a secondary underlying condition complicates the issue. This is the case with the management of the infectious patient.

Infectious diseases are common during infancy and childhood but not exclusively so. The anaesthetist may encounter infants and children who require urgent surgical treatment related to infectious disease, or more often this disease may be present in a child who requires surgery for an unrelated lesion. Here, the risks of anaesthesia in the presence of the infectious disease must be balanced against the urgency of the surgical procedure. Some judgements will be difficult but in all these patients the technique of anaesthesia used must be modified to adapt to the particular aspects of the infectious disease. Some childhood infectious diseases are extremely contagious and anaesthetists must be familiar with the mode of transmission if they are to take adequate precautions to prevent the spread of infection to other patients or to hospital staff. Infectious diseases in adults may include those in children but more commonly are diseases that have resulted from antibiotic resistant pathogens or blood borne viruses. Such infections in medically compromised patients can significantly increase the risk of morbidity and mortality.

FEVER

Fever is defined as an elevation of the body temperature above normal. When fever is associated with infection, this elevated temperature is part of the patient's response to that infection. There is some evidence that fever may assist the body in fighting the infectious agent. Certainly during an infection the patient's thermoregulatory mechanisms tend to maintain the elevated core temperature.

Fever is generated as the infecting agent stimulates the production of pyrogens by leucocytes, macrophages and other cells. The pyrogen, a polypeptide, acts directly upon the hypothalamus. Alternatively it may act on the hypothalamus via a prostaglandin, catecholamine and the cyclic adenosine monophosphate pathway. The result is a hypothalamic-induced increase in heat production centred in skeletal muscle in older children and adults. Young children may become febrile from non-shivering thermogenesis. Low birthweight infants may not develop a fever in response to sepsis but may become hypothermic. This lack of febrile reaction may contribute to the increased mortality associated with infection in newborn infants.

The increase in body temperature most commonly associated with fever results in an

Short Practice of Anaesthesia. Edited by M. Morgan and G. M. Hall. Published in 1997 by Chapman & Hall, London. ISBN 0 412 71890 1

increased metabolic rate and a raised oxygen requirement. In adults, this increase is approximately 13% for each degree centigrade rise above normal body temperature. In infants and small children the raised energy costs due to fever will be higher due to the greater heat loss from a relatively larger body surface area.

The clinical manifestations of fever include chills, headache, rigours and tachycardia. Sweating may occur as the fever resolves. Delirium and coma may occur during high fever and convulsions sometimes occur in children. Fluid losses via the skin and respiratory tract are increased and can result in dehydration if fluid intake is reduced due to associated anorexia, vomiting or iatrogenic fluid restriction.

The treatment of fever should generally be directed at the underlying infectious process. Active measures to reduce the body temperature of a febrile infected patient may cause harm; if a child is placed in a cool environment, for example a modern operating theatre, this may increase thermogenesis unless the hypothalamic set point is lowered. This increased thermogenesis will then be accompanied by a further increase in metabolic demand for oxygen and a vicious cycle is established resulting in a deteriorating condition.

Treatment to reduce fever can be justified if it benefits the general comfort of the patient, improves the outcome of the illness or the associated pathology, or reduces the incidence of febrile convulsions in children. However, a favourable response of a fever to antipyretic therapy does not indicate that the illness is trivial and it may lead to a false optimism in the carers. More seriously, such a response may mask the early signs of a developing serious illness. There is little evidence that antipyretic therapy for fever improves outcome. In children antipyretic drugs may cause toxicity but there may be clinical indication for their prescription, for example febrile convulsions or pre-existing heart disease.

None the less care must be taken when taking the drug; salicylates that have been known for many years as extremely effective antipyretics, are now implicated in the induction of Reye's Syndrome in children.

When anaesthetizing patients with a fever care must be taken to recognize the increased metabolic rate for oxygen and carbon dioxide and that this increase is directly related to the extent of the pyrexia. Special consideration must be given to ensure a high concentration of inspired oxygen and an increase in alveolar ventilation. Any interruption of oxygenation is poorly tolerated in the pyrexial patient and should this hypoxia proceed to cardiac arrest, the resulting neurological damage is more severe than that seen in the normothermic patient. Inability to ensure an adequate alveolar ventilation will also result in a respiratory acidosis due to the accumulation of carbon dioxide. This will not only adversely affect the patient but may affect the pharmacodynamics of the anaesthetic drug being used.

Atropine should not be given as a premedicant to the pyrexial patient as it will reduce sweating and so may enhance a preoperative increase in body temperature. If atropine is required, it is better administered during anaesthesia when temperature control is more easily achieved. Volatile anaesthetic agents such as halothane and isoflurane may be used to produce vasodilation of the skin vessels and so increase the heat loss from a pyrexial patient but neuromuscular blocking drugs must be given to prevent shivering and thus the associated increased metabolic demand for oxygen.

SEPTICAEMIA

Septicaemia implies a severe and overwhelming infection with bacteria. This severe infection is accompanied by fever, shock, debility and may lead to a disseminated intravascular coagulation in a patient who is susceptible to, or has a likely source of, infection.

Staphylococcal septicaemia is usually related to a focal site of infection but occasionally occurs without an identifiable focus. Osteomyelitis, arthritis and wound infections are common primary foci but staphylococcal infection can occur as a complication of a simple venous cannulation. The patient with staphylococcal septicaemia appears ill and toxic. A petaechial or purpuric skin rash may be seen together with haematuria, jaundice, seizures and cardiac murmurs as the disease progresses. Disseminated intravascular coagulation is common. Treatment is aimed at active fluid replacement and aggressive antibiotic therapy with the drainage of localized infections and the resection of grossly infected or infarcted tissues.

Streptococcal sepsis may complicate cellulitis or wound infection but is occasionally seen without an obvious focal point. Pneumococcal sepsis is usually seen in severely debilitated patients or in those who have undergone splenectomy. The pneumococcus is an encapsulated bacteria and the activity of the spleen is believed to aid phagocytosis of such organisms by its production of opsonins. Pneumococcal sepsis is a critical illness in which widespread purpura and disseminated intravascular coagulation frequently occur. A peripheral blood smear that has been Gram stained may demonstrate the bacterium. Although a pneumococcal vaccine is available for patients undergoing splenectomy, (Pneumovax, 0.5 ml by subcutaneous or intramuscular injection) a conservative approach to splenectomy is considered the more favourable option. Prophylactic antibiotics (phenoxymethylpenicillin) are often recommended for splenectomized patients undergoing surgery, but their value in preventing sepsis is unproven. Patients with sickle cell disease are often regarded as having impaired splenic function and are usually given prophylactic antibiotics.

Meningococcal septicaemia is a fulminating disease characterized by a high fever, a petaechial or purpuric rash, arthritis, vomiting and diarrhoea; meningitis may occur. The characteristic rash becomes widespread with involvement of the mucous membranes. The disease may progress extremely rapidly with circulatory failure and death within a few hours. Further complications are a myocarditis, disseminated intravascular coagulation and adrenal insufficiency due to bilateral adrenal haemorrhage (Waterhouse–Friderichsen syndrome). These are extremely sick patients and the initial management is often supportive to restore the circulating blood volume. Invasive haemodynamic monitoring is required and a urinary catheter must be inserted. Plasma, albumin and blood with appropriate electrolyte solutions must be infused to achieve optimal filling pressures. Inotropic support may be required. A low urine output despite adequate fluid input and a normal blood pressure may indicate the onset of renal failure. Corticosteroids are controversial but many advise their use even in the absence of defined evidence-based practice because of the unpredictable severity of this illness. Antibiotics, usually benzyl penicillin, chloramphenicol or cefotaxime, are an essential part of the therapy of these patients and if given early enough may halt the progression of the septicaemia to its more serious stages. Rifampicin is recommended for the prevention of secondary cases of meningococcal infection (where a second or third party has been in close contact with a patient infected with the meningococcus) but the side effects of this drug's administration, namely gastrointestinal symptoms, renal failure and alterations in hepatic function, must be considered carefully. Those taking rifampicin should be warned that their urine and saliva may become orange-red coloured.

SEPTIC SHOCK

The progression of acute sepsis to septic shock is associated with a rapid increase in mortality. The increasing complexity of surgery, the prolongation of the lives of patients with defective immunity, the widespread uses of antibiotics and the increase in invasive techniques providing portals of entry for infection are all responsible for the increase in the incidence of septic shock seen in modern medicine. The Gram negative organisms *Escherichia coli* and *Neisseria meningitidis* are especially frequent, but *Streptococcus pneumoniae* is commonly implicated. Septic shock is an unpredictable pattern of circulatory insufficiency with inadequate tissue oxygenation. Endotoxins are the mediators of the initial disturbances of septic shock. Activated macrophages produce cytokines – leucotrines IL1 (endogenous pyrogen), IL2 and IL6. The release of prostaglandins, tumour necrosing factor and thromboxanes then specifically damages the capillary endothelium of target organs. The appearance of free oxygen radicals and eicosanoids (PGE_2, 6-Keto-PC_1F_1, TXB_2) leads to endothelial dehiscence, leakage, pericapillary oedema, abnormal platelet deposition, white cell plugging and microvascular thrombosis. The early stages of septic shock are characterized by tachycardia, tachypnoea, bounding pulses and normotension and hypotension, with a decreased systemic vascular resistance and a high cardiac index. Later the tachycardia persists but is accompanied by hypotension, reduced cardiac index and systemic vascular resistance. Hypoxaemia is present throughout and in the latter stages is accompanied by a mixed respiratory and metabolic acidosis and oliguria. Progression of the septicaemia leads on to a coagulopathy and finally multiple organ failure unless the process can be reversed.

The treatment of septic shock must be aimed at preserving myocardial, renal and central nervous system function. These patients should be managed in an intensive care environment where extensive cardiovascular monitoring, accurate fluid therapy and detailed drug administration can occur. The detailed treatment of septic shock is beyond the scope of this chapter and is somewhat controversial. Nevertheless, the following important therapeutic steps should be considered.

- Cardiorespiratory support to attain maximum cellular oxygenation and thus maintain major organ function.
- Meticulous intravenous fluid therapy managed by appropriate intravascular monitoring.
- Correction of acid–base and electrolyte disturbances.
- Cardiovascular support with inotropic drug infusions to reverse hypotension and oligura.
- Corticosteroids may be considered.
- Surgical treatment of localized infections.

When anaesthesia is required for a patient in septic shock, it is important that the optimal therapy for the shocked state is already in progress. If it is not, it should be begun before the commencement of anaesthesia but the surgical treatment should not be delayed unduly. Hypovolaemia and acidosis should be corrected and fever reduced before surgery. Hypoxia should be reversed as much as possible and hypoventilation, if present, treated by establishing controlled ventilation. Corticosteroid therapy should be augmented and inotropic therapy optimized. The anaesthesia itself is difficult and should only be carried out by those with adequate experience. The technique chosen should selectively spare the cardiovascular system and ketamine is often chosen as the induction agent with fentanyl and oxygen for maintenance, supported by a neuromuscular blocking drug. Intensive care facilities, often in an isolation bay, are nearly always mandatory and must be available before the start of surgery for the effective postoperative management of patients.

Neonatal sepsis affects one in 230 preterm infants and one in 1200 term infants. Several factors predispose the newborn to sepsis and despite advances in antibiotic therapy the mortality and morbidity remains high. Cellular and humoral responses to infection are limited as leucocytes have impaired chemotactic, phagocytic and bactericidal activity. Immunoglobulin deficiency is also present, especially in the preterm infant, as transplacental transfer of globulins varies with the length of gestation. The organisms that most commonly cause neonatal septicaemia are the Gram positive group B streptococci and the Gram negative *Escherichia coli*. The risk of infection is high in the neonatal nursery. Tracheal intubation, intravenous infusions and invasive monitoring lines, now part of the routine practice of premature baby units, all provide routes for infection to enter these vulnerable bodies. Preterm infants who undergo urgent procedures are especially at risk. Failure to observe strict hand washing before handling of infants is a leading cause of spread of these infections. Although the clinical signs are similar to that seen in the older patient, temperature instability, abdominal distension, jaundice and apnoea are more classical signs in this age group. Changes in activity, feeding patterns and muscle tone are often noted in the early stages. Aggressive antibiotic and meticulous fluid therapy under careful full invasive cardiovascular monitoring conditions in a properly equipped special care baby unit are essential for survival. The infant must be nursed in a thermoneutral environment to minimize any further homeostatic changes. The anaesthetist may be involved in the surgical care of such infants. As in the adult the preoperative cardiorespiratory, metabolic, acid–base, electrolyte and haematological status must be accurately evaluated and optimized. Meticulous care must be directed at maintaining all established therapies during the transportation of the infant and in the intraoperative period to avoid physiological stress. Cold stress, hypoglycaemia and fluid overload must be prevented and it is therefore recommended that surgery on these infants is only carried out by experienced medical teams with the full support of the neonatal staff. Asepsis must be assured in all anaesthesia related procedures.

VIRAL INFECTIONS

Anaesthetists are exposed to a variety of viral infections during their normal working practice. Amongst the most common is the common cold (coryza) and the infectious diseases of childhood that may also be seen in adolescents or adults.

THE COMMON COLD

This is probably the most common infectious disease encountered by medical staff and accounts for more loss of working time than any other infectious disease. The problem for anaesthetists is that although they may accept the cross infection risk as part of an overall occupational hazard, the patient may suffer undue complications, morbidity and mortality having undergone anaesthesia when suffering from this infectious condition. In the emergency situation the symptoms and signs are often overlooked in an effort to proceed, with all due expediency, towards the required operative procedure. The problem arises in the non-urgent, elective case whose surgery has been planned and booked in that there may be a conflict between need and requirement. Some authorities have recommended that where a patient is suffering from a 'runny nose' with no secondary infection or increase in temperature that there may be no reason to delay surgery. Others take the opposite view, that this is subjecting the patient to an unnecessary, or even unknown, risk for the sake of an elective procedure. In favour of the latter argument is quoted the increased number of postoperative chest infections, the occurrence of the irritable airway and the incidence of intra- and postoperative airway complications that occur in these patients. If anaesthesia is delayed, the question must then be asked as to how long should the postponement period last. Furthermore, is there any intercurrent therapy that should be offered to the patient to alleviate their current symptoms and to improve their recovery? Commonly the decision is made on purely subjective grounds using the anaesthetist's clinical assessment of the overall status of the patient with the final arbiter being the patient's temperature.

INFECTIOUS DISEASES ASSOCIATED WITH CHILDHOOD

One of the most difficult decisions for an anaesthetist to make is to decide as to whether the child presented to him as a potential patient who is slightly 'off colour' with a runny nose that is beginning to improve is simply recovering from a common cold, has an upper respiratory tract infection or is in the prodromal phase of a more serious infectious disease. Although the disease itself may present little inherent risk to the child, it could have profound consequences for those with whom the child comes in contact. They could expose the pregnant anaesthetist, nurse and operating theatre attendant inadvertently to the rubella or herpes virus thus placing the young fetus at risk; they may expose the adult male to mumps; the immunocompromised patient in hospital could receive, by the most informal of contact, a dose of a simple viral infectious disease that will result in a serious or even fatal illness.

Rubella

This is a mild infectious disease with an incubation period of 10–21 days. The systemic signs are very mild and are often missed. They include a fever, sore throat, lymphadenopathy in the sternomastoid and occipital regions and a maculopapular rash that develops initially on the face and hands but spreads to the trunk and limbs. Occasionally arthritis or thrombocytopenic purpura develops and rarely encephalitis is reported as a complication. The rubella syndrome (low birth weight, deafness, congenital heart disease, eye defects, microcephaly) follows intrauterine infection during early gestation (less than 12 weeks) and is the most serious complication of the disease. It is currently recommended that a single dose antigen rubella vaccine be given to all girls between their 10th and 14th birthdays and to non-immune women before pregnancy and after delivery. Younger children are now given MMR or MR vaccine at the end of their first year of life.

Measles (rubeola)

This is a very infectious viral disease spread by droplet infection. Since the introduction of an active vaccination programme, measles notifications have steadied at about 10 000 per year but, more significantly, in the years 1990 to 1991 no single child died of acute measles-related illness in England and Wales. Nevertheless, measles does still present a serious risk to those from outside vaccination programme areas and to those who are poorly nourished, the chronically ill and the immunocompromised child where complications are more common. The incubation period is about 10 days, with a further 2–4 days before the rash appears. It is highly infectious from the beginning of the prodromal period to 4 days after the appearance of the rash. Clinical factors include Koplik spots, coryza, conjunctivitis, bronchitis, rash and fever. Complications have been reported in one in fifteen notified cases and include otitis media, bronchitis, pneumonia, convulsions and encephalitis (incidence of one in 5000 cases, 20–44% residual neurological consequences). Respiratory infections are common and pneumonitis is present in 20% of patients. Pleural effusions may appear and pneumomediastinum, pneumothorax and subcutaneous emphysema have occurred in association with measles. Laryngitis is a frequent complication in some countries and is a leading cause of death in young malnourished children. In the abdomen lymph node hyperplasia may result in abdominal pain that is occasionally mistaken for acute appendicitis. Muscle weakness and depressed tracheal reflexes may appear one or two weeks after appearance of the measles rash and progress to the typical clinical picture of Guillain–Barré syndrome. There are no specific treatment recommendations as, in the vast majority, the course of the infection is short and uncomplicated. Some doctors prescribe antibiotics to prevent secondary bacterial pneumonic infection. In hospital the infected patient should be isolated from the onset of the catarrhal stage until the third day of the rash to reduce exposure and contamination of those patients at risk.

Varicella (chicken pox) and Herpes Zoster

Varicella is a common, extremely contagious disease transmitted by direct personal contact or droplet spread. It is most common in children below the age of 10 years in whom the illness is relatively mild. Vesicles appear without prodromal illness on the face and scalp, spreading to the trunk, abdomen and eventually the limbs. The vesicles dry out to a granular scab in 3–4 days and are usually followed by further scabs. The disease can be more serious in adults, particularly for pregnant women, neonates and the immunosuppressed patient. The reactivation of the patient's varicella virus causes Herpes Zoster and is therefore transmissible to susceptible individuals as chickenpox. Vesicles appear in the dermatome representing cervical or spinal ganglia where the virus has been lying dormant. The affected area may be intensely painful with associated paraesthesia. In the immunocompromised patient varicella may rapidly progress to haemorrhagic disseminated infection with death ensuing from pneumonia or encephalitis. Varicella has also been associated with Reye's syndrome; 15% of patients with this syndrome give a history of an associated varicella infection.

Mumps (epidemic parotitis)

A viral infection most commonly seen in school aged children though it may occur in adults. The disease is characterized by fever, malaise and swelling of the parotid glands. The incubation period is 14–21 days but the virus is transmissible for several days before the parotid swelling to several days after it appears. Complications include pancreatitis, oophoritis, (which on the right side may resemble appendicitis) and orchitis. Meningoencephalitis is associated with mumps. It has been suggested that mumps might be implicated in the aetiology of juvenile diabetes mellitus.

Infectious mononucleosis

A disease of children, adolescents and young adults caused by the Epstein–Barr virus. It is characterized by lassitude, fever, pharyngitis, lymphadenopathy and hepatosplenomegaly. It usually runs a benign course and can be so insidious that it may resemble repeated coryzal infections. Complications which directly involve the anaesthetist include airway obstruction due to massively enlarged tonsils, splenic rupture and Guillain–Barré syndrome. Hepatic function may be impaired and jaundice may occur. Abnormal liver isoenzymes are found in the majority of patients.

OTHER INFECTIOUS DISEASES

DIPHTHERIA

This acute infectious disease is caused by the club shaped Gram positive rod *Corynebacterium diphtheriae* that invades the nose and throat causing a nasopharyngitis. The organism produces a powerful exotoxin that causes major myocardial and neurological damage. Although the disease has virtually disappeared in Western world countries due to the active immunization programme there have been a few outbreaks of the disease among recent immigrants spreading into the unimmunized population. During the disease the nasopharyngitis develops into white spots which coalesce to form a thin adherent membrane. This membrane thickens and darkens in colour and any attempt to remove it results in bleeding. The symptoms develop into severe upper airway obstruction and in cases of laryngeal diphtheria close observation must be maintained by an expert in emergency airway support in case a fragment of the membrane is dislodged and obstructs the upper airway. Anaesthetists are usually closely involved with the physicians and paediatricians in the management of the patients as they may require emergency tracheal intubation or tracheostomy. Cardiac and neurological damage resulting from the endotoxin may occur after even a mild infection and needs careful monitoring and appropriate therapy. Cardiac arrhythmias may require rapid treatment including pacing for heart block. Severe diphtheria interferes with oral feeding and therefore intravenous therapy, including parenteral feeding is required.

TETANUS

This is caused by infection of a wound with spore bearing, anaerobic Gram positive *Clostridium tetani*. The neurotoxin produced by this organism is responsible for the clinical picture including muscle rigidity, with tonic and clonic spasms of skeletal muscle triggered by sensory stimuli of touch, noise and bright light. As the spasms become more prolonged, they affect the ventilatory muscles and together with laryngeal spasms may lead to respiratory failure and death. The autonomic nervous system is also involved and there are changes in heart rate, labile hypertension, cardiac arrhythmias and disordered temperature control. Neonatal tetanus is seen from infection of the umbilicus. It has a short incubation period, presents in an inability to suck rapidly followed by a generalized stiffness and convulsions. Ventilatory muscle spasm leads to apnoea.

Treatment includes the administration of antitoxin and appropriate antibiotic therapy. The patient is best managed in a quiet area where all external stimuli are kept to a minimum. Diazepam has been used to sedate and control mild cases but more serious cases may require neuromuscular blockade and mechanical ventilation. Cardiovascular instability due to 'autonomic storms' may require antihypertensive therapy and it is suggested that tubocurarine has the ideal neuromuscular blocking properties for this disease. Isoflurane has been suggested to be the volatile agent of choice in that it can be administered to achieve good blood pressure control and arrhythmias may be less troublesome than with halothane. Hyperkalemia leading to cardiac arrest has been reported in patients with tetanus following the administration of suxamethonium.

TUBERCULOSIS

Infection by *Mycobacterium tuberculosis* or *Mycobacterium bovis* is usually by the airborne spread of the bacillus. There has been a rapid decline in the incidence of tuberculosis in the UK and it has now steadied at just over 5000 cases per year. The incidence varies widely between areas but is generally higher in areas where a high proportion of the population come from the Indian subcontinent. Although the majority of cases involve the respiratory system, non-respiratory forms are more commonly seen in immigrant ethnic groups and in those who are immunocompromised. The anaesthetist may become involved in many aspects of the tuberculosis infected patient. The multiplicity of organs that can be involved and may require surgical intervention dictates that a great variety of critical problems may present. Contamination of the anaesthetic equipment is a possible hazard and therefore disposable equipment is recommended to be used whenever possible. Anaesthetic ventilator breathing systems should, in addition, be protected by bacterial filters. Non-disposable equipment should be placed immediately in an antiseptic solution (0.1% chlorhexidine) for one hour and then they can be cleaned and scrubbed with soap and water with no danger to other personnel. Sterilization by boiling or autoclaving can then occur. Boiling for 3 min will destroy the tubercule bacillus. Other, more delicate items, can be treated with ethylene oxide and larger items in the operating theatre should be washed with a chemical disinfectant (70% alcohol in water). The operating theatre should be 'rested' for a period of time, to allow for an adequate number of air exchanges before being used again. Unfortunately the diagnosis of tuberculosis infection is often not made until after surgery has started but these simple precautions must be implemented and followed as soon as the diagnosis is suspected.

HOSPITAL-ACQUIRED INFECTION

Methicillin-resistant staphylococcus aureus (MRSA) and vancomycin-resistant enterococcus (VRE) are two organisms which have, in recent years, required careful infectious disease control measures. MRSA is resistant to many antibiotics as well as methicillin and some strains of this organism have a particular propensity for spread. These are termed epidemic MRSA (EMRSA). VRE is also resistant to many antibiotics as well as vancomycin. It is important to realize that these organisms are not dangerous to healthy adults but they may cause serious infections in susceptible hospitalized patients. Infected or colonized patients therefore require isolation by barrier nursing to prevent the spread by transient colonization of staff and other patients and to prevent contamination of equipment and the environment.

The precise procedures to be followed in the management of a colonized or an infected patient vary from hospital to hospital. The policy of the local Control of Infection Committee must be followed and there can be no exceptions by any medical, nursing or technical staff. Visitors must also adhere to the regimen that may require them donning plastic aprons and gloves. Hands must be washed immediately before leaving the isolation room and disinfected with an alcohol-based skin rub once outside the room. Relatives should be carefully counselled about why these procedure are taking place.

In the operating theatre these infectious patients must again be isolated. Careful planning of the operating list can place these patients who require surgery at a time when they will not contact other patients. All infected equipment must be properly labelled, washed and sterilized or more ideally disposed of as infected medical waste. Medical specimens, including blood, should be carefully sealed and labelled as coming from an MRSA- or VRE-positive patient. The operating room must be carefully cleaned with Hycolin 1% and left empty for at least 30 min before reuse. Some authorities require the patient to have anaesthesia induced in an operating theatre, thereby bypassing the anaesthetic room and for the patient to recover in the operating theatre, thus not contaminating the recovery area.

The implementation of isolation and barrier procedures must not compromise the patient's medical care or safety. The proper procedures are staff intensive and usually require a dedicated 'runner' to serve the 'infected' medical team with the equipment and drugs required from the non-infected external environment. The 'runner' must be an experienced professional member of staff so that there are no undue delays in the provision of essential supplies. Care in the operating theatre environment should be to the same standard as for any routine patient. If the patient is placed at the end of the operating session they should not be cancelled because of the shortage of operating time, nor should they be treated by the emergency team because the routine staff have finished. Finally the antibiotic prescribing policy within a hospital must be strictly followed. Frequent audits of prescriptions will prevent the indiscriminate prescribing of antibiotics that has led to the development of these multiresistant organisms. It is only by careful and meticulous infection control that these infectious diseases can be isolated without compromising patient care.

BLOOD-BORNE VIRUSES

The importance of blood-borne viruses has become increasingly apparent over the last decade. There are several viruses recognized for being occupationally transmitted to or by anaesthetists.

- Human immunodeficiency virus (HIV), where the majority of those infected will eventually develop acquired immune deficiency syndrome (AIDS).
- Hepatitis viruses. Hepatitis B poses the most serious threat. Hepatitis C and D viruses are also blood borne and up to 50% of those infected with Hepatitis C will develop chronic liver disease.
- Human T-cell leukaemia virus (HTLVI): infection which causes adult T-cell leukaemia and is also associated with tropical spastic paresis.

HUMAN IMMUNODEFICIENCY VIRUS (HIV)

Despite desperate efforts to control the AIDS epidemic the infection has continued to spread. In 1992, 5894 cases of AIDS were reported of whom 3686 have died. It is currently suggested that approximately three new cases of AIDS are reported each day. In spite of preconceived ideas about the sexuality of this illness, 19% of cases have occurred in heterosexual adults and there have been 69 known cases in children of whom 31 have died. Of more of a problem to anaesthetists is the fact that the actual number of HIV-positive individuals in the UK is not known. The distribution of infected individuals is not regular and there is a higher prevalence in certain areas, notably London, Edinburgh and Dublin. None the less the occurrence of HIV-positive cases cannot be assumed and proper sensible precautions against cross infection by contaminated blood must always be taken.

HIV is transmitted by blood, sexual contact and transplacentally from mother to fetus. Various body fluids have been designated as high risk and they are: amniotic fluid, pericardial fluid, pleural fluid, synovial fluid, cerebrospinal fluid, peritoneal fluid, semen and vaginal secretions. Faeces, nasal secretions, sputum, saliva, sweat, urine and vomit are not considered to present a significant risk of transmission **unless** they are visibly contaminated with blood. Anaesthetists are therefore considered at occupational risk from their routine exposure to blood and blood-stained body fluids. Of the 146 cases of occupational transmission of HIV, 51 documented seroconversions were following specific exposure. Of the 2475 cases of exposure to the virus from percutaneous injury (needle stick injury) nine have seroconverted, an occupational exposure risk of 0.36%.

Although there are effective screening tests for HIV antibodies, interpretation is complicated by the three-month window between infection and the appearance of antibodies. Therefore there will always be some patients who do pose a risk of infection but will not be identified by routine screening for antibodies. Where antibody screening is requested, it must only be carried out with the explicit consent of the patient. This should only be obtained after a careful explanation has been given to the patient and the patient offered special counselling as to the implications of his decision. If the patient is unconscious and the test is required for therapeutic reasons, consent via the next of kin must be sought. Only in their absence can it be considered reasonable to test without consent.

HEPATITIS

Infection with the Hepatitis B virus (HBV) is a major problem throughout the world. The number of overt cases of hepatitis B in the UK is low and there has been a marked decrease of reported cases in recent years. In addition to the overt cases is the carrier state. The carrier state, which is defined as 'the persistence of hepatitis B surface antigen in the circulation for more than 6 months' occurs in 5–10% of infected adults. It is estimated that about 1:500 of the adult population in the UK are carriers.

The illness usually has an insidious onset with anorexia, vague abdominal discomfort, nausea and vomiting. Arthralgia and a rash may occur with or without fever and the disease often progresses to jaundice. The incubation period is 40–160 days (but can extend to 9 months) and there is a 1% fatality rate of those admitted to hospital.

The most infectious patients carry the hepatitis Be antigen (HBeAg). These carriers have high concentrations of the virus in their blood. A proportion of these antigen carriers will progress to develop chronic hepatitis, cirrhosis and primary liver cancer. HBV is found in nearly all body fluids but occupational transmission has only been established where there has been contamination with blood, serum or vaginal secretions. The risk of transmission through occupational inoculation with HBV is higher than with HIV with a reported range of 5–30%.

All anaesthetists (and other health care workers) should be immunized against HBV. The vaccine contains 20 $\mu g\ ml^{-1}$ of hepatitis B surface antigen; 80–90% of individuals mount a response to the vaccine and an antibody level of 100 mUnits ml^{-1} is generally considered protective. Those individuals who do not reach this antibody level may not be effectively protected and may require Hepatitis B immunoglobulin for protection if exposed to infection. Antibody titres should be checked following immunization and poor or non-responders considered for booster or repeat vaccination. Vaccination produces antibody levels considered adequate for 3–5 years but retesting of antibody levels is required to establish the level of protection. Most health authorities and trusts have a strict hepatitis policy. These policies include screening for markers prior to immunization and then establishing an adequate hepatitis B antibody titre before staff are allowed to perform clinical work.

PRECAUTIONS AGAINST INFECTION WITH BLOOD-BORNE VIRUSES

There has been much discussion as to the role of the anaesthetist and whether an anaesthetist is considered an 'at risk' person by performing 'exposure prone procedures' (formerly known as an invasive procedure). The latest definition from the UK Department of Health defines exposure prone procedures as 'those procedures where there is a risk that injury to the health worker may result in the exposure of the patient's open tissues to the blood of the worker. These procedures include those where the worker's gloved hand may be in contact with sharp instruments, needle tips or sharp tissues (spicules of bone or teeth) inside a patient's open body cavity, wound or confined anatomical space where the hands or finger tips may not be completely visible at all times'. An expert advisory group of anaesthetists, the Blood Borne Viruses Advisory Panel of the Association of Anaesthetists, currently recommend that although anaesthetists put their fingers into patients' mouths during the course of their clinical work, anaesthesia should not be regarded as an exposure prone speciality. Nevertheless, the panel do recommend the following.

- It should be mandatory for anaesthetists to wear proper surgical gloves (non-sterile) when carrying out procedures which involve putting their fingers into the patients' mouths. These gloves should be

discarded once the procedure has been carried out.
- Gloves should also be worn during the induction of anaesthesia, inserting intravenous cannulae, setting up intravenous infusion, and inserting or removing airways and tracheal tubes.
- Where substantial blood spillage may occur, for example in setting up an intra-arterial monitoring line, a plastic apron, mask and eye protection should be worn.
- Equipment, notes and other articles must not be handled with contaminated gloves.
- Intact skin is impermeable to blood-borne viruses, but the anaesthetist with eczema, chapping or several scratches is at risk of being infected. Skin wounds must be covered with a waterproof dressing.

Prevention of percutaneous inoculation injury is very important. Needles that have been in contact with a patient must not be resheathed. All needles and sharps should be disposed of immediately after use in the appropriate 'Sharps Disposal Bin'. Any needle or sharp which has been uncovered must be considered the responsibility of the operator who uncovered it and it should be disposed of by that person. Sharps must not be handed from one person to another; where a second person is involved, the sharp should always be placed in a container to be picked up by the other person.

All contaminated equipment should be disposed of in appropriately labelled containers and, where possible, non-disposable contaminated equipment should be autoclaved. Where autoclaving is not possible the equipment should be carefully washed with detergent and water and then left for a time in 2% freshly prepared glutaraldehyde as recommended by local infection control policies. Floors and surfaces contaminated with blood or blood stained fluids should be washed with a solution containing 10 000 p.p.m. available chlorine. They should then be washed with detergent and water.

In May 1994 a report was published in the New South Wales Public Health Bulletin of an investigation of possible patient-to-patient transmission of Hepatitis C Virus (HCV) in a hospital. The report hypothesized that a single patient infected with HCV had contaminated the re-usable part of the breathing system. The virus was then transmitted to four other patients via areas of the upper airway traumatized during the insertion of a laryngeal mask airway. In view of this report, and considering other pertinent evidence, the Blood Borne Virus Advisory Panel recommended the following.

- Either an appropriate filter should be placed between the patient and the breathing system, a new filter being used for each patient, or that a new breathing system is used for each patient.
- Where expired gas sampling is used, the sample should be taken from the breathing system side of the filter.
- In paediatric practice where the use of a filter would increase deadspace and/or resistance unacceptably, filters should not be used but the breathing system should be changed between patients.

MANAGEMENT AFTER EXPOSURE

Accidents do occur, and while it is accepted that all necessary precautions are taken it is inevitable that contamination via inoculation and splashing with body fluids will occur. Local guidelines will determine the precise action to be taken when contamination occurs and these should be followed completely. All such incidents must be properly recorded and reported via an accident report form.

It is important that a medical adviser is identified to provide up-to-date advice on such occupational exposures. Such advice may require an investigation of the HIV or hepatitis status of the patient based on a risk assessment of the level of contamination. Where the HIV status is known to be positive, a prescription of zidovudine (AZT) may be considered, but careful counselling as to the side effects of this drug must accompany its prescription. If the patient is hepatitis positive, specific immunoglobulin can be given. Anti-tetanus immunization should not be forgotten. Finally the storage of a serum sample or follow-up testing should be discussed in addition to consideration of a temporary change of life style to minimize possible infectious risk to others.

As recognizing those patients infected with HIV or HBV is extremely difficult, the above precautions should be regarded as universal precautions. They should not only be applied to those with a proven or suspected infection.

THE HIV INFECTED ANAESTHETIST

Anaesthesia is not considered an exposure prone speciality. Therefore it is possible that an individual infected with HIV could continue in clinical anaesthetic practice provided that he or she follows special guidelines. The infected doctor must:

- practice cross infection precautions routinely,
- understand the routes of occupational transmission of HIV,
- seek advice and follow this advice about his or her practice,
- be familiar with the guidance of the General Medical Council, and
- be under regular medical supervision.

There has only been one case report of transmission of infection from a health care worker (a dentist) to his patients. There have been several studies of HIV positive doctors treating patients with no evidence of transmission of the virus. The risk is therefore present but extremely small and should be minimized by adherence to the guidelines enumerated above.

To ensure compliance it is important that any anaesthetist who suspects that he or she may have become HIV infected must be assured absolute confidentiality when they seek medical advice and care. In the UK the 'Sick Doctor Scheme' is available for those who feel that the local arrangements are not satisfactory.

THE HBV INFECTED ANAESTHETIST

HBV transmission from health care workers to patient is well documented. It is not recommended that anaesthetists who are HBeAg positive or HBsAg positive with no e markers carry out procedures which could be considered exposure prone.

FURTHER READING

Association of Anaesthetists of Great Britain and Ireland (1992). *HIV and Other Blood Borne Viruses – Guidance for Anaesthetists.* (Including Update January 1996). AAGBI, London.

Campbell, A. G. M. and McIntosh, N. (eds) (1992) *Forfar and Arneil's Textbook of Paediatrics* (4th edn). Churchill Livingstone, London.

General Medical Council (1995) *Guidance to doctors on HIV and AIDS.* GMC, London.

Jeffries, D. J. (1991) *Zidovudine after occupational exposure to HIV.* British Medical Journal, **302**, 1349–1350.

O'Donnell, N. G. and Asbury, A. J. (1992) *Anaesthesia*, **47**, 923–928.

Nunn, J. F., Utting, J. E. and Brown, B. R. Jr, (1989) *General Anaesthesia*, (5th edn), Butterworths, London.

UK Health Departments. (1994) *AIDS/HIV-Infected Health Care Workers: Guidance for the Management of Infected Health Care Workers.* Department of Health, London.

Zideman, D. A. and Steward, D. J. (1993) in *Anaesthesia and Uncommon Pediatric Diseases* (2nd edn) (eds J. Katz and D. J. Steward) Saunders, Philadelphia, 52–73.

DIABETES MELLITUS

J. Dinsmore and G. M. Hall

Diabetes has been known to physicians since ancient times. Its dominant features were noted to be polyuria and wasting, the word diabetes literally means a siphon. The sweet tasting urine was noted by Thomas Willis, 1621–75, and glycosuria demonstrated by Mathew Dobson in 1776. However, the source of this excess glucose was not known until 1889 when von Mering and Minkowski demonstrated that pancreatectomy caused diabetes. The discovery of insulin was made in Canada by Banting and Best in 1921 and insulin was isolated by Abel in 1926.

Diabetes mellitus is the most frequent endocrine disorder encountered by anaesthetists. It is common, affecting 5–7% of the population in Europe and North America. Byyny estimated in 1980 that 1 in 2 diabetic patients will require surgery at some stage in their lives and, with advances in surgical techniques, the number of diabetic patients presenting for surgery today is increasing. Therefore all anaesthetists need to be able to manage diabetic patients competently.

CLASSIFICATION

Diabetes mellitus consists of a heterogeneous group of disorders in which the hallmark is hyperglycaemia. This hyperglycaemia is due to an absolute or a relative lack of insulin. The most widely accepted classification of diabetes mellitus is the WHO classification which was first adopted in 1980 and then subsequently modified in 1985. It consists of three major clinical classes.

- **Diabetes mellitus**. This term is reserved for those who meet the diagnostic criteria: a fasting blood glucose of 7.8 mmol l^{-1} or a 2 h post-load blood glucose of 10 mol l^{-1}.
- **Impaired glucose tolerance**. The diagnosis of impaired glucose is reserved for those whose glucose tolerance is above the conventional boundaries of normality but does not meet the diagnostic criteria for diabetes mellitus.
- **Gestational diabetes**. The third group is gestational diabetes. This is defined as diabetes which is first recognized during pregnancy.

The majority of patients with diabetes mellitus fall into two main groups. Those with insulin-dependent diabetes mellitus or IDDM and those with non-insulin-dependent diabetes mellitus or NIDDM. This nomenclature has replaced the earlier terms type 1, or juvenile onset, diabetes and type 2, or maturity onset, diabetes.

Less commonly, diabetes may be associated with other conditions and rare syndromes, see Table 35.1.

INSULIN-DEPENDENT DIABETES MELLITUS

This accounts for approximately 20% of the diabetic population and it tends to present at a younger age. Patients are usually under 30

Short Practice of Anaesthesia. Edited by M. Morgan and G. M. Hall. Published in 1997 by Chapman & Hall, London. ISBN 0 412 71890 1

Table 35.1 Diabetes associated with other conditions

Diabetes	Associated conditions
Pancreatic disease	Pancreatitis
	Pancreatectomy
	Carcinoma of the pancreas
	Haemochromatosis
	Fibrocalculus pancreatitis
Hormone induced diabetes	Acromegaly
	Cushing's syndrome
	Phaeochromocytoma
	Glucagonoma
Drug induced diabetes	Corticosteroids
	ACTH
	Diazoxide
	Thiazide diuretics
Intensive care patients	Sepsis
	Burns
	Multiple trauma
Genetic syndromes	e.g. Prader–Willi syndrome

years of age and are prone to ketoacidosis. The diagnosis is usually obvious, with a rapidly progressive onset of symptoms over a period of weeks or months. There is polyuria, polydipsia and an elevated blood glucose. IDDM appears to be a T-cell mediated autoimmune disease. Its onset is triggered by an environmental agent, the nature of which is still unknown. It is characterized by infiltration and destruction of the pancreatic islets, leading to an absolute dependence on exogenous insulin. The HLA region on the short arm of chromosome 6 is probably responsible for 60% of the genetic susceptibility to IDDM. There is a strong association with the class II alleles DR3 and DR4. The DQ locus is also thought to be important with a single amino acid substitution at position 57 of the DQ chain greatly increasing susceptibility.

There are three main types of insulin available for treatment. Soluble insulins, which are typically short acting; protamine insulins, which are medium or long acting; and insulin zinc preparations with widely ranging durations of action. Various proprietary mixtures of these are available. The choice of which insulin preparation to use is based on the duration of action. The effects of different preparations tend to vary considerably from one patient to another. Insulin of three species is available: human insulin, porcine insulin and bovine insulin. Most patients now receive human insulin.

NON-INSULIN-DEPENDENT DIABETES MELLITUS

NIDDM is more common. It accounts for 80% of the diabetic population and affects 5–7% of the population in general. Patients tend to be older and many are obese. They are relatively resistant to ketoacidosis but are prone to a non-ketotic hyperosmolar state. The treatment of NIDDM hinges on dietary measures. These are backed up with oral hypoglycaemic drugs; sulphonylureas, biguanides and, if necessary, insulin. Sulphonylureas act primarily by stimulating pancreatic insulin secretion, although they may also increase insulin sensitivity at the post receptor level. Because of this they are only useful in patients with some residual insulin reserve. There are many sulphonylureas available, some are mentioned in Table 35.2. Selection is largely a matter of personal preference. They all have similar side effects which include hypoglycaemia and a tendency for weight gain. Hypoglycaemia is often mistaken for transient neurological or

Table 35.2 Sulphonylureas for treatment of non-insulin-dependent diabetes mellitus

Sulphonylurea	Dose range (mg)	Duration of action (h)
Glipizide	2.5–30	0–3 h
Tolbutamide	500–2000	3–6 h
Tolazamide	100–750	
Glibenclamide	2.5–15	6–12 h
Gliclazide	40–320	

cardiac events in the elderly. It can be prolonged and carries a worse prognosis than insulin-induced hypoglycaemia. It is most often seen with glibenclamide and chlorpropamide and is underdiagnosed. For this reason these drugs are best avoided in the elderly or in those with renal failure. Chlorpropamide is now almost obsolete.

The only biguanide commonly used is metformin. This acts mainly by decreasing intestinal glucose absorption and inhibiting hepatic glucose production. It is useful in overweight NIDDM patients when dietary measures have failed or as an adjunct to sulphonylureas. It has several unpleasant side effects, which include nausea, diarrhoea and it may cause a metallic taste.

Major advances have been made in understanding the pathogenesis of NIDDM. Like IDDM, both genetic and environmental disorders contribute. A strong genetic component is suggested by the high concordance of 60–90% in identical twins. The lifetime risk for first degree relatives of white patients with NIDDM to develop the disease is increased (20–40%) compared with age and weight matched subjects (6%). However, the mode of inheritance and the molecular basis for this remain unclear. Although specific genetic defects have been identified in a limited number of patients, it is probable that several different genes contribute.

Environmental causes are undoubtedly related to the sedentary lifestyles of westernized societies. There is evidence that age, obesity and physical inactivity contribute. Obesity seems to be an independent variable resulting in impaired insulin sensitivity in both normal and diabetic individuals. Its impact depends on a family history of NIDDM, the body fat distribution and the duration of obesity. Android obesity (upper body fat distribution) is more common in patients with NIDDM than in equally obese non-diabetic patients. Increased physical activity is inversely related to the prevalence of NIDDM, independent of a family history of NIDDM. Its beneficial effects seem to be mediated by enhancing insulin sensitivity rather than by reducing weight.

Prospective studies indicate that NIDDM is preceded by insulin resistance. The increased beta (B) cell demand induced by this period of hyperglycaemia is associated with a progressive loss of B cell function. Why this occurs, and whether or not there is a primary B cell lesion, is still unknown. Several major hypotheses have been proposed in an attempt to explain why. These include the following.

- **Glucose toxicity**. Both *in vitro* and *in vivo* studies support the suggestion that chronic hyperglycaemia is detrimental to insulin secretion. As chronic hyperglycaemia also induces insulin resistance, it may in itself, perpetuate the diabetic state leading to progressive loss of B cell function.
- **Inherited defects in insulin secretion**. Studies of inheritance of the glucokinase gene (responsible for glucose phosphorylation in B cells) have shown linkage in some early onset NIDDM patients. This group is known as maturity onset diabetes of the young (MODY). Several mutations have been identified and some of these may well have functional significance. However they do not explain the loss of B cell function in the wider diabetic population.
- **Islet amyloid polypeptide (IAPP)**. IAPP was identified in 1987. It is stored with insulin in the secretory granules in the B cells and it is secreted along with insulin in response to appropriate stimuli. Amyloid is found in the pancreas of more than 90% of patients with NIDDM. However, whether this in itself impairs insulin or whether it is a secondary phenomena is not known.
- **'Thrifty phenotype' hypothesis**. Poor fetal and early postnatal nutrition results in poor development of the pancreas, especially the B cells. These are then unable to compensate for insulin resistance in later life.

INSULIN AND METABOLISM

Insulin is synthesized, stored and then secreted from the beta cells of the pancreatic islets. Insulin is a polypeptide hormone with a molecular weight of 5800. It consists of an A chain with 20 aminoacids and a B chain with 31 aminoacids. The two chains are linked by two disulphide bridges and there is a third disulphide bridge within the A chain. It is initially synthesized as the short-lived precursor, pre-proinsulin which is then converted to proinsulin, an 86 aminoacid polypeptide. Proinsulin is, in turn, converted to insulin, by cleavage of the connecting peptide (C-peptide) which links its A and B chains. After cleavage, insulin and C-peptide are packaged together, in equimolar quantities, in storage granules until a suitable stimulus allows secretion. Secreted insulin reaches the liver via the portal system and about 40% is cleared by a first pass metabolism. C-peptide is cleared by the kidneys. In the normal individual insulin is continuously secreted at a basal level. Daily secretion is of the order of 50 units per day. After ingestion of food, a number of stimuli combine to cause a rapid increase in insulin release of 5–10 times the basal level. The plasma half-life of insulin is about 5 min.

Metabolic homeostasis requires an appropriate energy substrate for all tissues. This is achieved by a complex interplay of various hormones. A simplified approach is to consider the actions of insulin as principally anabolic and the other major hormones such as glucagon, cortisol, growth hormone and catecholamines as catabolic. These catabolic hormones have a combined action which oppose that of insulin. Under normal circumstances catabolism and anabolism are finely balanced. Food intake usually exceeds immediate metabolic requirements and, under the influence of insulin, glucose is stored for later use in the form of glycogen and triglycerides. Insulin also stimulates protein synthesis whilst inhibiting protein breakdown, lipolysis, ketogenesis and gluconeogenesis. During starvation, mobilization of stored energy depends initially on decreased insulin secretion, allowing the liver to release glucose from stored glycogen. As glucose reserves become depleted, gluconeogenesis occurs from lactate, alanine and glycerol. In prolonged starvation, there is an increase in lipolysis with a rise in circulating free fatty acids. These are partially oxidized by the liver to acidic ketone bodies, acetoacetate and 3-hydroxybutyrate. If food deprivation continues, ketone bodies become the main energy substrate for all tissues; although nervous tissues continues to require glucose for some time until 'ketoadaptation' occurs.

The basic structure of insulin that confers metabolic activity is common to all species. Bovine insulin was the mainstay of treatment for many years. It differs from human insulin by three amino acids and consequently antibody formation was common. Porcine insulin differs by only 1 amino acid and is, therefore, less antigenic. Preparations have been markedly improved and purified over recent years. Human insulin is available as enzyme modified porcine and also produced biosynthetically by insertion of genetic material into *E. coli*. More recently proinsulin has been synthesized and insulin produced from it by cleavage of C-peptide.

METABOLIC RESPONSE TO SURGERY AND ANAESTHESIA

Trauma or stress disturbs the fine balance between anabolic and catabolic activity. Hyperglycaemia occurring perioperatively is not uncommon in the non-diabetic patient. There is increased secretion of catecholamines, cortisol and growth hormone, all of which oppose the effects of insulin. In addition, there is relative hyposecretion of insulin together with insulin resistance. The net result is increased gluconeogenesis, peripheral lipolysis and decreased protein synthesis. If the process persists, the continued catabolism results in progressive tissue breakdown. Many electrolyte changes also occur including increased loss of potassium, calcium, magnesium and phosphate. When a diabetic state is superimposed upon this 'stress response' the situation is compounded, and there is a risk of an uncontrollable catabolic response and metabolic decompensation.

Anaesthesia itself can also modify the 'stress response'. Nearly all anaesthetic agents have some metabolic effects. There is some evidence to suggest that volatile agents may suppress insulin secretion *in vitro*. However this still remains to be substantiated by *in vivo* studies. Epidural and spinal anaesthesia seem to have the least effects on metabolic function.

COMPLICATIONS OF DIABETES

The complications of diabetes are well known and of great importance. Both macro- and micro-vasculature are affected and result in premature morbidity and mortality from cardiovascular disease, renal failure, retinopathy and neuropathy. The incidence of complications is different in the two groups, but unfortunately few studies distinguish between them. Most complications probably relate to the duration of the disease. Short-term complications include those of hypoglycaemia and hyperglycaemia, dehydration, acidosis, electrolyte and metabolic abnormalities.

Cardiovascular disease

This includes hypertension, ischaemic heart disease (IHD), peripheral and cerebrovascular disease. A specific diabetic cardiomyopathy has also been described. The risk of developing IHD is three times greater in diabetics than in non-diabetics, and there is some evidence to suggest that this increased risk occurs mainly in IDDM. Large epidemiological studies have shown that IHD is the main cause of morbidity and death in diabetics. Its presence also seems to be the major determinant factor in terms of outcome after surgery. Mortality from IHD increases in the presence of microalbuminuria. One study suggests that mortality is increased 37-fold in diabetic patients with microalbuminuria, in comparison to non-diabetic patients with IHD. Silent ischaemia may occur in up to 60% of patients and autonomic dysfunction is common. A lack of symptoms should not be enough to reassure the anaesthetist. Sudden deaths, without post-mortem evidence of myocardial infarction, have been described in patients with autonomic neuropathy and there is an increased incidence of perioperative hypotension and bradyarrythmias.

Renal disease

About 30–40% of patients with IDDM will develop overt diabetic nephropathy. The onset of clinical nephropathy is preceded by a period of increased urinary albumin excretion or microalbuminuria. This is defined as a value exceeding 30 μg min^{-1}. Once microalbuminuria has developed it is associated with hypertension, IHD and proliferative retinopathy.

Neuropathies

Both peripheral and autonomic neuropathies occur in as many as 50% of patients. In addition to the classical diffuse peripheral neuropathy, mononeuropathies and acute painful neuropathies also occur.

Retinopathy and blindness

After 30 years of diabetes over 80% of patients will have developed retinopathy, of these, 7% will be blind.

Infections

Hyperglycaemia interferes with granulocyte chemotaxis, opsonization and phagocytosis. Diabetic patients therefore have an increased incidence of infection. There is also evidence that there is impaired wound strength and delayed wound healing.

Additional complications which may present problems to the anaesthetist include:

Gastroparesis

Gastric stasis occurs in up to 50% of patients. This results in an increased volume of gastric contents and consequently a greater risk of aspiration. Patients are frequently asymptomatic.

Limited joint mobility syndrome

This is characterized by the 'Prayer sign', which is an inability to approximate the palmar surfaces of the phalangeal joints. Joint rigidity may also involve the laryngeal and cervical regions and may be associated with difficulty in intubation. It occurs in up to 30–40% of patients with long-term IDDM. The cause is disputed, but may be due to tissue glycosylation from chronic hyperglycaemia.

COMPLICATIONS AND HYPERGLYCAEMIA

There has been much debate about the link with chronic hyperglycaemia in the pathogenesis of complications. However a causal association now seems established. The diabetic control and complications trial ended prematurely in 1993 having found that there was substantially less risk of the development of, and the progression of diabetic retinopathy, microalbuminuria and abnormal nerve function in IDDM patients treated intensively. There are few data, as yet, about the effect of intensified blood glucose control in patients with NIDDM, or in those from ethnic minorities. However, as the pathogenesis of the microvascular disease is probably similar in all types of diabetes, the same principles may well apply. Despite this the potential risks and benefits of intensively treating the elderly NIDDM patient will obviously differ from those of a young IDDM patient.

In the short term, poor perioperative glycaemic control can lead to ketosis, acidosis, volume depletion from osmotic diuresis and the risk of electrolyte abnormalities. In addition, there is evidence from both human and animal studies that hyperglycaemia excerbates ischaemic damage to both the myocardium and the brain.

PERIOPERATIVE MANAGEMENT

Diabetic patients are twice as likely to need surgery as non-diabetic individuals and, although the management of diabetics has greatly improved, perioperative mortality has still been quoted as up to five times greater. However, this appears to be related more to the presence of complications than to the disease itself. In epidemiological studies, where the presence of diabetes *per se* was segregated from its complications (including IHD), this greater mortality has been questioned. The aim of the anaesthetist should be to achieve the same outcome, in terms of morbidity and mortality, as in the non-diabetic patient. It has been suggested that normal metabolic control should be mimicked as closely as possible, without running the risk of hypoglycaemia.

Both insulin and glucose are necessary. Insulin, for its anabolic effects and glucose to satisfy both the basal requirements and the additional demands of surgery. In the past it was thought that hypoglycaemia could be avoided by giving no insulin at all, but this simply leads to unrestrained catabolism. It must be remembered that it is possible for a patient with IDDM to have an only marginally elevated blood glucose, but for clinically important lipolysis to still occur, leading to ketosis and acidosis. The optimum, dose of glucose is not known. However, it should be sufficient to prevent unnecessary fat and protein catabolism during and after surgery. Recommendations are in the range 5–10 g per hour. The prevention of ketone body and free fatty acid accumulation in surgical patients is theoretically important. Elevated values have been shown to increase myocardial oxygen consumption and to increase the risk of cardiac arrhythmias. The ideal blood glucose is, likewise, uncertain. The advantages gained by avoiding hyperglycaemia must be balanced against the potentially disastrous effects of hypoglycaemia. A target range of 6.7–10 mmol l^{-1} has been proposed by Alberti. Many regimens have been suggested in order to achieve this. However, there is no universally accepted method and there appears to be little difference in outcome between the different regimens. What does appear to be important is the regular monitoring of blood glucose and its accurate interpretation by well trained staff, regardless of the method used.

PREOPERATIVE ASSESSMENT

Many earlier reviews recommended the routine admission of most diabetic patients, especially those with IDDM, 48 h before surgery. This was done to maximize their metabolic control and to assess the anaesthetic risk. However, this is costly and is now usually considered unnecessary. The clinical assessment of both diabetic control, and complications, can be done on an outpatient basis. Reasonable control of blood glucose can usually be achieved at home before admission, or even in a few hours before surgery. The measurement of a glycosylated haemoglobin (HbA$_1$C) value gives an indication of the overall glycaemic control over the previous 3 months (normal range: 3.8–6.4%). A value of greater than 10% indicates poor control and perhaps the need for admission and stabilization preoperatively, especially for major surgery. However, each patient should be assessed on an individual basis. The optimum control for a young IDDM patient will obviously differ from that of an elderly NIDDM patient, where the benefits of tight glycaemic control are not, as yet, proven.

The long acting bovine ultralente should be stopped several days before surgery and substituted with either human ultralente or an intermediate duration insulin. There is no evidence to suggest that intermediate duration insulins need to be stopped the night before surgery. Many patients now use injection pens with multiple doses of short acting insulin in combination with an intermediate duration insulin at night. This regimen can be continued up until the day of surgery. Oral hypoglycaemic drugs also need to be reviewed. Metformin should be stopped 2 days before surgery as it can result in lactic acidosis. The longer action drugs, such as chlorpropamide, must be stopped at least 3 days before surgery and shorter acting drugs substituted. Glibenclamide has been implicated as a cause of recurrent hypoglycaemia in the elderly.

Preoperative assessment also involves detection of the clinical complications. As the majority of anaesthetic morbidity associated with diabetes is due to IHD, much emphasis should be placed on examination of the cardiovascular system. Patients are frequently asymtomatic, and so a negative systemic enquiry is not enough. Routine investigations include: urinalysis to look for glycosuria, ketonuria and proteinuria; a full blood count; an electrolyte profile; and in adult patients, an ECG. Routine screening for the presence of autonomic neuropathy is more controversial. Despite its apparent association with an increased perioperative risk, it is rarely undertaken. It can be assessed by measuring respiration rate variation or the heart rate response to a Valsalva manoeuvre. However, a quick and useful bedside test is to look for the presence of postural hypotension.

MAJOR SURGERY

There is no question that patients with IDDM require insulin for major surgery and few would dispute that this also applies to those with NIDDM. Whether this is best administered by the intravenous route, or subcutaneously, has been queried. The subcutaneous route may be associated with erratic absorption. Absorption depends on the site chosen for injection and, in addition, there is marked intra- and interpatient variation. This is potentially even more of a problem during the perioperative period, when variations in blood flow and fluctuations in blood pressure will invariably occur. However there are few studies which compare the two methods of administration and, despite the risks, there is still quite widespread use of the subcutaneous route. In centres where it is used routinely, it appears to provide reasonable metabolic control.

The intravenous route seems a more logical approach for the administration of such a short acting hormone and its safety has been repeatedly demonstrated. There are several regimens available and, as might be expected, some debate as to the most appropriate. There has also recently been a resurgence in interest in the use of intravenous boluses, although these have been criticized as irrational and unphysiological. Despite this, with intensive monitoring, reasonable metabolic control can be achieved. However, the main choice rests between the combined infusion of glucose–insulin–potassium (GIK regimen) and the use of the variable rate separate glucose and insulin infusions.

Glucose–insulin–potassium (GIK) regimen

This is also known as the Alberti regimen and was described by Alberti and Thomas initially in 1979, although it has subsequently been revised. It consists of 500 ml 10% glucose to which is added 15 units soluble insulin and 10 mmol potassium chloride. This is infused at a rate of 100 ml h^{-1} and the blood glucose monitored every 2 h. The amount of insulin is adjusted by 5 units if the blood glucose drops below 5 or rises above 11 mmol l^{-1}. This regimen has been used successfully and achieved popularity because of its simplicity and apparent safety. It is theoretically impossible for the patient to receive insulin without glucose and it does not necessitate an infusion pump. One of its disadvantages is that there is a fixed insulin concentration in the bag, hence the need to change the entire infusion bag if the blood glucose falls outside the target range.

Variable rate (sliding scale) regimen

A continuous infusion of glucose is administered, as either a 5 or 10% solution at 100 ml h^{-1}, and a variable amount of insulin infused depending on the measured blood glucose (see Table 35.3). The insulin is usually made up as a concentrated solution of 1 unit per ml (e.g. 50ml soluble insulin in 50ml 0.9% sodium chloride solution). The potential problem of insulin adsorption by tubing is now thought unimportant, as the quantities involved are so small. The insulin dose for optimal control will obviously vary, but provided the preoperative control is reasonable, it is usually started at a rate of 1 ml h^{-1}. Blood glucose should be monitored every hour for the first 4 h and then every 2 h. It is recommended that in the operating theatre this should be undertaken every hour. It was originally thought that this regimen might be too complicated for some smaller hospitals. However, it does allow greater flexibility, especially with the wide variation in insulin

Table 35.3 Typical intravenous sliding scale regimen

Blood glucose	Infusion rate of insulin
<3 mmol l^{-1}	0.3 ml h^{-1} and increase glucose infusion
3–5 mmol l^{-1}	1.0 ml h^{-1}
6–9 mmol l^{-1}	1.5 ml h^{-1}
10–12 mmol l^{-1}	2.0 ml h^{-1}
13–16 mmol l^{-1}	4.0 ml h^{-1}
>16 mmol l^{-1}	6.0 ml h^{-1} and check infusion pump

requirements both within and between patients, and seems to be gaining in popularity, particularly in the UK. In a recent review by Hirsch and colleagues of perioperative management of diabetic patients, they concluded that it was the method of choice in IDDM patients undergoing in-patient surgery.

INTERMEDIATE AND MINOR SURGERY

IDDM

This is a more contentious area. Some authors maintain that all patients with IDDM require insulin for all types of surgery, while others still advocate a 'no insulin, no glucose' rule. With the latter, although changes in blood glucose values may not be marked, there is still the risk of exacerbating the metabolic disturbances of surgery, starvation and anaesthesia, and this is not to be recommended. The choice of route for administration of insulin is between the intravenous and subcutaneous routes. Alberti achieved better blood glucose control with the GIK regimen than with subcutaneous insulin in patients undergoing minor surgery. He claimed that his regimen was simple and flexible enough to be useful even in short procedures. Many patients feel nauseated for some time postoperatively even after minor surgery, and this regimen can be continued until the patient is ready to eat when the usual subcutaneous insulin can be restarted. Other authors advocate separate insulin and glucose infusions using sliding scale regimens. Again, this may be continued in recovery and on the ward until the patient is ready to eat, when the usual subcutaneous insulin is given. The insulin infusion is usually stopped 1 h later.

Subcutaneous insulin regimens need to be able to achieve adequate plasma insulin concentrations to avoid excess catabolism. Various regimens exist, all of which involve giving fractions of the normal insulin dose subcutaneously and then commencing a glucose infusion. Blood glucose needs to be monitored hourly and supplemental insulin may well be necessary. When the patient is able to eat, the remainder of the morning insulin is given subcutaneously. However, all of these regimens need to be used only as guidelines and tailored to the individual patient's requirements. Retrospective studies have shown that in the USA subcutaneous insulin regimens are the most commonly used.

NIDDM

Well controlled, diet-treated NIDDM patients need no special treatment in the perioperative period, except for monitoring of blood glucose. Appropriate therapeutic options for other patients with NIDDM depend upon their usual medication and their glycaemic control. Most authors advise stopping oral hypoglycaemic drugs on the morning of surgery, or even 72 h preoperatively in the case of the longer acting chlorpropamide. Normal medication is then recommenced with the first meal. Some, however, give well controlled patients their morning oral hypoglycaemic together with a glucose infusion.

It has been shown that there is no advantage of the GIK regimen over no treatment in this group. Most experts advocate no specific treatment unless the blood glucose is > 10 mmol l^{-1} when insulin therapy should be considered. Blood glucoses of this value reflect an absolute insulin deficiency and, in addition, are associated with the metabolic and electrolyte disturbances of hyperglycaemia. Whether insulin is given as a variable infusion, or as a GIK regimen, comes down to personal preference. If neither of these is used, the alternative is, regular subcutaneous insulin. However, it can be difficult to predict the quantity of insulin necessary in a patient not previously treated with insulin. Significant hyperglycaemia always calls for an intravenous infusion. NIDDM patients who are normally treated with insulin need to be managed as IDDM patients.

GENERAL PRINCIPLES

There is general agreement that elective surgery on diabetic patients should be scheduled for as early in the day as possible in an effort to minimize the metabolic disturbance. If perioperative intravenous fluids are required, those containing lactate, e.g. Hartmann's solution should be avoided. Lactate is a gluconeogenic precursor which, particularly in the starved or catabolic state, may lead to hyperglycaemia. Electrolyte replacement is often required in patients receiving insulin, especially by continuous infusion, and some authors advise the addition of potassium chloride to each litre of glucose. Potassium status should be regularly assessed during the perioperative period. In the longer term, significant decreases in plasma phosphate and magnesium can occur and this should be considered in patients undergoing major surgery or in intensive care.

Postoperative nausea and vomiting can significantly delay the return to eating and drinking and consequently normal diabetic control. This is particularly inconvenient if it follows a minor surgical procedure. Postoperative nausea should therefore be treated aggressively and the use of prophylactic antiemetics considered.

SPECIAL SITUATIONS

OBSTETRICS

Pre-existing diabetes occurs in about 1% of pregnancies and gestational diabetes complicates about another 1%. Fifty years ago almost one quarter of diabetic pregnancies ended in fetal death. Improvements in diabetic, obstetric and paediatric care mean that almost all are now successful. Fetal blood glucose closely mimics maternal values. The fetus is therefore at risk of both hyperglycaemia and hypoglycaemia. Tight glycaemic control during antenatal care and labour has dramatically improved both fetal and maternal outcome. Previously elective Caesarian section at 35–36 weeks was standard practice. Most pregnancies now continue to as close to term as possible and vaginal delivery is the aim.

During labour, glycaemic control is best achieved by insulin and glucose infusions. Maternal blood glucose must be closely monitored. Insulin requirements are often dramatically reduced following delivery and this must be anticipated. Blood glucose values should be checked in the baby immediately after delivery but also over the first 48 h, as it is at greater risk of hypoglycaemia. Epidural blockage is recommended for analgesia during labour, and as anaesthesia for operative delivery. This minimizes the metabolic disturbances of labour and surgery.

CARDIAC SURGERY

An increasing number of diabetic patients are presenting for cardiac surgery. Obtaining good glycaemic control in these patients is often extremely difficult. Even non-diabetic patients become hyperglycaemic and blood glucose values >32 mmol l^{-1} have been reported in these patients. Hyperglycaemia results from a combination of the stress of surgery and the adrenergic agents used perioperatively. Insulin resistance may occur with hypothermia. In addition, glucose may be present in the cardioplegic solution and the cardiopulmonary bypass pump is often primed with Hartmann's solution. The lactate contained in this is a gluconeogenic precursor. For these reasons insulin infusions and half-hourly blood glucose monitoring are essential.

DAY-CASE SURGERY

This is still a contentious area with some authors feeling that all patients with IDDM should be managed as inpatients, no matter what the surgery. However, with an increasing demand for day surgery from both patients and surgeons various protocols have been suggested. Many authors now take the view that with careful selection and preparation, many patients can be managed as day cases. At the preoperative assessment clinic, well controlled patients should be selected and the presence of any diabetic complications assessed. Appropriate investigations can be arranged at this time and the results documented in the notes ready for admission. Patients need to be provided with written instructions as to any changes necessary in medication before admission and on the morning itself, as well as instructions on the duration of starvation. Suitable domestic circumstances and necessary home support are, of course, essential. Postoperative nausea and vomiting and pain should be treated aggressively. If the patient remains nauseated, or unable to eat, then facilities for admission must be available.

EMERGENCY SURGERY

In 1963 Galloway and Shuman estimated that 5% of all diabetic patients would require emergency surgery. It seems likely that this estimate has changed little over the years. The most common indications for surgery are infections, appendicectomies and lower extremity amputations. All diabetic patients presenting for emergency surgery must be carefully assessed and stabilized before theatre. Urinalysis for ketones, blood glucose, electrolytes and either pH or bicarbonate are mandatory. Most patients will be complicated, and about one third of patients will have a blood glucose > 11 mmol l^{-1} on admission. As hyperglycaemia is often due to the coexistent condition necessitating surgery, it may be difficult to control. However, an attempt should be made, and fluid deficits and electrolyte abnormalities treated before surgery. Diabetic ketoacidosis can present with acute abdominal pain and vomiting; these symptoms disappear after treatment of the ketoacidosis. In contrast, it has also been noted that an acute abdomen may initially appear benign in diabetics. This is thought to be due to the presence of a diabetic neuropathy and is extremely rare. If diabetic ketoacidosis is confirmed, then this must be treated, and surgery postponed.

DIABETIC EMERGENCIES

DIABETIC KETOACIDOSIS

Ketoacidosis results from a lack of insulin. In practice it usually occurs in association with infections where there is often increased resistance to insulin. It also may occur as the result of poor compliance, or as the first presentation of a previously undiagnosed diabetic patient. In about 25% of patients there is no obvious precipitating cause. Despite advances in treatment, hospital admissions from ketoacidosis appear to be increasing. The overall mortality rate is 2–5%. Morbidity and mortality are related to length of time between the onset of ketoacidosis and initiation of treatment, the presence of infection and the patient's age. In the over 65 age group mortality rises to $> 20\%$. Complications arise from a combination of organ damage from hypoperfusion and thromboembolic episodes. One of the most serious problems is cerebral oedema. This occurs predominantly in children and usually following initiation of treatment. The pathophysiology is poorly understood, but the mortality rate is about 70%. The most obvious clinical feature in a patient with ketoacidosis is usually dehydration. The fluid deficit can be estimated by subtracting the patient's weight from their last known stable weight, but it is often about 100 ml kg^{-1} body weight. The patient is frequently drowsy and their breath may smell of ketones. They are often described as having 'air hunger', typically overbreathing, but not breathless. More severe cases are hypotensive and may be hypothermic.

Diagnosis is confirmed by laboratory tests. The severity of hyperglycaemia is variable, glucose values from <11.1 mmol l^{-1} to >55.6 mmol l^{-1} have been reported. Plasma osmolality (osmolality = glucose + urea + [Na^+ + K^+]) is raised, but is generally less than 320 mOsm l^{-1}. Arterial pH is reduced, as is the plasma bicarbonate concentration. Ketonaemia must be present by definition, and can be detected by the Ketostix test. One set of diagnostic criteria is: the presence of ketonaemia and a pH < 7.30. However, there is no universal consensus as to what actually constitutes diabetic ketoacidosis. Despite this a prompt diagnosis and initiation of treatment is imperative.

The management of ketoacidosis comprises the following.

- **Supportive measures**. The patient is best managed in a high dependency area where appropriate monitoring is available. The airway should be secured and O_2 administered and a urinary catheter, nasogastric tube and central venous cannula inserted.
- **Fluid management**. Restoration of the extracellular volume is critical to maintain adequate organ perfusion. However, fluid replacement at rates exceeding $4 \, l \, m^{-2}$ per 24 h is associated with cerebral oedema. Available data suggest that, in the absence of significant circulatory insufficiency, there is no advantage in rapid fluid replacement. In fact, slower rates appear to be more beneficial in treating the metabolic disturbances associated with ketoacidosis. Many regimens exist but most need to be modified according to age, the presence of cardiac disease and the patient's general condition. Central venous pressure is invaluable, especially in the elderly, in monitoring fluid replacement. The type of fluid to be used for resuscitation has been the subject of much debate, but the use of hypotonic fluids is not recommended. Too rapid a fall in plasma osmolality predisposes to the development of cerebral oedema, especially in children. The fluid of choice is 0.9% sodium chloride solution at rates which will restore fluid deficits in 12–24 h (48 h in children). If the serum sodium is >150 mmol l^{-1} 0.45% sodium chloride solution may be used. Colloid solutions are indicated if there is significant circulatory failure. When the blood glucose falls to 10–15 mmol l^{-1} 5% glucose solution should be started.
- **Potassium replacement**. Potassium needs to be measured regularly, every 2 h initially and then every 4 h. Serum potassium should be maintained at >4.0 mol l^{-1}. Potassium 10–30 mmol l^{-1} should be given when the insulin infusion is initiated if the potassium is <5.0 mmol l^{-1} and renal function is good. In hyperkalaemia this can be delayed temporarily.
- **Insulin**. Insulin should be given intravenously. There is no place for subcutaneous insulin in ketoacidosis. The intramuscular route has been used successfully but absorption will be unreliable if tissue perfusion is poor. Continuous infusion of moderate doses of insulin (5–6 units h^{-1} in adults and 0.1 units $kg^{-1} \, h^{-1}$ in children) gives the best results. Glucose needs to be monitored hourly and a reduction of 5 mmol l^{-1} per hour is aimed for. Insulin treatment should be continued until there is no ketoacidosis and the pH is normal.
- **Bicarbonate therapy**. Most authors suggest that bicarbonate is given when the pH is <7.1. However there are no valid reasons for this view. Potential disadvantages of bicarbonate therapy are an increased incidence of hypokalaemia, paradoxical CSF acidosis and hypoxia. In studies looking at bicarbonate replacement in ketoacidosis, the rate of correction of metabolic defects was either unchanged, or even delayed. In his review, Lebovitz now recommends that it should be reserved for when there is imminent cardiovascular collapse.
- **Phosphate replacement**. Ketoacidosis is associated with severe total body phosphate depletion, although at presentation, phosphate values may be high, normal or low. However, there is no evidence that phosphate supplementation is beneficial. If clinically significant depletion occurs, then replacement at 5–20 mmol h^{-1} has been suggested.
- **Heparin**. Much of the morbidity and mor-

tality associated with ketoacidosis is as a result of thromboembolic disease. Low-dose heparin is usually recommended for high-risk patients.
- **Antibiotics**. There is no need for the routine prescribing of antibiotics. However, precipitating infections need to be looked for, especially urinary tract or respiratory tract infections. These should be treated appropriately.

HYPEROSMOLAR NON-KETOTIC COMA

This tends to occur in older, often West Indian patients, usually with NIDDM. It is of more gradual onset than ketoacidosis, with polyuria, progressive dehydration and metabolic derangement. Blood glucose and osmolality are very high and there is no ketonuria. Treatment is with low-dose insulin (3 units h^{-1}) and 0.45% sodium chloride solution i.v. very slowly. Cerebral oedema may complicate attempts to correct the osmolality too quickly. Central venous pressure monitoring is mandatory for these patients and some may benefit from insertion of a pulmonary artery catheter.

LACTIC ACIDOSIS

This usually occurs in elderly patients and they are often profoundly ill. The cause of the acidosis must be urgently sought. It is usually associated with biguanides or renal impairment. The blood glucose may be normal with little or no ketones. These patients are often extremely insulin resistant.

CONCLUSIONS

There have been major developments in understanding diabetes, its causes and approaches to its management, over the past 10 years. The anaesthetist's goal should be to achieve the same morbidity as with non-diabetic patients. However, despite advances in treatment, diabetic patients are still high-risk patients. Much has been written about the management of anaesthesia in diabetes but there are still many unanswered questions. The best regimen to achieve optimum control perioperatively has not established. Although we strive to avoid hyperglycaemia, ketogenesis and proteolysis, there are no studies which show that this achievement will directly affect surgical outcome. Whether perioperative care is best provided by anaesthetists, or by diabetologists, is likewise a matter of debate.

However, it is becoming increasingly obvious that it is not the actual regimen itself, but its careful usage, with the frequent monitoring of blood glucose by well-trained staff and its accurate interpretation, that matters.

FURTHER READING

Alberti, K. G. M. M. (1991) Diabetes and surgery. *Anesthesiology*, **74**, 209–211.
Alberti, K. G. M. M. and Thomas, D. J. B. (1979) The management of diabetes during surgery. *British Journal of Anaesthesia*, **51**, 693–710.
Diabetic Control and Complications Trial Research Group (1993). The effect of intensive treatment of diabetes on the development and progression of long-term complications in insulin-dependent diabetes mellitus. *New England Journal of Medicine*, **329**, 977–986.
Hall, G. M. (1994) Insulin administration in diabetic patients – return of the bolus. *British Journal of Anaesthesia*, **72**, 1–2.
Hirsch, I. B., McGill, J. B., Cryer, P. E. and White, P. F. (1991) Perioperative management of surgical patients with diabetes mellitus. *Anesthesiology*, **74**, 209–211.
Lebovitz, H. E. (1995) Diabetic ketoacidosis. *Lancet*, **345**, 767–771.
McKenzie, C. R. and Charlson, M. E. (1988) Assessment of perioperative risk in the patient with diabetes mellitus. *Surgery, Gynecology and Obstetrics*, **167**, 293–299.
Milaskiewicz, R. M. and Hall, G. M. (1992) Diabetes and anaesthesia; the past decade. *British Journal of Anaesthesia*, **68**, 198–206.
Williams, G. (1994) Management of non-insulin dependent diabetes mellitus. *Lancet*, **343**, 95–100.
Yki-Jarvinen, H. (1994) Pathogenesis of non-insulin dependent diabetes mellitus. *Lancet*, **343**, 91–94.

TOTAL INTRAVENOUS ANAESTHESIA

N. P. Sutcliffe and G. N. C. Kenny

Anaesthesia has advanced over the course of the last century into a form of specialized medical practice with a low mortality. This is largely due to advances in the technology of anaesthetic equipment, the availability of new drugs, and improved training for anaesthetists. Sophisticated technology related to the delivery and on-line measurement of inhalational anaesthetic drugs has led to an increased accuracy of delivery, and ease of use for such agents. Are there, therefore, any clinical benefits to the patient and anaesthetist from the use of total intravenous anaesthesia (TIVA)?

There are some clinical situations where it is desirable, or even essential, to avoid the use of inhalational anaesthesia. During operative procedures such as laryngoscopy, bronchoscopy or thoracic surgery where it may be difficult or impossible to use inhalational anaesthesia effectively, TIVA is a more suitable option. Because of the overall safety of modern anaesthesia, attention has focused on postoperative morbidity and those rare occurrences of idiosyncratic reactions to anaesthetic drugs and it is in these areas where TIVA may have significant advantages. Volatile agents are among those which must be avoided in patients who suffer from malignant hyperthermia and TIVA has been reported as a safe alternative. Although safe in the majority of patients, halothane has been implicated as a cause of hepatitis, and cross-reactivity has been reported between different volatile anaesthetics in respect of hepatotoxicity. Postoperative nausea and vomiting (PONV) is more often seen after volatile anaesthesia compared with TIVA and propofol has been reported to have a specific anti-emetic effect. Postoperative recovery has been shown to be superior with propofol anaesthesia compared with volatile agents making the technique particularly suitable for day-case surgery.

There is also concern about the possible effect of inhalational anaesthetics on patients and staff exposed to the operating theatre environment.

Thus, there is a need for an alternative to conventional inhalational anaesthesia in certain circumstances. Unfortunately, TIVA is not widely practised and therefore trainee anaesthetists find it difficult to gain the appropriate skills.

PHARMACOKINETICS OF INTRAVENOUS DRUG ADMINISTRATION

When administered intravenously, a drug undergoes metabolism and distribution to other tissues of the body, its concentration in the blood and other tissues can be described by a pharmacokinetic model. A three-ompartment model can be used to describe this relationship for many intravenous anaesthetic agents (Figure 36.1). This model is a mathematical concept and the individual compartments do not represent any specific tissue, although the blood concentration is

Short Practice of Anaesthesia. Edited by M. Morgan and G. M. Hall. Published in 1997 by Chapman & Hall, London. ISBN 0 412 71890 1

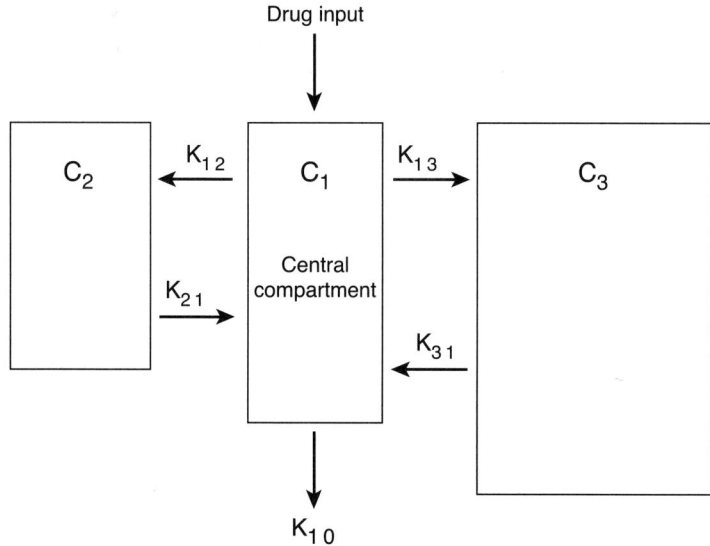

Figure 36.1 Three compartment pharmacokinetic model describing the distribution and elimination of an intravenous drug.

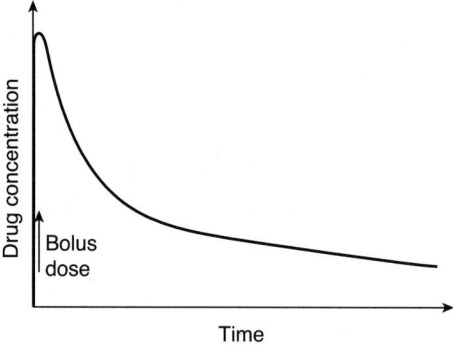

Figure 36.2 Changes in drug concentration with time within the blood following a single bolus dose of drug.

considered to reflect the concentration within the central compartment.

The administration of a single dose of drug causes a peak blood concentration which then decreases rapidly with time. This may lead to drug toxicity coincident with the peak blood concentration (Figure 36.2). Repeated single doses can be given to maintain drug effect, but this will result in alternating peaks and troughs in the drug concentration within the central compartment, with the potential for both toxic and sub-therapeutic effects (Figure 36.3). This may be acceptable when using drugs with a wide therapeutic window and low toxicity. However, this is not an appropriate delivery method for drugs with a narrow therapeutic window and clinically significant toxicity.

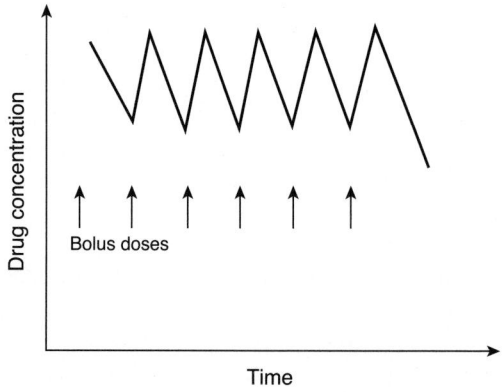

Figure 36.3 Changes in drug concentration with time within the blood during repeated bolus dosing of drug.

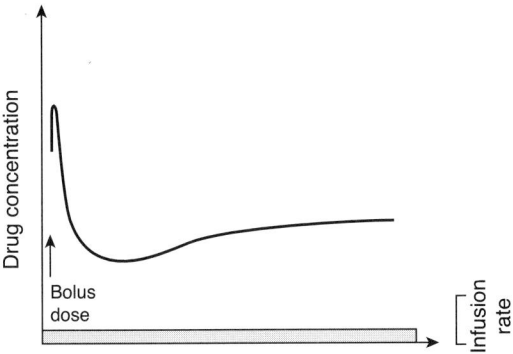

Figure 36.4 Changes in drug concentration with time within the blood following a single bolus dose followed by a continuous infusion of drug.

During intravenous infusion at a constant rate, a period of 4–5 times the distribution half-life of a drug would be required to achieve a steady-state concentration and is clearly unacceptable for the induction of anaesthesia in the clinical setting. Alternatively, the central compartment can be loaded by administering a single bolus dose whilst starting a continuous infusion at the same time. This results in a potentially high, peak blood concentration after the bolus dose, followed by a reduced concentration which gradually increases towards steady-state (Figure 36.4) with the potential for sub-therapeutic drug concentration. Such a regimen can be modified by giving a smaller bolus dose followed by a stepped infusion regimen to rapidly achieve and maintain a fixed blood concentration of a particular drug. However, such regimens do not offer the flexibility of changing the infusion in response to a perceived need for a change in level of drug effect.

Clearly, the optimal infusion regimen would produce a bolus designed to achieve rapidly the desired drug concentration, followed by a continuously-adjusting infusion rate calculated to maintain this 'target' drug concentration, and allow this concentration to be changed as appropriate. Such regimens exist, but require specialized computer-controlled infusion equipment not generally available at present.

AVAILABLE HYPNOTIC AGENTS

Just as with inhalational anaesthetic drugs, none of the current intravenous agents has the ideal profile for TIVA. Some of the newer agents approach this ideal. While any intravenous anaesthetic agent may be used for TIVA, drugs which are most suited for delivery by infusion are those with a rapid offset of action once the infusion is stopped. This property is usually described in the literature by the elimination half-life of the drug in question. This pharmacokinetic parameter is based on calculations derived from measured blood drug concentrations following drug bolus doses or short infusions. However, it must be appreciated that the speed of elimination of an infused drug from the central compartment will vary with the duration of that infusion. This can be illustrated by referring to Figure 36.1; the longer the infusion of a drug continues, the more compartments C2 and C3 become filled with drug. On cessation of the infusion, as drug is eliminated from the central compartment (C1) there will be a degree of redistribution between it, and the peripheral compartments, which will alter the half-time for that particular drug infusion. The factors which determine the speed of elimination from the central compartment are the duration of infusion (thus the quantity of drug within the various compartments), the clearance of the drug and the speed of movement of drug between the various compartments which is described by the rate constants $K_{2\,1}$, $K_{1\,2}$, $K_{1\,3}$, $K_{3\,1}$ (Figure 36.5). This time dependence of elimination of infused drugs has been referred to in recent literature as the 'context sensitive half-time'. With short infusions the concentration of drug in the peripheral compartments is lower than in the central compartment, and on cessation of the infusion the drug is cleared from the blood by both elimination and redistribu-

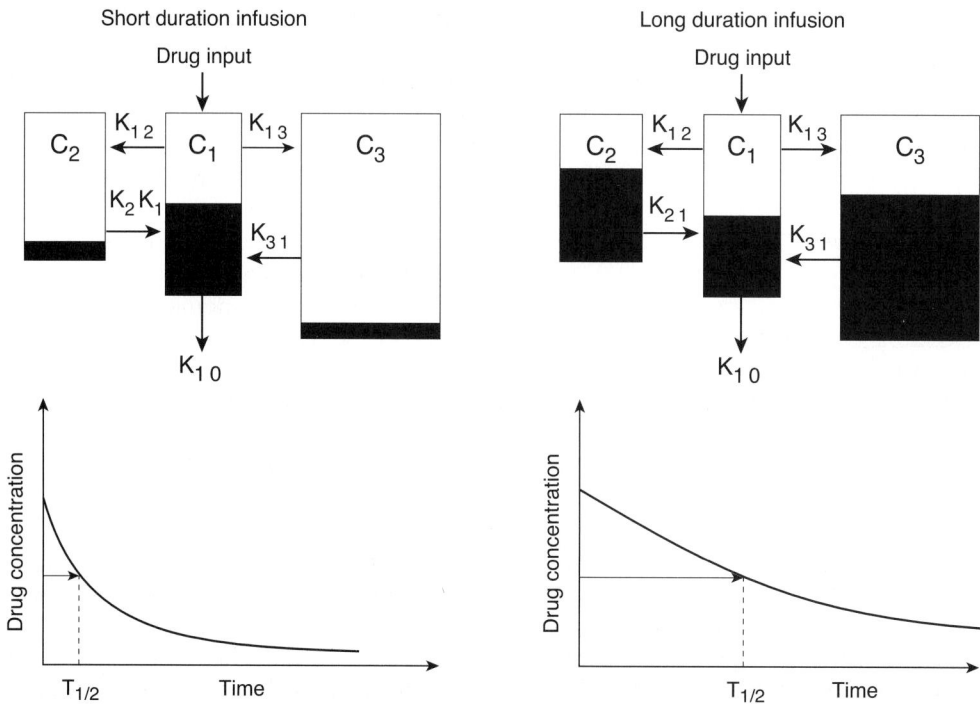

Figure 36.5 Schematic representation of the concentration of drug within the various compartments during a short, and a prolonged infusion of drug, and the effect on context sensitive half time.

tion resulting in a short half time. However, following a prolonged drug infusion there is increased filling of the peripheral compartments. As the concentration of drug falls in the blood due to elimination, there is a degree of refilling from the peripheral compartments, prolonging the blood half life of the drug. This time dependence of the 'context sensitive half-time' is less apparent for drugs with a high clearance, and slow movement of drug between the compartments, so that elimination of drug from the blood occurs at a much faster rate than redistribution between the compartments.

Several drugs with a pharmacokinetic profile suited to TIVA have been investigated. Propanidid and althesin were promising but are no longer available for use due to a high incidence of allergic reactions associated with the vehicle in which they were formulated. Etomidate has also been investigated for TIVA but has been found to interfere with steroid synthesis and should not be used for maintenance of anaesthesia. Methohexitone and thiopentone have also been used to provide TIVA but, because of their low clearance, use of these agents results in a prolonged recovery phase. Propofol has a satisfactory pharmacokinetic profile for the maintenance of anaesthesia and it has been shown also to have a specific anti-emetic action. In contrast to volatile agents, there appears to be no adverse effect on the hypoxic pulmonary vasconstriction reflect with propofol. The dual effect of a reduction in intracranial pressure and reduction in the cerebral oxygen requirement seen with this agent make it suitable for neuroanaesthesia in patients with decreased intracranial compliance. Eltanolone (pregnanolone) is a naturally occurring metabolite of progesterone, like propofol it is formulated in 10% Intralipid. Eltanolone is prepared as a

0.4% emulsion and is approximately three times as potent as propofol, with less pain reported on injection. There appears to be a similar degree of cardiovascular and respiratory depression compared with propofol. However, there is evidence that cardiac and splanchnic perfusion is better preserved, and that recovery from anaesthesia is more rapid with propofol than with eltanolone.

Currently, propofol is the agent most suited to be given by intravenous infusion for the maintenance of anaesthesia because of its short elimination half-life and high clearance.

INFUSION REGIMENS

MANUALLY ADJUSTED REGIMENS

For short surgical procedures in healthy patients, such as dilatation and curettage, a single dose of propofol may suffice. Longer procedures may be performed while the patient is anaesthetized with repeated bolus doses of propofol. However, this may result in alternating under- and over-dosing. Several manual infusion schemes have been developed empirically to maintain anaesthesia with propofol. A stepped infusion regimen based on approximations to a computer-generated infusion profile can be designed to achieve and maintain a particular blood propofol concentration. Roberts and colleagues have described such a regimen intended to maintain a blood propofol concentration of 3 $\mu g\ ml^{-1}$ (Table 36.1). Such regimens offer no facility to alter the targeted blood propofol concentration, and thus lack the flexibility to respond to different levels of surgical stimulation and differing patient requirements. In order to avoid the possibility of awareness such regimens should be supplemented. The technique described by Roberts and colleagues targets a relatively low blood concentration of propofol and is supplemented with nitrous oxide. One study using this regimen, with an opiate premedication, showed that 25% patients also required supplementation with a volatile agent.

TARGET CONTROLLED INFUSIONS (TCI)

The aim of TCI systems is to make the delivery of TIVA as simple and flexible as the administration of inhalational agents via a calibrated vaporizer. A TCI system consists of two key components: a delivery device (usually a motorized syringe driver) and a microprocessor equipped with appropriate control software, these two components have now been combined in a single delivery system (Figure 36.6). The control software contains a pharmacokinetic model for the particular drug to be infused. The anaesthetist inputs relevant patient data such as weight, age and sex, so that the system can match the pharmacokinetic model to an individual patient. The anaesthetist then selects the desired target

Table 36.1 Propofol infusion regimen designed to give a blood propofol concentration of 3 $\mu g\ ml^{-1}$

Propofol infusion regimen	
1. Bolus	1 mg kg^{-1}
2. Infusion rate 1	10 mg kg^{-1} h^{-1} for 10 min
3. Infusion rate 2	8 mg kg^{-1} h^{-1} for 10 min
4. Infusion rate 3	6 mg kg^{-1} until the end of the surgery

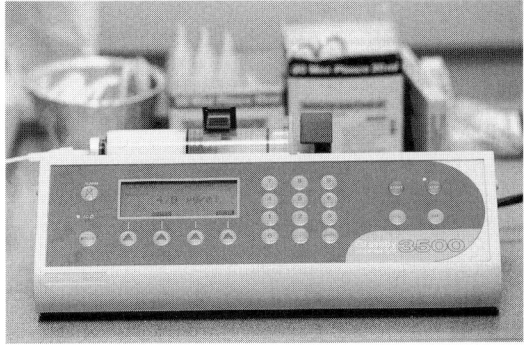

Figure 36.6 Prototype commercial target controlled infusion device.

blood concentration. The system will infuse at a rapid rate until it has calculated that the selected target concentration has been achieved. The control software then calculates the rate of infusion required to maintain this target concentration and controls the delivery device automatically without further adjustment by the operator. However, a new target can be selected at any time. The system will shut off the infusion if a lower target is entered or deliver a rapid infusion to achieve a higher target concentration. Once the control software has calculated that the new target has been reached, it will institute a new infusion regimen to maintain this different target concentration. Thus, in a manner analogous to the use of the calibrated vaporizer, the anaesthetist can easily alter the target concentration to suit any individual patient and level of surgical stimulation.

ASSESSMENT OF TCI

TCI may be assessed from a clinical point of view with respect to the perceived quality of anaesthesia and ease of use. Alternatively, it may be assessed in terms of how well the pharmacokinetic model fits an individual patient.

Improved cardiovascular and respiratory stability during induction of anaesthesia has been demonstrated with a target-controlled propofol infusion system compared with single doses or manually controlled infusions. Similarly, improved cardiovascular stability during maintenance with TCI administration of fentanyl and alfentanil has been described.

A study has been reported of 31 UK anaesthetists who evaluated TCI equipment over a 12 week period. Twenty seven of the 31 respondents indicated that the system had changed their use of propofol for maintenance of anaesthesia. The reasons given included ease of use and more confidence in the predictability of anaesthetic effect provided with TCI compared with manually controlled infusions. All participants found the concept of TCI acceptable. A cross-over study between manually adjusted and target controlled infusions of propofol has shown that anaesthetists not previously familiar with TIVA found both techniques easy to master, but expressed a clear preference for the TCI system.

The pharmacokinetic model on which a TCI system is based is derived from population pharmacokinetics, therefore, the model will not be an exact match for each individual patient being anaesthetized. It is possible to assess the accuracy of a system by taking blood samples during a target controlled infusion and retrospectively comparing the predicted with measured blood propofol concentrations. Such studies have been performed and show that the variation between target and measured blood propofol concentrations is similar to that seen between blood and end-tidal isoflurane partial pressures. It would be possible to improve the accuracy of such systems if circulating drug concentrations were measured on-line and this information fed back to the TCI system. This would allow the pharmacokinetic model to be tailored to suit each individual patient. Probes are under development which may allow real-time measurement. However, it is not the blood concentration which determines the action of an intravenous anaesthetic, but the concentration of drug at the site of action (effect site) and the current level of afferent input into the CNS.

EFFECT SITE CONCENTRATION

Since the effect site for anaesthetic agents is within the brain it is not possible, with current technology, to measure the effect site concentration. It is possible, however, to measure the drug effect. This can be performed using parameters derived from the raw EEG such as spectral edge, or from the recording of evoked potentials. This allows construction of a blood concentration versus

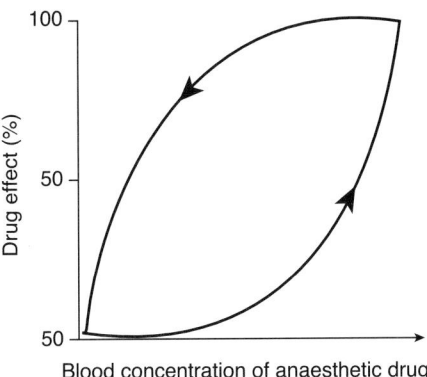

Figure 36.7 Schematic representation of drug effect plotted against blood concentration of anaesthetic drug.

drug effect plot, which shows a degree of hysteresis related to the disequilibrium between the blood and effect site concentration of anaesthetic drug (Figure 36.7). Mathematical modelling can then be used to estimate the rate constant for the movement of drug between the blood and effect site. Given this information the effect site concentration can be estimated at any point during administration of the drug. Future developments in intravenous anaesthesia may include the ability to target more effectively the sites within the brain where anaesthetic drugs exert their action. But a knowledge of the effect site concentration in itself will still not allow the anaesthetist to deliver a given level of anaesthesia. As well as these pharmacokinetic considerations there are pharmacodynamic factors to take into account. Factors such as age, physiological reserve, concurrent drug administration and level of surgical stimulation will all affect the level of arousal for a given effect site concentration of anaesthetic agent (Figure 36.8). However, the ability to target the effect site concentration would allow the anaesthetist to 'fine tune' drug delivery to an individual patient and level of surgical stimulation using clinical signs and physiological monitoring to gauge the depth of anaesthesia.

CLOSED-LOOP ANAESTHESIA

With any form of anaesthesia the anaesthetist uses his clinical skills to assess the depth of anaesthesia; the delivery of drug is then adjusted as appropriate. Given a measure of the depth of anaesthesia the process can be automated. An index of depth of anaesthesia is used to control the delivery system thus closing the loop and automating the process. A number of closed-loop systems have been described, but none are currently available for clinical use. One system, using the auditory evoked potential (AEP) as an index of anaesthesia depth, has been used to administer intravenous anaesthesia completely automatically in patients breathing spontaneously during surgery. The AEP is obtained by delivering auditory stimuli in the form of clicks to earphones at a frequency of 6–12 Hz. The EEG activity is recorded after each click from three electrodes placed on the scalp and several hundred EEG sweeps are filtered and averaged to produce the AEP. The AEP appears to provide a reproducible guide to the depth of anaesthesia obtained with a wide variety of different anaesthetic agents and to respond appropriately to varying levels of surgical stimulation. It is possible that similar systems will be available in the future to assist the anaesthetist in the delivery of anaesthetic agents.

DRUGS USED TO SUPPLEMENT INTRAVENOUS HYPNOTIC AGENT

When ketamine is used as a single agent for anaesthesia, it can lead to dysphoria in the recovery phase, but has been reported to be successful when combined with midazolam or propofol. Benzodiazepines act in synergism with opioids, and midazolam has been used successfully combined with fentanyl or alfentanil. However, recovery from midazolam may be prolonged after infusion because of its low clearance. Newer synthetic opioids, such as fentanyl, alfentanil, and remifentanil have a rapid onset and offset of action mak-

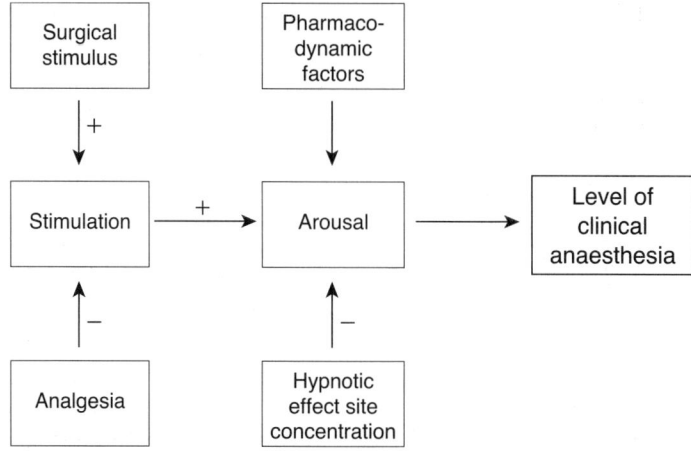

Figure 36.8 Schematic representation of the interaction of factors affecting the clinical level of anaesthesia.

ing them particularly suitable for infusion. Infusions of such agents offer the potential for a stable level of analgesia throughout surgery. Rapid offset of action allows titration against adverse drug effects in spontaneously breathing, anaesthetized patients, and rapid reversal of sedative effects following cessation of the infusion. Clinical studies have shown that during propofol anaesthesia, the response to skin incision is decreased when patients receive a concurrent infusion of fentanyl. Alfentanil can be delivered as an infusion to supplement the hypnotic effect of propofol. Alfentanil and propofol can be mixed together without loss of effect. However, this reduces the flexibility of the regimen to respond to the variations in anaesthetic requirements of patients breathing spontaneously during surgery. TCI systems delivering alfentanil have also been described both, for the supplementation of propofol anaesthesia, and for the provision of postoperative analgesia. Remifentanil is a newly synthesized opioid of the fentanyl family. It has a short context sensitive half life which attains a plateau after 3–4 min of infusion. It is metabolized rapidly by blood and tissue esterases, the major metabolite is eliminated more slowly but has little clinical significance due to its low potency. Remifentanil causes dose dependent analgesia and respiratory depression with a potency of 20–30 times that of alfentanil. The half time for equilibration between plasma and effect site was calculated as 1.3 min. Its rapid onset and short duration of action, even after prolonged infusion, may make this agent suitable for titration of infusion rate against clinical effect.

PERCEIVED PROBLEMS WITH TIVA

COMPLEXITY OF DOSING

Improved monitoring has presented the anaesthetist with a wealth of data so that information overload is a real concern. We must consider therefore, if it is justified to introduce yet more technology to allow the delivery of the complex, infusion regimens required for TIVA. Clearly, such technology would only be warranted if it results in improved and simplified delivery of TIVA so that its ease of use is comparable to that of inhalational anaesthesia. Recently the introduction of TCI systems has allowed such flexibility and ease of use to be allied to TIVA.

'IS THE PATIENT ANAESTHETIZED?'

One of the most frequent concerns about TIVA is the issue of awareness. How does one gauge the depth of anaesthesia when using TIVA? The simple answer is that the same skills are used as when administering volatile agents. Lack of experience and confidence with the newer technique of TIVA leads to a sense of insecurity. However, one study has shown that the introduction of TCI leads to better confidence in, and increased use of, TIVA by anaesthetists not previously familiar with the technique.

INFECTION

The vehicle in which propofol is formulated is an excellent culture medium and propofol in the form of Diprivan contains no preservatives. There have been reports of infection in the postoperative period which appear to have been associated with the use of Diprivan. However, all these cases seem to have occurred due to poor aseptic technique and failure to follow the manufacturer's guidelines for drug preparation. A procedural review amongst anaesthetic personnel involved in the outbreaks showed that many of them prepared syringes of propofol up to 24 h in advance, and the practice of re-using syringes or infusion catheters on different patients was common.

COST

The issue of the cost of TIVA is difficult to assess since it depends on the mode of delivery, the individual practice of anaesthetists, as well as drug costs. For instance, propofol maintenance with TCI is approximately equivalent to open circuit isoflurane in anaesthesia in the UK. However, the use of isoflurane in a circle circuit would result in a lower drug cost for long cases. The reduction in cost would be much less for short cases, since a period of high fresh gas flow is required at the start of each case. There are also the costs of theatre time, nurse time and hospital stay to be considered as well as antiemetic costs. These costs may be lower using TIVA with propofol administered via a target controlled infusion.

CONCLUSIONS

Currently the potential benefits of TIVA are not made available to the vast majority of patients undergoing anaesthesia. This is because of the complexity of dosing schedules, the lack of widespread experience with the technique and the inertia of many anaesthetists. The Royal College of Anaesthetists may in future require trainees to have knowledge and experience of TIVA. This requirement, combined with the imminent availability of TCI systems within the clinical environment, has the **potential** to revolutionize the way anaesthesia is delivered.

FURTHER READING

Brown B. R. (1991) Inhalational anaesthetics and hepatoxicity: an update. *Anaesthesiologica Scandinavica*, **35**, 42–43.

Carpenter, R. L. and Eger, E. I. (1989) Alveolar-to-arterial-to-venous anesthetic partial pressure differences in humans. *Anesthesiology*, **70**, 630–635.

Chaudhri, S., White, M. and Kenny, G. N. (1992) Induction of anaesthesia with propofol using a target-controlled infusion system. *Anaesthesia*, **47**, 551–553.

Davidson, J. A., McLeod, A. D., Howie, J. C., White, M. and Kenny, G. N. (1993) The effective concentration for propofol with and without 67% nitrous oxide. *Acta Anaesthesiologica Scandinavica*, **37**, 458–464.

Kenny, G. N., McFadzean, W. A. and Mentzaridis, H. (1993) Propofol requirements during closed-loop anesthesia. *Anesthesiology*, **79**, A329.

Marsh, B. J., White, M., Morton, N. and Kenny, G. N. (1991) Pharmacokinetic model driven infusion of propofol in children. *British Journal of Anaesthesia*, **67**, 41–48.

Russell, D., Wilkes, M. P., Hunter, S. C., Glen, J. B., Hutton, P. K. and Kenny, G. N. (1995) Manual compared with target-controlled infusion of propofol. *British Journal of Anaesthesia*, **75**, 562–566.

Schüttler, J., Kloos, S., Schwilden, H. and Stoeckel, H. (1988) Total intravenous anaesthesia with propofol and alfentanil by computer-assisted infusion. *Anaesthesia*, **43**(Suppl), 2–7.

White M. and Kenny, G. N. (1990) Intravenous propofol anaesthesia using a computerised infusion system. *Anaesthesia*, **45**, 204–209.

Kenny, G. N. and Sutcliffe, N. P. (1996) Target-controlled infusions – stress free anesthesia. *Journal of Clinical Anesthesia*, **8**, 15S–20S.

PART FOUR
SPECIAL SITUATIONS

POST-ANAESTHETIC RECOVERY ROOM

J. P. Millns and G. M. Cooper

The need for close surveillance in the early postoperative period was recognized in the first two decades after the beginning of modern anaesthesia in 1846. However, the role of specific recovery areas did not develop at the same rate as anaesthetic practice itself. It was not until the 1940s that a number of events provided the impetus to develop recovery units. These included increased numbers of patients having had more complex surgical procedures, a shortage of nurses and the need to centralize the use of limited and expensive resources. Intensive care units were developing with the provision of better monitoring and care of the critically ill and it was realized that half the deaths related to anaesthesia occurring in the postoperative period were preventable. It also became apparent that in institutions where recovery areas existed there were fewer post-anaesthetic deaths. Thus, it is only relatively recently that the invaluable contribution of good postoperative management has been understood and that recovery areas have been appropriately staffed and equipped. The introduction of recovery units differs between countries and only since 1993 has a recovery unit been mandatory in France in hospitals where surgery is performed. The presence of recovery units is one of the criteria used by the Royal College of Anaesthetists to assess the nature of training in anaesthesia.

The rationale for the provision of recovery areas lies in the fact that the early postoperative period is a dangerous time: two surveys, encompassing over 40 000 patients passing through the recovery rooms of district hospitals, showed that 1 in 5 patients develop a complication at this time. In another prospective survey of complications associated with anaesthesia, 40% were found to occur after anaesthesia and in the recovery period. The Medical Protection Society has also commented that serious sequelae after anaesthesia can be avoided if continuous skilled observations are made, correctly interpreted and acted upon. The importance of good postoperative care is also emphasized in the Confidential Enquiries into Maternal Deaths in England and Wales (1979–81, 1985–87 and 1988–90).

After major surgery it is only to be expected that a frail, unfit patient needs careful monitoring and treatment to avoid serious complications. However, it is equally important to look for the unexpected and avert tragic disasters in young, fit patients who may have undergone only minor surgery. Close monitoring immediately after surgery ensures that the benefits of good surgery and safe anaesthesia are not compromised by lack of attention in the recovery period. For this to occur, there has to be appropriate space, equipment and number of staff with relevant skills. Teamwork is essential, and clear instructions must be given to the recovery staff.

Short Practice of Anaesthesia. Edited by M. Morgan and G. M. Hall. Published in 1997 by Chapman & Hall, London. ISBN 0 412 71890 1

THE RECOVERY ROOM

The ideal features of a recovery room are itemized in Table 37.1, and are mostly self-explanatory. They should be achievable in a purpose-built unit, but it is recognized that existing facilities may have to compromise on some aspects, such as the availability of pipeline outlets (oxygen and suction are nevertheless essential), and ventilation systems.

The importance of close proximity to the operating theatre cannot be overemphasized because of minimizing the risks involved in the transport of potentially unstable patients and the ready availability of the anaesthetist to assist when required. Proximity to the intensive care unit is also highly desirable.

Access and space requirements need to consider the type of surgery performed, especially in the case of orthopaedic beds with devices for traction etc. There are advantages in having well-separated entrance and exit doors so as to guarantee an undisturbed flow of patients who are arriving and leaving at frequent intervals. The recommended floor space needs to be increased from that described in Table 37.1 to 18.6 m^2 (200 sq ft) per bay whenever ventilatory support has to be provided; the additional space permits movement of personnel and trolleys. When designing new facilities, computer simulations of movement of beds and trolleys through doors and round corners are useful. The number of recovery bays required will vary according to the type of surgery, and will be more when there is a rapid turnover, or when theatres are used as day-care facilities.

Adequate cupboard space is essential. The location of items of equipment should be known to all who work there. An overall list is useful, in addition to clear labelling of cupboards. A consistent approach is helpful to find things quickly. It must be emphasized that cupboards, rubbish bins, etc. should be placed so as not to impede free movement of beds and trolleys. Thus, essential equipment should be kept at the head end and is mostly suitable for wall mounting. Sense must prevail about the height at which this is done, remembering that oxygen and sucker tubing require frequent changing and that sucker bottles need to be emptied. It is clearly undesirable for ladders to be needed to perform these tasks!

Table 37.1 Ideal features of the recovery room. (Adapted from *Immediate Postanaesthetic Recovery* (1993), Association of Anaesthetists of Great Britain and Ireland, with permission.)

Close to operating theatre
1.5 bays per theatre
Curtains for some bays
Ability to segregate children
Floor space of 9.3 m^2 (100 sq feet) per bay
Clearance side-to-side 1.2 m
Sufficient wide doors
Temperature 21–22°C
Relative humidity 38–45%
Well ventilated (15 air changes per hour)
Well lit (preferably natural light augmented) with individual lighting for each bay
Ceiling hooks for hanging infusion bags
At least six 13A power points per bay
Sufficient telephone sockets
Adequate provision of sinks and clinical waste bins
Flat surface on which to write notes
Pipeline outlets for suction, oxygen, nitrous oxide and air
Waste gas scavenging points

EQUIPMENT

In order that each patient is monitored and cared for appropriately, each recovery bay needs a certain amount of basic equipment and this is listed in Table 37.2. It is inappropriate for the items to be shared between bays, as they all need to be immediately accessible, and the person looking after the patient must not leave the patient to find them. This obviously requires an efficient restocking system and regular checks that everything is in working order. This should be done daily before the arrival of the first patient.

Table 37.2 Basic equipment for each recovery bay. (Adapted from *Immediate Postanaesthetic Recovery* (1993), Association of Anaesthetists of Great Britain and Ireland, with permission.)

Emergency bell
Oxygen outlet with twin flow meters
Oxygen face masks (fixed and variable performance types)
Mapleson C breathing system or self-inflating bag
Anaesthetic face masks
Suction unit
Supply of suction catheters and Yankauer ends
Pulse oximeter
Automated blood pressure machine or sphygmomanometer
Stethoscope
Range of blood pressure cuffs
ECG monitor
Sharps disposal box
Store of swabs, adhesive tape, syringes, needles and cannulae
Range of oropharyngeal and nasopharyngeal airways
Bin for contaminated re-usable equipment
Vomit bowl and tissues
Rubbish bin

Table 37.3 Additional equipment required to be available in recovery. (Adapted from *Immediate Postanaesthetic Recovery* (1993), Association of Anaesthetists of Great Britain and Ireland, with permission.)

Paediatric equipment
Cardiorespiratory
   Anaesthetic machine
   Ventilator with disconnection alarm
   Equipment for intubation
   Intravenous infusion sets
   Blood warmer
   Pressure infusion bags
   Central venous cannulae and manometers
   Combined ECG monitor/defibrillator with recorder
   Wright respirometer
   Bronchoscope
   Cricothyroid puncture set
   Chest drain set
   Trolley with battery-operated monitors
Miscellaneous
   Thermometer
   Peripheral nerve stimulator
   Insulating blanket
   Electric fan
   Electric blankets for pre-heating beds
   Clock with sweep second hand clearly visible
   Refrigerator for drugs
   Storage for intravenous fluids
   X-ray viewing screen
   White boards and marker pens
   Stable platforms to facilitate chest compression by staff less than 170 cm tall
   Wedge for resuscitation of pregnant women
   Linen
   Fire extinguisher
Drugs
   Appropriate drugs for routine use
   Drugs for treatment of cardiac arrest, anaphylaxis and malignant hyperthermia
   Range of crystalloid and colloid solutions
   Access to blood bank refrigerator

Further equipment needs to be available within the recovery unit and the location of every item should be known to staff. This is detailed in Table 37.3 and highlights the need to be prepared for diverse situations and emergencies. Because some of this equipment is only required infrequently, but nevertheless urgently, it is vital that its availability and current working order are checked regularly. The futility of a malfunctioning defibrillator for a patient in ventricular fibrillation does not require elucidation. A common problem which calls for firm management is the borrowing of items for use in areas distant from recovery and the failure to return these items. A system needs to operate where a log is kept of loaned articles and their location and time of return recorded.

The drugs required in recovery vary with individual practices and medical advances but call for regular appraisal to ensure that drugs are not wasted because of infrequent use. It must be recognized that drugs which are required only for emergencies, such as those used in resuscitation, or for the treatment of malignant hyperthermia, may legitimately exceed their expiry date without being used and yet be essential stock. Whilst not itemizing individual drugs, suitable drugs for the treatment of complications must be available, also those for the management of pain. Thus, drugs for the treatment of arrhythmias, hypotension, hypertension, ventilatory depression and bronchospasm are essential. Suitable locked facilities for keeping drugs controlled by the Misuse of Drugs Act need to be at hand and it is useful to have oral preparations available, in addition to injectable analgesics. Drug stocks should be checked daily to ensure availability.

STAFFING

The performance and quality of the work in the recovery room are dependent on the knowledge and competence of the nurses who must be present in sufficient numbers. Clinical experience from work on surgical wards is not sufficient for the challenges of the recovery room. National courses such as post-basic courses for anaesthetic (ENB 182) and operating department (ENB 183) nursing are available. Other operating department personnel can also contribute to patient care in recovery. Operating Department Assistants who possess a City and Guilds 752 certificate will have received limited training in recovery skills, but will have knowledge and competence in anaesthetic and surgical matters which can be supplemented by local training. The recently introduced National Vocational Qualification in Operating Department Practice, at Level 3, ensures knowledge and competence in recovery care with the exception of the administration of drugs. Thus there is potential flexibility in staffing arrangements.

Nevertheless, all staff in the recovery room need to be educated and trained to the highest professional standards, so that they may provide optimum care for patients, and respond to the potentially life-threatening circumstances that frequently arise. A basic understanding of anatomy, physiology and pharmacology relevant to anaesthetic and surgical procedures must be supplemented by practical training in airway management and resuscitation. Full understanding of monitoring requirements and equipment, as well as the nursing needs of patients in a range of specialities, is mandatory. Where specialized procedures are undertaken, additional training will be required for a proportion of the staff. Wherever possible training and experience should encompass a full range of patient groups including pregnant and parturient women, children and the elderly. The recovery nurse should know how to initiate postoperative pain treatment. After completion of basic training, all staff should participate in regular in-service training and education designed to maintain proficiency in skills which are only used infrequently. Support for study leave is also essential.

TRANSFER TO THE RECOVERY ROOM

After general anaesthesia, the unconscious patient should normally be placed in the lateral position on a tipping trolley or bed and escorted to the recovery area by the anaesthetist. The important features of recovery trolleys are outlined in Table 37.4. It is possible for complications to arise during this transfer (and later to the ward) and hence the availability of oxygen, tilt and suction is important. It is always worthwhile checking that the trolley is brought in the right way round, with these facilities at the head end! Padded sides and locking wheels are features

Table 37.4 Features of recovery trolleys. (Adapted from *Immediate Postanaesthetic Recovery* (1993), Association of Anaesthetists of Great Britain and Ireland, with permission.)

Oxygen cylinder
Rapid head down tilt
Suction equipment
Padded cot sides
Adjustable back rest
Comfortable easily cleanable mattress
Locking wheels on steerable castors
Infusion poles and mounting sites
Tray for notes and ancillary equipment

to aid safety, preventing the patient from falling to the floor. The need for a comfortable mattress and adjustable back rest requires no further explanation. Infusion poles secure intravenous infusions and allow flow to be maintained during transfer.

The patient should not be moved from the operating table until the anaesthetist is satisfied that the following criteria are present:

- the physiological and, in particular, cardiorespiratory status of the patient is satisfactory;
- the recovery bed or trolley is correctly positioned with the wheel brake applied;
- suction equipment is available;
- equipment for airway and ventilatory support is to hand;
- monitoring equipment that may be required during transfer is available and functioning.

Transfer of the patient should take place avoiding direct lifting and without tension placed on items attached to the patient. Chest drains connected to an underwater seal may be clamped for the move to the bed, but at the earliest opportunity should be positioned below the patient and reopened.

From this moment, a continuum of care begins, the aims of which are highlighted below.

ARRIVAL IN RECOVERY

Basic monitoring equipment should be attached to the patient, namely pulse oximeter, non-invasive blood pressure and ECG. Oxygen therapy should be commenced.

The handover to recovery personnel should include identification of the following.

- The nature of the surgery that has taken place, including any complications which have occurred that may affect recovery care, e.g. potential bleeding sites
- Skin sutures, dressings and surgical drains used
- Important factors about the patient's preoperative condition, e.g. the presence of ischaemic heart disease or neuromuscular disorder
- Nature of the anaesthetic used, including any local anaesthetic procedures undertaken
- Complications occurring during the anaesthetic, e.g. arrhythmia/prolonged hypotension
- Acceptable physiological parameters for the recovery period.

CARE IN RECOVERY

Before the patient can be transferred back to the ward, certain criteria must be met. The patient must be able to maintain, and protect, their airway. The breathing pattern should be quiet and unlaboured, an effective cough must be present and the patient should be a good colour. The cardiovascular system should be stable and peripheral perfusion good. The patient should be fully conscious and orientated; comfortable and warm.

This next section identifies problems that may occur in achieving these endpoints and the remedies needed to correct them.

RESPIRATORY CARE

Ideally, the patient will have been extubated before transfer. If a tracheal tube is still in place, spontaneous ventilation should be occurring with supplemental oxygen administered via an anaesthetic circuit (e.g. Mapleson C) or a T-piece. In general, the tube will be removed once the patient is showing adequate ventilation and oxygenation, and to be waking. If a laryngeal mask is in place, this should not be removed until the patient objects to it.

In most patients, the adequacy of ventilation is assessed on clinical grounds, in particular a respiratory rate of 10–24 breaths a minute associated with good colour and absence of distress. The degree of movement of a reservoir bag when a close-fitting mask is applied to the face gives an indication of tidal volume. Some degree of hypoventilation, after general anaesthesia especially, is common and acceptable but it is important that the trend is towards improvement. If the respiratory rate is changing to values outside the suggested limits, and signs of reducing tidal volume and hypercapnia (tachycardia, hypertension and altered consciousness) are becoming apparent, a remedy must be sought.

Airway problems

Airway obstruction

Obstruction of the upper airway may be caused by the tongue, blood or secretions in the pharynx and may also occur as a result of laryngeal muscle hypotonia. If the obstruction is partial, there is stertorous breathing; as complete obstruction threatens, the effort of breathing increases as shown by use of the accessory muscles and tracheal tug. With complete obstruction of the airway, there is no longer any noise, but extreme ventilatory effort is obvious by the paradoxical movement of the chest and abdominal wall.

The patient should be in the lateral recovery position to aid drainage of secretions and the airway cleared with a sucker. Continuing obstruction may be alleviated by extending the head and lifting the chin forward. In the unconscious patient, an oropharyngeal airway may be inserted, although this procedure can cause gagging in a patient who is regaining consciousness. Sometimes, pushing the mandible forward can ease the obstruction, but this causes discomfort if the patient is almost awake. A nasopharyngeal airway may be helpful and is often inserted before extubation if the jaws are wired together at surgery. It should be lubricated with a suitable gel and care taken at insertion so that nasopharyngeal trauma and haemorrhage do not occur. This complication is more likely in pregnant women.

If the obstruction cannot be cleared by these means, and especially if hypoxaemia is ensuing, reintubation will be necessary until consciousness has returned. Rarely, reintubation will not be possible; then either cricothyroid puncture, or cricothyrotomy, will be necessary.

Situations in which airway obstruction is a potential problem include postoperative haemorrhage into the neck after thyroid and other neck operations, inadvertent retention of a throat pack after intraoral surgery, after surgery on intraoral tumours, after operations where the jaws have been wired together and in obese patients.

Laryngeal obstruction

Laryngeal oedema secondary to intubation can occasionally cause laryngeal obstruction which may be severe enough to warrant reintubation. The small diameter of a child's larynx relative to that of an adult means that even a small amount of oedema may cause trouble in a child. In adults, if the larynx is already oedematous, as is seen occasionally in pre-eclampsia, then the likelihood of a problem is increased. Treatment may be with dexamethasone and/or nebulized adrenaline.

Partial or complete laryngeal spasm is more common than oedema after extubation. Partial spasm is recognized by a high-pitched inspiratory stridor; complete obstruction can be difficult to differentiate from other causes of airway obstruction. Spasm may be precipitated by blood or secretions on the vocal cords, or irritation from an oral airway. It may also accompany inadequate reversal of neuromuscular blockade. If the methods to clear obstruction outlined above do not solve the problem, 100% oxygen should be administered until the spasm subsides and reintubation undertaken, after administration of suxamethonium, if hypoxaemia threatens.

After thyroid surgery on the contralateral side of the neck where there is previously damaged vocal cord innervation, or in primary surgery on both sides of the neck, the other/both recurrent laryngeal nerves can be damaged surgically. This leaves the superior laryngeal nerve supply to the cricothyroid muscle (adductor to the vocal cords) unopposed. Acute laryngeal obstruction results usually with the need for reintubation and formation of a tracheostomy.

Acute hypocalcaemia resulting from inadvertent removal of the parathyroid glands during surgery can also cause stridor.

Bronchospasm

Although it may arise occasionally as part of an anaphylactic reaction to a drug, in the recovery room bronchospasm is more likely to be seen as a response to the presence of a tracheal tube in a known asthmatic or chronic bronchitic patient. As consciousness returns, particularly if there is carinal irritation from the tip of the tube, coughing may also cause wheezing. If the patient is able, despite the spasm, to take an occasional large breath as evidence of adequate reversal from neuromuscular blockade, then it is better to remove the tube, administer 100% oxygen and wait for the coughing/spasm to subside. If the wheezing continues to cause respiratory distress bronchodilator drugs, such as nebulized salbutamol, should be administered.

Bronchospasm may also occur as a result of aspiration of gastric contents.

Hypoventilation

Although all the problems listed above cause alveolar underventilation, there are other causes of inadequate ventilation to consider. One of the more common scenarios is that of the unconscious patient who will not breathe. The possible reasons are listed in Table 37.5 of which the most common is residual depressant effect of drugs given during anaesthesia, or in the early postoperative period.

The majority of induction agents, the vola-

Table 37.5 Causes of hypoventilation in the unconscious patient

Persistent effect of drugs that are respiratory depressants
Persistent neuromuscular blockade
Intraoperative hyperventilation
Preoperative metabolic disorder, e.g. hypothyroidism, metabolic alkalosis
Hypothermia
Preoperative cerebral pathology
Intraoperative cerebral event, e.g. haemorrhage
Unrecognized total spinal anaesthesia

tile anaesthetic agents and opioids all depress ventilation and their effects are additive. The presence of residual volatile agent can be confirmed by exhaled gas analysis where this is available, and after a short period of ventilation spontaneous breathing resumes. When opioids are the main reason for not breathing the pupils are pinpoint. The two options are either to stimulate breathing with doxapram (1 mg kg^{-1} over a minute) or to antagonize the opioid with naloxone (bolus doses of 0.5–1.0 µg kg^{-1}). Unlike doxapram, naloxone will antagonize the analgesic effect of opioids. Both these drugs have a relatively short duration of action and consequently, patients should continue to be observed for at least half an hour in case further doses are necessary.

Drugs such as suxamethonium and mivacurium, which rely for their metabolism on plasma cholinesterase, will produce persistent neuromuscular blockade in the patient who has an abnormal enzyme, or reduced quantity of normal enzyme. In the former situation the prolongation of block may be for as little as 20 min or for several hours, depending on the genetic variant present. Peripheral nerve stimulation will show equal, but reduced, twitches in response to repeated stimuli and a train of four stimulus.

In the patient who is semi-conscious or indeed conscious, residual paralysis is manifest as anxiety (in both patient and recovery personnel) and jerky muscle movement together with hypoventilation and tachycardia. Peripheral nerve stimulation will show progressively decreasing twitches in response to repeated stimuli. A tetanic stimulus would show fade, but should be avoided in the conscious patient since this is painful. Clinical observation of strength of hand grip and ability to sustain a lift of the head from the pillow are cruder indices of reversal of neuromuscular blockade. Further neostigmine (total 5 mg) may be given but if the response to this is inadequate, then reintubation, sedation and ventilation will be needed. Factors which prolong neuromuscular block are listed in Table 37.6.

Excessive intraoperative ventilation removes the major stimulus to breathe and monitoring of the end-tidal carbon dioxide concentration will allow the diagnosis (and prevention) of this problem. Hypocapnia is particularly important if the patient has a preexisting metabolic alkalosis (e.g. due to gastric outlet obstruction).

An anaesthetic technique which raises intracerebral pressure in the presence of a pre-existing cerebral tumour, or mild cerebral oedema produced as a result of trauma, may damage the respiratory centre. Intracranial haemorrhage or infarction occurring as a result of cardiovascular disturbance during anaesthesia is also a possible cause of hypoventilation. Gross hypoxic episodes may also damage the respiratory centre and are likely to result in impaired consciousness.

Inadvertent spread of local anaesthetic drugs from an epidural, used as a supplement to general anaesthesia, sufficient to cause a total spinal anaesthetic will prevent breathing and is associated with severe hypotension as a result of sympathetic blockade. More unusually, subarachnoid injection can occur with some local anaesthetic blocks performed in the head and neck region.

Other causes of hypoventilation include pain, the presence of tight dressings, obesity and abdominal distension. In addition, one should not forget to look for causes within the chest, such as pneumo/haemothorax: thus knowledge of the patient's preoperative state and the procedures undertaken in theatre is vital.

Hypoxaemia

On arrival in the recovery room, absence of cyanosis suggests that there is no **gross** defect in cardiorespiratory status. Reliable detection of cyanosis is notoriously difficult and pulse oximetry has revolutionized practice in this area. While pulse oximetry is not infallible, or without limitations, evidence is provided of adequate oxygenation. More importantly, a small decrease in oxygen saturation serves as a trigger to observers to seek the cause before a major problem arises. Such changes are not diagnostic, but only reflect the final outcome of oxygen delivery from atmosphere to peripheral tissues. However, oximetry may alert staff to major problems such as pneumothorax and pulmonary oedema which may not be evident on clinical grounds alone. It is important not to rely on adequate oxygenation as evidence of adequate ventilation.

Table 37.6 Factors which can abnormally prolong non-depolarizing neuromuscular blocking agents

Neuromuscular disorders
Hepatic disease
Renal disease
Age
   Neonates (increased sensitivity)
   Elderly (reduced clearance)
Acid–base disorders
   Respiratory acidosis
   Metabolic alkalosis
Electrolyte disorders
   Decreased calcium
   Decreased potassium
   Increased magnesium
Hypoxia
Hypothermia
Drugs
   Aminoglycosides and polymixin antibiotics
   Local anaesthetics
   Quinidine

Hypoxaemia in the postoperative period may be due to:

- diffusion hypoxia;
- hypoventilation;
- ventilation/perfusion abnormalities;
- increased physiological shunt.

The use of nitrous oxide for general anaesthesia is associated with diffusion hypoxia as the patient is allowed to breathe room air again at the end of the procedure. This arises as the more soluble nitrous oxide diffuses into the lungs from the blood in larger amounts than nitrogen moving in the opposite direction. This results in a lower partial pressure of the other gases in the lungs and, as a consequence, transient hypoxaemia.

Hypoventilation has been discussed above. Application of the alveolar gas equation shows that as the alveolar partial pressure of carbon dioxide rises, the partial pressure of oxygen falls with resultant hypoxaemia.

General anaesthesia is associated with a reduced functional residual capacity. After an operation closing volume may impinge on normal tidal volume. Cardiac output changes are not infrequent, so ventilation/perfusion abnormalities are a common sequel to anaesthesia.

In the early postoperative period, intrapulmonary shunting is most likely to arise in patients with preoperative pulmonary consolidation or oedema.

Oxygen therapy may be administered by variable or fixed performance devices. In the case of variable performance devices such as the Hudson and MC masks and nasal cannulae, the inspired oxygen concentration will depend on several factors which include:

- the flow of oxygen into the mask;
- the volume of the mask;
- the respiratory variables of the patient: respiratory rate, tidal volume and peak inspiratory flow rate.

For the majority of patients, oxygen delivery at flow rates of 2–4 l min^{-1} will produce an adequate inspired oxygen concentration to overcome the effects of mild hypoventilation, diffusion hypoxia and minor ventilation/perfusion abnormalities. Patients who are dependent on hypoxic drive for normal ventilation, or those with increased shunt (e.g. due to pulmonary consolidation), require a high air flow oxygen enrichment device such as a Ventimask.

For alert patients with adequate carbon dioxide clearance, continuous positive airways pressure (CPAP) from a mask may correct persistent hypoxaemia, although it is best used when the cause of hypoxaemia can be corrected rapidly e.g. pulmonary oedema. Intubation and ventilation will be required if the Pa_{O_2} is not maintained above 9 kPa, or if hypoventilation results in a concomitant rise in Pa_{CO_2}.

CARDIOVASCULAR CARE

For the majority of patients, this entails monitoring of heart rate and blood pressure with appropriate therapy to maintain acceptable values, and observation and treatment of important arrhythmias. In some, continuous assessment of central venous pressure and even cardiac output will be required.

Blood pressure abnormalities

Hypertension

In the recovery room, this occurs most frequently due to pain or in a patient with pre-existing hypertension. It can also occur in response to hypoxaemia, hypercarbia and fluid overload. Patients with vascular disease exhibit hypertension as a result of increased cardiac output because of their inability to alter vascular resistance. Hence postoperative hypertension is a common problem after abdominal aortic and carotid artery surgery.

Persistent hypertension increases left ventricular work and myocardial oxygen consumption; left ventricular failure, myocardial ischaemia and arrhythmias may ensue. Cerebral oedema and haemorrhage can result from persistent hypertension. Acceptable limits of arterial pressure are decided bearing in mind the preoperative value and responses during anaesthesia. Initial treatment of hypertension should be to ensure adequate analgesia and to exclude hypoxia and hypercarbia. Specific therapies include labetalol and hydralazine, given in incremental doses until the desired blood pressure is achieved. If these are inadequate nitroprusside or glyceryl trinitrate will be needed, in which instance it is recommended that intra-arterial monitoring of blood pressure is undertaken.

Hypotension

Hypotension in the recovery room may be due to:

- decreased ventricular preload;
- diminished myocardial contractility;
- reduced systemic vascular resistance.

It is important to identify the cause quickly since a period of prolonged hypotension will lead to ischaemic damage in vital organs.

Decreased ventricular preload Usually, this means that either fluid replacement in the operating theatre has been inadequate or that loss from the circulation is continuing. The latter may be due to bleeding (inspection of the wound, drainage tubes or abdomen may point to this), continuing loss of fluid into the third space, as after major bowel surgery, prolonged diuresis or, less commonly, leakage out of the circulation in a septic patient. While a search for a cause is initiated, a fluid challenge of 5–10 ml kg^{-1} should be started; a colloid solution is preferable. Elevation of the legs may help to raise the blood pressure. If the situation does not resolve, the tachycardia and hypotension persist and particularly if the patient is elderly, subsequent fluid infusion should be aided by central venous pressure measurement. If myocardial depression is suspected, a pulmonary artery catheter is indicated. It should be remembered that the residual effects of anaesthetic drugs and normal preoperative medication such as β-adrenergic blocking drugs and calcium channel blocking drugs may affect adversely the situation. Surgical bleeding will usually require reoperation. However, if the patient has a known coagulopathy, surgery has required major transfusion or the administration of anticoagulants, or there is any reason to suspect a cause for disseminated intravascular coagulopathy such as septicaemia or amniotic fluid embolus, then a check of coagulation status should be undertaken. Bleeding due to this cause may be highlighted by the presence of bleeding from other sites, such as venepuncture sites.

Rarely, an acute pulmonary embolus will obstruct right ventricular outflow and cause severe hypotension.

Diminished myocardial contractility The two common causes of acute left ventricular failure are myocardial ischaemia and over-transfusion. It may be seen in patients who have had central neural blockade using local anaesthetics when the vasodilation produced by these drugs is waning and the effect of fluid given as a vascular preload to avoid hypotension persists. As with hypovolaemia, the patient is tachycardic and hypotensive with cold, poorly perfused peripheries. The presence of pulmonary oedema and/or a raised jugular venous pressure may aid diagnosis; often, though, it is treated in error as hypovolaemia. Invasive vascular monitoring will assist the diagnosis; evidence of myocardial infarction should be looked for. Treatment requires the administration of oxygen, fluid restriction, diuretics and on occasion inotropic or vasodilator therapy. Patients should be nursed in the sitting position.

Reduced systemic vascular resistance Residual effects of anaesthetic agents may result in reduced vascular resistance, especially if the patient is pain-free. Central neural blockade is an obvious cause and even if the patient is normotensive when supine, sitting the patient up in recovery may precipitate hypotension. For this reason, intravenous accesss should be maintained until the block recedes.

An important complication to recognize is septicaemia, where warm peripheries are associated with hypotension and tachycardia.

Arrhythmias

The more common arrhythmias seen in the recovery room are described.

Sinus tachycardia

This is seen frequently. It may be due to residual effects of anticholinergic drugs used to reverse neuromuscular blockade. In association with hypertension, it may indicate pain, hypoxia, hypercarbia or sympathetic stimulation, e.g. after aortic surgery. Treatment of the underlying cause is the first manoeuvre; if this has been addressed and the tachycardia persists, then in the patient with ischaemic heart disease the heart rate should be slowed, e.g. with a β-adrenergic blocking drug.

If the tachycardia is associated with hypotension, management should be directed towards treatment of hypovolaemia or cardiac failure, as appropriate.

Sinus bradycardia

This may be due to prolonged action of neostigmine or preoperative medication with β-adrenergic blocking drugs. Bradycardia is seen often in the trained athlete and also may occur as part of a high spinal or epidural block. Vagal stimulation as with vomiting, or in the insertion of a suction catheter, can cause bradycardia. Raised intracranial pressure is an unusual cause of bradycardia. Only if hypoxia is severe does bradycardia occur.

A heart rate less than 40 beats per minute requires treatment. Atropine 10 $\mu g\ kg^{-1}$ is the first choice. In the range 40–50 beats per minute, treatment may be withheld unless there is concurrent hypotension. Bradycardia unresponsive to atropine needs isoprenaline intravenously and where bradycardia is due to complete heart block, transvenous pacing will be necessary.

Ventricular ectopic beats

These may be present preoperatively and persist into the recovery room. They are more frequent when halothane has been used as the volatile anaesthetic agent. Provided that they remain unifocal, and no more frequent than one in every five beats, treatment is unnecessary. If they become multifocal, or more frequent, lignocaine given intravenously in a dose of 1 $mg\ kg^{-1}$ is first-line treatment.

It must be remembered that in the patient with ischaemic heart disease, the onset of ectopic beats, especially if this is in association with hypertension, should be viewed more seriously; it may herald the onset of myocardial infarction.

FLUID AND ELECTROLYTE BALANCE

Postoperative renal failure remains an important cause of death in the surgical patient. Although death occurs long after leaving recovery, careful attention to fluid balance and observation for oliguria in the early postoperative period is vital. Thus, an indwelling urinary catheter should be used in at-risk groups, e.g. those having heart and major vascular surgery; patients with obstructive jaundice, pre-existing renal disease and sepsis; and those who have had major blood transfusions or suffered major trauma. Prerenal oliguria is the most common type of oliguria seen and usually occurs following hypovolaemia. Otherwise, cardiac failure should be considered. More rarely, postrenal causes, such as division of the ureters at operation, result in oliguria.

The main electrolyte disorders that merit consideration in the recovery room are those relating to sodium, potassium and calcium ions. Hyponatraemia is caused by inadvertent administration of large volumes of glucose solution, or may occur as a result of instillation of large volumes of glycine solution during protracted endoscopic prostatic surgery or after endometrial resection. It presents as confusion often in association with pulmonary oedema. Treatment requires diuretics, oxygen and consideration of the use of hypertonic saline.

Hypokalaemia as an acute event may arise as a result of glucose/insulin therapy or a large diuresis. It is associated with cardiac arrhythmias especially ventricular disturbances. Hyperkalaemia is most likely to arise when renal failure occurs, especially if there is also significant tissue damage, e.g. in association with major trauma or sepsis. Once the serum potassium is above 5.5 mmol l^{-1}, treatment may be indicated with a combination of glucose/insulin, calcium and resonium, depending partly on the absolute value and also the rate of rise of the serum potassium concentration.

Hypocalcaemia predisposes to problems with reversal of neuromuscular blockade, cardiac contractility and cardiac conduction. It is caused by major transfusion, pancreatitis and hyperventilation; it is evident in hypoparathyroidism. Treatment requires infusion of calcium chloride and monitoring of ionized calcium levels.

CEREBRAL STATUS; CONFUSION AND AGITATION; COMMUNICATION

It is common for patients to be unconscious on arrival in the recovery room. This is most usually due to the residual effects of drugs given during the operation such as volatile agents, opioids, benzodiazepines and intravenous anaesthetic agents. Although these drugs may cause prolonged unconsciousness, other causes should be remembered: glucose disturbance in a diabetic patient; electrolyte abnormalities, e.g. hyponatraemia; hypothermia; intracerebral pathology, e.g. haemorrhage/oedema; postictal state.

It is not uncommon to see agitation in postoperative patients. Pain is the most frequent cause. However, hypoxaemia, hallucination (due to ketamine for example), inadequate reversal of neuromuscular blockade, gastric distension, bladder distension and irritation from an indwelling urinary catheter may also cause agitation. Milder cases of conditions mentioned under prolonged unconsciousness will also produce confusion.

PAIN CONTROL AND ANTI-EMETIC THERAPY

This is discussed in full in Chapter 38. However, one or two points are worth highlighting. Inadequate pain relief is a potent cause of disturbance and physiological upset in the recovery room. Prompt treatment is possible and bolus intravenous opioid treatment is preferable to intramuscular administration. The stay in recovery provides an ideal opportunity for the patient to accustom themselves to using a patient-controlled analgesia system. Local anaesthetic blocks provide excellent analgesia.

Some pain relief methods utilized in theatre produce unwanted side-effects: intercostal nerve block may produce a pneumothorax; epidural local anaesthetic may cause hypotension and spinal opiates may result in respiratory depression and itching.

Anti-emetic therapy is best administered early in the course of an anaesthetic rather than waiting for nausea to occur in the recovery room. Many factors contribute to the frequency with which this complication is seen. However, the recovery staff can help to relieve the problem by treating hypotension promptly and aspirating nasogastric tubes.

After intraoral surgery, encouragement to expel blood from the mouth will mean that less is swallowed.

The aim should be to have the patient comfortable before leaving recovery: once back on a busy ward one-to-one contact between nurse and patient, and thus opportunity for good relief of pain, is less likely.

TEMPERATURE CONTROL

Although hyperthermia is encountered, hypothermia is far more common and may contribute to slow awakening. After lengthy, intra-abdominal or intrathoracic operations, patients are often cold. This is distressing and produces peripheral vasoconstriction and hypertension. Conservation of body heat must be started in the theatre; once in recovery, re-warming can be helped by the use of warm blankets, hot air blankets and fluid warmers. Attention to continual covering of the patient is vital. Oxygen should be administered until any shivering ceases.

RECOVERY CHART

Accurate record keeping is essential, including the timing of observations. All events and physiological variables must be recorded in a clear and legible manner. A suitable flow chart, often on the reverse of the anaesthetic record, allows the trend of information to be assimilated at a glance. Drug and fluid administration should be included.

CONCLUSIONS

During the postoperative period vigilance is required. A wide variety of clinical problems may occur, many often manifesting themselves in similar ways. Anticipation and prompt response to problems is required if major morbidity at the time, or later, is to be avoided.

FURTHER READING

Association of Anaesthetists of Great Britain and Ireland. (1993) *Immediate Postanaesthetic Recovery.* AAGBI, London.

Cooper, G. M. (1994) Monitoring the recovery from anaesthesia in: *Monitoring in Anaesthesia and Intensive Care.* (eds P. Hutton and C. Prys-Roberts) Saunders, London. 350–364.

Frost, E. A. M. and Thomson, D. A., eds. (1994) *Post-Anaesthetic Care.* Baillière's Clinical Anaesthesiology, London.

CONTROL OF POSTOPERATIVE PAIN, NAUSEA AND VOMITING

M. Harmer

The past decade has seen increased interest in the management of postoperative pain, partly due to heightened awareness caused by the joint Colleges' report *'Pain after Surgery'* and partly by a natural progression of the anaesthetists' role in perioperative management. The heightened awareness of the inadequacy of postoperative pain management and subsequent improvements, has led to an appreciation of other troublesome perioperative symptoms; of these, the most unpleasant to the patient is nausea and vomiting. It is for this reason that the two topics are considered in a single chapter.

Although the existence of pain dates back into ancient history, the specific problem of postoperative pain really only came to prominence after anaesthetics had been introduced. Until then surgery was of very limited extent and the pain after surgery was as nothing compared to the pain during the surgery! So whilst one may blame the surgeon for having inflicted pain, the anaesthetist has historically been an accessory to the crime.

In 1806, Friedrich Wilhelm Adam Sertürner isolated the active constituent of opium, although the pain relieving properties of the opium poppy had been known for centuries. Sertürner first named his new alkaloid *principium somniferum* but later changed it to *morphine* after Morpheus, the god of dreams. However, it was not until the development of the hypodermic syringe and hollow needle in the 1850s that morphine could be administered in a measured manner. Cocaine was recognized as a powerful local anaesthetic in 1884 but the role of local anaesthetics in postoperative pain management has only been appreciated in recent decades.

Considering the changes that have occurred in general anaesthetic practice and the ready availability of powerful opioid analgesics, it is astonishing that there have been so few advances made in the management of postoperative pain. Behind this paucity of change would appear to be a number of fundamental misunderstandings about the use of opioids to control pain: it is recognized that pain is difficult to measure; postoperative pain management is often delegated to trainee staff; there is fear of addiction and side effects (particularly respiratory depression); and the adjustment of dosage to achieve optimal effect has, until recently, been difficult.

For many years, clinicians have looked for new agents that would provide analgesia without any side effects; to date this 'holy grail' is still awaited. In more recent years, efforts have concentrated on the delivery method used for traditional opioid analgesics rather than the use of new agents. It is this strategy, along with the development of structured acute pain services, that has done much

Short Practice of Anaesthesia. Edited by M. Morgan and G. M. Hall. Published in 1997 by Chapman & Hall, London. ISBN 0 412 71890 1

However, as improvements in postoperative pain management have occurred, it has highlighted the inadequacy of other symptom control, especially nausea and vomiting. Just as pain has in the past been considered an inevitable consequence of surgery, so nausea and vomiting have been associated with anaesthesia. The variability of effect and relatively common occurrence of unwanted side effects of the anti-emetics has been a source of discouragement for those considering therapy for the prevention and treatment of postoperative nausea and vomiting. Unlike postoperative pain though, it has been the development of newer agents that has led to an overall improvement, though often by a more rational use of older agents.

PRINCIPLES OF POSTOPERATIVE PAIN

RELEVANT PHYSIOLOGY

A basic understanding of the physiology associated with pain sensation and appreciation helps to provide a rational approach to its management. Most acute pain originates when specific nerve endings are stimulated. The nerve endings consist largely of two types: mechanoceptors and polymodal nociceptors. The mechanoceptors are mainly present in the skin and respond to strong pressure, pinprick or heat and the signal is transmitted through small myelinated $A\delta$ fibres. They warn of potential damage and are associated with withdrawal reflexes. The polymodal nociceptors are the nerve endings of unmyelinated C fibres. They are widely distributed throughout most tissues and respond to tissue damage (mechanical, thermal and chemical insults). The transmission of impulses from these receptors is relatively slow and they are responsible for the dull, prolonged, aching pain after injury.

Both $A\delta$ and C fibres enter the spinal cord through the dorsal root where their cell bodies are located. After entering the spinal cord, most of the $A\delta$ and C fibres terminate in one of the laminae of the grey matter of the dorsal horn. The $A\delta$ fibres terminate in lamina I and the C fibres immediately beneath in the substantia gelatinosa (lamina II). The majority of both fibres synapse, either directly or via intermediate neurones in the deeper layers of the dorsal horn, with ascending fibres which cross the midline to join the spinothalamic tract.

Pain transmission can be inhibited at the spinal cord level by inhibitory interneurones or from descending inhibiting fibres. This interrelationship was described as the Gate Control Theory by Melzack and Wall, whereby the 'gate' can be closed by stimulation of non-painful sensory mechanoceptors whose impulses are carried in large myelinated fibres. This is also proposed as the theory behind transcutaneous electrical nerve stimulation and the more basic 'rubbing it better' response to injury.

In the dorsal horn of the spinal cord the principal neurotransmitter is thought to be the peptide substance P, although other transmitters have been identified (angiotensin II, somatostatin, cholecystokinin, 5-hydroxytryptophan and noradrenaline). Also present in the dorsal horn, particularly in the substantia gelatinosa, are the opioid receptors with enkaphalins acting as neurotransmitters in the inhibitory interneurones.

The ascending pain impulses are transmitted mainly through the spinothalamic tract to the lateral and medial parts of the thalamus before further transmission to the sensory and motor cortex. Impulses may also travel via the spinoreticular tract to terminate in the pontomedullary reticular formation. These impulses have a major role in the arousal/motivational aspects of pain sensation due to the links with the limbic system.

Descending pathways are mainly inhibitory in nature. Stimuli are produced in response to cortical and subcortical activation caused by sustained 'pain' input. These descending impulses are thought to interact in the 'gate control' of ascending pain impulses.

It can be seen that the sites at which pain impulses can be modified or blocked are: in the periphery at the receptors; in the nerves prior to transmission to the spinal cord; at a spinal cord level; and at a central level. In many circumstances, a multiple approach is needed to provide satisfactory analgesia.

BENEFITS OF ADEQUATE POSTOPERATIVE ANALGESIA

The first, and possibly most important, reason for the provision of adequate analgesia after surgery must be the humanitarian desire to alleviate pain wherever possible. However, there are clinical benefits from providing good pain relief. Following trauma or surgery to any part of the body, the natural response is to attempt to immobilize the area concerned. There was a belief (and perhaps it still exists) among some surgeons that this 'splinting' of the operative site is invaluable for the repair of tissues and for this reason pain should be encouraged as a protective process against possible wound or tissue damage. This immobility will certainly reduce the pain perceived by the patient but may in itself be detrimental. For peripheral surgery, the immobilization of limbs may encourage poor venous return with a subsequent development of a deep venous thrombosis which might have disastrous consequences if part is dislodged. After abdominal surgery, the limited movement of the abdominal wall will restrict ventilation leading to basal atelectasis and subsequent chest infection and, possibly, respiratory failure. Far from aiding tissue healing, the subsequent hypoxia caused by the chest condition may lead to tissue hypoxia and poor wound healing. Adequate analgesia and ventilatory function is more likely to provide a satisfactory healing outcome than a dependance on the pain to prevent movement.

Increased sympathetic stimulation from pain increases the risk of myocardial ischaemia in susceptible patients as a consequence of the resulting tachycardia, hypertension and increased circulating catecholamines. The stress response to surgery and pain increases the secretion of catecholamines and catabolic hormones. This increases metabolism and oxygen consumption and promotes sodium and water retention. Pain may also cause decreased bowel motility and urinary retention.

The benefits to be gained are not only clinical, as a reduction in serious sequelae will lead to a reduced stay in hospital and a decrease in the need for intensive care management after major surgery. These both have cost-saving implications.

FACTORS INFLUENCING POSTOPERATIVE PAIN

Site of surgery

As a general rule, 'the more it moves, the more it hurts'. This is as a consequence of the movement of injured tissues being the cause of postoperative pain. Thus, any wound that moves with respiration is likely to result in more severe pain (e.g. thoracotomy, upper abdominal), while those where the wound does not 'move' may be less severe (e.g. craniotomy).

The surgery

It is often held by surgeons that wounds heal from side-to-side and thus the length of the wound has no relevance to healing. However, the length of an incision is very relevant to the ability to be able to provide analgesia, particularly if regional techniques are employed. Although difficult to prove, it is a long held belief that some surgeons are 'gentler' than others; it is not hard to imagine that tissues torn apart will cause more pain than those carefully divided.

Pain tolerance

It is often stated that patients have a different pain 'threshold' when what is really meant is that although patients will interpret a stimulus as pain at a similar level, the degree of pain that an individual can tolerate shows wide variability. The precise reasons for this are unclear but may relate to nervous interactions occurring in the spinal cord as such factors may influence the 'gate' or the sensitivity of opioid receptors.

Psychological factors

The central connection of the pain afferent input near to the limbic system suggests that emotion is likely to have an important role to play in the pain perceived after surgery. Patients with an inherent coping nature may be better able to tolerate pain while those with an 'inadequate' personality may be less able to cope. The patients' surroundings may also influence the ability to tolerate pain; it has been shown that a 'caring' nurse with close attention has a positive analgesic effect. Finally, the prognosis following surgery may have an influence. The woman who has undergone a lower abdominal incision for an elective Caesarean section is likely to complain of less postoperative pain than the woman who has undergone a laparotomy for an inoperarable tumour.

Variability of response to analgesics

This is as a consequence of a combination of pharmacokinetic and pharmacodynamic factors. The main pharmacokinetic factor is the route of administration of an opioid but others include concomitant drug therapy, the age, sex and health of the patient, altered organ blood flows consequent on surgery and anaesthesia and alterations in drug-protein binding. The pharmacodynamic variables are evidenced by the differing responses to a given plasma concentration of the drug. Such variability may be similar to that encountered in pain tolerance. The combination of the variability in pain tolerance and response to analgesics means that there is a very wide variation between patients in the amount of analgesic drug that is necessary to provide acceptable pain relief.

ASSESSMENT OF POSTOPERATIVE PAIN

Pain is a sensation which is difficult to express and quantify. Methods of measuring pain can be considered as subjective or objective. Subjective measurements rely mainly on the patient's perception of their pain. The simplest method is a descriptive scale ranging from 'no pain' to 'severe pain'. This type of scale is very simple to use but is often too crude to differentiate minor differences in pain. An alternative method is the use of a visual analogue scale (a 10 cm line marked at one end with 'no pain' and 'the worst pain possible' at the other). The patient is asked to consider the severity of the pain and place a single mark on the line. This is then measured from the 'no pain' end and expressed in millimetres. This method has been well validated for research in pain but is not always easily understood by the patient, particularly in the early postoperative period. Some workers have added either numbers or words/pictures along the scale to make them more user-friendly. The use of a number of points on the scale means that this is no longer an analogue scale and becomes a digital ranking score. For routine use, the simpler verbal rating scale may be preferable. As well as the method of subjective assessment, what the patient is doing at the time the assessment is made is important. Pain relief at rest is relatively easy to attain and is in part due to the 'splinting' effect already described. However, what is really important is an assessment of pain either when an injured limb is moved, or when the patient takes a deep breath or coughs. For this reason, measurements of postoperative pain should be either 'pain on movement' or 'pain on deep inspiration or cough'. These are much better measures of the adequacy of pain relief.

In addition to the patient's subjective assessment, it is possible for the attending nurse or doctor to give a subjective view of the pain as judged by the physiological responses to pain (e.g. pallor, sweating, behavioural reactions).

Objective measurement of pain is not widely used as it is more complicated and there is little evidence to suggest that it is superior to the much more simple subjective assessment. Most objective methods of pain measurement use physiological measurements that are known to vary with pain: most frequently these are respiratory volume and flow measurements. These are particularly relevant to thoracic and upper abdominal surgery as reduced ventilatory capacity may lead to lung collapse and hypoxia. The most commonly measured parameters are peak expiratory flow and forced expired volume. It has been shown that decreased values of these measurements can be corrected by adequate analgesia. One other major consideration in the use of these objective methods is that the actual measurement, by causing additional movement, will alter pain for the patient. However, a subjective score recorded after such an objective measurement may be a useful indication of 'pain during deep breathing or coughing'.

The timing of assessments is also important. For research purposes, pain may be recorded at regular intervals and, in addition, an overall 24 h score is obtained. It has been shown that these two systems (contemporaneous and daily) provide similar pain scores. For routine nursing observations, a simple pain assessment scale is best. This can be combined with a measure of sedation and be presented on a modified postoperative observation chart (Figure 38.1).

METHODS OF PAIN MANAGEMENT

OPIOID-BASED THERAPY

Opioids suitable for use in the postoperative period

An extensive explanation of the pharmacology of the agents currently used to treat postoperative pain is inappropriate in such a broad-based chapter but a brief overview of the drugs most commonly used and a few main points may be helpful in the appreciation of their use.

Morphine

Morphine is the mainstay of opioid-based therapy because few newer drugs have been found to be superior. Morphine is associated with 'opioid-induced' side effects: sedation, respiratory depression, nausea, dysphoria, itching, decreased bowel motility and urinary retention. Morphine is metabolized principally in the liver to morphine 3-glucuronide and morphine 6-glucuronide; the latter is pharmacologically active and may be an analgesic drug of the future.

Papaveretum

This is a mixture of alkaloids of opium. The original preparation was withdrawn due to concern over the possible tetratogenic effects of noscapine contained within the mixture; a reformulated compound is now available. Although much favoured by some anaesthetists, particularly as part of a premedicant regimen, there is little evidence to favour it over morphine.

Diamorphine (heroin)

Diamorphine closely resembles morphine structurally, the only difference being the substitution of two hydroxyl groups by acetyl groups. In the body, diamorphine is de-acetylated to morphine. The addition of the

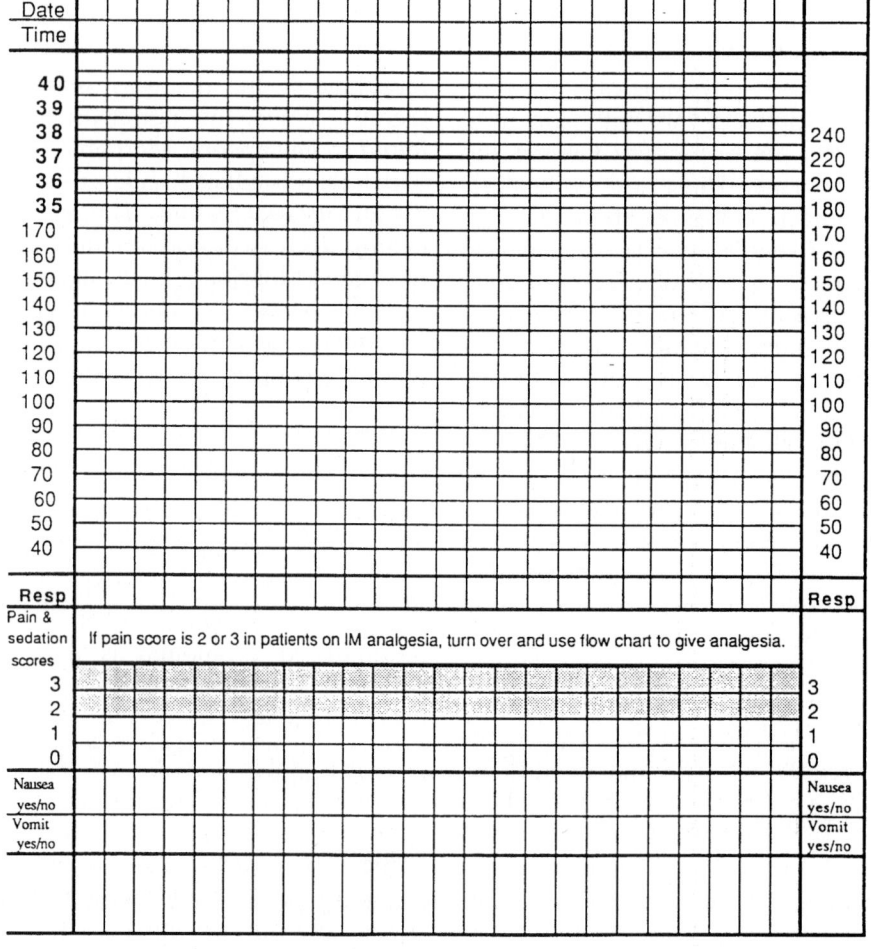

Figure 38.1 A postoperative operation chart incorporating a section for pain and sedation assessment.

acetyl groups does carry the advantage of making the drug more lipid soluble. It is said to produce less 'opioid-induced' side effects than morphine, though recent research does not confirm this.

Pethidine

This synthetic opioid has been in clinical use since the 1940s. One of its metabolites, norpethidine, is a central nervous system stimulant and may accumulate in patients with impaired renal function or in patients receiving prolonged administration, resulting in convulsions. Pethidine, contrary to other opioids, has atropine-like effects on the cholinergic nerve endings and is therefore not associated with bradycardia or smooth muscle contraction.

The fentanyl group

This group of synthetic opioids is chemically related to pethidine and produce little cardiovascular depression. Fentanyl has a relatively short duration of clinical action which makes it unsuitable for intermittent injections but it can be used by infusion or patient-controlled analgesic systems. Alfentanil has an even shorter duration of action and whilst useful as a peroperative opioid, there is little place for it in the management of postoperative pain. Sufentanil has characteristics that make it potentially useful for 'spinal' administration; at present it is not available in the UK. Remifentanil is an ultra short-acting opioid that must be given by infusion. It is rapidly eliminated by esterase metabolism. It probably has little or no place in routine postoperative pain management.

Buprenorphine

This is classified as a partial agonist and has a high affinity for μ receptors, but a low intrinsic efficacy. As a result, moderate analgesia of long duration and poor reversibility is produced.

Table 38.1 Intermittent intramuscular injection of opioid

Advantages	Disadvantages
Time-honoured and familiar	Painful injections
Perceived as safe	Delayed onset of analgesia
Inexpensive	Fixed dose does not allow for variability
No equipment required	Variable uptake from muscle
Anti-emetic usually given with analgesic	Can lead to wide 'swings' in pain

Tramadol

Tramadol has a dual mode of action both at opiate receptors centrally and monoamine transmission in the spinal cord. It is claimed to have analgesic properties similar to pethidine but, to date in the UK, there has been insufficient experience to ascertain its place in the management of postoperative pain.

Intermittent intramuscular injection

This is probably the most commonly used method of postoperative analgesic administration. It is usually prescribed as a standard dose of drug given as required with a minimum interval between doses. An inherent fear by staff of addiction and respiratory depression has ensured that this method is, in its traditional form, largely ineffective. As shown in Table 38.1, the advantages of the intermittent intramuscular injection centre about its time-honoured use and its perceived safety. The disadvantages are mainly related to the frequency of administration and concerns over the variability in response. Consideration should also be given to the blood flow to a muscle as an exercising or well perfused muscle will lead to a more rapid uptake of the drug. This element of variability may be important in the severely ill patient with poor muscle perfusion.

It has long been appreciated that the intermittent intramuscular injection technique could be improved if patients were given the drug as it was needed and not on a '4–6 hourly p.r.n.' basis (p.r.n. = pro re nata, when required). Evidence based on the pharmacokinetics and pharmacodynamics of intramuscular opioid administration has shown that the peak clinical effect of morphine and pethidine occurs within 1 h of its injection. This would suggest that analgesia could be improved if the minimum interval between doses was decreased to 1 h, with certain guidelines employed to ensure patient safety. Such a dosing regimen was proposed by Gould et al. who developed an algorithm (Figure 38.2) to be used in conjunction with a pain assessment chart (Figure 38.1) to allow the safe and improved administration of intramuscular analgesia.

The results of this combination are shown in Figure 38.3. It is worth remembering that this improvement is attained with minimal capital outlay.

Concern over the use of a 1-hourly intramuscular regimen has centred around the feasibility and desirability of such frequent injections. The need for frequent dosing is to allow the patient to attain, as quickly as possible, an effective plasma concentration of analgesic. Once this level is achieved, the dosing interval is likely to increase with injections only being necessary every 3–4 h. In order to overcome the objection of repeated injections, it is possible to insert an intramuscular cannula during anaesthesia and use it to administer the repeated doses of analgesic. Although there is some evidence that if this technique is used for pethidine the change in local pH will alter the bioavailability of the drug, there seems to be no such problem with morphine. Such a technique may also be suitable for use with children.

Suitable dosing regimens:

Adults Morphine 7.5–10 mg hourly p.r.n*.
Pethidine 75–100 mg hourly p.r.n*.
Children Morphine 0.1 mg kg^{-1} 3-hourly p.r.n.
Pethidine 1 mg kg^{-1} 3-hourly p.r.n.

*If supported by regular assessment and given according to a protocol. Otherwise 3-hourly.

Subcutaneous administration

Concerns about the variability of intramuscular uptake can be overcome if the subcutaneous route is used. The blood flow in the subcutaneous region is fairly constant in most patients though may be effected in the severely shocked patient. The favoured drug for subcutaneous administration is diamorphine on account of the low volume required and its limited pain at the site of injection. A small-bore cannula can be sited anywhere on the body and the drug given either as boluses or an infusion.

Suitable dosing regimen:

Adults Diamorphine 2.5–5 mg 3-hourly p.r.n. (bolus)
Diamorphine 1–2 mg h^{-1} (infusion)

Continuous intravenous infusion

In the 1970s, interest developed in the use of continuous intravenous infusions of opioid. The dosing regimens were largely derived from those in use at the time for intramuscular injections and consisted of giving a predetermined dose spread over 24 h. As shown in Table 38.2, the advantages are based upon rapid attainment of analgesia with minimal discomfort to the patient. However, the disadvantages relate predominantly to patient variability and the safety of the technique; in view of the recognized wide variability of analgesic requirement between patients, it is necessary to titrate the dose for the individual patient. However, once an analgesic dose has been achieved, it is known that the pain stim-

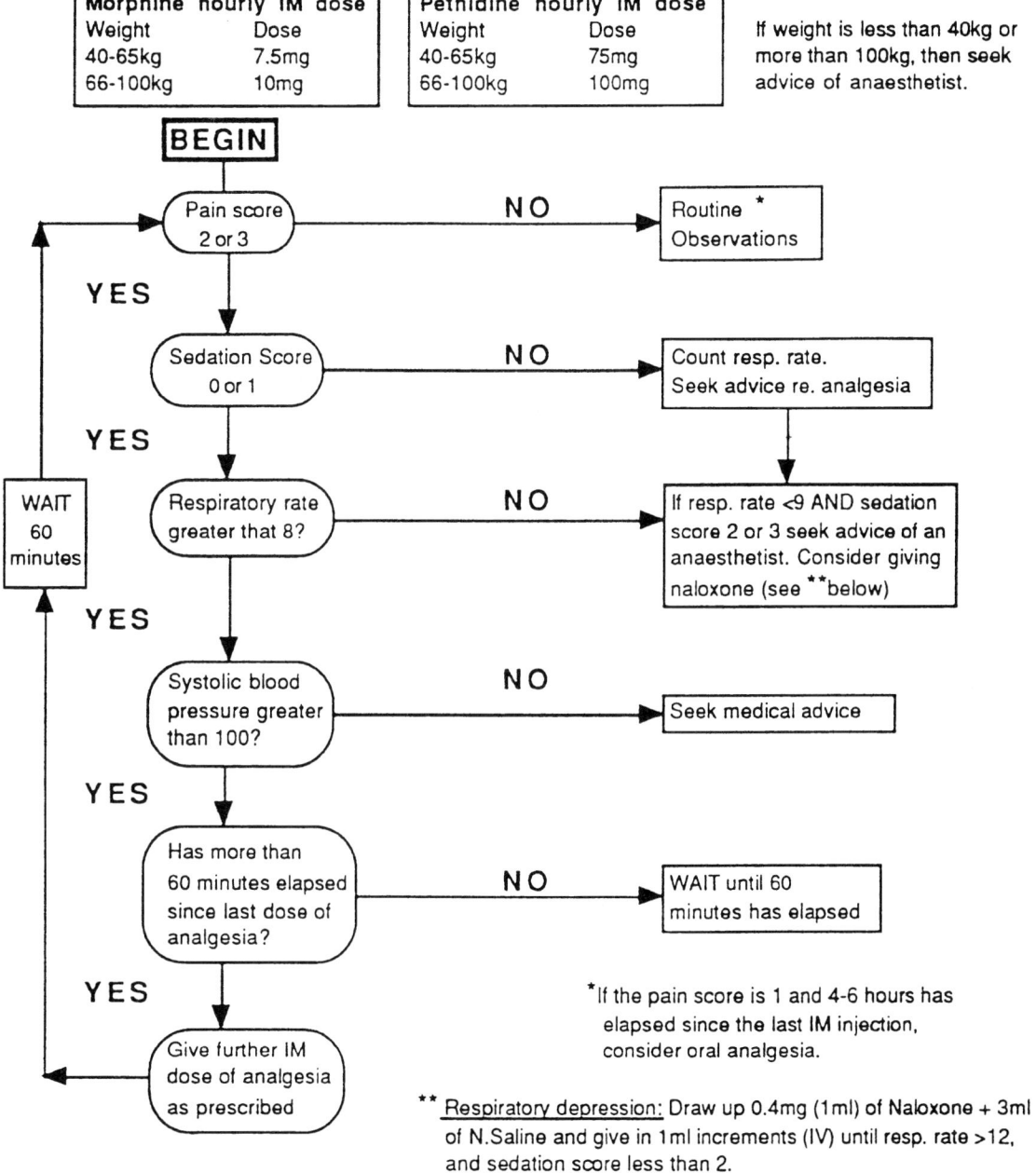

Figure 38.2 An algorithm for the intermittent intramuscular administration of opioids. (Reproduced, with permission, from Gould et al. 1992.)

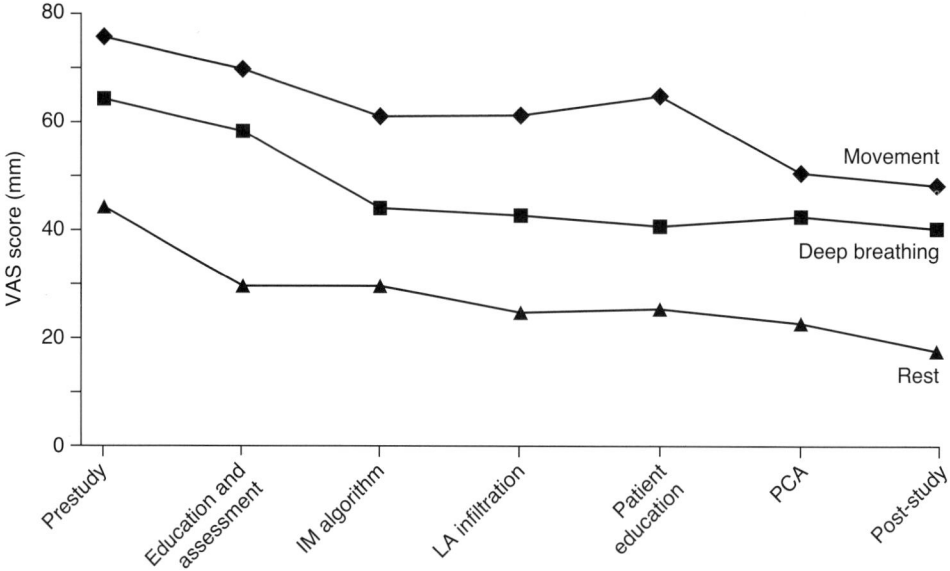

Figure 38.3 Changes in three types of pain in patients who have undergone major surgery. (Reproduced, with permission, from Gould *et al.* 1992.)

Table 38.2 Continuous intravenous infusion of opioid

Advantages	Disadvantages
Painless administration	Equipment required
Rapid onset	Need for regular assessment and adjustment
Titratable to patient	Errors can be life-threatening
'Smooth' analgesia	

ulus will diminish with time and so too will the analgesic requirements. The infusion rate must therefore be regularly reassessed and adjusted to ensure that analgesia is adequate without being excessive and producing unwanted and potentially life-threatening side effects.

This need for constant attention and adjustment has led to this technique being used predominantly in the intensive care or high dependency unit where the risk of overdose can be minimized. The technique should be used with great caution in the general ward situation.

Suitable dosing regimen:

Adults Morphine 2–4 mg h^{-1}
Pethidine 20–40 mg h^{-1}

Intravenous bolus administration.

In view of the wide variability in the patient's response to analgesics, it would seem logical to use the patients themselves to judge how much analgesia is required. In its simplest form, a nurse or doctor can administer repeated small boluses of analgesic in response to the patient's assessment of the pain. This technique has many advantages in achieving good levels of analgesia quickly at doses that are appropriate for the individual patient (Table 38.3). The method is most suitable for the patient in the immediate postoperative period as it allows rapid control of pain. Ideally, this should be routine practice

Table 38.3 Intravenous bolus administration of opioid

Advantages	Disadvantages
Simple method	Labour intensive
Allow titration to patient's needs	Problems with nurse-administration of i.v. drugs
Constant patient contact	Not suitable for general wards
Regular assessment of pain and other symptoms	

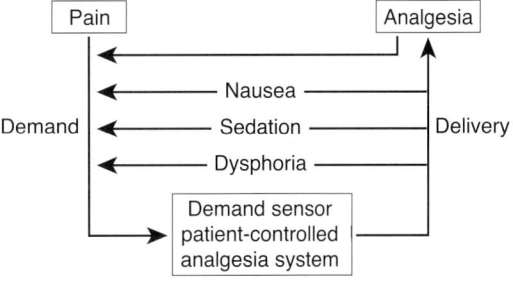

Figure 38.4 The principle of patient-controlled analgesia and how inhibitory factors will influence demands.

in the recovery area of all acute hospitals. However, outside of the recovery area (and possibly the intensive care unit), this technique is too labour-intensive to be used routinely in the postoperative period.

Suitable dosing regimen:

Adults Morphine 1–2 mg 5-minutely until comfortable
Pethidine 10–20 mg 5-minutely until comfortable

Patient-controlled analgesia

The principle and benefits of intermittent bolus administration have already been outlined. The major disadvantage of labour-intensity could be overcome if the technique were provided by a piece of equipment replacing the attending doctor or nurse. This is the basis of patient-controlled analgesia where a pump system stores a reservoir of analgesic which can be delivered in small boluses as requested by the patient but with a minimum interval between doses. As such this represents a feedback system with other factors apart from the patient also having an influence on demands and drug consumption (Figure 38.4).

The first patient-controlled analgesia machines were developed in the late 1970s and the original design features have changed little over the years. Machines have a number of variables that can be adjusted to suit the patient. There may be some misunderstanding over the terminology used for patient-controlled analgesia and it is important to understand the correct meaning of these terms (Table 38.4).

Although a variety of dosing regimens have been proposed for patient-controlled analgesia, the important element is self-titration whereby the patient is able to attain an adequate level of analgesia with only a minimum of dose restrictions. With this in mind, the practice of limiting drug administration by the use of a prolonged lockout time or a frugal dose limit is to be discouraged as it removes the vital patient-control element. The only benefit that can be conferred from the use of a dose limit is to alert the clinician to the patient that requires a large dose of analgesia to control the pain. This may necessitate a change in the standard prescribed regimen.

A potential disadvantage of patient-controlled analgesia is that during sleep the patient will receive no analgesia and as a result will awaken in pain. To overcome this, some have advocated the use of a concomitant infusion of analgesia. However, the effects of such infusions have been shown to be minimal on the overall analgesia attained but, by increasing the overall dose of drug used, cause an increase in unwanted side effects. As a result, there is little support for the use of

Table 38.4 Terminology used with patient-controlled analgesia

Bolus dose	The dose delivered with each successful demand. This should be large enough to be appreciated by the patient but not so large as to cause unwanted side effects.
Lock-out time	The time following a successful demand when the system will not respond to another demand. This should be of sufficient duration to allow the patient to appreciate one dose before demanding another. It should depend upon the drug and the route of administration used.
Background infusion	A constant infusion on which the bolus dose is superimposed. In general, its use is not recommended, but if it is used, it must not form the major part of the total drug administration.
Dose limit	The maximum dose that can be given in a set period. This should not be used to limit the amount of drug available to the patient but can be used to identify a 'high' drug consumer.

patient-controlled analgesia with a background infusion, except in children where it does seem to be advantageous without causing an increase in unwanted side effects. If a background infusion is to be used it should not form the major part of analgesic administration.

Although the actual bolus dose size is not vital, it should be of sufficient size to allow the patient to appreciate the dose being given but not be so great as to cause excessive side effects on each bolus. Recently, the patient's preference for bolus dose size has been studied using a modified patient-controlled analgesia machine which allows different bolus doses to be administered. Although this did allow better control for the patients at the extremes of dose requirement, it is reassuring that the majority of patients settled for the 'standard' prescribed dose (morphine 1 mg). As shown in Table 38.5, the clinical advantages of patient-controlled analgesia outweigh the disadvantages but unfortunately it is the financial aspect that has been largely responsible for its limited use.

The major hazards with patient-controlled analgesia relate to faulty programming and the use of inappropriate equipment. The former should be avoidable by having a system of double-checking of all programming before allowing the patient to use the system. Although such checks may be thorough before the commencement of therapy, most documented mishaps have arisen during the changing of the reservoir (syringe or bag) when it is possible that such stringent checks may not have been made. The danger of back flow into the intravenous fluid line and siphoning are well documented and proper infusion sets containing a one-way valve and an antisyphon valve must always be used; the only exception being that a one-way valve is not needed if a dedicated intravenous cannula is used (but this does not eliminate the need for an antisiphon valve).

Patient-controlled analgesia can be used for virtually all ages with children as young as 5 years old being able to manage the system. The system can deliver drugs through almost any route (intravenous, intramuscular, subcutaneous, epidurally).

Table 38.5 Patient-controlled analgesia

Advantages	Disadvantages
Patient in 'control'	Expensive equipment
Adjustable to patient needs	Needs patient cooperation
Small boluses limit fluctuation in plasma concentration	Not suitable for all ages
Painless	Must be able to use the demand button
Reduced nurses' workload	Potential hazards due to problems with programming or delivery system

Suitable dosing regimens:
Morphine 1 mg bolus, 5 min lockout, no background infusion
Pethidine 10 mg bolus, 5 min lockout, no background infusion

Oral, buccal and sublingual administration.

Most of the opioid drugs can be administered orally but all undergo a significant first pass effect as they are absorbed into the portal system and metabolized by the liver before they reach the systemic circulation. This effect, plus the problems of giving oral medication to patients with disturbed gastrointestinal function, has limited the usefulness of the oral route for the routine management of postoperative pain. Indeed, oral opioids may be hazardous in the postoperative patient if there is gastric stasis as repeated dosing may have little therapeutic effect as uptake from the stomach is poor. However, with the return of gastric motility there may be a large amount of opioid suddenly absorbed from the small intestine leading to an overdose. In view of the unpredictability of the route, it is best avoided except for patients with normal gut function who have undergone peripheral surgery, where it may have a limited place.

Buccal and sublingual administration have a theoretical advantage as the drug is absorbed directly into the systemic circulation and hence eliminates the 'first-pass' problems of oral administration. Preparations of buccal morphine have been investigated in the past but have been of limited efficacy. The only analgesic available in a sublingual formulation is buprenorphine. Given by this route it is as effective as when given parenterally but its prolonged action and high incidence of nausea and dysphoria limits its use in the postoperative period. However, both buccal and sublingual routes of administration carry a degree of safety in that if the drug is accidentally (or deliberately) swallowed, the absorption from the gastrointestinal tract is limited.

Rectal administration

The rectal route also provides access to the systemic circulation. While it would be possible to administer opioids by this route, the only analgesic drugs regularly administered thus are mild analgesics (paracetamol) and NSAIDs. The importance of informing the patient that this route of administration will be used has been clearly illustrated in the past.

Transdermal administration

Although drugs such as glyceryl trinitrate, and hormone replacement therapy have been available for administration through the skin for some time, it is only recently that a preparation of fentanyl has become available. The patches are available according to the dose administered per hour (25, 50 and 100 $\mu g\ h^{-1}$). Although this route can be very useful for chronic and palliative pain relief, the delay in onset makes it an unsuitable route for postoperative pain management. The few studies that have been performed have shown that transdermal fentanyl can only provide a background level of analgesia and is insufficient to be used alone.

A development of transdermal administration is the iontophoretic transfer of drugs through the skin by the charging of their molecules. This method may allow rapid transit through the skin of analgesics, particularly those with a high lipid solubility. Although still experimental, such delivery systems may allow the administration of both infusions and boluses through the skin and may have an important role to play in the future management of postoperative pain.

'Spinal' opioid administration

The discovery of opiate receptors in the spinal cord and the subsequent use of opioids delivered into the epidural or subarachnoid spaces, has been one of the major recent advances in the management of postoperative pain. The spinal effects of opioid drugs are thought to result from alterations in pain transmission at the level of the first- and second-order neurones in the dorsal grey matter. Receptors for opioids are present in the substantia gelatinosa near the termination of the primary afferent fibres. The effect of the opioid is to inhibit transmitter release and thus reduce nociceptive transmission.

The major benefit of 'spinal' opioids over local anaesthesia used at a spinal level is that analgesia can be achieved without sensory or motor deficit and, because there is no autonomic blockade, without the risks of hypertension. However, it should be borne in mind that unlike local anaesthetics, opioids are not licensed for use by the 'spinal' route.

Although virtually every opioid has at some time been used in the epidural or subarachnoid space, there are a number of factors that influence their use via this route. The main factor is lipid solubility of the drug as this will determine the rate of penetration through lipid membranes and thus the onset of analgesia. However, the duration of action will be reduced for the more lipid-soluble drugs as they are rapidly cleared after absorption into the blood-stream. The less lipid soluble drugs, such as morphine, have a slower onset but a prolonged action. Elimination of exogenous opioids is dependant upon absorption into the bloodstream and there is little evidence of local peptidase metabolism as occurs with endogenous opioids.

The theoretical advantages of 'spinal' opioids are slightly tainted by some of the unwanted effects. The central effects of opioids still occur with 'spinal' administration; this may be as a consequence of either systemic absorption, particularly from the epidural space, or by direct spread through the cerebrospinal fluid. Pruritis is a common finding when 'spinal' opioids are used and occurs with all the drugs, but is most pronounced with morphine. The itching is unrelated to histamine release or the dose of the

Table 38.6 'Spinal' opioid administration

Advantages	Disadvantages
Good analgesia	Possible respiratory depression
No motor blockade	? Need to nurse in special area
No autonomic blockade	Some systemic opioid effects
Limited systemic opioid effects	Insufficient for some pain
	Itching
	Urinary retention
	Equipment required
	Time-consuming to insert

drug used and most commonly affects the head and neck. It can be relieved by small doses of the opioid antagonist, naloxone (0.1 mg). Urinary retention is variable but is more common in males and after intrathecal administration. The main concern with 'spinal' opioids is respiratory depression which may be delayed in onset by as much as 24 h after administration. At particular risk are the elderly and patients who have received systemic opioids or other central nervous system depressant drugs. The less lipid-soluble opioids (e.g. morphine) are more prone to this problem since a large reservoir of drug remains in the CSF and may be distributed to higher centres. Intrathecal placement is said to increase the risk of respiratory depression but experience with low doses of intrathecal morphine (0. mg) given for pain after Caesarean section suggests that fears of a major problem may not be founded. The advantages and disadvantages of spinal opioids are summarized in Table 38.6.

In general, the more lipid soluble agents (fentanyl, diamorphine) are used by infusion into the epidural space, while the less lipid soluble agents (morphine) are used for intrathecal administration. Pethidine which is of intermediate solubility is of particular interest as it has inherent local anaesthetic qualities which may further enhance its opioid action.

Although the evidence regarding serious problems occurring with the use of 'spinal' opioids in clinical practice is scant, care must be taken with this technique and clear guidelines and protocols must be available. Such protocols must cover patient selection, site of nursing, assessments to be used, and actions in the event of unwanted effects. Such protocols should be underpinned by an effective educational programme and regular follow-up and is best achieved by an acute pain service.

The early promise of perfect analgesia with minimal side effects has not really been fulfilled and it is accepted that 'spinal' opioid alone is often insufficient to manage severe postoperative pain. The tendency has therefore been to combine the opioid with a very weak solution of local anaesthetic in an attempt to improve the analgesia without causing additional unwanted effects.

Suitable dosing regimens:

Bupivacaine 0.125%, fentanyl 10 µg ml^{-1} at 6–8 ml h^{-1}

Bupivacaine 0.125%, diamorphine 125 µg ml^{-1} at 6–8 ml h^{-1}

LOCAL ANAESTHESIA-BASED PAIN RELIEF

Infiltration

This is by far the simplest method of using local anaesthesia to provide pain relief. Although the duration of analgesia provided will be relatively short-lived, there is still benefit to be gained from a patient emerging from general anaesthesia in a pain-free state. Traditionally, wound infiltration is performed at the end of surgery, but there are some who would suggest that the pre-emptive use before surgery is more beneficial in reducing the pain after surgery. To be most effective, infiltration should include both deep and superficial layers and therefore lends itself to being performed during the layered closure of the wound. Even such simple single dose techniques can provide analgesia for up to 10 h if a longer-acting agent such as bupivacaine is used. In extensive surgery, this technique may be limited by the large dose that is required as it may approach toxic levels.

Nerve blocks

Surgery may be performed under nerve blocks which will also provide postoperative analgesia. However, postoperative analgesia can be provided by simple nerve blocks combined with general anaesthesia. Typical of such blocks would be ring blocks for surgery to digits, ilioinguinal/iliohypogastric block for herniorrhaphy and penile block for circumcision. These specific nerve blocks provide good analgesia at a low dose and without extensive additional blockade. As a rule such blocks can be rapidly administered.

For more extensive surgery, it is normally necessary to block either a number of nerves or a nerve plexus. Although the procedure to perform such blocks takes time, there is also the opportunity to place a catheter next to the nerve or plexus that will allow the continuous administration of local anaesthetic. Such a technique can be particularly useful for brachial plexus or lumbar plexus blocks. A description of all the possible nerve blocks is beyond the scope of this chapter, but, in general, if a nerve block can be used to provide surgical anaesthesia, it can equally be used to provide postoperative analgesia.

Epidural blockade

Considering how commonly used epidural analgesia is in obstetric practice, it is perhaps surprising how little it has been used to treat postoperative pain. The reason most often given is the time taken for epidural catheter insertion, though that argument should now be discounted.

Epidural analgesia for pain relief is provided through three routes: caudal, lumbar and thoracic. The caudal route is simple and quick to perform. It uses a single injection through an easily identifiable landmark and can be very useful for perineal surgical pain. In children, it is possible to pass a catheter upwards into the thoracic region but concern regarding the contamination of the insertion site limits this approach. When used for operations such as haemorrhoidectomy or circumcision, a caudal provides very good analgesia lasting for about 6 h; however, the concomitant motor block can be a disadvantage and certainly limits its use for day care surgery. The choice between the lumbar or thoracic approach depends largely upon the site of surgery. For lower abdominal surgery, a lumbar epidural is adequate, while for upper abdominal and thoracic surgery, a thoracic epidural is essential. The objective in siting the epidural is to choose a level comparable to the dermatomal distribution of the surgical incision. By doing this, it is hoped that the block produced can be limited to the specific dermatomes and therefore produce less unwanted effects.

The main problem associated with epidural local anaesthetic is that in addition to providing sensory blockade, there will also be motor and autonomic blockade (Table 38.7). The motor blockade is a problem with patient mobility and is often adversely commented upon by the patient. The autonomic blockade produces cardiovascular changes and hypotension is a common association of local anaesthetic epidural analgesia, especially if the thoracic route is employed. However, once established and any initial hypotension has been compensated for, subsequent falls in blood pressure should not be considered as due to the epidural, the cause much more likely being hypovolaemia or improving peripheral circulation (patient 'warming up').

There are clear contraindications to the use of epidurals and these relate to risks of haemorrhage or infection. In the presence of full anticoagulation or a significant coagulopathy, epidural placement of a needle or catheter

Table 38.7 Epidural local anaesthesia

Advantages	Disadvantages
Very good analgesia	Motor blockade
No opioid effects	Autonomic blockade
No central effects in normal dose	Urinary retention
	Risk of toxicity
	Equipment required
	Time-consuming to insert

would be unwise as haemorrhage may lead to haematoma formation within the vertebral canal which may lead to spinal cord ischaemia. The use of low-dose heparin does not carry such risk nor does heparinization once the catheter is *in situ*. As great care is taken with regard to bleeding for the insertion, similar concern should be taken for its removal. Infection of the skin at the site of needle insertion should also be a contraindication to epidural insertion but epidural abscess formation, which is fortunately rare, is often unrelated to the catheter insertion and either arises from bacteria 'tracking' along the catheter or as a secondary focus in the septic patient.

As already mentioned with 'spinal' opioids, care of patients with epidurals *in situ* must follow tight guidelines and protocols. Used correctly, epidural analgesia can revolutionize the recovery of patients after extensive thoracoabdominal surgery. Used carelessly, they can produce a large number of clinical problems and may even be life threatening.

Combined local anaesthetic and opioid administration.

As already mentioned epidural opioids alone do not seem to provide sufficient analgesia for major surgery, whilst local anaesthetics used in sufficient dose to give analgesia produce unwanted motor and autonomic blockade. The combination of weak solutions of both opioid and local anaesthesia is now commonly used to provide the best of both drugs profiles whilst eliminating the main problems. The usual combination is a lipid soluble opioid (fentanyl, diamorphine) and bupivacaine. This mixture can be given either as a continuous infusion or by a patient-controlled epidural system. The latter has the same principles as the intravenous PCA system but usually has a steady background infusion on which boluses can be superimposed.

Non-steroidal anti-inflammatory drugs (NSAIDs)

These agents predominantly act peripherally at the site of injury rather than in the central nervous system where the opioid drugs principally act. They work by inhibition of cyclo-oxygenase dependent prostaglandin synthesis. Prostaglandins are released in almost all forms of tissue damage and are thought to sensitize pain receptors. Non-steroidal anti-inflammatory drugs have a ceiling on their analgesic effect and are most suitable as a sole analgesic for mild or moderate pain but have also been shown to have a morphine-sparing effect in the management of severe postoperative pain.

The adverse effects of these agents include the following.

- *Gastrointestinal effects*: irritation, dyspepsia and ulceration are the most frequently reported side effects. Whether these are a problem with single or short-term use is not clear but treatment for up to 7 days has not been associated with serious side effects.
- *Renal tract*: interstitial nephritis can occur and lead to renal failure. Patients with impaired renal function, cardiac failure or shock are particularly at risk of renal damage.
- *Haematological effects*: NSAIDs reduce platelet aggregation. Although this may be considered beneficial in the prevention of cardiovascular disease, there is concern over their use in patients undergoing delicate reconstructive surgery where postoperative 'oozing' may be disastrous.

The NSAIDs most commonly used for postoperative pain management are diclofenac and ketorolac.

Diclofenac, an aryl acetic acid derivative, is available in a number of formulations. It can be given orally or rectally with good effect. Parenteral use is by either deep intramuscular injection or slow intravenous infusion. Problems including sterile abscesses have been associated with the intramuscular route and in view of the drug's availability in other formulations, is best avoided.

Ketorolac, a pyrolle acetic acid derivative, is available in both oral and parenteral formulations. Ketorolac, given parenterally, is claimed to have analgesic efficacy similar to opioids. Recent restrictions on the licence in the UK for parenteral administration has prevented its use in the presence of any anticoagulant therapy, including low-dose heparin. However, in other parts of the world it is still used widely without such restrictions. Given intravenously during anaesthesia, ketorolac is a useful NSAID with good morphine-sparing effects.

Longer-acting NSAIDs such as piroxicam have yet to prove their benefit in postoperative pain management.

The advantages and disadvantages of NSAIDs are summarized in Table 38.8.

Table 38.8 Non-steroidal anti-inflammatory drugs (NSAIDs)

Advantages	Disadvantages
Effective for mild/moderate pain	Can cause renal problems
Multiple routes of administration	Can cause bleeding problems
No respiratory effects	Can cause gastric problems
No gastric stasis	i.m. injections painful
No physical dependence	i.v. preparations not readily available

INHALED ANALGESIA

The only readily available agent in the UK is Entonox (premixed cylinder containing 50% oxygen and 50% nitrous oxide). This gas, widely used for the relief of pain in labour, has only a limited role in the management of postoperative pain. Its use long term is inadvisable as the nitrous oxide can, with extended exposure, lead to bone marrow depression and the scavenging of exhaled gases can pose technical problems. However, for a short, painful procedure, such as dressing change or drain removal, Entonox has a role. Inhaled for a few minutes before the procedure it can be most effective and because it is rapidly eliminated, there is no 'hangover' effect as might be seen if opioids are used for such short procedures.

PHYSICAL AND ADJUNCT METHOD

Transcutaneous nerve stimulation

Based upon the 'gate control theory' for pain transmission, transcutaneous nerve stimulation uses the hypothesis that stimulation of surface mechanoceptors will close the 'gate' to the transmission of pain in the small $A\delta$ and C fibres. It is used in obstetric practice and seems to help a number of women in that setting. However, in the management of postoperative pain, its efficacy has yet to be proven. There does seem to be a placebo effect in that patients even with an inactive system have been shown to benefit.

Cryotherapy

This can be performed either percutaneously or open at the time of surgery. The most popular use has been after thoracotomy when, at surgery, it is possible to isolate and freeze the intercostal nerves at the level of, as well as two above and two below, the incision. The analgesia produced is good but the nerves can take up to 6 months to recover and even then, painful neuroma formation is an unacceptable complication. The final problem relates to the loss of abdominal muscle tone on the side of the cryotherapy.

Antidepressants

These drugs modulate the response to pain within the brain and spinal cord and can be of use in the postoperative patient who seems resistant to traditional analgesic therapy. The accompanying relief of tension, anxiety and insomnia may also be beneficial. The standard drug to use is amitriptyline starting at a dose of 10–25 mg given at night.

Clonidine

The α_2 adrenoceptor agonist, clonidine, can be useful when given epidurally. Its effects result from pre- and postsynaptic activation in the spinal cord which is thought to inhibit the release of the pain transmitter, substance P. It is only really of value if more traditional opioid/local anaesthetic combinations have been unsuccessful.

Acupuncture

This is seldom used for postoperative pain but there have been case reports that suggest that it can be of value, particularly in patients where drugs or certain methods of analgesia are contraindicated. However, a skilled operator is necessary if this technique is to be considered.

Aromatherapy and reflexology

These techniques may also have a role to play in postoperative pain management but to date very few studies have explored these methods in a proper scientific manner. There can be no doubting though the psychological benefits to a patient of having a caring attendant and the element of massage is also likely to be beneficial.

POSTOPERATIVE PAIN MANAGEMENT IN THE 'AT-RISK' PATIENT

The techniques of postoperative pain management previously outlined are all suitable for healthy adults. However, certain drugs and techniques should be used with care in 'at-risk' patients. The following 'special cases' may influence the choice of analgesic employed.

Renal impairment

Even relatively mild renal failure can decrease the metabolism and elimination of opioids and lead to an accumulation of the drug. Although only 10–15% of a morphine dose is excreted unchanged by the kidneys, 90% of the metabolites, some of which are active, depend upon renal excretion. Pethidine should be avoided in renal failure because of the accumulation of the neurotoxic metabolite, norpethidine. Other shorter acting opioids appear to be acceptable. Non-steroidal anti-inflammatory drugs (NSAIDs) should be avoided in patients with pre-existing renal impairment.

Hepatic impairment

The metabolic clearance of all analgesics will be affected by hepatic impairment. Although opioids appear to be safe in patients with mild liver disease, morphine should not be given to patients with hepatic encephalopathy, ascites or severe jaundice. The half-life of morphine may be doubled in severe hepatic impairment. Shorter acting opioids (fentanyl, alfentanil) would seem to be relatively safe in these patients. Morphine can cause spasm of the sphincter of Oddi and thus increased intrabiliary pressure. This may predispose to leaks after biliary surgery and may worsen, rather than relieve, pain of biliary origin.

NSAIDs should be used with care as in patients with cirrhosis there may be an increased risk of gastrointestinal bleeding. If used, ketorolac would seem to be the most suitable agent.

Respiratory problems

Systemic opioids should be avoided, if possible, in patients with severe respiratory disease. There is also some concern regarding the 'spinal' use of opioids in these patients and a regional technique using local anaesthetic may be the safest option. However, this desire to avoid opioid analgesics must be balanced against the limitation of respiratory function caused by pain. Non-steroidal anti-inflammatory drugs should be avoided in patients with asthma.

Cardiovascular problems

Inadequate analgesia will cause an increase in circulating catecholamines which will be detrimental to the cardiovascular system but the treatment of pain may also have adverse effects as most opioids produce a bradycardia (with the exception of pethidine) and can induce hypotension. In contrast to systemic opioid administration, there are indications that 'spinal' opioids not only treat the surgical pain effectively but are beneficial to the coronary circulation, possibly by a reduction in myocardial oxygen demand. Non-steroidal anti-inflammatory drugs appear safe for use in the patient with cardiovascular problems though should be used with caution if the maintenance of cardiac function depends on prostaglandin production as may be the case in shock or myocardial ischaemia.

The elderly

Elderly patients are more opioid-sensitive than younger patients both in analgesic and side effects. Non-steroidal anti-inflammatory drugs are generally effective and appropriate in the elderly, but the risk of gastric erosion and renal toxicity is increased.

Children

Opioids are currently the mainstay of postoperative pain management in children. Young children and especially neonates, are more susceptible to the sedative and respiratory depressant actions of the opioids because of their immature respiratory control mechanisms. However, this should not lead to denigration of the treatment of pain in the very young. Over the age of about 2–3 months, the pharmacokinetics of morphine are similar to adults and certainly over 1 year, similar drugs can be used. In the very young, intermittent injections of opioid may be most suitable, but with regular monitoring, opioid infusions can be safely used. Over the age of about 5 years, patient-controlled analgesia can be used. Below this age, a system of nurse-controlled analgesia (the use of a PCA pump activated by the nurse) can be a useful method for the delivery of intermittent boluses of opioid. Non-steroidal anti-inflammatory drugs appear to be safe in children (although there is no licence for their use in postoperative pain in children). Local anaesthesia should be employed as often as possible, particularly for smaller procedures.

Opioid-dependent patients

Current opioid addicts are tolerant to the effects of opioids and so require larger doses to provide good analgesia. Opioids can be given by any route but an increased dose regimen should be used. If patient-controlled analgesia is used, a background infusion to provide the 'regular' opioid intake can be used. Opioid antagonists and partial agonist/antagonist agents should be avoided for the risk of causing withdrawal symptoms. The postoperative period is not the time to initiate a programme of drug withdrawal. Additional analgesic therapy with NSAIDs, local anaesthetics and physical methods may also be of value.

A similar approach should be considered in the patient who has been on therapeutic long-term opioid therapy and any postoperative opioid therapy should be superimposed on the existing analgesic regimen with the route suitably adjusted to cover the perioperative period. Particular caution should be observed if regional blockade is used for the operative procedure as it also removes the long-term pain and an opioid-induced respiratory depression can easily occur.

In contrast to current opioid users, patients who are former addicts are often highly motivated to avoid opioid treatment and postoperative management should utilize non-opioid methods as far as possible.

ACUTE PAIN SERVICES

One of the major factors that has led to improvements in the management of postoperative pain has been the establishment of acute pain services. These have allowed a multidisciplinary approach to pain management. The joint Colleges' report *'Pain after Surgery'* stresses the need for such services in all acute hospitals. Experience to date suggests that acute pain services are of importance in the improvement of postoperative pain management.

POSTOPERATIVE NAUSEA AND VOMITING

RELEVANT PHYSIOLOGY

Postoperative nausea and vomiting has a multifactorial aetiology which accounts for its variability in occurrence and the difficulty encountered in its prevention and treatment. The process of vomiting is controlled by the vomiting centre. A specific anatomical centre has yet to be identified and the term 'vomit-

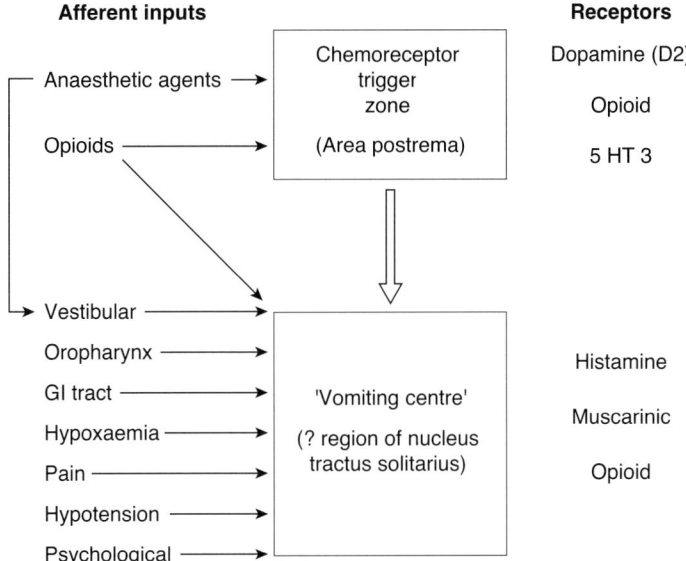

Figure 38.5 The afferent inputs effecting and the relevant receptors involved in the vomiting reflex.

ing centre' is used to describe the overall central mechanisms involved in the coordination of vomiting and so is physiological in origin rather than anatomical. However, there is some evidence that this physiological process occurs in the region of the nucleus tractus solitarius. Better understood is that the 'vomiting centre' receives afferents from a variety of sources. These act either directly or via the chemoreceptor trigger zone which has been identified as the area postrema situated in the caudal part of the fourth ventricle (Figure 38.5).

The chemoreceptor trigger zone appears sensitive to opioids and anaesthetic agents and once stimulated acts upon the 'vomiting centre'. Other afferents include inputs from the vestibular and gastrointestinal systems, inputs secondary to hypoxaemia, pain and hypotension and inputs from higher centres such as the limbic system.

The area postrema and the nucleus tractus solitarius are rich in dopamine, opioid, histamine, muscarinic cholinergic and 5-hydroxytryptamine receptors. This complexity of receptors explains the wide variety of drugs that have been shown to have antiemetic actions.

HARMFUL EFFECTS OF NAUSEA AND VOMITING

Much as for postoperative pain, the major reason for trying to prevent or treat postoperative nausea and vomiting is humanitarian as most patients find it more distressing than the pain after surgery. However, there are also good medical and even economical reasons for the improvement in the management of postoperative nausea and vomiting. These are outlined in Table 38.9.

FACTORS INFLUENCING POSTOPERATIVE NAUSEA AND VOMITING

As already mentioned, postoperative nausea and vomiting has a multifactorial aetiology. There are a range of patients, surgical, anaesthetic and drug related factors. These are outlined in Table 38.10.

Patient factors aside, probably the most important factor predisposing to postoper-

Table 38.9 The harmful effects of postoperative nausea and vomiting

Effect on patient	
Discomfort and distress	May be perceived by the patient as worse than the pain
Shame and embarrassment	Unlike pain, it is hard to 'suffer in silence' when vomiting
Exhaustion	Persistent vomiting can be physically draining
Psychological	Fear of future surgery
Medical effects	
Disruption of wound	Caused by strong abdominal contractions. Also vitreous extrusion and bleeding behind skin flaps
Electrolyte disturbance	Persistent loss of gastric fluids
Fluid and nutrition disturbance	Inability to maintain adequate intake may slow recovery
Interference with drug therapy	Oral medication will need to be converted to parenteral preparation
Oesophageal injury	Forceful vomiting can cause rupture
Aspiration of stomach contents	Only really a problem in patients with depressed level of consciousness or with jaws 'wired' after surgery
Economic effects	
Nursing time	Costs of nursing time and disposables and laundry
Delay in discharge	Particularly a problem after day-case surgery (overnight stay is not included in the cost)

Table 38.10 Factors that affect the incidence of postoperative nausea and vomiting

Patient factors	
Age	Risk is lower at extremes of age
Sex	Females three times the risk of males
Weight	Risk increased by obesity
Starvation	Prolonged starvation increases risk
History of motion sickness	May be related to mobilization
History of previous PONV	Very strong correlation
Physiological	Pregnancy
GI tract disorders	Obstruction, biliary colic, delayed gastric emptying
Surgical factors	
Gastrointestinal	Possible due to mechanical stimulation of autonomic afferents
Gynaecological	Related to hormonal effects
Otolaryngological	High incidence with ear surgery and tonsillectomy
Ophthalmic	High incidence with strabismus surgery
Anaesthetic and drug factors	
Premedication	Opioid premedication increases risk
i.v. induction agents	Etomidate and methohexitone have increased risk
Inhaled agents	Older agents were very emetogenic. Nitrous oxide may cause vomiting by bowel distension
Opioid agents	All opioids are emetogenic
Reversal agents	Neostigmine is emetogenic
Other anaesthetic factors	Hypotension, duration of anaesthesia, and oropharyngeal stimulation

ative nausea and vomiting is the perioperative use of opioid analgesics.

METHODS OF PREVENTION AND TREATMENT

Most anti-emetic drugs have adverse effects which make their routine use for prophylaxis debatable except in those patients or for those procedures with a recognized predisposition to postoperative nausea and vomiting. The anti-emetic drugs available relate to the receptors present in the 'vomiting centre' or the chemoreceptor trigger zone. They will therefore include: antidopaminergics, anticholinergics, antihistamines and 5-hydroxytryptamine antagonists.

Antidopaminergics

Butyrophenones

These are neuroleptic agents with potent antidopaminergic activity. Droperidol is particularly popular for the prophylaxis of nausea and vomiting but concern regarding disturbing dysphoric side effects as well as extrapyramidal reactions and sedation may call its use into question. The dose when given intravenously to obtain anti-emetic activity is relatively small (0.5–1 mg). The substituted butyrophenone, domperidone, does not readily cross the blood–brain barrier and so does not exhibit such unpleasant side effects. Concern over cardiac arrhythmias lead to the withdrawal of the intravenous preparation and domperidone is best given either orally or rectally.

Substituted benzamide

In the form of metoclopramide, this is widely used but the evidence of its effectiveness in the prevention or treatment of postoperative nausea and vomiting is scant. Its extrapyramidal reactions are more common in young women which may weigh against its prophylactic use in this group of patients. Its prokinetic action may be of benefit preoperatively but could be considered a relative contraindication after gastrointestinal surgery.

Phenothiazines

Phenothiazines, of which the most commonly used is prochlorperazine, are associated with the same unwanted effects as other antidopaminergic agents. The available preparation of prochlorperazine should be given intramuscularly and is only licensed for the treatment of nausea and vomiting.

Anticholinergic drugs

Hyoscine has proven efficacy in the prevention of motion sickness and postoperative nausea and vomiting. However, its use is limited by the sedation, confusion and dry mouth produced. Transdermal hyoscine, applied behind the ear, may be of value but must be applied several hours before surgery.

Histamine H_1-receptor antagonists

Cyclizine has proven efficacy in the treatment of both motion sickness and postoperative nausea and vomiting. The incidence of sedation may make it unsuitable for use in day-case surgery but this may be countered by its relatively short duration of action.

5-Hydroxytryptamine antagonists

These drugs (ondansetron, granisetron, tropisetron, dolasetron) were developed for the prevention and treatment of emesis associated with anti-cancer therapy which appears to be particularly linked to $5HT_3$ stimulation. Ondansetron has been shown to be effective in the prevention and treatment of postoperative nausea and vomiting. However, comparative studies against established antiemetics have been somewhat contradictory and it is not yet certain the role that ondansetron will play in the future. Of all the drugs with anti-emetic activity, the $5HT_3$ antagonists would appear to have the least incidence of serious side effects.

Other methods

Propofol

Propofol has been shown in subhypnotic doses to have anti-emetic properties. However, the extent and significance of this finding remains uncertain.

Ephedrine

Ephedrine, widely used to prevent or treat the nausea associated with acute hypotension occurring during spinal anaesthesia, has also been reported as being as effective as droperidol in the treatment of postoperative nausea and vomiting after general anaesthesia.

Cannabinoids

Cannabinoids have been used with good effect to reduce chemotherapy-induced emesis but the high incidence of side effects (dizziness, visual disturbances and confusion) has limited their usefulness in the postoperative period.

Ginger (Zingiber Officinale)

Ginger has been shown to be as effective as metoclopramide in the prevention of postoperative nausea and vomiting after day-case surgery.

Acupuncture and acupressure

Applied at the P-6 acupuncture point, these have been shown to reduce postoperative nausea and vomiting but other studies have not been confirmatory. The use of acupuncture and acupressure may be most suitable for the patient who is unable to be treated pharmacologically.

CONCLUSIONS

It is now clear that postoperative pain can be managed better by using a combination of established agents administered by an effective route and newer adjunctive agents. The establishment of acute pain services has done much to raise the profile of postoperative pain and to educate the staff who are responsible for its management. There have been clear improvements over the past decade but there is still room for further improvements. As part of the closer supervision of postoperative patients, other unpleasant symptoms such as nausea and vomiting have been identified and present a challenge. It may be that the future will see the expansion of the acute pain service into a postoperative care service responsible for pain, nausea and fluid therapy.

FURTHER READING

Ferrante, F. M. and VadeBoncouer, T. R. (1993) *Postoperative Pain Management*, Churchill Livingstone, London.

Gould, T. H., Crosby, D. L., Harmer, M., Lloyd, S. M., Lunn, J. N., Rees, G. A. D., Roberts, D. E. and Webster, J. A. (1992) Policy for controlling pain after surgery: effect of sequential changes in management. *British Medical Journal*, **305**, 517–522.

Park, G. and Fulton, B. (1991) *The Management of Acute Pain*, Oxford University Press, Oxford.

Report of a Working Party of the Commission on the Provision of Surgical Services (1990) *Pain After Surgery*. The Royal College of Surgeons of England and The College of Anaesthetists, London.

Smith, G. and Rowbotham, D. J. (1992) Supplement on postoperative nausea and vomiting. *British Journal of Anaesthesia*, **69** (Suppl 1).

Watcha, M. F. and White, P. F. (1992) Postoperative nausea and vomiting. Its etiology, treatment and prevention. *Anesthesiology*, **77**, 162–184.

THE DIFFICULT AIRWAY

B. A. Sutton

The ability to maintain a patent airway and allow adequate gas exchange to occur is the corner stone of practical anaesthesia. Failure to supply oxygen to a patient during anaesthesia rapidly leads to hypoxaemia, brain damage and death. Increasing levels of monitoring, especially pulse oximetry and capnography, have resulted in earlier recognition of ventilatory problems, and have reduced adverse outcome. Despite this, hypoxaemia during anaesthesia is responsible for a third of all anaesthetic-related deaths, and approximately 600 people per year worldwide die as a result of inadequate oxygenation during anaesthesia. It is worth noting that a large proportion of these people were previously healthy and undergoing elective surgery.

Anaesthetists learn to master the skills of airway management early in their training, and continue to use them throughout their working life. Experience is gained rapidly, and with increasing expertise comes the ability to manage the more difficult airway. However, no matter how experienced the doctor, the difficult airway is only a patient away, and may occur with no warning. The ability to control and manage the airway is the difference between successful anaesthesia, and severe patient morbidity or mortality.

WHAT IS THE DIFFICULT AIRWAY?

Following induction of anaesthesia, inspired gases, particularly oxygen, are delivered to the lungs via a firmly applied face mask, or by a tracheal tube. Mask ventilation and intubation are closely allied procedures, but difficulty in achieving one does not necessarily mean difficulty with the other. For example, edentulous patients are often awkward to ventilate by mask, but rarely difficult to intubate. Conversely, patients with cervical ankylosis may be easy to ventilate by mask, but impossible to intubate.

There is a spectrum of effort required to ventilate with a mask, or insert a tracheal tube. At one extreme, the effort is minimal and accomplished in seconds, at the other, mask ventilation or intubation may be impossible. In addition to patient characteristics, factors which determine the degree of difficulty encountered include: level of experience, position of patient, choice of technique and equipment.

An important point to appreciate is that the situation is not static, but dynamic. What begins as a difficult situation may become an impossible one. Progressive muscle relaxation, secretions, vomitus, repeated laryngoscopies producing bleeding and oedema all conspire against the unwitting anaesthetist.

The difficult airway therefore consists of two distinct elements, difficulty in mask ventilation and difficulty in tracheal intubation. The occurrence of one should not result in an adverse outcome for the patient. It is only when both problems are present that the patient's well-being is at risk.

Short Practice of Anaesthesia. Edited by M. Morgan and G. M. Hall. Published in 1997 by Chapman & Hall, London. ISBN 0 412 71890 1

Table 39.1 Factors which suggest that mask ventilation may be difficult

Large tongue
Heavy jowl and bull neck
Cricoid pressure
Edentulous
Reduced cervical mobility
Full beard
Limited access to face
Previous craniofacial surgery

DIFFICULT MASK VENTILATION

Although there is a considerable literature on the prediction and management of difficult intubation, much less attention has been given to difficult mask ventilation (Table 39.1). The presence of these features does not necessarily mean difficulty with mask ventilation, neither does their absence guarantee ease. They should simply serve as warning signs to possible difficulty, with the understanding that difficult mask ventilation can occur unexpectedly.

Anticipated difficult mask ventilation

If difficulty with mask ventilation, but not intubation, is suspected, the need for mask ventilation can be reduced by the use of a rapid-sequence induction, namely preoxygenation followed by a sleep dose of an intravenous agent and suxamethonium. Intubation can be achieved without the need for hand ventilation, and should intubation prove to be impossible a failed intubation drill can be followed.

Unexpected difficult mask ventilation

If difficulty with mask ventilation is unexpectedly encountered after induction of anaesthesia and the use of long acting neuromuscular blocking drugs, the following sequence is advocated.

- check oral cavity is unobstructed by secretions/vomitus
- check head is in optimum 'sniffing' position
- check appropriate size of face mask is being used
- give 100% oxygen
- consider using oro/nasopharyngeal airway
- slide mandible forward at temporomandibular joint: 'jawthrust'
- use two hands to maintain 'jawthrust' and airtight mask fit, assistant squeezes reservoir bag
- insert laryngeal mask airway (LMA) or attempt intubation

The use of the LMA is of great value in this situation, anaesthetists frequently opt for its use early, rather than persevere with airways and 'jawthrust'.

If it is possible neither to ventilate nor intubate, then the situation will rapidly deteriorate. There are a number of options open to the anaesthetist, and if a disaster is to be averted, the anaesthetist must remain in control. He/she will need to consider the various options available, and select the most appropriate. The following is designed to enable the trainee anaesthetist to appreciate and recognize potential and actual problems, to know what techniques are available, and to choose the most appropriate to the individual situation.

THE DIFFICULT INTUBATION

There is no precise definition of the difficult airway, but the American Society of Anesthesiologists has defined a difficult intubation as, 'proper insertion of a tracheal tube with conventional laryngoscopy requiring more than 3 attempts and/or proper insertion of an endotracheal tube requiring more than 10 min.'

This definition is useful, but over simplified. An inexperienced anaesthetist may require several attempts to successfully place the tracheal tube, compared with an experi-

What is the difficult airway? 677

Table 39.2 Cormack and Lehane grades at laryngoscopy. (Reproduced from Cormack and Lehane (1984).)

Grade 1	Most of glottis visible.
Grade 2	Posterior of glottis visible. Light external laryngeal manipulation usually brings arytenoids, if not cords, into view.
Grade 3	Epiglottis only visible. No part of glottis can be seen.
Grade 4	Not even the epiglottis can be visualized.

Cormack and Lehane (1984) suggest the approximate frequencies of each view to be: Grade 1, 99%; Grade 2, 1%; Grade 3, 1:2000; Grade 4, <1:10^5.

enced colleague who accomplishes the task swiftly. Equally, an experienced anaesthetist, on finding a truly unfavourable laryngoscopy, may decide not to attempt intubation but to abandon the procedure and wake the patient, well before 10 min has elapsed.

Cormack and Lehane have graded the degree of difficulty in tracheal intubation, based on the view at laryngoscopy. It assumes optimum conditions with regard to the patient position and equipment used, and no pre-existing neck pathology (Table 39.2).

CORRECT POSITION FOR INTUBATION

The human eye can only see in a straight line, therefore, to accomplish tracheal intubation using a conventional Macintosh laryngoscope it is necessary to align the axis of the mouth, pharynx and larynx. This alignment is achieved in the supine position by flexion of the lower cervical spine, and extension of the head at the atlanto-occipital joint. A pillow should be placed under the head, but not the shoulders. This has traditionally been described as the 'sniffing' position. Horton and colleagues have more precisely defined this position as: lower neck flexion of 35° and extension of the plane of the face by 15°, each angle measured relative to the horizontal plane. Alignment is completed by forward

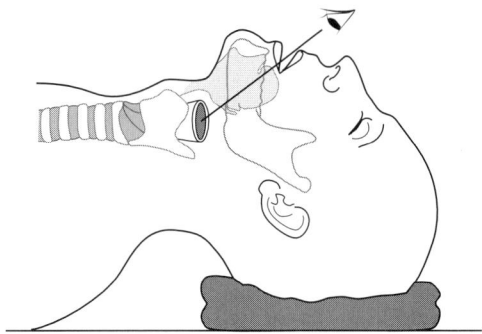

Figure 39.1 Correct position for intubation. (Modified and reproduced with permission from Cormack and Lehane (1984).)

displacement of the tongue into the mandibular space (Figure 39.1).

Factors which may inhibit alignment

Classical predictors of difficult intubation such as congenital (Down's syndrome, Klippel–Feil syndrome), infective (Ludwig's angina) and degenerative (rheumatoid arthritis) conditions, have tended to focus on the individual pathology, rather than its mechanical effect on intubation. As a classification it represents an incomplete list, rather than a useful guide to understanding the mechanics of the problem. In addition, a large proportion of patients, who are difficult to intubate, exhibit no abnormal pathology, merely a variant of normal morphology.

Figure 39.1 is a useful diagram as it illustrates how failure to obtain the optimum position and bring about correct alignment of the mouth, pharynx and larynx, may result in difficulty in tracheal intubation. Such factors include the following.

- Reduced cervical mobility, especially at the atlanto-occipital joint.
- Prominent maxilla, upper incisors and canine teeth.
- Restricted mouth opening.
- Large or posteriorly placed tongue.
- Anteriorly placed larynx.

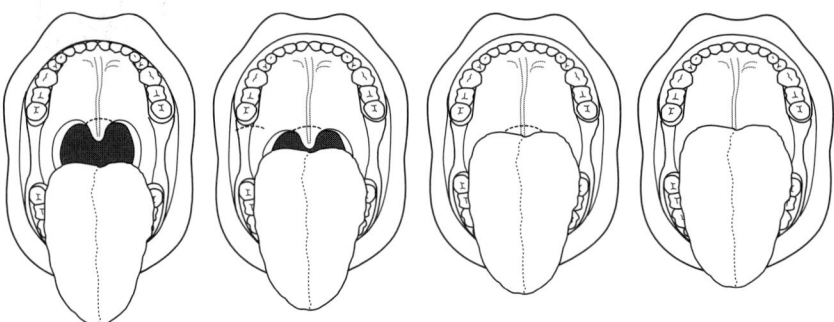

Figure 39.2 Mallampati classification of view of pharyngeal structures. (Modified and reproduced with permission from Samsoon and Young (1987).)

- Oral, pharyngeal or laryngeal pathological lesion.

PREDICTION OF DIFFICULT INTUBATION

Ideally, there should be a test which will predict those patients who are difficult to intubate. Such a test would need to be simple, quick, cheap, objective and performed at the bed side. It would need to be **sensitive** (sensitivity less than 100% produces false negatives), **specific** (specificity less than 100% produces false positives), and have a high **positive predictive value** (i.e. the proportion of patients predicted to be difficult, who actually are difficult).

From various studies, the prevalence of difficult intubations (Cormack and Lehane Grade 3 and 4 laryngoscopy), is estimated to be about 1–3%. When the prevalence of a phenomenon is low, tests with a sensitivity and specificity only slightly less than 100% will generate unacceptable large numbers of false positives and false negatives. In addition, when applying a test to a population, large numbers of subjects are required to validate the results. Retrospective studies tend to be flawed by incomplete data and lack of standardization. Prospective studies are superior, but require hundreds, if not thousands of subjects.

Various features have been investigated as predictors of difficult intubation. These have included tongue size, size of the mandibular space, cervical mobility, mouth opening, and mobility of the temporomandibular joint. They have been studied in isolation and in combination.

TONGUE SIZE

Mallampati and colleagues suggested a positive correlation between the visibility of the pharyngeal structures and exposure of the glottis. They graded the visibility of the faucial pillars, soft palate and base of uvula, when the patient opened their mouth and maximally protruded the tongue. The authors found a strong correlation between visibility of these structures and ease of intubation. Unfortunately subsequent studies have failed to replicate the original results. Despite this, more than ten years after publication, the Mallampati scoring system is probably the best known, and most widely used predictor of difficult intubation (Figure 39.2).

THE MANDIBULAR SPACE

The mandibular space is the area bounded by the line of vision of the glottis and the part of the mandibular arch in front of this plane. The size of the mandibular space is increased when the mandible is protruded. This is the area into which the tongue is displaced anteriorly during laryngoscopy. If this space is small there is less room to accommodate the

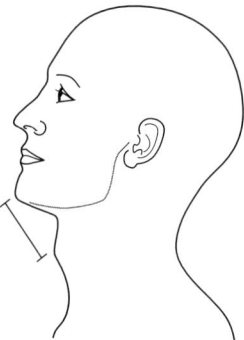

Figure 39.3 Measurement of thyromental distance from mental prominence to thyroid notch. (Reproduced with permission from Frerk (1991).)

base of the tongue, the line of vision is therefore obscured, and intubation difficult. A small mandibular space may be suspected by the presence of a receding jaw or retrognathesia.

This space can be estimated objectively by the thyromental distance. The head is extended and the straight line distance from the thyroid notch to the mental prominence is measured. A thyromental distance less than 6.5 cm is associated with a difficult intubation, and intubation is likely to be impossible with a distance less than 6.0 cm. As with Mallampati assessment of tongue size, measurement of the thyromental distance lacks the sensitivity, specificity and positive predictive value to make it a reliable preoperative test (Figure 39.3).

CERVICAL MOBILITY

To attain the correct 'sniffing' position, the head needs to be extended on the neck. The majority of this movement occurs at the atlanto-occipital joint, with up to 35° of extension possible in a normal joint. Reduced movement at this joint is likely to make intubation difficult. Assessment of joint mobility can easily be misjudged and patients may be unaware of a marked reduction of movement. Correct assessment is with the patient sitting with their head in the neutral position, such that the occlusive surfaces of the upper teeth are horizontal and parallel to the ground. The patient then extends their head as much as possible and the examiner estimates the angle traversed by the teeth (Figure 39.4).

Reduced atlanto-occipital movement results from degenerative changes and ankylosis, or may result from a congenitally small occipital–C1 gap. Normal extension at this joint is reduced in some obese patients due to deposition of fat pads over the neck and upper thoracic vertebrae. The presence of a reduced atlanto-occipital movement suggests intubation may be difficult, and should be regarded as a serious warning sign. Conversely, good atlanto-cervical movement does not necessarily mean intubation will be easy (Table 39.3).

In some patients movement in all the cervical vertebral joints is reduced, occasionally to the point of complete fixation. Such patients are usually difficult to intubate. Attempts to extend the head during laryngoscopy can produce anterior bowing of the rigid cervical vertebrae, which may displace the larynx anteriorly. Forceful extension of the head can cause damage to the neck itself and exacerbate an already difficult intubation.

THE TEMPOROMANDIBULAR JOINT

Limited movement of the temporomandibular joint has a well recognized association with difficult intubation. There are two movements at this joint, which are of significance. Depression of the mandible results in mouth opening, protrusion increases the mandibular space. Movement at this joint can be reduced by disease of the joint, and/or associated muscle spasm, especially masseter spasm. Reduction of movement may be acute or long-standing.

Decreased movement due to chronic pathology of the temporomandibular joint with ankylosis will not appreciably improve with

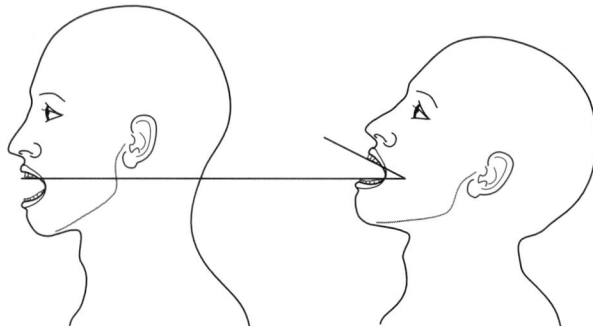

Figure 39.4 Estimation of atlanto-occipital extension. (Reproduced with permission from Bellhouse and Doré (1988).)

Table 39.3 Grading of reduced atlanto-occipital extension. (Reproduced with permission from Bellhouse and Doré (1988).)

Grade	Reduction of atlanto-occipital extension
Grade 1	Nil
Grade 2	1/3
Grade 3	2/3
Grade 4	Complete

induction of anaesthesia and neuromuscular blockade. Acute pathology is invariably associated with muscle spasm, which is often the main limiting factor in mouth opening, and usually resolves with induction of anaesthesia. An important exception is fractures of the condyle, where mechanical obstruction to mouth opening may be present. Muscle spasm present for more than a week may be associated with fibrotic changes within the muscles and contracture of the capsular ligaments. Improved mouth opening will therefore not occur with onset of anaesthesia and muscle paralysis.

The presence of a reduced interdental space should alert the anaesthetist to potential difficulty, and it is very unwise to assume that limited mouth opening will improve with onset of anaesthesia.

It is disappointing, but not surprising, that no single test is able to differentiate those patients who will be difficult to intubate from those who will be easy. Several investigators have looked at a combination of tests to see if this proves a more useful approach.

Clinically it has been shown that combining the Mallampati classification and thyromental distance improves the sensitivity and specificity to 81% and 97% respectively. This compares favourably with either test when used alone, but a sensitivity of 81% will still produce large numbers of false negatives, and so subject some patients to unnecessary, overcomplicated methods of airway management.

Wilson and colleagues looked at a large number of variables and produced a risk index score combining weight, head and neck movement, jaw movement, receding mandible and buck teeth. Scoring was from zero to ten, with ten representing the greatest risk. Difficulty arose in deciding above what score warranted special attention. If set too low, so as not to miss any difficult intubations, large numbers of false positives were produced. If the action score was elevated, less false positives were identified, but at a cost of increased false negatives.

The possibility of identifying difficult intubations has also been investigated radiologically. Bellhouse confirmed that reduced atlanto-occipital extension, decreased mandibular space and increased anteroposterior thickness of the tongue, were all associated with intubation difficulties, but was still unable to pin-point individuals who would be difficult to intubate. Radiological imaging will obviously never be suitable as a bedside test, but is an interesting research tool and may provide information which can be extrapolated to a simple clinical test.

Despite extensive work in this area we are no nearer the simple test required to identify at risk patients. However we do know which features **tend** to be associated with difficult intubation, and the more of these features present, the greater the risk. Before surgery, all patients should receive an assessment of their airway by an anaesthetist who appreciates the potential problems. The best that can be hoped for is to identify patients who are low, moderate or high risk. Based on this assessment a plan of action must be determined. Probably more important is the appreciation that a difficult/impossible intubation may occur in the absence of any warning features.

A PRACTICAL APPROACH TO THE AIRWAY

As we are unable to identify accurately patients who will be difficult to intubate, an alternative approach to airway management is required. In 1990, The American Society of Anesthesiologists convened a Task Force to develop guidelines, in the form of an algorithm, for management of the airway. If followed it takes the anaesthetist through a logical sequence of options available to allow intubation, or if this is impossible to facilitate oxygenation of the patient, and prevent hypoxic damage. This was the first time a body of experts had formally considered the situation, with the aim of producing a practical answer to a perennial problem. It is still undergoing a period of refinement, but has much to commend it (Figure 39.5).

It is important to appreciate that this algorithm is not suitable for referral after difficulties have arisen, but is best considered as an aid for teaching and learning. All trainee anaesthetists should be aware of it and have discussed and considered it at length during their training.

There are some points in the algorithm which are worth considering. Firstly, there is little emphasis on the advice to call for help early, even though a difficult airway nearly always requires additional help, even for an experienced anaesthetist. Second, the option to abandon the procedure sooner, rather than later, and awaken the patient, is not stressed. For inexperienced anaesthetists this is nearly always the correct course of action.

Thirdly, the role of the laryngeal mask (LMA) airway is under exploited. This probably reflects the more recent introduction of the LMA in the USA, compared with the UK and Europe. Finally, the algorithm includes techniques which some anaesthetists may never have seen, let alone performed, such as transtracheal jet ventilation or the retrograde technique. Anaesthetists attempting such procedures for the first time, should seriously question whether they are taking the correct course of action, rather than awakening the patient, and seeking senior help. None the less, the ASA algorithm provides excellent advice, in a simple and succinct manner, and should provide a basis for extensive discussion amongst all anaesthetists.

As shown in the ASA algorithm there are a number of methods by which intubation can be achieved, or if this proves impossible, means by which oxygenation of the patient is assured. Each has its own merits, indications and disadvantages, and it is important to appreciate the role of each technique in the management of the difficult airway.

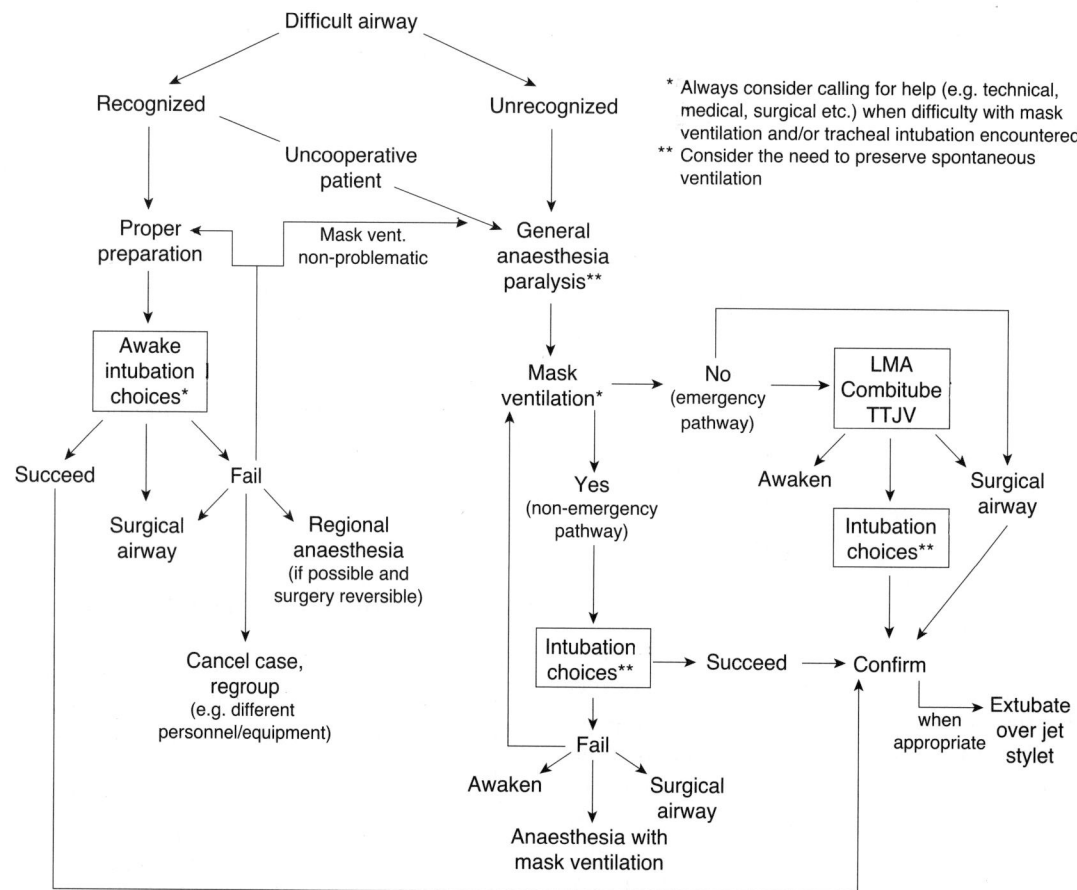

Figure 39.5 The ASA (American Society of Anesthesiologists) difficult airway algorithm. (Reproduced with permission from Biebuyck (1991).)

CONVENTIONAL LARYNGOSCOPY AND INTUBATION

The correct position of the patient and alignment of the mouth, pharynx and glottis have already been described. The tongue is swept to the left and anteriorly into the mandibular space, by means of a laryngoscope, most commonly the Macintosh, with its curved blade. This reveals a Grade I or II view of the glottis in the vast majority of patients, facilitating intubation, with no additional assistance. In a small number of patients intubation cannot be immediately accomplished, and a number of simple manoeuvres or aids are available to assist conventional intubation.

External laryngeal manipulation

A Grade III view of the glottis is occasionally encountered, often in association with a large 'floppy' epiglottis or relatively anterior larynx. Once correct positioning of the patient is assured, the view of the glottis can often be improved by external manipulation of the larynx by the anaesthetist or assistant. The manoeuvre can improve the view by a single grade, i.e. a Grade IV to a Grade III, a Grade III to a Grade II, etc. This is probably the most simple adjunct to conventional intubation used regularly by experienced anaesthetists, but its value needs to be emphasized to the trainee.

Laryngoscopes

Over the past 50 years a considerable number of laryngoscopes have been developed, each designed to improve the view at laryngoscopy, or to deal with specific difficulties. Most fall out of favour after a period of use, leaving a small number that have proved their worth and stood the test of time. For adult intubations these include the Macintosh, the Magill and the polio laryngoscopes.

The Macintosh is the most widely used adult laryngoscope, and will provide an excellent view of the glottis in most patients. The blade sweeps the tongue to the left and forward into the mandibular space. At the same time, the epiglottis is elevated out of the line of vision by pressure exerted on the hyoepiglottic ligament by the tip of the blade.

The straight bladed Magill laryngoscope remains popular for use in patients with a large 'floppy' epiglottis which overhangs the glottis regardless of the pressure exerted on the hyoepiglottic ligament. The tip of the blade is placed under the epiglottis, which is then physically lifted forward. Although this manoeuvre can be performed with a Macintosh laryngoscope, the curve of the blade obscures the view preventing insertion of the endotracheal tube, unlike the straight blade of the Magill.

The polio laryngoscope, despite the implication of its name, remains a valuable piece of equipment. The blade and handle are set at an angle of greater than 90°, unlike any other laryngoscope. This configuration makes it especially useful in the intubation of pregnant or morbidly obese patients, where insertion of the blade is difficult because the handle abuts on the patient's chest. When a polio laryngoscope is not available, an alternative is to use a short stumpy handle, with a regular Macintosh blade.

A new laryngoscope, is the McCoy. This laryngoscope has a moveable, angulated tip activated by a mechanism on the handle. It is used in the manner of a Macintosh laryngoscope, but when the occasional Grade III view is obtained, the activation of the angulated tip will usually improve the view by at least one grade.

There is a great temptation amongst trainee anaesthetists to make the situation more complicated than it really is. The correct selection and use of the standard laryngoscopes will allow sufficient view of the glottis to enable intubation in the vast majority of patients. This concept cannot be emphasized too strongly.

Gum elastic bougie

The gum elastic bougie is an invaluable aid to difficult intubations. It is useful in a variety of situations, such as the 'floppy' epiglottis, or the presence of an awkward configuration of dentition (e.g. missing or 'peg-like' right upper incisor or canine teeth). The bougie is passed under the epiglottis and into the trachea, blindly if necessary. Correct placement is suggested by: feeling clicks as the bougie slides over the tracheal rings; rotation of the bougie as it enters a main bronchus; and arrest of the bougie as it reaches the small bronchi. The tracheal tube is then 'railroaded' over the bougie into the trachea.

Success with inserting the tracheal tube in the trachea is increased by retaining the laryngoscope in the mouth during the procedure and rotating the bevel of the tube a quarter anti-clockwise, just before it passes through the cords. The use of a bougie with awkward dentition reduces the risk of damage to the teeth, as well as facilitating intubation.

Stilettes and lighted wands

Occasionally, although the glottis can be visualized with ease, there is difficulty in passing the tracheal tube into the trachea. This is particularly likely when using one of the softer, more pliable tubes, such as armoured or microlaryngeal, or again with an awkward dentition. A malleable stilette passed through the tube will provide a sufficiently rigid structure for easy manipulation. To prevent trauma to the trachea it is important to ensure that the stilette does not protrude beyond the end of the tracheal tube.

There is a variety of illuminated, intubating wands available on the market, of varying complexity and price. The most useful are the relatively inexpensive disposable wands. The tracheal tube is mounted over the wand. The shaft of the wand is malleable and can be bent to the desired shape for the patient. The wand is then passed through the mouth to the base of the tongue. With the room lights dimmed, the skin over the neck is observed as the wand is advanced towards the glottis. The procedure is performed blindly, with or without the aid of a laryngoscope. It can also be undertaken with an awake patient providing there is adequate anaesthesia of the upper airway. As the tip of the wand passes into the trachea the light is seen passing down the length of the neck and into the chest. The tracheal tube is then simply railroaded over the wand into position. If the wand is passed into the oesophagus, no transillumination is visible in the neck. The advantages of lighted wands are their portability and relatively low cost. The disadvantage is the necessity for considerable practice before it can be relied upon in a difficult case.

Blind nasal intubation

Blind nasal intubation has long been an option for difficult intubations, especially in times when other aids were not available. There are a few anaesthetists who are extremely skilled in this technique, but unfortunately, it appears to be a skill rarely perfected by todays trainees. In theory, the procedure can be performed on an awake patient, providing the nasal passage, and upper airway have been adequately anaesthetized, but in practice the patient is usually anaesthetized. Often carbon dioxide was added to the inspired fresh gas flow, encouraging large tidal volumes such that the patient practically inhaled the tracheal tube!

The main disadvantages of blind nasal intubation are the risk of trauma to the nasal and pharyngeal mucosa, avulsion of nasal polyps and adenoids, and damage to the glottis and vocal chords. It is easy to provoke brisk haemorrhage, which in an unsuccessful intubation complicates the position further.

Gas induction and intubation under deep anaesthesia

For many years the conventional management for intubation of patients with upper airway obstruction, or suspected difficult intubations, was to induce anaesthesia with a volatile agent in a high concentration of oxygen. Laryngoscopy was performed under deep anaesthesia, when pharyngeal/laryngeal reflexes were absent. The aim was to keep the patient breathing throughout, and if intubation proved to be impossible, anaesthesia was discontinued and the patient allowed to wake up. This practice is still widely used. The main problem with the technique is airway obstruction due to loss of pharyngeal muscle tone, and the main problem with the anaesthetist is failure to wait until sufficient depth of anaesthesia is attained before attempting laryngoscopy, thereby provoking laryngospasm. Unfortunately, it is a technique unsuitable for non-fasted patients.

Gas induction and intubation is the method of choice in children who are unlikely to tolerate an awake procedure of any kind. It is suitable for adults in whom the suspicion of difficulty is low, or who refuse an awake procedure. Because of the risk of airway obstruction, it is not one of the safest methods by which to secure the airway, and a plan of action should be decided in advance if difficulties should occur.

Rapid-sequence induction

All patients who require intubation and who have a full stomach, or are at risk of gastric reflux and pulmonary aspiration, should have anaesthesia induced by a rapid sequence technique with cricoid pressure. This procedure is familiar to all anaesthetists. In the case of a suspected difficult intubation a modified rapid sequence induction without cricoid pressure (assuming the patient to be fasted), can be very helpful.

The patient is allowed to breath 100% oxygen for several minutes before induction. Anaesthesia is induced with a short acting agent followed immediately by suxamethonium. Conventional laryngoscopy is then performed. An assessment of the degree of difficulty and a swift decision about the patient's airway should be made. The patient is intubated if possible, but if not, the decision to abandon the procedure should be made early rather than late. The patient is given 100% oxygen, and a failed intubation drill is followed. Although intubation has not been achieved the anaesthetist is in a good position to plan how best to proceed.

Conventional intubation may be complemented by a number of manoeuvres, many of which are overlooked by the inexperienced anaesthetist when under pressure. They should be taught and practised under supervision in conditions of an easy airway, where there is no reliance on their success. Using a new technique or piece of equipment for the first time in a difficult situation is unlikely to have a beneficial outcome.

THE LARYNGEAL MASK AIRWAY

The laryngeal mask airway (LMA) probably represents the most significant advance in airway management in recent years. It is a reusable, pharyngeal airway which is inserted blindly, with the patient anaesthetized. It has an inflatable cuff which helps hold it in the correct position, with the aperture facing the glottis. The device was developed by Dr A. I. J. Brain as a means of securing the airway in fasted patients. It can be used for spontaneous or controlled ventilation.

The LMA was not developed as an aid in the management of the difficult airway. However, it has been found to be an invaluable piece of equipment in such situations, and has probably saved many lives. It is surprising that in many cases of 'can't ventilate – can't intubate', a LMA can be inserted with minimal difficulty producing satisfactory ventilation and oxygenation. In many patients, if there is no contraindication to its use, surgery can continue with no further manipulation of the airway.

The LMA serves several purposes in the management of the difficult airway. It allows oxygenation and so prevents hypoxaemic damage. It provides time for a more considered approach to the problem; either seeking expert assistance or additional equipment. It can also act as a guide to intubation in its own right.

A 6 mm internal diameter tracheal tube can be passed blindly through the aperture of the LMA, and into the trachea. Ventilation can continue through the tracheal tube with the LMA remaining *in situ*. Alternatively, a gum elastic bougie can be passed through the LMA into the trachea. The LMA is then removed, and a standard size tube is 'railroaded' into position. If the blind insertion of a tube into the trachea is not possible, a fibreoptic scope, with a pre-mounted 6 mm tube can be passed under direct vision.

So successful has the LMA been in cases of difficult intubation, that Dr Brain has developed an intubating LMA, which is currently under evaluation. It consists of a wider and shorter inner tube, through which a 9 mm tracheal tube can be passed. In addition, it will have a handle to allow manipulation of the whole device.

The LMA has been successfully used in conjunction with cricoid pressure in patients at risk from reflux of stomach contents. If ventilation is not possible with cricoid pressure, it should be released. In an emergency situation every anaesthetist should remember that aspiration of stomach contents is not an inevitable consequence of an unprotected airway, but hypoxaemic damage is an inevitable consequence of prolonged failure to oxygenate. Where possible anaesthesia should be terminated as soon as possible. Only life-saving surgery should continue with a LMA on patients at risk of aspiration.

Correct insertion of the LMA is quickly learned by trainee anaesthetists. Paramedics and nurses have been successfully trained in its use for purposes of resuscitation. It has quickly become an invaluable piece of equipment, such that no anaesthetic should be administered without the ready availability of a LMA.

FIBREOPTIC INTUBATION

In recent years there has been an increase in the use of intubating fibrescopes. The introduction of the fibrescope into anaesthetic practice has significantly altered management of the difficult airway, and in certain situations is now the technique of choice. However, the role of the fibrescope should be put into perspective, it is not the answer to all difficult airways. The advantages of the fibrescope are best seen in cases of suspected or known difficult intubation, where intubation is performed electively by a skilled operator on an awake patient with sufficient airway anaesthesia. In these conditions the procedure is accomplished smoothly, with little or no distress to the patient. To be able to undertake this task, the anaesthetist needs to be prepared to spend a considerable length of time learning, under supervision, on anaesthetized patients with normal anatomy. For anaesthetists of limited experience, there is no point attempting fibreoptic intubation in a difficult situation, as they are likely to fail with potentially dangerous consequences. Far better to awaken the patient or use other techniques with which they are more familiar.

Awake or under anaesthesia?

Fibreoptic intubation can be performed with the patient awake, or anaesthetized. In the anaesthetized patient spontaneous respiration may be preserved or neuromuscular blockade employed. The choice depends on a number of factors. Awake fibreoptic intubation is by far the safest technique in cases of known, or suspected, difficult intubation.

Some patients may be reluctant to undergo awake fibreoptic intubation, but should be encouraged to do so, with the reassurance of adequate sedation, topical anaesthesia, and the knowledge that this is the safest technique. Even so, some patients will refuse. They should be left in no doubt that they have rejected the safest option, and when proceeding with a fibreoptic intubation under general anaesthesia the most experienced personnel available should be present, with a clear plan of action decided.

Fibreoptic intubation under general anaesthesia is indicated in uncooperative patients, those with learning and communication difficulties, and in children. Many experts in the field also recommend intubation under anaesthesia in patients with an unstable neck, because of the risk of severe coughing when performed awake.

Probably the most common indication for fibreoptic intubation under anaesthesia is for teaching purposes. In this situation maintenance of spontaneous ventilation has the added benefit of allowing the trainee more time. It also bears a greater resemblance to the view obtained in the awake patient, compared with the paralysed patient. The main disadvantage of this technique is the depth of anaesthesia necessary to tolerate the procedure, consequently care should be taken in the selection of patients for teaching purposes.

Fibreoptic intubation under general anaesthesia in patients with a full stomach should only be undertaken in the most exceptional circumstances. Only very experienced practitioners should attempt this, as the procedure is very difficult in the presence of cricoid pressure.

Premedication

It is unwise to prescribe sedative premedication to a patient with airway obstruction. Although anxious, the patient should be reassured that sedation will be given, but only immediately before the procedure. Those patients who have a difficult airway due to limited mouth opening, or simply because of an unusual variation of normal morphology, can safely be given sedative premedication.

Antisialogogues are essential. The efficacy of topical anaesthesia is enhanced and the reduction in secretions assists in providing a clear view through the scope. Hyoscine is useful in providing both good drying qualities and sedation. Where sedation is to be avoided, atropine or glycopyrrolate are effective.

Marked oedema, associated with tumours or infection, responds well to nebulized adrenaline. It can reduce stridor in the short term, improve the view, and lessen the risk of contact haemorrhage. Nebulized adrenaline should never be used in association with halothane or cocaine, as dangerous arrythmias may be provoked by the concomitant use of these drugs. Local anaesthetic lozenges, or nebulized local anaesthetic, may be given as premedication if desired.

Sedation

Clinicians should use sedative drugs with which they are most familiar. Opioids, benzodiazepines and propofol are all suitable. Opioids and benzodiazepines have specific antagonists, which make their use more attractive. Small, incremental doses are titrated to produce a relaxed, cooperative patient.

Oral or nasal intubation

Clinical circumstances may dictate whether the nasal or oral route is used. When either is suitable, the nasal route is usually preferred. Although the oral route may appear simpler, in reality the angle of approach to the glottis is more acute, and difficulty in insertion of the scope and tube is frequently encountered. In addition the patient may bite the scope, and use of a bite block or dental prop is necessary to prevent expensive accidents! To be able to deal with all situations, experience with both routes is necessary.

Local anaesthesia of the airway

Adequate local anaesthesia is imperative for an atraumatic, awake, fibreoptic intubation. Nerve blocks such as bilateral block to the lingual branch of the glossopharyngeal nerve, bilateral superior laryngeal nerve block and transtracheal injection of local anaesthetic via the cricothyroid membrane, undoubtedly give excellent anaesthesia and conditions for awake intubation. Unfortunately they are unpleasant and technically difficult to perform in many pathological conditions, such as trismus or laryngeal/pharyngeal tumours. Topical anaesthesia, if correctly performed, is all that is necessary in the majority of patients.

The pharynx, epiglottis, larynx including the vocal cords, and the trachea all require surface anaesthesia, in addition to the oral cavity (for oral intubations) or the nasal cavity (for nasal intubations). It is usually quite easy to produce good surface anaesthesia in the airway. Lack of success is commonly due to failure to allow sufficient time for the local anaesthetic to work.

The simplest, but probably the least effective method, is the use of nebulized lignocaine. Alternatively, local anaesthetic can be applied to the mucosal surface of the nose, mouth and pharynx by a combination of topical gel, spray or lozenge. In addition, aqueous lignocaine can also be injected down the suction channel of the scope. Application of local anaesthetic onto the epiglottis and trachea under direct vision obviates the need for cricothyroid membrane injection. Coughing is common during the procedure especially when local anaesthetic makes contact with the epiglottis, cords and trachea. If it is desirable to minimize coughing, premedication with nebulized lignocaine will desensitize these structures to direct application.

Vasoconstriction

Vasoconstriction of the mucous membranes is crucial for nasal intubation. When omitted, contact haemorrhage is frequently seen, making visualization through the scope very difficult. More worryingly, profuse bleeding in the upper airway in a difficult intubation can be disastrous. Cocaine paste or solution has the advantage of producing excellent mucosal vasoconstriction in addition to local anaesthesia, although toxic side effects reduce its usefulness.

Conduct of the procedure

Before attempting fibreoptic intubation, appropriate monitoring and intravenous access should be secured. Supplementary oxygen via a nasal catheter is recommended. Passing the tracheal tube over the scope and into the trachea is usually the most unpleasant part of the procedure for the patient, and frequently the most difficult part for the trainee anaesthetist. It is made easier by selection of the more patent nostril, gentle dilation of the nasal passage with increasing sizes of soft latex nasal airways, tracheal tube size no greater than 7.0 mm, and generous use of a suitable lubricant. With the scope held in position the tube is gently advanced through the nasal cavity and into the trachea. No force should be necessary. It is common for the bevel of the tube to catch on the epiglottis and rotation of the tube, so that the bevel faces anteriorly, overcomes this problem. The correct position of the tube is established by direct visualization of the carina distal to the tracheal tube.

The most important preparation to facilitate fibreoptic intubation is adequate surface analgesia, and an appropriate level of anxiolysis/sedation. Once correct placement is confirmed, general anaesthesia can be induced.

TRANSTRACHEAL AIRWAY

Oxygen can be delivered directly to the lower respiratory tract, by-passing the upper respiratory tract. There are a variety of methods by which this can be achieved including transtracheal jet ventilation, cricothyrotomy minitracheostomy, and formal surgical tracheostomy. Such procedures can be performed on awake or anaesthetized patients, as elective or emergency procedures.

These means of securing an adequate airway are often overlooked with preference given to fibreoptic intubation, laryngeal mask airway, or surgery under regional techniques. It is unfortunate that they tend to be used as a last resort in the most dire of emergencies, and consequently are associated with a high failure and complication rate. As a result they have gained a reputation for being difficult techniques, fraught with problems. This need not be the case. With the correct selection of procedure, patient and clinical condition, all can be accomplished with minimum discomfort to the patient and few complications.

These techniques are particularly valuable in cases of known difficult intubation when a fibrescope is not available and there are obstructive neoplasms of the upper airway. In the case of airway tumours, attempts to intubate the trachea from above are difficult due to the physical presence of the tumour which obstructs the view and distorts the normal anatomy. Repeated attempts to pass scopes, bougies or tubes through, or around, a tumour can result in bleeding or dislodgement of friable tumour tissue into the larynx.

These patients can deteriorate rapidly. Bleeding and hypoxaemia, progressing to the need for an emergency transtracheal airway is a recipe for disaster. Far better to secure a transtracheal airway in a patient who has been properly prepared, received appropriate premedication and local anaesthetic, and concomitant supplementary oxygen.

Disposable kits for transtracheal jet ventilation, and cricothyrotomy mini-tracheostomy are readily available and inexpensive in comparison with the financial outlay for a fibreoptic scope. A formal surgical tracheostomy requires no additional equipment, other than the tracheostomy tube, and a simple 16 G venous cannula can be used very successfully for jet ventilation. Therefore, a transtracheal airway maybe of particular value in centres with limited resources, who should not feel disadvantaged by their lack of expensive equipment.

Attempts to gain access to the lower airway via the cutaneous route is not advocated in certain situations. These include a coagulopathy, and gross distortion of the local anatomy by tumour, swelling or obesity. With limited neck extension, including an unstable neck, this approach to airway management is less advantageous. However, there is practically no absolute contraindication to a transtracheal airway.

Transtracheal jet ventilation

Satisfactory oxygenation and elimination of carbon dioxide can be achieved by the delivery of jets of oxygen directly into the trachea, via a cannula, at pressures of $2.6-4 \times 100$ kPa. Gas exchange is achieved by a combination of bulk flow, Venturi effect and fluid friction. The tidal volume delivered will depend on the size of cannula, duration of inspiration, driving pressure of gas, upper airway patency (for entrainment of air), and lung compliance. One second of gas at 3.3×100 kPa through a 16 G cannula will deliver approximately 500 ml.

The most convenient and safest site to place the cannula is through the cricothyroid membrane. A 16 G cannula or larger is necessary in an adult. The trachea is fixed between the fingers of one hand, and the head extended (if possible). The cannula is introduced in a caudal direction, at an angle of 30°. The catheter is advanced over the needle. Correct placement is confirmed by the aspiration of air into a saline-filled syringe. The hub of the needle is connected to the ventilation system via a luer lock.

A variety of systems are available, including a jet insufflator which can be controlled by a hand trigger. The emergency oxygen flush on some anaesthetic machines can be used for this purpose. A length of non-compliant tubing is connected to the common gas outlet via a 15 mm tracheal tube adaptor (from a 4 mm internal diameter tube). The other end of the tubing is connected to the cannula via a luer lock.

The cannula can also be connected by way of adaptors to a breathing circuit or AMBU bag, but such a system is very inefficient. Oxygenation can be maintained in the short term, but carbon dioxide elimination is unpredictable. This arrangement is only suitable in an emergency to prevent hypoxaemic damage.

Upper airway patency is essential to allow both the entrainment of air and the elimination of expiratory gases. It is unusual for upper airway obstruction to be complete, but in this event a second cannula must be inserted via the cricothyroid membrane, or between two rings of cartilage below this level.

A variety of commercial kits is available, and although not essential, have the advantage of containing all necessary equipment to insert a cricothyrotomy cannula. It is prudent to have such kits readily available on any site where anaesthetics are given.

The main complications associated with cricothyrotomy cannulation and jet ventilation are bleeding, damage to adjacent structures and barotrauma. Pre-existing lung pathology increases the risk of complications, and the lowest driving pressure to obtain adequate chest expansion should be used.

Mini-tracheostomy

Commercial kits are now available which contain all the necessary equipment to perform a small percutaneous tracheostomy, via the cricothyroid membrane. In the same manner as transtracheal jet ventilation, the cricothyroid membrane is identified and a cannula inserted. A guide wire is passed through the cannula, the cannula is then removed. Using a Seldinger technique, a 6 mm diameter tracheostomy tube is inserted with the assistance of a curved dilator.

The advantage of the mini-tracheostomy is that the tube is of sufficient size to allow either controlled or spontaneous ventilation to occur via conventional breathing systems. The size of tube also permits suction and clearance of secretions.

Just as the size of tube conveys its advantages, so it brings disadvantages. The increase in size necessitates a larger incision of overlying tissues and a greater force for insertion, which together increase the potential for trauma.

To perform a mini-tracheostomy a commercial kit is essential, as unlike jet ventilation, adaptation of available equipment is not possible.

Surgical tracheostomy

Performing an awake, surgical tracheostomy is not undertaken lightly. It requires considerable experience on the part of the surgeon, and a cooperative patient. However, in the right circumstances it may be the simplest and safest option. When anaesthetic experience and/or equipment are lacking, and a proficient surgeon is available, then this approach to a difficult airway should be considered seriously. In these circumstances, with the generous use of local anaesthetic, the procedure is less unpleasant than a poorly conducted, awake, anaesthetic technique. With the increasing number of options available, awake tracheostomies are rarely performed, but should at least be considered in all cases of difficult airway management.

A surgical tracheostomy performed as an emergency in a hypoxaemic 'can't ventilate – can't intubate' patient is extremely difficult, even for an experienced surgeon. This situation happens occasionally, but nearly always as a result of failing to recognize the problem initially and use an appropriate technique.

THE COMBITUBE

The Combitube® (Sheridan Catheter Corp., NY, USA) is a double lumen construction, which can be positioned in the trachea or the oesophagus. It is a relatively new addition to the anaesthetists' armoury for the management of a difficult intubation.

The tracheal lumen has an open distal end, and the oesophageal lumen has a blind distal end with perforations at the pharyngeal level. There are two cuffs, one distal and one proximal to the perforations. The proximal cuff seals the oral and nasal cavities, and the distal cuff seals either the trachea or the oesophagus. The tube is inserted with the head in the neutral position. The tongue and mandible are lifted with one hand, and the tube is inserted up to a preset mark on the tube. Both the larger proximal and smaller distal cuffs are inflated. The tube will have entered the trachea or the oesophagus. The anaesthetist must determine whether tracheal or oesophageal intubation has occurred. If tracheal intubation, then ventilation is via the open-ended tracheal lumen. If oesophageal intubation has occurred, ventilation is via the perforations in the blind ended oesophageal lumen (Figure 39.6).

The main advantages of the Combitube are its portability, lack of need for additional equipment, minimal skill required for inser-

A practical approach to the airway 691

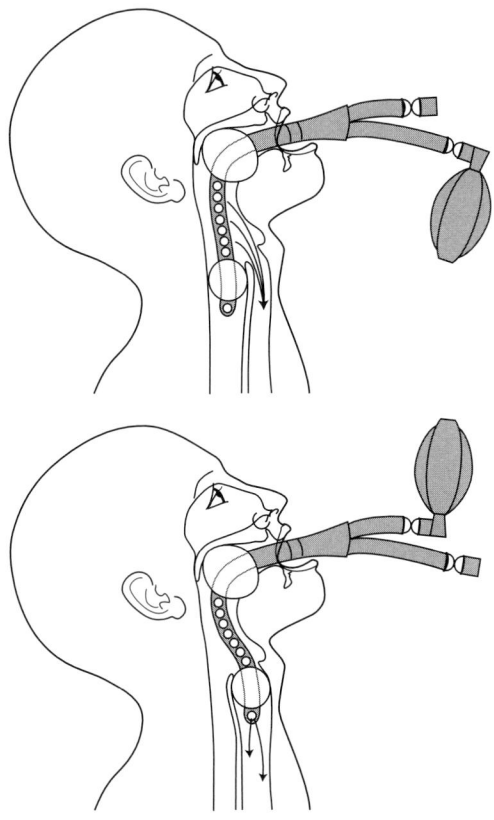

Figure 39.6 The Combitube: (a) insertion in the oesophagus, with ventilation via the pharyngeal perforations; (b) insertion in the trachea, with ventilation via the distal opening.

tion, isolation of the trachea from the oesophagus so reducing the risk of aspiration, and insertion with no neck movement. The main disadvantages are the need to be absolutely certain whether tracheal or oesophageal intubation has occurred, which is particularly difficult during resuscitation with no cardiac output. Failure to recognize where the tube has been placed will clearly have devastating results. In addition, it cannot be used on subjects less than 150 cm (five feet) tall, or in the presence of a gag reflex.

In clinical trials the Combitube has performed well, with ventilation comparable to conventional tracheal intubation. It has an established role in trauma and resuscitation, and although not fully evaluated, a place in the management of difficult intubations is emerging. It is likely to be most useful in the anaesthetized patient with an unexpectedly difficult airway, particularly where there is a risk of aspiration, or an unstable neck. In such cases it would appear to have an advantage over the laryngeal mask airway.

RETROGRADE INTUBATION

Retrograde intubation is a means by which an oral or nasal tracheal tube is passed over a guide wire which has been introduced, in a retrograde manner, through the cricothyroid membrane. It can be performed as an elective procedure, on either an awake or anaesthetized patient, or in an emergency. In the awake patient, local anaesthesia of the airway is required (see fibreoptic intubation).

A needle, attached to a saline filled syringe, is inserted through the cricothyroid membrane, in the mid-line, in a cephalad direction. Correct position in the trachea is confirmed by aspiration of air. A guide wire is passed through the needle, between the cords and into the mouth. Protruding or pulling forward of the tongue assists with this manoeuvre. A tracheal tube is then 'railroaded' over the guide wire until it makes contact with the wall of the trachea, at the point where the guide wire goes through the cricothyroid membrane. The guide wire is then withdrawn through the mouth, as the tracheal tube is advanced into the trachea.

The vertical distance between the vocal cords and the upper border of the cricoid cartilage is less than 2 cm. This leaves only a very short length of tube in the trachea when the guide wire is removed, and posterior displacement of the tube into the oesophagus can easily occur. To reduce the chances of this happening, a number of manoeuvres can be used. First, the needle through the cricothyroid membrane should be as low as possible, preferably placed by walking the needle off the upper border of the cricoid cartilage.

Second, passing the guide wire through the Murphy's eye of the tracheal tube will add approximately 1 cm to the length of tube in the trachea, when the guide wire is removed. Commercial kits have included a stiff catheter, to be placed over the guide wire in an antegrade direction. The catheter is sufficiently rigid to make posterior displacement unlikely when the wire is removed. Probably the most successful method is to use a fibreoptic scope, with a pre-mounted tracheal tube. The guide wire can be passed through the suction port of the scope, which is then 'railroaded' over the wire into the trachea. When the guide wire is withdrawn the tip of the scope hopefully remains in the trachea, and can be advanced towards the carina, before positioning the tube under direct vision.

Nasal intubation, if necessary, can be achieved by passing a catheter through the nose to the oropharynx. When visible at the back of the mouth, it is retrieved with the assistance of forceps, and brought out of the mouth. The tip of the nasal catheter is securely tied to the guide wire, which is then drawn back into the mouth, up into the nasopharynx and out through the nostril. The nasal catheter is discarded, and the nasal tracheal tube positioned over the guide wire.

The presence of a laryngeal tumour at the level of the cricothyroid membrane, a mass overlying the cricothyroid membrane, and coagulopathy are all contraindications to retrograde grade intubation. The procedure is very difficult to perform when the interdental space is less than 2 cm, and severely reduced mouth opening should be regarded as a relative contraindication.

The main advantage of retrograde intubation is the ability to perform the procedure with a minimum amount of additional equipment. Although commercial kits are now available, the technique can be adequately performed with a Tuohy needle and an epidural catheter. This method has long been an established means of intubating difficult airways in centres and countries of limited resources, and large series of cases testify to its success.

Complications of retrograde intubation include vocal cord damage, oesophageal perforation, haemorrhage and trauma to the larynx and epiglottis. As with all transtracheal methods of securing a patent airway, retrograde intubation has unjustly earned a reputation as a high-risk procedure. All complications are more common if the procedure is performed in an emergency. In expert hands, when performed electively, retrograde intubation has a good safety record and much to commend it.

REGIONAL ANAESTHESIA

When a patient is suspected or known to have a difficult airway, the alternative of surgery under local anaesthesia appears very attractive. Obviously, certain surgery is feasible only under general anaesthesia, but many operations can be performed in a totally pain free and safe manner with the use of regional techniques. Before embarking on such a line of management, it is important to consider a number of points. These include how resuscitation would be performed in the event of a complication, such as the unexpectedly high subarachnoid block or the management of insufficient neural blockade in mid-operation. What began as an apparently adroit answer to a difficult problem, can easily degenerate into a disaster.

Before contemplating a regional technique the anaesthetist should consider the likelihood of a major complication during surgery, and how easy it will be to stop the surgery. The balance of the risk of complications, against the advantages of a regional technique, must be carefully assessed. If the risk of complications is high, surgery difficult to terminate, or access to the patient's head likely to be poor, an alternative approach to the problem of the airway would be wise.

FIBREOPTIC LARYNGOSCOPES

A new generation of laryngoscopes is appearing, which incorporates fibreoptics and a rigid laryngoscope blade. By virtue of fibreoptics, the anaesthetist can, in effect, see round corners, and there is no longer the need to bring the axis of the mouth, pharynx and larynx into line. The curve of the blade approximates that of the oropharynx, which it naturally follows towards the larynx. These scopes allow visualization through the fibreoptic eye-piece of both the glottis that cannot be seen by conventional laryngoscopy, and the tracheal tube as it passes between the cords. Intubation can be achieved without movement of the neck, which is an advantage in cases of cervical trauma and instability. Some of these scopes are battery operated and portable, unlike intubating fibrescopes which rely on an external light source. The designs vary, but some have large cumbersome blades which can make insertion difficult, especially in patients with limited mouth opening.

Extensive experience with these scopes is not yet available, and at present they represent expensive pieces of equipment, whose future role in the management of the difficult intubation is promising but not fully evaluated.

THE DIFFICULT EXTUBATION

Extubation is a neglected area, yet mismanagement at this time can have as devastating consequences as a failed intubation. Difficulties at extubation may be predicted, or arise unexpectedly.

PROBLEMS AT EXTUBATION

Laryngospasm following extubation, though common, is usually mild. It is more prevalent in smokers, and often precipitated by blood or secretions irritating the cords. Minor laryngospasm is very noisy, whilst complete spasm is silent and more sinister. Treatment is by removal of any offending stimuli and administration of 100% oxygen under sustained pressure. If necessary, a small dose of a intravenous anaesthetic agent will break the spasm. Alternatively suxamethonium, with or without reintubation, may be used.

Laryngeal oedema frequently follows a traumatic intubation, where there have been many attempts to pass laryngoscopes, bougies and the tracheal tube. It can occasionally follow an apparently uneventful intubation. Laryngeal oedema should be suspected if stridor develops within a few hours of surgery. Treatment depends on severity and includes: a head-up position, humidified oxygen, nebulized adrenaline, steroids, helium/oxygen mix and, occasionally, re-intubation. When the oedema is severe enough to cause marked respiratory difficulty, re-intubation and ventilation may be necessary until the swelling has subsided.

Vocal cord palsy is unusual, but can occur following thoracic, thyroid and other neck surgery. Partial palsy results in a hoarse voice, but does not endanger the airway. Paralysis of the abductor muscles results in complete airway obstruction. Clinically it will resemble complete laryngospasm, but will fail to resolve with return of consciousness. Direct inspection of the cords will reveal no abductor movement. The patient requires re-intubating and a tracheostomy.

Some patients who were easy to intubate at induction of anaesthesia, may by virtue of their surgery, be difficult to reintubate after extubation. For example, wiring of the mandible to maxilla, application of external fixators, major head and neck surgery, or simply oedema as a result of a prolonged head-down position. All warrant careful consideration of how their airway is managed in the immediate postoperative period.

EXTUBATION OF THE DIFFICULT INTUBATION

In general, patients who were difficult to intubate once, will be difficult to intubate again.

In fact, any patient requiring re-intubation shortly after extubation, is likely to be more difficult the second time. This is because of oedema, blood and secretions, obtunded level of consciousness and cooperation, and decreased respiratory reserve. As a rule, patients with difficult airways should be extubated when awake, and those who experienced some degree of upper airway obstruction preoperatively (e.g. obese patients, laryngeal tumours), cope better when extubated sitting up.

When an intubation has been difficult, careful consideration of extubation is essential, if it is to be accomplished in a safe and orderly manner. The use of an airway exchange catheter is particularly helpful. This consists of a narrow catheter which is passed through the tube into the trachea and positioned just above the carina. The tube is then removed. Oxygen can be supplied down the catheter, which is blunt-ended and sufficiently rigid to prevent it being coughed out of the trachea. It is left in position until the patient is fully awake and there is no evidence of upper airway obstruction, at which time it can be withdrawn.

If airway obstruction occurs and re-intubation is necessary, the catheter acts as a guide over which a new tracheal tube can be 'railroaded'. In an emergency, or before re-intubation, jet ventilation down the catheter can be employed. To prevent barotrauma when using jet ventilation, it is imperative the catheter is within the trachea and not a bronchus. If an airway exchange catheter is not available, a nasogastric tube can be used as an alternative. The disadvantage of a nasogastric tube is its pliancy, which can result in it being coughed out of position.

In certain rare cases, such as a large laryngeal tumour, extubation would be unsafe and it is necessary to perform a surgical tracheostomy. Close cooperation and consultation between anaesthetist and surgeon is crucial in the management of these cases.

SPECIAL CIRCUMSTANCES

THE CERVICAL SPINE

As discussed above, to intubate the trachea the head is extended on the neck. In the presence of fractures, dislocations and joint instability in the cervical spine, excessive movement can easily occur during intubation. Compression and transection of the spinal cord will have a catastrophic outcome. Instability of the cervical spine is most commonly associated with trauma and degenerative changes, such as occur with rheumatoid arthritis.

Trauma

Trauma victims who may have sustained cervical injury must be treated as having a cervical fracture, until radiographically proved otherwise. Care of the airway in these patients can be challenging. The cervical spine should be immobilized by use of a rigid collar, or by sand bags and head strapping. The conscious patient with adequate respiration requires no intervention, other than administration of oxygen. If the patient is apnoeic, or respiration inadequate, mask ventilation by hand is the correct, first-line of management.

If intubation becomes necessary a number of options are available. Conventional intubation with an assistant maintaining in-line traction of the head is the preferred choice of most anaesthetists. If this cannot be accomplished, alternatives include the use of a LMA, Combitube, fibreoptic intubation, blind nasal intubation or cricothyrotomy. The correct choice will depend on the individual circumstances, experience of the anaesthetist and equipment available. Each case should be judged on its merits and common sense must prevail. Oxygenation is paramount and mask ventilation must not be forgotten in the enthusiasm to employ other techniques.

Rheumatoid arthritis

Cervical involvement affects up to 86% of patients with adult rheumatoid arthritis. Involvement may be present in the absence of any signs or symptoms. Difficulty with airway management may arise as a result of subluxation or ankylosis of the cervical joints. Initially, subluxation and instability occur and patients risk neurological and/or vascular damage during laryngoscopy, or perioperative positioning of the neck. Subluxation may progress to ankylosis and immobility. Those with poor neck mobility may be difficult to intubate, due to poor visualization of the larynx.

C1–C2 is the most commonly affected cervical joint. Subluxation may be in any direction, and is assessed by lateral, cervical spine radiographs in flexion and extension, plus odontoid views through the open mouth. Anterior C1–C2 subluxation is by far the most common abnormality. It is present when the distance between the atlas and odontoid process in the lateral, flexion view exceeds 3 mm in patients over 44 years, or 4 mm in younger patients. Anterior C1–C2 instability is exacerbated by flexion, which should be avoided throughout the perioperative period, but direct laryngoscopy is tolerated.

In contrast, vertical and posterior C1–C2 subluxation, whilst uncommon, are the most dangerous. Vertical subluxation is potentially life threatening due to cervical medullary compression, and posterior C1–C2 subluxation can produce irreversible spinal cord damage. In both instances the neck should be immobilized in a rigid collar. Direct laryngoscopy must not be attempted, and awake fibreoptic intubation is the method of choice. Patients with other forms of subluxation may be intubated with help of direct laryngoscopy and appropriate neck stabilization.

Preoperative assessment of patients with rheumatoid arthritis should include a history, examination and radiological assessment. In an emergency, when a full assessment is not possible, the anaesthetist should assume the presence of life-threatening cervical instability and approach the airway appropriately.

LARYNGEAL TUMOURS

Laryngeal tumours may be very small, whilst others are large, friable and bleed easily on contact. Patients with tumours of the larynx and supraglottic region often prove to be difficult to ventilate by mask, and difficult to intubate. Potential problems are rarely suggested by external appearance, and the presence of hoarseness bears little relationship to the size of the tumour. Stridor, dyspnoea and respiratory distress suggest a large tumour, but absence of these features does not guarantee a small lesion.

These patients require very careful assessment. In contrast to most other difficult airways, indirect laryngoscopy and CT/MRI scanning can provide useful information. Indirect laryngoscopy is simple and quick to perform, and if the vocal cords are clearly visible, intubation is unlikely to be difficult.

Conversely, if the cords cannot be seen, a difficult intubation is likely. The view obtained at direct laryngoscopy is rarely as good as that seen at indirect laryngoscopy, due to decreased muscle tone under anaesthesia. It is easy to fall foul of this discrepancy, and as a general rule, a difficult intubation should be anticipated if the cords are not clearly visualized. CT or MRI scanning will help to identify the upper and lower level of the lesion, the presence of laryngeal/tracheal narrowing, and the extent of structural distortion by tumour.

If there is any doubt about airway management, awake fibreoptic intubation, trans-tracheal jet ventilation, retrograde intubation and awake tracheostomy are all suitable means of securing the airway. The choice depends on several factors, including the extent of the tumour as judged by CT/MRI scans. When attempting intubation under anaesthesia, tracheal tubes of differing sizes, stilettes, bougies and suction must all be readily available. It is prudent to use a high inspired oxygen concentration and to avoid long-acting neuromuscular blocking drugs.

Once intubated, it is crucial that appropriate consideration is given to the conduct of extubation (see above).

CONCLUSIONS

A variety of techniques has been described which are suitable when encountering a difficult airway. These range from simple adjuncts to conventional management, to the highly invasive. Unfortunately, it is not possible to say which technique should be used in certain circumstances, as each situation is different. To be able to select the correct line of management, and be able to perform that technique, is best learned by case history discussion groups, practice on manikins and cadavers and finally, under supervision on patients. If training follows this plan, the incidence of mismanaged difficult airways should be reduced.

FURTHER READING

Bellhouse, C. P. and Dore, C. (1988) Criteria for estimating likelihood of difficulty of endotracheal intubation with Macintosh laryngoscope. *Anaesthesia and Intensive Care*, **16**, 329–337.

Benumof, J. L. and Scheller, M. S. (1989) The importance of transtracheal jet ventilation in the management of the difficult airway. *Anaesthesiology*, **71**, 769–778.

Biebuyck, J. F. (1991) Management of the difficult airway. *Anaesthesiology*, **75**, 1087–1110.

Cormack, R. S. and Lehane, J. (1984) Difficult tracheal intubations in obstetrics. *Anaesthesia*, **39**, 1105–1111.

Horton, W. A., Fahy, L. and Charters, P. (1989) Defining a standard intubation position using 'angle finder'. *British Journal of Anaesthesia*, **62**, 6–12.

Macarthur, A. and Keiman, S. (1993) Rheumatoid cervical joint disease – a challenge to the anaesthetist. *Can J Anaesth*, **40**, 154–159.

Mallampati, S. R., Gugino, L. D., Desai, S. P. et al. (1985) A clinical sign to predict difficult tracheal intubation: a prospective study. *Canadian Anesthetic Society Journal*, **32**, 429–434.

Ovassapian, A., Krejcie, T. C., Yelich, S. J. et al. (1989) Awake fibreoptic intubation in the patient at high risk of aspiration. *British Journal of Anaesthesia*, **62**, 13–16.

Samsoon, G. L. T. and Young, J. R. B. (1987) Difficult tracheal intubation: a retrospective study. *Anaesthesia*, **42**, 487–490.

Wilson, M. E., Spiegelhalter, D., Robertson, J. A. et al. (1988) Predicting difficult intubation. *British Journal of Anaesthesia*, **61**, 211–216.

FLUID THERAPY

P. G. Roe

The importance of fluid and electrolyte balance was first described in the 1830s with the arrival of the second cholera pandemic to the UK. William Brooke O'Shaughnessy, a young Edinburgh graduate, not only accurately described the signs of extracellular fluid (ECF) depletion and reduced plasma volume but discovered, by chemical analysis of the blood, a severe shortage of water, salt and alkali, He achieved remarkable success with intravenous administration of fluids to replace these deficiencies and noted the importance of monitoring therapy on the basis of physical signs. Little more is heard about intravenous therapy until reports in 1891 of fluids being used to treat haemorrhage. It was not, however, until the 1930s that it became accepted that the picture of haemorrhagic shock was in fact a result of a loss of plasma volume. Treatment of haemorrhage with intravenous fluids became widespread during the Second World War and has thrived ever since. Concerns over salt and water retention, the need to 'resuscitate' the interstitial space and the relative merits of crystalloids and colloids have added interest to the subject over the second half of the 20th century. The management of fluid balance in the critically ill patient with leaky capillaries remains a challenge.

PHYSIOLOGY

BASIC DEFINITIONS OF TERMS USED IN FLUID BALANCE

Molarity

A mole of a substance is its molecular weight expressed in grams. The molarity of a solution is the number of moles dissolved in a litre of solvent and is dependent on temperature. Molality is the number of grams dissolved in 1000 g of solvent and is independent of temperature.

Osmosis

A membrane is semi-permeable if it allows free passage of small molecules (e.g. solvent, water) but not of larger molecules (e.g. solute, protein). If the large molecules are restricted to one side of the membrane, they reduce the concentration of small molecules on this side by occupying space. The small molecules diffuse along a concentration gradient from the other side. The pressure required to counter this effect is the osmotic pressure.

Osmolality

An osmole is a mole of a substance multiplied by the number of particles it forms in solution. Sodium chloride in an 'ideal' solution dissociates into two ions and therefore one millimole gives rise to two milliosmoles. This effect is, however, reduced by both incomplete ionization and ionic interactions in plasma which is not an 'ideal' solution. This results in one millimole of sodium chloride giving rise to 1.86 mosmol.

Plasma osmolality is a measure of the total number of particles in a given weight of plasma water. Osmolality and osmotic pressure are quite different. It is important to appreciate that the osmolality of a solution refers to the total number of particles in a given weight of solvent *in vitro*. *In vivo* at a biological membrane the osmotic pressure developed will depend upon the permeability of the membrane to the solutes. For example, at vascular endothelium, electrolytes, which contribute a large part of the osmolality of plasma, do not in isolation result in osmotic pressure as this membrane is permeable to them. Plasma proteins, to which the vascular endothelium is impermeable, contribute only a very small part of the total osmolality of plasma but are the main providers of the osmotic pressure at this membrane.

Tonicity

Substances which are restricted to the ECF, principally sodium and its associated anions, chloride and bicarbonate, are important in determining the volume of this compartment and are said to provide 'effective osmoles'. The concentration of effective osmoles is known as the tonicity. Substances such as urea pass into cells and therefore do not provide effective osmoles although they contribute to the osmolality of plasma. Glucose does provide effective osmoles as long as it remains in the plasma. An isotonic solution does not result in a net movement of water in and out of cells when administered intravenously.

Colloid osmotic pressure

The term colloid refers to large gelatinous molecules with molecular weights in excess of an arbitrary figure of 10 000, for example, plasma proteins. If a semi-permeable membrane restrains the passage of these molecules but allows ionic salts to pass, the osmotic pressure developed by the colloid molecules is the colloid osmotic pressure (COP). Van't Hoff predicted that by analogy with the ideal gas laws, in an 'ideal' solution of infinite dilution, colloid osmotic pressure should be proportional to the colloid's concentration and inversely proportional to its molecular weight. However, if the theoretical colloid osmotic pressure of both albumin and non-albumin plasma proteins are calculated in this way, the result obtained is only half of the measured plasma COP. This is because of deviations from Van't Hoff behaviour which increase with colloid concentration and are the result of several mechanisms. Firstly, plasma proteins have a negative charge and this alters the distribution of otherwise permeable ions across the membrane (Gibbs–Donnan equilibrium) which then are able to exert osmotic effect. Second, large colloid molecules occupy a large volume of the available space hence increasing the apparent concentration of other molecules (excluded volume effect). Finally, other solute and solvent interactions occur in plasma.

Oncotic pressure

This is often used synonymously with colloid osmotic pressure but there is a distinct difference. Oncotic pressure is the osmotic pressure developed at the vascular endothelium by whatever means. It results in large part from the plasma proteins (COP) but also from osmotic effects of electrolytes held in the plasma by the negatively charged proteins (Gibbs–Donnan effect).

BODY FLUID COMPARTMENTS

Total body water

In a 70 kg man, total body water (TBW) is approximately 40 l, which is 60% of total body weight. In women it is reduced to 50% of total body weight as there is generally more fat which contains less water. In infants with very little fat, TBW is greater than 60% of total body weight. As muscle mass (with high water content) declines with age, both sexes have a reduction in TBW to less than 50% of total body mass. TBW can be divided into intracellular and extracellular compartments. The extracellular compartment can be further divided into interstitial and intravascular compartments.

Intracellular compartment

The intracellular compartment has a volume of 30 l; its principal cation is potassium. As the intracellular compartment contains twice the number of osmotic particles as the extracellular fluid (ECF), it has twice the volume. The cell membrane is impermeable to electrolytes which therefore contribute to the osmotic forces here. Because intracellular fluid (ICF) and ECF are isotonic, there is osmotic equilibrium at the cell membrane. ICF volume is sensitive to changes in the sodium concentration of the ECF.

Extracellular compartment

The size of the extracellular compartment is determined by homeostatic control of both its tonicity and volume. Alterations in tonicity, detected at osmoreceptors, affect both thirst and levels of arginine vasopressin (AVP) altering both the intake and output of water. Altered ECF volume can be detected by volume receptors in the circulation and by renal mechanisms. The total amount (not concentration) of sodium in the ECF determines its volume and consequently, homeostatic mechanisms controlling volume are mainly concerned with the retention or excretion of sodium. If a sodium load is added to the ECF such that tonicity increases, thirst will be stimulated and renal water retention occurs. The ECF volume therefore increases and this stimulates a loss of sodium (with water) which eventually returns the ECF volume to normal.

The microvascular endothelium

The intravascular and extracellular compartments are separated by the microvascular endothelium which is freely permeable to water and electrolytes but is relatively impermeable to proteins. Fluid fluxes at this membrane can be described by the Starling–Landis equation.

$$\dot{Q} = K\left[(P_{mv} - P_{pmv}) - \sigma(\Pi_{mv} - \Pi_{pmv})\right]$$

or

$$\dot{Q} = K\,\Delta P - \sigma\Delta\Pi$$

where $\dot{Q}$ is the net fluid flux, P is hydrostatic pressure and Π is osmotic pressure in the microvascular (mv) and perimicrovascular (pmv) compartments respectively. K is the hydraulic conductivity of the membrane (how permeable it is to water). σ is the Staverman reflection coefficient which is an indication of how semi-permeable the membrane is. If σ is less than unity, solute (protein) will to some extent pass through the membrane and there will be a fractional reduction in the osmotic pressure generated by a given concentration of protein on one side of the membrane.

It is important to appreciate that the protein concentration of interstitial fluid is 20–40% (70% in the lung) of that of plasma and with a reflection coefficient of 0.8 in health, the contribution of osmosis to opposing fluid egress is small. Consequently, there is a net flux of fluid and protein out of the vascular compartment into the interstitial compartment. This excess fluid is taken up by lymphatics which have a total flow of 1–3 l per day. This has the capacity to increase greatly without oedema formation.

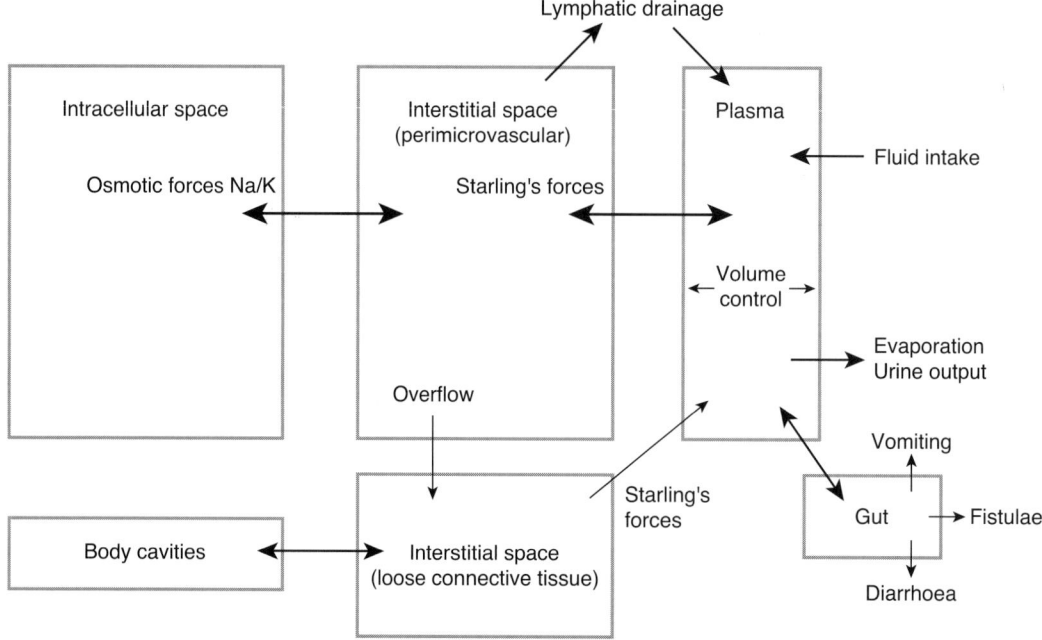

Figure 40.1 Schematic representation of fluid compartments and the fluxes between them.

The interstitial compartment

The interstitial compartment contains 33% of the total body water. It is the *milieu interieur* and has important transport functions between plasma and cells. It has two subcompartments, parenchymal (perimicrovascular) and loose binding connective tissue. Fluid filtered from the plasma passes into the perimicrovascular compartment which contains functional space between vessels and cells and is immediately taken up by the lymphatics which act as an overflow for small rises in pressure and volume. In health these lymphatics have a high capacity. If the capacity of lymphatic drainage is exceeded, fluid overflows into the loose binding connective tissue which is normally dry but which has a high capacity. Lymphatics are unable to remove excess interstitial fluid from this compartment and accumulation (oedema) occurs. This fluid no longer has the normal physiological function of interstitial fluid and is temporarily 'lost'. It has been referred to as the 'third space' and remains in place until reabsorbed into the vasculature by Starling forces and may overflow out of the tissues into body cavities, for example as pleural effusions, ascites and alveolar flooding. Figure 40.1 shows the fluid fluxes between the various compartments.

The interstitial compartment in the lung

In the normal lung, a reduced COP will result in increased fluid flux from the plasma to the interstitial compartment but will not result in an increase in extravascular lung water because of the high capacity lymphatic drainage. This effect of reduced COP is particularly marked at higher intravascular hydrostatic pressures. Indeed, crystalloid resuscitation of burns (which will reduce COP) does not lead to an increase in extravascular lung water provided that pulmonary capillary wedge pressure (PCWP) is maintained below 15 mmHg.

When fluid egress into the perimicrovascular space of the lung exceeds the capacity of lymphatic drainage, pulmonary oedema occurs. Initially this fluid is confined to the distensible interstitial space which occurs between layers of loose alveolar epithelium away from the pulmonary capillary. The closely applied capillary endothelium and alveolar epithelium, which is the principal site of gas exchange, is largely spared at this stage and consequently there is little effect on gas exchange. As extravascular lung water increases, further interstitial distension occurs, and fluid begins to leak out into the alveoli. Hydrophobic surfactant creates forces which minimise this leakage but eventually alveolar flooding occurs. It is only at this stage that a significant impairment of gas exchange occurs.

Renal threshold

Substances will be filtered through the glomerulus when their molecular weight is below a certain threshold value. As different substances have molecules of different shape, the value of this threshold will vary with the substance. In addition, the charge of a molecule will affect renal filtration as the glomerular basement membrane has a negative charge. This explains the low filtration from plasma of albumin, which has a negative charge.

PHARMACOLOGY OF FLUIDS

CRYSTALLOIDS

Crystalloids are solutions of ions (Na^+ and Cl^-) and/or small sugars (glucose) in water. They are cheap and easy to manufacture. Most are approximately iso-osmotic with plasma (see Table 40.1). They pass freely through the microvascular endothelium and do not, by themselves, contribute to oncotic pressure. After intravenous administration, the distribution of these fluids is determined by their sodium concentration. As sodium is largely restricted to the extracellular compartment, solutions containing isotonic concentrations of this ion will distribute through the whole of this compartment. Solutions containing less sodium, and whose osmotic activity is maintained with glucose, contain 'free water' (free of sodium) which is able to distribute into the intracellular compartment (Figure 40.2). The amount of 'free water' in a crystalloid preparation is determined by its

Table 40.1 Electrolyte concentrations of normal plasma and common crystalloid solutions

	Na^+ (mmol l^{-1})	Cl^- (mmol l^{-1})	K^+ (mmol l^{-1})	Mg^{2+} (mmol l^{-1})	Ca^{2+} (mmol l^{-1})	Gluconate (mmol l^{-1})	HCO_3^- (mmol l^{-1})	Glucose (mg dl^{-1})	Calculated osmolality (mOsm l^{-1})
Plasma	142	103	4.5	0.9	2.5	–	26	90–110	290
0.9% sodium chloride	154 (150)	154 (150)	–	–	–	–	–	–	308
5% glucose	–	–	–	–	–	–	–	50	278
4% glucose–0.18% sodium chloride	31 (30)	31 (30)	–	–	–	–	–	40	284
Hartmanns solution	131	111	5	–	2	–	29 (as lactate)	–	278
Lactated Ringer solution (USA)	130	109	4	–	1.5	–	28	–	273
Ringer solution for injection (UK)	147	156	4	–	2.2	–	–	–	311
Plasmalyte 148	140	98	5	1.5	–	23	–	–	296
Plasmalyte M	40	40	16	1.5	2.5	–	12	50	406

702 Fluid therapy

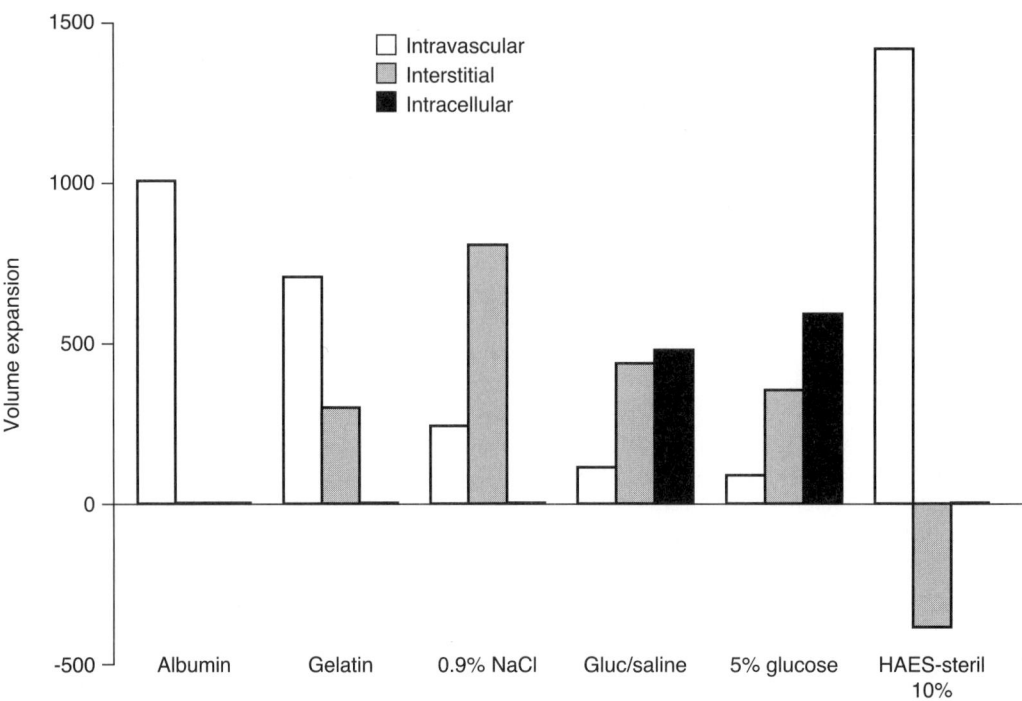

Figure 40.2 Distribution through body fluid spaces of one litre of different fluids one hour after intravenous administration.

sodium content with respect to normal saline: 1000 ml of 5% glucose solution contains 1000 ml of free water and will be distributed evenly throughout the total body water; 0.9% sodium chloride solution contains no free water and will be restricted to the extracellular compartment; 1000 ml of 4% glucose–0.18% sodium chloride contains 30 mmol of sodium which is 0.2 of that of normal saline, 0.2 of the litre may be considered to be normal saline and the remaining 0.8 (800 ml) to be free water.

Sodium chloride, 0.9%

This solution contains 154 mmol of both sodium and chloride ions and is isotonic with plasma. (In the UK, 150 mmol appears on some products, but this is in fact an approximation of labelling.) It is used to treat sodium depletion; 154 mmol is, however, well above the daily requirement and sodium overload (with increased ECF volume) may result from indiscriminate use of this product in the absence of a sodium deficit. It is primarily distributed in the extracellular compartment. It may be used for volume resuscitation in crystalloid-based regimens but has the potential to produce hyperchloraemic acidosis, when used in large volumes, particularly in patients with renal impairment. As with balanced electrolyte solutions, administration of three times the volume of blood loss is required to replace plasma volume.

Glucose, 5%

This is essentially free water. The glucose is added simply to render it iso-osmotic, although its calorific value may be exploited.

Glucose contributes to the tonicity of plasma but this is short lived in the presence of insulin when it is rapidly taken up by cells. The water is then distributed throughout the TBW and produces negligible plasma volume expansion. Severe hyponatraemia will result if this product is infused rapidly. It is usually administered slowly, alternating with normal saline for maintenance therapy.

Glucose saline solutions

A variety of mixtures of glucose and saline are available with considerable international variation. Depending on the precise combination, these solutions can be considered to be a combination of normal saline and free water. The most commonly employed mixture in the UK is 4% glucose–0.18% sodium chloride which is isotonic. This may be used as a maintenance fluid at a rate of 2–3 l per day in an adult. Care is needed in the perioperative period when both sodium and water are retained. As 1000 ml of this product only contains 30 mmol of sodium, dilutional hyponatraemia may result. In the USA, mixtures of 5% glucose–0.45% sodium chloride, and 5% glucose–0.9% sodium chloride are common and avoid the problem of hyponatraemia encountered with 4% glucose–0.18% sodium chloride. These solutions are, however, hyperosmotic. One litre of 5% glucose–0.45% sodium chloride contains 500 ml of free water. One litre of 5% glucose–0.9% sodium chloride contains no free water.

Balanced electrolyte solutions

These isotonic solutions contain potassium and calcium in addition to sodium and chloride ions. Certain brands also contain lactate which is metabolized to bicarbonate. It is important to appreciate that this bicarbonate is not immediately available. The purpose of these solutions is to maintain the composition of the extracellular environment when large volumes of intravenous fluids are required.

They form the basis of volume resuscitation in the crystalloid based regimens which are standard in the USA and in advanced trauma life support (ATLS) protocols. They are also useful in the intraoperative period when several litres of fluid may need to be administered rapidly. In the USA, a preparation of Ringer's lactate is available with 50 g of glucose per litre; 5% dextrose in Ringer's lactate (D5RL). This is a hyperosmotic solution. It does not contain free water.

COLLOIDS

Solutions of colloids, substances of large molecular weight > 10 000, are also used in fluid therapy. They will contribute to oncotic pressure at the microvascular endothelium. Unlike crystalloids, they are initially confined to the plasma and will produce a greater expansion of this compartment. It is important to appreciate that this effect is temporary with all available colloids and a wide variation in efficacy is found between different types. Some colloid preparations, for example 20% albumin and 40% dextran, have a greater oncotic pressure than plasma and tend to draw water into the plasma (plasma expanders) at the expense of the interstitial space.

ALBUMIN

Albumin has a molecular weight of 69 000. It is the primary oncotic particle in the plasma accounting for 70–80% of oncotic pressure. Each molecule has a charge of -17 at physiological pH which contributes to the Gibbs–Donnan effect, greatly increasing the oncotic pressure. Five per cent of intravenous albumin escapes each hour (transcapillary escape) and of this, 10% is metabolized and the remainder returns to the circulation. Two thirds of the exchangeable albumin pool is extravascular but the majority is held away from the perimicrovascular compartment and therefore does not contribute to the Starling

Table 40.2 Properties of colloid solutions

	Concentration (g l^{-1})	MW_w	MW_n	DS	COP (mmHg)
Hespan 6%	60	450	70	0.7	27
HAES-steril 6%	60	200	70	0.5	34
HAES-steril 10%	100	200	70	0.5	80
EloHAES 6%	60	200	60	0.62	25–30
Pentaspan 10%	100	264	63	0.45	55–60
Gelofusine	40	30	22.6	–	40–45
Haemaccel	35	35	15	–	25
Dextran-40	100	40	25	–	160
Dextran-70	60	70	39	–	78

MW_w = mean (weight average) molecular weight
MW_n = number average molecular weight
DS = degree of substitution
COP = colloid osmotic pressure

forces. Fifty per cent of extravascular albumin is in the skin and accounts for the large protein losses seen in burns. Solutions of human albumin solution are available for intravenous administration in 4.5% (isooncotic) and 20% (hyperoncotic) concentrations. One gram of albumin expands the plasma by approximately 18 ml regardless of its concentration on administration. The hyperoncotic 20% solution will draw fluid into the plasma from the interstitial compartment. When administered intravenously, albumin declines according to two half lives: the first, of 5–15 h, represents transcapillary escape and the second, of 17 days, represents metabolism. In the clinical situation the kinetics vary with the volume status of the patient. Apparent advantages of albumin as a replacement colloid include binding toxic substances and scavenging free radicals. However, it has not been shown to improve outcome in critically ill patients when compared to synthetic colloids and as solutions of intravenous albumin are very expensive they are not justified for routine volume replacement. Treatment of hypoalbuminaemia with intravenous albumin, although widespread, is now questioned as merely treating the result and not the cause of the pathophysiology. Indeed, serum albumin concentrations correlate poorly with COP and congenital an-albuminaemia is compatible with life.

Synthetic colloids

Whereas albumin is a monodisperse colloid with molecules of equal size, synthetic colloids (gelatins, dextrans and etherified starches) are all polydisperse, consisting of a wide range of molecules of different size (Figure 40.3). The mean (weight average) molecular weight (MW_w) of these dispersions is the sum of the number of molecules divided by the total weight of molecules at each molecular weight. It tends to be distorted by the larger molecules, some of which may have molecular weights as high as 10 000 000, but which have little osmotic effect. A different measure of these dispersions is the number average molecular weight (MW_n) which is the median of the distribution of molecular weights and indicates the average size of the majority of the osmotically active particles. As the distributions of these preparations are skewed towards lower molecular weight, values of MW_n are smaller than MW_w. Figures for available colloids are given in Table 40.2. Approximate relative volume expansion effects of various colloids are given in Figure 40.4. A hypovolaemic patient will have a

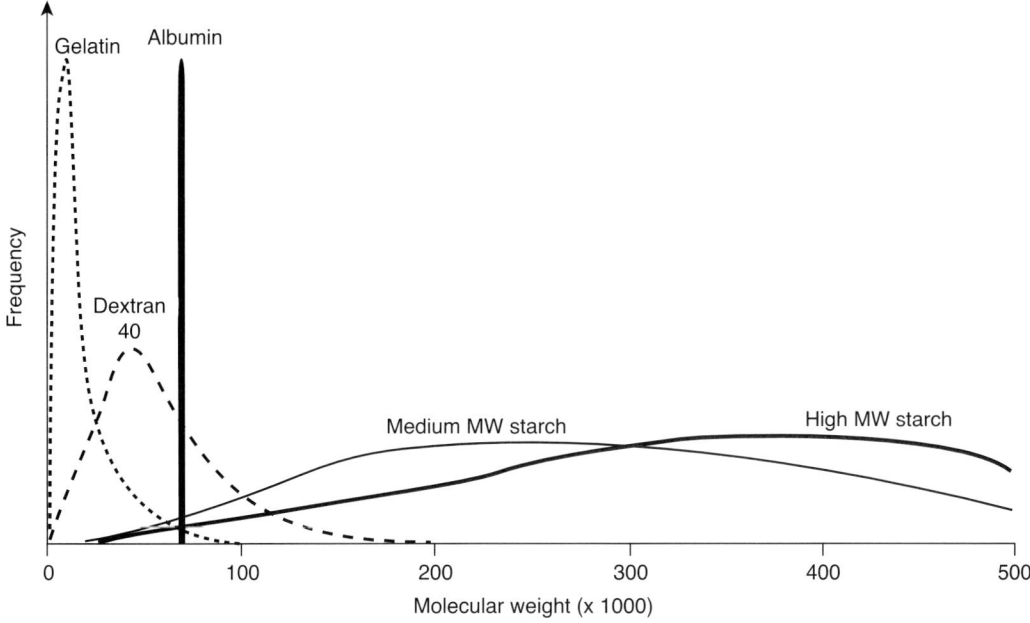

Figure 40.3 Molecular weight dispersion of gelatins, albumin and starch solutions.

greater volume expansion with a given quantity of colloid than a normovolaemic patient. Percentage volume expansion will be less with larger infusions. In patients with critical illness, the duration of the volume expanding effect is reduced.

Modified fluid gelatins

Two types of gelatins are available. Succinylated gelatins, e.g. gelofusine and urea linked gelatins, e.g. Haemaccel. Gelatins are the product of the degradation of animal collagen which is then modified to increase the size of the molecules and to improve vascular retention. With succinylated gelatins, NH_3 groups are replaced by charged COO^- groups causing conformational change which increases the size of the molecules. With urea linked gelatins, smaller molecules are linked to produce molecules of suitable size. These modified gelatins are polydipserse colloids. The low molecular weight (MW_w) of 35 000, which is well below the renal threshold, means that vascular retention is short (half-life of 3 h). Rapid excretion via the kidneys occurs, where they act as osmotic diuretics. They are of use in situations where short term volume expansion is required, for example to overcome the vasodilatation associated with spinal blockade or the administration of anaesthetic agents. They have the largest incidence of severe anaphylaxis of all the synthetic colloids although it remains infrequent ($\approx$ 1:5000 to 1:10 000). Histamine release increases the microvascular endothelial pore size which decreases further the volume expanding effect. Gelatins are administered in 0.9% sodium chloride, which represents a large sodium load when administered in quantity. In view of the rapid excretion of gelatin molecules, the remaining sodium and water will behave as normal saline and pass into the ECF. Haemaccel contains calcium ions which leads to clotting when blood is infused in the same giving set.

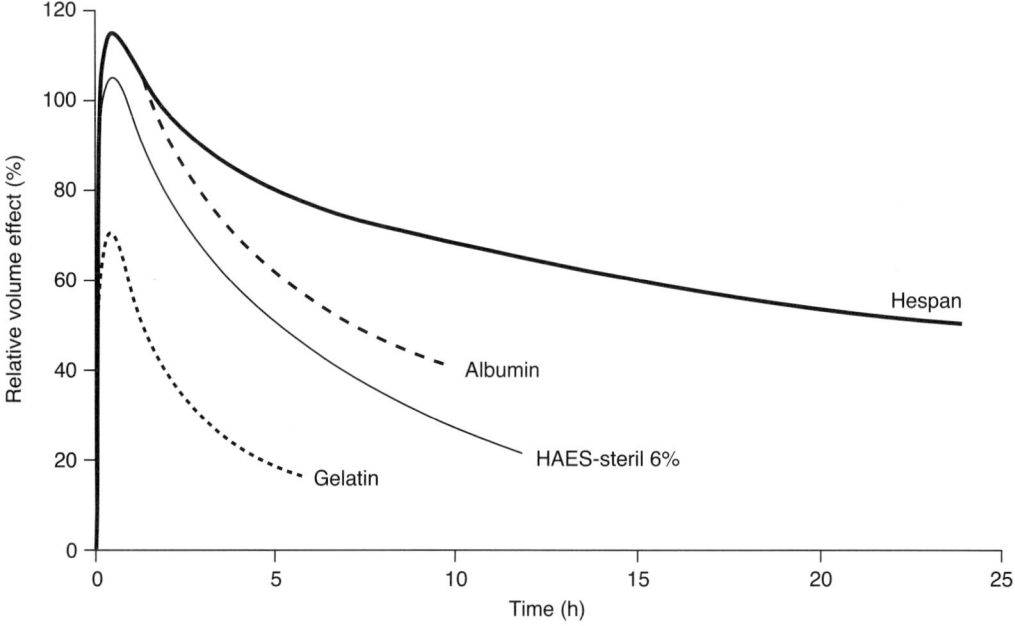

Figure 40.4 Approximate relative time courses of plasma volume expansion with different colloid solutions. Reported values vary widely and are affected by the initial volume status, renal function and the degree of microvascular endothelial damage.

Dextrans

Dextran is a naturally occurring glucose polymer which, unlike other synthetic colloids, is unmodified in manufacture. It is produced from sucrose by *Leuconostoc mesenteroides*. It is available in preparations of MW_w 70 000 (Dextran 70) 6% solution and MW_w 40 000 (Dextran 40) 10% solution. Both types of solution are available in either 0.9% sodium chloride or 5% glucose. Molecules of dextran are eliminated by the kidneys when the molecular weight is below the renal threshold for dextrans of 55 000. Before administration, 30–40% of dextran 70 and 60–70% of dextran 40 molecules are below this figure. Larger molecules are broken down by dextranases and are then eliminated by the kidneys. Some uptake of larger molecules can occur in the reticuloendothelial system (RES). When infused intravenously, dextran 70 has a half-life of 6 h. Dextran 40, because of the smaller molecular weight, is rapidly eliminated from the plasma with a half-life of 1–2 h. However, as a 10% solution, dextran 40 is hyperoncotic and draws fluid out of the interstitial space, leading to a short plasma expansion. This removal of interstitial fluid is undesirable in dehydrated patients and renal failure may be precipitated. Dextrans interfere with clotting and have been used in the treatment of post-surgical thromboembolic disease although they are probably less effective than low molecular weight heparin. Early use of high molecular weight dextrans was associated with a high incidence of anaphylaxis. This was found to be related to the size of the side chains, which have been reduced. Dextrans now have a similar incidence of allergic reactions to other colloids.

Etherified starch (hydroxyethyl starch)

A range of colloid products based on hydroxyethyl starch (HES) is available, differing on the basis of their molecular weight distribution and the length of their persistence in the plasma. Amylopectin, derived from corn wax starch, is a branch chained glucose polymer. It is subject to rapid hydrolysis by α-amylase and unmodified would be destroyed in the plasma within ten minutes. It is also insoluble in water. Addition of hydroxyethyl groups to the glucose subunits increases both solubility in water and resistance to hydrolysis by α-amylase. This increased solubility in water is a result of an increased water binding capacity of the molecule which in turn increases its osmotic activity (Partially dissolved, semi-hydrophobic molecules do not act as effective solutes as far as osmosis is concerned). The extent of this process of adding hydroxyethyl groups is indicated by the degree of substitution (DS) which represents the proportion of glucose units which have been etherified. A DS of one represents full substitution. Clinically available HES products have DS in the range 0.45–0.7. The higher the DS, the slower the α–hydrolysis. HES solutions have a very wide range of molecular weights. Following intravenous administration, individual molecules with a molecular weight below the renal threshold for HES (70 000) will be excreted. Molecules with a molecular weight of greater than this will not initially be excreted but will be hydrolysed by α-amylase at a rate proportional to the degree of substitution. Products of hydrolysis with molecular weights below the renal threshold will then be excreted. All molecules, whilst in the plasma, will contribute to oncotic pressure, with the smaller molecules contributing most. Although the larger molecules have very little oncotic activity in their original state, their products of hydrolysis contribute a large number of fresh medium molecular weight molecules at a time when the original medium MW molecules have been broken down to below renal threshold size and excreted. This mechanism also contributes to the volume expanding profile of HES. The extent and duration of volume expansion of HES solutions therefore depends on concentration, molecular weight and degree of substitution.

Larger molecules do pass into the RES by vacuolation and are metabolized. Many are re-released after breakdown. The extent of RES uptake is difficult to ascertain and accordingly, discrepancies exist in reported figures. This probably reflects a large (15%) but transient initial passage through the RES which is not sustained. Animal studies indicate that very small quantities are present at one week ($< 3\%$). This persistence is thought to be of little significance. Passage into the RES is not a major route of elimination of HES.

Hespan, 6% (hetastarch)

This has both a high MW_w (450 000) and DS (0.7) and is therefore charaterized by a long persistence in plasma. There is a very wide distribution of molecular weights ranging from 10 000 to 10 000 000. The larger molecules are either broken down rapidly by α-amylase in the plasma or more slowly by γ-amylase which is intracellular. Larger molecules are taken into the RES in the liver and spleen. Vacuolation and transient storage in hepatic parenchymal cells also occur. Hespan has an effect on clotting similar to dextrans.

HAES–steril, 6% (pentastarch)

This has a medium MW_w (200 000) and DS (0.5). The lower DS results in a shorter duration of plasma expansion as α-hydrolysis occurs more quickly than with Hespan or EloHAES (hexastarch solution).

HAES–steril, 10% (pentastarch)

This is a hyperoncotic preparation of HAES–steril. It is a plasma expander and results in an increase in plasma volume of 130% of the volume infused. This effect is short-lived, however, and after 3–4 h the plasma expansion profile is little different from HAES–steril 6%.

EloHAES, 6% (hexastarch)

This has a medium MW_w (200 000) but has a higher DS (0.62) than HAES-steril or pentaspan. The importance of the DS in determining the plasma volume expansion properties of starches during the first 24 h after administration is illustrated by the similar time course of both hespan and EloHAES. EloHAES had fewer of the very large molecules present in hespan and there will be less prolonged accumulation. It also has less effect on clotting than hespan.

Pentaspan, 10% (pentastarch)

This has a medium MW_w (264 000) and a low DS (0.45) and is presented in a hyperoncotic solution which results in some initial plasma expansion. It has a plasma profile similar to HAES-steril but may be eliminated faster. There is an effect on clotting by this is less than with hespan.

Pentrafraction

This is a special preparation of hydroxyethyl starch which remains under experimental evaluation. All small molecules (< 50 000) are removed and the majority of molecules are within a range of 100 000 to 500 000 (MW_n 120 000). It should be noted here that with all other colloids (including hespan), the majority of osmotic activity will result from molecules that are smaller than this. The purpose of this particular distribution is that the majority of molecules will be retained within the plasma even when injury has given rise to increased microvascular permeability. It has also been postulated that plugging of leaky capillaries may occur. The future possibilities of this preparation are considered further below.

FLUID BALANCE DERANGEMENTS AND FLUID THERAPY

Intravenous resuscitation became widespread during the Second World War. In the years after the war it was realized that salt and water were retained after trauma and surgery and it became customary to restrict them. Blood alone was given to replace blood loss. In the 1960s Shires showed that patients who received crystalloids and blood did better than those who received blood alone. Shires demonstrated a contraction of the interstitial compartment during haemorrhage using radioactive tracers. This was then also shown to occur in trauma and during major surgery. As crystalloids are distributed thought the ECF, their value was attributed to the resuscitation of this contracted compartment. Three possible mechanisms are proposed to explain the contraction of the interstitial compartment. Firstly, after moderate haemorrhage, a shift of fluid into the plasma (plasma volume refill) occurs from the interstitial compartment at rate of 90 to 120 ml h^{-1}. This is partly a result of altered Starling forces (low P_{mv}) and is also a result of sympathoadrenally mediated increase in pre-post capillary resistance ratio. Second, increases in intracellular osmolarity, secondary to cell hypoxia, result in a movement of fluid and electrolyte from the extracellular compartment to the intracellular compartment resulting in intracellular overhydration. Third, movement of fluid away from the parenchymal subcompartment into non-exchangeable subcompartments within the interstitial compartment (third space) is thought to occur. It remains here as oedema but its extracellular physiological function is lost. In this situation it would be logical to use crystalloids to resuscitate both the intravascular and interstitial compartments. The initial controversy that this caused in the 1960s was with those who believed that water and electrolytes were retained during the perioperative period with an expansion of the interstitial compartment, and should therefore be restricted. Retention of water and electrolytes undoubtedly occurs in relation to stress-mediated hormonal changes associated with surgery and anaesthesia. However, plasma deficits in these patients are greater than was then realized, and the benefits of restoring plasma volume and maintaining delivery of oxygen and nutrients to the tissues with large volumes of crystalloid are overwhelming. Fluid restriction is now no longer an issue in perioperative patients.

A major concern with the administration of large volumes of crystalloids is that it will lead to pulmonary oedema. In a healthy lung this will only occur when very large amounts are given that exceed perimicrovascular lymphatic drainage, which is extremely efficient in the lung. In addition, administration of crystalloids will lead to parallel changes in both Π_{mv} and Π_{pmv} and therefore crystalloids are more likely to remain in the vascular compartment after haemorrhage. Consideration of the equation above shows that alterations in hydrostatic pressure (ΔP) are then of greater importance than changes in oncotic pressure ($\Delta \Pi$) in determining fluid flux across the pulmonary microvascular endothelium. Administration of crystalloids in critical illness and adult respiratory distress syndrome (ARDS) is more problematic and is considered further below.

The controversy which followed in the 1970s related to whether deficits in plasma volume were better treated with colloids, which were believed to expand better that compartment. Colloids certainly now have an important place in plasma volume expansion although their use varies widely internationally depending on the prevailing practice. The main argument for the use of colloids is that they rapidly result in plasma expansion with a return of haemodynamic stability and tissue perfusion, hopefully preventing release of organ injury mediators which result in increases in microvascular permeability. It is important to appreciate, however, that not all colloids are equally effective in this regard. The use of large volumes of gelatins, for example, to replace blood loss on a volume for volume basis will result in late hypovolaemia as the volume expanding effect has a half-life of only 2–3 h.

The question of the contracted interstitial space remains unresolved. It is regarded as vitally important in the USA, where balanced electrolyte solutions (and blood when necessary) are used in quantity for resuscitation in trauma, haemorrhage and perioperatively with the explicit aim of restoring the interstitial compartment. Many authorities subscribing to the 'colloid school of thought' regard this as unimportant and, therefore, view crystalloid regimens as irrational. Shire's findings that the functional interstitial space is contracted have been disputed by others. It is obviously difficult to apply steady state measurements of tracer distribution to what is clearly a very non-steady-state situation.

If the interstitial space becomes depleted it is likely to do so in previously healthy individuals during the acute insults of haemorrhagic shock or trauma/major surgery. Even if colloids are preferred for rapid plasma volume expansion, one must still ask if the interstitial space needs resuscitation. In later stages, as fluids are given and as water and electrolytes are retained, extravascular fluid and electrolyte depletion is less likely to be a problem.

The crystalloid/colloid controversy remains important as practice varies widely throughout the world depending upon which view is taken. A balanced appraisal is difficult as most of the available research and reviews on this subject fall strongly into one camp or the other. Both types of fluid when used appropriately are, however, highly effective. It is commonly believed that the rapidity of effective resuscitation is far more important than the type of fluid used.

ABNORMALITIES OF WATER BALANCE

These are primarily a result of a deficiency or an excess of water and result in changes in the tonicity, but not necessarily the volume, of the ECF.

Water deficit

A primary deficit of water is commonly the result of a reduced intake, secondary to an inability to drink. Increased losses may also occur in central and nephrogenic diabetes insipidus. Water deficiency results in cellular dehydration as a result of increased ECF tonicity. Plasma volume remains normal until late. Water deficit is the commonest cause of hypernatraemia. Treatment is with 5% glucose solutions, although care is required if hypernatraemia is present as rapid rehydration will lead to cerebral oedema. Diagnosis is difficult and deficits may be up to 10 l.

Water excess

Water excess (increased TBW) is most commonly a result of administration of free water (5% glucose, 4% glucose–0.18% sodium chloride or 1.5% glycine irrigation during transurethral surgery). It causes hyponatraemia which is rarely a result of sodium loss. Hyponatraemia may also occur with the syndrome of inappropriate antidiuretic hormone secretion which occurs with certain tumours, central nervous system disorders and pulmonary sepsis. Excessive ADH secretion also occurs in the perioperative period.

The treatment of hyponatraemia depends on its duration. Asymptomatic chronic hyponatraemia of greater than three days duration is treated with fluid restriction aiming to correct the sodium level slowly (< 12 mmol l^{-1} day^{-1}). Central pontine myelinolysis is a complication of rapid correction of chronic hyponatraemia. Acute hyponatraemia of less than three days duration is usually iatrogenic. Treatment may proceed more rapidly and increase in the plasma sodium level of 24 mmol l^{-1} day^{-1} is acceptable: 0.9% sodium chloride is given and diuretics are used to excrete the water excess. Hypertonic sodium chloride solutions have been used, not because sodium is deficient, but to increase plasma tonicity and reduce the development of cerebral oedema. Complications of acute restoration of plasma sodium levels are of fluid overload (increased ECF volume) secondary to excessive sodium administration.

ABNORMALITITES OF SODIUM BALANCE

These are primarily a result of a deficit, or an excess, of salt and result in changes in the volume, but not necessarily the tonicity of the ECF. The concentration of sodium in the plasma indicates the amount of water relative to the amount of sodium. Hypernatraemia results in contracted ICF volume and hyponatraemia results in an expanded ICF volume.

Salt deficit

A primary deficit of salt is usually a result of increased loss of either salt alone, or salt and water with water replacement. It may occur with diarrhoea, Addisons disease, diabetic ketoacidosis, with ascites and in cases of chronic renal failure. Salt deficiency results in an early reduction in the volume of the ECF, and consequently the circulating blood volume, with haemoconcentration and increased blood urea. Intracellular dehydration does not occur. The clinical picture is of early circulatory failure. It is important to appreciate that it is the total amount of salt in the ECF which is of importance here. There may be little change in the plasma sodium concentration. Sodium deficiency leads to water loss as a compensatory mechanism, whereas sodium excess leads to water retention and oedema. Treatment is with 0.9% sodium chloride solution and losses may be up to 10 l, although considerable circulatory disturbance will occur with losses in excess of 4 l.

Changes in arterial pressure and heart rate are late signs and visual impressions of perfusion and hydration (skin turgor) are non-specific and difficult to quantify as signs of hypovolaemia. The use of central venous monitoring should be undertaken when in doubt, although this is insensitive with relatively large changes being required to show an effect. Where hypovolaemia is suspected, it is important to assess the response of the patient to repeated fluid boluses rather than to consider a single set of signs or values. Over a timescale of days sequential measurement of the patient's weight is an invaluable aid to the assessment of overall fluid balance.

Salt excess

This is usually the result of intravenous administration of hypertonic sodium chloride or 8.4% sodium bicarbonate. The ECF is expanded and intracellular dehydration occurs.

PERIOPERATIVE FLUID BALANCE

Preoperative fluid balance

Many patients will present for anaesthesia with an existing fluid deficit. Preoperative starvation without intravenous supplementation will result in a deficit equal to the maintenance requirements for the time involved (approximately 115 ml h^{-1} in adults). Despite recent trends to reduce times of preoperative fasting, many patients still present having starved for considerably longer than 6 h. Patients receiving 'bowel prep' may have lost large volumes of both fluid and electrolyte in addition to the preoperative fast. The condition for which the patient requires surgery may also have an effect on fluid balance. Gastrointestinal losses may be both external (vomit, fistulae and diarrhoea) and internal, for example into the gut lumen in intestinal obstruction. Careful preoperative assessment is required to identify and anticipate these losses. Sick patients with peritonitis or bowel obstruction are often seriously depleted and will need resuscitation before surgery in a high dependency environment with close monitoring and repeated evaluation of their response. Patients with lesser degrees of deficit are often missed, however, and are at risk of hypotension with intravenous induction of anaesthesia and/or epidural anaesthesia. Many of these situations will have evolved over hours allowing some plasma refill to occur. Consequently, an extracellular deficit may exist in addition to a deficit of plasma volume.

Intraoperative fluid balance

The salient points of intraoperative fluid management are to ensure that pre-existing deficits have been corrected, to continue with maintenance requirements and to replace on-going losses. Baseline water is required. The following formula has been used: 4 ml kg^{-1} h^{-1} for the first 10 kg, plus 2 ml kg^{-1} h^{-1} for the second 10 kg, plus 1 ml kg^{-1} h^{-1} for each kilogram thereafter. This results in an hourly rate of 115 ml h^{-1} in a 75 kg adult. This is sufficient to account for an insensible loss of 500–1000 ml day^{-1} and a urine output in excess of 1000 ml day^{-1}. Requirements of sodium and potassium are 50–150 and 40–80 mmol day^{-1} respectively. Intraoperative infusion of 120 ml h^{-1} of 4% glucose–0.18% sodium chloride solution will achieve this aim for water and sodium. Quite apart from replacement of coincidental blood loss, surgical trauma will increase the amount of fluid required by increasing tissue losses and other sequestration of fluid. This deficit will be manifest in both interstitial and intravascular compartments. Replacement of 3–4 ml kg^{-1} h^{-1} is suggested for minimal surgical trauma increasing to 5–6 ml kg^{-1} h^{-1} for moderate surgical trauma and 7–8 ml kg^{-1} h^{-1} for severe surgical trauma. In many USA centres these amounts will be give as balanced electrolyte solution as resuscitation of the interstitial space is considered paramount. If colloids are used to replace the plasma volume, losses that will occur as a result of fluid sequestration, smaller volumes than these will be required.

Intraoperative fluid losses may be overt of covert. Operative blood loss is usually obvious, but is notoriously difficult to measure, and is often underestimated. Large volumes may lie undetected in body cavities, on large swabs or under drapes. Large losses of fluid also occur into the gut during laparotomy, particularly when the gut is operated on. There will also be losses into tissues as oedema (third space losses).

Postoperative fluid balance

Again in the postoperative period, pre-existing fluid deficits must be corrected, maintenance fluid requirements must be administered, and ongoing losses must be identified and treated. Pre-existing fluid requirements will arise from inadequate replacement in the operating theatre. In practice it is difficult for these to be accounted for after the event by surgical house staff on the ward and they are a common cause of difficulty. In order to minimize this problem, intraoperative fluid deficits should be corrected as far as possible before the patient leaves the recovery room and careful recording of intraoperative fluid balance including urine output and blood loss is imperative. Even so, to those not accustomed to fluid balance problems during major surgery, the patients will invariably appear on paper to be in a large positive balance whilst often being hypovolaemic. The problem is compounded by the unreliability of clinical signs. Water and electrolytes will be lost both in urine, which must be measured hourly, and as insensible losses. Losses of fluid will occur into the gut particularly following laparotomy if an ileus is present. Measured nasogastric, faecal and fistulae losses may be only a small part of fluid sequestered in this way. The development of 'third space' oedema is usually an intraoperative event but may account for 'lost' fluid in the postoperative period.

Another cause of postoperative hypovolaemia, which may not be obvious to the surgical house staff, is the limited persistence of the plasma volume expansion of colloids administered intraoperatively. Gelatins have a volume expansion half-life of only 3 h and even etherified starches have a limited duration of action. Consequently, large deficits in plasma volume which were apparently well corrected in the recovery room may reappear several hours later.

Retention of sodium and water occurs in the perioperative period as a result of the stress response to major surgery. In practice, the main problem that commonly results is hyponatraemia consequent on administration of low sodium crystalloid solutions, for example 4% glucose–0.18% sodium chloride, which only contains 30 mmol of sodium per litre. Even though two litres of this solution given over 24 h contains more (60 mmol) than the maintenance requirement (50 mmol) of sodium, 80% (1600 ml) of the water is free and as this is also retained, dilutional hyponatraemia results. Careful monitoring of the plasma sodium level is clearly important in the perioperative period.

HAEMORRHAGE

The effect of haemorrhage depends on both the quantity and rate of blood loss. Acute haemorrhage can be divided into four classes. Class I (up to 15% of blood volume) produces minimal physiological changes and does not require treatment in isolation. Class II (15–30% of blood volume) is associated with a slight increase in heart rate, mild tachypnoea, postural hypotension and a narrow pulse pressure. Cardiac output is reduced but a compensatory increase in systemic and pulmonary vascular resistance occurs. Fluid therapy is required. Class III (30–40% of blood volume) is associated with tachycardia, tachypnoea, reduced systolic blood pressure and changes in mental status. Fluid and blood will be required. Class IV (> 40% of blood volume) is associated with tachycardia, marked hypotension, anuria, depressed conscious level and poor peripheral perfusion. Immediate fluid and blood transfusion with surgical intervention will be required. In all the above cases, pre-existing or ongoing fluid deficits will reduce the amount of blood loss required to elicit the above signs. Oedema and 'third space' losses following certain types of injury will increase the fluid requirement.

As a result of the risk of transmitting infection, transfusion of blood and blood products is now minimized wherever possible. This is particularly the case in USA although practice is rapidly changing in the UK also. Initial therapy in haemorrhage is with fluids (either crystalloid or colloid), blood (or red blood cells) only being required in class III and IV haemorrhage. In cases where blood loss is rapidly curtailed, some cases of class III haemorrhage can be managed without blood, although the haematocrit may fall as low as 20%.

The prime objective of fluid therapy is rapidly to restore organ and tissue perfusion. In the USA where trauma management was pioneered, balanced electrolyte solutions are used. These are distributed throughout the extracellular compartment and three or more volumes per volume of shed blood will be required (three to one rule). When crystalloids are given in large volumes to treat haemorrhagic shock, the parenchymal (perimicrovascular) interstitial subcompartment becomes saturated and lymph drainage becomes maximal. Massive losses into the loose binding connective tissue then occur without effective lymphatic salvage. As a result of this, the volume of crystalloid required to replace a given blood loss becomes much greater than three to one when the blood loss is greater than 40% of blood volume (Class IV).

Trauma with blood loss is often accompanied by hypotension, hypothermia and massive transfusion. It is not surprising, therefore, that widespread tissue injury may occur as a result. The effect of mediators released in response to injury and sepsis is to increase microvascular permeability, whereupon fluid flux will be much greater at lower hydrostatic pressures. The capacity of the perimicrovascular lymphatics will be exceeded after the administration of smaller amounts of crystalloids with accumulation of fluid as both systemic and pulmonary oedema. Colloids, unfortunately, offer little advantage in this situation as most molecules will pass through the leaky capillaries. A logical approach would be to use a mixture of crystalloids and long acting colloids (starches). This would enable the interstitial space to be resuscitated without excessive contribution to third space losses. Long acting colloids would restore plasma volume more rapidly and effectively, particularly with large volume losses (> 40% of blood volume). Again it cannot be over emphasized that rapid resuscitation with continuous re-evaluation and assessment of continuing losses is far more important than the type of fluid used.

FLUID BALANCE IN THE CRITICALLY ILL PATIENT

Fluid balance in the critically ill patient follows principles outlined earlier with respect to correcting deficits, treating ongoing losses and maintenance requirements. Fluid therapy will, however, be required for longer periods of time in the face of cardiovascular and renal insufficiency. Close monitoring and frequent reassessment is therefore required. The effect of fluid overload on pulmonary function is also of concern. Losses of water and electrolytes may be treated with crystalloids. Colloids are more appropriate for replacement of plasma volume deficit.

The major difference affecting fluid therapy

in this group of patients is the development of 'leaky capillaries'. Increased permeability of the microvascular endothelium is common as critical illness progresses. It occurs, for example, as part of the systemic inflammatory response syndrome and also in acute lung injury which are final common pathways to a variety of insults, in particular, sepsis and impaired oxygen delivery. Histamine, bradykinin, leukotrienes, platelet activating factor and endotoxin are among the many mediators involved. There may be direct receptor mediated activation of endothelial cell contractile elements which opens up gaps. Tumour necrosis factor, a prominent mediator in sepsis, produces a reversible change in pore size by a G-protein transduction mechanism. Also, acting in synergy with changes in permeability, alterations in local haemodynamics occur resulting from impaired autoregulation. This negates the 'shutdown' of certain capillary beds and thus increases the total surface area of leaking endothelium.

Leaky capillaries result in the passage of colloid molecules through the microvascular endothelium. This affects the Starling equation as $\Delta\Pi$ and σ will both be reduced to the extent that oncotic pressure becomes increasingly unimportant in determining fluid fluxes. Consequently, the hydrostatic pressure gradient becomes of primary importance. The control of fluid fluxes in the lung is of particular interest in view of its effect on gas exchange which must be maintained to avoid pathophysiological processes which will exacerbate microvascular leakage (see above).

In the critically ill patient the use of crystalloids is justified for maintenance and when a deficit of water and/or electrolytes is present, for example after gastrointestinal losses. Most patients in the intensive care unit will not have an interstitial fluid deficit and indeed oedema is common. Administration of large volumes of crystalloid in an attempt to increase plasma volume will result in overloading of the perimicrovascular zone and its lymphatic drainage with flooding of the loose connective tissue. However, the use of colloids in the critically ill patient also presents problems. The leak of colloid molecules into the interstitium may result in fluid trapping with the development of unresolving oedema. However, it has been shown that when resuscitating critically ill patients, haemodynamic variables are improved with colloids in preference to crystalloids, increasing oxygen delivery and minimizing the pathophysiological changes associated with unresolved shock.

An exciting development in fluid therapy in the presence of 'leaky capillaries' has been the use of pentrafraction starch solutions where the majority of osmotically active particles are larger than pore size, even in the critically ill patient. It has been suggested that they may be able to plug the holes in the microvascular endothelium. They are not, however, currently in clinical use.

BURNS (Chapter 26)

Thermal injury results in a reduction in blood volume secondarily to loss of plasma at the site of the burn. This loss is proportional to the size of the area burned. In addition there is increased capillary permeability with sequestration of intravascular fluid, electrolytes and protein into the interstitium with oedema and haemoconcentration. Attention to fluid resuscitation is vital, particularly when the area of the burn is greater than 20% of body surface area. A variety of regimens have been suggested but all may underestimate losses. There is a need to monitor the cardiovascular response closely and attempt to maintain the urine output at 50 ml h^{-1}. Invasive monitoring is vital to avoid persistent hypovolaemia. Maintenance fluids are required in addition to the plasma deficit replacement. The extent of evaporative water loss is dependent on how the burn is dressed, but may be up to 2 ml kg^{-1} h^{-1}. This should be given as 5% glucose and be sufficient to prevent hypernatraemia.

Most regimens suggest a volume of fluid replacement in the first 24 h after the burn of 2–4 ml kg^{-1} × percentage burn surface area. Half of this volume is given in the first 8 h with the remainder given in the next 16 h. Whether crystalloid or colloid are given depends upon prevailing practices. Many centres in the UK and Europe use entirely human albumin solution for this purpose. The value of colloids has, however, been questioned during the early post-burn period as capillary leakage is maximal in the first 8–12 h. It has been suggested that plasma volume resuscitation with colloids should start towards the end of the 24 h period with crystalloids used before this. Initial haemoconcentration will give way to haemodilution as resuscitation proceeds, particularly with full thickness burns. Red blood cells are transfused to a haematocrit of 30% and are usually necessary in proportion to the amount of full thickness burn. After the first 24 h, normal principles of fluid balance apply and a large diuresis is often seen.

FURTHER READING

Baron, J.-F. (ed) (1992) *Plasma Volume Expansion* Arnette, Paris.

Carrico, C. J., Canizaro, P. C. and Shires, G. T. (1976) Fluid resuscitation following injury: rationale for the use of balanced salt solutions. *Critical Care Medicine*, **4**, 46–54.

Halperin, M. L., and Goldstein, M.B. (1994) *Fluid, Electrolyte, and Acid–Base physiology*. WB Saunders Company, Philadelphia.

Harrison, R. A. and Rampton, A. J. (1988) Colloid–crystalloid controversy, in *Anaesthesia Review 5* (ed. L. Kaufman) Churchill-Livingstone, London, pp 101–118.

Ledingham, I. M. A. and Ramsey, G. (1986) Hypovolaemic shock *British Journal of Anaesthesia*, **58**, 169–189.

Soni, N. (1995) Wonderful albumin? Not all it is cracked up to be *British Medical Journal*, **310**, 887–888.

Twigley, A. J. and Hillman, K. M. (1985) The end of the crystalloid era? *Anaesthesia*, **40**, 860–871.

MASSIVE HAEMORRHAGE, BLOOD CLOTTING AND REPLACEMENT

D. Royston

Bleeding remains a considerable cause of mortality and morbidity. This is related to both the effects of loss of blood and also the effects of infusions of products aimed at compensating for the loss. This chapter will focus on the early problems associated with the loss of blood volume and constituents associated with massive bleeding, and transfusion practice to replace these losses. It will only mention briefly the late effects of blood transfusions.

DEFINING THE PROBLEM

Bleeding after surgery is not unusual: it is a integral part of any surgical procedure. A definition of abnormal bleeding will depend upon the surgeon and type of surgery. It is obvious that 2 or 3 ml loss in middle ear surgery may compromise the success of the operation, and an intracerebral bleed of less than 1% of the blood volume will have a significant, usually catastrophic, effect on the patient. This article will focus on those situations in which substantial volumes of fluid or red cell replacement are likely to be required over a few hours as a result of major bleeding that may prove difficult to control surgically.

Massive transfusion is usually defined as transfusion of blood, blood products and fluids equivalent to the circulating blood volume in any 24 h period. This definition will obviously encompass both patients who have a slow, but continuous, loss over the 24 h period and those who lose their circulating volume within minutes. Although similar physiological, haematological and biochemical changes will occur in response to this loss and its replacement, the most profound effects occur in those who have the most rapid loss and replacement therapy.

MORTALITY AND BLEEDING: THE 'AT RISK' POPULATION

The need for massive transfusion in non-surgical patients is most often seen during losses from the gastrointestinal tract. Bleeding due to ulceration of the mucosa and vascular–enteric fistula are most common, and bleeding from oesophageal varices following hepatic failure is particularly difficult to control. The major problem for the anaesthetist in such cases is that the patient is usually referred for a surgical intervention when they have depleted compensatory systems with no further physiological responses to protect them during the period of anaesthesia and surgery.

Major bleeding and the need for massive transfusions is remarkably rare during most routine, elective surgery. However, three groups of other procedures are recognized as being associated with an increased likelihood of bleeding.

The first group comprises patients with normal haemostatic control having elective major surgery such as orthopaedic or vascular surgery. These procedures are usually performed in patients who can be 'optimized' before surgery in terms of circulation volume, oxygen carrying capacity and haemostatic functions.

In the second group are patients undergoing urgent operations and/or procedures that are causally associated with abnormalities of haemostasis and coagulation. Examples of this include the following.

- Abnormal activation of platelets and deranged coagulation and fibrinolytic systems following cardiopulmonary bypass.
- Patients requiring liver transplantation have decreased concentrations of procoagulant factors and possibly thrombocytopoenia. In addition, in these patients there is a period of profound activation of the fibrinolytic system during the anhepatic phase of transplantation.
- Patients with malignant disease.

The most common alteration of haemostasis in malignancy is that of haemorrhage associated with thrombocytopenia, either drug- or radiation-induced, or from bone marrow invasion. However, thrombotic complications are also extremely common with malignancy. An active thrombotic tendency may present clinically as a consumptive coagulopathy or disseminated intravascular coagulation (DIC). Haemorrhage resulting from DIC is quite common and may present as bleeding, thrombosis, thromboembolus, or any combination. Certain tumour types give a greater risk of a haemorrhage as a consequence of a consumptive coagulopathy. For example, about 40% of patients with prostate cancer and one in fourteen women with ovarian carcinoma will show evidence of a coagulopathy on biochemical analysis. In these women, there was significant bleeding in about two-thirds of those with evidence of consumption.

The third group comprises patients who represent the true emergency of the rapidly bleeding patient requiring resuscitation before any intervention. In this category are patients with trauma, rupture or dissection of the aorta, and during pregnancy and the puerperium. These patients represent an enormous challenge and are associated with a poor outcome. For example, emergency surgery for rupture of the aorta carries an overall mortality of about 50%. Motor vehicle trauma has certainly decreased in its prevalence but the mortality remains high. More commonly urban violence associated with knife and gunshot injuries is a significant cause of acute bleeding. Bleeding associated with pregnancy, while representing a small total number, remains a significant cause of maternal mortality which has obvious huge social implications for the child(ren) and partner of the deceased.

QUANTIFYING THE LOSS

MEASUREMENT OF BLOOD LOSS

During surgery, blood loss is traditionally estimated by methods such as weighing swabs and measurement of blood aspirated into the suction apparatus. With major haemorrhage, the value of these methods is questionable. A considerable amount of blood is inevitably spilled onto the drapes, floor and surgeons. In traumatized patients, a large loss of blood may have occurred before arrival in hospital, or more likely will be concealed in the limbs and pelvis at the site of fractures, or in the chest or abdomen. All this will result in a gross underestimate of the true blood loss, with consequent inadequate replacement.

Rather than relying on such estimates of blood loss, patients should be transfused according to measured cardiovascular variables such as heart rate, arterial pressure, central

Table 41.1 Physiological effects of blood loss

	Blood loss (ml)			
	≤750	750–1500	1500–2000	≥2000
Loss as percentage of blood volume (%)	≤15	15–30	30–40	≥40
Heart rate (b.p.m.)	<100	>100	>120	≥140
Blood pressure	Normal	Normal	Decreased	Decreased
Pulse pressure	Normal	Decreased	Decreased	Decreased
Capillary 'blanch'	Normal	Slowed	Slowed	Slowed
Respiratory rate (breaths per min)	14–20	20–30	30–35	≥35
Urine output (ml h^{-1})	>30	20–30	5–15	Negligible
Mental status	Slightly anxious	Mild Anxiety	Confused	Lethargic
Suggested volume replacement	Crystalloid	Crystalloid/colloid	Blood	Blood

venous pressure, pulmonary capillary wedge pressure, cardiac output, oxygen delivery and oxygen consumption. As a simple rule of thumb, a young patient with an unexplained tachycardia is hypovolaemic. The measurement of PCV (packed cell volume, haematocrit) and blood lactate concentrations may also be helpful.

PHYSIOLOGICAL EFFECTS OF HAEMORRHAGE

Loss of circulating blood volume is compensated for by a number of physiological mechanisms. There is activation of the sympathetic and hypothalamic–pituitary–adrenal axis to increase vascular tone and decrease the size of the venous reservoir. There is some contraction of the splanchic blood volume and a redistribution of blood flow away from nonvital organs. These compensatory mechanisms will maintain the blood supply to vital organs initially, but unless adequate and appropriate corrective measures are taken, these mechanisms will decompensate. Compensatory mechanisms, which are brisk and sustained in young, healthy adults, will be less efficacious at the extremes of life and may be impaired by disease or medication.

At later stages, and with increasing volumes of loss, there is an increase in heart rate, decrease in stroke volume, reduced pulse pressure, increased respiratory rate and reduction in cerebral blood flow leading to a reduction in conscious level. An estimate of when these changes in vital signs may occur in relation to the volume loss from the circulation is shown in Table 41.1.

A number of other physiological events occur during the period of haemorrhage which may be of importance to the anaesthetist. In particular, animal studies show that a significant reduction in tone of the lower oesophageal sphincter occurs with haemorrhagic shock.

PRINCIPLES OF MANAGEMENT

For operations where increased blood loss is anticipated, replacement therapy should be available in advance of surgery. A variety of protocols and check lists have been designed and published to suggest appropriate quantities of blood and blood products to crossmatch and order before elective procedures. Management is more difficult in situations where rapid transfusions of substantial volumes of fluids, red cells and blood products are likely over a short time as a result of major bleeding which cannot be controlled immediately.

The five steps in the management of blood loss are the following.

- Restore and maintain a circulating fluid volume and maintain organ perfusion: classically shown as a continuing urine output.
- Call for the help of colleagues appropriate to the case.
- Achieve surgical control of bleeding.
- Maintain adequate blood oxygen transport capacity.
- Perform a coagulation screen to help guide blood component therapy should bleeding persist after attempted surgical haemostasis.

CONSEQUENCES OF MASSIVE BLEEDING

There are three principal consequences of major bleeding which will be considered in more detail in this section. These are loss of circulating volume, loss of circulating oxygen carrying capacity, and loss of haemostatic function.

Each aspect produces its own effects and requires different algorithms and approaches to therapy. In the clinical setting, however, these problems, and the appropriate reaction to them, occur simultaneously.

LOSS OF CIRCULATING VOLUME AND ITS REPLACEMENT

The rapid and effective restoration of an adequate circulating blood volume (to maintain tissue perfusion and oxygen delivery) is an important part of the early management of major haemorrhage. However, recent evidence has suggested that the duration of shock, at least in younger patients following blunt trauma or gunshot wound, is not related to a worsening of outcome. Indeed, there are now suggestions that fluid resuscitation is best delayed until surgical control of bleeding is established in these circumstances.

With major, but planned surgery, it is obviously mandatory to replace all losses from the intravascular space as quickly as possible. This is especially true in the anaesthetized patient as the compensatory mechanisms outlined above are reduced or prevented by the anaesthetic agents and adjuncts, and the patient will decompensate more quickly. This is especially true in elderly patients who tolerate blood loss extremely poorly.

Venous access and other monitoring

The first requirement is to establish adequate venous access by placing a large-bore cannula to allow rapid fluid administration. The diameter of the cannula and the ability to apply a continuous pressure of about 300 mmHg, via a pressurized infusion system, are the most important pre-determinants of the flow rate of fluid. With a 14 G cannula and 300 mmHg pressure a flow rate of crystalloid of 600 ml min^{-1} can be achieved.

There is little evidence that the use of manual compression of the ball chamber on a giving set or the use of manual roller pumps (Martins pump) significantly accelerates the flow rate of fluid. If a dedicated pressure infusion system is not available then the author has used a series of blood pressure cuffs inflated with the automatic tourniquet found in most orthopaedic theatres as a makeshift device.

When a massive transfusion is anticipated during surgery, at least two large-gauge venous cannulae (12 G if possible) should be inserted, solely for transfusion purposes. In addition, an arterial cannula and central venous catheter may prove useful, allowing rapid blood sampling, for acid–base and potassium status, and direct measurement of arterial and central venous pressures, respectively. There is little evidence to suggest that the insertion of a central venous pressure catheter is helpful in the initial stages of any resuscitation, or blood loss. However, there is no doubt that such monitoring can be useful in certain planned procedures where blood loss is going to be a major factor, for example transplant procedures (heart, lung, liver) and also major orthopaedic and certain neurosurgical operations.

The central venous catheter also provides access for intermittent bolus administration of drugs, or drug infusions. If massive uncontrolled loss is anticipated, such as from a ruptured aorta or during transplantation, it may be prudent to establish the central venous access with either the sheath introducer normally used for insertion of flow-directed pulmonary artery catheters or the catheter normally inserted to allow continuous haemofiltration. This latter catheter has two 12 G lumina and flow rates of 2 l min^{-1} can be achieved using a rapid infusion device or mechanical roller pump. The sheath introducer will allow a pulmonary artery catheter to be inserted, when indicated. As in the case of the central venous pressures the use of complex cardiovascular monitoring with flow directed catheters from the outset of surgery has had no discernible impact on the outcome after major blood loss and trauma.

In the acutely hypovolaemic patient the same rules apply: at least two large-gauge i.v. cannulae should be inserted into appropriately sized veins, usually in the antecubital fossae. If peripheral venous access is difficult, a cannula may be inserted into a large, central vein such as the subclavian, internal jugular or femoral vein. Alternatively, a venous cut down may be performed on the saphenous vein at the ankle.

There are obviously other consequences of the rapid infusion of large volumes of fluid and these should be anticipated. The solutions should be warmed, and regular measurements of acid–base and potassium concentrations in arterial blood may be needed. Unless contraindicated by pelvic or urethral injury, a urethral catheter should be passed and urine output monitored. In addition, central temperature should be recorded.

A separate, and clear, set of guidelines has been described for obstetric bleeding. The report of the confidential enquiry into maternal death 1988–1990 (published in 1994) has the following paragraphs of relevance to the anaesthetist.

- Summon all the extra staff required, including obstetricians, midwives and nurses. In particular the duty anaesthetic registrar should be contacted immediately as in most obstetric units the anaesthetists will take over the management of the fluid replacement. Alert the haematologist and the blood transfusion service who should be asked to be fully involved in the case as soon as possible. Make sure porters are available and warned that they will be required at short notice.
- At least two peripheral infusion lines should be set up using cannulae of not less than 14 G. Central venous pressure (CVP) monitoring should immediately be set up since it helps ensure that therapy is safely controlled. Central venous pressure should be continuously displayed and a display of intra-arterial pressure is also extremely useful.

This second paragraph sets out a standard of care which is ideal but not always attainable. In particular, the provision of invasive monitoring in obstetric units is not usually a high priority. Similarly the duty anaesthetist, while taking responsibility for the fluid management, is also usually busy with the processes of anaesthesia and airway protection.

Blood warming and rapid infusions

The requirements of a transfusion system for the management of major haemorrhage include the ability to transfuse blood at fast flow rates (up to 500 ml min^{-1}) and at temperatures greater than 35°C. Some systems use a constant-pressure infusion device combined with an efficient blood warmer and a purpose-designed blood-warming coil. Counter current aluminium heat exchangers have also been found to be effective. Priming or flushing blood through the system following fluids containing calcium (such as compound sodium lactate and Haemaccel) should be avoided, as this has been suggested as a cause of blood clot formation in the tubing by reversal of the anticoagulant effect of citrate.

The Haemonetics Rapid Infuser device is a purpose built, specialist instrument not available in most centres. It has a 3 l reservoir into which cell-saved or banked blood and blood products can be stored, warmed and infused at rates of up to 2 l min^{-1}. The system also incorporates a blood filter, air detector and heat exchanger, and in expert hands can be prepared for use in a short time, typically 5–10 min.

Initial resuscitation: crystalloid or colloid?

The success of initial resuscitation in the acutely hypovolaemic patient probably depends more upon adequacy of repletion than upon which fluids are used: anaemia is better than hypovolaemia. This is especially true in the anaesthetized patient who will have reduced tissue oxygen consumption as a consequence of the anaesthetic, but tolerates hypovolaemia poorly for the same reason.

The debate continues as to the best fluid for initial resuscitation. It is accepted that for a given blood volume expansion about 1.5–2 times the volume of crystalloid compared to colloid is required. There are no controlled trials to show that the outcome in patients resuscitated with albumin is superior to other colloid solutions (gelatins, dextrans or hydroxyethyl starch). Indeed in the majority of studies, the type of fluid administered did not influence outcome. It is not known, however, if there are any identifiable subgroups of patients in whom the choice of replacement fluid is important. Several such groups have been suggested including the elderly, those with low colloid osmotic pressures and poor wound healing, patients suffering from anaphylactic shock and those with non-cardiogenic pulmonary oedema. In practice, however, combined therapy using both crystalloids and colloids is often used, and has been shown to produce better results in experimental shock models than the use of either colloid or crystalloid alone.

Synthetic colloid solutions suffer from two potential drawbacks. First there is a small, but well documented, incidence of anaphylactic reaction to these agents. The incidence is higher for the modified gelatins than the starch-based agents. Since 1979, the manufacturers of the gelatin solutions have reduced the amounts of hexamethylene diisocyanate in their preparations and claim a reduction in the incidence of allergic reaction. However, there have been no studies large enough to prove that the incidence of these reactions has fallen and severe allergic reactions continue to be reported.

The second problem is the effects of these agents on the haemostatic and coagulation systems. Administration of large volumes of colloid will decrease the concentration of clotting factors by haemodilution. Manufacturers of Haemaccel recommend that only 1500 ml of this colloid is given in any 24 h period. If more is infused then there should be regular measurement of clotting function. In addition, dextran solutions interfere with normal platelet functions. Both hydroxyethylstarch and dextran reduce factor VIII concentration to a greater extent than haemodilution, and both are incorporated into the fibrin fibres during their formation. This has been suggested as a possible cause of increased bleeding as the resulting large, bulky clots are subject to enhanced fibrinolysis and easier breakdown.

Haemodilution may have effects on the anaesthetic also by altering the pharmacokinetics of the drug or by modification of protein binding. Of especial interest is the effect of haemodilution on the neuromuscular blocking drugs. (Table 41.2).

Table 41.2 Effects of haemodilution (haematocrit <22%) on the potency of neuromuscular blocking drugs (mg kg^{-1})

	Control ED$_{50}$	Haemodilution ED$_{50}$
Suxamethonium	0.236+0.092	0.085+0.024
Pancuronium	0.027+0.006	0.011+0.003
d-Tubocurarine	0.270+0.062	0.126+0.037

LOSS OF CIRCULATING OXYGEN CARRYING CAPACITY

Red cell transfusions are given to increase the haemoglobin concentration and thus increase, or normalize, the delivery of oxygen to the tissues. The question to address at this stage is what would be an appropriate haemoglobin value to ensure this process. Is there such an ideal as 'the transfusion trigger'.

Although reduction of red cell mass results in decreased oxygen carrying capacity, compensatory mechanisms exist:

- increased venous oxygen extraction
- a shift of the oxygen dissociation curve to the right
- increased red cell 2,3-diphosphoglycerate (2,3DPG)
- increased cardiac output and tissue flow, in part due to decreased blood viscosity at lower haematocrit values.

In conditions such as the anaemia of chronic renal failure, many patients function relatively normally even at a concentration of haemoglobin which might impair the acutely anaemic.

Two factors should be considered in assessing a patient's tolerance to a reduced haemoglobin value. These can be broadly divided into discussing the lower and upper haemoglobin levels.

The lower haemoglobin level

The concentration of haemoglobin at which the patient's life, or well being, may be put at risk will guide the lower level. This will depend on the prejudices of the clinicians involved, the type of surgery and the presence or absence of anaesthesia. Clinical studies and reports suggest that the mortality from haemodilution is low in otherwise fit patients whose haemoglobin falls to around 5 g dl^{-1}, provided other aspects of supportive management such as fluid volume replacement and oxygen supply are correctly provided. Published experience on the results of surgery in Jehovah's Witnesses show that many patients, including the elderly, can survive major surgery with extremely low haemoglobin values. There are also reports from a number of centres where patients are allowed to become profoundly anaemic, but have anaesthesia maintained to minimize oxygen consumption. In this way the oxygen delivery, albeit at a very low haemoglobin concentration, is sufficient to meet the needs of the body.

If the patient is unable to compensate by raising cardiac output, if respiratory insufficiency impairs adequate oxygenation, or if metabolic changes due to systemic factors such as sepsis increase tissue oxygen requirements, life may well be jeopardized and transfusion warranted. Recent clinical studies with newer monitoring techniques indicate that ventricular function, haemodynamics and oxygen transport parameters can be maintained during haemodilution to 5 g dl^{-1}, even in elderly patients. Notwithstanding this evidence, older patients are more likely to have cardiorespiratory problems that could make haemodilution hazardous, and have less risk of reduced life expectation from late-onset complications of transfusion. It is therefore important to be cautious about setting very low haemoglobin thresholds for transfusion of elderly patients, as the risks of anaemia could well outweigh the risks of transfusion. For example, in patients having elective repair of abdominal aortic aneurysm a moderate haemodilution to haemoglobin ≤ 8.5 g dl^{-1} was associated with evidence of ischaemia. Higher haemoglobin values may therefore be needed if other variables (e.g. cardiac output), which determine tissue oxygen delivery, are jeopardized, or if tissue oxygen requirements are increased, for example by sepsis. There is currently little evidence to support the use of red cell transfusions unless the haemoglobin concentration falls below 8.5 g dl^{-1}, which is equivalent to an haematocrit of about 25%. It would therefore seem prudent to have this as the lower 'intent to transfuse' limit in all apart from the younger, fit patient.

The upper haemoglobin level

The concentration of haemoglobin at which the patient functions optimally will guide the upper limit for stopping administration of red cells. Perhaps the most complete data in this regard are from studies on the dose of erythropoietin required to achieve optimal well-being and quality of life indicators in chronic renal failure patients. A haemoglobin around 10 g dl^{-1} appeared to provide optimal function for most of these patients; further increases provided no extra benefits.

A postoperative haemoglobin of around 10 g dl^{-1} at the time of discharge is widely accepted as a general guideline figure in adult, surgical patients. However, it is more appropriate to base transfusion decisions on a clinical assessment of the patient. In the absence of any other change in practice, accurate targeting of red cell transfusion to a final, pre-discharge haemoglobin of 10 g dl^{-1} could lead to a substantial reduction in the use of red cells by surgical units without exposing patients to unconventionally low haemoglobin values.

There are some special circumstances where increasing the haemoglobin concentration may contribute to improving haemostasis. It is well recognized that patients with uraemia, in which platelet function is deranged, have less haemostatic defects (shown by a normalization of their bleeding time) if their haemoglobin concentration is increased.

Table 41.3 Guidelines for red blood cell transfusions

Symptomatic anaemia in a normovolaemic patient, regardless of Hb value
Preoperative haemoglobin ≤8.5 g dl^{-1} together with a procedure associated with major blood loss
Acute blood loss ≥15% of estimated blood volume
Acute blood loss with evidence of inadequate oxygen delivery

It is possible that patients with low platelet counts, or those taking platelet-active medication before surgery, may benefit from an increase in haemoglobin concentration above that necessary purely to increase oxygen delivery. There are no data, however, to support this notion apart from those patients with renal impairment.

All the above statements assume that normovolaemia is maintained by infusion of fluids, other than blood, and that necessary supportive therapy is given.

Guidlines for the transfusion of red blood cells are shown in Table 41.3.

Red cell production and crossmatching

Red cells are available in a variety of forms, but are usually supplied as plasma reduced or 'packed cells', of whole blood. Blood is collected from the donor into bags containing an anticoagulant and cell preservation agents. The anticoagulant mainly used relies on removing ionized calcium from the plasma, thus inhibiting thrombin generation. This anticoagulant action does not, however, preserve platelet or certain clotting factor activity as discussed later. Transfusion of blood is not without hazard. Many blood bank personnel quote the adage that the best transfusion is no transfusion. Included in the short to medium term hazards associated with the administration of blood are clerical and administration errors, infection, febrile reactions, anaphyl-

Table 41.4 ABO compatibility for whole blood, red cells and plasma: ●=compatible

Recipient	Donor					
	A	B	O	AB	Rh+ve	Rh−ve
Whole blood						
A	●					
B		●				
O			●			
AB				●		
Rh+ve					●	●
Rh−ve						●
Red blood cells						
A	●		●			
B		●	●			
O			●			
AB	●	●	●	●		
Rh+ve					●	●
Rh−ve						●
Plasma						
A	●			●		
B		●		●		
O	●	●	●	●		
AB				●		
Rh+ve					●	●
Rh−ve						●

axis, haemolytic transfusion reactions and immunosuppression.

The supply of blood and blood products has been put into the same stringent production category as ethical pharmaceutical manufacture by the regulatory authorities in North America. Currently mandated testing or screening of donor blood includes antibodies directed against HIV-I, HIV-2, HTLV I/II, hepatitis B core antigen (anti-HBc) and hepatitis C (anti-HCV), as well as hepatitis B surface antigen (HBsAg), alanine aminotransferase (ALT), and a serologic test for syphilis. These tests have been introduced gradually, mostly during the 1980s.

Patients should receive ABO- and Rh-identical blood whenever possible. Whole blood, which contains both red cells and plasma, must always be ABO-identical. For other components, transfusion of ABO- and Rh compatible, but not identical, blood is a reasonable transfusion option. ABO compatibility considerations differ for red cells and plasma, Table 41.4. Type O donor red cells, because they lack both the A and B antigen, are not susceptible to haemolysis from either anti-A or anti-B. If necessary, type O red cells can be given to any patient with major trauma or other life-threatening bleeding when there is not enough time to wait for pretransfusion testing. Type O patients, however, can only receive type O blood products, because their natural anti-A and anti-B will destroy red cells of any other ABO type. Rh compatibility depends on the patient's Rh type and whether anti-D is present. Rh-positive patients can receive either Rh-positive or Rh-negative blood products. Rh-negative patients who have formed anti-D must receive Rh-negative blood. In an emergency, Rh negative patients who lack anti-D can be given Rh positive blood, although anti-

D sensitization of female children and women of childbearing age could cause haemolytic disease of the new-born with obstetric complications. Rh-immune globulin (RhIG) can prevent the formation of anti-D if administered within 72 h after exposure to Rh-positive red cells. Rh-negative patients should receive Rh-negative blood.

When major bleeding occurs, blood samples for measurement of haemoglobin concentration, platelet count, prothrombin time (PT), activated partial thromboplastin time (APTT) and fibrinogen concentration should be sent immediately to the laboratory, together with a warning of the urgent need for blood for transfusion. When unexpected major haemorrhage occurs and blood is required rapidly, uncrossmatched blood may be requested urgently (this assumes the patient's blood group is known and the presence of atypical antibodies has been excluded). In this situation compatibility testing simply involves checking the ABO and D group of the units before transfusion. However, in cases where the blood group of the patient is not known, O Rhesus Negative blood may be infused initially, before changing to ABO-specific blood when the patient's blood group has been identified.

This is especially relevant in obstetric emergencies. The confidential enquiry into maternal mortality for the years 1988–1990 showed that haemorrhage was responsible for about 10% of the deaths (22/238) during that period. In some of the deaths attributed to haemorrhage, delay in transfusion of red cells had been an important contributing factor. Both delay in delivery and reluctance to transfuse unmatched red cells, even in a desperate situation, seem to play a part. Reluctance to give uncrossmatched Group O negative blood to an exsanguinated patient, even when the blood is immediately available, presumably reflects an exaggerated perception of the risk of a severe reaction. Military experience involving transfusion of large numbers of casualties has shown that in young men, transfusion of uncrossmatched Group O Rh negative blood is reasonably safe. Even though young women are more likely to have red cell antibodies from previous pregnancies, the risks of uncrossmatched red cells are small when life is threatened by a massive bleed.

If at crossmatch, antibodies are known to be present and major haemorrhage is anticipated, sufficient antigen negative blood should be crossmatched in advance and reserved. However, if large supplies of antigen negative blood are not readily available, it may be necessary to use only ABO-compatible blood during the massive transfusion period. The antigen negative blood should then be given when the rate of blood loss has been substantially reduced. A record should be kept of the amount of blood and fluid given, including each unit number and blood group, as any transfusion reaction or transfusion-related infection requires identification and retrieval of the units responsible. In clinical practice, immunologically-mediated reactions to blood or blood products are rarely reported in patients having massive transfusions. The reason for this is not clear. The most likely reason is that a reaction may be overlooked in a critically ill patient or attributed to other causes. It is also conceivable there is dilution in the plasma resulting in low concentrations of circulating antibodies. Nevertheless, ABO-incompatible, haemolytic, transfusion reactions are the most common cause of acute fatalities because of blood transfusion. Clerical error is by far the most common cause for these reactions.

With regard to clerical errors, a recent survey of 245 hospital blood banks in the UK identified 111 incidents over a 24 month period in which patients were known to have received whole blood or red cells intended for another patient. Twelve of these incidents resulted in morbidity and six resulted in the patient's death. The principal error was reported to have occurred at the time of blood administration in 83: at the time of blood sample-taking in 23 and in the blood bank laboratory in 6. Two events were not reported and three cases were reported in more than one category. Another recent study in a large Scottish blood bank has revealed a minimum error rate of 5% in completion of request forms and labelling of sample tubes for compatibility testing. Published papers on transfusion errors report rates of error and mortality in other countries similar to those found in the UK.

This evidence of persisting problems in the implementation of procedural guidelines, leading to an unacceptable incidence of avoidable death and morbidity, provides compelling evidence to ensure that all procedures are followed in the handling of the unit(s) of blood product from the moment they leave the blood bank until transfusion to the patient is completed. Accurate recording of the transfusion of blood and products to the patients is an absolute necessity. During the early phase of a major bleeding episode there is often a conflict in priorities for the attention of the anaesthetists. In this case the task of checking and recording the fluids administered may be best delegated to other theatre personnel or assistants to ensure adequate recording and reduce the likelihood of a clerical error. It is normal practice for two people to check all blood when it first arrives in the operating theatre.

Intraoperative autotransfusion

If a major surgical procedure is planned then it is possible to decrease the amount of donor blood transfusions by reinfusing the patient's shed red cells. Autotransfusion, or autologous transfusion, is defined as the reinfusion of blood or blood products derived from the patient's own circulation. The main advantage of autotransfusion is that it avoids the complications associated with homologous transfusion. In addition, autologous blood may be the only option for some patients, especially those with rare blood phenotypes or those with rapid blood loss. It may also be acceptable to some patients who refuse transfusion of homologous blood on religious grounds, as systems have been described which ensure that the blood never leaves the 'circulation'.

Blood for reinfusion may be obtained from the patient either, by preoperative donation, or during operation by a process of blood salvage. In continental Europe this is a commonly practised method of blood conservation. However, because of fiscal restraint on the part of the government, there is no funding to support such endeavours inside the Health Service of the UK. Preoperative donation, involving either pre-deposit programmes or preoperative haemodilution, is an elective procedure and is not, therefore, of benefit in the management of unexpected, major haemorrhage.

Intraoperative autotransfusion using an automated cell saver system is of great value in decreasing the transfusion requirement for bank blood when a large blood loss occurs. In addition, the blood is compatible, has normal red cell concentrations of 2,3-diphosphoglycerate, is already warm and is available quickly. With such systems 'blood' is aspirated from the surgical field and collected via double-lumen suction lines where it is mixed with heparinized saline before transfer to a reservoir. The blood is filtered, centrifuged and washed with saline before resuspension in saline and transfer to a reinfusion bag at a haematocrit of usually more than 50%. The discarded supernatant solution contains debris from the surgical field, white blood cells, platelets, activated clotting factors, free plasma haemoglobin and anticoagulant. On average such systems can process about three units of blood automatically in approximately 10 min. Although the disposable part of these systems can be assembled quickly, technical help must be available in the operating theatre if the cell saver is to be used safely and efficiently. An alternative manual method of intraoperative blood salvage is the Solcotrans Autologous Collection System, although its capacity is limited. Blood is drained or sucked through a 40 μm blood filter into a specially designed reservoir containing acid citrate glucose; this anticoagulated whole blood is then reinfused.

There are many serious, potential complications of blood salvage systems. The most important is the risk of infection from the shed blood. To minimize this infection risk, the time elapsing between the start of collection and reinfusion should ideally not exceed 6 h. It could be argued that if bleeding is so slow that it takes 6 h to collect sufficient blood for processing then the system was not required. The second most obvious problem with these systems is that the material prepared for reinfusion contains red cells only. This may produce a coagulopathy from infusion of residual anticoagulant and, more likely, from dilution of coagulation factors and platelets. Hypocalcaemia (when citrate is used with the Solcotrans system) may also contribute to the coagulopathy. These aspects of the use of such devices in routine surgery have lead to recent studies showing that bleeding postoperatively, and especially after open heart surgery, may be more prolonged and heavier. Relative contraindications to the use of the cell saver include blood contamination by bacteria, intestinal contents or tumour cells.

LOSS OF HAEMOSTATIC FUNCTION: COAGULOPATHY OF MASSIVE TRANSFUSION

HAEMOSTASIS, COAGULATION AND FIBRINOLYSIS

A brief description of the normal processes involved in haemostasis, coagulation and fibrinolysis will assist in understanding the factors that may lead to a coagulopathy or its treatment.

The aim of the haemostatic system is to ensure that blood remains in a fluid state inside the intravascular compartment unless trauma occurs. Clot formation should occur only when and where it is needed, at the site of microvascular injury. Later the goals of the system are to remove or digest this clot when it is no longer needed. It is convenient to describe separately the processes of haemostasis, coagulation and fibrino- or clot lysis. However it is obvious that the system is highly interdependent and all three processes are active at all times.

Haemostasis

Vessel wall injury causes contraction of the surrounding smooth muscle cells which will slow the blood flow. Vasoconstrictor substances such as catecholamines are released from the vessel wall and other substances are released from platelets.

The first part of the haemostatic process relies on the platelet and the reaction between the platelet and the underlying microvascular endothelium, Figure 41.1. Platelets play a pivotal role in haemostatic plug formation by adhering to the sub-endothelium at the site of vessel damage. Such platelets then attract further platelets to form an aggregate which blocks the blood flow from the wound site. Platelets also act as an organizing surface for the plasma phase of coagulation leading to the formation of thrombin. This thrombin formation allows the platelet plug to be strengthened by a network of interlacing fibrin strands.

Circulating platelets will recognize and stick to an injured area by means of receptors on their surface. The major receptors are able to recognize and bind to collagen and also to von Willebrand Factor (vWF) by the Gp1b receptor. Neither collagen or vWF are expressed on the normal anticoagulant endothelial cell surface. However, these factors are bound to sub-endothelium. By this means the platelet is immobilized at the site of injury to the microvasculature. Also at this time, the platelet undergoes a change in shape to

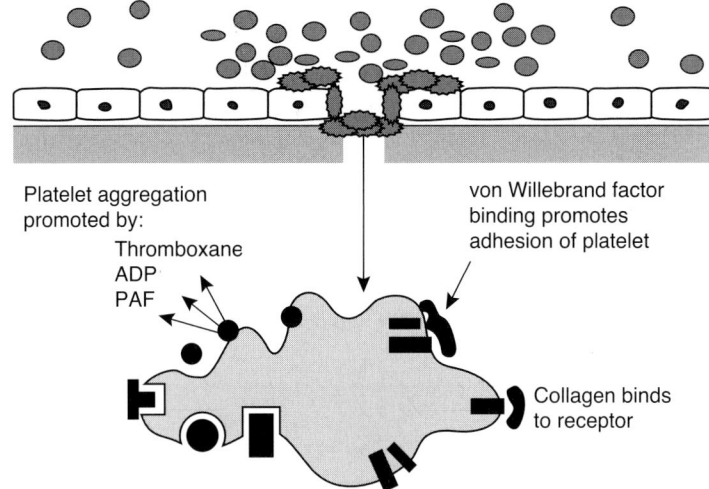

Figure 41.1 Platelet shape change and platelet/endothelium reaction to produce the haemostatic plug. Collagen and von Willebrand factor are found in exposed sub-endothelium shown as the shaded area. Once exposed these initiate biochemical changes within the platelet which amplify the process of haemostatic plug formation.

become flattened and 'sticky', and reverses the expression of acidic glycoproteins on its surface to present a negatively charged surface to the exterior.

A change in configuration also occurs at a specific receptor, the IIb/IIIa or fibrinogen receptor, on the platelet surface to bind fibrinogen and provide a loose meshwork, or bridge, between the platelets as part of the haemostatic plug formation.

A further amplification step takes place at this stage with the platelet undergoing attraction to and aggregation with other platelets; this aggregatory process forms the basis of the routine, if complex, laboratory tests of platelet function. Aggregation is associated with release of ADP and adhesive proteins which stimulate the adhesion and aggregation of nearby platelets. Pre-formed substances such as serotonin are also released from granules to promote platelet aggregation and microvascular constriction. The platelet also synthesizes thromboxane A2 from arachidonic acid to induce a powerful, local vasoconstriction which assists the fragile haemostatic plug to develop a more solid hold on the wound edges. The enzyme responsible for the *de novo* synthesis of thromboxane (cyclo-oxygenase) is inhibited by many drugs, but particularly by aspirin and other anti-inflammatory agents.

This loosely bound platelet plug will remain haemostatic for about 1–2 h. To augment the duration and strength of the plug requires the initiation and amplification of the second of the haemostatic processes, the so called plasma or coagulation stage. The aim of the coagulation phase is the generation of fibrin strands which will bind and stabilize the weak platelet haemostatic plug, Figure 41.2.

Coagulation

The process of fibrin formation has an initiation and amplification stage. A recurrent theme in the coagulation system is the formation of activation complexes involving a serine protease, a zymogen or substrate, a cofactor and the organizing surface provided by

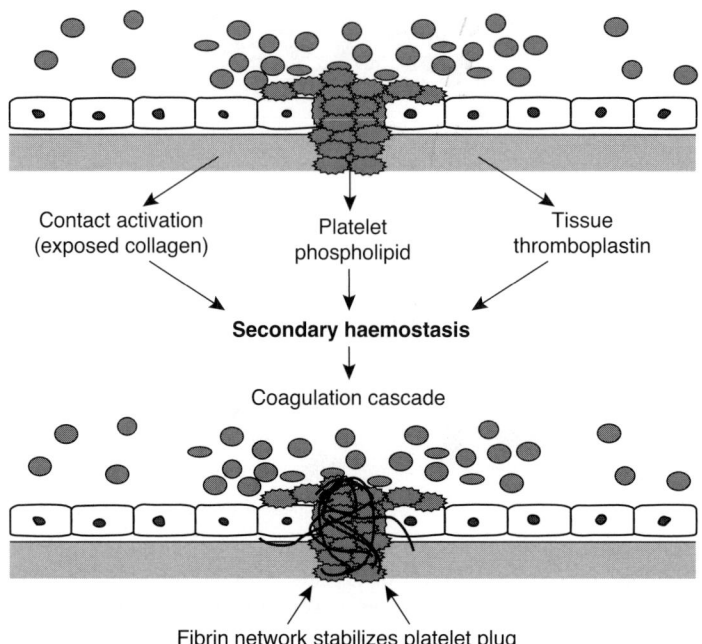

Figure 41.2 More permanent haemostatic plug formation relies on stabilizing the primary platelet plug. This requires the initiation and amplification of the next plasma or coagulation stage of the haemostatic processes. The coagulation phase will generate fibrin strands which bind and stabilize the relatively weak platelet haemostatic plug.

the platelet membrane. The primary function of the organizing surface is to act as a vice to hold the co-factors and clotting factors. The platelet will accept factors V and VIII into its surface and also bind other factors with the help of calcium ions as described below.

The coagulation system relies primarily on a group of soluble factors which circulate in the plasma. The majority of these factors are synthesized in the liver and released into the circulation. Of these factors some depend on the presence of Vitamin K for their activation. Vitamin K is a co-factor in the process involved in the attachment of the carboxy residue in glutamic acid to certain coagulation factors. This imparts a greater negative charge to one end of these factors. This part of the molecule attaches to the organizing surface of the platelet. As the platelet surface and circulating coagulation factors are negatively charged they will tend to repel each other.

The role of the calcium ion, with its positive charge, is to act as a buffer or sandwich between the two and allow the coagulation factor to 'attach' to the platelet surface in a specific orientation. This is important as these factors must be presented to each other in an absolutely specific and controlled way, otherwise the process of coagulation is not amplified or progressed.

This organization can be appreciated by considering the formation of thrombin from prothrombin shown in Figure 41.3. In this reaction factor Xa activates prothrombin to thrombin and involves a co-factor (factor V) on the platelet surface. Factor V is synthesized in the liver and has a half-life of ≈ 6 h in circulating or stored blood, leading to its description as Labile Factor.

The active Xa has exposed scissors but is unable directly to release the restraint, or bubble, over the scissors on prothrombin for two reasons (Figure 41.3). First the attachments of factor Xa and II to the platelet surface are mobile. These factors behave like a chair, or stool, on wheels (calcium ions) which can traverse around a room, but needs to collide with a specific object at a specific angle. The second problem is that to release the constraining bubble the scissors on the Xa must approach the factor II at a specific site to avoid steric hindrance.

Factor V overcomes these two problems by engaging itself into the organizing surface and then holding the two factors by a 'handle' which will align the proteins in the required configuration (Figure 41.3). An identical series of reactions occurs to produce activated factor X (Xa). In this case factor X is the zymogen, IXa is the serine protease and factor VIII is the co-factor. Factor Xa can also be produced by the action of factor VII. This factor is an active enzyme in the circulation and is held in the appropriate configuration to cleave factor X by tissue factor. This tissue factor is expressed from the surface of the endothelium by a large number of phlogistic agents and also during periods of hypoperfusion and relative hypoxaemia. This may have important effects in producing intravascular coagulation in shocked patients.

The pivotal importance of these co-factors is obvious when the kinetics of the reactions are considered. If we assume that the rate constant for the conversion of prothrombin to thrombin by factor Xa is unity, the addition of calcium ions makes the reaction rate 2.3 times faster. The addition of platelet phospholipid, calcium and factor Xa increases this rate 22 fold. The addition of factor V to this mixture accelerates the reaction by 278 000 fold. If similar kinetics are assumed for the activation of factor Xa then simple mathematics show a 7.7 million fold acceleration of thrombin generation in a fully active system. Put another way, what would take 1 s in the unrestricted intact system, would require 90 days in a system of enzyme and substrate alone (i.e. if blood clotted in plasma, not on the activated platelet surface with adequate supplies of factors V and VIII).

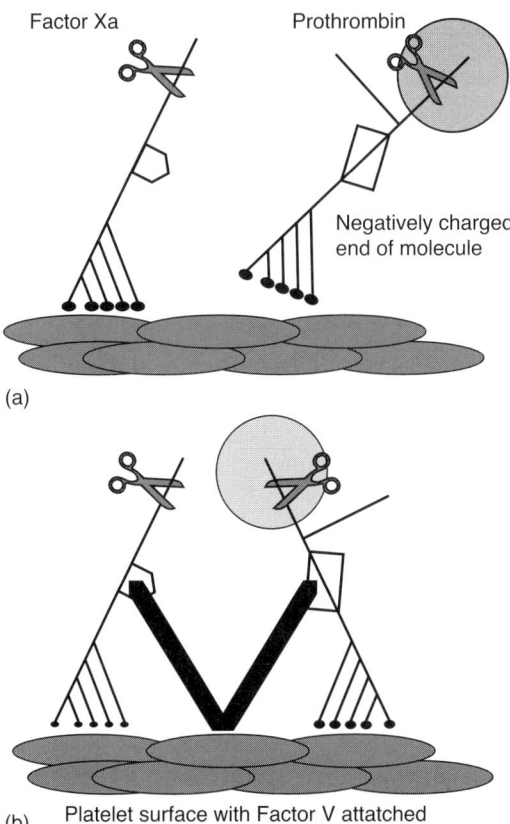

Figure 41.3 Panel A shows factor Xa and prothrombin without co-factor V. The shade area discs represent the negatively charged platelet surface. Filled circles on the lower extensions of the factors represent the positively charged calcium ions which allow the negative glutamate residues to approach the platelet surface. Xa cannot release constraint around active site of prothrombin (to release thrombin) as prothrombin is not correctly aligned. The bar protruding from prothrombin represents a portion of the molecule which gives steric hindrance and is intended to prevent unwanted activation of thrombin by other proteolytic enzymes. Site specific generation of thrombin is required.

Panel B shows the role of factor V to act as a co-factor to hold factor Xa and prothrombin in exact configuration to allow thrombin generation at its precise site of action.

Fibrinolysis

Once healing has occurred, the fibrin clot must be digested. As with haemostasis and coagulation, fibrinolysis must occur only when and where it is required. In addition, it must not occur too early in the repair process.

Both plasminogen, the zymogen precursor to plasmin, and tissue plasminogen activator (t-PA), the enzyme which acts to transform plasminogen to plasmin, are present in flowing blood. The t-PA in blood is an active enzyme. However, when blood is flowing the likelihood of t-PA encountering plasminogen with the right conformational alignment to permit their interaction is so improbable that virtually no plasminogen is converted to plasmin in the plasma. It is the fibrin surface itself that signals the system to activate fibrinolysis. When a fibrin surface forms, the amino acid lysine protrudes from the fibrin. Plasminogen contains a specific lysine binding site, which allows it to bind to this fibrin surface. Tissue plasminogen activator also has a fibrin binding site. When both plasminogen and t-PA bind to the fibrin surface, and are appropriately aligned, their interaction occurs readily and plasmin is generated.

The plasmin generated on a fibrin surface under physiological conditions is a highly active, broad spectrum, proteolytic enzyme which can digest fibrin, fibrinogen and most coagulation factors and co-factors. Plasmin may escape from its fibrin binding site because its binding affinity is not very strong, or it may be produced in the plasma by administration of clot lysing drugs such as streptokinase or t-PA. Consequently, there has to be a mechanism to neutralize plasmin when it dissociates from a fibrin clot. A good rule of biochemistry is that for every enzyme there exists a cognate inhibitor. The cognate inhibitor for plasmin is α_2-plasmin inhibitor (also known as α_2-antiplasmin). The plasmin on a fibrin clot is protected against inhibition by α_2-plasmin inhibitor; at this site, the inhibition process takes more than 5 min. But when plasmin escapes into solution, α_2-plasmin inhibitor exerts its inhibition in 0.01s, which is one of the fastest enzyme/inhibitor interactions in mammalian biology. The system thus protects plasmin when it is working where needed, but immediately neutralizes the enzyme when it escapes into solution where it might wreak havoc.

With exogenous streptokinase or t-PA, or if there is a pathological deficiency of the inhibitor of t-PA (plasminogen activator inhibitor-1), it is possible to have an excess of plasmin with no α_2-plasmin inhibitor to protect it. This occurs because the molar concentration of plasminogen in the blood is about 2 micromolar, but the concentration of α_2-plasmin inhibitor is only 1 micromolar. In this states the blood is 'hyperfibrinolytic'.

THERAPY WITH HAEMOSTATIC PRODUCTS

Coagulopathy is a clinical diagnosis. About 80% of patients who have massive bleeding will develop a diffuse ooze from raw or cut surfaces. The cause of this ooze is multifactorial, but includes relative hypothermia, abnormal platelet functions, dilution of clotting factors, consumption of factors and, in certain circumstances, enhanced fibrinolysis.

There is convincing evidence that the most important factors in this diffuse bleeding are abnormal platelet numbers or function, together with continuing, abnormal activation of coagulation and fibrinolysis. This latter effect is now thought to be due to the release of tissue thromboplastin and specifically tissue factor from the endothelium. This is able to act with circulating factor VII to activate factor X. Tissue factor and thromboplastin are released by surgery. More importantly this pathway is activated after tissue hypoperfusion and by inflammatory mediators and endotoxin. In other words, the coagulopathy may be a complication of shock and inadequate or delayed resuscitation (leading to hypoperfusion), or of the surgery itself (with release of tissue thromboplastin). In general terms, it is the disease (hypoperfusion) and not the treatment (transfusion) that leads to coagulopathy. Disseminated intravascular coagulopathy (DIC), causing thrombocytopenia and a reduction of plasma coagulation factors, is reported to occur in up to 30% of patients during major bleeding.

With massive transfusion there is no evidence that prophylactic replacement with FFP or platelet concentrates prevents the onset of abnormal bleeding or reduces transfusion requirements in patients requiring large-volume transfusions. Early laboratory assessment is needed to determine the precise nature of any disorders of coagulation which may have developed.

The clinical signs of coagulopathy in association with large-volume blood replacement include microvascular bleeding (oozing from the mucosae and skin puncture sites). This will usually be associated with thrombocytopenia due to dilution and consumption of platelets, with or without coexisting deficiency of soluble coagulation factors. Initial treatment to control bleeding should therefore include platelet concentrates. Whole blood that has been stored for 2 or 3 days is essentially devoid of functioning platelets. Massive transfusion leads to a decrease in platelet count, but not to the numbers predicted by the washout curve in mathematical and animal models of blood exchange. This implies a considerable reserve of platelets which can be synthesized or released rapidly from the spleen and marrow into the circulation when required.

Many studies of trauma patients have shown that the platelet count needs to fall to about $50 \times 10^9 \, l^{-1}$ before this contributes to increased bleeding. A higher figure of about $100 \times 10^9 \, l^{-1}$ is used when platelet function may be altered, for example after a period of extracorporeal support. Platelet functions and numbers are also altered by a large number of agents which are given during anaesthesia, surgery and in the intensive care unit. A list

Table 41.5 Drug therapies associated with thrombocytopenia

Alcohol	Nitrofurantoin
Aspirin	Paracetamol
Cephalothin	Penicillin esp. ampicillin
Chlorpropamide	Phenylbutazone
Cimetidine	Phenytoin
Digoxin	Quinine and Quinidine
Frusemide	Spironolactone
Heparin	Streptomycin
Isoniazid	Sulphonomides
Meprobamate	Thiazides

Table 41.6 Therapies which may affect normal platelet functions

Anti-inflammatory agents
   Aspirin
   Non-steroidal anti-inflammatory drugs
   Sulphinpyrazone
Antibiotics
   Penicillins such as carbenicillin and piperacillin
   β-lactam antibiotics such as cefoxitin and moxalactam
   Gentamycin
Anti-psychotic agents
   Phenothiazines
   Tricyclic antidepressants
Vasoactive compounds
   Phosphodiesterase inhibitors such as aminophylline, papaverine and enoximone
   Nitroso compounds such as nitrates and nitroprusside
   Propranolol
Others
   Frusemide
   Dextrans
   Some anti-histamines

of such agents is shown in Tables 41.5 and 41.6.

It is, therefore, critically important to monitor platelet numbers and the coagulation process during major bleeding and its resuscitation. The drawbacks to this approach are twofold. First, the majority of the microvascular bleeding is probably due to abnormal platelet function. In turn this may be related to hypothermia and tissue acidosis as a consequence of hypoperfusion. Platelet function, as opposed to numbers, is not readily monitored in blood transfusion laboratories. Therefore, it is not easy to determine if platelet functions are normal, and so define the transfusion trigger for effective platelet transfusion.

The second problem with trying to 'continuously' monitor coagulation is the time dependency of the system. Most major bleeding associated with trauma or obstetrics tends to occur outside normal laboratory hours and, the tests require a finite time to perform. Delays in acquiring the results of laboratory tests pose a formidable problem. If coagulation factors need to be administered, they take time to prepare and infuse. Efficacy of this therapy has to be measured to determine if further interventions are required. To counter this problem a number of bedside monitors of coagulation are available, but they are expensive and may not be cost effective for institutions without considerable experience of major haemorrhage such as trauma and transplant units.

Hepatic transplantation presents special problems. Normal hepatic function is required for all steps in the coagulation system. A decrease in platelet count is observed in about 70% of patients presenting with end-stage disease despite a normal or increased rate of production. The reasons for the thrombocytopenia include hypersplenism and a decreased platelet survival time. Patients with alcoholic cirrhosis may have folic acid deficiency and ethanol has a direct toxic action on the megakaryocyte. All coagulation factors except factor I and VII are deficient. Factor VIII is increased because of the increase in von Willebrand factor antigen and activity. Although fibrinogen concentrations may be normal, there is evidence to show that the quality is poor due to excess incorporation of sialic acid residues in the fibrinogen preventing effective polymerization during haemostatic plug formation. Altogether these deficiencies lead to a prolonged prothrombin time (PT) and activated partial thromboplastin time (APTT). If the coagulopathy is severe it may require correction with platelets, fresh frozen plasma and cryoprecipitate before operation to reduce bleeding associated with the insertion of intravascular, monitoring catheters.

PLATELETS

Platelet concentrates ('random donor' platelets) are prepared from whole blood by centrifugation. Each concentrate usually contains at least 5.5×10^{10} platelets in 50–70 ml plasma. Single-donor platelets are obtained by apheresis and contain in excess of 3×10^{11} platelets in 200–400 ml of plasma, the equivalent of approximately six platelet concentrates. The plasma volume of each concentrate should be considered when administration of FFP is indicated. There is little or no evidence of differences in clinical effectiveness in patients who are not immunized. Infusion of a single unit of platelets should increase the platelet count by 6–$8 \times 10^9 \, l^{-1}$. This effect should be monitored by measuring the platelet count about 30 min after transfusion. Failure to increase the platelet count implies continuing activation, or consumption, and the need for appropriate measures to reduce this and to give more platelet concentrates. Indications for infusion of platelets are shown in Table 41.7.

Table 41.7 Guidelines for platelet transfusion

Platelet count $<20 \times 10^9 \, l^{-1}$ in a non-bleeding patient with failure of platelet production
Platelet count $<50 \times 10^9 \, l^{-1}$ and impending surgery or invasive procedure
Diffuse microvascular bleeding and transfusion ≥ 1 blood volume and platelet count $\leq 50 \times 10^9 \, l^{-1}$, or result not available
Diffuse microvascular bleeding following cardiopulmonary bypass and platelet count $\leq 100 \times 10^9 \, l^{-1}$, or result not available
Bleeding in a patient with a qualitative platelet defect, regardless of platelet count

The primary advantage of single-donor platelets is reduced donor exposure. Platelet concentrates, like whole blood, are capable of transmitting HBV, HCV, HIV and CMV (cytomegalo virus) infection, and causing graft versus host disease in certain individuals.

ABO-compatible platelets should be used whenever possible as platelet recovery and survival may be superior. Rh(D) compatible platelets should be used for children and for women with a possibility of pregnancy in the future, to avoid the risk of developing anti-Rh(D) antibody.

Platelets should be infused via a special giving set provided by the transfusion service. Administration of platelets via standard blood giving sets, or through 'old lines' will result in activation and a significant loss of numbers and function.

Platelet concentrates contain donor white cells that lead to certain problems. First, the CMV status of donor and recipient may be important and must be matched if possible. Following liver transplantation graft failure is 8 times more common in patients who seroconvert to become CMV positive after transplant.

Second, multiple platelet transfusion results in alloimmunization to leucocytes. Up to two-thirds of regular recipients of random donor platelets become HLA alloimmunized and this may be associated with refractoriness to platelet transfusion. The management of these patients, either to attempt to prevent alloimmunization or to manage refractoriness, is extremely costly.

Finally, the white cells in platelet concentrates release large amounts of phlogistic agents such as cytokines and tumour necrosis factor. This is thought to be responsible for certain haemodynamic effects of transfusion of 'old' (> 7 day old) platelet concentrates.

There are UK guidelines for platelet transfusion. However these are related more to chronic administration rather than acute bleeding problems.

COAGULATION FACTORS

It is unusual for a significant reduction of plasma coagulation factors to occur solely as a result of massive transfusion of stored whole blood. Stored whole blood contains adequate amounts of coagulation factors I, II, VII, IX, X, XI and XII. Nevertheless, dilution of coagulation factors will occur when replacement therapy has largely consisted of fluid containing no coagulation factors, such as red cell concentrates or red cells re-suspended in additive solutions or saline–adenine–glucose–mannitol. Concentrations of factors V and VIII are significantly reduced in stored blood. However, plasma concentrations of about 25% of normal for factor V and 35% for factor VIII will produce normal clotting function. These two co-factors are in the final common pathway of the coagulation process and so a significant decrease in activity will be shown by prolonged prothrombin and activated partial thromboplastin times. Prolongation to more than 1.5 times control values, in the presence of a fibrinogen concentration of > 0.8 g l^{-1}, implies ineffective concentrations of these factors.

A significant reduction in concentrations of clotting factors follows certain therapies, such as the thrombolytic agents. These agents (t-PA, streptokinase and anistreplase) release plasmin which digests fibrin. Unfortunately, plasmin has a voracious appetite for all clotting factors and there may be significant decreases in concentrations of fibrinogen, and especially factor V, after administration of such agents. In these situations it may be necessary to administer an anti-plasmin agent. The most effective is aprotinin. This acts to enhance the natural anti-plasmin proteins in the blood. In addition, aprotinin binds to streptokinase to prevent it acting further.

A significant reduction in the activity of clotting factors occurs when patients are receiving vitamin K antagonists such as warfarin or coumadin. These drugs prevent the clotting factors receiving the glutamate residues to allow factor alignment and progression of coagulation. In other words, the plasma concentration of these factors is normal but their function is impaired. With normal liver function a dose of vitamin K will reverse this functional defect. Guidelines for the reversal of warfarin effects are well documented.

REVERSAL OF WARFARIN ANTICOAGULATION EFFECTS

Patients requiring immediate or rapid reversal of warfarin anticoagulation should be treated according to the following recommendations:

Life threatening haemorrhage

Immediately give vitamin K by intravenous infusion in a dose of up to 5 mg over 5–10 min. Remember vitamin K is solubilized in Cremophor and anaphylaxis may occur. Give prothrombin complex concentrate (PCC) (factor II, IX, X) together with factor VII concentrate at a dose of 50 units factor IX per kg body weight and 50 units factor VII per kg body weight. The prothrombin time should be monitored. If no concentrate is available, fresh frozen plasma should be infused (about 1 l for an adult), but this is not as effective.

Less severe haemorrhage such as haematuria and epistaxis

Withhold warfarin for 1 or more days and consider giving vitamin K, 0.5–2.0 mg i.v.

INR of > 4.5 without haemorrhage

Withdraw warfarin for 1 or 2 days, then review.

Unexpected bleeding at therapeutic levels

Investigate the possibility of an underlying cause, such as unsuspected renal or alimentary tract disease.

It is important to note that the use of PCC and factor VII concentrates for reversal of anticoagulation of liver disease are non-licensed indications and can therefore only be under-taken by a doctor at his/her own responsibility, using the 'named patient basis' procedure.

FRESH FROZEN PLASMA

Fresh frozen plasma is the component most often administered without an indication. It is prepared from whole blood by separating and freezing the plasma within 8 h of collection. In the UK, currently available fresh frozen plasma products for clinical use are prepared from fully screened blood donations but are **not** subjected to any virucidal process. When stored at −20°C the product is stable for 1 year but must be used within 24 h of being thawed. Storage in the liquid state results in significant losses of factors V and VIII. ABO compatible FFP should be used, but compatibility testing is not required. It is recommended to give Rh(D) compatible FFP to Rh(D) negative individuals, particularly women of child-bearing age. (Where this is not possible, anti-D immunoglobulin should be given at a dose of 50 units per pack (200–300 ml) of FFP transfused). There are relatively few indications for FFP administration. In 1992 the British Committee for Standards in Haematology published guidelines for the use of fresh frozen plasma. A summary of the guidelines is given in Table 41.8.

Table 41.8 Guidelines for fresh-frozen plasma transfusion

PT, APTT ≥1.5 times the mean normal value. This also applies to non-bleeding patients having surgery or an invasive procedure

Diffuse microvascular bleeding and transfusion ≥1 blood volume and PT, APTT not yet available

Reversal of warfarin before emergency surgery, if insufficient time for the effects of discontinuing therapy and administering vitamin K

Under-transfusion of FFP may be as common as over-transfusion. The dosage of FFP depends upon the clinical situation, but 12–15 ml kg^{-1} is generally an appropriate starting dose. Each unit contains 200–250 ml. It is important to monitor the response, both clinically and with laboratory tests. Plasma fibrinogen, PT and APTT should be monitored as a guide to additional replacement therapy along the following lines.

- PT or APTT prolonged **and** fibrinogen less than 0.8 g l^{-1}: **cryoprecipitate** is indicated.
- If the PT or APTT are prolonged and fibrinogen more than 0.8 g l^{-1}, then significant deficiencies of factor V and VIII are likely. In this case FFP 15 ml kg^{-1}, (3 to 4 units in an adult) is generally recommended as an initial dose.

Crystalloids or synthetic colloids are safer than plasma for the management of hypovolemia and are as effective. There is no indication for the use of FFP according to predetermined replacement schedules such as 1 unit of FFP for each 4–6 units of blood. This exposes the patient to additional risk for no proven benefit.

CRYOPRECIPITATE

Cryoprecipitate is prepared from FFP and is a concentrated source of plasma proteins (factor VIII, fibrinogen, factor XIII, and fibronectin). Cryoprecipitate contains no red blood cells and only 10–20 ml plasma. Each bag of cryoprecipitate concentrate contains about 250 mg of fibrinogen, 80–120 units of factor VIIIc, 40–70% of the factor VIII vWF and 20–30% of the factor XIII from the original FFP unit. Cryoprecipitate is used for treating both congenital and acquired coagulation disorders, and also for preparing fibrin sealant or 'glue' for use during surgery. Administration of ABO compatible cryoprecipitate is preferable, but not essential. Diffuse microvascular bleeding with a fibrinogen level > 1 g l^{-1} is usually considered an indication for cryoprecipitate in the surgical patient receiving massive transfusion. Other indications are haemophilia A, congenital or acquired fibrinogen deficiency, and von Willebrand's disease.

The dose is 1 concentrate per 7–10 kg. Once thawed, cryoprecipitate can be stored no longer than 6 h at 1–6°C.

COMPLICATIONS AND HAZARDS ASSOCIATED WITH MASSIVE BLEEDING AND TRANSFUSION

HYPOTHERMIA

Administration of unwarmed blood that has been stored at 4°C will decrease the recipient's temperature. Hypothermia represents the most common, and most easily preventable, complication of massive trauma and haemorrhage. Problems attributable to hypothermia include the following.

- An increased tendency to cardiac arrhythmias. If the temperature decreases to less than 30°C, ventricular irritability and even cardiac arrest may occur. This irritability is exacerbated by the use of certain anaesthetics agents such as halothane and after injection of calcium salts.
- Reduction in citrate and lactate metabolism (thereby increasing the probability that the patient will develop hypocalcaemia and a metabolic acidosis during transfusion). This may contribute to the arrhythmia potential, and acidosis will depress myocardial performance.
- Shift of the oxygen–haemoglobin dissociation curve to the left. The resulting increase in the affinity of haemoglobin for oxygen will lead to decreased tissue oxygenation. This will be at a time when peripheral oxygen consumption is increased due to shivering. A decrease in body temperature as small as 0.5 to 1.0°C may induce shivering. Shivering may increase oxygen consumption by as much as 400%.

- Impairment of red cell deformability, platelet and coagulation functions leading to coagulopathy. Numerous studies have shown that the primary haemostatic process (the platelet endothelial reaction) is impaired in cold skin. There is a paradoxical activation of platelets with cooling. This platelet activation occurs in inappropriate sites and may contribute to thrombocytopenia. The process of coagulation is an enzymatic process and thus slows with lowering of temperature.
- Impaired stress and immune responses.

All these factors can be reduced by ensuring warming of all fluids during administration.

ACID–BASE BALANCE AND MASSIVE TRANSFUSIONS

After transfusion, the citrate used as anticoagulant to prepare stored blood products is readily metabolized in the liver and cleared by the kidney. The pH of citrate solution is approximately 5.5. When this solution is added to a unit of freshly drawn blood, the pH of the blood immediately decreases to approximately 7.0–7.1. As a result of accumulation of lactic and pyruvic acids by red blood cell metabolism and glycolysis, the pH of bank blood continues to decrease to a value of about 6.9 after 21 days of storage. However, a considerable portion of the acidosis can be accounted for by the P_{CO_2} of 150 to 220 mmHg (20–29.3 kPa). The P_{CO_2} is high because the plastic container does not provide an escape mechanism for carbon dioxide. Bubbles seen in the tubing of blood transfusions are largely of carbon dioxide. With adequate ventilation in the recipient, this high P_{CO_2} should be of no consequence. When the P_{CO_2} is returned to normal a metabolic acidosis is still present in citrated blood, and some clinicians empirically recommend giving alkalinizing agents. However, this approach has little to support its use. The reasons for this are two-fold. First, relatively well controlled studies have shown that the acid–base response to blood transfusion is extremely variable. Second, blood transfusions provide citrate which is a substrate for the endogenous generation of bicarbonate. This accounts for the significant incidence of metabolic alkalosis after blood transfusions. Therefore, there is no logic in the empirical administration of bicarbonate for prophylactic treatment of an unpredictable acid–base abnormality. Bicarbonate therapy should be initiated when metabolic acidosis is diagnosed on an arterial blood sample. Large doses of bicarbonate (> 1 mmol kg^{-1}) can interfere with coagulation with a prolonged prothrombin and thrombin clotting times. Alkalosis augments a left shift of the oxygen dissociation curve thereby augmenting any tendency towards tissue hypoxia.

Infused citrate binds ionized calcium. The signs and symptoms of citrate toxicity are those of hypocalcaemia: hypotension, narrow pulse pressure with elevated intraventricular end-diastolic pressure and central venous pressure, suggesting impaired myocardial performance, muscle tremors, tetany, and Q–T interval prolongation on ECG. Citrate toxicity due to the binding of ionized calcium may occur with very rapid transfusion (1 unit of red blood cells every 4–5 min in adults), in patients with hypothermia, in infants undergoing exchange transfusion, or in patients with severely depressed hepatic function, particularly during liver transplantation. Because the citrate anticoagulant remains in the plasma fraction, single units of fresh frozen plasma or platelets (approximately 250 ml of plasma) contain as much citrate as 5 units of plasma reduced red blood cells (50–70 ml plasma per unit). This high citrate load should caution against the use of frozen plasma or platelet transfusions in patients at greater risk of developing 'citrate toxicity' as outlined above. In particular, in children with haemorrhage, volume expansion with crystalloid, albumin, or even red cells may be preferable to the use of fresh frozen plasma.

ELECTROLYTE IMBALANCE

Hypocalcaemia

As outlined above, calcium plays an essential part in both the extrinsic and intrinsic coagulation pathways. However, a bleeding diathesis associated with hypocalcaemia is uncommon, as cardiac arrest will usually occur before the plasma concentration decreases to a value that affects coagulation. In addition, and again outlined above, administration of calcium alone is associated with an insignificant increase in the rate of fibrin formation. If a haemorrhagic diathesis starts after administration of citrated blood or blood products, low calcium values are not part of the differential diagnosis.

Infusion of more than 1 unit of blood every 4–5 min is necessary for ionized calcium values to begin to decrease. Even at these rates of infusion, low calcium levels do not cause bleeding. Hypothermia, liver disease, liver transplantation, and hyperventilation increase the possibility of hypocalcaemia. Administration of calcium is rarely needed, but should be considered in high-risk patients, particularly infants undergoing exchange transfusion and during liver transplantation. The occurrence of hypocalcaemia during liver transplantation is well documented. For example, studies have shown that the plasma citrate concentration rose to about 10 times normal during the dissection period and 30 times normal during the anhepatic period. This was associated with a decrease in ionized calcium to about two thirds of normal during these periods of a high plasma citrate. Citrate metabolism, and thus calcium concentration, returns rapidly following adequate hepatic revascularisation.

The empirical administration of calcium on the basis of blood product transfusions cannot be recommended. Guidelines recommending routine administration of calcium after a certain number of units transfused, such as those contained in the maternal mortality reports, were based on the use of whole blood with a higher citrate load than the red cell products currently used in most transfusions. It is now recognized that calcium administration may impair cardiac relaxation, increase energy costs of enhanced contractility, and even hasten myocardial death. Hypercalcaemia can occur in seriously ill patients which makes these adverse effects more likely.

The deleterious effects of hypocalcaemia can be treated, either empirically by administration of calcium chloride, if the patient becomes hypotensive and is not hypovolaemic, or on the basis of a measured, decreased, plasma concentration of ionized calcium.

Although it is reported to be irritating to veins, 10% calcium chloride provides three times more calcium (0.91 molar calcium) than an equal volume of 10% calcium gluconate (0.22 molar calcium), because the chloride has a molecular weight of 147 and gluconate salt a molecular weight of 448.

Hypomagnesaemia

Hypomagnesaemia may be noted after multiple transfusions, but is rarely clinically significant. However, there are reports of long Q–T syndrome with recurrent **torsade de points** and ventricular fibrillation due to low magnesium concentrations after massive transfusion.

Hyperkalaemia

As a simple rule of thumb the potassium concentration in stored blood increases by about 1 mmol per litre per day. The potassium concentration in stored blood will thus increase to approximately 30 mmol l^{-1} after 3 weeks of storage although values up to 100 mmol l^{-1} have been documented. After transfusion, viable red blood cells re-establish their ionic pumping mechanism and intracellular re-uptake of potassium occurs. While transient hyperkalaemia has been observed during massive transfusions, more commonly hypokalaemia is noted. Risk factors for the development of hyperkalaemia include rapid transfusion (up to 500 ml h^{-1} with high capacity volume infusions), small children transfused rapidly, and pre-existing renal failure.

It follows that ECG monitoring is mandatory during massive blood transfusions. Peaked T-waves in the inferior and lateral leads occur at serum potassium values of 6–7 mmol l^{-1}. With increasing hyperkalaemia (> 6.5 mmol l^{-1}), the P-wave is lost as atrial conduction is suppressed. Widening of the QRS complex due to decreased interventricular conduction is seen at potassium values of 7–8 mmol l^{-1}. At 8–9 mmol l^{-1}, the widening QRS fuses into the T-wave, creating a sine wave pattern. Ventricular tachycardia and fibrillation, or asystole, occur at values greater than 9–10 mmol l^{-1}.

Acute hyperkalaemia is most rapidly treated with bicarbonate, or glucose and insulin, which promote entry of potassium into cells. Calcium may be given to modify the arrhythmogenic effects of high potassium. As with citrate intoxication, hyperkalaemia is rare, and this again rules against the routine administration of calcium. Tissue hypoperfusion with acidosis in shock states and the increase in citrate values found after rapid blood transfusion both contribute to the toxic effects of hyperkalaemia and hamper effective treatment. Calcium administration should be based on diagnostic signs of hyperkalaemia (peaked T-wave).

FURTHER READING

American Society of Anesthesiologists. (1996) Practice Guidelines for Blood Components Therapy. A report by the American Society of Anesthesiologists task force on blood components therapy. *Anesthesiology*, 84, 732–747.

Bick, R. L. (1992) Coagulation abnormalities in malignancy: a review, *Seminars in Thrombosis and Hemostasis*, 18, 353–372.

Brimacombe, J. and Berry, A. (1994) Haemodynamic management in ruptured abdominal aortic aneurysm. *Postgraduate Medical Journal*, 70, 252–256.

Carson, J. L., Poses, R. M., Spence, R. K. and Bonavita, G. (1988) Severity of anaemia and operative mortality and morbidity. *Lancet*, 1, 727–729.

Furie, B. and Furie, B. C. (1992) Molecular and cellular biology of blood coagulation. *New England Medical Journal*, 326, 800–806.

Kottke Marchant, K. (1994) Laboratory diagnosis of hemorrhagic and thrombotic disorders. *Hematology and Oncology Clinics of North America*, 8, 809–853.

Kruskall, M. S., Bodner, M. S., Dzik, W. H., Friedman, K. D., Gerber, L., Gould, S. A., Gravlee, G., Schoenleber, D. G. and Yomtovian, R. (1992) An annotated bibliography on autologous transfusion. *Transfusion*, 32, 286–290.

Mackie, I. J. and Bull, H. A. (1989) Normal haemostasis and its regulation. *Blood Reviews*, 3, 237–250.

Phillips, G. R. R, Kauder, D. R. and Schwab, C. W. (1994) Massive blood loss in trauma patients. The benefits and dangers of transfusion therapy. *Postgraduate Medicine*, 95, 61–2, 67–72.

Strauss, R. (1988) Volume replacement and coagulation: a comparative review. *Journal of Cardiothoracic Anesthesia*, 2, 24–32.

ANAPHYLAXIS TO ANAESTHETIC DRUGS

M. Fisher

The systemic inflammatory response, a defence mechanism, is regulated by the release and formation of mediators which interact in a complex fashion. In certain circumstances this mechanism becomes hostile. Anaphylaxis is one such example. Endogenous mediators have a range of effects in anaesthesia. The non-immunological release of histamine in response to drugs, or surgical or anaesthetic stimuli, occurs commonly but is transient and rarely life threatening. At the other end of the spectrum is the massive allergic release of histamine associated with the activation of other, longer acting mediators, which produce a sustained effect: anaphylactic shock.

Severe reactions resembling the classic descriptions of anaphylaxis were rarely described in anaesthesia before the 1970s. The incidence then appeared to rise in many countries. Early studies emphasized reactions to induction agents. This was partly due to the high frequency of reactions to the cremophor-based drugs Althesin and propanidid but probably also because reactions were often mis-attributed to thiopentone simply because of documented previous exposure (integral to the classical concept of anaphylaxis). Neuromuscular blocking drugs (NMBs) were disregarded because previous exposure was absent and because the non-immunological histamine-releasing effects of the NMBs were well known.

The use of skin testing, leucocyte histamine release and radioimmunoassays (RIA) for specific IgE to NMBs, while not escaping controversy, established the role of IgE antibodies to anaesthetic drugs and the likely anaphylactic nature of severe reactions.

MEDIATOR RELEASE IN ALLERGY

HISTAMINE

Histamine is released from mast cells in response to noxious stimuli, drugs and antigen–antibody reactions. There is considerable variability in individual release. Measurement of histamine release due to drugs and studies with histamine infusion show a correlation between plasma levels and cardiovascular, cutaneous and subjective symptoms but not bronchospasm. Indeed, intravenous histamine infusion usually only produces bronchospasm in β-blocked patients. Histamine may produce all the individual clinical features of anaphylaxis and has been shown to produce adverse effects during anaesthesia. Such effects can be prevented by pretreatment with H_1 and H_2 blockers. The plasma histamine levels produced by direct release rarely exceed 5 nmol l^{-1}. In anaphylaxis levels ten- to a hundredfold greater are common.

The degree of histamine release produced by a particular drug correlates with its ability to produce minor, but not severe, reactions. Potent histamine releasers such as morphine are not commonly associated with severe adverse events while weak releasers such as suxamethonium and alcuronium are 'common' causes. Lorenz believes that some patients may be identified who are 'super responders' to NMB's histamine-releasing effects and suffer severe reactions which are non-immunological.

Recent studies have shown that mast cells from different parts of the body show a different response to histamine-releasing drugs and basophils show a different response to mast cells. Morphine, for example, causes histamine release from skin mast cells but not lung, intestinal or cardiac mast cells or basophils. Morphine has been traditionally suggested to produce asthma due to direct histamine release but there is no evidence to support this. Although a potent releaser, very little histamine released from skin will reach the lungs. In contrast, we appear to be seeing an increased incidence of non-allergic asthma from drugs which release histamine directly from lung mast cells such as atracurium, vecuronium and propofol although it must be emphasized that such reactions are rare.

OTHER MEDIATORS

Most of the inflammatory mediators, leucotrienes, prostaglandins, thromboxane, bradykinin, chemotactic factors and platelet activating factor, have been shown to have a role in acute anaphylaxis.

ANAPHYLACTIC MEDIATORS AND THE HEART

The heart contains histamine and histamine receptors and IgE antibodies to suxamethonium have been isolated in cardiac tissue from a patient who died of suxamethonium anaphylaxis. Histamine, prostaglandins, leucotrienes and platelet activating factor also have adverse effects on the heart, although the effects of histamine in man usually require previous β-blockade in the experimental situation. Studies *in vitro* and animal models clearly demonstrate that the heart is a potential target organ in anaphylaxis. Evidence implicating the heart in human anaphylactic shock is limited and it is difficult to separate mediator effects from the effects of endogenous hypovolaemic shock. It is probable that the endogenous catecholamine release during anaphylaxis opposes the deleterious cardiac effects of anaphylactic mediators. Only two detailed cases of profound myocardial depression in human anaphylaxis in patients with normal cardiac function have been described. In aggregate anaphylaxis and some reactions to protamine, however, the heart appears to be an important target organ.

As with other forms of shock the underlying state of the myocardium is a key determinant of the effects of anaphylaxis on the heart.

ALLERGY AND ATOPY

There is an increased incidence of a history of allergy, atopy or asthma in patients who undergo anaphylactic reactions during anaesthesia compared with non-reacting controls, typically a three- to fivefold increase. However, in a French study where reactors and non-reactors were matched for age, sex and social class and atopy was measured by antigen testing, there was no significant difference between reactors and non-reactor. This increased incidence of anaphylaxis in people with a history of atopy and allergy is commonly raised in medicolegal cases and has been used by some to suggest that such a history should influence choice of drugs. It should be remembered that the majority of patients in all series of anaesthetic anaphylaxis do not have such a history, the majority of patients with such a history have uneventful anaesthesia and such a history is a poor predictor of a reaction.

PREVIOUS EXPOSURE

With thiopentone, multiple uneventful exposures (usually more than five) are usual. With NMBs a history of previous exposure is attainable in less than 50% of cases, in spite of the demonstration of an allergic basis to the reaction which, traditionally, requires previous exposure to form the antibody. It is likely that the antibody which binds NMBs is formed in response to some antigen other than the NMB. NMBs such as suxamethonium are of such simple structure that it is unlikely they could cause antibody formation.

MEDIATOR RELEASE

The clinical effects of mediator release have variable clinical expression relating to the mediator released, the mechanisms, the quantity and the timing. As a general principle, the effects are on smooth muscle cells producing bronchoconstriction in the airway and vasodilatation in peripheral blood vessels, increased capillary permeability and increased secretion of exocrine glands.

Minor skin changes are the most common manifestation of histamine release, particularly with atracurium, and changes in blood pressure during anaesthesia which correlate with histamine release and can be blocked with H_1 and H_2 blockers are well documented. Minor skin changes do not suggest risk of anaphylaxis at subsequent anaesthesia.

The role of direct histamine release in major reactions is less clear. Reactions requiring intervention may occur with histamine release alone, especially in β-blocked patients with cardiac disease and with preoperative haemodilution with Haemaccel®. Direct histamine release, however, is usually transient and not associated with severe reactions. Persistent reactions usually require the release of other vasoactive mediators. From the point of view of subsequent anaesthesia it should be assumed that all severe reactions persisting greater than 10 min are immune mediated. This almost certainly leads to overdiagnosis, but overdiagnosis only restricts anaesthetic options: underdiagnosis may lead to fatal subsequent reactions.

INCIDENCE

The incidence of life threatening anaphylactoid reactions during anaesthesia is unknown. Most published figures, with the exception of those from Sheffield, are encompassed by the Boston Collaborative Drug Surveillance Study of 1:900 to 1:20 000. The largest study, from France, gives an incidence of 1:6000. Studies in two local areas showed incidences of 1:1200 to 1:1700 reactions to NMBs. About 30 million patients would need to be studied to establish an incidence with 5% confidence limits. Thus reported incidences to specific drugs are relatively meaningless. Suxamethonium is the most common cause worldwide. Suxamethonium, alcuronium and atracurium appear to carry a greater risk than pancuronium or vecuronium, although the vecuronium appears to be a high risk drug in the French population. Rate of usage is a major determinant of incidence of reactions to specific drugs.

DRUGS PRODUCING ANAPHYLAXIS

The drugs producing reactions in our series are shown in Table 42.1. The neuromuscular blocking drugs are the most common. The patterns of anaesthetic anaphylaxis appear to be changing and this is probably largely related to usage.

PROPOFOL

The introduction of propofol was followed by reports of life threatening reactions. The incidence is unknown. Positive skin tests and RIA tests have been documented. Suggestions that a relationship between allergy to egg and

Table 42.1 Causes of life threatening clinical anaphylaxis during anaesthesia 1974–1995, n=548[a]

Induction agents (n=85)		Cephamandole	1
Thiopentone	46	Cephazolin	5
Alfathesin	29	Cefotaxime	2
Propanidid	6	Cefotetan	1
Methohexitone	1	Penicillin	1
Propofol	2	Ampicillin	2
Midazolam	1	Flucloxacillin	4
		Vancomycin	2
Induction agent and relaxant (n=3)		**Muscle relaxants** (n=318)	
Thiopentone/suxamethonium[b]		Alcuronium	123
Thiopentone/alcuronium[b]		Suxamethonium	93
Thiopentone/atracurium[b]		Atracurium	32
Colloid solutions (n=33)		d-Tubocurarine	22
Haemaccel®	22	Gallamine	17
Dextran 70	7	Pancuronium	12
Dextran 40	1	Vecuronium	10
SPPS	1	Decamethonium	1
NSA	1	Suxamethonium/atracurium	1[b]
Plasma	1	Suxamethonium/gallamine	2[b]
Other drugs (n=23)		Suxamethonium/alcuronium	4[b]
Protamine	9	Suxamethonium/d-Tubocurarine	1
Contrast media	4	**Local anaesthetics** (n=4)	
Neostigmine	1	Prilocaine/lignocaine	1[c]
Atropine	2	Bupivacaine	2
Platelets	1	Lignocaine	1
Ondansetron	1		
Latex	1	**Narcotics** (n=11)	
Gortex	1	Morphine	5
Patent blue	1	Fentanyl	2
Fragmin	1	Omnopon	1
Ergometrine	1	Pethidine	3
Antibiotics (n=24)			
Cephalothin	6	**No drug detected** (n=47)	

[a]Patients referred to author for investigation. Includes patients from New Zealand, Australia and Europe
[b]Both drugs received prior to reaction and positive skin and/or RAST tests
[c]Two reactions on separate occasions

the vehicle for propofol have not been supported by the literature. Propofol appears in our series to have a higher incidence of non-allergic asthma than thiopentone, but there are no studies confirming this.

NEUROMUSCULAR BLOCKING DRUGS

The NMBs still provide the major cause of life threatening anaphylactic reactions in all large series. The majority if not all severe reactions are IgE mediated. Suxamethonium is the most common cause throughout the world with the exception of Australia, where alcuronium was the most common until recently when suxamethonium and atracurium have become more common. In New South Wales suxamethonium is the commonest cause of death due to anaesthetic anaphylaxis. The important and unusual characteristic of reactions to NMBs is that they often occur on first exposure, suggesting sensitivity is not caused by the NMB. Cross sensitivity to NMBs occurs in at least 60% of reactors with suxamethonium and gallamine, alcuronium and tobocurarine, and pancuronium and vecuronium the most common pairs.

ANTIBIOTICS

Antibiotics are an increasing source of acute anaphylactic reactions during anaesthesia, with cephalosporins the most common. There is variable cross-sensitivity between cephalosporins and skin testing and RIA testing usually allows detection of a 'safe' cephalosporin. Cephalosporin administration in patients with a history of penicillin allergy is an increasing source of litigation in Australia. It it is felt that a cephalosporin is indicated in such a patient, the patient should be informed of the risks and reasons for a perceived cephalosporin advantage and the consent documented.

NARCOTICS

Reactions to morphine, codeine phosphate, pethidine, Omnopon® and fentanyl have all been described, but such reactions are rare, with less than twenty cases in total in the literature.

PROTAMINE

Protamine produces reactions by a number of mechanisms which may involve IgE, IgG and complement. A classical anaphylactic pattern may occur or a syndrome producing acute pulmonary hypertension and right ventricular failure. A prolonged and persistent massive capillary leak syndrome after bypass has been attributed to both protamine and plasma products although a cause and effect relationship has not been proven. Protamine from insulin, fish allergy and vasectomy have been suggested as predisposing factors but there is no convincing association.

COLLOID SOLUTIONS, BLOOD PRODUCTS

All the synthetic colloids produce anaphylactoid reactions and there is no clearcut evidence showing a higher incidence with a particular colloid. The reactions are very uncommon during shock. There is little convincing evidence of IgE involvement. Pretreatment with high molecular weight dextran reduces the incidence to dextrans but reactions have occurred after pretreatment and to the pretreatment. Surprisingly, reactions to blood have not been reported to our unit with any regularity, although such reactions are well documented.

LATEX

Recently attention has been drawn to reactions to the latex in gloves worn by surgeons and anaesthetists and in tracheal tubes and masks which caused, in one unit, 10% of all anaphylaxis during anaesthesia. These reactions are characteristically delayed more than 15 min and there is a high incidence of health care workers among reactors. Cross-sensitivity with food, particularly exotic fruits such as kiwi fruit, avocados and bananas occurs, is documented in Europe and the diagnosis is confirmed by skin testing and radioimmunoassay for latex specific IgE using commercial kits.

LOCAL ANAESTHETICS

Genuine allergy to local anaesthetics is extremely rare. The reactions tend to be painful swelling on the side of the dental block, collapse (usually related to dental injection) and bizarre neurological symptoms. The important clue to determining a vasovagal cause of collapse is that the patient recovers with minimal or no treatment. In many patients with bizarre neurological symptoms, or cardiovascular collapse, the syndrome may be precipitated by saline solution. Cross-sensitivity between amide local anaesthetics and less commonly between amide and esters

Table 42.2 Anaphylaxis to anaesthetics, severe reactions, clinical features (n=460)

	n	Sole feature	Worst feature
Cardiovascular collapse	406	53	365
Bronchospasm	174	14	82
Transient	74		
Asthmatics	78		
Cutaneous			
Rash	59		
Erythema	206		
Urticaria	38		
More than one	129		
Angiooedema	112	5	13
Generalized oedema	30		
Pulmonary oedema	13	1	1
Gastrointestinal	35		

Table 42.3 Anaphylaxis to anaesthetics, severe reactions, first clinical feature (n=460)

No pulse detected/fall in blood pressure	125
Difficult to inflate	121
Flush	95
Coughing	29
Rash	20
Desaturation	24
Cyanosis	12
ECG change	9
Subjective	9
Urticaria	8
Swelling	6
No bleeding	2
Total	460

has been described. Progressive challenge is used to confirm, or more usually exclude, the diagnosis. Every effort should be made to exclude spurious histories of local anaesthetic allergy. In genuine allergy, antihistamines may be used for local anaesthesia.

CLINICAL FEATURES OF ANAPHYLAXIS

Reactions may occur at any time during anaesthesia, but usually occur during induction (90%). In our series two reactions have occurred to premedication. The clinical features are shown in Table 42.2.

The following points are important.

- Cardiovascular collapse is the most common severe manifestation and is the only feature in 10% of patients. In such cases the diagnosis may be missed.
- Asthmatics who get anaphylaxis always get bronchospasm; severe bronchospasm is the most difficult feature to treat.
- The pulmonary oedema is a membrane oedema, associated with low filling pressures and a volume deficit; it is rare.
- Two different types of skin changes may occur in a single patient.

The first clinical feature noted in 460 patients is shown in Table 42.3. These figures show that reactions are usually well advanced by the time they are detected. Pulse oximetry has changed the initial signs of anaphylaxis. The commonest presenting feature since 1990 has been desaturation or loss of pulse waveform, or transient difficulty in inflation.

Factors which increase the severity of reactions and risk of death are a history of asthma, β-blocker therapy, epidural anaesthesia and cardiac disease.

MANAGEMENT

The spectrum of severity of anaphylactoid and anaphylactic reactions during anaesthesia is wide. Some patients respond to crystalloid infusion and corticosteroids, both of which are ineffective in severe cases. At the other end of the spectrum are patients who die in spite of early and excellent management. Successful litigation in anaesthetic anaphylaxis is usually related to poor treatment.

There are no randomized, controlled, trials of the treatment of human anaphylaxis and the nature of the disease probably precludes rigorous scientific study.

CARDIOVASCULAR COLLAPSE

IPPV and 100% oxygen should be commended and external cardiac compression instituted if the patient is pulseless, irrespective of rhythm. The assistance of a colleague should be obtained and elective surgery abandoned.

Adrenaline is traditionally regarded as the treatment of choice. However, German workers suggest colloid is better to treat anaphylactic cardiovascular collapse, as the major deficit is a reduced circulating blood volume on the basis of vasodilation and plasma leakage. In support of this approach these workers note that adrenaline, may produce infarction and ventricular arrhythmias.

In our series, sympathomimetic drugs appear to enable more rapid stabilization and offer obvious advantages when bronchospasm or angio-oedema occur concurrently. Failure to use adrenaline makes the defence of allegations of inadequate treatment very difficult.

Adrenaline is the drug most likely to produce a response in terms of blood pressure and bronchospasm and usually halts the progression of angio-oedema. In monitored patients, 3–5 ml of 1:10 000 adrenaline should be given intravenously and an infusion established. This should be followed by the rapid infusion of 1–2 l of colloid solution. While crystalloid solutions have been used successfully, the literature suggests much greater volumes are necessary and what literature there is, favours the use of colloids.

Most patients respond rapidly. Some do not. In particular patients taking β-blockers, or who have epidurals in place may be refractory. In the β-blocked patient massive doses of adrenaline may be necessary and drugs with α-effects such as metaraminol or noradrenaline should be tried. If there is no response after 2 l of colloid in a patient receiving an adrenaline infusion, a noradrenaline infusion may be successful. Angiotensinamide was successful in one patient refractory to noradrenaline. The heart should be imaged if there is further failure to respond and if myocardial dysfunction is present balloon counterpulsation may be necessary. H_2-blockers have been advocated as first line drugs, but have limited value early in severe cases. When given late in some protracted cases of hypotension they may make the management easier.

BRONCHOSPASM

Severe bronchospasm is the most difficult manifestation to treat. Adrenaline is the drug of first choice. In addition, continuous nebulization of a $β_2$-agonist such as salbutamol should be commenced and steroids, i.e. methylprednisolone 1 g given. Anaesthetic vapours may be effective: isoflurane is the agent of choice if adrenaline is being administered. Ketamine may produce a dramatic response, particularly in children.

The major hazard of bronchospasm is barotrauma. Initial ventilation should be at a slow rate (less than 6 breaths a minute). There is no need to lower CO_2 if the pH is above 7.0 and oxygenation is adequate. Minute volume should be allowed to remain low until improvement in airways resistance occurs.

In the extreme situation wherein the airways resistance exceeds the elastic recoil of lungs and chest wall and expiration does not occur, manually assisting expiration by squeezing the lateral chest wall at the end of expiration may be lifesaving.

Pneumothorax should be suspected and treated promptly if any sudden deterioration occurs. When all else fails, and mechanical ventilation is impossible, barotrauma has occurred and cardiac arrest is imminent, consideration should be given to cardiopulmonary bypass.

ANGIO-OEDEMA

The tracheas of the patients should be intubated and adrenaline given intramuscularly or intravenously, as well as an H_1-blocker.

PULMONARY OEDEMA

This is usually controlled by increasing PEEP until airway flooding is controlled and saturation adequate. The pulmonary oedema of anaphylaxis is a membrane oedema and is associated with a volume deficit. Diuretics are contraindicated. Rarely, at the end of cardiopulmonary bypass, a severe pulmonary oedema may occur in which losses of high protein oedema fluid of up to 35 l may occur over 24 h and massive replacement and invasive monitoring are required. In these patients, increasing PEEP to stop flooding may lead to oedema fluid exudating through the lung surface into the thoracic cavity and thoracotomy may be necessary to prevent tamponade of the lungs and heart.

FOLLOW-UP

The treatment of acute anaphylaxis does not end with the acute episode.

When a severe reaction occurs it is important to endeavour to determine whether the reaction is allergic or not, which drug is responsible and which alternative drugs may be safe. In Western countries, a second anaesthetic reaction in the absence of testing and provision of information to the patient would be indefensible.

The history is of vital importance and a history of previous exposure of little value in determining the drug responsible. Cutaneous testing must be carried out. The findings should be clearly documented and explained to the patient and the patient be instructed to carry a letter at all times in addition to a warning device. The letter is a vital adjunct because it gives subsequent practitioners the opportunity to assess the evidence for accuracy. Details of safe subsequent anaesthesia should be added to the letter. Such information is the best information upon which to base subsequent drug selection.

There has been great controversy over the precise value of different tests. Skin testing, whether by prick or intradermal routes, is the most valuable test and is mandatory in severe reactions. It detects a limited number of mechanisms (IgE and possible IgG mediated reactions) but has the overwhelming advantage that it can be performed by anybody in any hospital without special facilities. Although fatal reactions have been described in such tests (not in anaesthetic testing) severe adverse reactions are very rare: we have seen three easily treatable reactions in over 1200 tests, 500 of which were performed in extremely sensitive patients. The data supports safe subsequent anaesthesia using skin test negative drugs in patients skin test positive to other drugs, but this is not an absolute guarantee; we have seen two second reactions to skin- and RIA-negative drugs.

With minor reactions restricted to the skin, reactions of short duration and intermediate severity and delayed reactions, the available tests provide little help. It is extremely rare, however, for such reactions to lead to more severe subsequent reactions and in minor reactions the high incidence of negative tests may be because an allergic mechanism is not present.

Tests performed during the reaction

Histamine

This is a difficult assay in blood and needs to be performed within 10 min when resuscitation is the priority. Very high levels suggest an allergic cause. Urinary methylhistamine collected over an hour is easier but of less value.

IgE levels

Changes in serum total IgE levels after a reaction have been suggested as evidence that IgE is involved in such reactions. There is no evidence to support this contention and as the IgE involved in the reaction is cell bound, little logic to support serum levels being of use. However, drug specific IgE can be detected in blood taken during a reaction or before a reaction and postmortem and usually reflects the results shown in delayed sampling at the time of skin testing.

Complement

Changes in serum complement levels and activation of the classical alternate pathways of complement have been demonstrated after clinical anaphylaxis particularly due to Althesin, contrast media and protamine. As a diagnostic tool in clinical anaphylaxis complement levels have limited value although there is insufficient information published to enable a valid assessment and it appears that considerable experience is a prerequisite to interpreting them.

Mast cell tryptase

This test appears of importance in the diagnosis of anaphylactoid reactions during anaesthesia. Tryptase is a protease in mast cell granules and elevated serum mast cell tryptase levels are evidence of activation of mast cells. In anaphylactic reactions the levels are elevated for 1–5 h after the beginning of the reaction, enabling the delay of sampling until resuscitation is over. The assay is robust and requires no special handling of serum samples. Reliable results can be obtained in specimens taken postmortem. In anaesthesia, elevated mast cell tryptase levels appear highly specific and sensitive for IgE mediated reactions, although they are elevated in some states where IgE is unlikely to be involved such as reactions to contrast media, severe direct reactions to vancomycin and in mastcytosis (unpublished data). An elevated level of mast cell tryptase indicates that testing to determine the drug responsible is both mandatory and likely to be successful. All patients with elevated cell tryptase levels should be assumed to have a severe allergy and investigated further. We have not found a positive skin test or RIA test in a patient whose mast cell tryptase is not elevated.

Tests after the reaction

Skin testing

Skin testing is performed 4–6 weeks after the reaction. Although skin testing only detects reactions due to IgE, or possibly IgG, the high yield of positive results in published series reflects the high incidence of IgE involvement in severe reactions. Two forms of skin testing are used, intradermal tests in which the drug is diluted and injected into the dermis and prick testing in which the drug is introduced into the dermis by pricking the patient's skin through a drop of undilute drug. It is usual to use controls such as histamine and a high concentration of a narcotic to determine that histamine responsiveness and histamine releasability are normal.

Prick testing has the advantages of less trauma to the skin, ease of preparation and probably safety. Prick tests are more likely to be successfully completed in children. Their disadvantage is that although they may be inherently more accurate than intradermal tests, they tend to produce false negatives whereas intradermal tests tend to produce false positives. The consequences of a false negative test for subsequent anaesthesia are obviously greater than a false positive. However, agreement as to the drug implicated between the tests is greater than 90%. It is in establishing cross sensitivity of NMBs that the agreement between these tests (and RIA tests) is less reliable. Skin tests are of little value in reactions to colloids, contrast media and blood products.

With local anaesthetics the incidence of genuine reactions is so rare that the philosophy of diagnosis is changed and the goal is to exclude allergy. A progressive challenge is used. Unless there was a clear cut history suggestive of anaphylaxis and a clear cut positive wheal and flare reaction at 1:100 dilution of 0.5% local anaesthetic, the dosage should be increased up to 2 ml of undilute drug. Before skin testing, patients should be aggressively challenged with 2 ml subcutaneous saline, which will often reproduce the symptoms.

In spite of some controversy regarding skin testing, the literature clearly supports it use.

Radioimmunoassay tests

More recently radioimmunoassay tests have been used to detect IgE-drug specific antibodies. These tests are only performed in a few laboratories although a commercial version of the test for suxamethonium is available. Use of these tests in over 300 patients has shown the following.

- RIA tests will detect the drug responsible for a reaction with about the same frequency as skin tests if there is an RIA available for that drug. However, RIAs are only available for propofol, thiopentone, suxamethonium and alcuronium, vecuronium, pancuronium, gallamine and d-tubocurarine.
- A combination of RIA and skin tests will detect a drug responsible better than either test alone.
- There is generally agreement between the tests for the drugs responsible, but 50% disagreement for tests for other NMBs when a battery of tests is used. Cross-sensitivity as determined by RIA is greater than for cutaneous testing and those patients positive by RIA and negative on skin testing comprise both false positive RIAs and false negative skin tests.
- There is significant *in vitro* cross-sensitivity between thiopentone and NMBD radioimmunoassays. Because some patients are allergic to both thiopentone and an NMBD and skin tests or RIA inhibition are necessary to distinguish these patients.

In patients selected by any one test and studied with any alternative test the specificity of the alternative test increases. In practice when the results of tests disagree the patients should be warned off all positive drugs.

Other tests

Leucocyte and basophil histamine release tests have been used in specialized laboratories and give results similar to RIA. Recent evidence suggests that significant histamine release from leucocytes is highly suggestive of an immune mechanism. The disadvantages of the tests are the few laboratories with the expertise to perform them and that the patient rather than a blood specimen must go to the laboratory.

In severe reactions a combination of available tests will determine the drug responsible in 95% of patients. In patients with severe reactions in whom no drug is detected alternative forms of anaesthesia (regional volatile) should be considered.

Anaesthetic allergy has been shown to persist up to 27 months and few patients lose their sensitivity.

Preoperative testing

It has been argued that patients presenting for anaesthesia should be preoperatively screened by RIA testing to reduce the risk of anaphylaxis to NMBs. The case for such testing is poor. First, the commercial version of the RIA which is less accurate (80% specific) than laboratory RIAs is advocated. Second, the high incidence of cross-sensitivity between NMBs would mean that the alternative drugs which may be given to a positive cannot be guaranteed as safe without secondary cutaneous testing.

The selection of an at-risk group such as women of child bearing age with or without a history of allergy or atopy will improve the cost effectiveness of the testing but lead to a major reduction in reactors detected. As stated earlier, if 40% of patients who react have a history of allergy, atopy or asthma then the majority (60%) do not and that it is unlikely at the low prevalence of reactions reported that there is a statistically significant different in the incidence of life-threatening anaesthetic allergy between allergic and non-allergic patients.

If screening was to be performed, prick testing would be the only feasible and sufficiently reliable test. In areas in France where the incidence of allergy to NMBs is high, there is evidence that this screening has a high yield. As it could easily be done by the anaesthetist before anaesthesia to test the relaxant to be used at virtually no cost, it is likely to be a topic of future debate and medicolegal importance.

In spite of the limitations of diagnostic tests, the data show that when patients are investigated using skin testing and RIA testing where available, subsequent anaesthesia is usually safe, irrespective of whether the reaction was diagnosed as anaphylactic or not or whether the drug responsible was detected. We have records of subsequent anaesthesia in 290 patients diagnosed, with four subsequent reactions due to cross-sensitivity and one bradycardic reaction and in 70 subsequent anaesthetics in whom a diagnosis was not reached there has been one subsequent reaction.

The concept of pretreating patients allergic to NMBs with monoquaternary compounds to competitively block the IgE receptors without bridging has been accomplished successfully in two French studies.

FURTHER READING

Fisher, M. (1986) Clinical observations on the pathophysiology and treatment of anaphylactic cardiovascular collapse. *Anaesthesia and Intensive Care*, **14**, 17–21.

Fisher, M. (1984) Intradermal testing after anaphylactoid reaction to anaesthetic drugs: practical aspects of performance and interpretation. *Anaesthesia and Intensive Care*, **12**, 115–120.

Fisher, M. M. and Baldo, B. A. (1993) The diagnosis of fatal anaphylactic reactions during anaesthesia: Employment of immunoassays for mast cell tryptase and drug-reactive IgE antibodies. *Anaesthesia and Intensive Care*, **21**, 353–357.

Fisher, M. and Baldo, B. A. (1994) Anaphylaxis during anaesthesia: current aspects of diagnosis and prevention. *European Journal of Anaesthesia*, **11**, 263–284.

Laroche, D., Vergnaud, M. C., Sillard, B., Soufarapis, H. and Bricard, H. (1991) Biochemical markers of anaphylactoid reactions to drugs. Comparison of plasma histamine and tryptase. *Anesthesiology*, **75**, 945–949.

Laxenaire, M. C. Moneret-Vautrin, D. A., Widmer, S., Mouton, C. and Gueant, J. L. (1990) Substances anesthesiques responsables de chocs anaphylactiques. Enquete multicentrique francaise. Anaesthetic drugs responsible for anaphylactic shock. French multi-center study. *Annales Francais Anesthesie et Reanimation*, **9**, 501–506.

Leynadier, F. and Dry, J. (1991) Allergy to latex. *Clinical Reviews in Allergy*, **9**, 371–377.

Lorenz, W., Duda, D., Dick, W., Sitter, H., Doenicke, A., Black, A., Weber, D., Menke, H., Stinner, B. and Junginger, T. (1994) Incidence and clinical importance of perioperative histamine release: randomised study of volume loading and antihistamines after induction of anaesthesia. Trial Group Mainz/Marburg. *Lancet*, **343**, 933–940.

Moneret Vautrin, D. A., Motin, J., Mata, E., Gueant, J. L., Kanny, G., Widmer, S. and Laxenaire, M. C. (19??) Preventing muscle relaxant anaphylaxis with monovalent haptens. A preliminary study. *Annales Francais Anesthesie et Reanimation*, **12**, 190.

Snidel, L. J. and deShazo, R.D. (1991) Accidents resulting from local anesthetics: true or false allergy?*Clinical Reviews in Allergy*, **9**, 379–395.

Stelleto, C., de Paulis, A., Cirillo, R., Mastronardi, P., Mazzarella, B. and Marone, G. (1991) Heterogeneity of human mast cells and basophils in response to muscle relaxants. *Anesthesiolgy*, **74**, 1078–1086.

AWARENESS IN ANAESTHESIA

J. Andrade and J. G. Jones

Waking up during surgery can be a terrifying experience. A report by Moerman, Bonke and Oosting (1993) reveals some common themes in accounts of awareness during anaesthesia. Most patients said they were aware of people talking or of their inability to breathe, and felt extremely anxious or powerless when they tried to attract attention and found they were paralysed. For example, a woman undergoing Caesarean section said she, 'Heard much noise and voices, felt the mask pressed on her face, could not move, tried to warn but was unable to do so, no pain but was afraid this would come, felt anxiety and panic, felt like suffocating, thought she was dying'. Another patient, during an operation for a leg fracture, 'Felt and heard being manipulated on his leg, heard drilling and tightening of screws, could see people, heard people talking about his leg, tried to warn anyone but was unable to do so, completely paralysed, unable to open mouth, pain in his jaws, afraid to feel more pain, panicked, thought he might never get out of it and might become comatose'.

How common are experiences like this? The question is addressed in the second part of this chapter. We then discuss the potential consequences of awareness during anaesthesia, and end with a consideration of various preventative measures. We begin, however, with a brief account of the relationship between memory and awareness, as this is central to the rest of the chapter.

MEMORY AND AWARENESS: SOME DEFINITIONS

The term **awareness during anaesthesia** is in some ways a blanket expression referring to the various possible experiences of a patient who is inadequately anaesthetized during surgery. In the most extreme case, the patient may wake up and be fully aware that they are undergoing an operation. Awareness here is essentially the state of consciousness that is a property of normal, waking life. The patient may, or may not, be in pain, depending on the adequacy of analgesia provided by the anaesthetic and supplementary analgesics.

However, consciousness is not an all-or-none phenomenon. We equate full consciousness with full awareness, but someone may be less than fully conscious and still have some residual awareness. For example, if someone is drowsy, they may close their eyes and be unaware of visual stimuli or of the passage of time, but still hear a doorbell or alarm clock ringing. Similarly, a patient who is lightly anaesthetized may be unaware of pain or the visual aspects of their environment, yet still be able to hear and comprehend operating theatre conversation. A patient who has slightly deeper anaesthesia combined with poor analgesia may be unaware of environmental sights and sounds, but intensely aware of pain when surgery begins. Only someone who is fully unconscious will be unaware of all these things.

Short Practice of Anaesthesia. Edited by M. Morgan and G. M. Hall. Published in 1997 by Chapman & Hall, London. ISBN 0 412 71890 1

These different levels of awareness are summarized in Table 43.1.

Psychologists typically divide memory into two or more components. **Short-term, or working, memory** refers to brief retention of a small amount of information. This is the sort of memory you would use to retain a telephone number before dialling. It is thought to be essential for consciousness, in that it enables us to keep track of our experiences from one moment to the next. In contrast, **long-term memory** refers to our more permanent storage of a practically infinite amount of information. Memory for intraoperative events is long-term memory if it is still detectable on recovery. This long-term memory may be **explicit** (conscious) or **implicit** (unconscious). If someone is aware of remembering something then their memory is explicit. Thus, recall of surgery is an instance of explicit memory. Implicit memory does not involve a feeling of remembering. It can be demonstrated if the person's behaviour has changed in some way because of the learning episode. For example, someone may be unable to recall or recognize the word KAYAK from a recent study list. If they nonetheless show a better than usual ability to use the word to complete the fragment ___Y__K, then we say they have implicit memory, but not explicit memory, for the word.

The relationship between the state of consciousness at learning and the type of memory at some later time is not straightforward.

Table 43.1 Possible levels of awareness during anaesthesia

Conscious	Fully aware of surroundings, may or may not be in pain
Partially conscious, or semi-conscious	Not fully awake but aware of some things, e.g. may hear voices or feel pain
Unconscious	No awareness

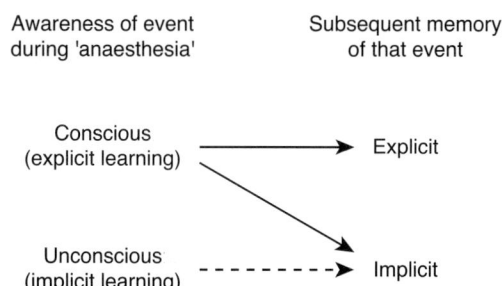

Figure 43.1 Learning during anaesthesia. Note that implicit memory may result from implicit or explicit learning, hence implicit memory of intraoperative events may be a sign that the patient was conscious during anaesthesia.

Someone may be fully conscious at learning and later have explicit or implicit memory. As consciousness is lost, it is possible that implicit memory persists for longer than explicit memory, but this has not been conclusively demonstrated. Psychologists disagree about whether unconscious learning is possible, but it is assumed that it would lead only to the formation of implicit memory and not to explicit memory. Note that implicit memory of intraoperative events is **not** evidence for implicit learning. It may also arise from explicit learning by a patient who woke up during surgery. These relationships are illustrated in Figure 43.1.

INCIDENCE OF AWARENESS DURING ANAESTHESIA

RECALL OF SURGERY

Until the 1970s, the incidence of awareness during surgery was thought to be around 3%. This has declined in recent years, presumably because volatile agents and opioids are now used to supplement nitrous oxide anaesthesia. Also, in the UK at least, anaesthesia based solely on opioids is less common than previously. Jones (1994) reviewed the literature on the incidence of awareness during anaesthesia. In one study he cites only 2 out of 7306 patients (0.03%) were awake and in pain during general anaesthesia for various surgical procedures. In another study more than 3000 women were questioned between 1982 and 1989 about their experiences during Caesarean section. Fewer than 1% were able to recall something of their operation. None complained of pain at the time of the interview, although one person did so subsequently. Overall, Jones concluded that 1 patient in every 10 000 recollects waking during surgery and feeling pain, whereas 3 patients per thousand have some recollection, but no memory of pain. Although this incidence is low, it should be remembered that every year around 2.5 million people have an operation under general anaesthesia in the UK alone, hence awareness during surgery may be experienced and remembered by hundreds, if not thousands, of people each year.

These figures probably underestimate the incidence of awareness during anaesthesia, because memory of surgery is not always reported. In 1987, Hargrove reported that the Medical Defence Union receives only four or five complaints of awareness a year. This is probably less than today's figures, but it is difficult to obtain exact numbers. There is a considerable under-reporting of awareness – for example, 31% of Moerman's patients did not mention their experience to their anaesthetist, or to other hospital staff. Of those who did report their experience, six were met with scepticism or disbelief. Fear of this sort of response may prevent some patients reporting awareness during surgery, whereas other patients may consider their experience insufficiently traumatic to justify a complaint, particularly if they were not in pain at the time. However, there is another reason why people may not report waking during surgery, and that is that they may not remember it happening. In this instance, they may none the less have some implicit memory for the event and this point will be considered next.

IMPLICIT MEMORY FOR INTRAOPERATIVE EVENTS

We have so far discussed only those examples in which the patient can recall details of their operation. However, recall is actually quite a difficult activity and it is often impossible even to recall things which we have seen or heard many times (for example, try drawing a coin from memory). One might argue that someone who wakes up during surgery is bound to recall such a salient experience, but there are several reasons why this may not occur.

One reason is that much lighter anaesthesia is needed for conscious or explicit memory formation than is sufficient for awareness. We have demonstrated this in volunteer studies with low doses of isoflurane and propofol. For both drugs, there was a depth of anaesthesia at which people could respond to verbal stimuli and remember them for brief periods, and yet, on recovery, they could not recall those stimuli or identify them on an easier recognition memory test. In other words, there was a depth of anaesthesia at which people were conscious but amnesic.

Another reason someone may not recall waking up is if they have been premedicated with drugs such as midazolam. Midazolam and other benzodiazepines are amnesic agents and impair conscious recollection. It is sometimes argued that they should be given to patients before surgery specifically for the purpose of preventing recollection in the event of inadequate anaesthesia. However, these drugs do not always prevent the formation of **implicit** memories, and these unconscious memories may have an adverse influence on behaviour and, potentially, on recovery from surgery.

A third reason for a patient failing to recall an episode of awareness during surgery is that successful recall requires retrieval cues, that is, something to trigger a memory of the episode. These retrieval cues may be things that were quite incidentally associated with the remembered event. For example, the sound of a seagull, or the scent of pine trees, may trigger a recollection of a childhood holiday. Without the appropriate cues, a memory may never be retrieved : in other words it will be 'forgotten'. If someone wakes up during surgery, they will be surrounded by sights and sounds which are quite specific to the operating theatre. The recovery room or hospital ward may not, therefore, provide the retrieval cues necessary for them to recollect the event. It is possible that hypnosis may mimic the state of mind of someone who is lightly anaesthetized, and may therefore help them recollect surgery, but the strongest retrieval cue will be provided by a return to the anaesthetic room or operating theatre for a subsequent operation. This is probably the worst possible time for someone to recall a traumatic experience.

To summarize this section, we have discussed a number of reasons why someone may be unable to recall intraoperative events. They may have been aware during surgery but have formed no memory of the event, or they may have only implicit memory for surgery, or they may have explicit memory but be unable to recall it at present because of lack of retrieval cues. Thus, a patient's failure to recollect details of surgery is not proof that they remained unconscious throughout the operation.

CONSEQUENCES OF AWARENESS

Two case studies illustrate the potentially damaging effect of awareness during surgery. In the first of these, a patient complained of chronic insomnia dating from a hysterectomy operation. Under hypnosis, she recalled the anaesthetist saying, 'She will sleep the sleep of death' (the anaesthetist confirmed that this remark may indeed have been made). In the second case, a shy, obese student had undergone counselling which had increased her self-confidence and helped her keep to a healthier diet. However, shortly after a minor operation, she became depressed and reported suicidal thoughts. Hypnotic regression led her to recall the surgeon exclaiming 'She is fat, isn't she?'

It should be noted here that the status of hypnosis as an aid to memory is uncertain. Hypnosis seems to increase the amount of detailed information which someone can recall, and it may do this because it mimics a state of light anaesthesia. That is, it reinstates the internal environment in which the learning first occurred. It is known that recall of an event is better in a context which is similar to that in which the event took place. However, it has also been shown that hypnosis encourages people to 'fill in' the gaps in their memory, that is, to confabulate the details which they cannot genuinely recall. At best, therefore, hypnosis is an unreliable way of eliciting recall of intraoperative events, and may produce quite misleading results.

In Moerman's study of awareness during anaesthesia, 18 of 26 people reported disturbing after-effects. The most common of these were sleep disturbances, nightmares, and daytime anxiety, all of which are typical systems of **post-traumatic stress disorder**. These symptoms are easily attributable to other aspects of illness and hospitalization. For instance, sleep disturbances are common in a hospital environment and prolonged illness, time off work, or absence from one's family, may all contribute to anxiety and depression. Therefore, if an episode of intraoperative awareness is not reported, its consequences may be overlooked and untreated.

It is not only conscious recollection of awareness which may cause these symptoms. Implicit memory also (by definition) affects behaviour. This is well illustrated by Claparède's report in 1911 of an amnesic patient. One day, as was his habit, Claparède went to shake hands with this patient while conducting his ward round. On this occasion, he secreted a pin in the palm of his hand. The following day, the patient refused to shake hands with him, yet could not explain her reluctance to do so. In the anaesthesia literature, it has been claimed that implicit memory for positive suggestions (e.g. 'You will recover quickly') played during surgery may be beneficial for recovery. Conversely, implicit memory for a traumatic event such as waking paralysed and in pain could produce the symptoms of post-traumatic stress disorder described above. It is conceivable that lack of explicit memory for waking would actually exacerbate these symptoms, as the patient would be unable to reflect upon and rationalize their experience.

CAUSES OF AWARENESS DURING ANAESTHESIA

Why does intraoperative awareness occur? Hargrove categorized the cases of awareness reported to the Medical Defence Union according to their most probable cause. Faulty anaesthetic technique was thought to be responsible for 70% of the incidents. Most of these were patients in whom the anaesthetist had used the 'balanced' technique of combining nitrous oxide, opiate and neuromuscular blocking drug. Adding a volatile agent to this sequence should prevent awareness, but it may not do so if given in too low a concentration or administered intermittently during the operation. In particular, Hargrove noted a reluctance to use a volatile supplement during Caesarean section between induction of anaesthesia and delivery, even though this is the period of greatest risk of awareness. In one of the studies cited by Jones (1994), the overall incidence of awareness dropped from 1.3 to 0.4% when a 1% isoflurane supplement was introduced to their standard anaesthetic technique. Other examples of faulty anaesthetic technique include failure to attend to the patient (including leaving the operating theatre), and responding to a difficult intubation by increasing the dose of neuromuscular blocking drug, but not giving more induction agent.

Twenty per cent of cases of awareness are due to the anaesthetist failing to check the anaesthetic apparatus. With volatile agents, awareness has resulted from room air being drawn in through a faulty connection between the anaesthetic machine and the ventilator, and from dilution of the anaesthetic by oxygen when the emergency oxygen supply has accidentally been left on. Other causes include incorrectly attaching the ventilator and using an empty vaporizer. All these cases could have been prevented by meticulous checking of the apparatus.

The remainder of the cases reported to the Medical Defence Union fall into three categories: genuine apparatus failure, spurious claims, and justified risks. Under the heading of genuine apparatus failure are cases where vaporizers have been inaccurately calibrated, so that they deliver lower concentrations of vapour than are indicated on the dial, and malfunctioning ventilators which deliver too little nitrous oxide to the patient. These problems can be overcome by the use of anaesthetic agent monitors. Spurious claims may be prompted by media attention to the problem of awareness during surgery. In the eyes of the law, it is not enough simply to report that one was aware during surgery. Rather, the claimant must be able to give appropriate detail of the awareness episode to demonstrate that the anaesthetist was negligent, and many of these cases are therefore withdrawn before reaching the courts. Finally, the category of justified risks refers to cases where a very ill patient was aware, but the anaesthetist had reason to believe that deeper anaesthesia may have been fatal. Although patients in this situation tend not to sue, the traumatic effects of necessarily light anaesthesia can be offset by adequate analgesia and by reassurance before, during and after the operation.

To summarize, conservative estimates of the incidence of awareness during anaesthesia show approximately one patient in every 10 000 experiencing pain during surgery, and three in every 1000 having some recollection of intra-operative events. This incidence of awareness could be considerably reduced by the following measures:

- using volatile or intravenous anaesthetic agents in conjunction with nitrous oxide and opiates, rather than relying solely on nitrous oxide and narcotics;
- ensuring that the dose of induction agent is sufficient to prevent awareness during intubation and that its duration is sufficient for the surgical procedure in question;
- rigorously checking the apparatus used to deliver the anaesthetic, and having it regularly serviced and re-calibrated;
- monitoring volatile anaesthetic agents.

Note that premedicating patients with benzodiasepines is **not** a solution to the problem of awareness during anaesthesia. Although these drugs may prevent patients recollecting and reporting awareness, they do not abolish implicit memory for the episode of awareness and neither do they prevent its consequences for the patient's recovery.

The biggest advance in preventing awareness during surgery would be to introduce monitors of depth of anaesthesia into operating theatres. These would alert anaesthetists to potential equipment failures, for example, when the patient fails to reach the desired depth of anaesthesia, and would avoid the necessity of giving high doses of anaesthetics just to be on the safe side. Also, in cases where very light anaesthesia is unavoidable, a means of detecting awareness would enable anaesthetists to offer proper counselling to patients who wake up during surgery, including those who have no recollection of doing so. Unfortunately, however, there is no universally accepted way of monitoring depth of anaesthesia. The next part of this chapter will address the problems involved in monitoring depth of anaesthesia and will discuss some recent developments in this area.

MONITORING DEPTH OF ANAESTHESIA

THE PROBLEM

Depth of anaesthesia reflects the balance between the hypnotic effect of the anaesthetic agent and the arousal effect of intubation and surgery. The strength of these opposing effects varies throughout surgery. For example, with a constant level of surgical stimulation, anaesthesia will lighten as the effect of the induction agent wears off and deepen when a bolus of an intravenous maintenance anaesthetic is infused. Similarly, if the infusion rate or end-tidal concentration of the anaesthetic is constant, anaesthesia will lighten in response to intubation or surgical incision. Thus, a dose of anaesthetic which is sufficient to prevent awareness as the patient is wheeled into the operating theatre may be inadequate to maintain unconsciousness during surgery.

For the first century of anaesthetic practice, a major problem was deep anaesthesia, characterized by John Snow in 1847 as feeble and irregular respiratory movements, that is, the stage just preceding death. However, the problem altered in the 1940s when the neuromuscular blocking drug, curare, was introduced into clinical anaesthetic practice. Curare had two important effects: it meant that deep anaesthesia was no longer needed for producing muscle relaxation, and it meant that light anaesthesia could no longer be reliably detected by observing pupil size and respiratory movements. This remains a problem today; studies attempting to categorize the clinical signs of depth of anaesthesia found that this was difficult even for a single anaesthetic, let alone for inhalational agents in general.

There is now an even greater range of anaesthetics which vary hugely in their pharmacology and in the extent to which they relieve pain, impair memory, induce muscle relaxation, and abolish consciousness. Although anaesthetists still use changes in arterial pressure, heart rate, pupil dilation, sweating and tear production as indicators of anaesthetic depth, their value for detecting awareness is very limited. This is partly because the relationship between these physiological responses and consciousness probably varies from anaesthetic to anaesthetic, and from patient to patient.

The worthlessness of these clinical signs for detecting awareness is clear from studies by Moerman and by Russell. Moerman and her colleagues asked three experienced anaesthetists ('the raters') to examine the anaesthetic records of 12 people who were aware during surgery. Photocopies of the records were presented along with the photocopied charts of 24 similar cases, so that each case of awareness was matched with two cases in which there was no awareness. As far as possible, the cases were matched for anaesthetic technique, gender, type and duration of surgery, ASA score, premedication, and tracheal intubation. Relevant comments, such as 'The patient is awake', were of course removed from the photocopies (interestingly, these were present on only 3 of the 12 records). The raters were asked to score the records in three ways: first, they were asked to rate the possibility that awareness had occurred, on a scale of 1 ('very unlikely') to 5 ('very likely'); second, they were shown each record along with its two matched control records, and asked to select the record for the person who was aware during the operation; third, they were given more detailed information about the patients' recollections of surgery and were then asked to repeat their selection of one case from each group of three records. On all three tests, the raters were unable to reliably select the case of awareness from the two matched controls. Even on the third test, where most information was available, the raters correctly identified the case of awareness on only 5, 4 and 7 trials respectively. Given that, by guessing, they would select the correct record on an average of 4 out of 12 trials, this shows that the anaesthetic records were useless when deciding retrospectively whether patients had been awake during surgery.

DETECTING AWARENESS DURING ANAESTHESIA: THE ISOLATED FOREARM TECHNIQUE

Tunstall's isolated forearm technique is a means of assessing awareness by asking the patient to make a deliberate, and therefore conscious, response during anaesthesia. The technique involves inflating a blood pressure cuff around the patient's arm, after induction of anaesthesia, but before the neuromuscular blocking drugs are injected into the contralateral arm. The patient therefore remains able, if they become conscious, to move their arm in response to commands played to them over headphones or spoken by the anaesthetist. Typically, these instructions will ask the patient to 'Squeeze my hand' or to 'Squeeze once if you can hear me and squeeze twice if you are in pain'. Thus, a conversation can be conducted with the patient during the operation.

Research by Russell and colleagues, using the isolated arm technique, has produced some alarming findings. For example, a recent paper reports a study of 32 patients undergoing major gynaecological surgery with alfentanil–midazolam anaesthesia and neuromuscular blockade. Seventy two per cent of these patients responded to command using their unparalysed arm. Furthermore, twenty of these patients responded positively when asked if they were in pain. The arterial pressure, heart rate, sweating and tear (PRST) score gave no indication that these people were awake and in pain. Nobody in the study spontaneously recollected being in pain, or even aware, during surgery.

There are three important conclusions to be drawn from this study. Firstly (as many anaesthetists would presumably agree), opiates do not produce anaesthesia, whether used alone or in combination with benzodiazepines. Secondly, the autonomic signs on which the PRST score is calculated are, at best, unreliable indices of consciousness. Thirdly, someone can be awake and in pain during surgery and recollect nothing of their experience when they recover from the anaesthetic. This is unsurprising if one considers the deleterious effects on explicit memory of drugs such as midazolam and various anaesthetics, including isoflurane and propofol. However, the fact that **awareness cannot always be recalled** must be strongly emphasized, because many anaesthetists persist in assuming that their patients must have been unconscious throughout surgery, simply because they recollect nothing of the procedure on recovery.

Does the isolated forearm technique solve the problem of preventing awareness during anaesthesia? Unfortunately, it does not. There are practical problems with the technique if it is used for prolonged operations. The isolated arm may suffer ischaemic paralysis if the cuff is left inflated for more than about 20 min, and deflation of the cuff will enable an influx of neuromuscular blocking drug into the arm. Interpreting a patient's responses to command presents another problem. The anaesthetist must be able to distinguish purposive responses from spontaneous and reflex movements. Furthermore, the lack of response does not prove that the patient is unconscious, as people have sometimes recalled hearing commands but failed to respond to them. If someone was aware during surgery and in pain, then it is probably safe to assume that they would respond to the anaesthetist's commands. This, however, raises another issue; even if the isolated arm technique were a foolproof indicator of awareness, it could do no more than detect awareness. What is really needed is a graded measure of depth of anaesthesia, one which will enable the anaesthetist to **predict** awakening and hence to prevent it by increasing the dose of anaesthetic. Proposed measures of depth fall into two categories, which can be thought of as indices of body state and indices of brain state. These measures will be considered next.

PROPOSED MONITORS OF DEPTH OF ANAESTHESIA: MEASURES OF BODY STATE

Oesophageal contractility

When someone is awake, the contractility of their oesophagus increases during psychological stress. This increased contractility has been studied as a potential index of stress (awareness) during anaesthesia. Two types of contraction are important: contractions of the lower portion of the oesophagus which can be provoked by pressure on the wall of the oesophagus, and spontaneous contractions of the lower oesophagus which are non-propulsive and of unknown physiological function. These contractions are measured using two balloons placed in the lower oesophagus. One balloon acts as a sensor and the other is inflated at intervals to provoke contractions of the oesophagus. These contractions can not be elicited during deep anaesthesia, but they appear with increasing amplitude as anaesthesia lightens. The amplitude of the provoked contractions and the frequency of the spontaneous contractions are used to calculate the oesophageal contractility index. This technique gives some indication of depth of anaesthesia, but varies too greatly between patients and between different anaesthetic agents to be considered a reliable index of awareness during anaesthesia.

The facial electromyogram

Measurements of the activity of facial muscles have been proposed as an index of depth of anaesthesia. For example, at the Third International Symposium on Memory and Awareness in Anaesthesia held in Rotterdam in 1995, Bennett described facial muscle activity (FMA) in experimental studies of awareness. FMA responded well to loss and return of consciousness as indicated using the isolated forearm technique. Preliminary reports of this monitor sound promising, but further research is needed to evaluate its performance as a predictor, rather than detector, of awareness.

Sinus arrhythmia

The variability of cardiac function from one beat to the next may provide an index of depth of anaesthesia. For the present purposes, the most interesting aspect of this variability is respiratory sinus arrhythmia. As someone breathes in, the expansion of the lungs triggers a reflex signal via the vagal motor neurones to the heart, causing the heart rate to increase during inspiration. A corresponding decrease in heart rate is observed during expiration. This fluctuation in heart rate declines during anaesthesia and increases during recovery. It may provide, therefore, a useful measure of depth of anaesthesia, but it has yet to be shown to reflect psychological changes, i.e. awareness during surgery.

A drawback with all these 'body state' measures is that at best they give only indirect information about psychological function. Measures of brain function, via an electroencephalogram (EEG), potentially enable a more direct assessment of the level of consciousness during anaesthesia.

PROPOSED MONITORS OF DEPTH OF ANAESTHESIA: MEASURES OF BRAIN STATE

The resting EEG

The latencies of the various peaks in the EEG tend to increase as depth of anaesthesia increases. This alone does not provide a useful index of depth of anaesthesia, because the relationship between depth and changes in the EEG varies with the type of anaesthetic agent and with factors such as blood glucose concentration, body temperature and carbon dioxide levels. Also, interpretation of complex patterns of changes in the EEG requires a certain amount of expertise yet provides at best only a subjective index of anaesthetic depth. A number of computerized techniques have been developed to get around this problem of subjectivity. These techniques process the raw EEG to provide an easier to read and more sensitive measure of depth of anaesthesia. They include analysis of the EEG, by fast Fourier transformation, into a power spectrum of consecutive epochs. From this **spectral analysis** can be derived variables such as the frequency band power, the median (band) frequency and the spectral edge frequency. Changes in these variables indicate the relative depth of anaesthesia. However, derivatives of the processed EEG have the same disadvantages as the raw EEG when it comes to their potential use in the operating theatre: that is, different anaesthetic agents produce different changes. None the less, recent research using a mathematical approach known as bispectral analysis, a technique for quantifying the level of synchronization in the EEG, is producing more promising data (Sigl and Chamoun, 1994).

Evoked potentials in the EEG

Three types of evoked responses have been studied: somatosensory, visual and auditory. Of these, the auditory evoked response looks the most promising. Responses evoked by flashes of light are possible during anaesthesia as they do not require the patient to look at a complex visual stimulus, but they tend to vary too greatly between trials and between subjects to provide useful information about depth of anaesthesia. Somatosensory evoked responses either do not vary in any consistent way with anaesthesia (short-latency responses) or seem to reflect the analgesic properties of anaesthetics, but not their hypnotic properties (cortical responses). Thus, only auditory evoked responses will be considered here.

Auditory evoked responses (AER) are typically generated by playing 6–9 Hz clicks to patients over headphones, and the responses are extracted from the EEG by computer averaging. The resultant **transient AER** comprises a series of waves which are generated from different levels of the neuraxis. The first waves (I–VI) occur at 1–8 ms after the stimulus and reflect electrical activity in the acoustic nerve, pons, and mid-brain. Together they are known as the **brain stem response**. The next waves (No, Po, Na, Pa, Nb) occur at 8–50 ms after stimulation. These are collectively called the middle latency waves, or **early cortical response**. They reflect activity in the medial geniculate body (thalamus) and the primary auditory cortex. Waves occurring later than 50 ms after stimulation (P1, N1, P2, N2) comprise the **late cortical response** and reflect activity in the frontal cortex and association areas. These different areas of the brain are differentially sensitive to various drugs, but they are unaffected by neuromuscular blocking drugs. The brain stem response shows a dose-related slowing to volatile anaesthetics, but does not respond to intravenous agents such as propofol and etomidate. It is therefore unsuitable as a measure of depth of anaesthesia. The late cortical response is also unsuitable because it is excessively sensitive; drastically attenuated by sleep and sedation, as well as by general anaesthesia.

The early cortical response (middle latency waves), on the other hand, shows dose-related responses to various anaesthetics. Thornton and colleagues demonstrated increases in latency and decreases in amplitude of these waves in response to increasing doses of halothane, enflurane, isoflurane, althesin, etomidate, and propofol. In contrast, they are influenced to a negligible degree by opioids or benzodiazepines supporting the view that these agents do not produce the state of anaesthesia.

The problem with the middle latency of the transient AER is that it does not lend itself to automatic analysis and the signal to noise ratio is poor, even after considerable averaging (> 2000 sweeps). This is aggravated by the electrically noisy environment found in most operating rooms which can make acquisition of the AER impossible. An improvement in signal-to-noise ratio and reduction in averaging time can be achieved by increasing the stimulating frequency to about 40 Hz. This produces a standing wave phenomenon: the **steady state AER**, and improves the signal to noise ratio by increasing the resultant signal, narrowing signal bandwidth and therefore reducing the noise contribution. The best signal in the awake subject is attained at a stimulating frequency at 35–45 Hz.

We have used a steady-state, recording protocol by systematically changing the stimulating frequency. From previous studies we know that anaesthetics prolong the latency of the transient response and it was expected that the maximum amplitude in the steady state response would be achieved not at 40 Hz, but at progressively lower frequencies as anaesthetic concentration increased. Thus, we varied the stimulating frequency from 7–49 Hz and showed that increasing doses of isoflurane decreased the frequency of a distinctive response, called the coherent frequency, from about 40 Hz to around 15 Hz. Explicit memory of intra-anaesthetic events was abolished at a coherent frequency of 25 Hz and consciousness (defined in this instance as ability to raise thumb to command) was lost when the coherent frequency fell below 15 Hz. We have recently obtained similar results with propofol.

The potential usefulness of the steady state AER as a measure of depth of anaesthesia is tentatively supported by Crick and Koch's Neurobiological Theory of Consciousness. This proposes that consciousness is based on the brain generating coherent semi-synchronous oscillations which are probably in the 40 Hz range. These oscillations in turn activate a transient short term or working memory. It is possible that the coherent frequency is picking up changes in the frequency of these oscillations as consciousness is lost.

CONCLUSIONS

Awareness during anaesthesia affects a small proportion (under 0.3%) of surgical patients, but the large numbers of patients being anaesthetized means it is experienced by many people. Estimates of awareness are usually based upon patients' spontaneous recall of surgery. We suggest that an additional group of patients may be awake during surgery, but subsequently have only implicit memory for events during this time. This implicit memory may still influence recovery. To resolve this issue, there is a need for an objective measure of depth of anaesthesia, clinical signs are of no value. The most promising candidates for measuring depth of anaesthesia are median frequency, bispectral analysis, and the transient and steady-state auditory evoked responses.

FURTHER READING

Andrade, J. (1995). Learning during anaesthesia: A review. *British Journal of Psychology*, **86**, 479–506.

Andrade, J., Sapsford, D. V., Jeevaratnum, D., Pickworth, A. J. and Jones, J. G. (1996) The coherent frequency in the electroencephalogram as an objective measure of cognitive function during propofol sedation. *Anaesthesia and Analgesia*, **83**, 1279–1284.

Crick, F. and Koch, C. (1990) Towards a neurobiological theory of consciousness. *Seminars in the Neurosciences*, **2**, 263–275.

Cullen, D. J., Eger, E. I. and Stevens, W. C. (1972) Clinical signs of anesthesia. *Anesthesiology*, **36**, 21–36.

Hargrove, R. L. (1987) Awareness under anaesthesia. *Journal of the Medical Defence Union*, **3**, 9–11.

Jones, J. G. (1994). Perception and memory during general anaesthesia. *British Journal of Anaesthesia*, **73**, 31–37.

Moerman, N., Bonke, B. and Oosting, J. (1993) Awareness and recall during general anaesthesia: Facts and feelings. *Anesthesiology*, **79**, 454–464.

Russell, I. F. (1993) Midazolam–alfentanil: An anaesthetic? An investigation using the isolated forearm technique. *British Journal of Anaesthesia*, **70**, 42–46.

Sigl, J. C. and Chamoun, N. G. (1994) An introduction to bispectral analysis for the EEG, *Journal of Clinical Monitoring*, **10**, 392–404.

Thornton, C. and Jones, J. G. (1993) Evaluating depth of anesthesia: Review of methods, in *Depth of Anesthesia*, International Anesthesiology Clinics, Vol 31. No 4 (ed J. G. Jones), Little, Brown and Co., Boston, pp. 67–88.

CARDIOPULMONARY RESUSCITATION

M. E. Ward

The success of resuscitation, following a cardiac arrest, has been shown to be directly related both to the skill of the resuscitator in diagnosing and treating the cause of the cardiac arrhythmia and the speed with which the resuscitative efforts are applied.

A recent study has shown that the resuscitation skills of a group of British anaesthetists, tested according to the guidelines of the Resuscitation Council of the United Kingdom and the European Resuscitation Council, were of a high level and that this was independent of their grade. This study suggests that anaesthetists, by the nature of their work, maintain the skills and knowledge of cardiopulmonary resuscitation (CPR) as well as, if not better than, other hospital groups previously studied as cardiologists and Accident and Emergency physicians. However, other studies have shown that physicians presenting for their membership examination exhibit poor skills and knowledge of CPR. It is clearly appropriate that anaesthetists should be highly skilled in this area, as not only are they routinely involved in the resuscitation process outside the operating theatre, but within it they manipulate physiology on a regular basis and to such a degree as to be able to take patients almost as close to death as does cardiac arrest itself. Furthermore, the practical skills involved in resuscitation such as airway care, central and peripheral venous cannulation and ECG interpretation, are the very skills that they use routinely.

In order to achieve the optimum outcome, successful resuscitation in hospital therefore depends both on organization and training, which require the proper use of agreed protocols. A multidisciplinary resuscitation committee should meet regularly to review the hospital resuscitation policy, and should consist of representatives of senior medical staff (with specific interests in resuscitation), senior nursing staff (with particular involvement from those working in high dependency areas) and junior medical staff, who are the most likely to be involved in the advanced life support process. Those hospitals fortunate enough to have the benefit of resuscitation training officers must involve them on the resuscitation committee as they are the lynch pin for information acquisition and distribution, and training. The degree of involvement of the anaesthetist in this resuscitation committee will vary from hospital to hospital, but generally speaking the presence of an anaesthetist with the aforementioned special skills and knowledge can make a substantial difference to success at a cardiac arrest.

BASIC LIFE SUPPORT

It must always be remembered that the diagnosis of cardiac arrest is a clinical one. It must be suspected in a previously conscious patient who becomes suddenly unresponsive, and is confirmed by the absence of a major pulse on palpation. Electrocardiographic diag-

Short Practice of Anaesthesia. Edited by M. Morgan and G. M. Hall. Published in 1997 by Chapman & Hall, London. ISBN 0 412 71890 1

nosis alone is unreliable unless confirmed by pulselessness, and the other clinical features are equally unreliable. Fixed and dilated pupils, for example, may result from a number of causes (particularly during anaesthesia) and absent spontaneous respiration is frequently, and routinely, induced pharmacologically in the intensive care unit and operating theatre.

The management of basic life support in the pre-hospital or ward situation is well described elsewhere, but essentially depends upon a rapid response and enlistment of those trained in advanced life support. It has only recently been widely accepted that basic life support alone is unlikely to revive a pulseless patient, and recent changes in protocol emphasize the need to call for professional help once cardiac or respiratory arrest is diagnosed. Recommendations now agree that, having assessed responsiveness, the rescuer should call out for help and then check for breathing and pulse. If the patient is breathing, the rescuer should turn him to the recovery position and ensure the early arrival of assistance. If he is not breathing, and the rescuer has not already done so, someone must be sent for help. If no assistant is available, the rescuer must leave the victim, go for help, return and start rescue breathing. However, in the event that this is a primary respiratory arrest in a child, or in an adult as a result of trauma or drowning, then 10 rescue breaths should initially be given, either using expired air or some other ventilating device before the single handed rescuer leaves the patient. Where the event is presumed to be cardiac in origin (the majority of sudden adult collapse) the help should, immediately after assessment, be summoned even if this means leaving the patient for a short time, provided that, after a quick reassessment, 'rescue breathing' and, where necessary, chest compression is commenced on the rescuer's return. If the patient at first assessment, exhibits neither ventilatory efforts nor has signs of a circulation, then the patient must be left in order that the rescuer can summon help before committing him/herself to resuscitative efforts (Figure 44. 1).

EXPIRED AIR RESPIRATION (RESCUE BREATHING)

The airway should be opened using the techniques of head-tilt and chin-lift. Only minimal head extension should be used if there is any suspicion of cervical spine injury. The rescuer places his/her lips around the mouth ensuring a good seal. The nasal passages can either be obstructed by the side of the rescuers mouth, or the nares can be pinched by the rescuer's index finger and thumb. In the case of children or small adults some trained rescuers include the nose within the rescuer's open mouth. While supporting the airway in this manner the rescuer takes a deep breath and blows into the patient until the chest is seen to rise as with normal ventilation. Excessive pressure is not required and if the inflation is in any way difficult, or the airway appears obstructed, it may be necessary to modify the head-tilt, jaw-thrust position. In the event that inflation is still difficult the presence of a foreign body should be suspected and dealt with appropriately. This can be achieved with either finger sweeps, back blows or abdominal thrusts according to the clinical situation and presentation. Once inflation has occurred and chest movement has been seen, the rescuer removes his mouth allowing complete passive exhalation to occur before inflating the lungs again at a rate of 10 breaths a minute for adults, 20 per minute for children. Excessive inflation pressures should be avoided as this may result in gastric distension leading to passive regurgitation and pulmonary soiling.

Wherever possible expired air should be replaced by the use of simple ventilatory devices such as the pocket mask or the self-inflating bag/valve device, both of which have the advantage of allowing the addition

Basic life support 767

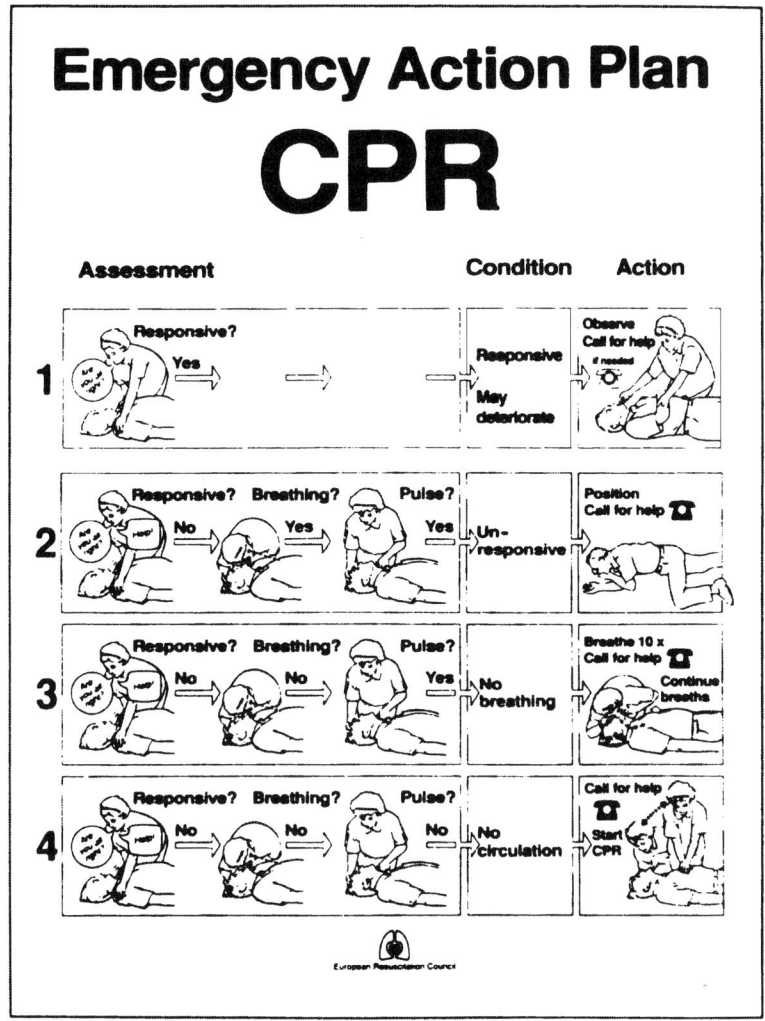

Figure 44.1 Emergency action plan for basic life support. (Reproduced with permission from *Resuscitation* 1992, **24**, 110, by courtesy of the European Resuscitation Council.) Now modified in line with the advisory statement from ILCOR 1997 (see text).

of oxygen to the ventilating gases. Indeed, concentrations of up to 90% can be achieved with high flows and oxygen reservoir systems. In properly trained hands manually triggered oxygen powered resuscitators can also be used, but these must only be used by authorized personnel who can time their use appropriately and when artificial circulatory support its also provided.

EXTERNAL CHEST COMPRESSION

The debate as to whether external chest compression provides an artificial circulation by a 'cardiac pump' (compression of the heart between sternum and backbone) or 'thoracic pump' (compression of the entire intra-thoracic structures) is on-going. In any case, it is largely immaterial provided that the technique used is appropriate and produces a circulation. Compression is achieved by placing the heel of the hand over the junction of the lower and middle third of the sternum, and then placing the second hand on top of the first. With the arms locked straight, compress vertically downwards 4–5cm in an adult. Compression should be rhythmical, with the compression phase lasting approximately as long as the release phase, and should be repeated at the rate of 100 compressions a minute.

External chest compression and expired air resuscitation are combined to provide an artificial circulation of oxygenated blood. A single rescuer should give 15 compressions followed by 2 inflations, and should repeat this until such time as he/she is relieved by another rescuer or a member of the emergency services or until exhaustion makes it impossible to continue. If two rescuers are present it is normal for one to be responsible for ventilation and the other for chest compression and in this situation every five chest compressions should be separated by a single ventilation.

RATIONALE BEHIND EXTERNAL CHEST COMPRESSION

Exactly what takes place during external chest compression remains unclear. The fact that this has not yet been fully elucidated is not surprising, particularly when it is remembered that closed chest compression was only described originally some 35 years ago.

Kouwenhoven's original hypothesis was that manual compression of the chest simply squeezed the heart between the spine and the sternum. This of course would depend upon the full functionality of the heart valves to close, preventing retrograde flow during compression, and open during relaxation, to allow the filling of the ventricles. Observations, however, that patients could remain conscious during episodes of ventricular fibrillation occurring in the cardiac catheter laboratory by being made to follow instructions to cough rhythmically, threw doubt on this simple explanation.

Production of a cardiac output by coughing and other methods of increasing intrathoracic pressure, led to the postulation of flow produced by a 'thoracic pump' mechanism of creating a pressure gradient from the cardiac chambers to the extra-thoracic vessels. It is likely that elements of both mechanisms play significant parts, but it is possible that both mechanisms contribute to the antegrade flow of blood but that direct compression of the heart is likely to be the most significant factor. However, the debate continues in spite of recent improvements in the techniques available for study of blood flow in the intact human chest.

One of the difficulties in coming to any of these conclusions arises in connection with the problems of studying the effectiveness or otherwise of chest compressions in humans. During closed chest compression cardiac output will rarely approach 25% of normal and in these situations perfusion of the myocardium may be no more than 5% of normal, so that prolonged periods of external chest compression will lead to severe myocardial hypoperfusion and deleterious metabolic consequences. Augmentation of these blood flow values can be achieved by the use of adrenergic drugs and this is the rationale behind the repeated administration of adrenaline (epinephrine) during the advanced life support cycle.

In an effort to improve on the performance achieved with simple external chest compression, a number of modifications to the basic technique and mechanical adjuncts have been developed and studied. 'High impulse CPR' (with compression rates of up to 150 per minute) or interposed abdominal compression are examples, but unfortunately, whilst these enhancements produce improvements in measuring of cardiac output during resuscitation, none of them have been effective in improving outcome from resuscitative efforts.

Mechanical CPR using machines with pistons, either with or without synchronized positive ventilation, has been available for some time but has not been widely used in clinical practice. Centres that have used them have been very enthusiastic in their praise, but the technique is limited by the need to have skilled operators available. Whilst the advantage of a tireless mechanical resuscitator is obvious, their relatively high cost and lack of proven efficacy have limited their widespread introduction.

Most recently the active compression–decompression device has been shown to enhance cardiac output significantly. This device uses a large suction cup which is applied to the lower part of the chest over the sternum and is used to compress the chest as in normal external chest compression. After each compression phase the cup is actively lifted, pulling the chest wall up and creating an intra-thoracic negative pressure decompression phase which has been shown to increase venous return and left ventricular filling. On-going studies in the USA of this device, the Cardio-Pump, have shown significant improvement in output and the early signs looked encouraging for survival. However, difficulties with the Federal Drug Administration (FDA) have led to a temporary cessation of the on-going clinical study.

RISKS TO THE RESCUER

Recent concern has been expressed about the fear of micro-organism transmission to rescuers, particularly the human immunodeficiency (HIV) and hepatitis B viruses during direct contact from mouth-to-mouth/expired air resuscitation. So far there has been no recorded case of direct transfer of HIV from casualty to rescuer or vice versa. Nevertheless, there is still an understandable concern and reluctance on the part of many to become involved in the resuscitation of patients whose HIV status may be unknown. For this reason a number of barrier devices have been developed which may be in the form of a thin filter membrane, or an interposed simple ventilation mask with valve mechanism. Provided that these devices are readily available and can be used by the rescuer to provide an adequate gas-flow then their use is recommended. Currently, however, the risk is considered to be exceedingly small provided that there is not a large amount of bloody contamination of the patients' airway.

HOSPITAL LIFE SUPPORT

The generally accepted definition of basic life support accepts only the limited use of equipment other than simple airway devices, whereas the term 'advanced life support' includes the full panoply of electrical defibrillation and drug intervention and embraces the extreme intervention of left thoracotomy and internal, or open, cardiac compression. Within the hospital environment there is now a recognition of an intermediate stage which should be employed by trained nursing, paramedical and medical personnel whilst awaiting the arrival of the full resuscitation team; this stage has been called 'hospital life support'. It may include the use, in appropriate patients, of the precordial thump, defibrillation (with the automatic external defibrillator), ventilation using bag-valve-mask adjuncts and the laryngeal mask airway, and could include the use of external chest compression adjuncts such as the active compression–decompression Cardio-Pump or automated chest compression devices. The recognition of arrest and peri-arrest rhythms, and familiarization with the arrest drugs and their delivery, are also parts of the training package used for this innovative area.

THE PRECORDIAL THUMP

There is evidence that a newly arrested heart can be restarted by a blow to the precordium. The current view is that the precordial thump should be used wherever the cardiac arrest is witnessed and the monitor shows ventricular fibrillation (VF) or pulseless ventricular tachycardia. It would appear that the blow acts by the conversion of the mechanical energy of the blow into an electrical impulse and as such the precordial thump can be considered as the lowest energy defibrillation that is currently available. Anxiety has been expressed in the past at the possibility of converting a low output state to ventricular fibrillation by the precordial thump. This is the reason for the proviso that the patient be monitored. This is now a widely accepted guideline, even though the risks of harmful conversion appear to be very low. As it also appears that the probability of successful cardioversion decreases with time, the current recommendation is that a single precordial thump should be given as rapidly as possible at the start of resuscitation.

ADVANCED LIFE SUPPORT

The sooner that advanced life support techniques can be employed, the more likely the survival of a patient suffering from cardiac arrest. Within the hospital environment a preplanned procedure for summoning suitably qualified personnel should exist, and everyone responsible for patient care should be familiar with the procedure and the emergency call number. It is to be hoped that a standard number will be introduced in all hospitals, thereby reducing confusion, particularly in the light of increasing mobility of medical and nursing personnel.

In general the prime aim of the advanced life support team is to convert ventricular fibrillation to an output-producing rhythm. Occasionally, a precordial thump (see above) may be all that is required.

Pulseless ventricular tachycardia (VT) will usually rapidly deteriorate to VF and the two conditions are treated identically (Figure 44.2). The BRESUS study showed that rapid resuscitation from VT or pulseless VT should be easily achieved where the appropriate facilities and trained personnel are available, but prospects for survival decrease by approximately 5% per minute even when effective basic life support is employed. Thus, defibrillation of a non-output rhythm to a spontaneous output rhythm is the first and overriding essential requirement for survival.

Other rhythms that may be encountered during the arrest sequence are asystole and pulseless electrical activity (previously known as electromechanical dissociation). Asystole is most commonly seen as an end result in patients with ventricular fibrillation where resuscitation has been unsuccessful. During anaesthesia short periods of asystole may occur as a result of high vagal activity; in this situation the immediate first aid measure is the stimulation of a pulse with 'thump pacing' (the administration of rhythmically repeated precordial blows). Vagolytic agents, such as atropine, will not find their site of action without an artificial circulation provided either by thump pacing or by external cardial massage. In any event, most episodes of vagal arrest are short-lived provided that the initiating stimulus is removed. Management should be according to the algorithm shown (Figure 44.3). Pulseless electrical activity implies the presence of an electrocardiographic trace and hence electrical activity within the myocardium, but the absence of functional mechanical activity. There are a number of specific causes of pulseless electrical activity which have to be considered and treated at the same time as the cardiac arrest itself is being managed (Figure 44.4).

The algorithms produced by the European Resuscitation Council Advanced Life Support Working Party for treating the three cardiac arrest rhythms are shown.

The algorithms are largely self-explanatory and an exposition of most of the elements can be found in the paper published at the time. It

Advanced life support

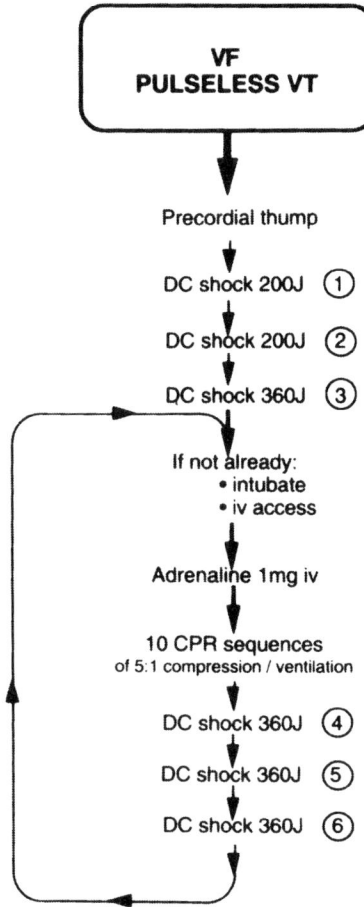

Figure 44.2 Algorithm for ventricular fibrillation or pulseless ventricular tachycardia. (Reproduced with permission from *Resuscitation* 1992, **24**, 115, by courtesy of the European Resuscitation Council.) But see Figure 44.5 for 1997 modifications.

must, of course, be remembered that as our knowledge and equipment advance there will be revisions in connection with the algorithms and it is also hoped that the few differences that currently exist between the American and the European and Australasian

772 *Cardiopulmonary resuscitation*

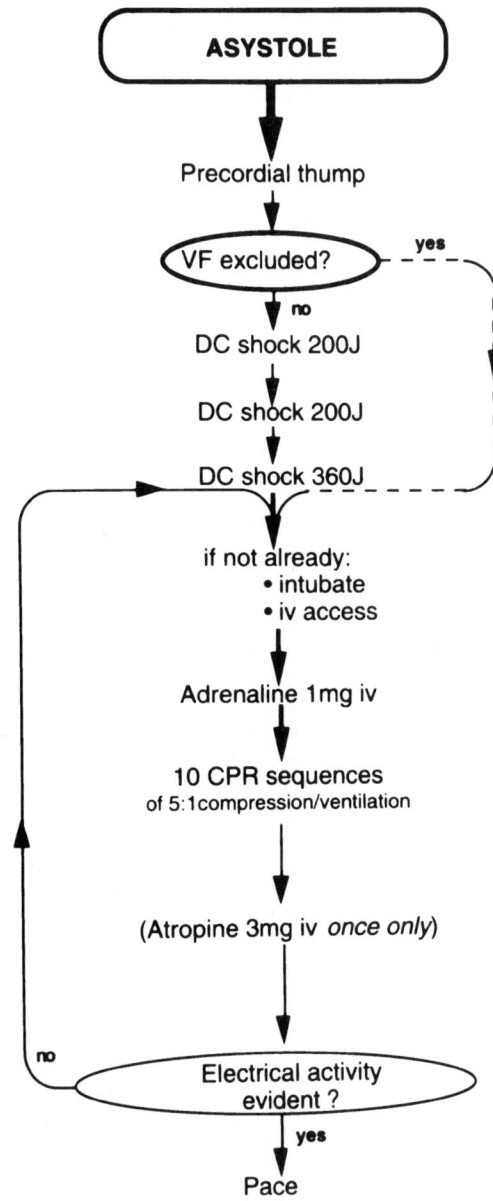

Figure 44.3 Algorithm for asystole. (Reproduced with permission from *Resuscitation* 1992, **24**, 118, by courtesy of the European Resuscitation Council.) But see Figure 44.5 for 1997 modifications.

protocols will shortly be reconciled. The guidelines were revised in 1992, reconfirmed in 1994 and are now to be reviewed regularly in the light of new research and clinical experience in their use. Through the medium of International Liaison Committees on Resuscitation (ILCOR), consisting of representatives from the world's resuscitation committees, it is hoped that a degree of merging will occur naturally and ultimately Global Guide-

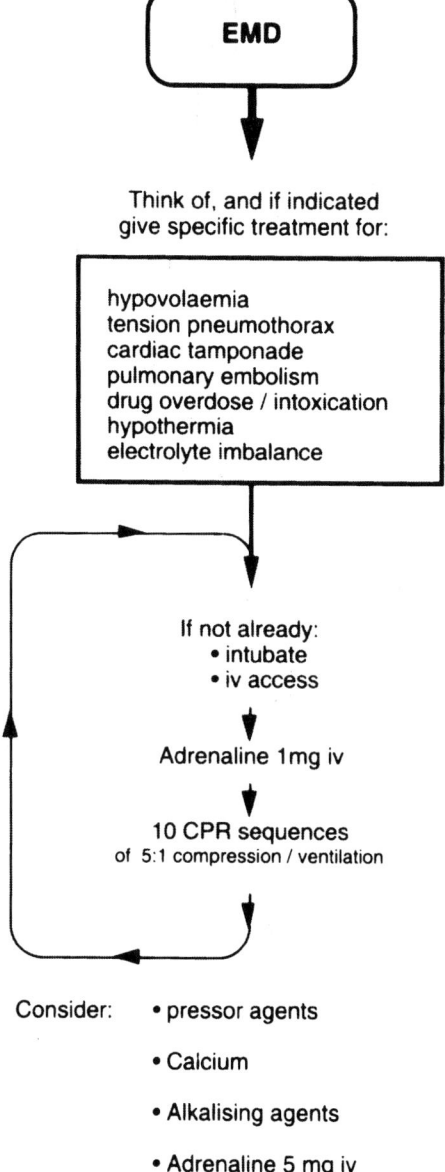

Figure 44.4 Algorithm for pulseless electrical activity previously known as electromechanical dissociation. (Reproduced with permission from *Resuscitation* 1992, **24**, 120, by courtesy of the European Resuscitation Council.) But see Figure 44.5 for 1997 modifications.

lines can be promulgated. ILCOR have now produced a series of Advisory Statements which attempt to simplify and streamline the management of both adult and paediatric, basic and advanced life support. These statements have been accepted, virtually in their entirety, by the Resuscitation Council (UK) as the guidelines to be followed in the United

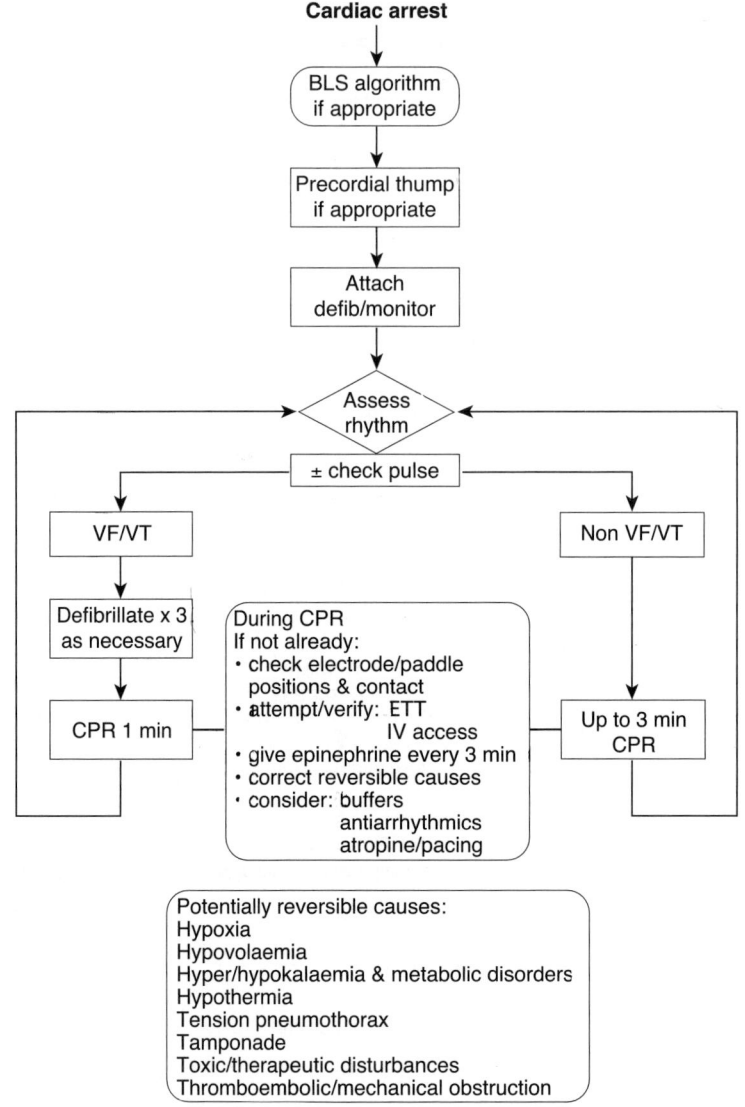

Figure 44.5 1997 Advanced life support algorithm for the management of cardiac arrest in adults. (Reproduced with permission of the International Liaison Committee on Resuscitation.)

Kingdom from April 1997. Copies of the protocols should be widely available within the hospital environment and it is recommended that they be followed unless there are overwhelming clinical reasons otherwise.

A number of controversies, however, still exist in the area of advanced life support and these will now be addressed.

USE OF ADRENALINE

Adrenaline is recommended to be given after the first sequence of defibrillatory shocks in order to improve the efficiency of basic cardial life support. It must be given either intravenously or via the tracheal tube. The rationale for the use of adrenaline is to improve the myocardial and cerebral perfusion pressures obtained during cardiopulmonary resuscitation. Other catecholamines have been suggested as alternatives because of their greater α-adrenoceptor activity, but in spite of their theoretical benefits have had no clinical improvements in the few studies published. Whilst there have been suggestions to use much larger doses of adrenaline during cardiac resuscitation (up to 15 mg), studies using such large doses have not shown any improved survival.

AIRWAY MANAGEMENT

There still remains little doubt that the gold standard for airway care during cardiopulmonary resuscitation is tracheal intubation, for which the claimed advantages include isolation, and therefore protection, of the lower airway from aspiration avoidance of gastric distension by ventilating gases, ease of mechanical ventilation and the ability to deliver a high oxygen concentration. Tracheal intubation also allows the use of the endobronchial route for drug administration and facilitates suction of the trachea and lower airways. However, the ability to intubate successfully requires considerable training and is therefore only available to experienced individuals. Furthermore, it is essential to confirm, without any shadow of doubt, the placement of the tube in the trachea rather than the oesophagus, and a number of different techniques have been developed to this end. Examples are the use of end-tidal CO_2 measurement, and the Wee oesophageal detector.

A number of other airway isolation devices have been described, such as the Esophageal Obturator Airway (EOA), the Pharyngo-Tracheal Lumen Airway (PTLA) and the Oesophago-Tracheal Airway, known as the Combitube. Whilst all these devices were reclassified in the 1992 American Heart Association Guidelines as 'acceptable and possibly helpful', and the Combitube is now accepted by the European Resuscitation Council as a suitable airway in adults, they have not achieved any measure of wide acceptance in the UK. Emphasis in the UK has, instead, focused on the increasing acceptance of the use of the laryngeal mask airway (LMA).

DRUG DELIVERY ROUTES

With recognition of the increasing importance of defibrillation as the most significant factor resulting in successful conversion of cardiac arrest, the emphasis on drugs and their delivery has lessened somewhat in recent years. Many of the drugs used in the resuscitation sequence are being subjected to a more stringent, critical examination, such as the current European Resuscitation Council International Multicentre study of the use of lignocaine and bretylium in patients failing to respond to early defibrillation.

The venous route is still recommended for drug delivery during cardiac arrest. Because of the ease of access for, and relative safety of, peripheral venous cannulation, and the ability to acquire access to this route without interrupting cardiopulmonary resuscitation, it is without doubt the most widely used. A large vein such as that situated in the antecubital fossa is the site of choice, but an as yet unanswered question is the volume of flushing solution needed to propel peripherally administered drugs into the central circulation to achieve their objective. Recommendation of the use of 20 ml solution are widely accepted, but the exact position of the extensive use of dextrose solutions in the resuscitation period is itself open to question, as a result of anxiety concerning the effects of high glucose levels on the eventual recovery of cerebral function.

Increasing emphasis is turning to the use of central venous cannulation which enables drugs to reach their site of action more directly. However, such procedures require considerably greater expertise and are associated with higher risks of complications such as inadvertent arterial puncture, haemothorax, pneumothorax and extravascular drug deposition.

Much attention has been placed on the use of the tracheal route of drug administration. In spite of now being accepted in some ambulance services in the UK as the route of first choice it should still be considered very much a second line approach for drug delivery. Where, however, peripheral or central venous access has not been rapidly achieved, the endobronchial route of administration may prove to be life saving. One method is for drugs to be either injected via the proximal end of the tracheal tube and then followed by rapid positive pressure ventilations in an effort to distribute the drug; alternatively a catheter, with multiple openings distally, can be introduced to aid generalized distribution and improve the rate of absorption. There is agreement that in order to achieve adequate blood levels at least twice the normal intravenous dose should be given and that the dose should be diluted with normal saline to a total volume of approximately 10 ml. Drugs which can be administered via the endobronchial route are adrenaline, lignocaine, atropine and with less reliability, diazepam and naloxone. The installations can be repeated after 10 min. Drug absorption via the bronchial tree may be impaired by atelectasis, pulmonary oedema and in the case of adrenaline by local vasoconstriction induced by the drug itself. Furthermore a marked decrease in Pao_2 may result from endobronchial drug administration caused by local variations in ventilation perfusion ratio and an increase in shunt.

Intraosseous route

Resurgence of interest in the use of the intraosseous route for drug administration and fluid resuscitation in infants has led to its increasing acceptance in children. All drugs suitable for intravenous administration can be given by the intraosseous route in the same dosages. Additionally, solutions of intravenous fluids can be administered by this route, including sodium bicarbonate. A special needle is required for safe access to the bone marrow, and this is inserted into the tibia proximal to the medial maleolus of the adult, of just below the tibial tuberosity in a child. Pressurized infusion of fluids is required.

Intracardiac

Whilst intacardiac injections have attracted much attention as providing the most rapid delivery of drugs to the central circulation, it requires considerable expertise to do and it is necessary to halt external chest compression to perform them. Other complications are haemothroax, pneumothorax, haemopericardium, direct damage to the coronary arteries and direct intramyocardial injection; 72% of so-called intracardiac injections at a recent postmortem study were actually intramural. As a result of these anxieties intracardiac administration of drugs should be considered only as a last resort when all other routes are unavailable. The same drugs and dosages can be used as for normal intravenous administration.

OPEN CHEST CARDIAC MASSAGE

Until Kouwenhoven's description of closed chest pulmonary resuscitation, open chest cardiac massage was the routine procedure in many hospitals. Whilst the closed chest technique was clearly superior in being available to a much larger number, suitable for out of hospital use, performable by all manner of resuscitators from the lay to the highly skilled technician, no study has shown any improvement in outcome compared with the open chest technique. Conversely, open chest cardiac massage has been shown to achieve much higher cerebral and coronary perfusion in both animal and human studies, with cardiac outputs of two and a half times greater and similar improvements in common carotid blood flow. Indeed, studies in man have shown a dramatic increase in survival following open chest cardiac massage compared with external chest compression, one study achieving survival as high as 58%. However, as the majority of these arrests occur during anaesthesia or surgery where the likely aetiology was considered to be hypoxia or myocardial irritability as a result of sympathetic or vagal stimulation aggravated by anaesthesia, part of this dramatic increase was due to the underlying disease process which may have had a considerable contribution to the outcome. In one randomized study where 52 patients suffering from cardiac arrest out of hospital were treated on arrival in the emergency room with either open or closed cardiac compression, there were no long-term survivors from either group, but all these patients had received out-of-hospital CPR for at least 20 min before arrival in the emergency room.

At the present time it would appear that the indications for open chest cardiac massage include cardiac arrest occurring during cardiothoracic surgery or upper abdominal surgery, cardiac tamponade from any cause, major intrathoracic or intra-abdominal haemorrhage following trauma, penetrating cardiac injuries, pulmonary embolism (when the opportunities for pulmonary embolectomy are available), patients with recent sternotomy, or patients where closed chest CPR is ineffective, either because of anatomical constraints or as a result of severe pulmonary pathology such as emphysema or status asthmaticus. Provided that there is a reasonable chance of successful resuscitation with closed chest CPR, defibrillation and drug treatment following up-to-date advanced life support protocols, it is presently unjustified to perform a thoracotomy.

A recent innovation in the USA has been the introduction of a mini-thoracotomy procedure providing access to the pericardium for the insertion of a small cardiac plunger. This is undergoing evaluation, but earlier reports suggest that it can enhance cardiac output during cardiac arrest.

PERI-ARREST ARRYTHMIAS

It is hoped that with the widespread adoption of the guidelines produced by the European Resuscitation Council and other similar bodies the toll of cardiac arrests can be reduced. Stabilization of patients with rhythm disorders will lead to a reduction in those patients suffering cardiac arrest. It is well known that ventricular fibrillation is often triggered by tachyarrhythmias. The European Resuscitation Council has therefore published guidelines for clinicians providing the initial management of a number of arrhythmias known to be associated with cardiac arrest. These guidelines were drawn up with the recognition that many of these clinicians will not be cardiologists and therefore areas of the algorithm recommend gaining expert advice. None the less, as such expert help may not be immediately available, the algorithms are designed to advise on appropriate treatments to be used until such time as more expert help can be found. The guidelines are presented as three algorithms (Figure 44.6). One is for bradyarrhythmias and intracardiac block, another for broad complex tachycardia (which could be equated in the area of resuscitation to ventricular tachycardia, recognizing that in this environment the distinction from less common varieties of supraventricular tachycardia may be impractical) and the third for narrow complex tachycardia which could also be equated with supraventricular tachycardia, but which may also include atrial fibrillation.

PAEDIATRIC RESUSCITATION

Overall, the outcome from cardiac arrest in children is worse than that from cardiac arrest in adults and this is largely a result in the

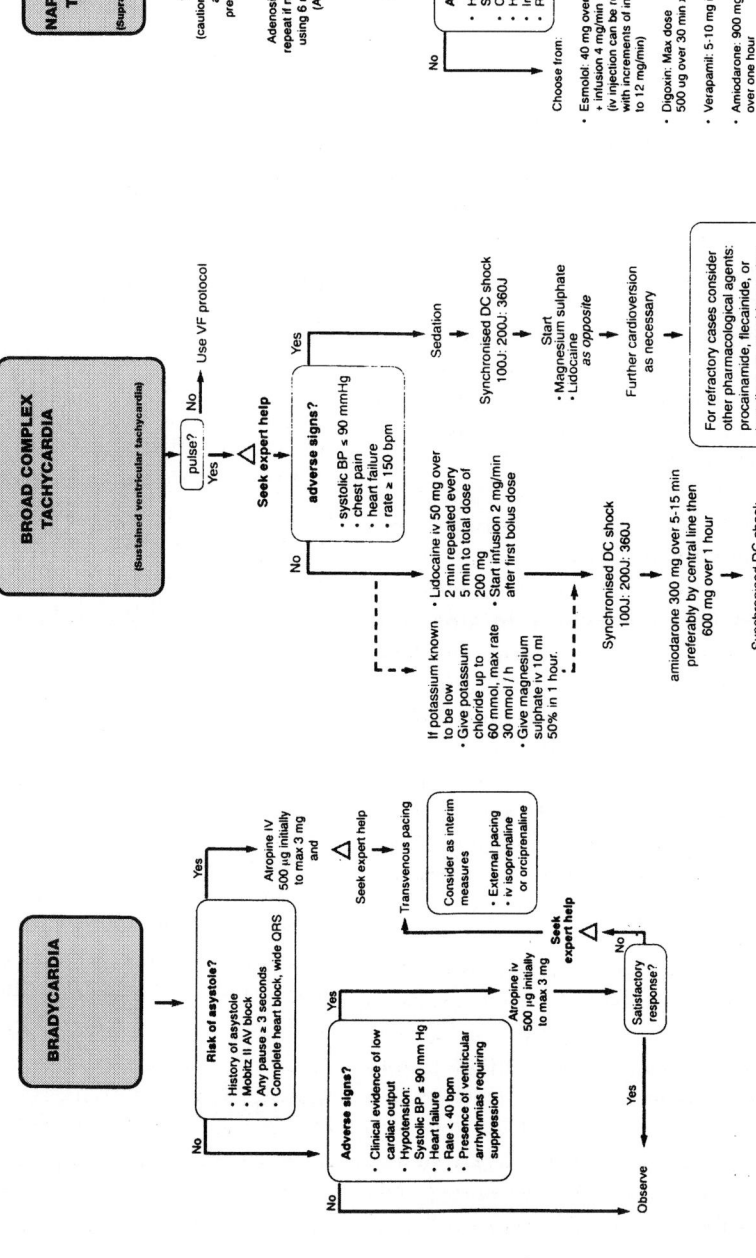

Figure 44.6 Algorithm for the management of peri-arrest arrhythmias. (Reproduced with permission from *Resuscitation* 1994, **28**, 153, by courtesy of the European Resuscitation Council.)

difference in the pathogenesis of cardiac arrest in the two groups. In adults the cause of cardiac arrest is primarily cardiac; this is unlikely to be true in children, where the most common underlying cause is respiratory failure, resulting either from lung or airway disease, or injury which can include foreign body inhalation or pneumothorax.

The poor long-term outcome from cardiac arrest could therefore be partly explained by an appreciation of the severity of cellular anoxia which has to occur, resulting in damage to the brain and other organs, before a direct affect on the myocardium producing cardiac arrest. Therefore it is unfortunate that cardiopulmonary resuscitation may restore cardiac output in a child who later dies from multisystem failure or survives with significant neurological damage. Recent emphasis has been on the recognition of pre-arrest pathology and its management to avoid cardiac arrest and this has resulted in the development of specialized paediatric courses, such as the Paediatric Advanced Life Support and the Advanced Paediatric Life Support courses available now in the UK.

Another problem is the need to divide children into at least two distinct groups because of variations in size and physiology. Resuscitation protocols have therefore been written specifically for infants, defined as patients in the first year of life and children from the end of their first to eighth year. In both groups, however, the early diagnosis and aggressive management of respiratory and cardiac insufficiency to avoid cardiac arrest are the keys to improving survival. Also in both groups it is generally true that the establishment of a clear airway and adequate oxygenation are of the highest priority (Figure 44.7). Children over eight years old may require resuscitation as adults but scaled appropriately and according to the aetiology of their arrest.

In the infant (i.e. less than one year old) a bradycardia of less than 60 b.p.m. should be regarded as cardiac arrest and should initiate the administration of circulatory support by chest compressions. Full cardiac arrest requires basic life support resuscitation and in this age group ventilations should occur immediately and even before the call for expert help, as so many cases of cardiac arrest in children are as a result of hypoxia which can be readily reversed.

If there is suspicion of foreign body aspiration, back blows or chest thrusts should be applied immediately and vigorously. Finger sweeps should never be used as these can impact foreign bodies further into the larynx. The importance of ventilation is emphasized further, with the recommended ratios of compressions to ventilation throughout the paediatric range being five compressions to each ventilation. After one minute of basic life support the emergency services should be activated. In the case of infants or small children it may be possible to carry the patient to the telephone rather that leaving the patient as is necessary with a larger child. Basic Life Support should, however, be recommended as soon as possible following the interruption to call the emergency services and continued thereafter with no further interruptions until more expert help arrives.

Advanced life support management in children follows guidelines and protocols similar to that in adults, but as ventricular fibrillation is so rare and as asystole is the final common pathway of respiratory or circulatory failure in a child, emphasis is placed in the asystole protocol (Figure 44.8).

One major problem in the management of cardiorespiratory arrest in children is in achieving confidence in the management of the correct dose of drugs and the sizes of equipment to be used in the various size patients encountered. A number of aids are now available, such as the Oakley chart available from the British Medical Association, or the Broselow Tape which is based on patient length using a specifically designed tape measure. It is important to become familiar with one system so that it can be referred to efficiently.

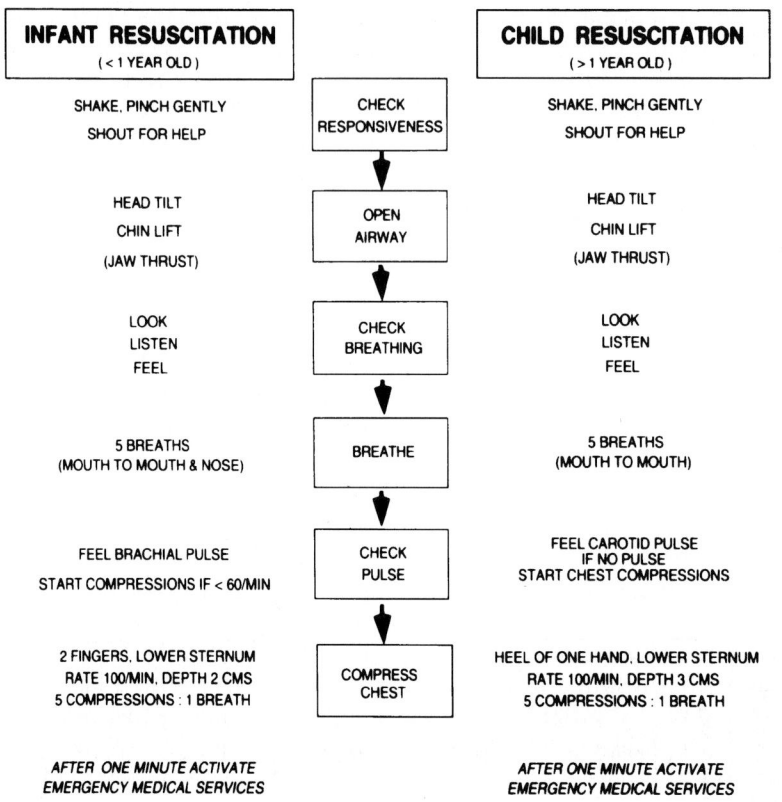

Figure 44.7 Paediatric basic life support. (Reproduced with permission from *Resuscitation* 1994, **27**, 93, by courtesy of the European Resuscitation Council.)

RESUSCITATION IN PREGNANCY

Cardiac arrest occurs approximately once in every 30 000 pregnancies. Survival from cardiac arrest in late pregnancy is exceptional and, as the latest report of the Confidential Enquiry into Maternal Deaths shows that most deaths are due to acute causes it is therefore important for all staff working in maternity units to be trained and familiar with resuscitation and the special requirements necessary in pregnancy.

There are a number of specific anatomical factors that make it difficult to maintain a clear airway and to intubate the tracheas of pregnant patients easily. There are also a number of pathological changes and physiological factors that mitigate against successful resuscitation, such as physiological laryngeal oedema in pregnancy, increased oxygen consumption, raised intragastric pressure and possible decreased barrier pressure at the gastro-oesophageal junction with an increased likelihood of regurgitation and pulmonary aspiration. However, the most significant factor of all is the presence of a large intra-abdominal mass compressing the inferior vena cava when the mother lies in the supine position. This impairment of venous return is a significant incumbrance against resuscitation.

The presence of a second 'intra-uterine' patient, together with the enhanced emotive response to cardiac arrest in late pregnancy, are further factors which must be considered. The approach to resuscitation in later preg-

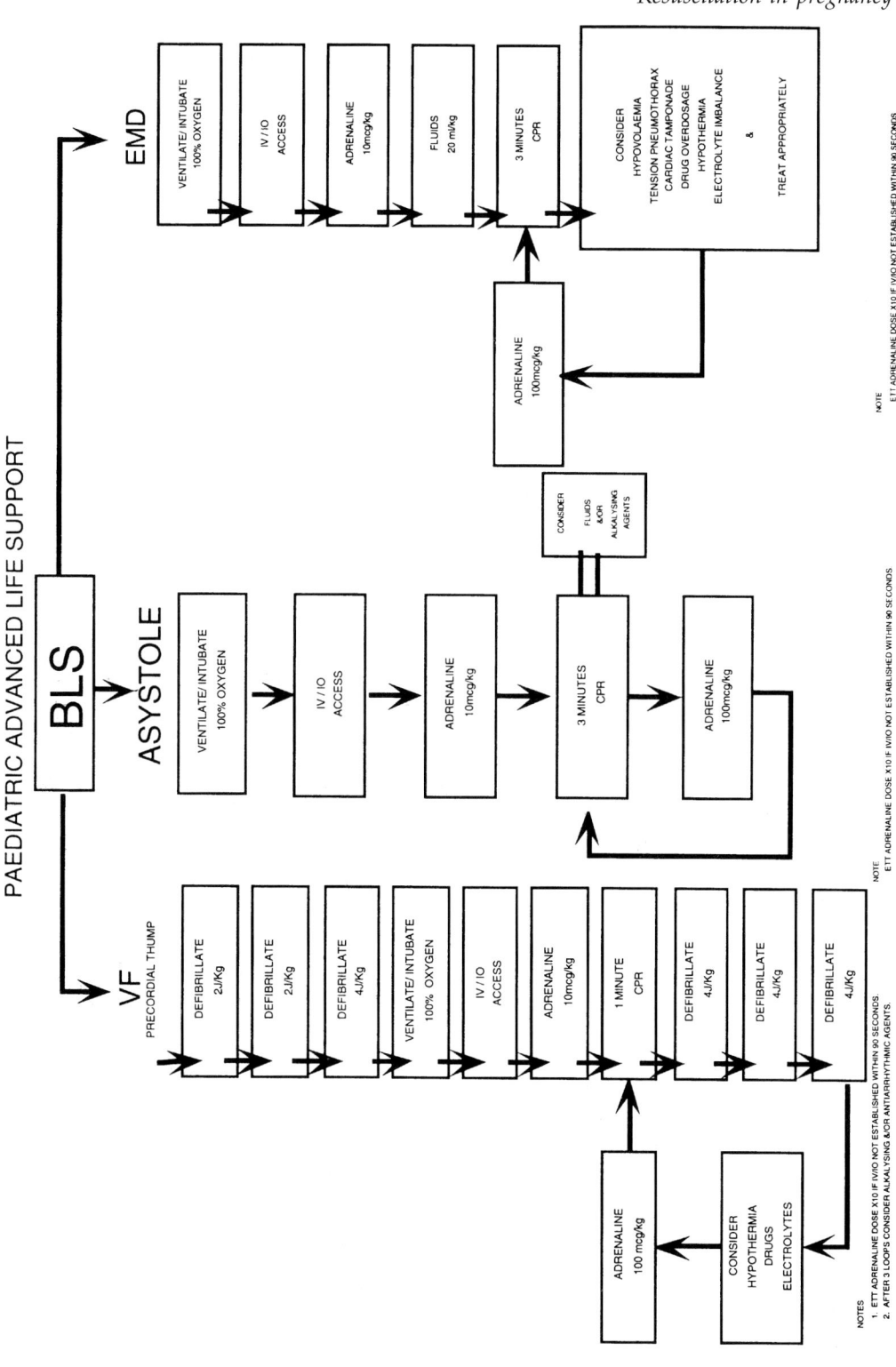

Figure 44.8 Paediatric advanced life support. (Reproduced with permission from *Resuscitation* 1994, **27**, 105, by courtesy of the European Resuscitation Council.)

nancy follows that of normal adulthood with the standard ABC sequence.

The airway may be difficult to maintain because of enlargement of the tongue from the oedema of pregnancy. Furthermore, when dealing with young patients, full dentition may make intubation more difficult than in the older, partly endentulous patients. Adequate ventilation must be started as soon as the airway has been cleared, but because of the increased risk of regurgitation and pulmonary aspiration cricoid pressure should be applied by a trained assistant until the airway can be protected by tracheal tube. Ventilation may be further complicated by the increased oxygen requirements and reduced chest compliance that occur in late pregnancy from the splinting of the diaphragm by the increased abdominal contents. Chest compression in pregnant women is rendered difficult by the flaring of the ribs and raised diaphragm and by breast hypertrophy. However, the greatest problem in producing an artificial circulation arises from inferior vena cava compression by the gravid uterus, which impairs venous return. All attempts at resuscitation will be futile unless caval compression can be relieved. This can be done by placing the patient in an inclined lateral position using a wedge such as that described by Rees and Willis (the Cardiff Wedge). In the absence of a custom-made wedge, a human wedge can be used where one person relieves caval compression using his knees placed under the right side of the pelvis. Manual displacement can be achieved by moving the uterus off the inferior vena cava by lifting it to the left and towards the patient's head.

Advanced life support guidelines of the Resuscitation Council should be followed with no special modifications in details of defibrillation and drug protocols. If maternal cardiac arrest managed with full attention being paid to the above factors does not achieve a successful return of spontaneous circulation within 5 min, a Caesarean section should be performed. Ventilation and artificial circulation must, clearly, be continued throughout the emergency Caesarean section and afterwards. There are many reports of successful resuscitations after prompt surgical intervention. It is likely that the improvement in outcome is as a result of the relief of the occlusion of the inferior vena cava achieved by emptying the uterus.

Clearly monitoring of a live baby delivered at such an emergency Caesarean section must be continued well into the neonatal period as there is likely to have been prolonged and severe hypoxia to the infant.

The majority of babies at normal delivery need no active resuscitation but a few will require airway clearance. A very few will need more robust tracheal intervention if ventilatory efforts are still inadequate. Here the airway should be controlled rapidly and ventilation with high concentration oxygen commenced. Any degree of bradycardia should be aggressively managed, and a heart rate below 60 b.p.m. should be treated as a cardiac arrest with external chest compression. Acidosis and hypoglycaemia should be corrected cautiously. It is recommended that resuscitation efforts should not be continued beyond half an hour in any neonate in asystole, unless the baby is making at least intermittent respiratory efforts.

DO NOT RESUSCITATE ORDERS

Resuscitation may not always be in the best interests of the patient or the proper use of scarce or limited resources. Resuscitation should be considered in the same way as other forms of treatment (such as antibiotic therapy, marrow transplantation), and wherever possible a decision on whether to apply this treatment made in advance of its urgent need. In some centres the use of the term 'Do Not Resuscitate' has been replaced by the phrase 'Ethical Resuscitation Decision' in an effort to shift the emphasis from a negative to a positive approach.

Many patients may have views of their

own which must be considered. There is no legal requirement to seek the consent from families or proxies, except in the case of minors, but their views may yield important information about the patient's previously held views or beliefs.

It is essential that any resuscitation decision (for or against) be made known to all those involved in the patient's care.

FURTHER READING

Advanced Cardiac Life Support Committee of the European Resuscitation Council (1994) Management of arrhythmias associated with cardiac arrest. *Resuscitation*, **28**, 151-159.

Advanced Life Support Working Party of the European Resuscitation Council (1992) Statement. *Resuscitation*, **24**, 111-121.

Airway and Ventilation Management Working Group of the European Resuscitation Council (1996) Guidelines for the advancement management of the airway and ventilation during resuscitation. *Resuscitation*, **31**, 201-230.

Airway and Ventilation Management Working Group of the European Resuscitation Council (1996) Guidelines for the basic management of the airways and ventilation during resuscitation. *Resuscitation* **31**, 187-200.

Baskett, J. F. (1993) *Resuscitation Handbook*, 2nd edn, Mosby, London.

Curran, J. W., Jaffe, H. W., Hardy, A. M., *et al.* (1988) Epidemiology of HIV infection and AIDS in the United States. *Science*, **239**, 610-616.

Fisher, J. M. and Handley, A. J. (1995) Basic Life Support, in *ABC of Resuscitation*, 3rd edn. (ed. N. C., Colquhoun, A. J. Handley, T. R. Evans), BMJ, London.

Gwinnutt, C., *et al.* (eds) (1997) *Advanced Life Support Course Manual*, 3rd edn. Resuscitation Council, London, UK (in press).

Holmberg, S., Handley, A., Bahr, J. *et al.* (1992) Guidelines for Basic Life Support. A Statement by the Basic Life Support Working Party of the European Resuscitation Council 1992. *Resuscitation*, 24, 103-110.

International Liaison Committee on Resuscitation (1997) Advisory Statements. *Resuscitation* (in press)

Kouwnehoven, W. C., Jude, J. R. and Knickerbocker, G. G. (1960) Closed chest cardiac massage. *Journal of the American Medical Association*, **173**, 94-97.

Paediatric Life Support working party of the European Resuscitation Council (1993) Statement *Resuscitation*, **27**, 91-105.

Pell, A. C. H., Guly, U. M., Sutherland, G. R., Steedman, D. J., Bloomfield, P. and Robertson, C. (1994) Methods of closed chest cardiopulmonary resuscitation investigated by transoesophageal echocardiography. *Journal of Accident and Emergency Medicine*, **11**, 139-143.

Rees, G. A. D. and Willis, B. A. (1998) Resuscitation in late pregnancy. *Anaesthesia*, **43**, 347-349.

Royal College of Physicians (1987) Resuscitation from cardio-pulmonary arrest. Training and Organisation. *Journal of the Royal College of Physicians*, **21**, 1-8.

Tunstall-Pedoe, H. Bailey, L., Chamberlain, D. A., Marsden, A. K., Ward, M. E. and Ziderman D. A. (1992) A survey of 3765 Cardio Pulmonary Resuscitations in British Hospitals (the BRESUS Study); Methods and overall results. *British Medical Journal* **304**, 1347-1351.

BRAIN DEATH

P. A. Razis and R. Rogers

> To himself every one is an immortal; he may know that he is going to die, but he can never know that he is dead.
>
> *Samuel Butler (1835–1902)*

The fact that the diagnosis of death is dependent on someone else's ability to recognize its features, has lead to the fear that somehow an error of judgement will be made. Although this has been a human concern well recognized throughout history, the development of artificial organ support with the advancement of medical technology has made these fears even more pertinent today. The classical diagnostic triad of death, i.e. loss of the ability to breathe, absent central pulses and an unconscious patient, cannot be used in intensive care where artificial ventilation and cardiac support may be employed to temporarily to prevent the first two features. As a result, the concept of brain death developed, and our perception of death as a physiological process has changed.

DEVELOPMENT OF THE CONCEPT OF BRAIN DEATH

PHYSIOLOGICAL CONCEPTS

The human body, as an integrated living organism, is not homogeneous in its requirements to maintain normal function. Conversely, the 'vital' organs show a variable ability to withstand and recover from extreme physiological derangement. The brain is not only extremely sensitive to deprivation of nutrients, it also has negligible powers of regeneration. From a physiological point of view it may be regarded therefore as the weakest link in life; that organ whose irreversible global damage signifies the disintegration of the living organism and the onset of the process of death. Like all the body's organs, the brain has a 'physiological reserve', so that minor degrees of anatomical damage may produce little or no neurological effects. The difficulty arises in defining which physiological deficits are important in determining that the brain has ceased to function as part of the rest of the body.

Observations on patients dying from increasing intracranial pressure have shown that consciousness is lost early, followed by progressive loss of the brain stem reflexes and terminating with apnoea (and the loss of vasomotor tone in ventilated patients). Although philosophical arguments are used by some to suggest that the loss of cerebral cortical function and, therefore, personal identity signify brain death, from a physiological point of view the sustained ability to breathe means that the brain remains part of the rest of the body. From this we can conclude the following.

- Before a diagnosis of brain death can be considered the patient must be both uncon-

---

Short Practice of Anaesthesia. Edited by M. Morgan and G. M. Hall. Published in 1997 by Chapman & Hall, London. ISBN 0 412 71890 1

Table 45.1 Brain stem functions

The brain stem is the hub of brain functions as it:
  determines level of consciousness – reticular activating system,
  determines the ability to breathe independently,
  determines the level of cardiovascular function,
  contains III–XII cranial nerve nuclei and central connections,
  connects forebrain to spinal cord,
  connects cerebellum to the rest of the brain.

scious and unable to breathe, that is reliant on artificial ventilation and making no respiratory effort when disconnected. Neither coma nor apnoea singly are sufficient to make the diagnosis.

- Not only does the brain stem act as the stimulus to many central and somatic functions, but it is also the anatomical and physiological link between the central nervous system and the rest of the body via the spinal cord (Table 45.1). The loss of brain stem function disconnects the entire brain, from a neurological point of view, from the rest of the body. This signifies the onset of the process of death.
- The diagnosis of brain death is dependent on the demonstration of loss of brain stem function and we should therefore call it brain stem death to be semantically correct. Unfortunately, as brain death was first used it remains the more common term.
- Because not all the cells in the brain stop functioning at precisely the same moment, it is theoretically possible to demonstrate isolated neuronal activity in the cerebral cortex in the presence of brain stem death. However, these neurones are not physiologically connected in any way to the body, because the link through the brain stem has been destroyed, so they are irrelevant.
- The spinal cord remains intact, and without higher control may occasionally be responsible for reflex movement in the limbs secondary to various stimuli. In addition, the hypertensive and tachycardic response to spinal, painful reflexes remains intact; this has been observed for many years in tetraplegic patients.
- Angiography and transcranial Doppler ultrasonography have demonstrated cessation of intracranial blood flow following brain death: further evidence that the brain is no longer an integrated part of the body.

Therefore, from a physiological point of view, death is a process rather than an immediate cessation of all cellular function. If the pathological process affects the brain primarily, the irreversible loss of brain stem function signifies irremediable damage, and therefore the onset of death.

PHILOSOPHICAL AND ETHICAL ARGUMENTS

Although theoretical and clinical arguments are very convincing in supporting the concept of brain death, the presence of a patient with a beating heart on a 'life-support' machine is not a picture of death as conceived by most of the public. In addition, the arbitrary timing with which the medical examination required to confirm the diagnosis is made, when there may have been no change in the patient's condition for many hours, does not inspire confidence in the concept. It is the equivalent of discovering a dead person and entering that as the time of death, even though there are signs of putrefaction suggesting that death occurred days previously. Indeed, many relatives view it as a confirmation of hopeless prognosis, and by accepting the doctor's diagnosis, they are agreeing to the 'death' of their relative by withdrawal of artificial ventilation.

It is a common misconception that the impetus to develop criteria for diagnosing brain death was as a result of the emergence of organ transplantation. This is not only historically untrue, but ignores the fact that it may still be necessary to diagnose brain death in patients who are not being considered for organ donation.

A clear and well established set of criteria are of benefit to the relatives and intensive care staff for the following reasons.

- Drug treatment which is of no benefit to the patient may be discontinued.
- The time from the brain stem becoming unresponsive to the moment of asystole, can be extremely variable, especially if the endocrine and cardiovascular systems are artificially supported. If brain death were not diagnosed, relatives may have unreasonable hopes despite what they are told, and in those who accepted the inevitability of the situation, it would unfairly prolong the grief of dying.
- It is damaging to the morale of intensive care staff to continue to treat a dead patient, especially in situations where demand for intensive care beds is greater than availability.
- To disconnect a patient from a ventilator who is known to be unable to breathe could be viewed as euthanasia. Once a diagnosis of brain death has been made, that becomes the time of death, so that the act of disconnection has as little significance as removing the tracheal tube from someone who has died.
- Permission from the relatives to disconnect the patient from the ventilator is not required. Although undesirable, it would be possible to go against a relative's wishes for ventilation to be continued. Every effort should be made to avoid this situation by explaining the concepts before testing, emphasizing that once death has been diagnosed, artificial ventilation is futile.

Despite some philosophical arguments, the criteria have at their core a desire to avoid unnecessarily prolonging inevitable death by the misplaced use of technology. Their development over many years, based on good physiological principles and widespread observation, ensure that they achieve this without being viewed as a self-fulfilling prophecy.

DEVELOPMENT OF THE CRITERIA

The development of the criteria for diagnosing brain death evolved over 10–15 years. The recognition of a state in which a patient with intracranial pathology remained in coma and was unable to breathe was first noted in 1959. The later demonstration on angiography that this was accompanied by cessation of intracranial blood flow contributed to the growing realization that brain death may precede cardiac arrest. In 1968 a committee at Harvard Medical School which included lawyers theologians as well as neurologists and neurosurgeons, developed the first criteria. The Conference of Medical Royal Colleges and their faculties in the UK responded to the growing need for criteria by issuing memoranda in 1976 and 1979 which formed the basis of the code in this country. This code differed from the early USA codes in the following respects.

- Between the 1976 and 1979 memoranda there was a shift in emphasis from defining brain death as the USA codes had done, to identifying brain stem death as the onset of death.
- A greater emphasis was placed on excluding other causes of coma and ensuring that irremediable, structural brain damage had occurred.
- Peripheral reflexes were abandoned, as they reflected spinal cord activity and not brain stem activity.
- The demonstration of an isoelectric EEG was not part of the UK criteria, as it did not reflect brain stem function. This caused great controversy at the time, but the EEG has now been abandoned by many countries.
- Testing for apnoea was much more strictly defined in terms of technique, and expected changes in arterial blood gases.

Crucial to their acceptance, was the demonstration that when patients fulfilled the criteria for brain death and artificial ventilation was none the less continued, all patients developed asystole. The only variable was the time it took, with the majority occurring within 24 h. Equally, all reports of patients 'waking up' after being declared dead, have not fulfilled all the criteria, especially the demonstration of irremediable, structural brain damage. When the physiological changes associated with brain stem death are examined, it is not surprising that the resultant deterioration leads to asystole.

PATHOPHYSIOLOGICAL CHANGES ASSOCIATED WITH BRAIN STEM DEATH

INTRACRANIAL EFFECTS

The principal causes of brain death are shown in Table 45.2. Of note, it is rare for extracranial pathology, such as hypovolaemia or cardiac arrest to cause brain death, as the brain stem is more resistant to hypoxaemia than the rest of the brain. The clinical result in such cases is often a patient in the persistent vegetative state in whom higher cortical function is irreparably damaged, but the brain stem, especially the ability to breathe unaided, remains intact.

Whatever the primary cause, there is a final common pathway leading to brain death through autonomic disruption. Much of the information on the pathological mechanisms of autonomic disruption has come from animal studies. In these experiments the intracranial pressure can be raised to produce ischaemia, which starts above the tentorium with progressive caudal extension to finally include all brain structures down to the spinal cord. Cerebral ischaemia alone increases vagal activity which reduces the heart rate, arterial pressure and cardiac output. As the ischaemia is extended down to the level of the pons, sympathetic stimulation is added to the pre-existing vagal stimulation. Consequently the bradycardia and reduced cardiac output continues, but the mean arterial pressure (MAP) rises. The combination of bradycardia and systemic hypertension is called the 'Cushing response' and is an indicator of significant brain stem compression or coning. As the ischaemia progresses further to the lower border of the medulla, vagal stimulation is blocked because of ischaemia of the vagal nucleus. Sympathetic stimulation is then unopposed, resulting in tachycardia, raised MAP and increased cardiac output. This occurs at the onset of brain stem death and is called the sympathetic or autonomic storm. It can be considered as a last desperate attempt to try to maintain brain stem perfusion and so reverse the process of ischaemia. But as a result of loss of autoregulation in the damaged areas of the brain, this increase in MAP produces worsening oedema and a rapidly rising intracranial pressure (ICP). Eventually ICP overtakes the increase in mean arterial pressure (MAP) and as the cerebral perfusion pressure (CPP) = MAP − ICP, the CPP falls to zero and intracranial blood flow ceases. Both sympathetic and parasympathetic control are then lost causing sudden vasodilatation, decreased cardiac output, systemic hypotension and tachycardia.

EXTRACRANIAL EFFECTS

Cardiovascular system

Hypotension is an almost universal consequence of brain death, resulting from hypovolaemia and ventricular dysfunction.

Table 45.2 Causes of brain death

Cause	Percentage
Head injury	50
Cerebrovascular accidents	30
Infection	8
Primary or secondary brain tumours	8
Extracranial causes, e.g. post cardiac arrest	4

Dehydration is often deliberately produced, by fluid restriction or diuretics, to decrease cerebral oedema. Diuresis also occurs from diabetes insipidus, secondary to brain death, or from hyperglycaemia. In addition, there may have been incomplete fluid replacement particularly following the initial trauma or bleeding. The loss of autonomic control after brain death reduces systemic vascular resistance, and pooling blood in capacitance vessels causes a relative hypovolaemia.

Hearts show extensive structural damage after brain death. Microinfarcts are seen throughout, particularly in the left ventricular subendocardium and in conduction tissues. These changes are produced by the massive sympathetic stimulation and high myocardial work induced during coning. In experimental animals the ECG passes through a sequence of changes during brain death. An initial bradycarda is followed by a tachycardia later with added ventricular ectopic beats, and lastly global, ischaemic changes. This is in keeping with the autonomic changes described during brain stem death. All of these factors together produce cardiovascular depression, which is compounded by low coronary perfusion pressures, resulting in multiorgan failure and, ultimately, in asystole.

Respiratory system

Since the centres for respiratory control are located in the brain stem, all brain stem dead patients will be ventilator dependent. Deterioration of lung function most frequently occurs as a result of accumulation of secretions, atelectasis, infection and aspiration of gastric contents.

The massive catecholamine release during the autonomic storm can be damaging to the lung. Catecholamine-induced vasoconstriction leads to a rise in right atrial pressure, and right ventricular output. Vasoconstriction also causes high left atrial pressures. As a result the left atrial pressure may temporarily exceed pulmonary artery pressures producing 'neurogenic' pulmonary oedema. The high pulmonary capillary pressures will also cause pulmonary capillary disruption and pulmonary haemorrhage. Pulmonary oedema can also be cardiac in origin, or from fluid overload, particularly with colloids.

Endocrine system

Destruction of the hypothalamus and pituitary results in loss of temperature regulation and endocrine control. Antidiuretic hormone (ADH) failure results in neurogenic diabetes insipidus. Low circulating thyroid hormones, cortisol, and insulin are thought to be responsible for disruption of cellular function producing the metabolic, hypoxic lesions which are found in all tissues.

During coning produced in experimental animals plasma catecholamine values may rise several hundred fold, and later drop below basal levels. Pituitary damage results in low circulating cortisol, thyroid hormones and insulin concentrations in animals, but the results of investigations of humans have not given such clear cut results.

Hyperglycaemia occurs as a result of the initial catecholamine and cortisol release and is sustained later by the low insulin values. Brain stem dead patients are known to show insulin resistance.

Kidneys

The kidneys are damaged by surges of high perfusion pressure during the autonomic storm, followed by hypoperfusion subsequently. Treatment of hypovolaemia, and the maintenance of organ perfusion after brain stem death, improves the function of kidneys after transplantation. In human kidneys the disruption of cellular function, such as low intracellular ATP and loss of normal transmembrane ionic gradients occurs after brain death has been demonstrated and correlates with the function of the kidneys after transplantation.

Loss of pituitary function produces neurogenic diabetes insipidus which may lead to hypovolaemia and electrolyte disturbances.

Liver

The liver, with its high blood flow, might be expected to be sensitive to the autonomic changes during brain stem death, but the high physiological reserve of the organ makes it relatively resistant to hypotension.

Coagulation

A variety of different factors may produce abnormalities of the clotting system. Fragments of ischaemic, cerebral tissue can pass into the circulation and trigger a consumptive coagulopathy. The high circulating catecholamine and cortisol concentrations have a procoagulant effect. Hypothermia is known to release tissue thromboplastins, inhibit platelet function and prolong bleeding times.

CLINICAL DIAGNOSIS OF BRAIN DEATH

During a 6 month audit of 5803 deaths in intensive care units in England in 1989, brain death was confirmed in 497 (8.6%) patients. There was wide variability in the number of cases seen, depending on the type of unit. A review of the criteria used in the diagnosis of brain death was published in October 1995, confirming that all published series had validated the original criteria produced in 1976 and updated in 1979. In addition, the criteria are included in Department of Health guidelines published in 1983, *Cadaveric organs for transplantation: a code of practice including the diagnosis of brain death*.

There are three necessary elements to the diagnosis of brain death: preconditions, exclusions, and tests (Table 45.3). The preconditions define which patients are suitable for testing. The exclusions are factors which could lead to a false diagnosis of brain death. The third element is the series of tests of brain stem function. Brain stem areflexia alone is not the same as brain stem death, so that the preconditions and exclusions, by ensuring that the cause of coma and respiratory depression are irreversible and irremediable, are essential to the diagnosis of brain stem death.

Table 45.3 Diagnosis of brain death from Conference of Medical Royal Colleges and their Faculties in the United Kingdom, 1976

Preconditions
All of the following should coexist.
1. The patient is deeply comatose.
2. The patient is ventilator dependent.
3. There should be a positive diagnosis of the cause of coma, which is known to lead to brain death and has caused irremediable, structural brain damage

Exclusions
The following should be excluded
1. Reversible causes of coma,
    e.g. drugs,
        metabolic, endocrine disturbances,
        hypothermia (<35°C).
2. Reversible causes of respiratory failure,
    e.g. drugs,
        neurological conditions.

Tests for confirming brain death
All brain stem reflexes should be absent.
1. Pupillary light reflex.
2. Corneal reflex.
3. Vestibulo-ocular reflex (caloric testing).
4. Motor response in cranial nerve distribution.
5. Gag/bronchial reflex.
6. Apnoea test.

PRECONDITIONS

There are three preconditions which should all coexist.

The patient is deeply comatose

The patient will lie in a neutral position with closed eyes and will not show any understandable response to the external world or inner needs. Coma is an unrousable, sleep-like, unresponsive state. If brain dead, there is no spontaneous movement, abnormal posturing or movement suggesting seizure activity.

The patient is being maintained on a ventilator

Apnoea is an essential condition. The brain stem contains respiratory centres, and as the ability to breathe is usually the last brain stem function to be lost, an apnoea test is an essential part of the testing for brain death. Therefore the patient should not make any effort to breathe while on the ventilator or during physiotherapy, otherwise a diagnosis of brain death cannot be considered.

There should be no doubt that the patient's condition is due to irremediable, structural brain damage

The diagnosis of a disorder which can lead to brain death should have been fully established. The demonstration of structural brain damage has been made much simpler by the widespread availability of CT and MRI scanning. The diagnosis should be commensurate with these findings. To satisfy the requirement that the damage is irremediable, observation over a reasonable period of time is necessary, ensuring that the Glasgow Coma Scale and brain stem reflexes remain unchanged. This time is not specified as it depends entirely on the underlying diagnosis, but the Department of Health Guidelines (1983) state: 'Diagnosis of brain death should not normally be considered until at least 6 h after the onset of coma or, if cardiac arrest was the cause of the coma, until 24 h after the circulation has been restored'. Patients therefore fall into one of three categories.

Testing within 6–12 h

This would be reasonable in most neurosurgical cases; as the diagnosis is well established and demonstrated on a scan, the neurological deterioration has been closely observed and documented, and there is a wealth of experience in dealing with the specific conditions and well established opinion on prognosis.

Testing within 12–24 h

This would include most of the neurological disorders such as encephalitis and meningitis, as the progression to coning is not as rapid as in the first group, and progression can be halted, or reversed by therapy. Also included in this group would be neurosurgical patients in whom short acting drugs or alcohol intoxication needs to be excluded.

Longer than 24 h

This would include all patients in whom an extracranial cause for the brain damage is suspected. This is because a vegetative state is a more common outcome than brain death. Furthermore, patients in whom drugs with a long half-life need to be excluded as a cause of coma may have to be observed for days.

The importance of satisfying the preconditions before moving on to the next diagnostic stage cannot be over emphasized. The establishment of a diagnosis and observation of the patient for a sufficient period of time is vital, and often the progression to brain death is clinically obvious, with the tests providing the confirmation as required by the code. A balance must be struck between unreasonably hasty diagnoses of brain death and unduly prolonging the grief of dying for the relatives and the staff.

EXCLUSIONS

The exclusions aim to ensure that there is no reversible contributory cause to the features of coma and apnoea required in the preconditions.

Coma

There should be no evidence that the patient's state could be due to drugs. Most drugs in high enough concentrations will produce either excitation, or depression, of the central nervous system. Alcohol, narcotics, sedatives and anaesthetic agents are obvious examples, but overdose of drugs such as bretyllium or amitriptyline has been reported to produce apnoeic coma with brain stem areflexia. Drugs administered in hospital will have been recorded, but ingestion of drugs before admission may not be so clearly defined. If there is suspicion of drug intoxication then adequate time should be allowed for drug metabolism. As a rule of thumb a delay before testing of four times the half-life has been suggested, but it must be remembered that concomitant hypothermia and hepato-renal failure may delay drug metabolism and excretion. Alternatively, toxicological screening and assessment of plasma drug concentration may provide valuable information.

Metabolic and endocrine disturbances can cause, or contribute, to coma. A list of the more common diagnoses is shown in Table 45.4. In the absence of a history or suggestive of an endocrine metabolic disturbance, the serum electrolytes, acid–base balance and blood glucose should be normal. This occasionally causes clinical problems as these variables may become slightly abnormal and difficult to correct as a result of the metabolic effects of brain death. Reasonable efforts should be made to treat these variables, but occasionally experienced clinical judgement may be required to decide whether these abnormalities are important in the overall clinical presentation.

As hypothermia causes depression of neuronal activity, core temperature should be greater than 35°C before brain stem testing. This may require active methods of warming.

Apnoea

Drugs, including neuromuscular blocking agents, narcotics and hypnotics, must be excluded as the cause of respiratory failure. The presence of neuromuscular blockade must be excluded, either by testing peripheral tendon reflexes or the use of a nerve stimulator (at low levels of neuromuscular blockade 5 s of sustained tetanus is a more sensitive test than the train-of-four).

TESTS OF BRAIN STEM REFLEXES

The Department of Health recommends that the tests should be conducted by 'a consultant, preferably the one in charge of the patient, and another consultant or senior registrar, clinically independent of the first, who shall assure themselves that the preconditions have been met before testing is carried out'. The question of experience is implicit in the seniority of those involved in the tests, and it is generally accepted that they should have been fully registered for longer than 5 years. They can carry out the tests separately, but more usually perform them together and neither should be involved in any transplantation programme. The tests are regarded as valid in all age groups down to the age of 2 months, beyond which there is insufficient information on the recognition and diagnosis of brain death. The presence of relatives during the testing is discretionary,

Table 45.4 Metabolic and endocrine causes of coma

Abnormal temperature regulation
   Hypo/hyperthermia
Organ failure
   Liver (hepatic failure)
   Renal (uraemia)
   Respiratory (carbon dioxide narcosis)
Endocrine dysfunction
   Panhypopituitarism
   Thyroid (hyperthyroidism, myxoedema)
   Parathyroid (hyper/hypocalcaemia)
   Adrenal (Addison's desease, Cushing's disease)
   Pancreas (diabetes)
Abnormalities in acid–base and electrolytes
   Hyper/hyponatraemia
   Hyper/hypo-osmolarity
   Hyper/hypocalcaemia
   Acidosis

and may be helpful especially in children, as even the most doubting relatives find the apnoea test convincing.

The five tests of brain stem reflexes and the apnoea test enable the layers of the brain stem to be examined in a simple, unambiguous way. Brain stem dead patients exhibit an absence of the normal response to all the tests.

Pupillary response to light

The eyes should be opened from a closed position and a bright light shone into each eye in turn. The normal reflex is constriction of the pupil and the eye should be observed for the period of a minute to ensure no pupillary constriction. Pupillary size is not diagnostic of brain stem death. Complete sympathetic and parasympathetic denervation results in mid-position, fixed pupils (3–5 mm), however denervation may be incomplete producing a wide range of pupil sizes. Potential pitfalls are pre-existing abnormalities such as the Holmes–Adie pupil (congenital absence of pupillary response to light) or previous eye surgery (e.g. iridectomy), eye trauma, or even glass eyes. Drugs may also interfere with the reflex, for example anticholinergics such as atropine used during resuscitation, mydriatics used to examine the fundi, or neuromuscular blocking drugs.

Corneal reflex

A stronger stimulus is needed in the unconscious, than in the conscious, patient to elicit this reflex. Firm, direct pressure is applied to each eye across the surface of the cornea using a throat swab or cotton bud. This should not be repeated unnecessarily, to avoid corneal abrasions. The normal response is blinking of the eyelids, either bilaterally, or more predominantly on the side stimulated, which is felt by the observer holding the eyelid open. Contact lenses, if present, should be removed.

Vestibulo-ocular reflex: caloric test

Before this test is performed, the tympanic membrane must be visualized by direct inspection to ensure that the cold water reaches the ear drum. Wax or blood should be removed by gentle irrigation. The eyes are watched whilst at least 20 ml of ice-cold water is injected in to each external auditory meatus in turn. The patient's head should be in the midline and elevated 30° from supine to obtain the maximum response. In brain stem death there is no movement of either eye during, or after, the cold water irrigation. In deeply comatosed patients with an intact brain stem, convection currents in the semicircular canals induce tonic deviation towards the irrigated ear after a delay of about 20s.

Problems may arise if there is a perforation of the ear drum. Injection of cold water through a perforation in the ear drum of a patient with an intact brain stem will cause a decrease in arterial pressure and a bradycardia. The injection of cold air has been suggested as an alternative, when a perforation is present. Rarely, failure to elicit this reflex may be due to pre-existing middle ear disease, or drug-induced middle ear damage such as with gentamicin. The central mechanism of the reflex may be suppressed by drugs such as sedatives, anticholinergics, anticonvulsants and tricyclic antidepressants.

Motor response in the cranial nerve distribution

There should be no grimacing in response to painful stimuli within the cranial nerve territory (firm supraorbital pressure). The absence of a cranial nerve response to a peripheral stimulus may be due to high cervical cord damage. The important part of this test is the absence of a cranial nerve motor response, so a peripheral motor response to peripheral painful stimuli is compatible with brain stem death. The ear is an unsuitable site for stimulus because it has mixed cervical and cranial sensory innervation.

Gag–Bronchial reflex

Pharyngeal, or palatal, movement should be looked for when both sides of the oropharynx are stimulated with a tongue depressor. Chest or diaphragmatic movement should be sought when a suction catheter is passed down the tracheal tube to stimulate the carina.

Apnoea test

There should be no respiratory movement when the patient is disconnected from a mechanical ventilator for long enough to ensure that the arterial carbon dioxide tension rises above the threshold for stimulating respiration (Pa_{CO_2} greater than 6.7 kPa, 50 mmHg).

It is important that the patient should not become hypoxic during the apnoea test. The patient should be preoxygenated before the apnoea test and then 100% oxygen at 6 l min^{-1} should be supplied, via a suction catheter, into the trachea. The additional safeguard of a pulse oximeter is sensible.

During the apnoea test arterial carbon dioxide tension will slowly rise. The rate of rise is usually in the range of 2–4 mmHg min^{-1} (0.25–0.5 kPa min^{-1}). The rate is dependent upon factors such as temperature, metabolic rate and carbon dioxide washout during diffusion oxygenation. The patient should be normocapnic (35–40 mmHg, 4.6–5.3 kPa) before starting the test, so that the apnoeic threshold can be reached within a period of approximately 10 min.

If blood gas analysis is not available, then the alternative procedure is to ventilate the patient for 10 min on 100% oxygen, then with 5% carbon dioxide in 95% oxygen for 5 minutes.

The ventilator should be disconnected for 10 min, while delivering oxygen at 6 l min^{-1} via a catheter, into the trachea. This procedure should allow adequate oxygenation during 10 min of apnoea.

The apnoea test requires a functioning phrenic nerve so the test cannot be performed on patients with high cervical cord injuries.

The recommendation for brain stem testing is that the tests are repeated by both doctors on a second occasion to ensure there is no observer error and that the neurological signs remain unchanged. The code of practice does not specify a fixed delay before repeat testing, but suggests this is a matter for medical judgement and a period of 2–3 h is reasonable. It is illogical to suggest different intervals between tests depending on the underlying diagnosis, as this should form part of the preconditions before any tests are performed.

The time of death is that moment when both sets of tests have been completed and have demonstrated brain death. This has some important implications.

- Disconnection from the ventilator does not constitute an act of euthanasia.
- The relatives should feel no responsibility in the decision to disconnect the patient as this is a post-mortem event.
- If consent for organ donation has been obtained, the death certificate can be issued and the relatives may leave the hospital without becoming involved in the delays that occur in organizing organ retrieval. This also emphasizes the fact that death is not the moment when asystole occurs.

CONTROVERSIES SURROUDING BRAIN DEATH

The clinical criteria surrounding the diagnosis of brain death are well established and accepted. None the less there are still observations which cause controversy.

EEG in brain dead patients

Various studies have looked at the EEG in patients fulfilling the clinical criteria for brain death. The principal conclusion of all studies is that, despite the technical difficulties of performing an EEG without external interference in these circumstances, even when EEG activity was demonstrated, all patients developed asystolic arrest usually within 4 days. The demonstration of EEG activity is, therefore, irrelevant.

Imaging of cerebral blood flow

The lack of intracranial blood flow on four vessel cerebral angiography, transcranial Doppler ultrasonography or radionucleide scanning has been used as proof that the brain can cease to be a viable part of the body before the onset of asystole. There have been reports though, that rarely a greatly reduced cerebral blood flow may persist following the clinical diagnosis of brain death. Again, when ventilation was continued, all these patients developed asystole, and it was felt that this observation had no prognostic significance.

Pituitary function

Although it is usually the case that pituitary function declines with the onset of brain death, this is not an invariable finding, and the assay of hormone concentrations cannot be used as a diagnostic test. This observation could be explained by the persistence of cerebral blood flow in some patients.

All of these areas of controversy attempt to demonstrate loss of function of the whole brain. It is important to emphasise that it is the **loss of brain stem function** that is essential to the diagnosis of brain death and within that concept it is rarely possible, although irrelevant, to demonstrate a temporary persistence of some intracranial activity.

CONCLUSIONS

Death is always an emotive subject, and brain death is even more so. But clinicians following the diagnostic steps can be confident that these have evolved from extensive, international experience and have withstood the test of time. Despite this, some relatives find it difficult to accept the finality of what has occurred. Although some authors argue that the diagnosis is clear enough not to warrant the seniority of medical personnel recommended, it is the experience of dealing with these difficult situations that is important. Adverse publicity about the handling of brain death, not only increases the grief felt by the relatives, but damages morale in the intensive care unit and can set back the transplant programme considerably. All relatives of patients who are brain dead should at some stage be asked about organ donation, unless they have already expressed opposition to the idea. The timing depends on assessing when they are coming to terms with the diagnosis of death, a good time is often before conducting the second set of tests. If organ donation has not been agreed to, the patient can be left disconnected from the ventilator after the second apnoea test.

The fact that the relatives often request to sit with the patient when artificial ventilation is discontinued, shows that although intellectually the concept of brain death has been accepted by the public, emotionally it is still the change in appearance with asystole that to them signifies the final moment of life. It is, therefore, essential that those in the intensive care unit have a clear idea of the concepts and criteria for diagnosing brain death so that they can provide authoritative support for the family.

FURTHER READING

British Paediatric Association. (1991) *Diagnosis of Brain Stem Death in Infants and Children*. BPA, London.

Cooper, D. K., Novitzky, D. and Wicomb, W. N. (1989) The pathophysiological effects of brain death on potential donor organs, with particular reference to the heart. *Annals of the Royal College of Surgeons of England*, **71**, 261–66.

Dobb, D. J. and Weekes, J. W. (1995) Clinical confirmation of brain death. *Anaesthesia and Intensive Care*, **23**, 37–43.

Gore, S. M., Ross Taylor, R. M. and Wallwork, J. (1991) Availability of transplantable organs from brain stem dead donors in intensive care units. *British Medical Journal*, **302**, 149–153.

Health Department of Great Britain and Northern Ireland. (1983) *Cadaveric Organs for Transplantation: a Code of Practice Including the Diagnosis of Brain Death*. HMSO, London.

Jennett, B. (1981) Brain Death. *British Journal of Anaesthesia*, **53**, 1111–1119.

Conference of Medical Royal Colleges and their Faculties in the United Kingdom. (1976) Diagnosis of death. *British Medical Journal*, **ii**, 1187–1188.

Conference of Medical Royal Colleges and their Faculties in the United Kingdom. (1979) Diagnosis of death. *British Medical Journal*, **i**, 332.

Pallis, C. (1983) *ABC of Brian Death*. BMA publications, London.

Power, B. M. and Van Heerden, P. V. (1995) The physiological changes associated with brain death – current concepts and implications for treatment of the brain dead organ donor. *Anaesthesia and Intensive Care*, **23**, 26–36.

MANAGEMENT OF HEAD INJURY

P. A. Razis

Head injuries account for 200–300 hospital admissions per 100 000 population per annum. On the basis of the Glasgow coma scale (Table 14.2) (GCS), 85% of those admitted will have a minor head injury (GCS 13–15), while 5% will have a severe head injury (GCS 3–8). In the severe group, 50% will have a haematoma or raised intracranial pressure (ICP) necessitating surgery, and 20% will have other significant injuries. The majority of head injuries result from road traffic accidents; 27% of the minor group but 70% of the severe group, with falls at work and assault accounting for most of the remainder. As head injury remains the main cause of death between 15 and 34 years of age in England and Wales, and is the cause of death in half of multiply injured patients, these patients are a particularly difficult challenge for anaesthetists involved in trauma care and neuroanaesthesia.

PATHOPHYSIOLOGY

MECHANISMS OF BRAIN DAMAGE

The mechanism of impact determines some of the pathological features seen.

Linear deceleration

This is usually associated with brain contusions at the site of impact; frontal and temporal poles, the inferior surfaces of the frontal and temporal lobes where the brain abuts on the irregular surface of the anterior cranial fossa, and occasionally contrecoup injury. Skull fractures and extra- or subdural haemorrhages may complicate the injury. As long as there are no major complicating factors such as uncontrolled intracranial hypertension, and the non-dominant hemisphere is affected, these patients often make a surprisingly good recovery.

Rotational injuries

These are often associated with diffuse, axonal injury characterized by punctate haemorrhages in central structures, and microscopically-varying degrees of shearing of white matter and the formation of axonal retraction balls. Clinically, this group of patients suffer prolonged coma, have diffuse cerebral oedema, often show abnormal breathing patterns on weaning from mechanical ventilation, exhibit sympathetic over-activity with hypertensive episodes and make a poor recovery.

Missile injuries

These may be classified as depressed, penetrating or perforating, and the amount of brain damage they produce is dependent on the track and energy of the missile.

Short Practice of Anaesthesia. Edited by M. Morgan and G. M. Hall. Published in 1997 by Chapman & Hall, London. ISBN 0 412 71890 1

INTRACRANIAL COMPLICATIONS OF INJURY

Haematomas

These are associated with skull fractures, occurring in one in 30 fully conscious patients, rising to one in four patients who are not fully orientated, especially if they have focal neurological signs or have had a fit.

Extradural haematomas (Figure 46.1) occur in 4–6% of severe head injuries and result from rupture of a meningeal artery, usually in association with a skull fracture. As 60% of patients have no underlying brain injury, the outcome is related to the adverse effects of a rapidly rising ICP and therefore to the GCS before surgical evacuation. A GCS of 9 or more has a mortality of 1% or less, and a GCS of 8 or less a mortality of 27%, rising to 60% if associated with cerebral contusions.

Acute subdural haematomas occur in 30% of severe head injuries and, as they result from venous or arterial haemorrhage in the cerebral cortex, are frequently associated with underlying brain injury. In general, subdural haematomas less than 3 mm thick are not evacuated, but larger ones with evidence of midline shift or uncal herniation are treated surgically. The mortality is often over 50% with few patients making a good recovery.

Intracerebral haematomas have an incidence of 4–23% depending on the series, with over 80% located in the white matter of the temporal and frontal lobes. These are associated with a mortality of over 60%.

Herniation

This occurs as a result of increasing cerebral oedema, or haematoma, forcing the brain substance through anatomical barriers, i.e. subfalcine, transtentorial or cerebellum tonsillar herniation. The physiological effect of this is to cause ischaemia, worsening cerebral oedema and occasionally hydrocephalus exacerbating the rise in ICP. The development of focal neurological signs such as the ipsilateral dilatation of the pupil (uncal herniation), or contralateral weakness with a rising arterial pressure, are warning signs of worsening herniation and the need to decompress the brain surgically if possible. Finally, if the ICP continues to rise unabated, eventually it exceeds the cerebral perfusion pressure (CPP) resulting in cessation of cerebral blood flow and the onset of brain stem death.

Infarction

Infarction results from hypoxia, spasm of the cerebral vessels or ischaemia caused by herniation for example posterior cerebral artery occlusion following transtentorial herniation.

EFFECTS ON CEREBRAL PHYSIOLOGY

Post-mortem studies consistently show that 85–90% of patients who die following head injury have evidence of significant ischaemia.

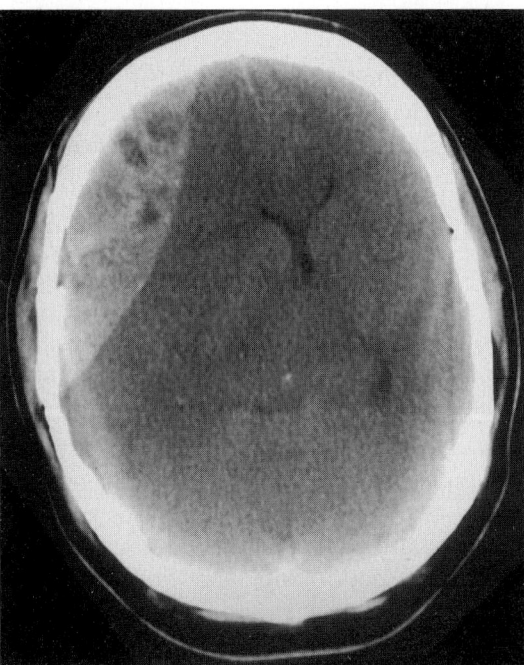

Figure 46.1 CT scan demonstrating an extradural haematoma.

This has led to the concept of secondary cerebral damage, that is a combination of systemic and cerebral consequences of the primary injury whose final common pathway is cerebral ischaemia.

Knowledge of the immediate physiological response to head injury is based on animal experiments and may not necessarily extrapolate to humans. There appears to be a variable rise in ICP, apparently dependent on the severity of the impact, and on arterial pressure. More severe trauma is required to alter conscious level than to affect cardiovascular stability. Disturbances of the normal breathing pattern, and apnoea, are common, and therefore hypoxaemia is an early feature of head injury. Temporary flattening of the EEG accompanies the respiratory effects, and returns within a minute of impact in survivors, with initially some slow wave activity.

A severe impact on the brain causes the normally stable cerebral haemodynamics to be thrown into disarray, producing the following effects.

Cerebral autoregulation

There is loss of cerebral autoregulation to an area of the brain greater than is obviously damaged by the injury. This area of the brain develops a linear dependence of cerebral blood flow (CBF) on mean arterial pressure (Figure 46.2). As the cerebral perfusion pressure (CPP) is governed by the relationship

CPP = MAP − ICP

where MAP is the mean arterial pressure, it is obvious that hypotension in the presence of increased ICP and lack of autoregulation can rapidly produce critical ischaemia. The mechanism for the loss of autoregulation is unknown, but it is suggested that a sudden hypertensive surge following impact damages the endothelium of the cerebral blood vessels. This triggers the release of prostacyclin and thromboxane A_2 locally affecting

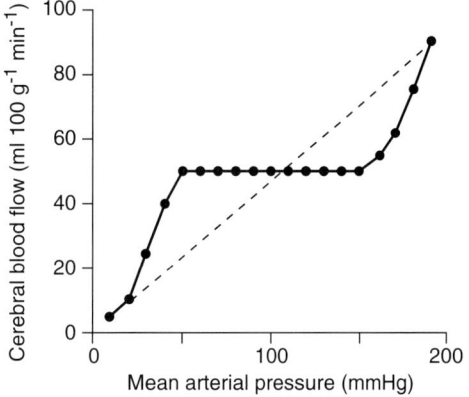

Figure 46.2 Alteration in autoregulation in the injured brain: CPP=MAP−ICP; −−=head injury.

the ability of cerebral blood vessels to react to changing transluminal pressures.

Cerebral blood flow

This is very variable, often reduced in adults during the first 8 h following impact, despite a normal CPP. The initial inability to raise CBF may be a potent cause of cerebral ischaemia, especially as the injured brain may be hypercatabolic due to the injury or uncontrolled fits, or if there is concomitant systemic hypoxaemia or hypotension. Serial measurements have shown that CBF gradually increases after this initial phase, and because cerebral metabolism is depressed during coma, CBF exceeds requirements during this time. Over the next few days the CBF becomes variable, decreasing in 20–40% of patients who develop vasospasm, and in others (especially children) entering into a hyperaemic phase. Both extremes of CBF carry a poor prognosis.

Hypocapnic response

The decrease in CBF in response to hypocapnia is preserved until just before death supervenes, even in severe head injuries, although this occurs probably in cerebral blood vessels unaffected by the injury. The resultant 'reverse steal' redirecting flow to the damaged areas of the brain has been demonstrated using Xe^{133}, but is not necessarily beneficial as occasionally shown by rapidly increasing cerebral oedema in those areas. A controversial topic is whether the decrease in CBF to hypocapnia is maintained for longer than the 24–36 h seen in the normal brain. It appears that hyperventilation can reduce cerebral blood flow to some degree for as long as it is used, therefore increasing the risk that it may produce cerebral ischaemia.

Hypoxic response

The hyperaemic response to hypoxia is also preserved, but because it only causes an increase in CBF when Pa_{O_2} decreases below 6.6 kPa, hypoxic brain damage may occur.

Cerebral metabolism

Although cerebral metabolism may be depressed because of coma, the decrease in cerebral blood flow and commonly associated hypoxaemia result in an increase in anaerobic metabolism of glucose. A rise in CSF lactate in the early phase of head injury has been well documented, and appears to resolve rapidly in those patients with a good clinical outcome.

The appreciation of the role of calcium in reperfusion injury and the deregulation of the excitatory amino acids (EAA), L-glutamate and L-aspartate, has generated much research recently. Ischaemia causes a decrease in adenosine triphosphate (ATP) which damages the cell's ability to maintain Ca^{++} homeostasis in the endoplasmic reticulum and at voltage-dependent Ca^{++} channels in the membrane. In addition, an imbalance of EAA to inhibitory neurotransmitters increases the influx of Na^+ and Ca^{++} via receptor-gated channels (e.g. N-methyl-D-aspartate or NMDA), both giving rise to lethal, intracellular Ca^{++} values.

Brain damage also causes the release of enzymes, e.g. creatine kinase BB isoenzyme (CKBB). CSF concentrations of CKBB rise for the first 36 h and rapidly decline to undetectable levels by 3 days. A further increase may signify secondary brain damage, but it only contributes to the clinical picture, and the prognosis.

Intracranial pressure

A major consequence of brain damage is the development of a raised ICP, either as a result of cerebral oedema, or intracranial haematomas. High ICP values in patients with brain injuries not requiring surgery carry a worse prognosis. Although it has been suggested that all this reflects is a bad primary injury, recent evidence suggests that raised ICP is an independent, adverse, prognostic feature. Until recently it was thought that good ICP control carried a better prognosis, but it has not been possible to demonstrate consistently an improved outcome. It is now recognized that hyperventilation may decrease ICP in some patients by causing critical hypoperfusion, and the balance between cerebral perfusion and ICP is not always possible to predict with the monitoring available.

EARLY MANAGEMENT OF HEAD INJURED PATIENTS

The most important finding in all studies of the early management and subsequent outcome of head injured patients, is that hypotension and hypoxaemia are associated with a worse outcome. Therefore, guidelines for care of the multiply injured patient emphasize the importance of airway management and fluid resuscitation before consideration of the head injury. It has also been demonstrated that the GCS often improves following resuscitation and is, therefore, a more accurate guide to the patient's true neurological condition.

Table 46.1 Indications for tracheal intubation

Inability to maintain an unobstructed airway
Glasgow coma scale, 8 or less
Absent, or reduced, cough or gag reflex
Separate indication for controlled ventilation
Facial injuries, or burns, that will compromise the airway

AIRWAY MANAGEMENT AND VENTILATION

It has been found that 25–30% of head-injured patients are hypoxaemic on arrival in the casualty department, so it is essential that all of them receive supplemental oxygen from the moment the ambulance team arrives. The role of pre-hospital intubation is dependent on the skill of those first attending to the patient, and may be associated with a decrease in early mortality, although the effect on overall outcome is unclear.

In securing the airway, the guidelines in Table 46.1 are useful in determining the need for tracheal intubation.

Tracheal intubation should form part of a rapid sequence induction with cricoid pressure, with specific consideration of the following problems.

- Positive pressure ventilation with a face mask should be avoided in patients with cerebrospinal fluid rhinorrhoea, as it is possible to force air into the skull and dramatically raise the ICP.
- The nasal route should be avoided as some patients will have a base of skull fracture, and there is a risk that the tracheal tube may cause further trauma and increase the risk of infection. Useful clinical signs of a base of skull fracture are CSF rhinorrhoea or otorrhoea, bilateral periorbital bruises (Racoon eyes), bruising over the mastoid bone (Battle's sign), haemotympanum and facial nerve palsy.
- If the patient is showing signs of a rapidly deteriorating GCS, mannitol 0.5 g kg^{-1} should be infused before induction of anaesthesia, or if intubation is urgent, mannitol should be started.
- As laryngoscopy may cause a large increase in ICP, a balance needs to be obtained between limiting the cardiovascular response to intubation but not producing hypotension, especially if the patient is hypovolaemic. Therefore, a small dose of an induction agent is required, even in patients who are deeply unconscious. Thiopentone 2–3 mg kg^{-1} or etomidate 1–2 mg kg^{-1} are the safest agents, with propofol 1–2 mg kg^{-1} used only in those patients who are haemodynamically stable, as it can cause marked hypotension.
- Coughing and straining raise the ICP, so good neuromuscular blockade is essential for intubation. Although suxamethonium has been shown to transiently raise ICP, the rapid onset and reliable effect make it the agent of choice in emergencies.
- The coexistence of cervical spine injuries must always be considered, but recent work suggests that they only occur in up to 3.5% of head injury patients. If possible, a lateral cervical spine X-ray down to the C7–T1 interspace should be performed to exclude any instability, but as the risk of hypoxaemia is much greater, the clinical condition should determine whether radiological examination should precede intubation. Manual in-line traction is useful in stabilizing the neck, and every effort should be made to intubate with minimal movement of the head and neck.
- The tracheal tube should be secured without any constriction of the neck, and hence rise in venous pressure which may increase ICP.

Once intubated, most patients require controlled ventilation (as outlined in Table 46.2).

Table 46.2 Indications for controlled ventilation

Pa_{O_2} <10 kPa breathing maximal oxygen therapy
Tachypnoea with a Pa_{CO_2} <3.5 kPa
Hypoventilation with a Pa_{CO_2} >6 kPa
Abnormal respiratory pattern
Spontaneous extensor posturing

The requirement for sedation depends on whether the patient is to be transferred, or going to theatre or ITU, and is dealt with in those Sections.

CIRCULATION

Hypotension is not a feature of isolated closed head injury, and therefore other causes for hypotension should be sought. The exceptions to this rule are the following.

- Children under the age of 4 years, who can lose a significant percentage of their circulating blood volume from scalp lacerations.
- Adults who have become brain stem dead after intubation and ventilation, and have therefore lost brain stem control of vasomotor tone.
- All patients with compound head injuries in whom a dural sinus is torn.
- All patients with a coexisting, high spinal cord injury.

The adverse effects of hypotension are evident from the fact that the overall mortality of severely head injured patients is approximately 45%, but this rises to 87% in those admitted to the neurosurgical unit with a systolic arterial pressure less than 90 mmHg. Glucose-containing solutions should be avoided in resuscitating these patients as they exacerbate the lactic acidosis associated with cerebral injury and result in a poorer outcome. The use of hypertonic saline has theoretical advantages as only 10% of the volume of isotonic saline is required for resuscitation with marked increases in arterial pressure without adverse effects on ICP. However, artificial colloid solutions are used commonly in conjunction with crystalloids for resuscitation. Blood is transfused to maintain the haematocrit above 30%.

CENTRAL NERVOUS SYSTEM

Assessment of the central nervous system should occur at the same time as resuscitation, and be repeated at regular intervals looking specifically for changes in pupil size and reaction to light, deterioration in the GCS and the development of focal neurological signs. The criteria for seeking urgent neurosurgical consultation or a CT scan, are summarized in Table 46.3.

As a CT brain scan is standard practice in the evaluation of moderate to severe head injuries, the benefits of skull X-rays have waned. The scan image may be varied to give a 'bone window', which is increasingly used to exclude skull and cervical spine fractures. The main problem during this time is monitoring the progress of resuscitation of the patient in a changing environment.

Finally, epileptic fits should be treated with either 5–10 mg diazepam to terminate the fit, or a loading dose of phenytoin 15 mg kg^{-1} as prophylaxis.

TRANSFER OF HEAD-INJURED PATIENTS

Neurosurgical services are often located in a centre some distance from the admitting hospital, so anaesthetists are often involved in the transfer of these critically ill patients. Several studies have shown that the major problems associated with transfer are unrecognized hypoxaemia and hypotension. In general, it is much safer to electively intubate patients if there is any doubt about their

Table 46.3 Criteria for urgent neurosurgical consultation

Coma: GCS <8
Deteriorating GCS despite normal blood pressure and Pao_2
GCS persistently 8–14 for 8 h
Skull fracture associated with any one of the following:
    GCS <15
    Focal neurological signs
    Unequally dilated pupils
    Epileptic fit
Depressed or compound skull fractures
Suspected base of skull fracture

ability to protect the upper airway. In addition, no patient should be considered ready for transfer if, after the initial resuscitation, there are still signs of cardiovascular instability suggesting uncontrolled blood loss.

The neurosurgeons often request that the effects of anaesthetic drugs are reversed on arrival in the neurosurgical unit to re-assess the patient's GCS. Bolus doses of 1–2 mg of midazolam and 25–50 μg fentanyl, and neuromuscular blockade with either atracurium or vecuronium, can be used. Basic monitoring of ECG, pulse oximetry and non-invasive BP are essential; invasive arterial pressure and capnography are useful, if available.

ANAESTHESIA IN HEAD-INJURED PATIENTS

Head-injured patients often require anaesthesia for a CT scan, a neurosurgical procedure, or for treatment of their extracranial injuries. Regional anaesthesia may be adequate for minor injuries and provides postoperative analgesia, but epidural and spinal anaesthesia are contraindicated in the presence of raised ICP, so most patients require general anaesthesia. The principles of induction of anaesthesia are the same as outlined in the section on airway management and ventilation.

In maintaining anaesthesia the following details need to be considered.

- Ventilation should be adjusted to produce mild hypocapnia with a Pa_{CO_2} of 3.5–4.0 kPa.
- Nitrous oxide must not be used in patients with base of skull fractures, as the CSF leak may allow air into the skull which would expand under anaesthesia.
- Drugs used for the maintenance of anaesthesia depend on the severity of the head injury as defined by the pre-induction GCS:
  a) Minor (GCS 13–15): isoflurane up to a maximum of 1% in nitrous oxide. Adequate analgesia must be provided; morphine or fentanyl are acceptable.
  b) Moderate (GCS 9–12): isoflurane in nitrous oxide may be used, unless there was a rapid deterioration in GCS before induction of anaesthesia. If so, a technique using fentanyl 5–7 μg kg^{-1} with droperidol 2.5–7.5 mg and nitrous oxide in oxygen is safer, although there may be a risk of awareness.
  c) Severe (GCS 3–8): isoflurane should be avoided. Fentanyl, droperidol and nitrous oxide have been used safely, although there is still controversy about whether nitrous oxide causes clinically significant cerebral vasodilation in the presence of hypocapnia in these patients. An alternative would a total intravenous technique using propofol, although there is a significant risk of hypotension with this technique if the patient is hypovolaemic, or large doses of fentanyl are given concomitantly. These patients are often electively ventilated postoperatively.
- Neuromuscular blockade should be maintained to avoid any coughing during anaesthesia. The choice of drug is not critical.
- Measurement of ECG, non-invasive BP, pulse oximetry and neuromuscular blockade are mandatory. Capnography is useful but should not be relied upon without arterial blood gas analysis, as there is often up to a 2.5 kPa difference between the end tidal CO_2 and Pa_{CO_2} concentrations. As these patients often have multiple injuries, invasive arterial and CVP monitoring are advisable, but urgent surgery should not be unreasonably delayed if this is technically difficult. Long catheters via the antecubital fossa or femoral vein are preferred, as not only may these be inserted during the neurosurgical procedure, but the dangers of obstructing the internal jugular veins or causing a haematoma in the neck are avoided.

The anaesthetist's aim is to maintain a stable arterial pressure avoiding hypotension at all costs. Estimation of blood loss is often difficult in these circumstances and the decision whether to administer blood may be helped by performing serial haematocrit estimations. Platelets and fresh frozen plasma may be necessary to promote haemostasis especially if there is a suspicion of disseminated intravascular coagulation. If the brain is herniating through the craniotomy, 50–100 mg thiopentone may alleviate the situation while a further dose of mannitol 0.5 g kg^{-1} or frusemide 1 mg kg^{-1} is given: it is essential that the bladder is catheterized if diuretics are used, because a full bladder may be a cause of unexplained hypertension and restlessness after operation.

The decision to extubate the patient depends on the degree of anticipated cerebral oedema and any extracranial reasons for artificial ventilation. As coughing and straining on the tracheal tube raise the ICP, a 'trial of extubation' is commonly used once the decision to extubate has been made. It is recognized, therefore, that many of these patients may require re-intubation if, after a reasonable trial, they still fulfil the criteria for intubation or ventilation (Tables 46.1 and 46.2). Admission to an intensive care unit is necessary in the first instance, so that progress can be closely monitored.

INTENSIVE CARE MANAGEMENT

The medical management of head injured patients is centred on the control of raised ICP and the provision of an adequate supply of oxygenated blood. Achieving these aims depends on manipulating the physiology of the intracranial contents, venous and arterial blood, CSF and the brain itself.

DECREASED VENOUS VOLUME

There are no venous valves between the right atrium and the dural sinuses. Therefore, any increase in venous pressure will distend the intracranial veins and produce a rise in ICP. To decrease intracranial venous volume the following measures are employed.

- The patient is nursed with at least 15–30° head-up tilt.
- The head is kept in alignment with the body at all times, and the tracheal tube ties are well padded so that the internal jugular veins are not occluded.
- In patients in whom it is difficult to control raised ICP, neuromuscular blockade may be used to prevent coughing and straining on the tracheal tube. The disadvantages of the use of such drugs are that they negate any useful neurological signs, may mask underlying epilepsy, prolong ICU stay and are associated with a higher incidence of pneumonia. Therefore, their use must be re-assessed daily and withdrawn as soon as ICP control improves.
- The use of positive end-expiratory pressure (PEEP) may increase ICP by raising intrathoracic pressure. If kept to the minimum value that achieves clinically acceptable oxygenation, PEEP does not usually cause problems in combination with a 30° head-up tilt.

DECREASED ARTERIAL VOLUME

Hyperventilation

This has been the cornerstone of ICP control by causing cerebral vasoconstriction in the small regulatory arteries in the brain. Its continuing use in ICU is surrounded by two controversial issues.

- Does the effect of hyperventilation wear off in 24 h in head-injured patients as it does in the normal brain?
- Does hyperventilation contribute to the ischaemic damage seen following head injury?

There is no doubt that the head-injured brain reacts differently from the normal one. Not only is there evidence that the vasoconstrictor response to hypocapnia is less than the vasodilator effect of an equivalent amount of hypercapnia, but that these responses are maintained for longer than 24 h. A prospective randomized trial of hyperventilation for 5 days showed that patients with a GCS of 4–5 had worse outcome scores at 3 and 6 months compared with a control group who were not hyperventilated. Although cerebral ischaemia was not demonstrated, other studies have shown that hyperventilation appears to cause some ischaemia which is related to the degree of hyperventilation. However, this assumes that all head injuries are the same, and that cerebral blood flow does not vary significantly. This is incorrect: it is known that children tend to have hyperaemic head injuries, and that adults may have a hyperaemic phase a few days after the head injury. In these cases hyperventilation may decrease ICP without causing ischaemia.

The current recommendations are that moderate degrees of hyperventilation (3.5–4.4 kPa) may be used early to try to control ICP, but that the Pa_{CO_2} should be allowed gradually to return to normal values after the first 24 h. Continuous jugular bulb oximetry provides some indication of global ischaemia if ICP is difficult to control and hyperventilation is required for a longer period.

Decreased cerebral metabolism

Sedation is now routinely used because it is known that a fall in cerebral metabolism decreases the cerebral blood flow and allows easier ICP control. High dose barbiturate therapy was abandoned because of the demonstration that the decline in ICP resulted from cardiovascular instability and that there was no decrease in mortality. Morphine (1–8 mg h^{-1}) and midazolam infusions (1–5 mg h^{-1}) are commonly used and do not cause significant cardiovascular instability. Propofol (100–250 mg h^{-1}) can be used safely as long as bolus doses are avoided and the patient is not hypovolaemic.

Cerebral metabolism appears to be more sensitive to the depressant effects of hypothermia than the rest of the body. There is renewed interest in the use of mild hypothermia (36.5–34°C) which has been shown to have a beneficial effect in decreasing ICP without the systemic problems associated with greater degrees of hypothermia.

Seizures greatly increase cerebral metabolism and therefore it is extremely important to control them rapidly and avoid secondary cerebral damage. The latest recommendation is that phenytoin is effective in preventing post-traumatic seizures only in the first seven days. It should be prescribed in those patients at risk: GCS < 10, haematoma, contusion, penetrating injury and depressed skull fractures.

Arterial pressure management

The deleterious effects of hypotension have already been mentioned. From a practical point of view there is increasing evidence that CPP must be maintained above 70 mmHg to avoid ischaemic episodes, as shown by jugular bulb oximetry. This should be possible by ensuring normovolaemia and it is rare that inotropic support is required.

Oxygen therapy

An increase in inspired oxygen before physiotherapy will ensure that hypoxaemia does not contribute to the rise in ICP seen during tracheal suction. In addition, patients with pneumocephalus are given high oxygen concentrations to try to accelerate the rate of absorption of the intracranial air.

DECREASED CEREBROSPINAL FLUID VOLUME

Cerebrospinal fluid is displaced out of the skull with rising ICP. There is growing evidence that both mannitol and frusemide decrease ICP by a combination of actions, one of which is to decrease CSF production. The mechanism is unknown, but for mannitol seems to be related to the increase in plasma osmolarity. This either causes a decrease in the movement of fluid into CSF (which is naturally hyperosmolar) or decreases fluid movement into the choroid plexus which produces CSF. A combination of mannitol 0.25–0.5 g kg^{-1} followed 15 min later by frusemide 1 mg kg^{-1} appears to be the most effective combination.

The possibility of the development of hydrocephalus must always be considered as a cause of neurological deterioration, and treated appropriately.

DECREASED BRAIN VOLUME

The development and progression of cerebral oedema is very difficult to predict. Oedema reaches its peak at about 48 h after injury and is slow to resolve, giving rise to the fluctuating conscious level often seen during recovery.

Mannitol has been found to have various effects which decrease ICP. The initial rapid decrease in ICP following a bolus dose is a result of decreased blood viscosity causing cerebral vasoconstriction and a decrease in CSF production. Its effect as an osmotic diuretic is seen with frequent administration (10–20 g 4–6 hourly) in combination with fluid restriction, aiming to produce a rise in plasma osmolality to 295–305 mosmol kg^{-1}. Care must be taken to monitor renal function as the risk of renal failure increases substantially if osmolality exceeds 310 mosmol kg^{-1}.

Because steroids decrease the cerebral oedema surrounding tumours, high dose dexamethasone was tried following head injury. Not only was this ineffective, but there was an increased incidence of infection in multiple trauma victims.

Craniotomy to excise a badly contused non-dominant frontal lobe is sometimes undertaken and can be life saving. In addition, decompressive craniectomy is used in some countries for refractory ICP, but the results in terms of outcome are disappointing.

NEUROLOGICAL MONITORING IN INTENSIVE CARE

ICP monitoring

The use of fibreoptic intraparenchymal monitors provides a reliable measurement of ICP. The indications for ICP monitoring are summarized in Table 46.4. A continuous printout is useful with events such as physiotherapy marked, as spontaneous rises in ICP carry a worse prognosis than those following physiotherapy or repositioning.

Jugular bulb oximetry

A fibreoptic catheter is inserted retrogradely into the internal jugular vein and positioned in the jugular bulb on X-ray. It is inserted either into the right jugular vein, or into the side which caused the greatest rise in ICP when compressed. Its value lies in the fact that in a sedated patient with stable systemic oxygenation, cerebral metabolism remains constant, so that high oxygen extraction is a sign of low cerebral blood flow. It is useful in patients who require to be continually hyperventilated to reduce ICP, those with CPP less than 70 mmHg and when the ICP trace shows frequent spontaneous peaks. The disadvantages are that it requires recalibration against an oximeter every 12 h, has a high incidence of movement-related changes and is only a crude measure of global ischaemia.

Table 46.4 Indications for intracranial pressure monitoring

All patients requiring sedation or muscle paralysis
GCS <8
Small subdural or intracerebral haematomas on CT scan
Evidence of brain shift on CT scan
Patients requiring non-neurosurgical major surgery

Cerebral blood flow

Transcranial Doppler ultrasonography (TCD) provides an easy, non-invasive monitor of CBF. Recently it has been shown that differences in the diastolic component of the waveform can help differentiate increased flow secondary to vasodilatation from that due to vasospasm, thus influencing medical management.

Other forms of CBF monitoring tend to be research tools, and disappointingly, the benefits of CBF monitoring in terms of outcome have been difficult to demonstrate.

Electroencephalogram

The possibility of undetected, epileptic activity must always be considered in patients requiring sedation and paralysis. The cerebral function monitor is helpful in detecting increased electrical activity which can be followed by a diagnostic EEG. The best monitor of neurological function remains the GCS, and therefore the use of neuromuscular blocking drugs should be kept to a minimum.

ASSOCIATED SYSTEMIC PROBLEMS

Pulmonary problems (Table 46.5)

Thoracic injuries occur in about 3% of all head injured patients, but account for 25% of trauma deaths.

As the cough and gag reflexes may be obtunded, aspiration of blood, pharyngeal secretions and gastric secretions is a common

Table 46.5 Pulmonary problems in head injury

25–30% patients are hypoxaemic because of associated chest injuries – 30% patients aspiration of blood and vomit – 35–40% increased P_{AO_2}–P_{aO_2} associated with head injury – 80%
neurogenic pulmonary oedema
fat embolism

complication of head injury, and is contributory in the 41% patients who subsequently develop pneumonia.

Of patients with a severe head injury, 80% have a $P_{AO_2} - P_{aO_2}$ of greater than 2.5 kPa. Although pulmonary shunting is the cause of the hypoxaemia, the mechanism is controversial. Some researchers have demonstrated a reduction in functional residual capacity (FRC) of similar magnitude to that which occurs with anaesthesia, and this may be related to sedative drugs used, or coma. Animal experiments have also demonstrated that hypoxic pulmonary vasoconstriction may be attenuated by a markedly raised ICP and others have shown increased pulmonary water without X-ray evidence of pulmonary oedema. Neurogenic pulmonary oedema is rare in blunt head injuries but more common in gunshot injuries. The rapidity of the increase in ICP and the height of the peak pressure following impact seem to determine the degree of sympathetic overactivity and therefore endothelial damage. These changes, in combination with the effects of brain thromboplastin released intravascularly, may determine where the patient lies on the spectrum from increased $P_{AO_2} - P_{aO_2}$ to pulmonary oedema. The increased $P_{AO_2} - P_{aO_2}$ resolves as the patient's neurological condition improves.

Abnormal respiratory patterns are frequently seen and are an important cause of hypoxaemia immediately following the injury. Tachypnoea is the most common pattern, and is thought to result from the CSF acidosis that accompanies the injury. Interestingly, those patients who have a P_{aCO_2} less than 4 kPa when breathing spontaneously have a worse prognosis. Irregular breathing patterns and Cheyne–Stokes respiration are also commonly seen.

Cardiovascular problems

Head injuries are associated with a massive increase in serum catecholamines in proportion to the severity of the injury. Hypertension and tachycardia are, therefore, a common feature of severe head injury, and may be paroxysmal in patients with brain stem injury. Occasionally bradycardia is seen with increasing arterial pressure (Cushing response) and is a sign of rising ICP and ischaemia of the brain stem.

Arrhythmias and ECG changes are commonly seen: 62% patients who die following head injury have areas of focal myocardial necrosis. The most ominous arrhythmia is the development of atrial fibrillation, or a supraventricular tachycardia resistant to intravenous adenosine, which occurs in patients with a rising ICP. In our experience this is a sign of impending brain stem death, and is followed by a return to sinus rhythm once brain stem function has ceased.

Fluid and electrolyte disturbance

Hypernatraemia is commonly seen as a result of fluid restriction and mannitol therapy. In addition, evidence from animal studies that hyperglycaemia increases cerebral infarct size has lead to the avoidance of glucose containing i.v. fluids, so that patients receive a high sodium load. The development of diabetes insipidus is usually a poor prognostic sign.

Occasionally hyponatraemia may occur, possibly related to increased atrial natriuretic peptide secretion, or the result of water retention secondary to elevated cortisol and aldosterone values. As hyponatraemia may itself cause cerebral oedema, all efforts should be made to treat it with fluid restriction or occasionally hypertonic saline.

Transient hyperglycaemia occurs frequently and results from greatly enhanced catecholamine and cortisol secretion. Several studies have shown that patients who remain hyperglycaemic have a worse prognosis. The role of lactate in causing reperfusion injury to ischaemic areas of the brain has now been well documented and probably accounts for this increased mortality.

Gastrointestinal tract and nutrition

Stress ulceration of the stomach is seen endoscopically in over 90% head injured patients within 12 h, and is not prevented by the use of H_2 receptor antagonists. The decrease in symptomatic bleeding from these lesions is probably related to the emphasis on early nasogastric feeding. Gastric mucosal barrier protection with drugs such as sucralfate is useful, but as they interact with food should be reserved for patients in whom gastric stasis persists.

The hormonal response to head injury, increased catecholamine, cortisol and glucagon secretion, renders the patient hypercatabolic. Damage to the hypothalamus (affecting temperature control) and paraparesis greatly accelerate the loss of muscle protein. In the absence of infection, these effects wane within a week. Attempts to achieve a neutral nitrogen balance in that time have failed and are accompanied by complications of the feeding regimens. Total parenteral nutrition is very rarely indicated because of its inherent risks, problems with fluid balance and high incidence of hyperglycaemia. Percutaneous endoscopic gastrostomy, or surgical jejunostomy, are gaining favour as routes of enteral nutrition because of the problems of sinusitis, difficulty in clearing secretions and discomfort caused by nasogastric tubes.

Coagulation problems

The brain is a rich source of thromboplastin which may be released into the circulation, especially after penetrating head injuries. The frequency of disseminated intravascular coagulation (DIC) is difficult to quantify, because of the inconsistency of the tests used, and the presence of other injuries requiring resuscitation. The DIC is usually self-limiting and does not need treatment unless the patient requires a surgical procedure, but should always be thought of in patients in whom haemostasis is difficult. Fibrin degradation products appear to be an independent predictor of outcome, especially in patients with a moderate head injury, very high values are associated with a poor outcome.

The risk of bleeding into intracerebral haematomas contraindicates the use of heparin prophylaxis in the initial period following a head injury. The incidence of symptomatic deep vein thrombosis (DVT) is unclear and of fatal pulmonary embolism (PE) about 1%.

OUTCOME

Most neurosurgical units report a mortality of 30–40% for severely head-injured patients. Of such patients, only about 10% make a good neurological recovery and 5–10% remain in a persistent vegetative state. The emphasis must always be on the primary prevention of brain damage. Once head injury has occurred, the welfare of these patients depends primarily on meticulous evaluation and rapid resuscitation, because the potential for secondary, cerebral damage is great, and the prospect of cerebral salvage is limited.

FURTHER READING

Cooper, P. R. (ed) (1993) *Head Injury*, 3rd edn, Williams and Wilkins, Baltimore.

Hicks, I. R., Hedley, R. M. and Razis, P. (1994) Audit of transfer of head-injured patients to a stand-alone neurosurgical unit. *Injury*, **25**, 545-549.

Hsiang, J. K., Chesnut, R.M., Crisp, C. B. et al. (1994) Early, routine paralysis for intracranial pressure control in severe head injury: Is it necessary? *Critical Care Medicine*, **22**, 1471–1476.

Jennett, S. (1985) Pulmonary function in the head-injured patient, in *Head Injury and the Anaesthetist*, (eds W. Fitch and J. Barker), Elsevier Science Publishers B.V. (Biomedical Division), pp. 53–82.

Lam, A. M. (ed) (1995) *Anesthetic Management of Acute Head Injury*, McGraw-Hill, Inc., USA

Miller, J. D. (1985) Head injury and brain ischaemia-implications for therapy. *British Journal of Anaesthesia*, **57**, 120–129.

Miller, J. D., Dearden, N. M., Piper, I. R. and Chan, K. H. (1992) Control of intracranial pressure in patients with severe head injury. *Journal of Neurotrauma*, **9** (Suppl 1), S317–S326.

Muizelaar, J. P., Marmarou, A., Ward, J. et al. (1991) Adverse effects of prolonged hyperventilation in patients with severe head injury: A randomized clinical trial. *Journal of Neurosurgery*, **75**, 731–739.

Sheinberg, M., Kanter, M. J., Robertson, C. S. et al. (1992) Continuous monitoring of jugular venous oxygen saturation in head-injured patients. *Journal of Neurosurgery*, **76**, 212–217.

Shiozaki, T., Sugimoto, H., Taneda, M. et al. (1993) Effect of mild hypothermia on uncontrollable intracranial hypertension after severe head injury. *Journal of Neurosurgery*, **79**, 363–368.

INDEX

(Page numbers in **bold** type refer to tables, those in *italic* type to figures)

A–D switches 80
Abdominal trauma 439
ABO compatibility **725**
Acid–base balance
  and transfusions 738
  see also Electrolytes; Fluid balance
Acoustic neuroma 332
Acromegaly 432–3
  clinical 432
  intraoperative 432
  pathophysiology 432
  postoperative 432–3
  preparation 432
  surgery 432
Activated partial thromboplastin time 170
Acupuncture
  as anti-emetic 674
  postoperative pain 668
Acute intermittent porphyria *see* Porphyrias
Acute pain services 670
Adenoidectomy 317–19
Adrenal surgery 424–31
  adrenocortical insufficiency 428
  corticosteroid therapy and surgery 428–9
  Cushing's syndrome 430–1
  phaeochromocytoma 425–8
  primary aldosteronism 429–30
Adrenaline
  epidural anaesthesia 510
  and life support 774–5
α-Adrenoceptor agonists, premedication 144
β-Adrenoceptor blocking drugs, and anaesthesia 136
Adrenocortical insufficiency 428
Air embolism 257–8
Airway 84–9
  assessment 157–8
  compromised, anaesthesia management 323–5
  contamination 379–80
  difficult *see* Difficult airway
  foreign body in 326
  laryngeal mask *see* Laryngeal mask airway
  nasopharyngeal *85–6*
  obstruction
    dental surgery 379
    paediatric surgery 354
    recovery room 642
    see also Difficult airway
  oropharyngeal *84–5*
  paediatric problems 354–5
    acute obstruction 354
    aspirated foreign body 355
    croup 354
    epiglottitis 354–5
  transtracheal 688–90
  upper
    laser surgery 321–3
      airway fires 323
      anaesthetic hazards 322–3
      safety 322
      theory and applications 321
    malignant disease 323
  see also Airway management
Airway management 83–100
  cardiopulmonary resuscitation 775
  dental surgery 375–6
  emergency 325–6
  facemasks 83–4
  head injury **801**–2
  spinal injuries 446
  thermal injury 460–1
  tracheal tubes 89–99
    catheter mounts 92
    connectors 92
    correct placement 98, *99*
    design *90*
    laryngoscopes *97, 98*
    material 89–90
    size 89
    specialist 92–7
      laryngectomy tubes *95*
      microlaryngeal tubes 93, *94*
      Oxford pattern tubes 95, *96*
      paediatric tubes 92–3
      RAE pre-formed tubes 93
      reinforced tubes 93, *94*
      tracheostomy tubes 94, *95*
      tubes for use with lasers 96, *97*
    tracheal cuff 90, *91*–2
  trauma surgery 437–8
  see also Airways
Alarms
  oxygen failure 8–9
  ventilators 57
Alberti regimen 618
Albumin 703–4
Alcohol and anaesthesia 136
Allergy *see* Anaphylaxis
Amniotic fluid embolus 565
Amoxycillin, antibiotic prophylaxis **143**
Anaesthesia workstation 16–18
Anaesthetic breathing systems *52, 53*–4, 69–81
  A–D switches 80
  classification of 72–8
  CO_2 removal systems 72, *73*
  coaxial systems 78–80
    Bain system 78, *79*
    Lack system 79–80
  enclosed afferent reservoir *80*–1
  filters 81
  flow requirements 70, *71*
  non-rebreathing systems 73, *74*, *75*
  paediatric surgery 349–50
  partial rebreathing systems 74–5, *76*–8
    Mapleson A 75, *77*
    Mapleson B and C 77
    Mapleson D, E and F 77, *78*
  resistance in 70–2
Anaesthetic machines 3–18
  anaesthesia workstation 16–18
  checking of 11, *12–13*, 14–15
  classification 15–16
  continuous-flow 3–4
  draw-over and portable 11
  flowmeters and restrictors 7–8
  filters 8

Anaesthetic machines (contd)
  flow restrictors 8
  flowmeters 7, 8
  gas supplies 4–5
    medical gas cylinders 4
    medical gas pipeline 5
    pin-index system 4
  safety devices 8–9
    direct oxygen flush valve 9
    oxygen failure alarm 8–9
    safety valves 9
  standards 3
  valves and gauges 5–7
    flowmeter needle valves 6–7
    one-way/backflow check valves 6
    pressure reducing valves (regulators) 6
  vaporizers 9, 11
Anaesthetics see Inhalational anaesthetics; Total intravenous anaesthesia
Analgesia
  dental surgery 378–9
  liver transplantation 482
  obese patients 594
  obstetric 552–3
  patient-controlled 661, **662**–3
  porphyria 169
  postoperative see Postoperative pain
  premedication 141–2
  recovery room 648–9
  renal transplantation 489
  route of administration
    continuous intravenous infusion 658, 660
    intermittent intramuscular injection **657**–8, 659
    intravenous bolus administration 660, **661**
    oral, buccal and sublingual 663
    rectal 663
    spinal 663, **664**–5
    subcutaneous injection 658
    transdermal 663
  thermal injury 463–4
  thoracic surgery 193
  trauma surgery 441–2
  see also individual analgesics
Anaphylaxis 741–51
  allergy and atopy 742
  clinical features **746**
  drugs producing 743–6
    antibiotics 745
    colloid solutions and blood products 745
    latex 745
    local anaesthetics 745–6

narcotics 745
neuromuscular blockers 744–5
propofol 743, **744**
protamine 745
heart and anaphylactic mediators 742
incidence 743
management 746–51
  angio-oedema 747
  bronchospasm 747
  cardiovascular collapse 746–7
  follow-up 748–51
  pulmonary oedema 748
mediator release 741–2, 743
previous exposure 743
Angicoagulation, see also Coagulation; Coagulation disorders
Angiooedema 747
Angiotensin converting enzyme inhibitors and anaesthesia 137
Ankylosing spondylitis, anaesthetic management 131–2
Antacids, premedication 142
Antibiotics
  and anaesthesia 137
  anaphylactic reactions **744**, 745
  prophylaxis **143**, 144
Anticholinergics
  as anti-emetics 673
Anticoagulation 213–14
  see also Coagulation; Coagulation disorders
Anticonvulsants and anaesthesia 136
Antidepressants, postoperative analgesia 668
Antithrombin III 174
Antithrombotic prophylaxis **144**
Anxiolytics, premedication **139**, **140**–1
Aortic reconstructive surgery 238–41
  anaesthetic considerations 238
  anaesthetic technique 240–1
  blood transfusion 238–9
  haemodynamic consequences of aortic cross-clamping 239
  renal function 239–40
  spinal cord 240
Aortic valve 219–21
  aortic regurgitation 221
  aortic stenosis 219–21
APACHE score 112, **113**
Apnoea
  and brain death 793, 794
  dental surgery 379
  sleep 347
Aromatherapy 668–9

Arrhythmias 380
  recovery room 647
Arterial blood gas analysis 154–5
ASA physical status 111, **112**
Ascites 293
Asthma
  anaesthetic management 128
  in children 346–7
Atmospheric pollution 101–8
  carbon dioxide absorbers 105
  global pollution 107–8
  local pollution 105–7
  nitrous oxide 101–2
  volatile anaesthetic toxicity 103–5
    kidney 104–5
    liver 103–4
Atropine, premedication **139**
Audit 118–20
  CEPOD and NCEPOD 119–20
Auditory evoked potentials 41
Autologous blood transfusion 390
Autonomic block 511
Autotransfusion 727–8
Awareness 753–63
  causes 757–8
  consequences 756–7
  definitions 753, **754**
  incidence 754–6
    implicit memory for intraoperative events 755–6
    recall of surgery 754–5
  monitoring depth of anaesthesia 758–62
    body state 760–1
      facial electromyogram 760–1
      oesophageal contractility 760
      sinus arrhythmia 761
    brain state 761–2
      evoked potentials in EEG 761–2
      resting EEG 761
    detection of awareness 759–60
    problems of 758–9
Axillary block 529–30

Babies
  magnetic resonance imaging 415
  ophthalmic surgery 307–8
  see also Children; Paediatric
Backflow check valves 6
Bag-in-bottle system 53, 64–5
Bain coaxial system 78, 79
Balanced electrolyte solutions 703
Bat ears 393–4
Bayesian model **115**–16
Bile 290
Bile duct obstruction 300
Bioartificial livers 486

Biochemistry, preoperative tests 160–1
  hypokalaemia 160–1
  renal function 161
  urinalysis and diabetes mellitus 161
Bladder
  temperature monitoring 43
  tumour, transurethral resection 274–5
Bleeding see Haemorrhage
Blood conservation **214**
Blood flow measurement 38
Blood pressure monitoring 32, **33**–5
  direct 34–5
  and MRI 413
  non-invasive 32–4
    automated monitoring 33–4
      versus manual 34
    Finapres 34
    oscillotonometer 33
    sphygmomanometer 32
  recovery room 645–7
Blood transfusion
  and acid–base balance 738
  aortic reconstructive surgery 238–9
  autologous 390
  autotransfusion 727–8
  and hypothermia 737–8
  liver transplantation 479–80
  platelets **734**–5
  preoperative 134
  red cells **724**, **725**–7
Blood-borne viruses 606–9
Body fluid compartments 698–701
  extracellular compartment 699
  interstitial compartment *700*
  lung 700–1
  intracellular compartment 699
  microvascular endothelium 699
  renal threshold 701
  total body water 698–9
Bone tumour surgery 455
Brachial plexus
  block 527, *527*
  formation 525, *525*, *526*
Brain death 267–8, 785–96
  causes **788**
  clinical diagnosis **790**–4
    brain stem reflexes 792–4
      apnoea test 794
      corneal reflex 793
      gag–bronchial reflex 794
      motor response in cranial nerve distribution 793
      pupillary response to light 793
      vestibulo-ocular reflex 793

exclusions 791, **792**
preconditions 790–1
controversies surrounding 794–5
  EEG in brain dead patients 794–5
  imaging of cerebral blood flow 795
  pituitary function 795
development of criteria 787–8
extracranial effects 788–90
  cardiovascular system 788–9
  coagulation 790
  endocrine system 789
  kidneys 789–90
  liver 790
  respiratory system 789
intracranial effects 788
philosophical and ethical arguments 786–7
physiological concepts 785, **786**
Brain stem reflex tests 792–4
  apnoea test 794
  corneal reflex 793
  gag–bronchial reflex 794
  motor response in cranial nerve distribution 793
  pupillary response to light 793
  vestibulo-ocular reflex 793
Brain tumour 255–7
  posterior fossa/brain stem surgery 256–7
  stereotactic surgery *256*
Brain volume, decreased in head injury 806
Breast operations 394–5
Brompton Pallister endobronchial tube *195*
Bronchopleural fistula 194–6
  anaesthesia 195, *195*
  induction techniques 195
  intubating techniques 196, *196*, *197*
Bronchoscopy 187–8
  adults 187, *188*
  children 188
Bronchospasm 643, 747
Bupivacaine
  epidural anaesthesia 510
  peripheral nerve block **522**, **523**
Buprenorphine 657
Burns see Thermal injury
Butyrophenones
  as anti-emetics 673

C1 esterase deficiency 174–6
  anaesthetic management 176
  clinical manifestations 174–5
  treatment 175–6
Caesarean section

general anaesthesia 559–62
  aspiration of gastric contents 560
  induction 561–2
  maintenance 562
  reversal and recovery 562
  tracheal intubation 560, **561**
regional anaesthesia 562–4
  combined spinal–epidural 564
  epidural 563
  spinal 564
Calcium channel antagonists and anaesthesia 136
Caloric test 793
Cannabinoids, as anti-emetic 674
Cape paediatric attachment 67
Capnography 413
Carbon dioxide
  absorbers 105
  monitoring **24**, *25*, *26*, *27*
  removal systems *72*, *73*
Carbonated solutions, epidural anaesthesia 510
Carcinoid syndrome 435–6
  clinical 435–6
  intraoperative 436
  pathophysiology 435
  postoperative 436
  preparation 436
  surgery 435
Cardiac arrhythmias and pacing 222, 223–4
Cardiac cycle *217*
Cardiac pacemakers, anaesthetic management **127**–8
Cardiac surgery 203–31
  anaesthesia 205–6
  cardiac arrhythmias and pacing 222–4
  cardiopulmonary bypass 206, *207*–8
    deep hypothermic circulatory arrest 208
    hypothermia 207–8
    weaning from 208
  complications 214–16
    central nervous system 215–16
    renal 215
    respiratory 214–15
  congenital heart disease **226**, *227*, *228*–31
    obstruction to flow 228–9
    shunts 228
    ventricular status *229*, *230*–1
  diabetic patients 620
  haematological aspects 213–14
    anticoagulation 213–14
    blood conservation **214**
    haemostasis 214

Cardiac surgery (contd)
　heart and lung transplantation
　　225–8
　　anaesthesia 226–7
　　donor 226
　　pathophysiology 227–8
　　recipient 226
　monitoring 203, 205
　myocardial protection 208–9
　　cardiac reserve 209
　　cardioplegia **209**
　　intermittent aortic cross-clamp
　　　and ventricular fibrillation
　　　208
　　limitation of demand 209
　　limitation of reperfusion injury
　　　209
　myocardial revascularization 216,
　　217, 218
　preoperative assessment 203, **204**
　re-operations 222
　risk analysis **204**
　thoracic aortic disease *223, 224,
　　225*
　trauma 438–9
　valve surgery 218–22
　　aortic valve *219*, 220–1
　　mitral valve *219*, 221–2
　ventricular dysfunction 209–13
　　assist devices 212
　　intra-aortic balloon
　　　counterpulsation 211–12, *213*
　　management 210, **212**
　　measurement of ventricular
　　　function 210
　　pathophysiology 210, *211*
　　right ventricle 212–13
Cardioplegia **209**
Cardiopulmonary bypass 206, *207*–8
　deep hypothermic circulatory
　　arrest 208
　hypothermia 207–8
　weaning from 208
Cardiopulmonary resuscitation
　　765–83
　advanced life support 770, *771*–4,
　　775–7
　　adrenaline 774–5
　　airway management 775
　　drug delivery routes 775–6
　　open chest cardiac massage
　　　776–7
　　peri-arrest arrhythmias 777
　basic life support 765–9
　　expired air respiration 766, *767*
　　external chest compression
　　　767–8
　　　rationale behind 768–9
　　hospital life support 769

　paediatric 777–8, *777–9, 781*
　precordial thump 769–70
　in pregnancy 780, 782
　risk to rescuer 769
Cardiovascular collapse 746–7
Cardiovascular disease
　anaesthetic management 126–8
　　cardiac pacemakers **127**–8
　　hypertension 127
　　ischaemic heart disease 126–7
　　left ventricular failure 126
　diabetic patients 615
　postoperative pain management
　　669
Cardiovascular drugs and
　　anaesthesia 136–7
　β-adrenoceptor blocking drugs
　　136
　angiotensin converting enzyme
　　inhibitors 137
　calcium channel antagonists 136
　clonidine 137
Cardiovascular system
　effects of brain death 788–9
　elderly patients 571–2
　epidural anaesthesia 511–12
　and head injury 807–8
　laparoscopic surgery 498–9
　in liver failure 471, 483
　monitoring 30
　　blood flow measurement 38
　　blood pressure 32, **33**–5
　　direct monitoring 34–5
　　non-invasive monitoring 32–4
　　　automated 33–4
　　　automated versus manual 34
　　　Finapres 34
　　　oscillotonometer 33
　　　sphygmomanometer 32
　　central venous pressure 35, 37
　　clinical observation 30
　　ECG 30
　　perfusion of individual organs
　　　38–9
　　pulmonary artery
　　　catheterization 37, *38*
　　pulse oximetry 30–2
　　transoesophageal
　　　echocardiography 39
　　zeroing and calibration 35, *36*
　obese patients 588
　postoperative care, thoracic
　　surgery 193
　in pregnancy 550
　preoperative tests 148–53
　　ambulatory ECG monitoring
　　　149–50
　　dipyridamole thallium
　　　scintigraphy 150

　　echocardiography 151
　　electrocardiography 148–9
　　exercise ECG 149
　　radionuclide ventriculography
　　　150–1
　renal failure 486
Carotid artery surgery 242–5
　anaesthetic considerations 242–3
　anaesthetic technique 244
　brain monitoring 243–4
　cerebral blood flow 243
　general anaesthesia 243
　postoperative complications 244–5
　preoperative assessment 242
　surgical procedure 242
Caudal block 355, *356*
　obstetrics 559
Central nervous system
　and cardiac surgery 215–16
　　awareness 216
　　emboli 215–16
　　metabolic 216
　　perfusion 215
　head injury **802**
　in liver failure 472
　monitoring 40, **265**–6
　in pregnancy 551
Central venous pressure 35, 37
Cerebral aneurysm 259–60
Cerebral autoregulation and head
　　injury 799
Cerebral blood flow *248, 249*
　head injury 799, 807
　imaging, and brain death 795
Cerebral ischaemia **262**–5
　anti-excitatory agents 264–5
　cerebral protection 263–4
　free radical scavengers 265
　haemodilution 264
　normoglycaemia 264
　normoventilation 264
　perfusion pressure 264
Cerebral metabolism, head injury
　　800, 805
Cerebral oedema, liver disease 484
Cerebrospinal fluid 248
　decreased volume in head injury
　　805–6
Cervical mobility, and difficult
　　intubation 679, *680*
Check procedures for anaesthetic
　　machines 11, *12–13*, 14–15
Chest drains 194
Chest X-ray 153
Chicken pox 603
Children
　asthma in 346–7
　bronchoscopy in 188

cardiopulmonary resuscitation 777–8, *777–9*, 781
dental procedures in 372
fluid balance in **341**
magnetic resonance imaging 415
pain in 342
postoperative pain management 670
preoperative preparation 134
regional anaesthetic block 355–7
respiratory system 337–8
temperature regulation *340*–1
see also Paediatric
Cholinesterase variants 177–8
Christmas disease 172
Chronic obstructive airways disease, anaesthetic management 129
Circulatory system
fetal and transitional 338, *339*
head injury 802
neonatal *339*–40
Cleft palate/lip 392–3
Clindamycin, antibiotic prophylaxis **143**
Clonidine
and anaesthesia 137
postoperative analgesia 668
Closed-loop anaesthesia 631
Clostridium tetani 445, 604
Clotting defects see Coagulation disorders
Coagulation 729, *730*, *731*
effects of brain death 790
and head injury 808–9
Coagulation disorders 170–4
classification 170
factor IX deficiency 172
haemophilia 171–2
inhibitors of coagulation 174
liver disease 292
liver failure 473
normal haemostasis 170
tests for clotting defects 170–1
Von Willebrand's disease 172–4
Coagulation factors 735–6
Coagulation inhibitors 174
Coaxial systems 78–80
Bain system 78, *79*
Lack system *79*–80
preferential flow system *79*
Cognitive function
elderly patients 576–7
recovery room 648
Colloid osmotic pressure 698
Colloids 703, **704**–8
albumin 703–4
anaphylactic reactions **744**, 745
rapid infusion 722
synthetic 704, *705*, 706–8

dextrans 706
EloHAES 6% 708
etherified starch 706–7
HAESsteril 6% 707
HAESsteril 10% 707–8
Hespan 6% 707
modified fluid gelatins 705
Pentaspan 10% 708
Pentrafraction 708
Coma, and brain death 792, **793**
Combitube 690, *691*
Common cold 601–2
Common peroneal nerve block 543
Complement, serum levels 749
Computed tomography, anaesthesia for *406*, *407*
Congenital abnormalities 391–4
bat ears 393–4
cleft palate and lip 392–3
hypospadias 393
syndactyly 393
Congenital diaphragmatic hernia 351–2
Congenital heart disease **226**, *227*, *228*–31
fetal circulation *230*
obstruction to flow 228–9
shunts 228
systemic/pulmonary vascular resistance **230**
ventricular status *229*, *230*–1
Congenital pyloric stenosis 353–4
Conn's syndrome 429–30
clinical 429
intraoperative 430
pathophysiology 429
postoperative 430
preparation 430
surgery 429
Continuous-flow anaesthetic machines 3–4
Contrast media 403–4, 411–12
Core temperature 42
Corneal reflex 793
Coronary angiography 234–5
Corticosteroids
and anaesthesia 137
and surgery 428–9
Corynebacterium diphtheriae 603–4
Cosmetic surgery 394–5
breast operations 394–5
liposuction and tumescent anaesthesia 395
local anaesthesia 397–8
rhinoplasty 395
Craniofacial reconstruction 397
Cricothyroid puncture 325
Crossmatching **724**, **725**–7
Croup, airway problems in 354

Cryoprecipitate 737
Cryotherapy 668
Crystalloids **701**, *702*–3
balanced electrolyte solutions 703
glucose 5% *702*–3
glucose saline solutions 703
rapid infusion 722
sodium chloride 0.9% 702
Cushing's syndrome 430–1
clinical 430–1
intraoperative 431
pathophysiology 430
postoperative 431
preparation 431
surgery 430
Cyclizine, premedication **139**

Dacrocystorhinostomy 308
Datex-Engstrom AS/3 Anaesthetic Delivery Unit 64–7
central electronic controls 64
pneumatic system 64–7
bellows assembly 64
driving gas system 64, *65*
fresh gas control unit 65, *66*–7
Day-care surgery 361–70
after-care 369
diabetic patients 620–1
drugs 366–8
future development 369–70
guidelines, protocols and reports 361–4
nasal surgery 335
postoperative care 368–9
preoperative preparation 364–6
Deep vein thrombosis 194
Demand valve *75*
Dental surgery 371–85
equipment 383–4
inpatient general anaesthesia 382–3
outpatient general anaesthesia 372–81
airway control 375–6
anaesthetic technique 374–5
complications 379–80
airway contamination 379–80
airway obstruction 379
arrhythmias 380
hypotension 380
respiratory depression and apnoea 379
contraindications 372–3
dental procedures in young children 372
indications for 372
monitoring 377–8
pain relief 378–9
patient assessment 373

816 Index

Dental surgery (contd)
    patient preparation 373–4
    pollution 380–1
    posture 376–7
    recovery 378
    sedation 381–2
Depth of anaesthesia 40–1
    see also Awareness
Dextrans 706
Diabetes insipidus 433
Diabetes mellitus 611–23
    anaesthetic management 129–30
    classification 611–13
        insulin-dependent 611, **612**
        non-insulin-dependent **612**–13
    complications 615–16
        cardiovascular disease 615
        gastroparesis 616
        hyperglycaemia 616
        infections 615–16
        limited joint mobility syndrome 616
        neuropathies 615
        renal disease 615
        retinopathy and blindness 615
    emergencies 621–3
        diabetic ketoacidosis 621–3
        hyperosmolar non-ketotic coma 623
        lactic acidosis 623
    insulin and metabolism 614–16
    metabolic response to surgery and anaesthesia 614–15
    perioperative management 616–20
        general principles 619–20
        intermediate and minor surgery 619
        major surgery 617–19
            glucose–insulin–potassium regimen 618
            variable rate regimen **618**–19
        preoperative assessment 617
    special situations 620–1
        cardiac surgery 620
        day case surgery 620–1
        emergency surgery 621
        obstetrics 620
    urinalysis 161
Diabetic ketoacidosis 621–3
Diabetic retinopathy 615
Diamorphine 655, 657
Diazepam, premedication **139**, **140**
Difficult airway 675–96
    Combitube 690, *691*
    conventional laryngoscopy and intubation 682, *682*–5
        blind nasal intubation 684
        external laryngeal manipulation 682

    gas induction/intubation under deep anaesthesia 684
    gum elastic bougie 683
    laryngoscopes 683
    rapid-sequence induction 685
    stilettes and lighted wands 683–4
    definition of 675, **676**
    extubation 693–4
    fibreoptic intubation 686–8
        conduct of procedure 688
        local anaesthesia of airway 687–8
        oral or nasal intubation 687
        premedication 687
        sedation 687
        timing of 686
        vasoconstriction 688
    fibreoptic laryngoscopes 693
    intubation 676, **677**
        correct position 677–8
    laryngeal mask airway 685–6
    mask ventilation 676
    predictive factors 678–81
        cervical mobility 679
        mandibular space 678, *679*
        temporomandibular joint 679, *680*–1
        tongue size *678*
    regional anaesthesia 692–3
    retrograde intubation 691–2
    special circumstances 694–6
        laryngeal tumours 695–6
        rheumatoid arthritis 695
        spinal trauma 694
    transtracheal airway 688–90
        mini-tracheostomy 690
        surgical tracheostomy 690
        transtracheal jet ventilation 689
    see also Airway; Airway management
Digital nerve block
    lower limb 544
    upper limb 531–2
Diphtheria 603–4
Dipyridamole–thallium scintigraphy 150, 234
Direct oxygen flush valve 9, *10*
Discriminant analysis model 115
Donor
    liver transplantation 474–5
    renal transplantation 491
Dorsal nerve block 537–8
Double-burst nerve stimulation *45*
Down's syndrome 347
Drager Divan ventilator *61*, *62*–4
    breathing system 62, *63*–4
Draw-over anaesthetic machines 11
Droperidol, premedication **139**

Drug delivery routes 775–6
Drug metabolism 290–1, *294*–5
Duchenne muscular dystrophy 181
Dural puncture 514, 517–18
Dystrophia myotonica 182

Ear, nose and throat surgery 318–35
    anaesthetic hazards 322–3
    compromised airway 323–5
    ear surgery 327–32
        acoustic neuroma and skull base surgery 332
        anaesthesia 328
        choice of anaesthetic technique 329–30
        facial nerve preservation 331
        mastoidectomy 332
        middle ear surgery 331–2
        myringotomy and ventilation tube insertion 331
        nitrous oxide effects 330–1
        patient positioning 331
        postoperative nausea and vomiting 331
        preoperative assessment 328–9
        preoperative medication 329
    foreign body in airway 326
    laryngoscopy and microlaryngoscopy 319–21
    laser surgery to upper airway 321–3
        safety considerations 322
        theory and applications 321
    malignant disease of upper airway 323
    management of airway fires 323
    nasal surgery 332–5
        anaesthetic techniques 334–5
        day-case surgery 335
        local preparation of noise 333–4
        preoperative assessment and investigations 333
        topical anaesthesia 545, *545*
        types of 332–3
    surgery for snoring 326–7
    tonsillectomy and adenoidectomy 318–19
        post-tonsillectomy haemorrhage 319
    tracheostomy and emergency airway management 325–6
Ear surgery see Ear, nose and throat surgery
Ecchymosis 313
ECG see Electrocardiography
Echocardiography 151, 234
Eclampsia 567
EEG see Electroencephalogram
Elderly patients 571–85

anaesthetic management 580–1
cognitive function 576–7
perioperative risk and outcome 577–9
pharmacology 574, *575*–6
physiology 571–4
  body composition 573
  cardiovascular system 571–2
  renal function 572–3
  respiratory system 572, *573*
  temperature regulation 573–4
postoperative management 582, *583*–4, 669–70
preoperative assessment 579–80
regional anaesthesia 581–2
Electrical nerve stimulation 43–4
Electrocardiography 30
  ambulatory monitoring 149–50
  exercise 149
  and MRI 412–13
  preoperative 125, **126**, 148–9
Electroencephalogram 40
  and awareness monitoring 761–2
  brain death 794–5
  head injury 807
Electrolytes 125
  in head injury 808
  imbalance 739–40
  liver failure 473
  liver transplantation 481
  recovery room 647–8
  renal failure 283–4
EloHAES 708
Emission computed tomography, anaesthesia for 407–8
Enclosed afferent reservoir *80*–1
Endocrine disorders, anaesthetic management 129–31
  diabetes mellitus 129–30
  obesity 130–1
Endocrine surgery 417–36
  adrenal 424–31
  gastrointestinal 435–6
  pancreas 433–5
  parathyroid 423–4
  pituitary 432–3
  thyroid 417–22
Endocrine system, effects of brain death 789
Endolymphatic sac decompression 328
Endoscopic surgery
  kidney stone removal 274
  transurethral 271–3
  ureter 273–4
Enflurane
  dental surgery 375
  toxicity 103, 105
Ephedrine, as anti-emetic 674

Epidemic parotitis 603
Epidural anaesthesia 356–7, 503–19
  anatomy 503–6
    blood supply 505–6
    epidural space 504, *505*
    meninges 504
    nerve roots 505
    vertebrae *503*–4
  care of patients 519
  catheters *508*
  caudal 515–16
  combined spinal–epidural anaesthesia 518
  complications 514–15
    accidental dural puncture 514
    accidental spinal anaesthesia 514
    neurological damage 515
    subdural block 514–15
    technical problems 514
    toxic reaction 515
  contraindications **513**–14
  epidural pressures 506
  factors influencing spread of injected solutions 508–9
    age 508–9
    arteriosclerosis 509
    gravity 509
    height 509
    pregnancy, intra-abdominal tumours or ascites 509
    site of injection 508
    volume of injectate 508
  indications for 512–13
  local anaesthetics used 509–10
  location of epidural space 506–7
  needles 507, *508*
  obstetrics 554–8
    Caesarean section 563
    complications 557–8
    failure 557
    placement of catheter 555
    techniques 555, **556**–7
  physiological effects 510–12
    autonomic block 511
    cardiovascular effects 511–12
    gastrointestinal effects 512
    respiratory effects 512
    somatic nerve block 510–11
    stress response 512
    thermoregulation 512
  postoperative pain control 665, **666**
  sites of action 509
  see also Local anaesthetics; Spinal anaesthesia
Epidural space 504, *505*
  location of 506–7

Epiglottitis, airway problems in 354–5
Epilepsy
  anaesthetic management 131
  surgery 260–1
Eschariotomy 459
Etherified starch 706–7
Etidocaine, epidural anaesthesia 510
Evoked responses 43
Exercise testing 156
Exomphalos 352–3
Expired air respiration 766, *767*
Explanator 113–14
External chest compression 767–8
  rationale behind 768–9
Extracorporeal lithotripsy 274
Extubation, difficult 693–4

Facemasks *83*–4
  paediatric surgery 348
Facial electromyogram, and awareness monitoring 760–1
Facial nerve block 311, *312*
Factor IX deficiency 172
Factor VIII deficiency *see* Haemophilia
Fascia iliaca block 541
Fasting, preoperative 134–5
Fat embolus 443
Femoral nerve block 541
Fentanyl 657
Fever 597–8
Fibreoptic intubation 686–8
  conduct of procedure 688
  local anaesthesia of airway 687–8
  oral or nasal intubation 687
  premedication 687
  sedation 687
  timing of 686
  vasoconstriction 688
Fibreoptic laryngoscopes 693
Fibrinolysis 732
Filters 8
  breathing systems 81
Finapres blood pressure monitor 34
First generation anaesthetic machines 15
Flow generation in ventilators *48*, 49
Flow requirements in breathing systems 70, *71*
Flow restrictors 8
Flowmeter needle valves 6–7
Flowmeters 7, *8*
Fluid balance
  in children **341**
  critically ill patients 713–14
  head injury 808
  intraoperative 711–12

Fluid balance (contd)
  paediatric surgery 341
  postoperative 712
  preoperative 711
  recovery room 647–8
  renal transplantation 489–90
  thermal injury 462, 714–15
  see also Fluid therapy
Fluid therapy 697–715
  body fluid compartments 698–701
    extracellular compartment 699
    interstitial compartment *700*
    in lung 700–1
    intracellular compartment 699
    microvascular endothelium 699
    renal threshold 701
    total body water 698–9
  colloid osmotic pressure 698
  colloids 703, 704–8
    albumin 703, **704**
    synthetic 704–8
      dextrans 706
      EloHAES 6% 708
      etherified starch 706–7
      HAESsteril 10% 707–8
      HAESsteril 6% 707
      Hespan 6% 707
      modified fluid gelatins *705*
      Pentaspan 10% 708
      Pentrafraction 708
  crystalloids **701**, *702–3*
    balanced electrolyte solutions 703
    glucose 5% 702–3
    glucose saline solutions 703
    sodium chloride 0.9% 702
  fluid balance derangements 708–15
    burns 714–15
    critically ill patients 713–14
    haemorrhage 712–13
    perioperative fluid balance 711–12
    sodium balance 710–11
    water balance 710
  molarity 697
  oncotic pressure 698
  osmolality 697–8
  osmosis 697
  physiology 697–701
  tonicity 698
  see also Fluid balance
Flunitrazepam, premedication **140**
Foreign bodies, bronchoscopy for 188
Free radical scavengers 265
Fresh frozen plasma **736**–7
Frontalis EMG 41

Gag-bronchial reflex 794
Galvanic cells 28–9
Gas analysers 25, 27–9
  galvanic and polarographic cells 28–9
  infrared spectroscopy 25, 27–8
  mass spectrometer 29
  paramagnetism 28
  Raman spectroscopy 29
Gas supplies 4–5
  medical gas cylinders 4
  medical gas pipelines 5
  pin-index system 4
Gases and vapours, monitoring of **24**–5, *26*, *27*
Gastrointestinal disorders, anaesthetic management 132–3
Gastrointestinal surgery 435–6
Gastrointestinal system
  epidural anaesthesia 512
  and head injury 808
  obese patients 589
  postoperative care, thoracic surgery 194
  in pregnancy 551
  renal failure 486–7
Gastroparesis 616
Gastroschisis 352–3
Gelatins 705
Genitourinary and renal surgery 269–86
  day-case surgery 270
  endoscopic removal of stones 274
  endoscopic ureteric surgery 273–4
  extracorporeal lithotripsy 274
  major pelvic surgery 277
  minor transurethral procedures 273
  open procedures on kidney 277, 278
  penile surgery 270, *271*
  radiological procedures 276–7
  renal failure 278–86
    clinical pathophysiology **278**–81
    drugs in 281–3
    fluid and electrolyte status 283–4
    induction 284–5
    intravenous cannulation 284
    intravenous fluids 285
    maintenance of general anaesthesia 285
    postoperative management 285–6
    premedication 284
    preoperative assessment 283
    regional anaesthetic techniques 285

surgery 283
testicular surgery 271
transurethral endoscopic procedures 271–3
  antibiotic therapy 273
  blood loss estimation 272
  lithotomy position 272
  spinal versus general anaesthesia 271–2
  temperature loss 273
transurethral resection of bladder tumour 274
transurethral resection of prostate (TURP) 274–6
  aetiology 275
  new methods 276
  pacemakers and diathermy 276
  pathophysiology 275
  presentation 275
  prevention 275–6
  treatment 276
Gentamicin, antibiotic prophylaxis **143**
Ginger, as anti-emetic 674
Glasgow Coma Scale 265
Global ischaemia 265
Glucose metabolism, in liver failure 472
Glucose saline solutions 703
Glucose solution 702–3
Goitre 418–21
  clinical 419
  intraoperative 420
  pathophysiology 418
  postoperative 420–1
  preparation 419
  surgery 418–19
Goldman risk index **112**
Gordon Green endobronchial tube *195*
Grommet insertion 331
Guedel airways *84*
Gum elastic bougie 683

Haematology 125
  preoperative tests 158–60
Haemoglobin, loss of see Oxygen carrying capacity, loss of
Haemoglobinopathies 163–6
  anaesthetic management 165–6
  sickle cell syndrome 163–4
  thalassaemias 164–5
Haemophilia 171–2
  clinical features 171
  diagnosis 171
  treatment 171–2
Haemophilia A see Haemophilia
Haemophilia B 172
Haemorrhage 298–9, 717–40

complications and hazards 737–40
  acid–base balance 738
  electrolyte imbalance 739–40
  hypothermia 737–8
and fluid balance 712–13
haemostatic therapy 732, **733**–7
  coagulation factors 735–6
  cryoprecipitate 737
  fresh frozen plasma **736**–7
  platelets **734**–5
  reversal of warfarin
    anticoagulation effects 736
loss of circulating oxygen
    carrying capacity 723–8
  intraoperative autotransfusion
    727–8
  lower haemoglobin level 723–4
  red cell production and
    crossmatching 724, **725**–7
  upper haemoglobin level **724**
loss of haemostasis 728–32
  coagulation 729–30, *731*
  fibrinolysis 732
  haemostasis 728, *729*, *730*
loss/replacement of circulating
    volume 720–3
  blood warming and rapid
    infusions 721–2
  initial resuscitation 722, **723**
  venous access 720–1
management 719–20
mortality 717–18
orbital 313–14
physiological effects **719**
in pregnancy 564–5
quantifying blood loss 718, **719**
see also Coagulation; Coagulation
    disorders
Haemostasis 214, 728, *729*
HAESsteril 707–8
Halothane
  dental surgery 375
  hepatitis 103
  toxicity 103
Head injury 252, *253*–5, 797–809
  anaesthesia 803–4
  clinical management 254–5
  early management 800–3
    airway and ventilation **801**–2
    central nervous system **802**
    circulation 802
    transfer of head-injured
      patients 802–3
  effects on cerebral physiology
    798–800
    cerebral autoregulation *799*
    cerebral blood flow 799
    cerebral metabolism 800
    hypocapnic response 799–800

hypoxic response 800
intracranial pressure 800
haematoma *798*
herniation 798
infarction 798
intensive care 804–9
  associated systemic problems
    807–9
    cardiovascular problems
      807–8
    coagulation 808–9
    fluid and electrolyte
      imbalance 808
    gastrointestinal tract and
      nutrition 808
    pulmonary **807**
  decreased arterial blood
    volume 804–5
    arterial pressure management
      805
    decreased cerebral
      metabolism 805
    hyperventilation 804–5
    oxygen therapy 805
  decreased brain volume 806
  decreased cerebrospinal fluid
    volume 805–6
  decreased venous volume 804
  neurological monitoring **806**–7
    cerebral blood flow 807
    electroencephalogram 807
    intracranial pressure **806**
    jugular bulb oximetry 806
intracranial complications *798*
linear deceleration 797
mechanisms of brain damage 797
missile 797
outcome 809
rotational 797
Heart and anaphylactic mediators
    742
Heart and lung transplantation
    225–8
  anaesthesia 226–7
  donor 226
  immunosuppressive regimen **225**
  pathophysiology 227–8
  recipient 226
  see also Lung transplantation
Heart murmur 347
Heparinization 238
Hepatectomy 485
Hepatitis 607
  in anaesthetists 609
Hepatobiliary and pancreatic
    surgery 287–302, 433–5
  anaesthetic management **295**–9
    haemorrhage 298–9

induction and maintenance
  296–7
maintenance of body
  temperature 298
monitoring 297
postoperative care **299**
renal function 297, **298**
risk assessment 296
anatomy 287–9
  arterial blood supply 287, *288*–9
bile duct obstruction 300
insulinoma 434
liver functions **289**, 290–1
  bile 290
  effects of disorders of 292–5
    ascites 293
    cardiopulmonary disorders
      292
    coagulation abnormalities 292
    drug metabolism *294*–5
    portal hypertension 292–3
    renal function 293–4
  metabolism
    in acinus 290
    drugs 290–1
  tests of **291**–2
liver resection 300–1
open cholecystectomy 300
pancreatectomy 301–2
portal hypertension 301
vipoma 434–5
Hereditary angioneurotic oedema
    see C1 esterase deficiency
Hereditary coproporphyia *see*
    Porphyrias
Heroin 655, 657
Herpes zoster 603
Hespan 707
Hip dislocation, congenital 450–1
Hip fractures 444–5
Hip replacement surgery 447
Histamine
  and anaphylaxis 741–2
  assay 748
  H_1-receptor antagonists, as anti-
    emetics 673
Hospital-acquired infection 605–6
Human immunodeficiency virus 606
  in anaesthetists 609
Hydrocephalus 260
5-Hydroxytryptamine antagonists
  as anti-emetics 673–4
Hyoscine
  as anti-emetic 673
  premedication **139**
Hypercalcaemia 424
Hyperglycaemia 616
Hyperkalaemia 739–40
Hyperosmolar non-ketotic coma 623

Hyperparathyroidism 423–4
  clinical 423
  intraoperative 424
  pathophysiology 423
  postoperative 424
  preparation 423–4
  surgery 423
Hypertension
  anaesthetic management 127
  pregnancy 565–7
  recovery room 645–6
  see also Blood pressure monitoring
Hyperventilation, head injury 804–5
Hypnotic agents 627–9
Hypocapnic response, head injury 799–800
Hypomagnesaemia 739
Hypospadias 393
Hypotension 380
  controlled 390–1
  recovery room 646–7
Hypothermia
  cardiopulmonary bypass 207–8
  cerebral protection 263–4
  transfusion-related 737–8
Hypothyroidism 421–2
  clinical 422
  intraoperative 422
  pathophysiology 421
  postoperative 422
  surgery 421
  treatment 422
Hypoventilation **643**, **644**
Hypoxaemia 644–5
Hypoxic response, head injury 800

Iliohypogastric block *357*
Ilioinguinal block *357*
Immunoglobulin E assay 748–9
Independence of variables 114
Induction of anaesthesia
  anaphylactic reactions **744**
  bronchopleural fistula 195
  Caesarean section 561–2
  induction agents, porphyria 169
  liver transplantation 476
  ophthalmic surgery 306
  paediatric surgery 344
  thermal injury 465, 466
  thoracic surgery 190
  trauma surgery 441
Infants see Babies; Children; Paediatric
Infection
  in diabetes 615–16
  in liver disease 484–5
  see also Infectious patients
Infectious mononucleosis 603
Infectious patients 597–609

blood-borne viruses 606–9
  hepatitis 607
    HBV infected anaesthetist 609
    human immunodeficiency virus 606
    HIV infected anaesthetist 609
    management after exposure 608–9
    precautions 607–8
  diphtheria 603–4
  fever 597–8
  hospital-acquired infection 605–6
  septic shock 599–601
  septicaemia 598–9
  tetanus 604
  tuberculosis 604–5
  viral infections 601–3
    childhood diseases 602–3
      infectious mononucleosis 603
      measles 602–3
      mumps 603
      rubella 602
      varicella 603
    common cold 601–2
Infiltration
  obstetric analgesia 559
  postoperative analgesia 665
Infrared gas analysers 25, 278
Inguinal hernia repair, field block 535, *536–7*
Inhalation injury 461–2
Inhalational anaesthetics
  paediatric surgery 342, *343–4*
  toxicity 101–8
    carbon dioxide absorbers 105
    global pollution 107–8
    local pollution 105–7
    nitrous oxide 101–2
    volatile anaesthetics 103–5
      kidney 104–5
      liver 103–4
  volatile anaesthetics
    porphyria 169
    toxicity 103–5
Inherited diseases 163–82
  C1 esterase deficiency 174–6
    anaesthetic management 176
    clinical signs 174–5
    treatment 175–6
  cholinesterase variants 177–8
  coagulation disorders 170–4
    classification 170
    factor IX deficiency 172
    haemophilia 171–2
    inhibitors of coagulation 174
    normal haemostasis 170
    tests for clotting defects 170–1
    Von Willebrand's disease 172–4

Duchenne muscular dystrophies 181
haemoglobinopathies 163–6
  anaesthetic management 165–6
  sickle cell syndrome 163–4
  thalassaemias 164–5
malignant hyperthermia 178–81
  anaesthesia for susceptible patients 180–1
  clinical presentation 179–80
  genetics 179
  preoperative diagnosis 179
  treatment 180
Marfan's syndrome 176–7
myotonias 181–2
  dystrophia myotonica 182
  myotonia congenita 182
porphyrias 166–9
  acute intermittent 167
  anaesthetic management 168–9
  hereditary coproporphyria 167
  management 168
  pathogenesis 167
  variegate 168
Insulinoma 434
Intensive care
  head injury 804–9
    associated systemic problems 807–9
      cardiovascular 807–8
      coagulation 808–9
      fluid and electrolyte balance 808
      gastrointestinal tract and nutrition 808
      pulmonary **807**
    decreased arterial blood volume 804–5
      arterial pressure management 805
    decreased cerebral metabolism 805
    hyperventilation 804–5
    oxygen management 805
    decreased brain volume 806
    decreased cerebrospinal fluid volume 805–6
    decreased venous volume 804
    neurological monitoring 806–7
      cerebral blood flow 807
      electroencephalogram 807
      intracranial pressure **806**
      jugular bulb oximetry 806
  neurosurgical 266–7
Intercostal nerve block *533*
Interscalene block 528–9
Interventional radiology 408–9
  anaesthetic practice 408–9
  equipment and patient set-up 409

monitoring 409
Intestinal obstruction 353
Intra-aortic balloon counter-
    pulsation 211, *213*
Intracranial pressure *248*
    head injury 800, **806**
    monitoring in liver failure 485
    raised 250–2
        anaesthesia in patients with
            251–2
Intraocular pressure 303–4
    drugs used to lower 305
Intravenous regional anaesthesia
    532
Intubating wands 683–4
Intubation
    blind nasal 684
    fibreoptic *see* Fibreoptic
        intubation
    retrograde 691–2
    see also Airway; Airway
        management; Difficult airway
Ischaemic heart disease, anaesthetic
    management 126–7
Isoflurane, dental surgery 375
Isolated forearm technique 41,
    759–60

Jaundice, postoperative **299**
Joint replacement 447–9
    methyl methacrylate cement 448
    pneumatic tourniquets 448–9
    thromboembolic prophylaxis 448
    total hip replacement 447
    total knee replacement 447–8
Jugular bulb oximetry 806

Kidney
    anaesthetic toxicity 104–5
    effects of brain death 789–90
    stones, endoscopic removal 274
    see also Renal disease; Renal
        failure
Knee replacement surgery 447–8

Labyrinthectomy 328
Lack coaxial system *79–80*
Lactic acidosis 623
Laparoscopic surgery 493–502
    anaesthetic management 500–1
    intra-abdominal procedures **495,
        496**–500
        cardiovascular effects 498–9
        CO_2 homeostasis 497
        creation of pneumoperitoneum
            496
        patient position 496–7
        pneumomediastinum and
            pneumothorax 497–8
        respiratory function 499–500

trocar insertion 496
    thorascopy and video-assisted
        thoracic surgery 493, **494**–5
Laryngeal mask airway *86–9*
    difficult intubation 676, 685–6
    indications 88–9
    insertion 86, *87–8*
    paediatric surgery 348
    removal 88
Laryngeal obstruction 642–3
Laryngeal spasm 326
Laryngeal surgery *see* Ear, nose and
    throat surgery
Laryngeal tumours, airway
    management 695–6
Laryngectomy 323
Laryngectomy tubes *95*
Laryngoscopes *97, 98*
    difficult airway 683
    fibreoptic 693
    paediatric surgery 348, *349*
    see also Laryngoscopy
Laryngoscopy 319–21
    difficult airway 682, *682*–5
        blind nasal intubation 684
        external laryngeal manipulation
            682
        gas induction/intubation under
            deep anaesthesia 684
        gum elastic bougie 683
        laryngoscopes 683
        rapid-sequence induction 684–5
        stilettes and lighted wands
            683–4
    see also Laryngoscopes
Lasers, tracheal tubes for use with
    96, 97
Lateral cutaneous nerve of forearm,
    block 530
Lateral cutaneous nerve of thigh,
    block 542
Lateral rhinotomy 333
Latex allergy 347–8, **744**, 745
Left ventricular failure, anaesthetic
    management 126
Lignocaine
    epidural anaesthesia 510
    peripheral nerve block **522, 523**
Limb trauma 439
Limited joint mobility syndrome
    616
Liposuction 395
Liver
    anaesthetic toxicity 103–4
    effects of brain death 790
    function **289**, 290–1
        bile 290
        drugs 290–1
        effects of disorders of 292–5

ascites 293
cardiopulmonary disorders
    292
coagulation abnormalities 292
drug metabolism *294*–5
portal hypertension 292–3
renal function 293–4
metabolism, acinar 290
tests of **291**–2
resection 300–1
see also Hepatobiliary and
    pancreatic surgery
Liver disease
    anaesthetic management 133
    fulminant hepatic failure 482–5
        cardiovascular instability 483
        cerebral oedema 484
        classification 482–3
        infection 484–5
        management **483**
        renal failure 484
    postoperative pain management
        669
    see also Liver transplantation
Liver transplantation 469–86
    anaesthesia 475–7
        induction 476
        maintenance 476
        premedication 476
        vascular access 476–7
    auxiliary 485
    bioartificial livers 486
    contraindications 470
    fulminant hepatic failure 482
        classification 482–3
        management 483
            cardiovascular instability 483
            cerebral oedema 484
            infection 484–5
            renal failure 484
    hepatectomy 485
    immediate postoperative care and
        complications 481–2
        analgesia 482
        bleeding and coagulation
            problems 481–2
        cardiovascular 481
        fluids and electrolytes 481
        infection 482
    indications for 469, **470**
    intracranial pressure monitoring
        485
    intraoperative management 475
    monitoring and management
        477–81
        cardiovascular and general 477
        coagulation 478–9
        haemodynamic instability 477–8

Liver transplantation (contd)
  management of massive
    transfusion 479–80
  metabolic function 478
  thermal balance 479
  venovenous bypass 480–1
  pathophysiology of end-stage
    liver disease 470–3
    cardiovascular 471
    central nervous system 472
    coagulation 473
    metabolic 472–3
    portal hypertension 471
    renal 472
    respiratory 471–2
  plasmapheresis 485
  preoperative preparation 473–5
    cardiac tests 473–4
    donor matching 474–5
    renal assessment 474
    respiratory assessment 474
Local anaesthetics
  adverse reactions to 372
  anaphylactic reactions **744**, 745–6
  cosmetic surgery 397–8
  failure of in dental surgery 372
  fibreoptic intubation 687–8
  obstetrics 553
  paediatric surgery **345**
  plastic surgery 399
  porphyria 169
  postoperative pain relief 665–7
  see also Epidural anaesthesia;
    Spinal anaesthesia
Lorazepam, premedication **139,
  140**–1
Lumbar plexus *540*
Lumbosacral plexus *538, 539*
Lung transplantation 198–201
  anaesthetic technique 199–200
  complications 201
  postoperative management 200
  pre-operative assessment 199
  see also Heart and lung
    transplantation

Magnetic nerve stimulation 44
Magnetic resonance imaging 409–16
  anaesthesia 413, *414*–15
  babies and infants 415
  basic principles 409–10
  biological effects 411
  contrast media 411–12
  critically ill patients *415*
  ferromagnetic attraction 411
  gradient noise 411
  magnetic field 410–11
  monitoring **412**–13
    blood pressure 413

capnography 413
ECG 412–13
pulse oximetry 413
stethoscopes 413
planning of unit 416
resuscitation 416
Malignant hyperthermia 178–81
  anaesthesia for susceptible
    patients 180–1
  clinical presentation 179–80
  genetics 179
  preoperative diagnosis 179
  treatment 180
Mallinckrodt Laser-flex tracheal
  tube *96*
Mandibular space, and difficult
  intubation 678, *679*
Manley Multivent ventilator 57,
  58–60
  E-model 60
  electronic system 60
  manual operation 60
  pneumatic system 58, *59*–60
Mapleson systems *see* Partial
  rebreathing systems
Marfan's syndrome 176–7
  anaesthetic management 177
  cardiac system 176–7
  ocular system 177
  skeletal system 177
Mass spectroscopy gas analysers 29
Mast cell tryptase 749
Mastoidectomy 328, 332
Measles 602–3
Median nerve block 531
Mediastinoscopy 189
Medical gas cylinders 4
Medical gas pipelines 5
Medical history 123–4
Meninges 504
Metabolic function
  central nervous system, cardiac
    surgery 216
  liver transplantation 472–3, 478
  renal transplantation 487
Methyl methacrylate cement 448
Metoclopramide
  as anti-emetic 673
  premedication **139**
Microlaryngeal tracheal tubes 93, *94*
Microlaryngoscopy 319–21
Microvascular surgery 395–7
Midazolam, premedication **139**, 141
Mini-tracheostomy 690
Miotics 305
Mitral valve 221–2
  mitral regurgitation 221
  mitral stenosis 221–2
Models 114

comparison of **117**, *118*
types of 114–17
  Bayesian model 115–16
  discriminant analysis 115
  multiple logistic regression
    114–15
  multiple regression 114
  neural networks *116*–17
Molarity 697
Monitoring 19–46
  cardiac surgery 203, 205
  cardiovascular system 30–40
    blood flow measurement 38
    blood pressure 32/**33**–5
      direct monitoring 34–5
      non-invasive monitoring 32–4
    central venous pressure 35,
      36–7
    clinical observation 30
    ECG 30
    perfusion of individual organs
      38–9
    pulmonary artery
      catheterization 37, 38
    pulse oximetry 30–2
    transoesophageal
      echocardiography 39
    zeroing and calibration 35
  CNS and depth of anaesthesia 40,
    265–6
    auditory evoked potentials 41
    clinical observations 40
    EEG 40
    frontalis EMG 41
    isolated forearm technique 41
    oesophageal contractility 41
  dental surgery 377–8
  depth of anaesthesia 758–62
    body state 760–1
      facial electromyogram 760–1
      oesophageal contractility 760
      sinus arrhythmia 761
    brain state 761–2
      evoked potentials in EEG
        761–2
      resting EEG 761
    detection of awareness 759–60
    problems of 758–9
  evidence 20–1
  hepatobiliary and pancreatic
    surgery 297
  human beings and machines 19
  interventional radiology 409
  intracranial pressure 485
  laparoscopic surgery 500–1
  liver transplantation 477–81
    cardiovascular and general 477
    coagulation 478–9
    haemodynamic instability 477–8

management of massive
    transfusion 479–80
  metabolic function 478
  thermal balance 479
  venovenous bypass 480–1
magnetic resonance imaging
    412–13
minimal standards 20, **21**
neuromuscular function 43–6
  clinical assessment 43
  evoked responses 43
  nerve stimulation 44
  patterns of 44–6
obese patients 592–3, *595*
respiratory system 21–9
  clinical observation 22–3
  gas analysers 25, 27–9
    galvanic and polarographic
      cells 28–9
    infrared spectroscopy 25,
      27–8
    mass spectrometer 29
    paramagnetism 28
    Raman spectroscopy 29
  gases and vapours 24–5
    carbon dioxide 25, *26, 27*
    oxygen 24–5
  pressure and flow 23–4
risk and benefit 20
special situations 39
spinal cord 453, *454*–5
temperature 41–3
  core 42
  sites of monitoring 42–3
    bladder 43
    nasopharyngeal 42
    oesphageal 42
    pulmonary artery 43
    rectal 42
    skin 42
    tympanic membrane 42
  types of thermometer 42
  thermal injury 462–3, 467
  trauma surgery 439–40
  vascular surgery **237**–8
  ventilators 57
Monoamine oxidase inhibitors, and
    anaesthesia 135
Morphine
  postoperative pain 655
  premedication **139**, 141
Multiple logistic regression model
    114–15
Multiple regression model 114
Multivariate analysis 114
Mumps 603
Muscle relaxants
  anaphylactic reactions **744**
  ophthalmic surgery 306–7

thermal injury 465–6
trauma surgery 441
see also Neuromuscular blocking
    drugs
Muscular dystrophies, anaesthetic
    problems 347
Mycobacterium tuberculosis 604–5
Mydriatics 304–5
Myotonia congenita 182
Myotonias 181–2
Myringoplasty 328
Myringotomy 331

Nasal polypectomy 333
Nasal surgery *see* Ear, nose and
    throat surgery
Nasopharyngeal airway 85–6
Nasopharyngeal temperature
    monitoring 42–3
Nausea/vomiting
  postoperative 670–4
    factors influencing 671, **672**–3
    harmful effects 671
    physiology 670, *671*
    prevention and treatment 673–4
      5-hydroxytryptamine
        antagonists 673–4
      anticholinergic drugs 673
      antidopaminergics 673
      histamine H_1 antagonists 673
Nazari tube *197*
Necrotizing enterocolitis 354
Neonatal ventilation *see* Paediatric/
    neonatal ventilation
Nerve stimulation 43–4
  electrical 43–4
  magnetic stimulation 44
  patterns of 44–6
    double-burst stimulation *45*
    post-tetanic count 45
    single twitch *45*
    tetanus 45
    train of four *44*
  stimulating electrodes 44
Neural networks *116*–17
Neurological diseases, anaesthetic
    management 131–2
Neuromuscular blocking drugs
  anaphylactic reactions 744–5
  haemodilution effects **723**
  hepatic failure 297
  paediatric surgery 344–5
  porphyria 169
  renal transplantation 489
see also Muscle relaxants
Neuromuscular function,
    monitoring 42–5
  clinical assessment 42–3
  evoked responses 43

nerve stimulation 43–4
patterns of 43–6
  double-burst stimulation *45*
  post-tetanic count 45
  single twitch *45*
  tetanus 45
  train of four *44*
Neuroradiology *261*–2
Neurosurgery 247–68
  air embolism 257–8
  brain death 267–8
  brain tumour 255–7
    posterior fossa/brain stem
      surgery 256–7
    stereotactic surgery *256*
  cerebral anatomy and physiology
    247–50
  cerebral aneurysm 259–60
  cerebral blood flow *248, 249*
  cerebral ischaemia 262–5
    anti-excitatory agents 264–5
    cerebral protection 263–4
    free radical scavengers 265
    haemodilution 264
    normoglycaemia 264
    normoventilation 264
    perfusion pressure 264
  cerebrospinal fluid 248
  CNS monitoring **265**–6
  epilepsy 260–1
  global ischaemia 265
  head injury 252, **253**–5
    clinical management 254–5
  hydrocephalus 260
  intensive care 266–7
  intracranial pressure *248*
    raised 250–1
      anaesthesia in patients with
        251–2
  neuroradiology *261*–2
  paediatric 258
  pharmacology 249–50
  pituitary 258–9
  see also Head injury
Nitrogen, monitoring **24**
Nitrous oxide
  effect on middle ear surgery
    330–1
  monitoring **24**
  toxicity 101–2
Non-rebreathing systems 73, *74, 75*
Non-rebreathing valve *74*
Non-steroidal anti-inflammatory
    drugs
  postoperative analgesia **667**
  premedication 141–2
Nutrition
  liver disease 473
  thermal injury 462

Obesity 130–1, 587–96
　access 590–1
　anaesthesia 592–4
　　monitoring 592–3
　　reversal and extubation 593–4
　coexistent disease 591
　measurement of 587, **588**
　movement of patient 590
　physiological changes 588–90
　　cardiovascular system 588
　　drug metabolism 590
　　endocrine abnormalities 589
　　gastrointestinal system 589
　　respiratory system 588–9
　postoperative care **594**–5
　　analgesia 594
　　intensive care and resuscitation 595
　　monitoring 595
　　oxygenation 595
　　resuscitation 595
　preoperative management 591
Obstetric anaesthesia/analgesia 549–69
　analgesia 552–3
　　inhalation 552
　　opioids 552–3
　　sedatives and tranquillizers 552
　Caesarean section
　　general anaesthesia 62
　　　aspiration of gastric contents 560
　　　induction 561–2
　　　maintenance 562
　　　reversal and recovery 562
　　　tracheal intubation 560, **561**
　　regional anaesthesia 562–4
　　　combined spinal-epidural anaesthesia 564
　　　epidural anaesthesia 563
　　　spinal anaesthesia 564
　diabetic patients 620
　regional anaesthesia 553–9
　　adjuvant drugs 554
　　caudal analgesia 559
　　epidural analgesia 554–8
　　　complications 557–8
　　　failure of 557
　　　placement of epidural catheter 555
　　　techniques 555, **556**–7
　　local anaesthetics 553
　　local infiltration 559
　　opioids 553–4
　　paracervical block 559
　　pudendal nerve block 559
　　spinal anaesthesia 558–9
　see also Pregnancy
Obturator nerve block 542

Oculocardiac reflex 308
Oesophageal atresia 351, *352*
Oesophageal contractility 41
　and awareness monitoring 760
Oesophageal detector device *99*
Oesophageal temperature monitoring 42
Oesophagoscopy 188–9
Oncotic pressure 698
One-lung anaesthesia 190–2
One-way check valves 6
Open chest cardiac massage 776–7
Open cholecystectomy 300
Ophthalmic surgery 303–15
　dacrocystorhinostomy 308
　general anaesthesia 305–9
　　emergency surgery 309
　　induction 306
　　maintenance 307
　　muscle relaxants and airway control 306–7
　　oculocardiac reflex 308
　　postoperative analgesia 307
　　premedication 306
　　preoperative assessment 305–6
　　preparation 306
　　recovery 307
　　small babies 307–8
　　strabismus surgery 308
　intraocular pressure 303–4
　oculoplastic surgery 308
　orbital decomposition and tumours 308
　preparation of eye 304–5
　　antibiotics 305
　　miotics 305
　　mydriatics 304–5
　　reduction of intraocular pressure 305
　regional anaesthesia 309–14
　　anatomy 310–11
　　assessment of block 313
　　care in operating theatre 313
　　choice of solution 311
　　combined retrobulbar/peribulbar block 311, *312*
　　complications 313–14
　　　amaurosis 314
　　　bruising 313
　　　central spread of local anaesthetic 314
　　　external ocular muscle palsies 314
　　　globe penetration or perforation 314
　　　haemorrhage 313–14
　　　optic nerve 314
　　　subconjunctival oedema 314
　　　systemic toxicity 313

　　contraindications 310
　　external ocular muscle palsies 314
　　peribulbar block 312, *313*
　　preoperative assessment 310
　　retrobulbar and facial nerve blocks 311
　　sub-Tenon's injection 311
　　subconjunctival injection 311
　　topical 311
　retinal detachment 308–9
Opioid analgesics
　addicted patients 670
　anaphylactic reactions **744**, 745
　obstetrics 552–4
　paediatric surgery 345, 357–8
　postoperative pain 655, 657
　thermal injury 465
　see also Analgesia; and individual opioid analgesics
Orbital decompression 308
Organ perfusion 38–9
Oropharyngeal airways *84*–5
Orthopaedic surgery 447–56
　bone tumours 455
　elective paediatric surgery 450–1
　elective spinal surgery 451–3
　intraoperative management 456
　joint replacement 447–9
　patients with rheumatoid arthritis 449–50
　spinal cord monitoring 453, *454*–5
Oscillotonometer 33
Osmolality 697–8
Osmosis 697
Outcome 113
Oxazepam, premedication **139**, **140**
Oxford pattern tracheal tubes 95, *96*
Oxygen carrying capacity, loss of 723–8
　intraoperative autotransfusion 727–8
　lower haemoglobin level 723–4
　red cell production and crossmatching 724, **725**–7
　upper haemoglobin level **724**
Oxygen failure alarm 8–9
Oxygen monitoring **24**–5
Oxygen therapy, head injury 805

Pacing 222, 223–4
Paediatric laryngoscope blades *98*
Paediatric surgery 337–59
　anaesthetic equipment 348–50
　　breathing systems 349–50
　　facemasks and laryngeal mask airway 348
　　laryngoscopes 348, *349*
　　tracheal tubes **349**

ventilators *350*
asthma 346–7
burns 464–5
circulation 338–40
   fetal and transitional circulation 338, *359*
   neonatal circulation *339–40*
Down's syndrome 347
fluid balance **341**
heart murmur 347
latex allergy 347–8
metabolism and coagulation 341
muscular dystrophies 347
neonatal anaesthesia 350–4
   congenital diaphragmatic hernia 351, *352*
   congenital pyloric stenosis 353–4
   exomphalos and gastroschisis 352–3
   intestinal obstruction 353
   necrotizing enterocolitis 354
   oesophageal atresia *351, 352*
   problems of 354–5
      acute airway obstruction 354
      aspirated foreign body 355
      croup 354
      epiglottitis 354–5
neurosurgery 258
orthopaedic 450–1
pain 342
pain management 355–8
   regional anaesthetic block 355, *356, 357*
   systemic opiates 357–8
pharmacology 342–5
   induction agents 344
   inhalation agents 342, *343*–4
   local anaesthetics **345**
   neuromuscular blocking agents 344–5
   opioids 345
premedication 348
preoperative preparation 345–6
respiratory system 337–8
resuscitation 358–9
retinopathy of prematurity 342
sickle cell disease 346
sleep apnoea 347
temperature regulation *340*–1
trauma 442–3
upper respiratory tract infection 347
Paediatric tracheal tubes 92–3
Paediatric/neonatal ventilation *67*–8
   conversion to pressure generator 67–8
   increasing internal compliance 67

introduction of leak 68
pressure controlled ventilation 68
modification to maintain flow generator characteristics
   reduction of internal compliance of tubing compartment 67
   separate paediatric attachment 67
   use of smaller bellows 67
   use of T-piece 68
Pain
   in children 342
      management 355
   postoperative *see* Postoperative pain
   see also Analgesia
Pancreatectomy 301–2
Pancreatic surgery *see* Hepatobiliary and pancreatic surgery
Pancuronium, haemodilution effects **723**
Papaveretum 655
Paracervical block 559
Paramagnetic gas analysers 28
Parathyroid surgery 423–4
   hypercalcaemia secondary to malignant disease 424
   hyperparathyroidism 423–4
Paravertebral block 540
Paravertebral nerve block 534
Parkinson's disease, anaesthetic management 131
Partial rebreathing systems 74–5, 76–8
   Mapleson A 75, 77
   Mapleson B and C 77
   Mapleson D, E and F 77, *78*
Patient-controlled analgesia 661, **662**–3
Pelvic trauma 439
Penile block 270, *271*, 357
Penlon Scoti device *99*
Pentaspan 708
Pentrafraction 708
Peribulbar block 312, *313*
Peripheral nerve blocks 521–47
   contraindications 521–2
   head and neck 544–6
      nasal cavity 545
         complications 546
         outer surface of nose 545, *545*
      superficial cervical plexus block 546
   lower limb 537–42
      ankle 543–4, *540, 544*
      digital nerve block 542
      hip 541–3

      femoral nerve 541
      lateral cutaneous nerve of thigh 542
      obturator nerve 542
      sciatic nerve 542–3
   IVRA 544
   knee 543
   lumbar plexus 538–41
      fascia iliaca block 541
      paravertebral block 540
      psoas compartment block 540–1
      three-in-one block 541
   lumbosacral plexus 538, *539*
peroperative phase 522–4
   asepsis 522
   drugs and doses **522, 523**
   environment 522
   location of nerve 524
   needles, cannulae and catheters 524
   toxicity 523
   vasoconstrictors 523–4
postoperative care 524
preoperative visit 521
thorax and abdomen 532–7
   dorsal nerve block 537–8
   field block for inguinal hernia repair 535, *536*–7
   innervation of trunk 533–4, *533*
   intercostal nerve block 534
   paravertebral block 534
upper limb 524–32
   brachial plexus 525–30
      axillary block 529–30
      block 527, *527*
      drugs and doses 527
      formation of brachial plexus 525, *525, 526*
      interscalene block 528–9
      subclavian perivascular block 528
   elbow and wrist 530–1
      digital nerve block 531–2
      lateral cutaneous nerve of forearm 530
      median nerve 531
      radial nerve 531
      ulnar nerve 530
   intravenous regional anaesthesia 532–3
Peripheral vascular surgery 241–2
Pethidine
   postoperative pain 657
   premedication **139**, 141
Phaeochromocytoma 425–8
   clinical 426
   intraoperative 427–8
   pathophysiology 425

Phaeochromocytoma (*contd*)
  postoperative 428
  preparation 426–7
  surgery 425–6
Pharyngeal surgery *see* Ear, nose and throat surgery
Pharyngolaryngectomy 323
Physical examination 124–5
Pin-index system 4
Pituitary function, and brain death 795
Pituitary surgery 258–9, 431–3
  acromegaly 432–3
  diabetes insipidus 433
Plasmapheresis 485
Plastic surgery 387–99
  autologous transfusion 390
  congenital abnormalities 391–4
    bat ears 393–4
    cleft palate and lip 392–3
    hypospadias 393
    syndactyly 393
  controlled hypotension 390–1
  cosmetic surgery 394–5
    breast operations 394–5
    liposuction and tumescent anaesthesia 395
    local anaesthesia 397–8
    rhinoplasty 395
  craniofacial reconstruction 397
  intravenous sedation 398
  local anaesthesia 399
  microvascular surgery 395–7
  multiple procedures 387
  multiple sites 387
  red cells 389
  reduction in blood loss 389
  skin expansion 394
  skin flaps 394
  skin grafts 394
  tissue perfusion versus blood loss 387–9
Platelet transfusion **734**–5
Pneumatic tourniquets 448–9
Pneumoperitoneum 496
Pneumothorax 497–8
Pneumomediastinum 497–8
Polarographic cells 28–9
Pollution, inhalational anaesthetics 107–8, 380–1
Popliteal fossa, nerve block 543
Porphyrias 166–9
  anaesthetic management 168–9
  clinical features 167–8
    acute intermittent porphyria 167
    hereditary coproporphyria 167
    variegate porphyria 168
  management 168
  pathogenesis 167
Portable anaesthetic machines 11
Portal hypertension 292–3, 471
Postoperative pain 651–70
  acute pain services 670
  assessment of 654–5, *656*
  benefits of analgesia 653
  factors influencing 653–4
  management 655–70
    acupuncture 668
    antidepressants 668
    aromatherapy and reflexology 668–9
    at-risk patients 669–70
      cardiovascular problems 669
      children 670
      elderly 669–70
      hepatic impairment 669
      opioid-dependent patients 670
      renal impairment 669
      respiratory problems 669
    clonidine 668
    combined local anaesthetic/opioid administration 666–7
    cryotherapy 668
    inhaled analgesia 668
    local anaesthesia 665–7
      epidural block 665, **666**
      infiltration 665
      nerve blocks 665
    non-steroidal anti-inflammatory drugs 667
    opioids 655–65
      buprenorphine 657
      continuous intravenous infusion 658, **660**
      diamorphine 655, 657
      fentanyl 657
      intermittent intramuscular injection **657**–8, *659*
      intravenous bolus administration 660, **661**
      morphine 655
      oral, buccal and sublingual administration 663
      papaveretum 655
      patient-controlled analgesia *661*, **662**–3
      pethidine 657
      rectal administration 663
      spinal administration 663, **664**–5
      subcutaneous injection 658
      tramadol 657
      transdermal administration 663
    transcutaneous nerve stimulation 668
  physiology 652–3
  see also Analgesia
Posture in dental surgery 376–7
Precordial thump 769–70
Pregnancy
  cardiopulmonary resuscitation 780, 782
  complications 564–8
    amniotic fluid embolism 565
    eclampsia 567
    haemorrhage 564–5
    hypertension 565, **566**–7
    maternal heart disease 567–8
    preterm delivery 565
  physiological changes during 549–52
    cardiovascular system 550
    central nervous system 551
    gastrointestinal and hepatic changes 551
    haematological changes 550
    renal changes 551
    respiratory system 550
    uterine physiology 551–2
  see also Obstetric anaesthesia/analgesia
Premedication 138, **139**–46
  alpha adrenoceptor agonists 144
  analgesia 141–2
  antacids 142
  antibiotic prophylaxis **143**, 144
  antithrombotic prophylaxis **144**
  anxiolysis 139, **139**–1
  fibreoptic intubation 686–7
  liver transplantation 476
  ophthalmic surgery 306
  paediatric surgery 348
  prevention of nausea and vomiting **142**–4
  recommended doses **139**
  renal surgery 284
  thoracic surgery 186
  vagal block 141
Preoperative evaluation 123–37
  blood transfusion 134
  cardiac surgery 203, **204**
  carotid artery surgery 242
  children 134
  concurrent medication 135–7
    antibiotics 137
    cardiovascular drugs 136–7
    corticosteroids 137
    psychoactive drugs 135–6
  day-care surgery 364–6
  documentation 133–4
  ear surgery 328–9
  fasting 134–5
  medical conditions affecting

anaesthetic management 126–33
cardiovascular disease 126–8
  cardiac pacemakers **127**–8
  hypertension 127
  ischaemic heart disease 126–7
  left ventricular failure 126
endocrine disorders 129–31
  diabetes mellitus 129–30
  obesity 130–1
gastrointestinal disorders 132–3
liver disease 133
neurological diseases 131–2
renal diseases 132
respiratory disease 128–9
viral infections 133
medical history 123–4
nasal surgery 333
ophthalmic surgery 305–6
paediatric surgery 134
physical examination 124–5
preparation for theatre 135
renal surgery 283
routine investigations 125–6
  electrocardiography 125, **126**
  electrolytes 125
  haematology 125
Preoperative tests 147–62
airway 157–8
biochemistry 160–1
cardiovascular system 148–53
  ambulatory ECG monitoring 149–50
  dipyridamole thallium scintigraphy 150
  echocardiography 151
  electrocardiography 148–9
  exercise ECG 149
  radionuclide ventriculography 150–1
haematology 158–60
respiratory system 153–7
  biochemistry
    hypokalaemia 160–1
    renal function 161
  cardiac surgery 157
  non-thoracic surgery 153–5
    arterial blood gas analysis 154–5
    chest X-ray 153
    spirometry 153–4
  thoracic surgery 155–7
    evaluation of tests 156–7
    exercise testing 156
    split lung function studies 155–6
Pressure generation in ventilators *48–9*
Pressure reducing valves 6

Preterm delivery 565
Prilocaine
  epidural anaesthesia 510
  peripheral nerve block **522**, **523**
Primary aldosteronism *see* Conn's syndrome
Prochlorperazine
  as anti-emetic 673
  premedication **139**
Propofol
  anaphylaxis 743–4
  as anti-emetic 674
Prostate, transurethral resection *see* Transurethral resection of prostate
Protamine, anaphylactic reactions **744**, 745
Protein C 174
Protein S 174
Prothrombin time 170–1
Psoas compartment block 540–1
Psychoactive drugs, and anaesthesia 135–6
  alcohol 136
  anticonvulsants 136
  monoamine oxidase inhibitors 135
  tricyclic antidepressants 135
Pudendal nerve block 559
Pulmonary artery
  catheterization 37, *38*
  temperature monitoring 43
Pulmonary oedema 748
Pulse oximetry 30–2
  and MRI 413
Pupillary response to light 793

Quality of practice 120–1
  professional performance and ethical responsibilities 121
  training and assessment of quality 120–1

Radial nerve block 531
Radioimmunoassay tests 750
Radiology, anaesthesia for 401–16
  anaesthetic procedure 405–6
  computed tomography *406, 407*
  contrast media 403–4
  emission computed tomography 407–8
  interventional neuroradiology 408–9
    anaesthetic practice 408–9
    equipment and patient set-up 409
    monitoring 409
  magnetic resonance imaging 409–16
    anaesthesia 413, *414, 415*
    babies and infants 415

basic principles 409–10
biological effects of high magnetic fields 411
contrast media 411–12
critically ill patients *415*
ferromagnetic attraction 411
gradient noise 411
magnetic field 410–11
monitoring **412**–13
planning 416
resuscitation 416
radiation hazards 402–3
sedation 404–5
work environment 401, **402**
Radionuclide ventriculography 150–1
RAE pre-formed tracheal tubes *93*
Raman spectroscopy gas analysers 29
Recovery chart 649
Recovery room 637–49
  arrival in 641
  care in 641–7
    cardiovascular system 645–7
      arrhythmias 647
      blood pressure 645–7
    respiratory system 641–5
      airway obstruction 642
      bronchospasm 643
      hypoventilation **643**, 644
      hypoxaemia 644–5
      laryngeal obstruction 642–3
  cerebral status 648
  equipment 638, **639**–40
  fluid and electrolyte balance 647–8
  ideal features **638**
  pain control and anti-emetic therapy 648–9
  recovery chart 649
  staffing 640
  temperature control 649
  transfer to **640**–1
Rectal temperature monitoring 42
Red blood cell transfusions **724**, **725**–7
Reflexology 668–9
Regional anaesthetic block
  in children 355–7
    caudal block 355, *356*
    epidural 356–7
    ilioinguinal and iliohypogastric blocks *357*
    penile block 357
    spinal 357
    wound infiltration 357
  difficult airway 692–3
  elderly patients 581–2
  hip fractures 444–5

Regional anaesthetic block (contd)
  obstetrics 553–9
  see also Epidural anaesthesia;
    Spinal anaesthesia
Regulators 6
Reinforced tracheal tubes 93, *94*
Remifentanil 657
Renal dialysis 488
Renal disease
  anaesthetic management 132
  and cardiac surgery 215
  diabetic patients 615
  and liver failure 472, 484
  see also Renal failure; Renal
    transplantation
Renal failure 278–86
  clinical pathophysiology **278**–81
    acid–base balance 281
    anaemia 279
    bleeding 279
    calcium and phosphate 281
    cardiovascular system 279–80
    gastrointestinal system 280–1
    nervous system 280
    potassium 281
    respiratory system 280
  drugs in 281–3
    anticholinesterases 283
    induction agents 282
    inhalational agents 283
    neuromuscular blockers 282
    opioid drugs 283
    premedication 282
  fluid and electrolyte status 283–4
  induction 284–5
  intravenous cannulation 284
  intravenous fluids 285
  and liver disorders 293–4, 297,
    298
  maintenance of general
    anaesthesia 285
  postoperative management 285–6
  postoperative pain management
    669
  premedication 284
  preoperative assessment 283
  regional anaesthetic techniques
    285
  surgery 283
  see also Renal transplantation
Renal function
  aortic reconstructive surgery
    239–40
  elderly patients 572–3
  pregnancy 551
Renal surgery see Genitourinary and
  renal surgery
Renal transplantation 486–92
  drug metabolism 489–90

analgesics 489
fluid management 489–90
neuromuscular blocking drugs
  489
vascular access 489
graft rejection 490–1
immediate postoperative care and
  complications 490–1
intraoperative management 488–9
management of living related
  donor 491
preoperative preparation 486–8
  cardiovascular complications
    486
  dialysis 488
  gastrointestinal complications
    486–7
  haematological features 487
  intercurrent disease 486
  metabolic factors 487
  neurological complications 487
  premedication 488
Rescue breathing 766, *767*
Reservoir bag **22**
Respiratory depression 379
Respiratory disease
  anaesthetic management 128–9
  and cardiac surgery 214–15
  postoperative pain management
    669
Respiratory system
  in children 337–8
  effects of brain death 789
  elderly patients 572, *573*
  epidural anaesthesia 512
  and head injury 807
  laparoscopic surgery 499–500
  in liver failure 471–2
  monitoring 21–9
    clinical observations **22**–3
    gas analysers 25, 27–9
      galvanic and polarographic
        cells 28–9
      infrared spectroscopy 25,
        27–8
      mass spectrometer 29
      paramagnetism 28
      Raman spectroscopy 29
    gases and vapours **24**–5, *26*, *27*
      carbon dioxide 25, *26*, *27*
      oxygen 24–5
    pressure and flow 23–4
  obese patients 588–9
  postoperative care, thoracic
    surgery 193
  in pregnancy 550
  preoperative tests 153–61
    cardiac surgery 157
    non-thoracic surgery 153–5

arterial blood gas analysis
  154–5
chest X-ray 153
evaluation of tests 155
spirometry 153–4
thoracic surgery 155–7
  evaluation of tests 156–7
  exercise testing 156
  split lung function studies
    155–6
recovery room care 641–5
  airway obstruction 642
  bronchospasm 643
  hypoventilation **643**, **644**
  hypoxaemia 644–5
  laryngeal obstruction 642–3
vascular surgery 235–6
Resuscitation
  dental surgery 384
  MRI unit 416
  obese patients 595
  paediatric *358*–9
Retinal detachment 308–9
Retinopathy of prematurity 342
Retrobulbar nerve block 311, *312*
Retrograde intubation 691–2
Rheumatoid arthritis
  airway management 695
  anaesthetic management 131–2
  surgery 449–50
Rhinoplasty 395
Risk evaluation 111–18
  APACHE score 112, **113**
  ASA physical status 111, **113**
  cardiac surgery **204**
  comparison of models 117, *118*
  definitions 113–14
    explanator 113–14
    independence 114
    model 114
    multivariate analysis 114
    outcome 113
    training data 114
    validation data 114
  future of 118
  Goldman risk index **112**
  hepatobiliary and pancreatic
    surgery 296
  scoring systems 137, **138**
  types of model 114–17
    Bayesian model 115–16
    discriminant analysis 115
    multiple logistic regression
      114–15
    multiple regression 114
    neural networks 116–17
Ropivacaine, epidural anaesthesia
  510

Rubella 602
Rubeola 602–3

Safety devices for anaesthetic machines 8–9, 10
  direct oxygen flush valve 9, 10
  oxygen failure alarm 8–9
  safety valves 9
Safety valves 9
Saphenous nerve block 543
Sciatic nerve block 542–3
Scoliosis 451, **452**–3
  anaesthesia 453
  postoperative care 453
  preoperative assessment 452–3
  surgical correction 453
Scoring systems for anaesthesia risk 137, **138**
Second generation anaesthetic machines 15
Septic shock 599–601
Septicaemia 598–9
Septoplasty 333
Sevoflurane, toxicity 103, 104–5
Sheridan laser tube 96
Sickle cell syndrome 163–4
  anaesthetic management 165, 166
  brain 164
  cardiovascular system 164
  in children 346
  kidneys 164
  liver 164
  respiratory system 164
Single twitch nerve stimulation 45
Sinus arrhythmia, and awareness monitoring 761
Skin expansion 394
Skin flaps 394
Skin grafts 394
Skin temperature monitoring 42
Skin testing 749–50
Sleep apnoea 347
Sleep nasendoscopy 326–7
Snoring, surgery for 326–7
  sleep nasendoscopy 326–7
  uvulopalatopharyngoplasty 327
Sodium balance abnormalities 710–11
Sodium chloride solution 702
Somatic nerve block 510–11
Sphygmomanometer 32
Spinal anaesthesia 357, 516–18
  accidental 514
  anatomy 503–6
    blood supply 505–6
    epidural space 504, 505
    meninges 504
    nerve roots 505
    vertebrae 503–4

  care of patients 519
  combined spinal–epidural anaesthesia 518
  complications 517–18
  continuous 518
  equipment 516
  obstetrics 558
    Caesarean section 563
  spread of solution 517
  see also Epidural anaesthesia; Local anaesthetics
Spinal cord
  aortic reconstructive surgery 240
  blood supply 505–6
  monitoring 453, 454–5
Spinal injuries 445–7
  airway management 446
  anaesthesia 446
  cardiovascular problems 446
  chronic 447
  gastrointestinal and urinary problems 446
  patient positioning 446–7
  temperature regulation 446
  ventilation 446
Spinal surgery 451–3
  cervical spine 451
  scoliosis surgery 451, **452**–3
  spinal cord decompression 451
  spinal fusion 451
  thoracic spine 451
Spirometry 153–4
Standards
  anaesthetic machines 3
  monitoring 20, **21**
Stapedectomy 328
Stereotactic surgery 256
Stethoscopes 413
Stilettes 683–4
Storz Hopkins intubating bronchoscope 196
Storz ventilating bronchoscope 188
Strabismus surgery 308
Stress response, epidural anaesthesia 512
Sub-Tenon's injection 311
Subclavian perivascular block 528
Subdural block 514–15
Submucous resection 333
Sufentanil 657
Superficial cervical plexus block 546
Suxamethonium
  apnoea 178
  haemodilution effects **723**
Syndactyly 393

Talipes equinovarus 450
Target controlled infusions 629–30
Temazepam, premedication **139**, **140**

Temperature monitoring 441–43
  bladder 42
  core temperature 42
  liver transplantation 479
  nasopharyngeal 42
  oesophageal 42
  pulmonary artery 42
  recovery room 649
  rectal 42
  skin 42
  spinal injuries 446
  trauma surgery 440–1
  tympanic membrane 42
  types of thermometers 41
Temperature regulation
  in children 340–1
  epidural anaesthesia 512
Temporomandibular joint, and difficult intubation 679, **680**–1
Testicular surgery 271
Tetanus 45, 604
  post-tetanic count 45
Tetralogy of Fallot 228
Thalassaemias 164–5
  anaesthetic management 165–6
Thermal injury 457–68
  airway management 460–1
  anaesthesia 466–7
  analgesia 463–4
  fluid balance 714–15
  inhalation injury 461–2
  monitoring 462–3
  nutrition and fluid balance 462
  operative procedures 458–60
    dressing changes 460
    escharotomy 459
    immediate excision and grafting 459
    primary excision and grafting 459–60
    reconstructive surgery 460
    removal of eschar 460
  paediatric burns 464–5
  pharmacokinetics and pharmacodynamics 465–6
  pathophysiological changes 457, **458**
  venous access 463
Thermometers 42
Thermoregulation 298
  elderly patients 573–4
Third generation anaesthetic machines 16
Thoracic aortic disease 223, 224–5
Thoracic surgery 185–201
  bronchopleural fistula 194–6
    anaesthesia 195, 195
      induction techniques 195

Index

Thoracic surgery (contd)
    intubating techniques 196, *196, 197*
    diagnostic procedures 187–90
        bronchoscopy 187–8
            adults 187, *188*
            children 188
        mediastinoscopy 189
        oesophagoscopy 188–9
        thorascopy 189–90
    investigations 185–6
    laparoscopic 493, **494**–5
    lung transplantation 198–201
        anaesthetic technique 199–200
        complications 201
        postoperative management 200
        pre-operative assessment 199
    major open procedures 190–4
        induction of anaesthesia 190
        introduction of double-lumen endobronchial tube 190, **191**
        one-lung anaesthesia 190–2
        pain relief 193
        postoperative care 193–4
        termination of anaesthesia 193
        underwater seal 192
    premedication 186
    preoperative assessment 185
    tracheal stenosis 196
    trauma 438–9
Thoracoscopy 189–90, 493, **494**–5
Three-in-one block 541
Throat surgery *see* Ear, nose and throat surgery
Thyroid surgery 417–21
    goitre 418–21
        clinical 419
        intraoperative 420
        pathophysiology 418
        postoperative 420–1
        preparation 419
        surgery 418–19
    hypothyroidism 421–2
        clinical 422
        intraoperative 422
        pathophysiology 421
        postoperative 422
        surgery 421
        treatment 422
Tibial nerve block 543
Tongue size, and difficult intubation 678
Tonicity 698
Tonsillectomy 317–19
    post-tonsillectomy haemorrhage 319
Total body water 698–9
Total intravenous anaesthesia 625–34

available hypnotic agents 627–9
closed-loop anaesthesia 631
effect site concentration 630, *631*
infusion regimens 629–30
    assessment of TCI 630
    manually adjusted **629**
    target controlled infusions 629–30
pharmacokinetics 625, *626, 627, 628*
problems with 632–3
    complexity of dosing 632–3
    cost 633
    infection 633
    patients awareness 633
supplementary drugs 631, *632*
Tracheal cuff 90, *91–2*
Tracheal stenosis 196–8
Tracheal surgery *see* Ear, nose and throat surgery
Tracheal tubes 89–99
    catheter mounts 92
    connectors 92
    correct placement 98, *99*
    design *90*
    laryngoscopes *97, 98*
    material 89–90
    paediatric surgery **349**
    size 89
    specialist 92–7
        laryngectomy tubes 95
        microlaryngeal tubes 93, *94*
        Oxford pattern tubes 95, *96*
        paediatric tubes 92–3
        RAE pre-formed tubes 93
        reinforced tubes 93, *94*
        tracheostomy tubes 94, *95*
        tubes for use with lasers *96, 97*
    tracheal cuff 90, *91–2*
Tracheostomy 325–6
    mini 690
    surgical 690
Tracheostomy tubes 94, *95*
Train-of-four nerve stimulation *44*
Training data 114
Tramadol 657
Transcutaneous nerve stimulation (TENS) 668
Transoesophageal echocardiography 39
Transtracheal airway 688–90
    mini-tracheostomy 690
    surgical tracheostomy 690
    transtracheal jet ventilation 689
Transtracheal jet ventilation 689
Transurethral endoscopy 271–3
    antibiotic therapy 273
    blood loss estimation 272
    lithotomy position 272

spinal versus general anaesthetic 271–2
temperature loss 273
Transurethral resection of prostate (TURP) 274–6
    aetiology **275**
    new methods 276
    pacemakers and diathermy 276
    pathophysiology 275
    presentation 275
    prevention 275–6
    treatment 276
Trauma surgery 437–47
    abdominal injury 439
    airway management 437–8, 694
    anaesthesia 439–42
        analgesia 441–2
        induction 441
        maintenance 441
        monitoring and intravenous fluid replacement 439–40
        muscle relaxants 441
        temperature control 440–1
    extremities 439
    fat embolus 443
    hip fractures 444–5
    paediatric trauma 442–3
    pelvic injury 439
    spinal injuries 445–7
    thoracic injury 438–9
    Volkmann's ischaemic contracture 443
Tricyclic antidepressants, and anaesthesia 135
Tuberculosis 604–5
d-Tubocurarine, haemodilution effects **723**
Tuohy needles 507, *508*
Turbinate reduction 333
TURP 274–6
Tympanic membrane, temperature monitoring 42
Tympanoplasty 328

Ulnar nerve block *531*
Underwater seal 192
Univent tube *197*
Upper respiratory tract infection 347
Ureteric surgery, endoscopic 273–4
Urinary output, postoperative, thoracic surgery 194
Uvulopalatopharyngoplasty 327

Vagal block 141
Validation data 114
Valve surgery 218, *219, 220*
    aortic valve 219–21
        aortic regurgitation 221
        aortic stenosis 219–21

mitral valve 221–2
  mitral regurgitation 221
  mitral stenosis 221–2
Valves and gauges 5–7
  demand valve 75
  flowmeter needle valves 6–7
  non-rebreathing valve 74
  one-way/backflow check valves 6
  pressure reducing valves
    (regulators) 6
Vancomycin, antibiotic prophylaxis **143**
Vaporizers 9, 11
Varicella 603
Variegate porphyria *see* Porphyrias
Vascular access
  liver transplantation 476–7
  renal transplantation 489
Vascular surgery 233–45
  anaesthetic procedure 236–7
  aortic reconstruction surgery 238–41
    anaesthetic considerations 238
    anaesthetic technique 240–1
    blood transfusion 238–9
    haemodynamic consequences of aortic cross-clamping 239
    renal function 239–40
    spinal cord 240
  cardiovascular assessment 233–5
    coronary angiography 234–5
    dipyridamole-thallium imaging 234
    echocardiography 234
    optimization 235
  carotid artery 242–5
    anaesthetic considerations 242–3
    anaesthetic technique 244
    brain monitoring 243–4
    cerebral blood flow 243
    general anaesthesia 243
    postoperative complications 244–5
    preoperative assessment 242
    surgical procedure 242
  heparinization 238
  intraoperative monitoring **237**–8

laboratory investigations 236
peripheral vascular system 241–2
respiratory system 235–6
risk factors 233
Vasoconstrictors 523–4
Venovenous bypass, liver transplantation 480–1
Ventilators 47–68
  Datex-Engstrom AS/3 Anaesthetic Delivery Unit 64–7
    central electronic controls 64
    pneumatic system 64–7
      bellow assembly 64
      driving gas system 64, *65*
      fresh gas control unit 65, *66*–7
  Drager Divan *61*, *62*–4
    breathing system 62, *63*–4
  effect of fresh gas flow on tidal volume 56–7
  modes of ventilation 56–7
  monitoring and alarms 57
  functional characteristics 47, *48*–51
    cycling from expiration to inspiration 51
    cycling from inspiration to expiration 50
    expiratory flow production 50–1
    inspiratory flow production *48*–50, *52*
  Manley Multivent 57, *58*–60
    E-model 60
    electronic system 60
    manual operation 60
    pneumatic system 58, *59*–60
  operational characteristics 51–6
    bag-in-bottle system 54–5
    breathing system *52*, 53–4
    internal compliance 55–6
    power source 51, *52*, *53*
  paediatric/neonatal ventilation 67–8, 350
    conversion to pressure generator 67–8
    increasing internal compliance 67

introduction of leak 68
pressure controlled ventilation 68
modification to maintain flow generator characteristics *67*
reduction of internal compliance of tubing compartment 67
separate paediatric attachment *67*
use of smaller bellows *67*
use of T-piece 68
Ventricular dysfunction 209–10, *211*, **212**, *213*
  assist devices 212
  intra-aortic balloon counter-pulsation 211, *213*
  management 210–11, **212**
  measurement of ventricular function 210
  pathophysiology 210, *211*
  right ventricle 212–13
Vertebrae *503*–4
Vestibular nerve section 328
Vestibulo-ocular reflex 793
Vipoma 434–5
Viral infections 601–3
  anaesthetic management 133
  common cold 601–2
  infectious mononucleosis 603
  measles 602–3
  mumps 603
  rubella 602
  varicella 603
Volatile anaesthetics *see* Anaesthetics, inhalational
Volkmann's ischaemic contracture 443
Von Willebrand's disease 172–4
  clinical features 173
  treatment 173–4

Warfarin, reversal of effects 736
Water balance abnormalities 710
Whole blood clotting time 170
Wound infiltration 357

Zopiclone, premedication **139**, 141